ORTHOPAEDIC KNOWLEDGE UPDATE-I

HOME STUDY SYLLABUS

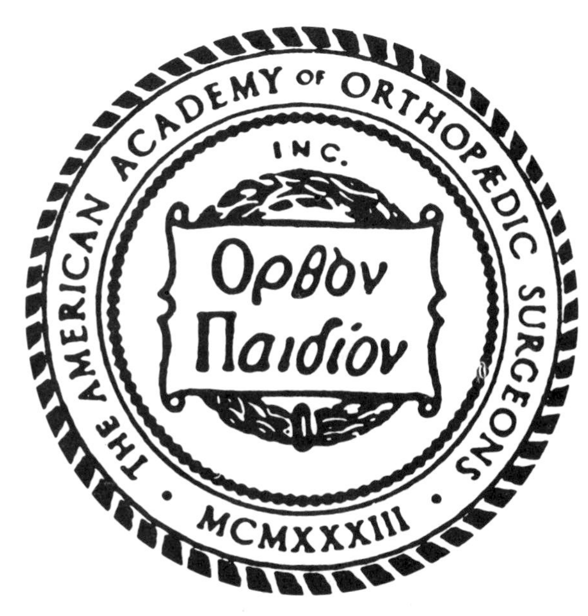

AMERICAN ACADEMY OF ORTHOPAEDIC SURGEONS

CHICAGO, ILLINOIS

1984

ORTHOPAEDIC KNOWLEDGE UPDATE I
Home Study Syllabus

Library of Congress Cataloging in Publication Data
American Academy of Orthopaedic Surgeons.
Orthopaedic knowledge update I.

Bibliography: p.
Includes index.
1. Orthopedia. 2. Orthopedia—Abstracts. I. Title.
[DNLM: 1. Orthopedics—Abstracts. 2. Orthopedics—Handbooks. W1 OR795]
RD731.A556 1984 617'.3 83-21332
ISBN 0-89203-000-3

Published by the American Academy of Orthopaedic Surgeons
444 North Michigan Avenue, Suite 1500
Chicago, Illinois 60611-3981
January 1, 1984

FIRST EDITION

To cite Syllabus:
Singer, K.: Section 1, Health maintenance of the musculoskeletal system. *In* Orthopaedic Knowledge Update I: Home Study Syllabus, pp. 1-8, Chicago, American Academy of Orthopaedic Surgeons, 1984.

HOME STUDY SYLLABUS
was composed in phototype Times Roman and Helvetica
by The Lowell Press of Kansas City, Missouri
and
was printed by George Banta Co. of Menasha, Wisconsin
on 60-pound Paloma Matte,
in an edition of 10,000 Smythe-sewn soft-cover volumes.

CONTENTS

Acknowledgments *iv*
Contributors *v*
Introduction *vii*

General Orthopaedics

MUSCULOSKELETAL

1. Health Maintenance of the Musculoskeletal System . . . 1
2. Congenital Abnormalities of the Skeleton . . . 9
3. Bone Metabolism: Normal Physiology and Disease . . . 15
4. Arthritis . . . 29
5. Musculoskeletal Neoplasms . . . 41
6. Infection . . . 49
7. Trauma: Special Pediatric Considerations . . . 59
8. Amputations and Prosthetics . . . 65

NEUROLOGICAL SYSTEM

9. Neuromuscular Disorders and Gait . . . 73

NONNEUROMUSCULOSKELETAL SYSTEMS

10. Circulatory, Respiratory, Hematopoietic, Gastrointestinal, Genitourinary, and Integumentary Systems . . . 79

NON-ORGAN SYSTEM ORIENTED

11. Metals Used in Orthopaedic Surgery . . . 89
12. Polyethylene in Total Joint Replacement . . . 99
13. Polymethyl Methacrylate . . . 103

Upper Extremity

SHOULDER AND HUMERUS

14. Pediatric . . . 109
15. Trauma . . . 115
16. Reconstruction . . . 125

ELBOW AND FOREARM

17. Pediatric . . . 133
18. Trauma . . . 143
19. Reconstruction . . . 153

WRIST AND HAND

20. Pediatric . . . 163
21. Trauma . . . 173
22. Reconstruction . . . 181

Spine

CERVICAL

23. Pediatric . . . 189
24. Trauma . . . 199
25. Reconstruction . . . 209

THORACOLUMBAR

26. Pediatric . . . 217
27. Trauma . . . 227
28. Reconstruction . . . 237

LUMBOSACRAL

29. Reconstruction . . . 245

Lower Extremity

PELVIS, HIP, AND FEMUR

30. Pediatric . . . 259
31. Trauma (Pelvis and Acetabulum) . . . 271
32. Trauma (Hip and Femur) . . . 287
33. Reconstruction . . . 297

KNEE AND LEG

34. Pediatric . . . 311
35. Trauma (Soft Tissue) . . . 319
36. Trauma (Bone) . . . 329
37. Reconstruction . . . 337

ANKLE AND FOOT

38. Pediatric . . . 349
39. Trauma . . . 359
40. Reconstruction . . . 369

Author Index . . . 377

Subject Index . . . 387

ACKNOWLEDGMENTS

There have been many persons involved with the inception and development of *Orthopaedic Knowledge Update I: Home Study Syllabus.* It seems inevitable that some will have been overlooked and for that we apologize.

Presidents
William R. MacAusland, M.D., 1980-1981
Robert E. Wells, M.D., 1981-1982
David G. Murray, M.D., 1982-1983
J. William Fielding, M.D., 1983-1984
Charles A. Rockwood, Jr., M.D., 1984-1985

Education Committee
William F. Donaldson, M.D., Chairman
J. Drennan Lowell, M.D., Secretary
William P. Bunnell, M.D.
Sherman S. Coleman, M.D.
Walter A. Hoyt, Jr., M.D.
Newton C. McCollough, III, M.D.
C. Dayton Riddle, Jr., M.D.
Augusto Sarmiento, M.D.
Taylor K. Smith, M.D.

Ad Hoc Committee on Home Study
Marc A. Asher, M.D., Chairman
James V. Luck, Jr., M.D., Secretary
Robert H. Fitzgerald, Jr., M.D.
William T. Green, Jr., M.D.
J. Drennan Lowell, M.D.
John J. Hinchey, M.D., Advisor
Robert H. Cofield, M.D., Advisor

Consultants
Norton J. Greenberger, M.D., General Chairman
Medical Knowledge Self Assessment Program VI
David T. Sisk, M.D., Chairman
Committee on Examinations and Evaluation

Staff
Janice M. Brunks, Project Secretary

American Academy of Orthopaedic Surgery
Charles V. Heck, M.D., Executive Director
Robert Napolitano, Associate Executive Director

CONTRIBUTORS

Editorial Board

MARC A. ASHER, M.D., Chairman, Kansas City, Kansas
JOHN J. GARTLAND, M.D., Philadelphia, Pennsylvania
WOOD W. LOVELL, M.D., Jacksonville, Florida
AUGUSTO SARMIENTO, M.D., Los Angeles, California
RICHARD N. STAUFFER, M.D., Rochester, Minnesota

Advisors

FRED V. FEATHERSTONE, M.D., Chicago, Illinois
BARBARA W. FUNK, M.A., Kansas City, Missouri
DOUGLAS M. REIMER, J.D., Chicago, Illinois

General Orthopaedics Task Force

ROBERT H. FITZGERALD, JR., M.D., Chairman Rochester, Minnesota	Infection Polymethyl Methacrylate
KENNETH M. SINGER, M.D. Eugene, Oregon	Health Maintenance of the Musculoskeletal System
RODNEY K. BEALS, M.D. Portland, Oregon	Congenital Abnormalities of the Skeleton
JOSEPH M. LANE, M.D. DANIEL D. BUSS, M.D. New York, New York	Bone Metabolism: Normal Physiology and Disease
ALLAN E. GROSS, M.D. Toronto, Ontario, Canada I. M. FARINE, M.D. Tel Aviv, Israel	Arthritis
JAMES O. JOHNSTON, M.D. Oakland, California	Musculoskeletal Neoplasms
HAMLET A. PETERSON, M.D. Rochester, Minnesota BEHROOZ A. AKBARNIA, M.D. St. Louis, Missouri	Trauma: Special Pediatric Considerations
NEWTON C. MCCOLLOUGH, III, M.D. Miami, Florida	Amputations and Prosthetics
MARK M. HOFFER, M.D. JACQUELIN PERRY, M.D. ROBERT L. WATERS, M.D. Downey, California	Neuromuscular Disorders and Gait
ROY WILLIAM PETTY, M.D. Gainesville, Florida	Circulatory, Respiratory, Hematopoietic, Gastrointestinal, Genitourinary, and Integumentary Systems
JORGE O. GALANTE, M.D. Chicago, Illinois	Metals Used in Orthopaedic Surgery
ROBERT M. ROSE, SC.D., P.E. Cambridge, Massachusetts	Polyethylene in Total Joint Replacement

Upper Extremity Task Force

DEAN S. LOUIS, M.D., Chairman Ann Arbor, Michigan	Wrist and Hand: Trauma
MARK NISSENBAUM, M.D. Abington, Pennsylvania	Shoulder and Humerus: Pediatric
ROBERT J. NEVIASER, M.D. Washington, D.C.	Shoulder and Humerus: Trauma

Anthony G. Gristina, M.D. — Shoulder and Humerus: Reconstruction
Lawrence X. Webb, M.D.
Winston-Salem, North Carolina

Thomas F. Kling, M.D. — Elbow and Forearm: Pediatric
Ann Arbor, Michigan

Samuel S. Kaplan, M.D. — Elbow and Forearm: Trauma
Scottsdale, Arizona

Roy A. Meals, M.D. — Elbow and Forearm: Reconstruction
Los Angeles, California

Thomas L. Greene, M.D. — Wrist and Hand: Pediatric
Tampa, Florida

Lawrence C. Hurst, M.D. — Wrist and Hand: Reconstruction
Stony Brook, New York

Spine Task Force

Robert B. Winter, M.D., Chairman — Thoracolumbar: Pediatric
Minneapolis, Minnesota

Robert N. Hensinger, M.D. — Cervical: Pediatric
Ann Arbor, Michigan

E. Shannon Stauffer, M.D. — Cervical: Trauma
Springfield, Illinois

John A. Hartwig, M.D. — Cervical: Reconstruction
Minneapolis, Minnesota

Francis Denis, M.D. — Thoracolumbar: Trauma
St. Paul, Minnesota

John E. Lonstein, M.D. — Thoracolumbar: Reconstruction
Minneapolis, Minnesota

Leon L. Wiltse, M.D. — Lumbosacral: Reconstruction
Long Beach, California

Lower Extremity Task Force

Eduardo A. Salvati, M.D., Chairman — Pelvis, Hip, and Femur: Reconstruction
Paul M. Pellicci, M.D.
New York, New York

Peter L. Meehan, M.D. — Pelvis, Hip, and Femur: Pediatric
Atlanta, Georgia
Robert E. Eilert, M.D.
Denver, Colorado

Dana C. Mears, M.D., Ph.D. — Pelvis and Acetabulum: Trauma
Harry E. Rubash, M.D.
Pittsburgh, Pennsylvania

Joseph S. Barr, Jr., M.D. — Hip and Femur: Trauma
Boston, Massachusetts

Robert E. Eilert, M.D. — Knee and Leg: Pediatric
Denver, Colorado

Bertram Zarins, M.D. — Knee and Leg: Trauma (Soft Tissue)
Victor A. Nemeth, M.D.
Boston, Massachusetts

Frederick W. Reckling, M.D. — Knee and Leg: Trauma (Bone)
Kansas City, Kansas

John N. Insall, M.D. — Knee and Leg: Reconstruction
Thomas P. Sculco, M.D.
New York, New York

Marc A. Asher, M.D. — Ankle and Foot: Pediatric
Kansas City, Kansas

Leland G. Hawkins, M.D. — Ankle and Foot: Trauma
Cedar Rapids, Iowa
William R. Pontarelli, M.D.
Iowa City, Iowa

Donald M. Mauldin, M.D. — Ankle and Foot: Reconstruction
Dallas, Texas

INTRODUCTION

In response to an increasing number of challenges to existing postgraduate educational techniques, the American Academy of Orthopaedic Surgeons conducted a continuing education workshop in May 1979. A major recommendation coming from that workshop called for the development of learner-centered educational programs. This recommendation was studied in detail by the Education Committee and the Ad Hoc Committee on Home Study. As a result of these studies and deliberations of the Board of Directors of the Academy, the development of a home study program, centering on the *Home Study Syllabus*, was approved in April 1982. This Syllabus is the product of intense work by many persons since that date.

Orthopaedic Knowledge Update I: Home Study Syllabus is a new learner-centered educational tool in the specialty. It consists of illustrated narratives and annotated bibliographies that are based primarily on the literature of the past four years (1979-1982). The Syllabus is designed to help orthopaedic surgeons and scientists remain current with the ever-expanding fund of information in this field. It differs from any other educational tool currently available in orthopaedic surgery.

The Syllabus is designed to present orthopaedic knowledge in a logical and easy-to-follow format. Information is considered to be of general interest or oriented by anatomical region. Thus, there are four major divisions: General, Upper Extremity, Spine, and Lower Extremity.

The General division is subdivided by organ system and also includes non-organ system related sections of general interest. The major organ system of concern (musculoskeletal) is further subdivided on the basis of etiology, including a section on health maintenance. Each of the three anatomical divisions is subdivided according to anatomy. Each subdivision is further categorized into sections on pediatrics, trauma, and reconstruction. In all, there are forty separate sections.

The Task Force Chairman for each of the four major divisions was selected on the basis of a recognized, comprehensive understanding of the subject material in that division. The writers represent a cross-section of orthopaedic practice and includes one nonorthopaedic scientist. Two writers' workshops were conducted to provide instruction about the concept, as well as the details of Syllabus preparation. Each author was provided a set of specifications and wrote from an outline with an allotment of allowable pages, illustrations, and bibliographic citations.

Considerable effort was expended to provide both medical and copy editing in an attempt to make the Syllabus as comprehensive and cohesive a review as possible.

In each illustrated narrative, recent basic and clinical information is synthesized with some older relevant information to provide a clear perspective of current thinking. To encourage information synthesis and readability, each narrative is not directly cross-referenced with a bibliographic citation. However, the bibliography is organized in the same sequence as the narrative and annotated to provide a source of additional information. The bibliography represents a selection of approximately 1,000 references from many thousands reviewed by the contributors.

The Syllabus is designed to be a benchbook, useful in daily practice as a narrative to be read, a reference to be consulted, and a guide providing direction to more detailed information. To assure maximum access to the information, the Syllabus includes a contents page, a tabular index staggered by division with section initials, and both an author and subject index. The contents of the Syllabus will be partially reflected in the 1984 Orthopaedic Self-Assessment Examination, since many of the questions will be taken from the Syllabus.

Orthopaedic Knowledge Update I: Home Study Syllabus is not intended to be a textbook and does not cover all the important information upon which the practice of orthopaedic surgery is based. Basic orthopaedic information is available in the many standard textbooks. It is not a yearbook or a periodical. Finally, it is not a statement of principle or a standard of practice.

Work on the Syllabus has been in progress for over a year. Although the contributors have made every effort to include the latest information, it must be recognized that the field of orthopaedic surgery is dynamic and, therefore, not susceptible to being capsulized at any given moment. For this reason the Academy must take the position that the Syllabus should not be regarded as all-inclusive.

Orthopaedic Knowledge Update I: Home Study Syllabus is an attempt, on the part of those entrusted with its development, to provide a useful, comprehensive, and accessible synthesis of the latest information and knowledge available in the literature related to orthopaedic surgery. Present plans call for a new edition in 1987 that will be based primarily on the literature of 1983-1985.

1 HEALTH MAINTENANCE OF THE MUSCULOSKELETAL SYSTEM

This section discusses some factors relevant to health maintenance of the musculoskeletal system. It includes the energy systems utilized in exercise, their accessibility to the body, neuromuscular concepts, functions of the oxygen transport system, and the effects of various training programs.

Exercise

Energy Systems Adenosine triphosphate (ATP), an intracellular biochemical compound, is the immediately usable form of chemical energy needed for muscle activity. All biological work performed by the cell requires energy directly released from the high-energy phosphate bonds when ATP is broken down into ADP and inorganic phosphate, as in the equation ATP = ADP + Pi + Energy. The body must then recreate ATP by reversing this reaction. This requires a source of energy, and the cells basically have three available energy sources.

Anaerobic Systems The most rapidly available source of energy is from the phosphagen system. Phosphocreatinine is enzymatically broken down in muscle cells and releases energy to swiftly reform ATP. Muscular stores of ADP and Pi are small, and the amount of energy available utilizing this system is limited. The important role this system plays is to make available to the body a very rapid source of energy, and, therefore, its primary use is in high intensity, short duration activities.

The second source of energy available to the body is the lactic acid system, also known as anaerobic glycolysis. Muscle cells will partially metabolize glucose, releasing energy and forming lactic acid as a by-product. Lactic acid accumulates in the muscle and blood causing symptoms of fatigue. Anaerobic glycolysis is also a limited source of energy for ATP resynthesis, providing muscle cells with a fairly fast supply of energy that lasts only a short duration, as fatigue becomes a limiting factor.

Aerobic Glycolysis In this third source of energy, glycogen is completely broken down to carbon dioxide and water in the presence of oxygen. This reaction occurs in the mitochondria of muscle cells and releases large amounts of energy for ATP resynthesis without forming fatiguing by-products. Aerobic glycolysis is the energy source utilized in prolonged endurance types of activities.

In aerobic glycolysis, the amount of oxygen available to the cell is the limiting factor. Carbohydrate, fat, and protein can be used as fuel sources, but the oxygen needs will vary with the energy source. For example, more oxygen is needed when fat is utilized and less with carbohydrate. At rest, approximately 0.2 to 0.3 liters per minute of oxygen is consumed, and with maximal exercise the amount increases to 3 to 6 liters per minute.

Energy Utilization During Exercise The body is quite versatile in that it can provide a major portion of ATP for any given activity in three distinctly different ways. The system it utilizes depends upon the specific activity. For example, in endurance types of activities the aerobic system is utilized, whereas in short duration, high intensity activities the phosphagen system is selected, and in intermediate activities, such as middle distance running, the lactic acid system is employed. But many activities require variable energy sources, and the body can adapt readily. For example, as a runner begins slowly, the aerobic system is utilized, but as the pace increases both the aerobic and lactic acid systems function. At the conclusion of the race, the "kick" utilizes predominantly the lactic acid and phosphagen systems. As the rate of ATP requirement increases, the amount of energy produced by the anaerobic systems increases, with the phosphagen systems supplying ATP at the highest rate. Similarly, the total energy requirements for a given activity in part determines the energy system utilized. The phosphagen system supplies less than 1 mole of ATP, the lactic acid system slightly greater than 1 mole, but the aerobic system can furnish over 10 moles. How the body makes these transitions, at what point the various systems are utilized, and in what proportion depends upon the type, duration, and intensity of the activity. The state of individual physical conditioning for various types of activities also plays a role.

This has been described as the energy continuum. This concept correlates the relationships with the activities involved. Figure 1 and Table I present examples of how the various energy systems are used in the performance of some specific activities.

Fuels Used for Exercise The basic fuel supply for exercise comes from carbohydrate and fat. Protein, used as an energy source only when other sources are unavailable, is not considered in the context of this discussion.

Carbohydrate Metabolism Glucose is the basic usable form of carbohydrate, and glycogen is the storage form. Almost all ingested carbohydrates are converted to glucose before utilization. Glycogen, a polymer of glucose, is stored primarily in the liver and muscle. Liver glycogen is broken down into glucose and is taken to muscle by the blood. The liver stores large quantities of glycogen, and when the blood glucose level drops, liver glycogen is broken down into glucose and released into the bloodstream to maintain the blood glucose level. Muscle gly-

Table I
Four Areas of the Energy Continuum

Area	Performance Time	Major Energy System(s) Involved	Examples of Type of Activity
1	Less than 30 seconds	ATP-PC	Shot put, 100-meter sprint, base stealing, golf and tennis swings, running plays of football backs
2	30 seconds to 1½ minutes	ATP-PC and lactic acid	200- to 400-meter sprints, speed skating, 100-meter swim
3	1½ minutes to 3 minutes	Lactic acid and O_2	800-meter dash, gymnastics events, boxing (3-min. rounds), wrestling (2-min. periods)
4	Greater than 3 minutes	O_2	Soccer and lacrosse (except goalies), cross-country skiing, marathon run, jogging

2
MS:H

(Adapted with permission from Sports Physiology, by E.L. Fox, p. 28. Saunders College Publishing/Holt, Rinehart and Winston. Reprinted by permission of Holt, Rinehart and Winston, CBS College Publishing, 1979.)

cogen is utilized only in the muscle, and its metabolism does not contribute to blood glucose levels. It is either metabolized to lactic acid by anaerobic glycolysis or completely utilized aerobically. Any lactic acid produced can be transported to the liver for conversion to glucose or glycogen storage.

Very little blood glucose is utilized by muscle tissue during rest. During exercise, glucose uptake from the blood increases markedly and can account for as much as 30 to 40 percent of the total fuel oxidized. The use of muscle glycogen during exercise is also high and is dependent upon a number of factors, including the type and intensity of exercise, stores available, and recent diet. As exercise continues, muscle glycogen is gradually used up, and, eventually, total glycogen depletion can follow.

Fat Metabolism Fat, the other form of metabolic fuel, exists as free fatty acid (FFA) in its usable form and triglycerides in its storage form. As with glycogen, there are fat stores both in the muscle itself and in remote areas, i.e., as adipose tissue. During prolonged exercise, triglycerides in adipose tissue are broken down into FFA and transported by the blood to skeletal muscle, representing a major source of fuel for ATP production by the oxidative system. The uptake of FFA by working muscles appears to be related to how much FFA is in the blood. Muscle triglyceride stores also are used considerably during prolonged endurance activities. However, depletion of muscle triglyceride stores does not appear to be related directly to the duration of the activity as does glycogen depletion. The depletion seems related to the amount of fat stores in the muscle prior to exercise. During exercise, glycogen is used preferentially as an energy source, but in the presence of fat, the latter is used to a variable extent, and its utilization causes glycogen sparing. This lower utilization of glycogen prolongs exercise tolerance in an individual. Carbohydrate stores in muscle can be directly influenced by diet and exercise over a relatively short period of time and can be manipulated by the athlete to have a beneficial effect upon endurance. But, muscle triglyceride stores are not nearly as directly influenced by diet or depleted by exercise and are more difficult to manipulate effectively.

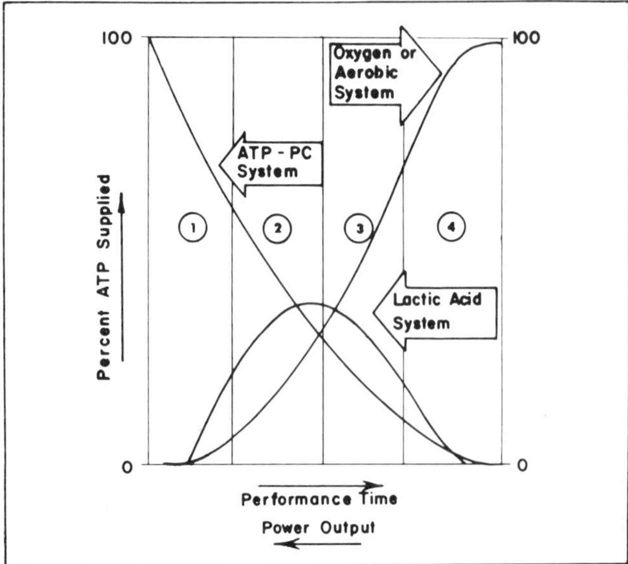

Figure 1: Division of the energy relationships into four areas of activity. The specific sports are covered by the energy continuum guidelines cited in Table I. (Adapted with permission from Sports Physiology, by E.L. Fox, p. 27. Saunders College Publishing/Holt, Rinehart and Winston. Reprinted by permission of Holt, Rinehart and Winston, CBS College Publishing, 1979.)

As an example of the utilization of the various forms of fuel during exercise, during 1 hour of bicycling 11 percent of the fuel comes from blood FFA, 13 percent from blood glucose, 32 percent from muscle triglycerides, and 44 percent from muscle glycogen. These ratios will vary with the sport, the intensity, conditioning, diet, and many other factors relevant to the athlete. In the preceding example of submaximal bicycle riding, 75 percent of the fuel is supplied by muscular stores of glycogen and triglyceride with the remainder coming from blood-borne fuels. In a shorter, more intense exercise, such as a moderately rapid 400-meter run, most food fuel would come from muscle glycogen, whereas in a 100-yard sprint the fuel would be phosphocreatinine, since there is insufficient time for either the blood-borne or stored fuels to be utilized.

Nutrition Much remains unknown about nutrition in athletes. If an individual is eating a reasonably balanced diet, the addition of a vigorous exercise program requires no vitamin, mineral, calcium, or protein supplementation. Since the major fuels utilized are carbohydrates and fats and since the former is much more accessible, adding carbohydrate to the diet should provide the additional fuel needed for strenuous exercise. There are no "quick energy" products, and athletes should be discouraged from engaging in any of the many dietary fads or gimmicks that are available.

Fluids are important during periods of strenuous exercise, and athletes should be encouraged to drink as much as they desire. Water is the important ingredient. There are no significant advantages to any of the combinations of electrolyte and carbohydrate products available. Fluid restriction of any sort during strenuous exercise is to be condemned.

The Recovery Process Following vigorous exercise, the body must be able to return to its preexercise state, and its ability to do this rapidly is a measure of how well conditioned one is. For recovery to occur, lactic acid must be removed from muscle, muscle glycogen must be replenished, phosphagen and ATP must be restored, and any remaining oxygen debt must be eliminated.

Lactic acid removal is hastened by light exercise, which is the basis for "warming down" after extreme exertion. Lactic acid removal is relatively rapid, owing in part to its conversion back to muscle glycogen and in part to its aerobic conversion through the pyruvate system to release energy for ATP production. Since this latter conversion requires oxygen, it further enhances the oxygen debt from the exercise. Recovery time for this to occur completely is about 1 hour in a well-conditioned athlete.

A significant amount of muscle glycogen can be resynthesized in 1 to 2 hours following moderate exercise, but complete muscle and liver glycogen replacement following long duration exercise requires dietary carbohydrate. Glycogen replacement is most rapid during the first 6 hours and usually is complete within 24 hours following short-term, high intensity exercise with a normal carbohydrate diet. Prolonged endurance activities may require 48 hours for replenishment accompanied by a high carbohydrate diet.

Muscle phosphagen store replacement is quite rapid, usually occurring within minutes. This is why sprinters can perform maximally several times during a competitive session.

Recovery from oxygen debt is a two-phase process. That component not related to lactic acid metabolism, the lactic acid debt, is repaid in a few minutes. This basically consists of replenishing the myoglobin with oxygen and the aerobic recovery of phosphagen stores. The lactic acid component of the debt, or the oxygen debt needed to assist with conversion of lactic acid, takes 1 to 2 hours to repay.

Thus, the recovery process is dependent upon the particular type of athletic endeavor, the duration and extent of activity, and the energy systems most involved. In short duration, high intensity activities, recovery would be mainly from oxygen replacement and phosphagen restoration and would, therefore, only take minutes. In long duration activities, muscle glycogen restoration can take from 8 to 48 hours depending upon the duration and intensity of the exercise. Playing a series of racquetball games, such as in a 1- or 2-day tournament, would require a rest period between each game of 1 hour or longer to repay the lactic acid oxygen debt, but during that time the shorter duration restorations would have occurred. Eventual glycogen replacement would need 1 or 2 days but would not be a sufficient deficit to interfere with performance. Conditioning can shorten all these recovery times.

Muscle

Structure and Function Each skeletal muscle consists of a number of muscle bundles, and each bundle, in turn, is composed of a variable number of muscle fibers. The muscle fiber is the individual cell of the muscle and contains protoplasm, nuclei, mitochondria, glycogen, ATP, and numerous other cellular components. The basic subcellular component distinguishing skeletal muscle is the myofibril. It consists of filaments of actin and myosin, the protein components responsible for muscle activity. The basic unit of the myofibril is the sarcomere (shown schematically, Fig. 2).

The sarcomere is the area from one Z-line to the next Z-line. Immediately inside the Z-line is a lighter I-band, composed only of the contractile protein actin. The A-band consists of interdigitating layers of actin and myosin. The H-zone in the center of the sarcomere represents an area where only myosin is present.

Muscle Contraction Muscles may contract isotonically, isometrically, eccentrically, or isokinetically.

During isotonic contraction, the myofibril generates tension and shortens. The actin filaments slide over the myosin filaments, and the H-zone essentially disappears. How this occurs is not completely understood, but it is likely that there are myosin cross-links extending toward the actin filaments that remain uncoupled when the muscle is relaxed. When the muscle is stimulated, the cross-links couple the actin with the myosin, and during contraction the cross-bridges swivel, sliding the myosin over the actin to effect shortening and develop tension. Contraction requires energy from ATP breakdown, and

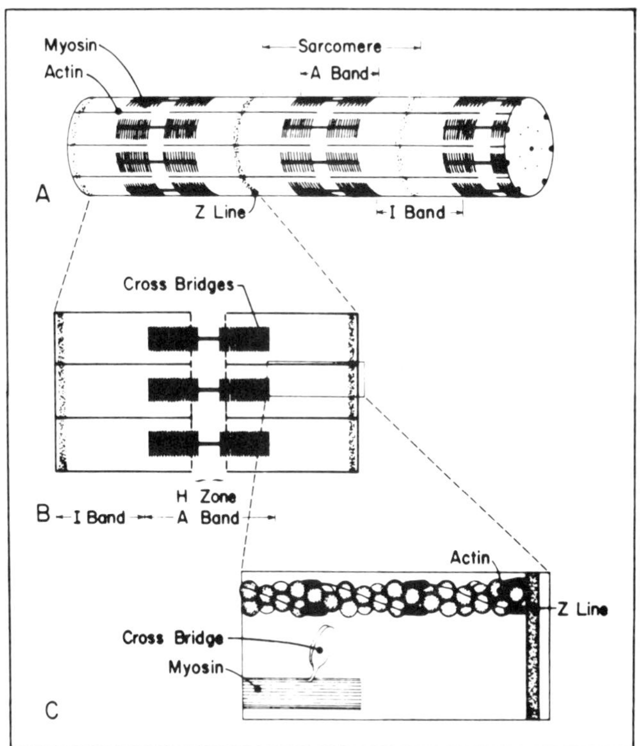

Figure 2: Detailed structure of the myofibril. (Adapted with permission from Sports Physiology, by E.L. Fox, p. 89. Saunders College Publishing/Holt, Rinehart and Winston. Reprinted by permission of Holt, Rinehart and Winston, CBS College Publishing, 1979.)

calcium is released. As the muscle relaxes, the cross-links become uncoupled, and the actin and myosin return to their previous positions, allowing the sarcomere to lengthen and the muscle to return to its resting length.

During isometric contractions (such as leg lifts), tension is generated, but the muscle does not shorten. In eccentric contractions, the muscle lengthens (as in slowly lowering a weight). Finally, isokinetic contractions occur when maximal tension is generated in a muscle contracting at a constant speed over the full range of motion.

Muscle Fiber Types A single motor nerve innervates multiple muscle fibers. The motor nerve and the muscle fibers it innervates are called the motor unit.

Two separate types of motor units, fast twitch (FT) and slow twitch (ST), can be identified anatomically and have significant metabolic and functional differences. The degree of specialization existing between FT and ST fibers has a special relevance for athletes.

FT fibers contract much quicker than ST fibers and generate maximal tension in approximately one-third the time. FT motor units are larger and, therefore, can generate more strength than ST units. Individual FT fibers have higher enzymatic activities for the phosphagen and glycolytic systems and, therefore, predominate during activities dependent upon anaerobic energy. ST fibers have a much greater aerobic capacity, with corresponding enzyme systems and increased mitochondria to facilitate oxygen utilization. Although the amount of glycogen is similar in both types, triglyceride stores are considerably higher in ST fibers.

Muscle fiber distribution in an individual is believed to be genetically determined. During any physical activity there is a selective recruitment of those fibers best suited to the specific activity. It is unlikely that the ratio of FT to ST fibers in an individual can be altered with specific training or conditioning. Instead, specific training can selectively improve the abilities of the individual fibers. Most world-class endurance athletes have a relatively high percentage of ST fibers, whereas FT fibers predominate in athletes involved in activities predominantly requiring strength. However, any athlete can differentially improve the performance of both fibers with training methods specific for either strength or endurance activities.

Muscle biopsy techniques are available to analyze the ratio of FT and ST fibers and determine various enzyme activities or glycogen stores. At the present time, these are research techniques and are not of value in specific clinical situations. However, they are adding considerably to our knowledge of exercise and muscle physiology under varying conditions.

Strength Training Increasing strength is a goal common to all athletes. To accomplish this, it is necessary to exercise the muscle group to be strengthened against maximal resistance. The resistance, or weight, must be increased as the strength improves. These principles of overload and progressive resistance are the basis of successful strength enhancement programs.

In DeLorme's original description of progressive resistance exercise programs, he defined a 10-RM load as the maximum amount of weight that could be lifted just ten times before the specific muscle group being exercised was fatigued. The program he advocated consisted of three sets of ten repetitions, using one-half of a 10-RM load for the first set, three-fourths of the 10-RM load for the second set, and the full 10-RM load for the third set, with a brief rest period between each set. When a 10-RM load could be lifted fifteen times, a new 10-RM load was established.

The ideal number of repetitions and sets for maximal strength improvement has not been determined, but probably three sets at from 6-RM to 10-RM loads are equivalent.

Isometric exercises can also significantly increase strength. For such a program to be maximally effective, a muscle group should be exercised at maximal strength for 5 seconds against resistance from five to ten times. Each muscle group should be exercised with the involved joint at three different angles.

There are numerous comparisons of isometric and isotonic programs. Isometric programs have an advantage in that they require no equipment and can be performed anywhere. However, isotonic exercises produce a more uniform increase in strength over the entire range of joint motion, and muscular endurance, as well as strength, is improved more effectively. Isometric exercises are sometimes desirable when an injured joint is involved and when the joint should not be loaded over a range of motion. Examples of this may be in the early phase of rehabilitation following knee ligament surgery or when attempting to strengthen the quadriceps and hamstrings in patients with patellofemoral disorders.

Isokinetic exercises produce the greatest strength improvement, as the muscle groups are exercised at maximal tension over the full range of motion. Thus, isokinetic programs are better at improving performance of specific patterned motor activities, such as those used in most competitive sports. However, these programs require special expensive equipment (e.g., Cybex or Nautilus). Exercises can be performed at different speeds, but training at rapid speeds of movement seems more effective in improving strength at all speeds than does training at slow speeds. Muscular endurance also can be enhanced to a greater degree than with isotonic or isometric exercise programs.

Individual exercises are specific in strengthening only those muscle groups and movement patterns used in the particular exercise. Strength programs should be designed with the individual exercises performed in a sequential manner so that the larger muscle groups are exercised before the smaller ones and arranged so that no two successive exercises involve the same muscle groups in order to allow adequate recovery time. A circuit can be established consisting of various stations, each with an exercise for a specific muscle group or action and separated by brief rest periods. Strength training workouts should be performed no more than three times weekly and probably only two times weekly during the athlete's competitive season.

The same principles apply for increasing strength and muscular endurance in both female and male athletes. However, because of low testosterone levels, females do not develop the muscle bulk of males, and the amount of strength improvement achieved is less. Similarly, preadolescent males do not develop the same muscle definition or the major strength increases as adults, although they can improve their strength to some degree. They are much

Table II

Fit or Fat?

Recommended Heart Rates During Exercise

Age	Maximum Heart Rate	85% of Maximum (Athlete-Training Rate)	80% of Maximum (Recommended Training Rate)	75% of Maximum (Heart Disease History) *Not to exceed*
20	200	170	160	150
22	198	168	158	148
24	196	167	157	147
26	194	165	155	145
28	192	163	154	144
30	190	162	152	143
32	189	161	151	142
34	187	159	150	140
36	186	158	149	140
38	184	156	147	138
40	182	155	146	137
45	179	152	143	134
50	175	149	140	131
55	171	145	137	128
60	160	136	128	120
65+	150	128	120	113

Based on resting heart rates of 72 for males and 80 for females.
Men over forty and people with any heart problem should have a stress electrocardiogram before starting an exercise program.
(Reprinted with permission from Fit or Fat?, by C. Bailey, p. 24, Houghton Mifflin, 1978.)

more susceptible to injury during strength training programs and must be carefully supervised.

Oxygen Transport Systems

Since oxygen is necessary for ATP energy production, it is important to understand its route from the environment to the muscle mitochondria. Oxygen transport involves the respiratory and circulatory systems.

Respiratory System Pulmonary ventilation is responsible for bringing oxygen into the lungs. Increasing oxygen needs are met by an increase in breathing rate, and since in reasonably healthy individuals there is a substantial reserve, pulmonary ventilation does not limit physical performance.

Oxygen, once inside the alveoli, must diffuse across the alveolar-capillary membrane. Conditioning can increase both the number of alveoli available by improving lung aeration and the diffusion capacity by enlarging the total surface area available for oxygen diffusion.

Circulatory System Once in the bloodstream, oxygen must be carried to the muscle. How efficiently this is effected greatly influences work capacity and athletic performance.

Cardiac output, the amount of blood pumped by the heart per minute, is the product of the volume of blood in each contraction, stroke volume, and heart rate. Cardiac output is about 4 to 6 liters/minute at rest but can increase to as much as 35 liters/minute during exercise. Stroke volume increases from its resting value by about 50 percent during submaximal exercise but no further during maximal exercise. Stroke volume values in an untrained individual vary from 60 to 70 ml/beat at rest to 110 to 120 ml/beat during exercise. Endurance training can increase stroke volume to as much as 100 to 110 ml/beat at rest and to 150 to 170 ml/beat during exertion. Heart rate, on the other hand, continues to rise during exercise in direct relation to the intensity of the exercise until an age-determined maximum is reached. Therefore, the major contribution to the increase in cardiac output during maximal exercise is from the rise in pulse rate.

As an individual becomes better conditioned aerobically, stroke volume increases requiring a lower heart rate at any given level of activity, from rest to maximal exertion. Monitoring the pulse rate can be used effectively to assess appropriate exercise intensity, recovery from exercise, and conditioning. To be more specific, an individual can effectively and safely monitor and modify a conditioning program at any level by performing exercise to raise the pulse to a predetermined age-related level and maintaining that level for 15 to 30 minutes. An example is given in Table II. When an individual is poorly conditioned, it may require only brisk walking to achieve the desired pulse rate, and as conditioning improves, running, bicycling, or another more strenuous activity is needed. If an individual can achieve and maintain the pulse at the desired level for the appropriate length of time three to five times weekly, significant improvements in aerobic capacity occur.

Oxygen Transport The crux of this transport system is how effectively oxygen can be provided to the muscle in a usable form. The arterial-venous oxygen difference is a measure of the amount of oxygen the muscle extracts from arterial blood. If cardiac output is multiplied by the arterial-venous oxygen difference, the result is the amount of oxygen utilized by the muscles. This is usually referred to as VO_2. If this is measured under conditions of maximum exercise, it indicates the maximal amount of oxygen capable of being transported to and consumed by the working muscles. This value, known as VO_2max, is usually expressed in milliliters of oxygen per kilogram of body weight per minute (ml/kg-min). It is possible to increase the VO_2max 15 to 20 percent with training. Some individuals are capable of achieving much higher values than others. It is probable that, even though the value can be improved by training, the ability to achieve a very high VO_2max is genetically determined. It has been noted that world-class athletes in endurance sports, such as cross-country skiing, distance running, and triathletes, have the highest VO_2max values measured.

6 MS:H **Oxygen Utilization** It is not only the magnitude of VO_2max that is important during performance of endurance activities but also how efficiently oxygen is utilized. The amount used during a given activity can be expressed as a percent of the VO_2max. Therefore, an activity requiring a fixed amount of oxygen will be performed more efficiently by an individual with a higher VO_2max, since the percent VO_2max will be lower. Thus, this is an indication of how stressful an activity is with respect to maximum capacity.

Conversely, if two individuals with the same VO_2max require different amounts of oxygen to run at a given pace, the one requiring less oxygen will be able to run faster to achieve an equal percent VO_2max.

Lactic acid begins to accumulate with increasing activity level, and the higher the percent VO_2max achieved before significant levels of lactic acid build up, the better the individual is able to perform endurance activities. While VO_2max is genetically determined, the ability to utilize a high percent VO_2max without significant lactic acid accumulation is almost solely determined by training.

Training Programs

Continuous submaximal training exerts the greatest effect upon the oxygen transport system, whereas high intensity and interval training affect primarily the structural and biochemical properties of the muscle.

Interval training has a theoretical basis in the knowledge that by interspersing short rest periods between bursts of high intensity exercise, the total accumulated exercise time can be increased. This is of particular advantage in improving performance times.

General Conditioning General conditioning programs, when appropriately implemented, increase cardiac efficiency and work capacity, decrease body fat stores, decrease appetite, increase high density lipoprotein levels without changing plasma triglyceride or cholesterol levels, and decrease fasting blood sugar and endogenous insulin requirements. All these effects are believed to be beneficial. They also are commonly associated with a perceptible increase in one's sense of well-being.

Exercise programs are of value in weight control and probably are effective in decreasing blood pressure. The increased skeletal load associated with exercise will increase bone density, and the involutional osteopenia occurring with aging can be decreased. Animal experiments have shown an increase in strength and stiffness of ligaments as a direct response to exercise, and other experiments have shown that there is no increase in the incidence of degenerative joint disease in exercised animals as compared with sedentary controls, provided that the joints are reasonably normal. In the presence of significant joint dysfunction, such as ligamentous instability or preexisting degenerative changes, repetitive impact loading exercises, such as running and jumping, may hasten the progression of degenerative arthritis in weight-bearing joints. This has never been well quantitated but must be considered when advising patients.

There also appears to be an association between early coronary artery disease and low levels of high density lipoprotein cholesterol. Several studies have shown that aerobic exercise programs will increase the levels of HDL cholesterol and, thereby, perhaps afford a measure of protection against cardiovascular risk factors.

For general recreational conditioning, an individual should select a program that gives a cardiovascular response, improves strength, and improves flexibility. Adding variety to the program will be helpful in maintaining individual compliance, and exercise circuits often are available that include all essential elements for an interesting workout.

For example, an individual could begin with a series of exercises designed to stretch all of the major muscle groups in the body, particularly emphasizing the posterior trunk and lower extremity musculature. An aerobic activity, such as running, swimming, or bicycling, would follow with the pulse rate monitored to determine the appropriate intensity. The initial length of the aerobic component should be 15 to 20 minutes, but as conditioning improves, it should become longer, depending upon individual goals. Aerobic activity can vary but should be accomplished from three to five times weekly to be effective.

Strength training may be added in a variety of ways but always should be under supervision. The program should be designed to strengthen the major muscle groups and done no more than three times weekly.

If improvement of performance times is desired, interval training can be added, depending upon the goals and involvement of the individual. Interval training is a necessary component of training in competitive and high performance athletes but often is eliminated in general or recreational conditioning. It should be alternated with an aerobic workout, and 1 or 2 days weekly is sufficient.

Specificity When designing programs for competitive athletes, it is important to emphasize that each component of any training program is highly specific and is effective predominantly for only those modalities and muscle groups being exercised. The most effective programs are those that are sport specific. Although there may be endurance and cardiovascular fitness benefits in putting a cross-country skier on a running program, the athlete is much more efficiently and effectively trained by doing the distance and interval workouts skiing. Strength workouts designed for the muscle groups most utilized in cross-country skiing, even to the extent of using the same patterns of movements, are also more effective.

Rehabilitation It is important to differentiate training and conditioning programs from rehabilitation. Efforts to restore function in a limb following injury or surgery must employ different techniques than will be utilized in conditioning. Supervisory personnel must be trained therapists or athletic trainers who are accustomed to working within the limitations present when poor strength or limited joint motion are present. To permit a patient to undergo rehabilitation in a fitness center without supervision by personnel trained in dealing with that specific injury or surgery would be inadvisable. The distinction between conditioning and rehabilitation must always be kept in mind. Conditioning the athlete may continue while the injured part is being rehabilitated, and following any rehabilitation program, a strong conditioning effort is mandatory prior to returning to competition.

Sex Differences

Females have greater body fat and lower strength than males, due to the higher estrogen and lower androgen levels. With training, females can achieve very low body fat content but often with attendant temporary amenorrhea.

Strength comparisons are quite interesting. Males are stronger than females at all ages, but when strength is broken down and expressed relative to body size, lower extremity strengths are nearly equal, whereas the female is 30 to 50 percent weaker in the upper extremities. This difference can be decreased significantly with strength training. Power and muscular endurance are more difficult to assess. Females show the same high correlation between the VO_2max and the percentage of ST fibers as do males, although males have a larger muscle fiber cross-sectional area on muscle biopsy specimens, probably reflecting the greater strength.

Cardiovascular endurance is usually lower in females, due largely to the decreased stroke volume and the lower blood hemoglobin concentration. Measured VO_2max levels are equal up to the age of 15 years. In the older groups the values in males are higher, probably due to the decreased maximum cardiac output in females. However, when expressed in terms of lean body weight, males and females are much closer to being equal at all ages.

Few sex differences are noted below the age of 12 years. Beyond this age, however, there are considerable differences in all parameters. In our society, until very recently, males were much more active than females after puberty. Assuming a sedentary lifestyle, the basic physiological components of general fitness deteriorate, and, therefore, much data may be available comparing active males with sedentary females. The dramatic biologic difference in the sexes may be related to cultural and social factors. Studies are in process which should clarify these observations.

ANNOTATED BIBLIOGRAPHY

Exercise

Exercise Physiology

Fox, E.L.: Sports Physiology. Philadelphia, W.B. Saunders, 1979.

A summary of the physiologic parameters as applied to sports.

Effects of Exercise

American College of Sports Medicine, Position Statement: The recommended quantity and quality of exercise for developing and maintaining fitness in healthy adults. Med. Sci. Sports 10: vii, 1978.

This outlines the recommended guidelines for prescribing exercise programs for basically healthy adults and uses background provided by the bibliography as the rationale. It is essential to utilize a rhythmical, aerobic activity that uses large muscle groups continuously, maintaining 60 to 90 percent of maximum heart rate for 15 to 60 minutes, with a frequency of three to five times weekly.

Bailey, C.: Fit or Fat? Boston, Houghton Mifflin, 1978.

A monograph with ideas about conditioning programs. This source of information for patients describes the rationale for sensible weight loss and conditioning for all ages.

Fox, E.L.: Methods and effects of physical training. Pediat. Ann. 7:690-703, 1978.

Methods of various training programs and the advantages of various types of activities for specific training are summarized.

Franklin, B.A., and Rubenfire, M.: Losing weight through exercises. J. Am. Med. Assn. 244:377-379, 1980.

A discussion of how weight can be lost with sensible exercise programs, particularly emphasizing the popular misconceptions often touted in advertising and the lay press.

Leon, A.S.; Conrad, J.; Hunninghake, D.B.; and Serfass, R.: Effects of a vigorous walking program on body composition, and carbohydrate and lipid metabolism of obese young men. Am. J. Clin. Nutr. 32:1776-1787, 1979.

Vigorous regular walking programs in six sedentary obese men produced a reduction in body fat stores, food intake, and endogenous insulin requirements. There was also a beneficial effect of increasing the high density lipoprotein cholesterol fraction.

Fuels for Exercise

Buskirk, E.R.; Hermansen, L.; Hultman, E.; Kaijser, L.; and Saltin, B.: Muscle fuel for competition. Physician Sports Med. 7:49-58, 1979.

A panel of experts discusses glycogen utilization and how athletes can manipulate it in their diet to maximum advantage in competition.

Herbert, V.: Megavitamin therapy. N.Y. State J. Med. 79:278-285, 1979.

This discussion of vitamin function in general and utilization by athletes with guidelines for advising athletes points out the hazards of vitamins in large dosages and what few benefits can accrue by supplementation.

Muscle

Smith, N.J.: Food For Sport. Palo Alto, CA, Bull Publishing Company, 1976.

This monograph describes the basics of nutrition and diet as they pertain to athletes of all ages. It has numerous specific examples of applications of the information to specific situations. Since it is non-technical, it is appropriate reading for physicians, patients, athletes, coaches, and trainers.

Salmons, S., and Henriksson, J.: The adaptive response of skeletal muscle to increased use. Muscle and Nerve 4:94-105, 1981.

This is a review of the morphologic, biochemical, and physiological changes that occur in muscle undergoing prolonged exercise.

Training Programs

Videman, T.: The effect of running on the osteoarthritis joint: An experimental matched pair study with rabbits. Rheumat. and Rehab. 21:1-8, 1982.

The only recent experimental study attempting to determine whether repetitive impact loading exercises (running) are detrimental to joints. Rabbits were used as the model, and no significant degenerative joint changes were observed in those subjected to vigorous running programs in matched pair studies.

Woo, S.L.-Y.; Kuei, S.C.; Amiel, D.; Gomez, M.A.; Hayes, W.C.; White, F.C.; and Akeson, W.H.: The effect of prolonged physical training on the properties of long bone: A study of Wolff's law. J. Bone Joint Surg. 63A:780-787, 1981.

Intense exercise training in pig models resulted in a major increase in the quantity of femur bone, principally due to replacement of the marrow bone with cortical bone. The mechanical properties of the cortical bone were unchanged, indicating that the exercise increased the quantity of bone without altering the quality.

Sex-Related Differences in Exercise and Training

Cox, J.S., and Lenz, H.W.: Women in sports: The Naval Academy experience. Am. J. Sports Med. 7:355-357, 1979.

Initial female Naval Academy entrants averaged three times the incidence of physical injuries as males; however, with each succeeding class, the incidence has decreased. The article concludes that as physical conditioning requirements for females are increased and met, the sex differences will be minimized and that current differences are societal rather than physiological.

8
MS:H

Frisch, R.E.; Gotz-Welbergen, A.V.; McArthur, J.W.; Albright, T.; Witschi, J.; Bullen, B.; Birnholz, J.; Reed, R.B.; and Hermann, H.: Delayed menarche and amenorrhea of college athletes in relation to age of onset of training. J. Am. Med. Assn. 246:1559-1563, 1981.

A group of swimmers and runners who began training prior to menarche were compared with a similar group who had not begun extensive training until after menarche. The former showed a delay of the average age of menarche of approximately 2.5 years and following menarche had higher incidences of oligomenorrhea and amenorrhea than did the postmenarchal-trained athletes. All irregularities cleared after training ceased, and therefore no long-term effects were postulated. The reasons for the delay in menarche are unclear, and possible hormonal and body fat content mechanisms are discussed.

Warren, M.P.: The effects of pubertal progression and reproductive function in girls. J. Clin. Endocrinol. and Metab. 51:1150-1157, 1980.

The author studied 15 ballet dancers ages 13 to 15 who had been involved in high levels of activity for several years. Significant differences were found in body fat content (lower), age at menarche (higher), and sexual development (slower) than age-matched controls. Progression of sexual development seemed to occur when activity levels were relatively low, such as during convalescence from injury or while on vacation. Criteria of prolongation of prepubertal state were documented and believed to be due to the stress of the physical activity.

Wilmore, J.H.: The application of science to sport: Physiological profiles of male and female athletes. Can. J. Appl. Sport Sci. 4:103-115, 1979.

Review of previous data regarding male-female differences and similarities in highly trained athletes reveals considerable similarities in strength per unit of body weight, cardiovascular endurance, body composition, and muscle fiber type.

2 CONGENITAL ABNORMALITIES OF THE SKELETON

This section is a review of advances in evaluation and management of congenital abnormalities of connective tissue, generalized bone dysplasias and the growth plate, and skeletal abnormalities with environmental cause.

Connective Tissue Disorders

The first disease regarded as a generalized disorder of connective tissue on clinical grounds was osteogenesis imperfecta. The prototype of "heritable disorders of connective tissue," the phrase popularized by McKusick, is the Marfan syndrome. The first human disorder of collagen in which the biochemical defect was identified is one of the forms of Ehlers-Danlos syndrome.

COLLAGEN: Many connective tissue disorders are believed to be caused by an abnormality in collagen, the major structural protein of connective tissue.

Collagen molecules consist of three polypeptide alpha chains, each having about 1,000 amino acids, arranged in helical form. The amino acid composition of the alpha chains determines which one of five types of collagen is produced (Table I). The system of production is complex, thus creating the possibility for errors in the raw materials, the enzymes required for assembly, and the assembly process.

CLASSIFICATION: Most connective tissue disorders can be grouped as Ehlers-Danlos, Marfan or Marfan-like conditions, and osteogenesis imperfecta.

Ehlers-Danlos Syndrome These diseases are characterized by skin that is hyperlax and which also may be thin, fragile, and bruisable; joint hyperextensibility; and hernia as well as other manifestations of connective tissue dysfunction. Nine forms of Ehlers-Danlos are delineated, and it is likely that additional forms will be recognized (Table II).

ORTHOPAEDIC MANAGEMENT: Patients with lax skin should be evaluated to determine the type of abnormality present. This diagnosis permits anticipation of special complications and appropriate genetic counseling. Incisions normally heal well, but care is required to minimize scarring. Several types of Ehlers-Danlos exhibit thin skin that creates "cigarette paper" scars with minimal trauma.

The most common orthopaedic problems associated with Ehlers-Danlos are scoliosis, joint dislocation, and clubfoot. The management of scoliosis is as in idiopathic scoliosis. Increased flexibility of the spine appears to contribute to a high incidence of progressive scoliosis, and early fusion often is indicated.

Joint dislocations occur principally at the patellofemoral and shoulder joints but may occur in the fingers, jaw, and hips. Recurrent shoulder dislocation in this syndrome may indicate universal joint laxity and respond poorly to conventional anterior repair. Joint laxity in the feet is often symptomatic and may benefit by the use of arch supports beginning in childhood.

Clubfoot, a paradoxical feature of Ehlers-Danlos, tends to be severe and is characterized by marked laxity of the overlying skin making manipulative and casting techniques difficult. Surgical management is commonly required.

Table I

Collagen

Type	Location
I	Skin, bone, tendon
II	Cartilage
III	Blood vessels, skin, spleen
IV	Basement membrane
V	Placenta, smooth muscle

The Marfan Syndrome This syndrome classically affects the skeleton, lens, and heart. Skeletal changes include tall stature (90 percent), disproportionate growth of extremities in comparison to the trunk (70 percent), disproportionate growth of phalanges in comparison to the metacarpals (80 percent), scoliosis (60 percent), and chest wall deformity (50 percent). The lens may be dislocated, and the heart affected by valvular abnormalities, aortic dilatation, and aneurysm.

DIAGNOSIS: This syndrome demonstrates considerable variation in expression, and no single clinical or biochemical feature defines it. Diagnosis of Marfan's syndrome implies dominant transmission of a condition associated with limited life span and considerable morbidity. Thus, this diagnosis should be made with caution. McKusick has indicated that, "diagnosis of the Marfan syndrome can usually not be made with complete confidence when ectopia lentis or a positive family history are not found." Other connective tissue disorders that resemble Marfan's include the various forms of Ehlers-Danlos, congenital contractural arachnodactyly, homocystinuria, the Stickler syndrome, hypermobility syndrome, and the mitral valve prolapse syndrome.

Congenital contractural arachnodactyly, a dominant disorder, is characterized by congenital peripheral contractures, gracile extremities, and ear deformity in the

Table II
Forms of Ehlers-Danlos Syndrome

		Major Clinical Features	Heritability	Biochemistry
	I Gravis	Skin: soft, fragile, lax, bruises, venous varicosities Hernia Joint dislocations	Dominant	Not known
10 MS:C	II Mitis	Skin: soft, lax, bruises Joints: moderately hypermobile Less severe than Type I	Dominant	Not known
	III Benign hypermobility	Skin: soft Joints: very hypermobile, dislocations common	Dominant	Not known
	IV Ecchymotic	Skin: thin, bleeds easily Joints: finger joints hypermobile Bowel rupture Arterial rupture Hernia common	Dominant and Recessive	Decreased Type III collagen
	V X-linked	Skin: striking peripheral hyperextensibility, bruises Joints: moderate hypermobility	X-linked	Not known
	VI Ocular	Skin: hyperextensible, bruises Joints: hypermobile, TEV, CDH Scoliosis Sclera and cornea ruptures Retinal detachment	Recessive	Lysl hydroxylase deficiency
	VII Arthrochalasis multiplex congenita	Skin: soft, lax, thin Joints: extreme hypermobility Short stature	Recessive	Variable
	VIII Periodontitis variety	Skin: fragile, loose, bruises Joints: moderately loose Teeth: severe periodontitis with early tooth loss	Dominant	Not known
	IX Occipital horns	Skin: fragile, loose, bruises Joints: mildly hypermobile, radial head dislocation Other: hernia, bladder diverticulitis Skull: occipital horns	X-linked	Not known

presence of normal height. The syndrome lacks lens dislocation and heart disease is rare.

Homocystinuria is a recessive disorder with mental retardation, osteoporosis, fracture, life-threatening thromboembolic phenomenon, and ectopic lens. Normal intelligence does not rule out this diagnosis. Isolated patients with lens dislocation and apparent Marfan's syndrome should have a urine screen for homocystine.

The Stickler syndrome, a relatively common dominant disorder, often is associated with micrognathia in infancy, myopia, thin extremities, mild scoliosis, and early degenerative arthritis.

The hypermobility syndrome is often familial and characterized by normal skin and lax joints which may dislocate. Affected patients lack heart disease and lens subluxation.

Mitral valve prolapse is a dominant disorder in which the patient may or may not be symptomatic, i.e., chest pain, palpitations, syncope, and easy fatigability. These patients have significant narrowing of the anteroposterior chest diameter, increased arm spans, and often have scoliosis and pectus excavatum. Patients with this condition commonly resemble those with Marfan's syndrome but have normal lens and lack aortic dilation.

Orthopaedic management: Young female patients anticipated to become very tall may be considered for estrogen treatment, causing early skeletal maturation. Children with Marfan's syndrome should be followed carefully for development of scoliosis and at its earliest onset be placed in an appropriate spinal orthosis. Established scoliosis may be progressive despite bracing, and early surgery after appropriate cardiac evaluation should be considered.

Connective tissue disorders, especially Marfan's, have a high incidence of protrusio acetabuli. Research indicates that closure of the triradiate cartilage in symptomatic patients will correct this abnormality.

Regular cardiac evaluation is desirable in Marfan patients. Participation in sports generally is not advisable.

Osteogenesis Imperfecta This connective tissue disorder is characterized by fragile bones and congenital osteoporosis. A new and tentative classification has been created by Sillence, who suggests that the prior classification of congenita versus tarda, broad bone versus thin bone, or mild versus severe is less useful. His classification of four groups (Table III) appears rational but unfortunately does not always permit classification at birth.

Clinical, histologic, and biochemical abnormalities found in osteogenesis imperfecta are variable. Abnormalities are present in connective tissue throughout the body and are not confined to bone. In all osteogenesis imperfecta there is decreased bone mass and often increased bone turnover. In some forms there is evidence of increased type III collagen and concomitant decreased production of type I collagen. Biochemical findings are not currently useful in diagnosis, and prenatal diagnosis is unreliable.

Orthopaedic management: No systemic treatment has proved effective in its management. Orthopaedic management deals with the treatment of fractures, bowing of long bones, and scoliosis.

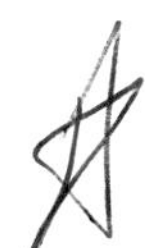

Fractures heal promptly in osteogenesis imperfecta. Bracing may help minimize bowing of the long bones and assist in mobility.

Bowing occurs in both upper and lower extremities. The use of intramedullary rods with multiple osteotomies has

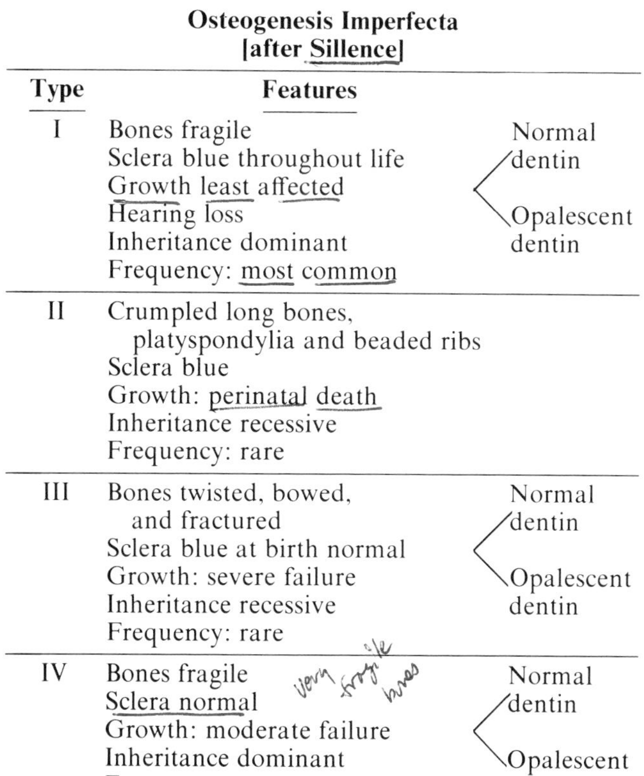

Table III

Osteogenesis Imperfecta [after Sillence]

Type	Features	
I	Bones fragile Sclera blue throughout life Growth least affected Hearing loss Inheritance dominant Frequency: most common	Normal dentin Opalescent dentin
II	Crumpled long bones, platyspondylia and beaded ribs Sclera blue Growth: perinatal death Inheritance recessive Frequency: rare	
III	Bones twisted, bowed, and fractured Sclera blue at birth normal Growth: severe failure Inheritance recessive Frequency: rare	Normal dentin Opalescent dentin
IV	Bones fragile Sclera normal Growth: moderate failure Inheritance dominant Frequency: rare	Normal dentin Opalescent dentin

been modified by the introduction of telescoping rods. These and other techniques of straightening bones have wide application for both upper and lower extremity deformities.

Scoliosis occurs in nearly one-half of patients with osteogenesis imperfecta and often is associated with vertebral collapse. Orthoses are typically ineffective except in mild forms, and early surgery to stabilize the spine often is indicated.

11

MS:C

Skeletal Dysplasias

During the past decade many advances have been made in clinical delineation of the numerous types of inherited skeletal dysplasias. These vary greatly in clinical presentation. The 1977 International Nomenclature of Constitutional Diseases of Bone included seventy-one osteochondral dysplasias and eighteen dysostoses syndromes. Ten additional chondrodystrophies were added recently. Despite increased knowledge of the various mucopolysaccharidoses, the orthopaedic management of the disorders remains limited awaiting advances in genetic engineering.

Accurate diagnosis is the most important step in management of skeletal dysplasias. This allows for anticipation of ultimate height, prognostication of the most likely deformities or other medical problems, and indication of the recurrence risks to the patient and family. Because of the complexity of diagnosis, patients with dysplasias of uncertain type should be referred to diagnostic centers.

Achondroplasia This most common bone dysplasia is a rhizomelic (short proximal portion of the extremity), short-limbed dysplasia resulting in an adult height of about 122 cm. It is transmitted by autosomal dominant inheritance. Diagnosis is certain at any age by evaluation of clinical and radiographic features. The biochemical defect is unknown, but there appears to be an abnormality of chondrocyte proliferation. Clinical features include a depressed nasal bridge, prominent forehead, trident hands, lax joints, and limb disproportion. Radiographic features include a failure of widening of the interpedicular distance in the lower lumbar spine, short iliac wings with a small sacrosciatic notch, and epiphyses appearing to be embedded into the metaphysis. Growth failure within a bone is roughly proportional to the area of the adjacent growth plate and produces disproportionate growth failure of the paired bones. There is, for example, greater growth failure of the tibia than the fibula.

Orthopaedic management: Orthopaedic management is directed primarily at deformities of the thoracolumbar spine and the lower extremities. Since there is a high incidence of increased lumbar lordosis and thoracolumbar kyphosis in achondroplasia, periodic lateral radiographs of the lumbar spine should be obtained. Kyphosis develops due to a combination of lax joints, weak muscles, large and heavy skull, and persistence of newborn hip contractures. Treatment in infancy involves the avoidance of weight transmission in the spine by the use of reclining infant seats and the delay of sitting. If kyphosis develops, it should be braced (Fig. 1). If progressive, surgery may be indicated. In the adult achondroplast, spinal stenosis and degenerative disc disease also may become symptomatic in the narrowed, lordotic lumbar spine. Genu varum, common in patients with achon-

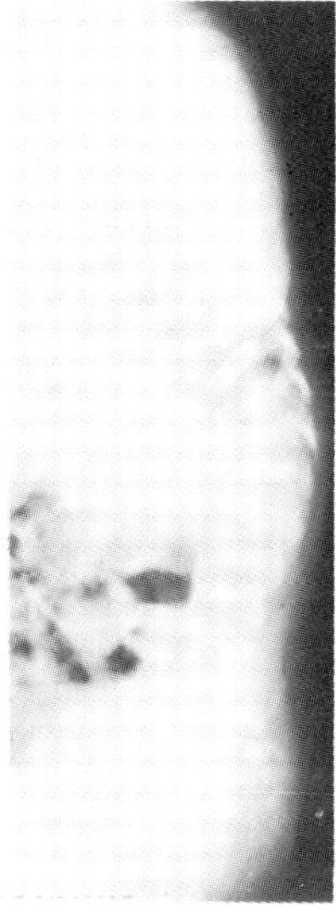
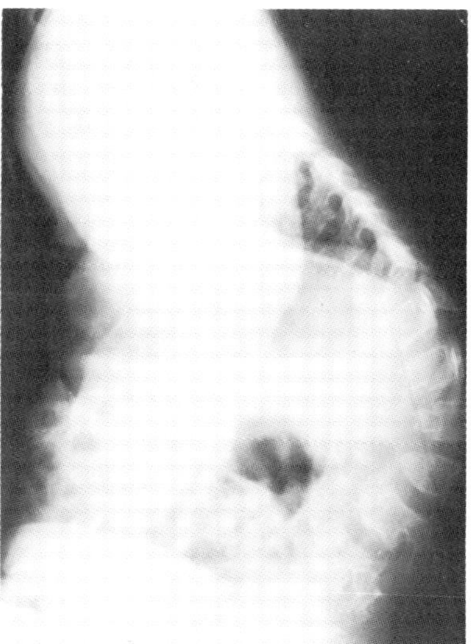
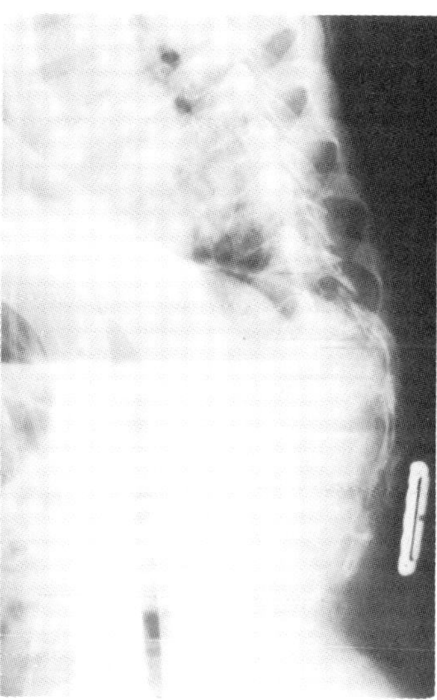

Figure 1: Sequence of lateral spine radiographs of an achondroplastic child demonstrating progression and improvement following application of a thoraco-lumbo-sacral orthosis.

droplasia, usually is associated with a relative overgrowth of both proximal and distal fibulae, but these features may not be etiologically related. Persistent deformity may require proximal tibial osteotomy.

Other Dysplasias Skeletal abnormalities associated with bone dysplasias include alteration in stature and proportion, spinal lordosis and kyphosis, scoliosis, contractures, joint laxity and mechanical instability, bowing and angular deformities, bony coalition, osteolysis, altered bone mass and density, and osteoarthritis. The most serious complications are kyphosis at the thoracolumbar junction and instability of the cervical spine.

Cervical instability occurs in so many dysplasias that screening cervical spine radiographs should be considered for most patients with skeletal dysplasias. Abnormalities include an absent odontoid, ligamentous laxity, and invagination of the cervical spine into the base of the skull (see Section 23, Cervical Spine: Pediatric).

Growth Plate

Current research focuses on clinical and genetic characterization of bone dysplasia. When appropriate, growth plate biopsies (usually from the iliac crest) are utilized to study the ultrastructure and histochemical features. An increasing number of dysplasias can be identified by these characteristics.

Additional research is directed toward the role of metabolites, oxygen, and vascular supply on the growth process. The effects of trauma and electrical current on the growth plate are also being studied.

Structure and Function The growth plate consists of several zones of cartilage cells that rest on a bony metaphysis and are surrounded by fibrous tissue, each of which has a separate blood supply (Fig. 2).

The growth cartilage is divided into zones of cells: reserve, proliferative, and hypertrophic, which is subdivided into maturating, degenerating, and provisional calcification (Fig. 3).

The function of the reserve zone is storage; the proliferative zone is cell proliferation and matrix production; and the hypertrophic zone is matrix calcification. The metaphysis transmits vessels for invasion of the calcified matrix and is the site of initial bone formation and remodeling.

Compression and Distraction of the Growth Plate One area of study with clinical relevance is the effect of pressure and distraction on the growth plate. For example, epiphyseal arrest by stapling produces pressure and stops growth. This process is generally reversible when compression is removed.

Partial epiphyseal closure by trauma often produces distorted growth. This also is reversible in many patients following resection of the offending bony bar and replacement by some interposing substance, such as fat, Silastic, cartilage, or methyl methacrylate (see Section 7, General: Trauma).

Distraction of the epiphysis and metaphysis at the distal portion of the growth plate theoretically should not

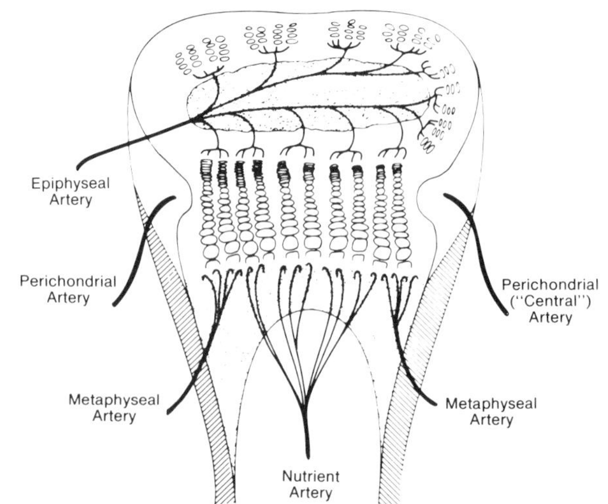

Figure 2: Drawing showing the blood supply of a typical growth plate. (Reprinted with permission from Structure and function of the growth plate, by C.T. Brighton, Clin. Orthop. 136:23, 1978.)

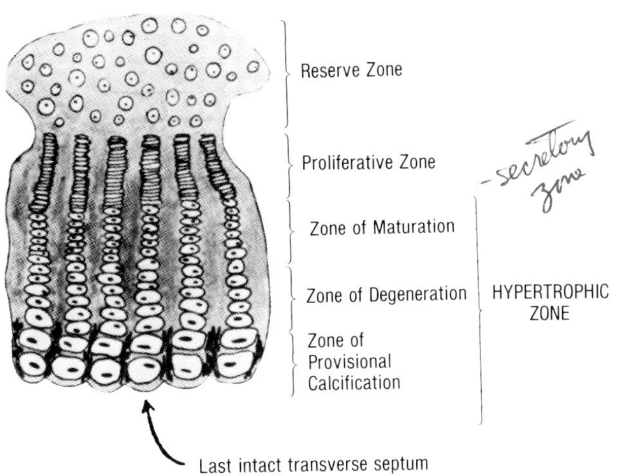

Figure 3: Cartilaginous component. Drawing depicting the various zones of the cartilaginous portion of the growth plate. (Reprinted with permission from Structure and function of the growth plate, by C.T. Brighton, Clin. Orthop. 136:24, 1978.)

interfere with the growth process and may promote increased cell column growth. Although this concept is being tested clinically to create increased length, the results have not been verified.

Congenital Skeletal Abnormalities With Environmental Cause

Three conditions appearing to have environmental causes are discussed to alert the clinician to the importance of including an evaluation of the prenatal environment as part of the work-up of congenital abnormalities and to suggest that some skeletal abnormalities may be preventable.

Arthrogryposis Studies of the incidence of classic arthrogryposis disclosed a worldwide "epidemic" in the 1960s. Retrospective maternal health data reveal increased medical problems in early pregnancy and suggest the possibility of viral etiology. In classic arthrogryposis, which is nonheritable, the upper limbs are internally rotated, the shoulders and elbows have limited voluntary motion, and there are severe peripheral contractures. The lower limbs tend to be externally rotated, and there is limited hip and knee motion. Clubfoot deformity is common. Intelligence is normal.

In contrast, there are many patients with congenital limb contractures often classified as arthrogryposis for lack of better terminology. A comprehensive study of these patients has led to a useful classification of "distal arthrogryposis." Type I is dominantly inherited, is not associated with other anomalies, has ulnar deviated, clenched fists at birth with positional foot deformities, and undergoes improvement with age. Type II has associated abnormalities ranging from cleft palate and facial anomalies to mental retardation, and it is divided into five subgroups. The study illustrates the value of separating a variety of similar conditions that have different cause, prognosis, and inheritance.

Foetal Alcohol Syndrome The search for environmental causes of congenital anomalies has defined a syndrome caused by maternal alcoholism during pregnancy. The main features of the syndrome are low intelligence, low birth weight, small head circumference, and facies characterized by blepharophimosis, absent nasolabial folds, and narrow upper lip. This syndrome now is recognized increasingly and may present with orthopaedic problems.

Radioulnar synostosis, fusion of the cervical spine, and coalition of the capitate and hamate occur in approximately one-half of these patients. Other skeletal abnormalities include clinodactyly, short fingers, and flexion contracture of the elbow.

Diabetic Embryopathy The incidence of diabetes is increasing, and about one of every 500 babies has a diabetic mother. Improved perinatal care, especially cardiorespiratory, has improved the survival rate to about 95 percent. Children of diabetic mothers have two to three times the incidence of congenital anomalies as do those of nondiabetic mothers. Congenital anomalies are now the most common causes of death in children of diabetic mothers.

These congenital anomalies affect, in decreasing order of frequency, the skeletal, cardiac, neural, genitourinary, and gastrointestinal systems. The skeletal malformation most associated with maternal diabetes is the caudal regression syndrome which occurs 200 times more commonly in children of diabetic mothers than in the general population. The caudal regression syndrome includes partial or total absence of the sacral elements with or without associated femoral and other lower limb anomalies. The considerable variability in limb anomalies ranges from sireniform (mermaid) deformities to "arthrogryposis." The sacrum may be spared, and the upper limbs may be affected.

The pathogenesis of these anomalies is not understood, but they occur in the first several weeks of gestation and are more common in the fetuses of mothers with poorly controlled diabetes.

ANNOTATED BIBLIOGRAPHY

Connective Tissue Disorders

Ehlers-Danlos Syndrome

Beighton, P., and Horan, F.: Orthopaedic aspects of Ehlers-Danlos syndrome. J. Bone Joint Surg. 51B:444-453, 1969.

This is a brief description of orthopaedic problems encountered in 100 patients with Ehlers-Danlos syndrome.

Bornstein, P., and Byers, D.H.: Collagen metabolism *In* Curr. Concepts. Upjohn, 1980.

This pamphlet is a review of the relationship between known biochemical abnormalities of collagen and the clinical states of connective tissue disorders.

Hollister, D.W.: Clinical features of Ehlers-Danlos Syndrome types VIII and IX. *In* AAOS Symposium on Heritable Disorders of Connective Tissue, pp. 102-113, edited by W.H. Akeson, P. Bornstein, and M.J. Glimcher. St. Louis, C.V. Mosby, 1982.

The clinical features of these last two types of Ehlers-Danlos are described.

The Marfan's Syndrome

Finsterbush, A., and Pogrund, H.: The hypermobility syndrome. Clin. Orthop. 168:124-127, 1982.

One hundred patients with generalized joint laxity who did not have increasing skin laxity or evidence of known connective tissue disorders were evaluated. It was found to be familial in over one-half of the patients. The most common orthopaedic problems were flat feet (48), patellar hypermobility (28), scoliosis (20), and recurrent ankle sprains (16).

McKusick, V.A.: Heritable Disorders of Connective Tissue. Ed. 4. St. Louis, C.V. Mosby, 1972.

This text forms the basis of clinical knowledge of all connective tissue disorders.

Pyeritz, R.E.: The Marfan phenotype: Pleiotrophy and variability as clues to genetic heterogeneity. *In* AAOS Symposium on Heritable Disorders of Connective Tissue, pp. 114-121, edited by W.H. Akeson, P. Bornstein, and M.J. Glimcher. St. Louis, C.V. Mosby, 1982.

A discussion with references of the differential diagnosis of Marfan's syndrome is included in this article.

Steel, H.H.: Protrusio acetabuli. Its occurrence as a constant in Marfan's syndrome and a surgical approach to the problem by closure of the triradiate epiphysis. Orthop. Trans. 4:353, 1980.

Early experience with surgical closure of the triradiate epiphysis in patients with symptomatic protrusio acetabuli demonstrates that the radiographic abnormality can be reversed.

Osteogenesis Imperfecta

Albright, J.A., and Miller, E.A.: Osteogenesis imperfecta. (Editorial Comment) Clin. Orthop. 159:2, 1981.

This symposium includes a review of current knowledge of medical and surgical management of osteogenesis imperfecta with special consideration of orthopaedic care. Sillence's classification is included.

Yong-Hing, K., and MacEwen, G.D.: Scoliosis associated with osteogenesis imperfecta. J. Bone Joint Surg. 64B:36-43, 1982.

A report of 121 patients with scoliosis and osteogenesis imperfecta documents the complications and problems associated with management.

Skeletal Dysplasias

Beals, R.K.: Orthopaedic care for patients with skeletal dysplasias. *In* AAOS Symposium on Heritable Disorders of Connective Tissue, pp. 362-368, edited by W.H. Akeson, P. Bornstein, and M.J. Glimcher. St. Louis, C.V. Mosby, 1982.

An overview of the types of problems encountered in skeletal dysplasia is presented. General strategies for management of deformities are discussed without technical details.

Bethem, D.; Winter, R.B.; Lutter, L.; Moe, J.H.; Bradford, D.S.; Lonstein, J.E.; and Langer, L.O.: Spinal disorders of dwarfism. J. Bone Joint Surg. 63A:1412-1425, 1981.

This review of eighty patients documents the frequency and type of spine problems found in short-statured patients with bone dysplasia. Kyphosis (71 percent), scoliosis (26 percent), and atlantoaxial instability (13 percent) were the most common.

Sillence, D.O., and Rimoin, D.L.: Chondroosseous morphology in the skeletal dysplasias. *In* AAOS Symposium on Heritable Disorders of Connective Tissue, pp. 333-351, edited by W.H. Akeson, P. Bornstein, and M.J. Glimcher. St. Louis, C.V. Mosby, 1982.

The authors present some of the newer techniques of study of bone dysplasias and review the histochemical and morphologic findings in many dysplasias. A list of the recently recognized bone dysplasias is included.

Spanger, J.W.; Langer, L.O.; and Wiedemann, H.R.: Bone dysplasias. *In* An Atlas of Constitutional Disorders of Skeletal Development, pp. 55-61. Philadelphia, W.B. Saunders, 1974.

Clinical and skeletal features that characterize achondroplasia at birth, during childhood and in adulthood are illustrated.

Growth Plate

Brighton, C.T.: Structure and function of the growth plate. Clin. Orthop. 136:22-32, 1978.

This is a review of structure and function of the various components of the growth plate.

Monticelli, G., and Spinelli, R.: Distraction epiphysiolysis as a method of limb lengthening. Clin. Orthop. 154:274-285, 1981.

Epiphysiolysis distraction was used in sixteen patients nearing the end of growth. Five to 10 cm length was obtained without major complication. Use of this technique in the younger child may lead to premature epiphyseal closure.

Congenital Skeletal Abnormalities With Environmental Cause

Dignan, P.St.J.: Teratogenic risk and counseling in diabetes. Clin. Obstet. and Gynec. 24:149-159, 1981.

There is a threefold increase in congenital malformation in infants of diabetic mothers. The skeletal system is most commonly affected, but the only consistent cluster of malformations is the caudal dysplasia syndrome. Altered fetal environment is the most likely mechanism, and early maternal metabolic control appears to lower the incidence.

Hall, J.G.; Reed, S.D.; and Greene, G.: The distal arthrogryposes: Delineation of the new entities—Review and nosologic discussion. Am. J. Med. Genetics. 11:185-239, 1982.

The authors studied 350 patients with congenital joint contractures. From these they identified forty-four kindreds with distal limb contractures who could be divided into those with or without associated anomalies. Five subtypes of those with associated anomalies were identified.

Wynne-Davies, R.; Williams, P.F.; and O'Connor, J.C.B.: The 1960s' epidemic of arthrogryposis multiplex congenita. J. Bone Joint Surg. 63B:76-82, 1981.

This survey of the incidence of classic arthrogryposis in Australia, Great Britain, and the United States documents an increased incidence worldwide in the 1960s.

Zaffer, Z.; Nelson, M.; and Beighton, P.: Bone fusion in the foetal alcohol syndrome. J. Bone Joint Surg. 63B:569-571, 1981.

The foetal alcohol syndrome is reviewed with particular attention to skeletal abnormalities.

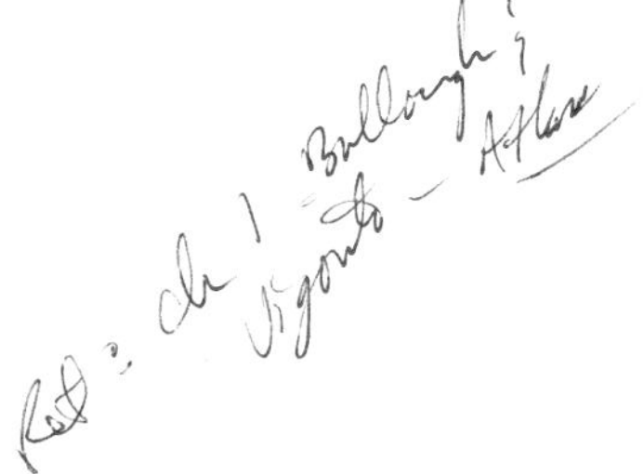

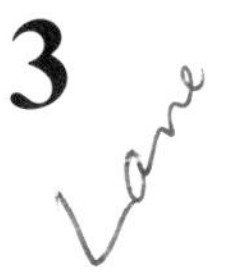

3 BONE METABOLISM: NORMAL PHYSIOLOGY AND DISEASE

Subjects considered in this section include endochondral bone formation, bone repair and fracture biology, bone grafting, osteoporosis, and Paget's disease.

Bone Formation and Turnover

Bone Cells

Osteoblasts and Osteocytes Three major physiologic functions of bone cells (osteoblasts, osteocytes, and osteoclasts) are calcium transport, biophysical or bioelectrical properties, and hormonal responses. Osteoblasts form bone, osteocytes contribute to mineral matrix homeostasis, and osteoclasts resorb bone. Much recent research on osteoblasts and osteocytes has been directed toward the role of the bone cell membrane. This membrane lines the bone mineral phase and controls the flow of ions between the bone fluid compartment (BFC) and the extracellular fluid (ECF). Some believe the term bone cell *envelope* is preferable to bone cell *membrane*. The term *membrane* has a fairly rigid biological definition that is not strictly met since the flow of ions between the BFC and the ECF can be intercellular as well as transcellular.

It is currently believed that all trabecular and cortical bone surfaces are covered with either osteoblasts, osteocytes, or thin fibroblastic cells. These cells make up the bone cell envelope, are responsive to calcitonin and parathyroid hormone, and are directly responsible for the ion concentration differences that exist between the BFC and the ECF compartments. Gaps in the bone cell envelope do occur, but a limited number of leaks between cells is still consistent with the concept of the bone cell envelope.

The membranes of bone cells (as distinct from the *bone cell membrane*, which is a layer of whole cells enveloping bone spicules) are similar to many other cell membranes when examined by electron microscopy. They have the typical trilaminar appearance seen in the lipid bilayer with a total thickness of 6 to 10 nm. The described fluid mosaic model for a cell's membrane showing potential for asymmetry on each side may have important implications in bone cells. The inner layer of the plasma membrane has a high content of phosphatidylserine, a phospholipid with a negative charge that potentially could bind significant amounts of calcium. In this respect, the membrane of osteoblasts resembles the matrix vesicle membrane.

Matrix vesicles are submicroscopic (30 to 100 nm) extracellular, membrane-invested particles that serve as the initial site of calcification in newly formed bone matrix, as well as in growth plate cartilage and in dental matrix. In matrix vesicles, phosphatidylserine can serve as a non-energy-requiring mechanism to attract calcium, whereas matrix vesicle phosphatases can localize phosphate for the formation of nascent calcium phosphate mineral within the matrix vesicle.

The electrical potentials in bone cells and bone derive from two sources: the piezoelectric effect generated by mechanical stress on bone and the "regeneration signal" produced in an area subjected to trauma. Some believe this regeneration signal is the basis of bone healing by electric stimulation and that the current may involve calcium movement conformational changes induced by the bioelectricity and secondary intracellular, kinetic, enzymatic changes partially mediated by prostaglandin and/or cyclic adenosine monophosphate (cAMP) synthesis.

Osteoblasts and osteocytes respond to several different hormones. Parathyroid hormone and calcitonin act directly via the second messenger, cAMP, in bone cells. When both hormones are present, their effect on cAMP production is additive, indicating the possibility of two sets of receptor sites, each responsive to one hormone. Osteoblasts also have nuclear receptors to glucosteroids. No direct receptor has been identified for any of the known estrogen or androgen metabolites.

Osteoclasts In the last 6 years much research has been performed on the origin and function of osteoclasts, and significant new knowledge has been gained. Osteoclasts are the multinucleated "giant" cells responsible for the resorption of bone. Osteoblasts and osteoclasts derive from two different cell lines. Progenitor cells of osteoclasts originate from hematopoietic tissues, not the surface of bones. Preosteoclasts are believed to closely resemble cells of the monocyte/macrophage system and are brought to the bone surface via the bloodstream.

There is considerable evidence supporting this origin including knowledge that osteopetrosis, a disease characterized by defective osteoclastic activity and, hence, failure of bone resorption, can be cured by bone marrow transplantation in humans and animal models.

Two intracellular areas of the osteoclast are clearly important to its function of resorbing bone. The names *ruffled* border and *clear zone* adequately describe their ultrastructural appearance. The ruffled border is a complex of plasma membrane infoldings found over the portion of the bone being resorbed.

In the space between the bone matrix and the ruffled border, dissociated collagen fibrils and free mineral crystals are found. These crystals are believed to be degraded in vacuoles within the cell; no collagen fragments ever have been found within vacuoles and so its final dissolution most likely occurs extracellularly. The extracellular digestion of the bone matrix by hydrolytic enzymes and collagenase has three major effects: it dislodges the mineral crystals which lie in contact with the collagen fibrils; it uncovers the collagen fibrils and makes them more susceptible to the collagenase; and it activates the collagenase which is originally released by the osteoclast in a procollagenase form.

The clear zone completely surrounds the ruffled border, and there are few cytoplasmic organelles located in this area. Electron microscopy shows it is in close contact with surface of the bone. Perhaps, it serves either to maintain a "seal" around the ruffled border to permit correct ion microenvironment or to act as a storage area for material to be used later by the ruffled border.

Parathyroid hormone (PTH) and osteoclast activating factor (OAF) stimulate the formation of the ruffled border. The amount of ruffled border present is directly proportional to the amount of bone being resorbed.

Since the resorption and remodeling of bone is a very specific spatial process, resorption must be under close local control, perhaps by the bone-lining cells. It is suggested that these lining cells initiate the resorptive process by initially exposing the bone surface. Osteoclasts or preosteoclasts, which fuse to become osteoclasts, recognize the exposed bone and then resorb it.

The longevity of osteoclasts is uncertain. Several studies have shown that they can acquire and shed nuclei; thus the life span could continue as long as the stimulus to resorb bone is present.

Endochondral Bone Formation and Mineralization The process of endochondral bone formation is now understood much better. The function and structure of the growth plate has been studied intensively at the cellular level. The growth plate can be divided into three parts: the actual cartilage of the growth plate; the metaphysis; and the fibrous periphery of the plate, consisting of the ossification groove of Ranvier and the perichondrial ring of LaCroix.

The actual cartilage of the growth plate is subdivided further into the reserve zone, the proliferative zone, and the hypertrophic zone. Cells in the reserve zone are not actively proliferating but appear to be storing nutrients to be used for later growth. The proliferating zone is the area where longitudinal growth occurs. Chondrocytes rapidly proliferate in this zone so that they are stacked in long columns separated by cartilage matrix. The matrix contains large amounts of aggregated proteoglycans that are significant inhibitors of calcification. The zone closest to the metaphysis is the hypertrophic zone, an avascular area in which the Po_2 is low. The cells first accumulate calcium here in their mitochondria, an energy-consuming process. Then, as the cell becomes depleted in glycogen and dies, calcium is released from the mitochondria. This calcium is believed to translocate to the extracellular matrix vesicles for incorporation into nascent mineral. Proteoglycans in the zone of provisional calcification are predominantly in a nonaggregated form which does not interfere with the sequential calcification of the matrix. This process proceeds to calcify fully the cartilage bars.

The metaphysis is where the blood vessels grow into canals formed by the dead chondrocytes. Osteoblasts follow the vessels and lay fibrous bone down on the calcified cartilage bars to form the primary spongiosum. The fibrous bone is remodeled gradually into secondary spongiosum (lamellar bone). The principal events in the metaphysis are vascular invasion, bone formation, and both histologic and anatomic remodeling (lamellar bone).

The last component of the growth plate is the fibrous structure encircling its periphery. It is subdivided into its two functional components: the ossification groove of Ranvier and the perichondrial ring of LaCroix. The ossification groove supplies chondrocytes to the periphery of the plate which fosters lateral growth. It also contains osteoblasts that are supplied to the surrounding perichondrial ring and fibroblasts that anchor it to the cartilage of the plate. The perichondrial ring is composed of dense, fibrous tissue encircling the total structure of the growth plate and provides mechanical support.

The process of mineralization, which occurs in many other tissues as well as bone, is very complex. The term mineralization (in mammals) is synonymous with calcification. Mature bone contains an analogue of the mineral compound hydroxyapatite [$Ca_{10}(PO_4)_6(OH)_2$] that is deficient in both Ca^{++} and OH^- with respect to true hydroxyapatite. It is doubtful that this compound is the first actual mineral formed in calcified tissue. The determination of the nature of the first crystal is a major question to be resolved.

Chondrocytes in the growth plate and osteoblasts and osteocytes in bone are the cells directly controlling the process of calcification in these tissues by altering the composition of the extracellular organic matrix. Macromolecules in the matrix potentially may control calcification by helping to form nucleators around which crystals may grow or by stabilizing crystals once they are formed and by controlling the orientation and size of the crystals. Collagen is believed to be very important in controlling the orientation of newly formed crystals. Two important noncollagen proteins located in the matrix are the phosphoproteins and the γ-carboxyl amino acid-containing (vitamin K dependent) proteins that avidly bind calcium.

Proteoglycans are molecules that may form aggregates of macromolecular size, which inhibit crystal nucleation and growth. Disaggregation is perhaps one of the key events occurring in cartilage in the hypertrophic zone when it calcifies.

Phospholipids are membrane-bound compounds widely distributed in calcified tissues. They are capable of forming calcium-phospholipid-phosphate complexes, a high concentration of which are found in the hypertrophic zone when calcification begins. Membrane-bound complexes may form a microenvironment suitable for crystallization of hydroxyapatite. Several enzymes (alkaline phosphatase, phospholipase A, C, and D) may have roles in calcification, but their exact function remains unclear.

Bone Repair and Fracture Biology Fracture healing is a complex process dependent upon many different factors. There are four types of fracture repair: primary callus response, external bridging callus, late medullary callus, and primary cortical healing. The type predominating in a fracture is determined by the alignment and apposition of the bone ends, the efficiency of the fracture immobilization, and the amount of associated soft-tissue damage.

The initial phase of all fracture healing is localized inflammation. Bleeding occurs from the ends of the fractured bone, and hematoma forms in the surrounding soft tissues. Leukocytes then migrate into the area to begin cleaning up the damaged tissue and debris. Increased cell division is evident after 8 hours and takes place in the soft tissue and the periosteum.

There are two current theories concerning the origin of the osteogenic cells which repair a fracture. In one, the cells originate from cells predetermined to form bone. The alternative view proposes that fibroblasts are able to form callus and repair bone. These theories, however, are not mutually exclusive.

The first type of repair occurring in all fractures that are not rigidly immobilized is the primary callus response. It takes place within 2 weeks after the injury. Exuberant amounts of callus are formed during this period with the ultimate goal of bridging the bone ends. If the bone ends are not apposed, perhaps due to interposition of soft tissue or due to a gap between the bone ends, the process stops and cannot be reactivated. This process is basically independent of environmental and hormonal influences and most likely arises from cells already present in bone tissues (Table I).

If the bony ends are not in continuity, the second type of healing is that of external bridging callus. This stage is under the control of mechanical (piezoelectric effect of bone) and humoral (local and systemic regeneration) factors and hormones. The cells involved most likely are derived from the surrounding soft tissues. This process is able to bridge gaps, is tolerant of movement, depends upon the availability of viable external soft tissues, and is not decreased by absolutely rigid fixation of the fracture.

The third type of bone repair is late medullary callus formation. Cartilage formation, found in the first two types of repair, is much less predominant in this type. This healing often occurs along with external bridging callus formation but is not inhibited by immobilization of the fracture as is external bridging. The osteogenic material seems to come directly from the ends of the bone fragments. This type of repair is a slow, progressive process that can continue for many months and is capable of bridging large gaps between the bone ends. The presence of two bone ends is required since this type of repair does not take place in the proximal end of a bone in an amputation stump.

Primary cortical healing, the fourth type of fracture healing, happens only when mechanical immobilization and apposition of the bone ends are almost perfect. When an extremely rigid system is obtained, the formation of external bridging callus is suppressed severely, and the fracture heals mainly by late medullary callus formation and primary cortical healing. This type seems to involve just the normal process of bone turnover and remodeling

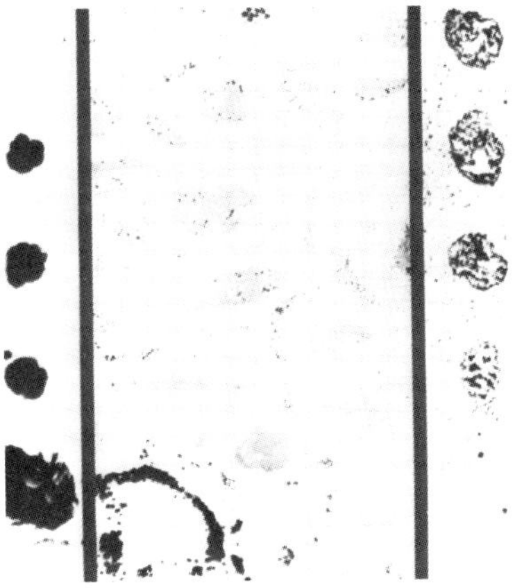

Figure 1: Mineralization in early fracture healing. This EM photograph represents a montage of early fracture healing. The slide has been subjected to pyroincineration and only the calcium remains. The column on the left represents matrix vesicles undergoing progressive mineralization. The column on the right represents chondrocyte mitochondria losing the calcium, and the center panel demonstrates the early mineralizing matrix from which these close-ups were taken.

which includes osteoclasts resorbing canals in the old bone and blood vessels and osteogenic cells following into these canals and laying down new haversian systems. This form of bone "healing" can be very protracted especially if there is much dead bone at the fracture ends.

When rigid immobilization and apposition of the ends of the fracture are not achieved, the process of callus formation and remodeling is very similar to that of endochondral bone formation occurring at the growth plate. Biochemical and histologic events appear to be similar in the two processes. Proteoglycan, calcium-phospholipid-phosphate complexes, and alkaline phosphatase are elevated in both processes in a similar temporal sequence. Matrix vesicles are present in both and may be the first site of calcification (Fig. 1).

The effects of several hormones are important in fracture healing. Calcitonin prevents disuse osteoporosis in the fractured limb. In the presence of normal vitamin D and calcium levels, augmented vitamin D, calcium, or growth hormone do not increase the final fracture healing outcome but may accelerate the normal process.

Indomethacin and aspirin decrease the rate of fracture healing in rats, as graded by histologic criteria. The effect of indomethacin is greater than that of aspirin. This decreased fracture healing may be due to alterations in prostaglandin metabolism. The potential for manipulating the rate of fracture healing by hormonal or pharmaceutical means is an area of great interest.

Table I
Comparison of the Four Types of Fracture Repair

Type of healing	Speed	Ability to bridge gaps	Tolerance of movement	Tolerance of total rigidity	Importance of external soft tissues
Primary callus response	+ + + +	+	+ + + +	+ + + +	–
External bridging callus	+ + +	+ + +	+ + +	–	+ + + +
Late medullary callus	+ +	+ + + + (slow)	+ +	+ + +	–
Primary cortical	+	–	–	+ + + +	–

(Reprinted with permission from The biology of fracture healing in long bones, by B. McKibbin, J. Bone Joint Surg. 60B:159, 1978.)

One study shows that electrically induced osteogenesis is dependent upon the charge and current density applied to the intramedullary canal. This relationship is directly proportional up to high current levels where cell necrosis occurs. Pulsed currents form a similar amount of bone only as the total charge delivered becomes equal to that of a similar constant current. Invasive, semi-invasive, and noninvasive bioelectrical stimulation have no significant effect on normal fracture healing but may have a potential role in fractures with poor healing environment (such as navicular fractures).

Bone Grafting There are several bone grafting techniques to bridge osseous gaps and failed union sites: (1) autologous cortico-cancellous bone; (2) transference of whole bone segments; (3) allograft osseous or osteochondral bone transplants; (4) free vascularized bone grafts; and (5) modified osteogenic products (bone matrix gelatin and bone morphogenic protein).

Osteoinduction is defined as the process of inducing bone formation locally or recruiting cells with the potential for osseous production. Osteoconduction furnishes a suitable environment upon which bone matrix can be deposited. Each of the bone grafting techniques has a varying ability to provide these two requirements for successful osseous synthesis and incorporation.

Classical autologous cortical and cancellous grafts provide both osteoinduction and osteoconduction. Cancellous bone yields 30 percent osteosynthetic cells and some osteoconductive surfaces. Cortical bone has less than 3 percent osteosynthetic cells but provides excellent osteoconductive surfaces. It is remodeled only slowly as compared to cancellous bone.

Whole segment grafting has been advocated by some. Although bony union is relatively easily achieved, the rate of stress fractures is over 58 percent if the gap is more than 12 cm. Successful union and remodeling after 2 years is high even in large defects. Mechanical strength is lowest from 6 to 24 months, and the limb must be protected during this period. Decreased strength is caused by imbalance between bone resorption and creeping substitution.

Vascularized bone grafts have distinct advantages over nonviable large autologous cortico-cancellous grafts when the anastomosed vascular pedicle remains patent. Viability is maintained in a significant proportion of the osteocytes, bone marrow elements, and osteoblasts. Union is obtained quickly, and stress fractures occur in less than 25 percent of large defects. These grafts have been used successfully to reconstruct large osseous defects even in the presence of osteomyelitis or inadequate soft tissue viability.

Demineralized and defatted allogenic bone (bone matrix gelatin, BMG) loses its antigenicity and is quite effective in osteoinduction and osteoconduction. A purified glycoprotein family within this material has been isolated, and it appears to have extremely potent osteoinductive properties. This glycoprotein, termed *bone morphogenetic protein,* as well as BMG are under experimental clinical trials as sources of bone graft.

Mineral Metabolism

Calcium and Phosphate Homeostasis Calcium homeostasis is a complex process. All calcium intake is via the diet, and significant calcium is lost via the kidneys and bowels. The average calcium requirement is unknown. It is estimated that in western countries 900 mg of calcium daily is required for 95 percent of the population. This total approximately matches the federal government recommendations for adults and, interestingly, is close to the amount of calcium in the average diet. Children require significantly more calcium during growth, but the minimum amount is undetermined. Pregnant women (1,500 mg), lactating women (2,000 mg), adolescents (1,300 mg), and postmenopausal women (1,500 mg) have the greatest calcium requirements.

In the average adult male, calcium makes up 1,050 g of the total weight. Only 1 percent of this is located outside the bones. Calcium in circulation is more than 50 percent bound to the plasma proteins with the majority bound to albumin. Calcium is crucially involved in many different processes in the living organism such as enzyme control, secretion of peptide hormones and other cellular products, blood coagulation, and membrane electrical potential.

Bones represent a potential reservoir for calcium and phosphate. Two different methods for the movement of calcium between bone and body fluids are known.

The first method is osteoclastic resorption and osteoblastic bone formation, i.e., the system by which bone is remodeled. It is relatively slow in causing changes in serum calcium levels. However, since theoretically the entire skeleton is available, this system has a huge capacity for supplying calcium. PTH is one of the factors controlling this process. The long-term effects of PTH are increased osteoclast activity and recruitment of more osteoclasts.

The other process is both rapid and reversible. It has the ability to control the minute-by-minute functions of calcium. The cells lining the bone surface are responsible for maintaining the plasma calcium concentration. Osteocytes and osteoblasts respond rapidly (within 5 minutes) to PTH injection by changing their shapes and the amount of intracellular organelles present (Golgi apparatus and endoplasmic reticulum). There is evidence that the perilacunar material surrounding osteocytes is a primary source of calcium on a short-term basis. It is this material that PTH causes to be rapidly transferred into the body fluid compartment from the bone surface. Calcitonin also may be important in the postprandial storing of calcium in these areas.

Vitamin D also seems essential in promoting bone mineralization and in the short-term storing of calcium supplies, but its role is undefined. 1,25 $(OH)_2$ vitamin D potentiates PTH in its bone resorptive function and activates calcium-binding protein in gut. 25(OH) vitamin D or another analogue may play a role in bone mineralization.

Calcium is absorbed mainly in the duodenum and jejunum. In the duodenum, its absorption is mediated by an active transport process. In the jejunum, calcium is absorbed via facilitated diffusion. Even though absorbed by an active process in the duodenum, most calcium is taken up in the jejunum because of the greater length of this portion of the bowel and the slower speed of content movement, thus providing more time for absorption. The normal intestine has a huge reserve capacity available for absorbing calcium.

A metabolite of vitamin D is necessary for calcium

resorption. The presence of 1,25 $(OH)_2$ vitamin D can enhance greatly the ability of the gut to transport calcium. The presence of PTH is unnecessary for this direct effect of vitamin D. This accelerated transport is caused by increases of the surface area available in the gut, the synthesis of proteins involved in transporting calcium, and the transport of calcium across the serosal surface of the intestinal cell.

The kidney is capable of resorbing over 98 percent of calcium filtered in the glomerulus. Less than 200 mg of calcium usually is present in a 24-hour urine collection (normal <2mg/kg/day). Calcium resorption is similar to that of sodium in that it occurs throughout the nephron. PTH closely controls the amount of calcium excreted. Administration of small amounts will increase significantly the amount of calcium resorbed. Interestingly, PTH seems to decrease resorption in the proximal tubule and increase resorption in the distal tubule.

Vitamin 1,25 $(OH)_2D_3$ increases calcium resorption in the kidney in states of hypocalcemia, low PTH, and during total body volume expansion. Early studies, which showed that vitamin D increased urinary excretion of calcium, were primarily the result of increasing intestinal absorption of calcium and, secondarily, increasing the amount of calcium filtered by the kidneys.

Phosphate metabolism is less well understood. It is now known that 1,25 $(OH)_2$ vitamin D stimulates active phosphate absorption across the gut. Phosphate is secreted in the renal tubules, and this process is augmented by elevated PTH.

Vitamin D

Metabolic Pathway Vitamin D is unique among vitamins in that it is formed in the skin when 7-dehydrocholesterol is exposed to ultraviolet light. One hour of sunlight supplies this daily requirement in a white person; more exposure is required for more heavily pigmented skin. This endogenous form of vitamin D is called cholecalciferol or vitamin D_3. The other major source of vitamin D is the diet. This form is named ergocalciferol or vitamin D_2. These two forms differ only at a point on a side chain and act the same endogenously. Both are stored in several tissues. The highest concentrations are found in adipose tissue and muscle.

In the liver, vitamin D is converted to 25-hydroxycholecalciferol, 25 (OH) D, by either of two vitamin D 25-hydroxylases. The enzyme that is active at normal physiologic levels of vitamin D is located in the microsomes. The other 25-hydroxylase is found in the mitochondria of hepatic cells and is active only at high levels (pharmacologic doses). 25(OH) vitamin D is the major circulating form of vitamin D. It is transported by and bound to an alpha-globulin.

The next and most important step in the metabolism of vitamin D is the 1-hydroxylation of 25-(OH) D to form the active form 1,25 $(OH)_2$ vitamin D. This reaction is catalyzed by 25-(OH)D-hydroxylase which is found in the mitochondria of kidney cells. The only other tissue in which this enzyme has been found is the placenta. The production of 1,25 $(OH)_2$ vitamin D is under very close controls: PTH, phosphate, Ca^{++} levels and the amount of 1,25 $(OH)_2$ vitamin D itself all regulate 1-hydroxylase activity.

1,25-dihydroxy vitamin D meets the criteria for a hormone. Its structure is similar to other steroid hormones, as is its mechanism of action at target tissues. 1,25 $(OH)_2$ D diffuses across the cytoplasmic membrane and becomes bound to a cellular protein that helps transport it into the nucleus where it enhances the production of specific mRNA and subsequently protein production.

Vitamin D Target Organs The major target tissues of 1,25 $(OH)_2$ D are bone, intestine, parathyroid gland, and kidney. In the kidney, it increases proximal tubular reabsorption of phosphate and, perhaps, calcium. It also increases 24-hydroxylase activity, which produces another metabolite of vitamin D-24,25$(OH)_2$ D, and reduces 1-hydroxylase activity thereby acting as a feedback inhibitor of its own formation.

In bone, the major role for 1,25 $(OH)_2$ D is in promoting the mobilization of calcium from bone. Most likely, it acts as a permissive agent and PTH causes the actual process of mobilization. It may also play a role in promoting bone mineralization but probably in another form such as 25(OH) vitamin D or 24,25$(OH)_2$ vitamin D.

There is some evidence that 1,25 $(OH)_2$ D has a negative feedback effect on the production of PTH since PTH hormone is known to stimulate 1,25 $(OH)_2$ D production. This point is unproven.

In the intestine, much is known about the action of 1,25 $(OH)_2$ D. Its major function is to promote intestinal calcium and phosphate absorption. It does this by increasing the active absorption of Ca^{++} in the bowel probably through stimulating the production of a calcium-binding protein.

24,25$(OH)_2$ D is another metabolite of 25(OH) D. As mentioned, high levels of 1,25 $(OH)_2$ D induce the hydroxylation of 25 (OH) D at the 24 position in several tissues besides the kidney. The function of 24,25$(OH)_2$ D has stimulated much research with no clear results as yet. It is perhaps involved in bone mineralization.

Several degradation products of vitamin D have been found, each of which has little in vivo activity. The main one is calcitroic acid which is produced in the liver and excreted into the bile.

Calcium-Binding Proteins At least three classes of calcium-binding proteins have been identified in the calcified bone matrix. They include phosphoproteins, gamma-carboxyglutamic acid-containing proteins (Gla-proteins), and osteonectin. The phosphoproteins attract Ca^{++} by virtue of acidic phosphate groups, often attached to serine. The Gla-proteins attract Ca^{++} by virtue of carboxyl groups on glutamic acid residues. Osteonectin was recently described as a binding protein between the collagen of bone matrix and associated hydroxyapatite mineral.

Phosphoproteins are believed to be localized within the "hole" region of collagen fibrils and, by the action of their phosphate groups, attract calcium to this particular area during formation of CaPO4 mineral nuclei.

The Gla-proteins that have been most studied are the vitamin K-dependent clotting factors (II, VII, IX, and X) and the Gla residues of both prothrombin and factor Xa phospholipid. This Gla-protein-phospholipid-calcium complex serves at least three functions in coagulation. It concentrates the factors in certain areas, allows certain conformational changes in the structure of the peptide, and exposes the correct part of the peptide for proteolytic cleavage.

A Gla-protein, osteocalcin, recently has been isolated in bone. It constitutes between 10 and 20 percent of all noncollagen protein present in bone matrix and 1 to 2 percent of total bone protein. Osteocalcin is synthesized by the bone cells and undergoes a similar vitamin K-dependent posttranslational modification as prothrombin. The amount of osteocalcin in bone is such that less than 1 in 1,000 calcium ions is bound to it, but the onset of mineralization of bone does coincide both in time and location with the formation of osteocalcin. Indeed, there is a linear relationship between osteocalcin content and the increasing density of bone.

Animals given Coumadin, which blocks Gla production, have a decreased amount of osteocalcin in their bones, but no other significant changes in bone structure. Furthermore, the Gla-proteins have actually been shown to inhibit apatite mineral deposition in in vitro systems suggesting that they are not necessary for mineral initiation in bone. Given their high affinity for the calcium of hydroxyapatite mineral, the Gla-proteins may accumulate in bone, at least to some extent simply because of an affinity for apatite. Although the role of Gla-proteins in bone metabolism is unknown at the moment, current thinking has led to the suggestion that it may function as a hormone, since Gla-protein recently has been shown to be elevated in serum in patients with Paget's disease, primary hyperparathyroidism, renal osteodystrophy, and osteoporosis.

Most of the Gla is excreted in nonmetabolized form in the urine. Approximately 25 percent of the urinary Gla comes from mineralized tissues and associated osteocalcin. Perhaps it will be possible to use urinary Gla excretion as an indicator for bone mineral turnover or even to monitor a patient's anticoagulation and vitamin K status.

Endocrine Effect

Parathyroid Hormone Parathyroid hormone (PTH), in association with 1,25 $(OH)_2$ vitamin D, controls the concentration of calcium in body fluids. Its three major target organs are the intestine, kidneys, and bone. Two areas of major new discoveries are the peripheral metabolism of PTH and its intracellular production.

Normally PTH is produced in and secreted exclusively from the parathyroid gland in humans. Intracellulary, PTH is preceded by two precursors. Preproparathyroid (preproPTH) is a 115 amino acid peptide and is produced directly from mRNA. Its half-life is less than 1 minute and in the rough endoplasmic reticulum it is cleaved to the other, proPTH, which contains 90 amino acids. In the Golgi apparatus, it is cleaved to the major secretion product, PTH, which contains 84 amino acids. The Golgi apparatus packages PTH in vesicles for secretion.

Secretion of PTH is a very tightly regulated, but sensitive, system. As small a change of the ionized calcium concentration as 0.1 mg/dl will stimulate release of hormone. Secretion control by calcium is apparently regulated via the second messenger system of adenylcyclase and cAMP. An increase in calcium flux results in an inhibition of cAMP formulation and a decrease in the amount of PTH secreted. Other than hypocalcemia, PTH release is stimulated by prostaglandin E_2, secretion, and β-adrenergic agonists. Interestingly, propranolol has the ability to block PTH release, and further studies indicate that the parathyroid gland probably has specific β_2 receptors.

There are at least three immunologically identifiable circulating PTH forms in the peripheral circulation. One is the intact 84 amino acid PTH that is secreted from the parathyroid gland. The other two forms result from the proteolytic cleavage in the liver of PTH into two parts. The carboxyl end is larger and exists as the predominant circulating form. It is not biologically active and is cleared by the kidney. The N-terminal fragment is smaller, has a short half-life, and has many of the same actions as PTH. Interestingly, this fragment is taken up almost completely by bone. The complete 84 amino acid PTH is much less active in bone than its N-terminal peptide. Consequently, immunologic assays of intact N-terminal and C-terminal PTH have different clinical interpretations and do not directly correlate consistently with biological effect.

The action of PTH or its N-terminal peptide on target tissues is via the activation of membrane-bound adenylcyclase to produce intracellular cAMP. The intracellular events taking place after this step are unclear, but the typical activation of protein kinases and elevation of intracellular cytoplasmic calcium are believed to occur. These kinases then further alter cellular metabolism.

Calcitonin The exact physiologic role of calcitonin is controversial. The theory that it is a vestigial or nonfunctioning hormone in humans probably is incorrect. It does have a significant calcium- and phosphate-lowering action at physiologic doses in humans.

Calcitonin is produced and secreted mainly by the "C" cells or parafollicular cells in the thyroid gland. These cells also are known to originate in the embryonic neural crest tissue. Other tissues believed to contain small amounts of calcitonin are thymus, pituitary, gut, liver, and the CSF. The significance of calcitonin in these tissues is unclear.

Biosynthesis of calcitonin is similar to other exported peptides. First synthesized in a large precursor form, it subsequently undergoes proteolytic cleavage at least two times to reach the final structure of 32 amino acids that weighs 3,500 daltons. Calcitonin isolated from many sources (pig, cow, rat, etc.) all have the same length of 32 amino acids. Salmon calcitonin, which is available as a drug, differs from human calcitonin at sixteen different sites in amino acid composition. This alteration is large enough to cause it to be immunogenic. Interestingly, it is several times more potent for patients than human calcitonin.

Secretion of calcitonin is controlled by serum calcium levels. Hypercalcemia stimulates secretion and low levels suppress its release. Several other divalent cations will influence secretion but only at superphysiologic levels and are probably not important in vivo. β_2-androgenic receptors are believed to exist that stimulate calcitonin release, an effect that can be blocked by propranolol. Pharmacologic doses of the intestinal hormones gastrin, cholecystokinin, and cerulein stimulate its release. This raises the interesting possibility that calcitonin is involved in some way with GI function.

Breakdown of calcitonin occurs almost totally in the kidney where it is filtered, resorbed, and then degraded. The half-life is approximately 10 minutes in a patient with normal renal function but increases significantly with renal failure. The best assays available for analysis of calcitonin levels are radioimmune techniques, but all existing assays have difficulty measuring very low levels of calcitonin. In addition, they are not selective for the biologically active hormone, but often react with breakdown products or other similar proteins.

Calcitonin exerts its effect by binding to specific membrane receptors and activating adenylcyclase which increases intracellular cAMP. Further information about its intracellular effects is unknown.

The major target tissues of calcitonin seem to be bone, kidney, and the GI tract. In the bone, its major defined action is the inhibition of osteoclastic bone resorption. Osteoclasts lose their ruffled borders and clear zones within 15 minutes in response to calcitonin. It has been proposed that calcitonin plays an important role in the rapid storage of calcium after meals in the perilacunar space. In the kidney, specific receptors are known to exist for calcitonin. It decreases tubular reabsorption of both calcium and phosphate. In the gut, pharmacologic doses of calcitonin increase secretion of Na+, K+, Cl, and water and decrease acid secretion.

Interestingly, hypercalcitonin deficiency states cause no known disorders of metabolism.

Though calcitonin has no proven important physiologic role, it is likely that it is involved in the long-term maintenance of calcium homeostasis and skeletal mass.

Calcitonin does have several proven pharmacologic uses. It is effective in treating Paget's disease, preventing disuse osteoporosis, and rapid lowering of serum calcium in severe hypercalcemic states.

Estrogens and Corticosteroids Bone loss associated with increasing age in both males and females has been documented (see Section 28: Thoracolumbar Spine: Reconstruction). However, the rate of bone loss in females increases in the postmenopausal years. This rate is correlated with decreasing amounts of endogenous estrogens at menopause. Several studies have shown that estrogen replacement therapy in the postmenopausal years blocks, or significantly decreases, the loss of bone stock.

Patients who undergo bilateral oophorectomy before menopause also respond to estrogen therapy. This group is especially at risk for development of osteoporosis, probably because greater parts of their lives are spent with low estrogen levels. Discontinuation of estrogen therapy can result in a greatly accelerated rate of bone loss in these patients. To obtain the maximum benefit from therapy, estrogens should be started shortly after menopause. If not, the effect is not substantial.

Two other symptoms of a low estrogen level are hot flashes and genitourinary problems, which are adequately treated with the low doses of estrogen given to prevent osteoporosis. Estrogen contained in topical creams that can be used to treat atrophic vaginitis are absorbed into the circulation. It is not known what effect this type of estrogen therapy has on the probability of developing endometrial cancer, but the occurrence of this carcinoma is believed to be approximately eight times higher in women on estrogen therapy. Therefore, any female on estrogen should be followed closely with serial Pap smears and an annual biopsy of endometrial tissue. Additional complications include increased risk of CVA, thrombosis, and uterine bleeding. In one study, 13 percent of patients on supplemental estrogen required hysterectomies.

The mechanism by which decreasing levels of estrogen causes bone loss or the mechanism by which estrogen therapy prevents bone loss is unknown. No receptors for estrogens have been demonstrated in osteoblasts. This has led some to believe that the effect of estrogen on bone is indirect.

One possible cause of the development of osteoporosis is an imbalance between corticosteroid and estrogen levels. Corticosteroids cause bone loss. After menopause, estrogen levels fall, and cortisol levels remain at premenopausal levels. Some patients who develop osteoporosis after oophorectomy have elevated levels of urinary cortisol excretion. Some believe that estrogens induce increased synthesis of cortisol-binding proteins in the liver. Hence, in estrogen-treated patients, there is a relative decrease in the amount of free cortisol in the body, and in females who develop osteoporosis, there is a relative excess of cortisol as compared to the level of estrogen.

Recently, one study has demonstrated the significantly decreased rate of vertebral fractures in a group of females with osteoporosis treated with estrogens and calcium supplements. The rate was approximately four times less in the treated group than in the control group. The prevention of fractures is one of the major goals in treating osteoporosis.

Several reports have indicated that estrogen therapy may cause a decreased incidence of breast cancer in treated patients. This is an interesting finding since this cancer has a very poor cure rate while endometrial cancer has a better cure rate and prognosis. Combination cyclic estrogen-progestin therapy is believed to decrease the occurrence of endometrial cancer.

Estrogen-progestin therapy could be offered to premature postmenopausal patients who have the following risk factors: slender build, smoking habit, disabling osteoporosis including fractures, glucocorticoid treatment, and/or a very inactive lifestyle. Close follow-up is essential for continuing therapy.

Corticosteroids may lead to bone loss by directly inhibiting calcium absorption across the gut, increasing renal calcium excretion, and indirectly stimulating secondary hyperparathyroidism. Very high doses of steroids decrease both bone formation and resorption. Moderately elevated levels predominantly affect bone formation. Alternate day programs have less osteopenic potential.

Thyroid Hormones The thyroid gland produces two hormones, thyroxine (T4) and 3,5,3'-triiodothyronine (T3). Both are bound extensively to proteins in the plasma. The major binding proteins in order of decreasing binding affinity are as follows: thyroxine-binding globulin, thyroxine-binding prealbumin, and albumin. T4 is bound approximately ten times more tightly to these proteins than T3.

T4 is the major secretory product of the thyroid, which is the only tissue source of T4 in the body. Approximately 80 percent of T3 is formed from T4 in nonthyroid tissue. The two major organs that convert T4 to T3 by 5-monodeiodination are the liver and kidney. Although there is less T3 in circulation, it is three to four times more active biologically than T4. T3 controls cellular function by binding to nuclear receptors that are nonhistone proteins. These complexes then regulate the synthesis or specific

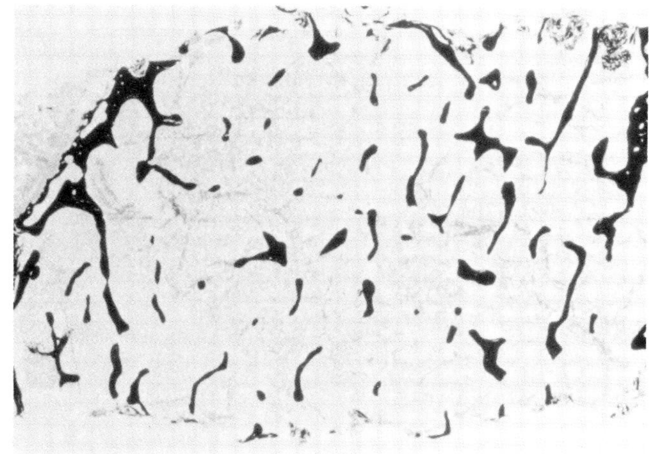

Figure 2: Transiliac bone biopsy from postmenopausal osteoporotic patient presenting with a subcapital fracture. The undecalcified slide stained with Von Kossa demonstrates the skimpy cortical and trabecular bone.

proteins by altering the rate of formation of an RNA that codes for these proteins.

The amount of T4 secreted by the thyroid is dependent upon the level of thyroid stimulating hormone (TSH) present. TSH is, in turn, released in response to thyroid regulating hormone (TRH). T3 and T4, respectively, feed back on both TSH and TRH release.

Patients with hyperthyroidism may develop osteoporotic bone disease. This osteopenic condition occurs in hyperthyroid, postmenopausal patients. The radiologic findings may be indistinguishable from "senile" osteoporosis. Bone resorption and bone formation are taking place at stimulated rates, but it appears that resorption occurs at a rate slightly faster than bone formation. High normal physiologic levels of thyroid hormone, particularly when given pharmacologically, may have a disproportionately augmented effect on bone metabolism. Consequently, chronic thyroid supplementation may contribute to osteoporosis.

Osteopenia

Osteoporosis It is estimated that approximately 15 percent of Caucasian females over the age of 65 years have evidence of significant osteoporosis. Up to 30 percent reaching 75 years of age have sustained fractures related to this problem. The short-term, direct cost of the treatment of hip fractures due to osteoporosis alone was estimated to be more than $1 billion in 1979. Thus, this condition is one of national significance. Typical fractures in osteoporotic individuals are located most frequently in the proximal humerus, lower forearm, hip, spine, and pelvis.

The amount of bone loss associated with aging has been the subject of numerous research projects. From 40 years of age until menopause, compact bone is lost at a rate of 3 percent per decade and from menopause until 70 years of age is lost at 9 to 10 percent per decade. At age 70 years, the rate of loss decreases to 3 percent per decade. The rate of loss of trabecular bone does not appear to differ between the sexes. It progresses at a steady rate of 6 to 8 percent per decade starting in early to mid-adulthood.

The typical patient with osteoporosis is a slender, sedentary, white female of northern European descent who smokes and has breastfed several children. She also usually has a diet deficient in calcium and vitamin D and has little exposure to the sun. Blacks or obese women experience this condition much less commonly. Obese women are believed to be "protected" from osteoporosis because of their increased levels of circulating estrogens and their greater bone mass at menopause.

The differential diagnosis of osteopenic conditions that must be ruled out before making the diagnosis of idiopathic or postmenopausal osteoporosis includes hyperparathyroidism, hyperthyroidism, a malignancy of the medullary cavity, osteomalacia, glucocorticoid excess, or, rarely, osteogenesis imperfecta tarda.

Appropriate laboratory tests should be performed to eliminate these other diagnoses. In addition, a general metabolic profile of the patient should be obtained to include calcium balance, creatinine clearance, urinary hydroxyproline, BUN, and phosphorus. Radiation absorptiometry as a single measurement is of marginal value due to site and individual variance and differences in what is occupying the marrow cavity. However, serial examinations are of value in following the response of patients to therapy or to progression of bone loss. Transiliac bone biopsy is very reliable as a diagnostic aid (Fig. 2) especially if the bone has been previously labeled with tetracycline.

The etiology of postmenopausal osteoporosis is not clearly delineated. The reduced levels of circulating estrogens often are implicated, but there is no evidence showing that estrogen receptors exist in bone cells. Estrogen is well known to block the loss of bone postmenopausally. Other studies show a blunted response of calcitonin secretion to calcium challenge. This has been postulated to play a role in osteoporosis. A significant number (50-60 percent) of females with osteoporosis are lactase deficient and, consequently, have a diet very low in calcium. This, perhaps, plays a role in its pathogenesis.

TREATMENT: The effects of several different treatments for postmenopausal osteoporosis have been studied. The criteria used for judging the efficacy of each treatment was the reduction in occurrence of vertebral fractures. The study groups received: (1) a placebo; (2) calcium +/- vitamin D (50,000 units per week); (3) fluoride and calcium +/- vitamin D; (4) estrogen and calcium +/- vitamin D; and (5) fluoride, calcium, and estrogen +/- vitamin D. The results showed that all treatment groups had a significantly reduced rate of vertebral fractures as compared to the control groups. The greater reduction occurred in group 5, followed by group 4, group 3, and group 2. In addition, group 3 (receiving fluoride and calcium) had a 30 percent lower rate than the group 2 (receiving calcium). Sixty percent of the patients treated with fluoride had radiographic evidence of increased vertebral bone mass. This concurs with a 75 percent response rate previously reported. In addition, it took approximately 1 year of treatment with fluoride before a significant decrease in the fracture rate occurred. Common side effects of fluoride treatment include GI symptoms (nausea, vomiting, and ulcers) and arthralgias. Thirteen percent of those patients receiving estrogen required hysterectomies. Other studies have achieved comparable reductions of fractures with sodium fluoride and calcium alone without estrogen.

Interestingly, the addition of large doses of vitamin D did not substantially alter the rate of fracture with any of the treatment regimens. It does appear that a physiologic

Table II

Treatment of Osteoporosis

	Estrogen .625 mg Premarin per day	**Calcium 1.5 /day**	**Vitamin D 400-800 units/ day**	**Sodium Fl. 1mg/kg/day**
Postmenopausal women at risk	–	X	X	–
Postmenopausal women at risk (<40 yrs. old)	X (only 6 yrs.)	X	X	–
Postmenopausal women with osteoporosis	–	X	X	X (2 + yrs.)
Postmenopausal women with osteoporosis/ osteomalacia	–	X	X	X (delay until osteomalacia corrected)

amount of vitamin D must be available for bone formation to occur normally. A summation of available data suggests that calcium supplementation and/or estrogen and/or androgens will halt or decrease bone loss, but only sodium fluoride can increase bone mass.

Sodium fluoride stabilizes the hydroxyapatite crystal and stimulates osteoblastic bone formation. Although the newly synthesized bone is slightly irregular (increased osteocytes, increased lacunar size, perilacunar basophilia, and slight irregularity of the collagen weave), the fracture rate significantly decreases and the mass of initial trabecular bone is increased on an average of 25 percent per year. Fluoride therapy, when given in the absence of calcium supplementation, leads to increased osteoid content and actual bone brittleness. Occasional indigestion and arthralgias about the feet (20 percent) are temporary and usually respond to nonoperative treatment.

One method treats postmenopausal osteoporosis initially with calcium carbonate (1,500 mg elemental calcium per day) and vitamin D (400-800 units per day) for 3 to 12 months until any preexisting undermineralization (osteoid excess) can be corrected. Estrogen (650 mg Premarin per day for 3 weeks with 1 week rest) is only utilized in women who have had premature menopause (40 years of age) or are within 6 years of menopause. Estrogen is terminated after 6 years of therapy. Sodium fluoride (1mg/kg/day) is only given to women with documented osteopenia and after some calcium/vitamin D pretreatment.

Any osteomalacia or excess osteoid must be corrected prior to sodium fluoride therapy (Table II and Fig. 3). Sodium fluoride is continued with calcium and vitamin D for at least 2 years or until the bone scan and radiographs show no new fractures for 2 years. On the average, most patients receive 3 years of combined therapy. Thereafter, calcium and vitamin D are continued indefinitely.

Heparin-induced osteoporosis is a rare cause of spinal fractures. It typically occurs in women who are taking heparin for antepartum thrombophlebitis. The cause is unknown, but it can be avoided if not more than 10,000 units are given daily and therapy is not continued past 120 days.

Osteomalacia Osteomalacia as well as its equivalent in children, rickets, has a multitude of causes. These causes can be grouped into the classic deficiency of dietary or endogenous vitamin D, intestinal malabsorption disorders, acquired and hereditary renal disorders, and a "miscellaneous" group. To obtain the correct diagnosis, all of these causes must be considered in an appropriate workup.

The clinical diagnosis of osteomalacia is often difficult. Patients usually have nonspecific complaints (such as muscle weakness or just diffuse aches and pains, symptoms common in older patients). Frequently, the diagnosis is not made until the disorder is far advanced with evidence of kyphosis or significant decrease in trunk height. The vertebral bodies are usually affected severely because bones made up of trabecular structure are more affected than bones having large amounts of cortical bone.

Radiographic evidence of osteomalacia is often not very specific and can mimic other disorders. The presence of pseudofractures or Looser's zones are good evidence that some degree of osteomalacia is present. Looser's zones are radiolucent areas of bones that are the result of multiple microstress fractures that heal by the formation of osteomalacic bone. Other radiographic signs of osteomalacia include biconcave vertebral bodies and the "trefoil"

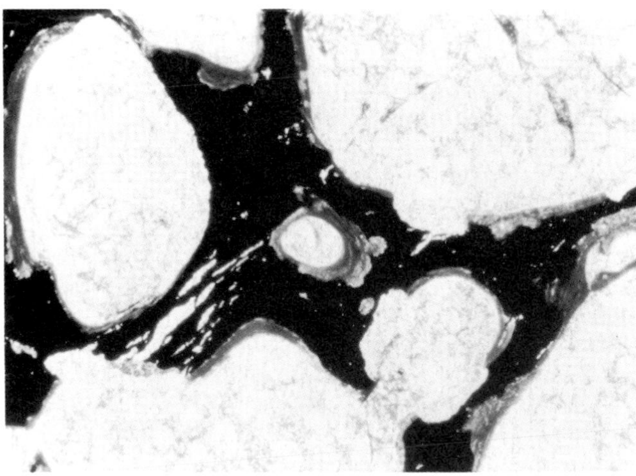

Figure 3: Transiliac bone biopsy from a female with osteomalacia. The undecalcified slide stained with Von Kossa demonstrated excessive unmineralized osteoid (light gray) on mineralized (black) trabecular bone.

Table III

Treatment of Common Forms of Osteomalacia

Nutritional and Vitamin D Deficient:
Vitamin D: 50,000 units 1-3/week
Elemental Calcium: 1,000-1,500 mg/day
Malabsorption (Sprue, Billroth II procedure):
Vitamin D 50,000 units 1-3/week
1,25 $(OH)_2$ Vitamin D .25-.50μg
Elemental Calcium: 1,500 mg/day
Drug Induced (Dilantin)
Vitamin D: 2,000-5,000 units/day
Elemental Calcium: 1,500 mg/day
Renal Osteodystrophy
Decrease Phosphate with Aluminum Hydroxide Gel
Elemental Calcium: 750-1,500 mg/day
1,25 $(OH)_2$ Vitamin D: .25-.50μg/day
and
25(OH) Vitamin D: 20-50μg/day
or
Dihydrotachysterol: .2-1 mg/day

Goal of treatment is mid-normal serum calcium and phosphate values, and if renal function is normal, a 24-hour urinary calcium .5mg/kg/day. As osteomalacia is corrected, the Vitamin D supplementation should be approximately diminished.

pelvis. The process of osteomalacia is far advanced when these findings are present.

In many patients, a transiliac bone biopsy is necessary to confirm the diagnosis of osteomalacia (Fig. 3). The histological hallmark of osteomalacia is an increase in the width and extent of the osteoid seams. Associated changes often encountered include decreased rate of mineral apposition as determined by tetracycline labeling and reduction in the surface extent of the mineralization front. Osteoblasts on the bone surface do not appear to be actively stimulated and show a low, flattened profile.

Osteomalacia is not a disease of rapid onset but appears gradually over a period of several years. Its development depends upon the quality and quantity of initial bone stock and the severity of the underlying disorder.

Following is a brief survey of the most common causes of osteomalacia and a description of some of the newer ideas about each of these disorders. Current treatment recommendations for the most common types are outlined in Table III.

Classic osteomalacia is caused by a decrease in the vitamin D present in the diet. These patients are easily identified because of their unusual dietary habits, i.e., strict vegetarianism or an extremely low-fat diet. Typically, classic osteomalacia occurs in patients who are elderly. It has been proposed that the "mild malabsorption of the elderly" predisposes these patients to bone disease. This disorder is easily treated with small amounts of vitamin D.

Gluten sensitive enteropathy is a common cause of osteomalacia due to a malabsorption syndrome. It is believed that the disease is present at birth, but it is not uncommon for patients to present as adults with osteomalacia due to gluten sensitivity. Treatment consists of a gluten free diet (mainly a wheat- and rye-free diet) and initially administering low doses of vitamin D.

Changes in gastrointestinal physiology secondary to abnormalities such as blind loops or Crohn's disease or changes secondary to surgery (60 percent of Billroth II procedures after 10 years) may alter vitamin D metabolism and calcium homeostasis enough to produce osteomalacia. A more common result, however, is osteoporosis. These changes in GI physiology may be very minor but over a period of years can cause significant disease.

Vitamin D metabolites are known to undergo enterohepatic circulation; thus, a biliary fistula may lead to depletion of vitamin D and osteomalacia. Bile salts are important in the process of vitamin D absorption in the bowel, and any disorder of the biliary system or liver may potentially affect vitamin D uptake by the intestine.

There are several known hereditary renal causes of rickets. Patients with these disorders (such as sex-linked dominant hypophosphatemic rickets) often will develop normally if the diagnosis is made early in life. Treatment with phosphate and 1,25 $(OH)_2$ vitamin D can maintain normal growth and usually is discontinued after a mature skeleton is achieved. It may need to be restarted as these patients age.

Albright in 1948 originally described the disorder termed distal renal tubular acidosis. It is characterized by a dominant gene mode of inheritance with a variable penetrance. When patients present, they usually show at least one of the three major complications of the disorder: renal stones, hypopotassemic paralysis, and osteomalacia. High dosages of vitamin D and sodium bicarbonate are usually unnecessary. It has been suggested that vitamin D deficiency and subsequent osteomalacia occur because of damage done to the renal tubular cells by calcium deposited within the kidney. The tubular cells slowly regain their function of vitamin D metabolism as the disorder is brought under control with bicarbonate.

Although the most common cause of bone loss in chronic renal failure (CRF) is hyperparathyroidism (due to low serum calcium levels), osteomalacia frequently is also a concomitant of renal osteodystrophy. This osteomalacia usually cannot be explained by diminishing CaxPO4 ion product in serum. (The CaxPO4 ion product is usually high in CRF because of elevated serum phosphate.) Recently, it has been shown that aluminum, taken in either as a contaminant of dialysis baths or by excessive ingestion of aluminum containing phosphate binders, will concentrate at the calcification front of bone spicules and prevent mineralization, thus allowing the accumulation of excessive osteoid.

Anticonvulsant osteomalacia occurs in patients on long-term Dilantin therapy. Patients who are immobile are especially at risk to develop this form of osteomalacia. Any of the anticonvulsant drugs that induce hepatic enzyme formation in the endoplasmic reticulum can cause the disorder (P 450 hydrolase). It is believed that the increased level of enzymes compete with 25-hydroxylase in metabolizing vitamin D and subsequently produce metabolites of vitamin D which are inactive. Therapy consists of moderate doses of vitamin D.

Mild forms of hyperosteoidosis are common in osteopenia (30 percent of patients). Bone biopsies and morphometric analyses of undecalcified specimens may be the only way to recognize these subtle forms of osteomalacia. Many recommend transiliac bone biopsies in all patients with osteopenia undergoing operative repair of hip fractures.

Increased Osteodensity

Paget's Disease of Bone Paget's disease of bone has been found to occur mainly in the United Kingdom, Germany, and France. It is rare in Scandinavian countries, Africa, the Middle East, and the Far East. Its incidence in the United States is roughly 3 percent. There have been reports of the disorder appearing in clusters in some areas. No genetic link and no increased incidence of specific HLA antigens have been found.

The possibility that it is caused by a viral agent has been raised. Intranuclear inclusion bodies have been found in the osteoclasts from areas of pagetoid bone of forty-one consecutive patients with Paget's. Control patients without the disease did not have the intranuclear bodies. The presentation is consistent with the etiologic agent being a slow virus, perhaps similar to the measles virus which is believed to be the cause of subacute sclerosing panencephalitis (SSPE). Interestingly, Sir James Paget was the first to propose that the disease was an inflammatory disorder of uncertain infectious origin. Mirra described a giant cell tumor occurring in bone which was also involved with Paget's disease. Intranuclear inclusion bodies similar to those seen in Paget's were demonstrated in the nuclei of the giant cells in the tumor. Giant cell tumors (and more commonly bone sarcomas) have been described as occurring more often in bone involved with this disease. This is due to either viral overstimulation of osteoclasts despite a normal PTH level or viral antigenic products activating the membrane-bound adenylcyclase and thereby stimulating osteoclastic activity.

Histologically, the initial event in Paget's disease is bone lysis by overly active osteoclasts. This creates the radiolucent zones seen on radiographs in the early phase of the disease. Later, osteoblasts become more active and start to form new bone rapidly. This causes the sclerotic areas present on radiographs. Some believe that the osteoblasts are only responding to the massive resorption of bone in a manner that allows calcium homeostasis to exist in the organism and are not abnormal cells. No inclusion bodies ever have been found in osteoblasts or osteocytes from bone involved with this disease.

The local rate of bone turnover is markedly increased in pagetoid bone. Estimates as high as twenty times the normal rate have been found in some studies using radioactive calcium. This hypermetabolic state causes increased amounts of alkaline phosphatase to be present in serum and an increased amount of hydroxyproline to be cleared in the urine. Alkaline phosphatase activity correlates with osteoblastic activity and, therefore, bone production. Hydroxyproline clearance is an indicator of bone resorption and osteoclastic activity because most of the hydroxyproline in the body is contained in collagen and type I collagen makes up most of the organic matrix of bone. Hydroxyproline, in addition to being cleared by the kidneys, is also degraded in the liver. Recently a large peptide containing hydroxyproline has been isolated in the urine. These peptides, perhaps, are not breakdown products of collagen but are short chains of amino acids cleaved off when procollagen is converted to collagen. If correct, it would indicate collagen production and, hence, bone formation. Metabolically, patients with Paget's disease typically have normal serum calcium, phosphate, and PTH levels and calcium clearance by the kidney is not elevated. These are all indications that the osteoclastic resorption is closely coupled to osteoblastic bone formation even though the rates of each are greatly increased.

Often, Paget's disease is initially discovered as an incidental finding on radiographs taken for other reasons. In patients who become symptomatic, bone pain and deformity are common complaints. Eighty-three percent of patients with the disease have some rheumatologic complaint. Back pain is the most common finding; usually some component of osteoarthritis is present. Only 2 percent of patients have bone pain in which the only cause is Paget's disease. This finding emphasizes the importance of looking for alternative sources of pain in patients with this disease.

25
MS:M

TREATMENT: There are three classes of drugs available: calcitonin, mithramycin, and the diphosphonates. Each of these drugs acts to decrease osteoclastic resorption of bone. As resorption decreases, so does osteoblastic activity. Typically, hydroxyproline clearance decreases first, and later alkaline phosphatase levels fall but not usually to normal values.

Calcitonin is effective initially in almost 100 percent of patients treated. It acts by decreasing both osteoclastic activity and the absolute number of osteoclasts present in bone. "Resistance" to calcitonin therapy does develop in a significant number of patients. This resistance is not necessarily due to the development of antibodies to calcitonin. Approximately 60 percent of patients given salmon calcitonin develop antibodies. To demonstrate antibody mediated resistance, it is necessary to return the disease to pretreatment levels by discontinuation of therapy and remission of the disorder when another nonimmune calcitonin, such as human calcitonin, is used.

Mithramycin action is believed to act via binding of the drug to DNA and thereby selectively inhibiting the synthesis of specific RNA sequences. The drug was initially developed as an antibiotic. Side effects include both hepatotoxicity and nephrotoxicity, especially at high dosage levels. It is primarily utilized to treat impending Paget's paraplegia.

The diphosphonate most commonly used is EHDP (diphosphonate disodium etidronate) which functions as an analogue of pyrophosphonate. This drug takes several weeks before its effectiveness can be documented. In vitro the diphosphonates also inhibit the formation of hydroxyapatite crystals. The in vivo significance of this effect is believed to be minimal at levels of 5mg/kg. Structural similarities shared by all diphosphonates are the presence of a P-C-P group in the molecule. An important property of the diphosphonates is their ability to be rapidly absorbed by bone. Approximately one-half of the amount of EHDP in circulation is absorbed by bone, especially bone which is turning over rapidly.

Paget's disease requires treatment when the disorder affects weight-bearing bones, hearing, spinal impingement, or osseous fractures, all with the alkaline phosphatase levels being elevated twofold. Treatment protocols usually suggest calcitonin 50 units three times a week for 6 months with, or followed by, diphosphonate 5m/kg/day. Alternatively, 20mg/kg/day of diphosphonate can be used cyclically for 1 month with a 3-month rest period.

Osteopetrosis There are two distinct forms of this relatively rare genetically transmitted disorder: a juvenile or "malignant" form and the more common adult or "benign" form. Recently, a third form has been reported that is midway between the two in severity.

The juvenile form is also known as infantile, precocious, or congenital osteopetrosis. The mode of transmission is autosomal recessive. It is characterized by anemia, hepatosplenomegaly, thrombocytopenia, cranial nerve palsies, and usually death at an early age. Radiographic studies show radiodense bone with obliteration of the medullary canal and widening of the metaphysis but no gross alteration in the secondary growth zones other than the increased radiodensity. Histologically, cores of calcified cartilage are seen surrounded by new bone and an increased number of osteoclasts are present. All knowledge of this disorder is consistent with the conclusion that the skeletal lesions are caused primarily by a markedly decreased rate of cartilage and bone resorption. There is no evidence that there is any alteration in the rate of cartilage or bone formation.

Evidence from studies of tissue obtained from humans with the disorder and several animal models that simulate the disease strongly implicate altered osteoclastic activity as the cause. Ultrastructural studies have shown that the number of osteoclasts in bone is increased but that they lack the characteristic ruffled border and clear zone of normal osteoclasts resorbing bone. The cells are responsive to PTH, but they are not able to form the ruffled border and clear zone. Tissue collagenase, which is important for resorption, cannot be detected in osteopetrotic bone.

Recently, several patients with juvenile osteopetrosis have been cured by bone marrow transplantation. After transplant, there is a progressive resolution of the osteopetrotic deformities with return to normal blood counts, decreased radiodensity of bone, and increased medullary cavity. The transplanted patients are found to be in a negative state of calcium balance as the excess bone is mobilized. These patients need to undergo vigorous hydration to allow the excess calcium to be excreted in the urine. Bone marrow biopsy of one patient has shown that the osteoclasts are now actively resorbing bone and indicates their origin is from the bone marrow donor.

Patients with osteopetrosis have also been shown to have deficient killer cell function and impaired thymic secretory activity. This has caused some researchers to believe that juvenile osteopetrosis is a more complex disorder than simply a dysfunction of osteoclasts. Following bone marrow transplantation, both the preceding alterations return to normal levels. It is now postulated that these alterations are caused by the decrease in hematopoietic activity associated with obliteration of the bone marrow cavity.

The adult type of osteopetrosis is also known as tarda osteopetrosis. It is inherited via autosomal dominant pattern and does not alter the life expectancy of the affected individual. It is usually an incidental finding on a radiograph taken for another reason. The radiographic findings are increased bone density but little or no disturbance of skeletal remodeling. Occasionally, these patients have bone pain, excessive fracturing, or cranial nerve palsies. Osteoclasts are found in increased number on bone biopsy, and the amount of bone present is increased with some remaining calcified cartilage present. Defective osteoclastic function is believed to be the cause, but the osteoclasts have retained enough function so that severe skeletal deformity does not occur.

ANNOTATED BIBLIOGRAPHY

Bone Formation and Turnover

Bone Cells

Baud, C.A., and Biovin, G.: Effects of hormones on osteocyte function and perilacunar wall structure. Clin. Orthop. 136:270-281, 1978.

This review presents the effects of all major hormones on perilacunar, osteocytic, and osteoblastic changes.

Bonucci, E.: New knowledge on the origin, function and fate of osteoclasts. Clin. Orthop. 158:252-269, 1981.

The osteoclast originates within the monocyte/macrophage system and is brought to the bone surface via the bloodstream.

Messer, H.H.: Bone cell membranes. Clin. Orthop. 166:256-276, 1982.

This review centers around the cellular membrane of "bone cells" and why the membrane is the site at which hormones, Ca^{++}, and electrical current affect cell function.

Growth Plate, Endochondral Bone Formation and Mineralization

Anderson, H.C.: Calcification processes. *In* Pathology Annual, edited by S.C. Sommers and P.P. Rosen. Part 2, vol. 15, pp. 45-75. New York, Appleton-Century-Crofts, 1980.

A complete description of matrix vesicle calcification plus review of calcification concepts and update on pathological calcification.

Boskey, A.L.: Current concepts of the physiology and biochemistry of calcification. Clin. Orthop. 157:225-257, 1981.

A review of the events of calcification discusses the mineral phases and the controlling factors including collagen, proteoglycan, noncollagen (vitamin K), phosphoproteolipids, and the cell organelles.

Brighton, C.T.: Structure and function of the growth plate. Clin. Orthop. 136:22-32, 1978.

Blood supply, reserve zone, proliferative zone, hypertrophic zone, metaphysis, and new information about the ossification groove of Ranvier and perichondrial ring are discussed.

Glimcher, M.J.: Composition, structure, and organization of bone and other mineralized tissues and the mechanism of calcification, pp. 25-116. *In* Handbook of Physiology: Section 7: Endocrinology, edited by R.O. Greep and E.B. Eastwood. Washington, D.C., American Physiological Society, 1976.

This article contains an in-depth discussion of mineralization.

Bone Repair and Fracture Biology

Brighton, C.T.; Friedenberg, Z.B.; Black, J.; Esterhai, J.L., Jr.; Mitchell, J.E.I.; and Montique, F., Jr.: Electrically induced osteogenesis: Relationship between charge, current density, and the amount of bone formed. Clin. Orthop. 161:122-132, 1981.

This article covers the various factors that specifically effect bone osteogenesis by electricity.

Enneking, W.F.; Eady, J.L.; and Burchardt, H.: Autogenous cortical bone grafts in the reconstruction of segmental skeletal defects. J. Bone Joint Surg. 62A:1039-1058, 1980.

Large autogenous fibular grafts have good or excellent results in 75 percent of patients. The length of the defect does not affect the incidence of nonunion, but it does adversely affect the number of fatigue fractures.

Lane, J.M.; Boskey, A.L.; Li, W.K.P.; Eaton, B.; and Posner, A.S.: A temporal study of collagen, proteoglycan, lipid and mineral constituents in a model of endochondral osseous repair. Meta. Bone Dis. 1:319-324, 1979.

The roles of collagen, proteoglycan, and mineralization in the fracture repair process are discussed.

McKibbin, B.: The biology of fracture healing in long bones. J. Bone Joint Surg. 60B:150-162, 1978.

A review of fracture healing breaks the healing process into stages and subdivides these by location.

Weiland, A.J.: Current concepts review. Vascularized free bone transplants. J. Bone Joint Surg. 63A:166-169, 1981.

A review summarizes the advantages and disadvantages of current methods of osseous reconstruction of massive bone defects, autogenous grafts, allografts, and vascularized bone graft.

Mineral Metabolism

Calcium and Phosphate Homeostasis

Lyles, K.W., and Drezner, M.K.: An overview of calcium homeostasis in humans. Urol. Clin. North America 8:209-226, 1981.

An overview of calcium metabolism includes a review of vitamin D and parathyroid hormone function.

Nordin, B.E.C.; Horsman, A.; Marshall, D.H.; Simpson, M.; and Waterhouse, G.M.: Calcium requirement and calcium therapy. Clin. Orthop. 140:216-239, 1979.

This is a review of calcium requirements and supplementation by an investigation of calcium homeostasis in hormonal and osteoporotic patients.

Vitamin D/Osteomalacia

Chesney, R.W.: Current clinical applications of vitamin D metabolite research. Clin. Orthop. 161:285-314, 1981.

A review of vitamin D metabolism with an extensive discussion of its role in various common and some rarer conditions of abnormal bone mineralization.

Ward, M.K.; Feest, T.G.; Ellis, H.A.; Parkinson, I.S.; Kerr, D.N.S.; Herrington, J.; and Goode, G.L.: Osteomalacia dialysis osteodystrophy: Evidence for a water-borne aetiological agent, probably aluminum. Lancet I:841-844, 1978.

The prevalence of osteomalacia after 1 to 4 years of hemodialysis seems to correlate with the concentration of aluminum in the dialysate.

Calcium-Binding Proteins

Gallop, P.M.; Lian, J.B.; and Hauschka, P.V.: Carboxylated calcium-binding proteins and vitamin K. New England J. Med. 302:1460-1466, 1980.

This review discusses vitamin D's participation in calcium-binding protein synthesis and where calcium-binding protein is found and how it functions.

Price, P.A.; Otsuka, A.S.; Poser, J.W.; Kristaphonis, J.; and Raman, N.: Characterization of a γ-carboxyglutamic acid-containing protein from bone. Proc. Nat. Acad. Sci. 73:1447-1451, 1976.

A γ-carboxyglutamic acid-containing protein was extracted from bovine cortical bone. It was found to bind strongly with hydroxyapatite and to inhibit hydroxyapatite crystalization.

Termine, J.D.; Kleinman, H.K.; Whitson, S.W.; Conn, K.M.; McGarvey, M.L.; and Martin, G.R.: Osteonectin, a bone-specific protein linking mineral to collagen. Cell 26:99-105, 1981.

When bound to type I collagen, this 32,000 dalton bone specific protein "binds synthetic apatite crystals and free calcium ions," and "nucleates mineral phase deposition from metastable balanced salt solutions."

Veis, A.; Stetler-Stevenson, W.; Takagi, Y.; Sabsay, B.; and Fullerton, R.: The nature and localization of the phosphophorylated proteins of mineralized dentin. *In* The Chemistry and Biology of Mineralized Connective Tissue, pp. 377-393. Elsevier/North Holland Press, 1981.

The authors suggest that a portion of newly secreted phosphophoryns is bound to the collagen fibril surface near the mineralization front and that it avidly binds calcium ions.

Endocrine Effect

Parathyroid Hormone

Habener, J.F.: Regulation of parathyroid hormone secretion and biosynthesis. Ann. Rev. Physiol. 43:211-223, 1981.

The article discusses PTH synthesis and metabolism.

Martin, K.J.; Hruska, K.A.; Freitag, J.J.; Klahr, S.; and Slatopolsky, E.: The peripheral metabolism of parathyroid hormone. New England J. Med. 301:1092-1098, 1979.

Various measurable immunoreactive forms of PTH and their clinical significance are discussed.

Calcitonin

Austin, L.A., and Heath, H., III: Calcitonin: Physiology and pathophysiology. New England J. Med. 304:269-277, 1981.

This review covers all recent information about calcitonin physiology as well as pathologic states and role in treatment of skeletal disorders.

Estrogen

Worley, R.J.: Age, estrogen, and bone density. Clin. Obstet. Gyn. 24:203-218, 1981.

Estrogens can decrease the fracture rate and bone loss vs. control in the postmenopausal population.

Osteopenia

Osteoporosis

Kleerekoper, M.B.; Tolia, K.; and Parfitt, A.M.: Nutritional, endocrine, and demographic aspects of osteoporosis. Orthop. Clin. North America 12:547-558, 1981.

A review of contributing factors to osteoporosis, includes multiple articles about the disease and covers the pathophysiology and available treatment strategies.

Lane, J.M., and Vigorita, V.J.: Current concepts review. Osteoporosis. J. Bone Joint Surg. 65A:274-278, 1983.

This is a review of the pathophysiology, diagnostic tests, and treatment of osteoporosis.

Riggs, B.L.; Seeman, E.; Hodgson, S.F.; Taves, D.R.; and O'Fallon, W.M.: Effect of the fluoride/calcium regimen on vertebral fracture occurrence in postmenopausal osteoporosis. New England J. Med. 306:446-450, 1982.

This study clearly demonstrates the efficacy of sodium fluoride and calcium in preventing spine fractures in osteoporosis.

Wallach, S.: Hormonal factors in osteoporosis. Clin. Orthop. 144:284-292, 1979.

An overview covers the effect of parathyroid hormone, gonadal steroids, calcitonin, thyroid hormone, and adrenocortical steroids on bone metabolism.

Osteomalacia

See Vitamin D.

Increased Osteodensity

Paget's Disease

Medsger, T.A., Jr., et. al.: Twenty-fifth Rheumatism Review: Paget's Disease. Arthrit. Rheumat. 26:281-283, 1983.

This is a review of the etiology, pathogenesis, clinical aspects, and therapeutic modalities for Paget's disease. There is a bibliography. Included in the review is a discussion of mithramycin, calcitonin and diphosphonate therapy and the newly discovered possible viral etiologies.

Nagant de Deuxchaisnes, C.; Maldague, B.; Malghem, J.; Devogelaer, J.P.; Huaux, J.P.; and Rombouts-Lindemans, C.: The action of the main therapeutic regimes on Paget's disease of bone, with a note on the effect of vitamin D deficiency. Arthrit. Rheumat. 23:1215-1234, 1980.

Calcitonin is more effective by improving osseous structure in Paget's disease.

Osteopetrosis

Sorell, M.; Kapoor, N.; Kirkpatrick, D.; Rosen, J.F.; Chaganti, R.S.K.; Lopez, C.; DuPont, B.; Pollack, M.S.; Terrin, B.N.; Harris, M.B.; Vine, D.; Rose, J.S.; Goossen, C.; Lane, J.; Good, R.A.; and O'Reilly, R.J.: Marrow transplantation for juvenile osteopetrosis. Am. J. Med. 70:1280-1287, 1981.

Two patients undergo marrow transplantation with successful reconstruction of marrow cavity.

Metabolic Bone Disease—Transiliac Bone Biopsy

Whyte, M.P.; Bergfeld, M.A.; Murphy, W.A.; Avioli, L.V.; and Teitelbaum, S.L.: Postmenopausal osteoporosis: A heterogeneous disorder as assessed by histomorphometric analysis of iliac crest bone from untreated patients. Am. J. Med. 72:193-202, 1982.

The paper covers role of bone biopsies and histomorphometry in defining several predominant disorders under the broad title of osteoporosis.

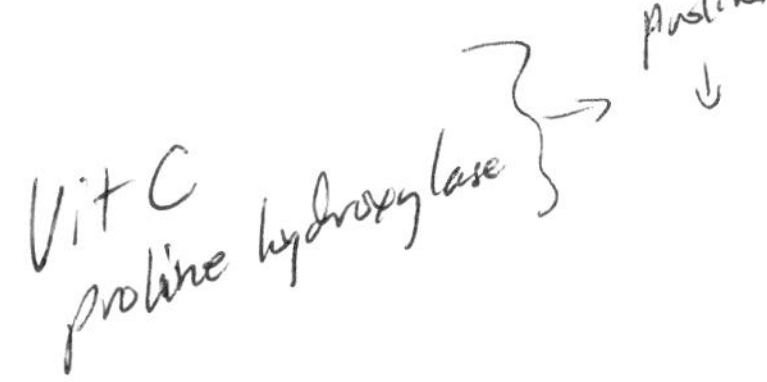

4 ARTHRITIS

Topics in this section include normal joint physiology and arthritis with an overview of its surgical treatment, including osteochondral grafting. Because of the prevalence of osteoarthritis in orthopaedic practice, it receives greatest emphasis; however, rheumatoid and traumatic arthritis also are discussed.

Normal Joint

Hyaline Cartilage Hyaline cartilage is composed of cells and matrix (Fig. 1). Macroscopically it appears opaque, smooth, shiny, and wet; but microscopically it is neither smooth nor uniform. The contour of the cartilage corresponds to the shape of the joint, but its surface contains undulations or "pits" having a role in the lubrication and loading of the joint.

Cells Chondrocytes produce the matrix (collagen and proteoglycans) and some enzymes responsible for normal cartilage metabolism (synthesis and degradation). Chondrocytes compose between 1 to 10 percent of the cartilage volume and range in size from 3 to 40 μ. Cell development is influenced by hormones, metabolites, and enzymes. In immature cartilage, chondrocytes multiply by mitosis but do not multiply in normal adult cartilage.

In the superficial layer (tangential zone) the cells are flat and parallel to the surface. In the second layer (transitional zone) the cells are randomly arranged. The cells are smaller and arranged in short columns perpendicular to the surface in the third layer (radial zone). In the fourth layer (calcified zone) the cells are pyknotic.

Matrix Matrix is composed of collagen, proteoglycans, and water.

COLLAGEN: Collagen represents 50 percent of the dry weight and 90 percent of the total protein of cartilage (Fig. 2). Synthesis of collagen starts in the chondrocytes. Three polypeptide alpha chains of amino acids (glycine, x [usually proline], y [usually hydroxyproline], etc.) with two sugars (galactose or glucosylgalactose) form the procollagen-3-helix, which leaves the chondrocytes and enters the matrix. The length of the procollagen is 300 nm (1 nm [nanometer] equals 1/1000 of a micron [μ]), and the weight of the molecules is 300,000 daltons (1 dalton equals 1/12 the atomic mass of carbon or approximately 1

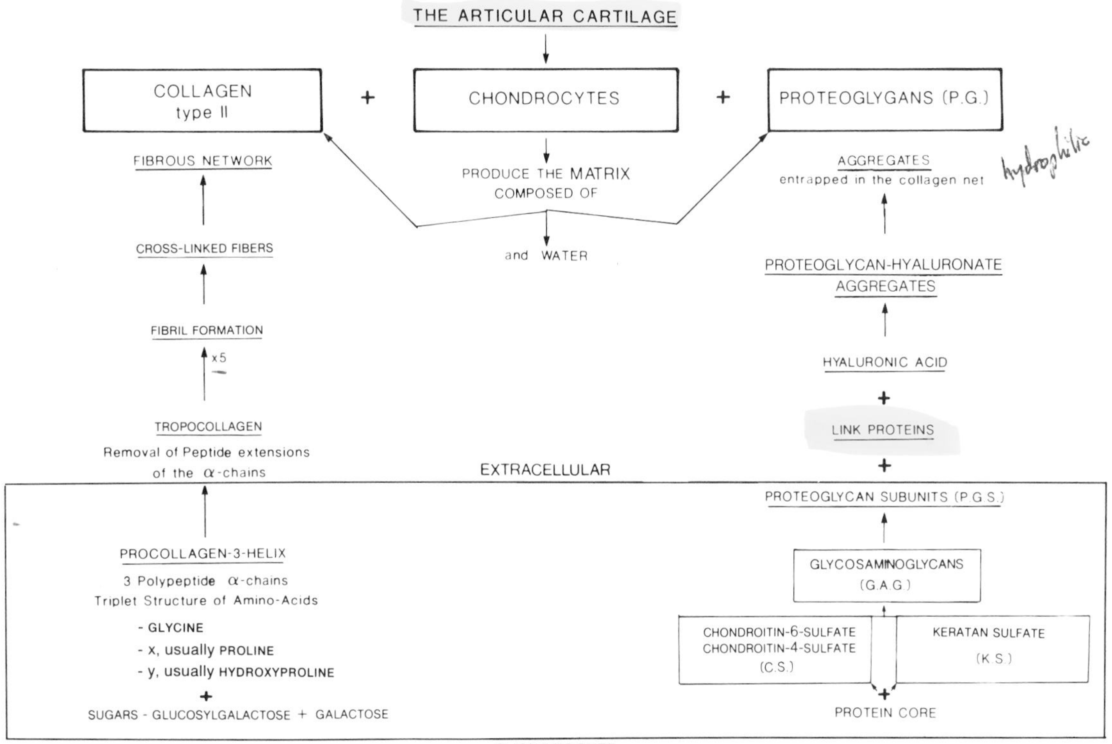

Figure 1: Articular cartilage components.

COLLAGEN

SUGARS = GLUCOSYLGALACTOSE and GALACTOSE
+ 3 POLYPEPTIDE α-CHAINS (GLYCINE, x, y*)
=
TRIPLET STRUCTURE of AMINO ACIDS
PEPTIDE EXTENSIONS
PROCOLLAGEN-3-HELIX
CHONDROCYTE MEMBRANE
PROCOLLAGEN
REMOVAL of PEPTIDE EXTENSIONS of the α-CHAINS by PEPTIDASE
TROPOCOLLAGEN
TROPOCOLLAGEN x5
COLLAGEN FIBRIL
CROSSLINKED FIBERS = COLLAGEN

*x IS USUALLY PROLINE; y IS USUALLY HYDROXYPROLINE

Figure 2: Collagen.

hydrogen atomic mass). The peptide extensions are removed from the alpha chains by peptidase. This results in a tropocollagen molecule, five of which bond together in a "quarter stagger" formation with intermolecular linkage to form the collagen fibril. These fibrils are then cross-linked to form the collagen fiber network.

In the most superficial layer of the articular cartilage (lamina splendens) the collagen fibers are quite fine, 4-10 nm in diameter. In the tangential zone the fibers are parallel to the surface and 30-32 nm in diameter. In the transitional zone the fibers are 30-32 nm in diameter but are oriented in different directions (arcades). In the radial zone the fibers are radial and 40-100 nm in diameter. In the calcified zone the fibers are perpendicular and may be up to 450 nm in diameter.

At least five types of collagen, as determined by the polypeptide alpha chain composition, have been identified. Hyaline cartilage contains exclusively type II collagen, which has more carbohydrate than type I (the predominant collagen of bone). The clinical implications of these collagen differences are not yet clear.

PROTEOGLYCANS: The proteoglycan (P.G.) subunit consists of a core protein (mw 200,000; length 0.2 nm) to which up to 150 chains of glycosaminoglycans (G.A.G.) are covalently linked (Fig. 3). G.A.G.'s consist of monosaccharides in repeating disaccharide units and are characterized by differences in monomer composition, sulfation, and glycosidic linkages.

After being secreted and entering the matrix, the proteoglycan subunits become noncovalently bound to another G.A.G., hyaluronic acid, thus forming proteoglycan-hyaluronate aggregates. These noncovalent bonds are stabilized by link protein. The degree of P.G. subunit binding to hyaluronic acid determines the hydrodynamic size of the aggregates.

The P.G. aggregates interact partially with the collagen fiber network so that about 25 percent of the P.G. cannot be extracted without degradation of the collagen (Fig. 4).

Proteoglycan-hyaluronate aggregates are hydrophilic macromolecules exerting a considerable swelling pressure which is resisted by the collagen network. The network is, as a result, under constant tension. Any weakening of this network allows more water to enter the tissue. Being

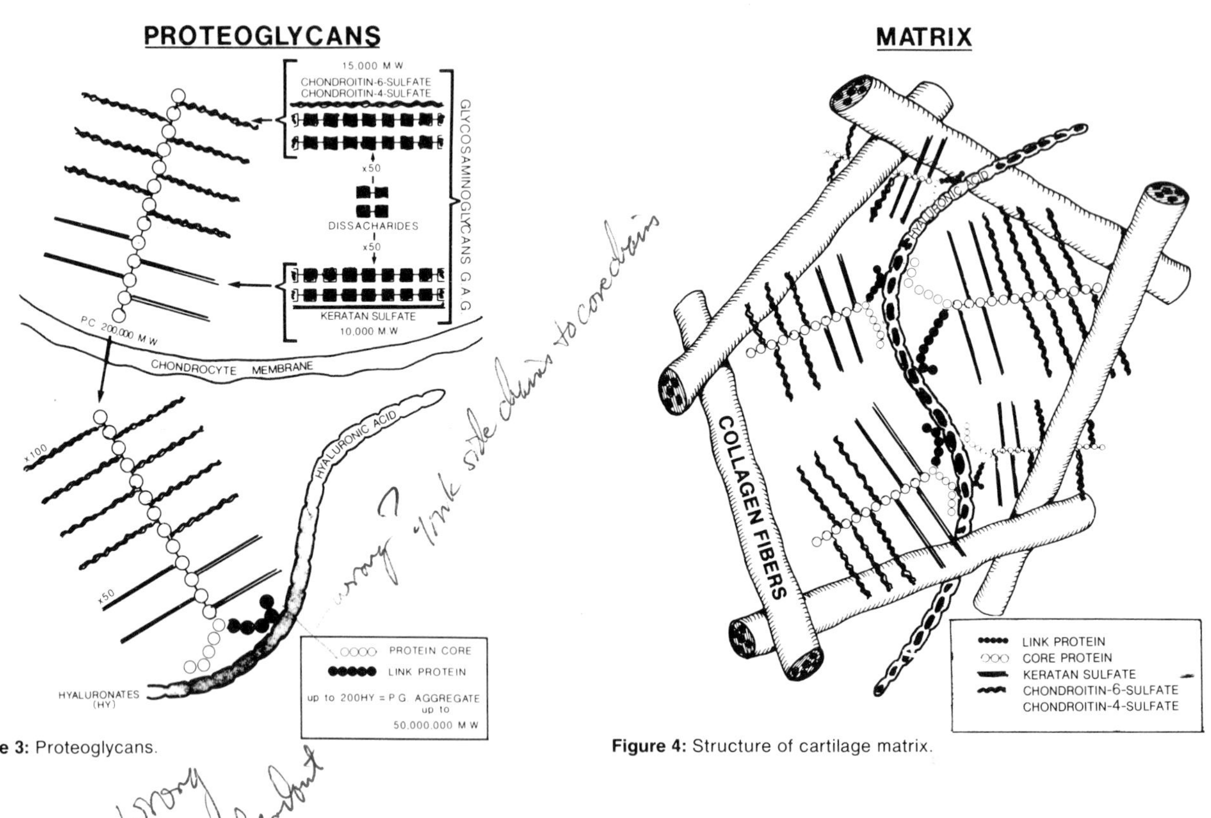

Figure 3: Proteoglycans.

Figure 4: Structure of cartilage matrix.

enmeshed in the collagen network, proteoglycan-hyaluronate aggregates also arrest the flow of interstitial water when an external load is applied. Thus, the compressive stiffness of cartilage is directly proportional to the aggregate content.

WATER: This fluid composes 70 percent of the matrix of articular cartilage in normal young adults and is important for nutrition and lubrication. It is bound to the proteoglycans and collagen by hydrostatic attraction produced by the dipole moment in water. The binding forces are weak, and molecular exchange readily occurs. The fluid movement from the cartilage into the joint fluid after prolonged loading is only about 30 percent because of the small pore size on the cartilage surface. More exchange occurs during standing than walking. Six percent of the water is so strongly bound that it cannot be extracted by any means.

Synovium and Synovial Fluid There are two cell types in the synovium: type A, a macrophage-like cell which phagocytizes; and type B, a fibroblast-like cell that produces multiple substances including proteinase, collagenase, hyaluronic acid, and prostaglandins. Synovial fluid is the product of the synovial membrane. This fluid is an ultrafiltrate of plasma plus the unique products of the synovial membrane.

Synovial fluid, like blood, has nonnewtonian characteristics, such that shear rate and shear stress are not proportional. Thus, increase in the velocity of joint movement is not accompanied by a proportional increase in joint friction.

Nutrition Growing cartilage is nourished by synovial fluid and by subchondral blood vessels. Mature cartilage is nourished by diffusion from synovial fluid. Cartilage is avascular, and the chondrocytes are isolated from direct blood supply. Thus, nutrition comes from fluid diffusing through the matrix. The intermittent impact loading of a joint has a sponge effect which helps to diffuse nutrients into the cartilage.

Lubrication In 1932 MacConail proposed that joint lubrication was *hydrodynamic*, i.e., fluid separates the surfaces under load. He was impressed with the incongruity of joint surfaces moving under load causing convergent wedges of fluid to separate the surfaces.

In 1959 Charnley described *boundary lubrication*, which implies that the surfaces are slippery but with no fluid between them. This may be because either the surfaces are intrinsically slippery or there are substances that react chemically with the sliding surface and function as a molecular film too thin to show viscosity in accordance with the laws of fluid mechanics. These observations are consistent with the fact that synovial fluid contains protein constituents which interact with the surfaces of the cartilage, acting as a boundary lubricant.

In 1959 McCutchen described *weeping lubrication*. Cartilage is permeable and fluid-soaked. Because it is not rigid, applying load pressurizes the fluid within the cartilage, causing it to flow to the surface under high pressure and carry load. McCutchen believed that joints were lubricated by the combined action of weeping and boundary lubrication.

In 1968 *boosted lubrication* was described. Since cartilage has undulations on its surface, when contact is made between two cartilaginous surfaces, contact is made at the peaks which are lubricated by the boundary mechanism. In the depressions between the peaks there are pools of trapped synovial fluid. These pools develop a high concentration of hyaluronic acid protein complex because of diffusion of water and low molecular weight proteins through the cartilage pores into the cartilage. Boosted lubrication is this mechanism of fluid entrapment and enrichment.

It is probable that the last three types of lubrication are utilized at some time during the gait cycle.

Of interest is that the coefficient of friction in a normal synovial joint is .002 and the best artificial joint is thirty times higher.

Aging of Cartilage Senescent chondrocytes are two to three times larger than normal and demonstrate increased quantity of the intracellular lysosomal enzymes which cause more degradation of matrix than is needed for normal remodeling. There is no mitosis and no synthesis of DNA in these aging cells.

The proteoglycans in cartilage decrease from 7 percent of the wet tissue at birth to about 3.5 percent in the adult. The protein content increases with age from about 6 percent at birth to 12 percent in the adult. The ratio of chondroitin sulfate to keratan sulfate ranges from about 12:1 at birth to 2:1 in the adult. With aging, the proteoglycan subunits become smaller, and the water content also decreases. All these changes diminish the elastic properties of cartilage. The fact that these changes occur equally in the knee and shoulder indicates that load-bearing is not the primary causative factor.

Osteoarthritis

Knowledge of osteoarthritis is based upon three sources: experimentally induced osteoarthritis in animals, osteoarthritis occurring naturally in animals, and human osteoarthritis.

The topic is complex and controversial not only because there are differences in cartilage structure between species but also because most experimental osteoarthritis is produced mechanically (i.e., joint immobilization, compression, partial joint resection, meniscectomy, cutting of ligaments, and osteotomy).

Experimental Osteoarthritis Chondrocytes in adult cartilage do not undergo mitosis, but in osteoarthritis, mitotic figures are identified. Chondrocytes are seen in clusters and even in columns. This appearance is termed *cloning*.

Chondrocyte proliferation and migration have been well documented in experimental osteoarthritis. That chondrocytes are more active and produce more proteoglycan has been interpreted as an abortive attempt by chondrocytes to repair cartilage. In more advanced osteoarthritis, chondrocytes appear to "give up" after their initial attempts to repair. In spontaneous murine osteoarthritis, inactive chondrocytes are identified before changes in the matrix can be seen. Thus, some believe that the primary problem is in the chondrocytes. Similar conclusions have been drawn when aging mouse cartilage was found to show decreased activity of the oxidative enzymes produced by chondrocytes.

The water content of osteoarthritic cartilage is increased. Alterations in the proteoglycans and collagen have been implicated.

Each proteoglycan-hyaluronate aggregate contains dozens of proteoglycan subunits. In normal cartilage there is variation in the length of the protein core and the number and length of the glycosaminoglycans, depending upon the age and site of the cartilage. This variability is more diffuse in osteoarthritic cartilage. There is also decreased binding of P.G. subunits to the hyaluronic acid chain which also may be shorter. Thus, the compressive stiffness of the cartilage, which depends upon the hydrophilic P.G. hyaluronate aggregates, is reduced.

Proteolytic damage may occur in the binding region of the P.G. subunit to hyaluronic acid, and even limited damage in this vulnerable region is sufficient to change the structure of the macromolecules and their physical properties. It has been suggested that the increased release of proteolytic enzymes may be due to increased prostaglandin E synthesis secondary to the increased availability of arachidonic acid. Anti-inflammatory medicines may exert their effect by inhibiting production of prostaglandins.

In some studies of advanced osteoarthritis, deficits of link proteins and hyaluronic acid have been demonstrated, suggesting decreased proteoglycan-hyaluronate aggregation rather than a decrease of P.G. subunits.

In experimental osteoarthritis, disruption of the collagen network also has been reported. This was believed not to be purely mechanical but rather due to increased amounts of collagenolytic enzymes (collagenase). Type II collagen normally is stabilized against disruption by an intermolecular cross-link of its fibers. An enzyme or enzymes that disrupt this cross-link could be responsible for the initial step in the degradation of the collagen. The resulting increase in the extensibility of the collagen network could explain the increase in the water content of osteoarthritic cartilage.

Following production of experimental cartilage mechanical defects, increased collagen formation has been reported. In the early stages type I predominates, whereas after 8 weeks type II does. However, after 1 year there is still some residual type I collagen. The collagen content is increased and the proteoglycan decreased.

Human Osteoarthritis

Some recent observations: Early in human osteoarthritis, chondrocytes are metabolically hyperactive (as assessed by radioactive tracers), and there are many immature chondrocytes. These changes are present both in the weight-bearing and nonweight-bearing areas. In advanced osteoarthritis there are three distinct cytopathological tissue types: hypocellular with spheroidal cells and lacunar halos (a sign of impaired matrix synthesis); cell clones of six to twelve small spheroidal cells arranged in columns or ovoid clusters; and numerous small fusiform cells with irregular matrix production. In normal cartilage of individuals over 50 years of age, the first type may be identified.

Cartilage matrix turns over very slowly and, therefore, may appear grossly normal even though histological and biochemical changes already have occurred. The proteoglycan synthesis by cartilage is increased in early osteoarthritis, especially surrounding clones of chondrocytes. Also, the ratio of chondroitin sulfate to keratan sulfate more closely resembles immature cartilage. These changes, as well as those mentioned for the cells, appear to be an attempt at repair. Even though the hyaluronic acid content nearly triples, protein aggregation is diminished. This indicates the inadequacy of repair. By the time the disease process has advanced to the point that fibrillation is visible, the total proteoglycan content is decreased. This occurs before the disease becomes visible on plain radiography, although arthrography demonstrates changes at the fibrillation stage.

There appear to be different types/phases of osteoarthritis. Chemical analysis of the cartilage, in one study of 90 patients, indicated three types/phases: inflammatory osteoarthritis with high enzymatic activity and loss of P.G.; mechanical osteoarthritis with less enzymatic activity and less loss of P.G.; and a mixed group. Heavy individuals illustrated greater loss of P.G. without necessarily high enzyme activity. That there often may be a systemic factor is supported by another series of 170 patients in which most showed osteoarthritis in more than one joint. However, if only one joint was involved, it was most likely to be the hip.

Because small focal areas of superficial subchondral osteonecrosis are common in advanced osteoarthritis, the relationship between osteonecrosis and osteoarthritis has been examined. It is believed that these entities are separate and independent of one another in that the cartilage overlying osteonecrosis is normal until secondary changes occur due to lack of bony support.

Etiology and pathogenesis of human osteoarthritis: In the European literature *arthrosis* (i.e., coxarthrosis refers to osteoarthritis of the hip and gonarthrosis refers to osteoarthritis of the knee) implies a purely degenerative process, whereas *arthritis* implies an inflammatory process. In the North American literature osteoarthrosis and degenerative joint disease often are used interchangeably. This confusion in terminology is indicative of our ignorance regarding the exact etiology of this condition. In fact, osteoarthritis likely represents a common clinical manifestation of a whole spectrum of diseases or conditions.

Osteoarthritis is still believed to be either *primary* (due to an intrinsic defect) or *secondary* (due to previous pathology, e.g., infection or trauma). Theories of etiology to explain primary osteoarthritis have included aging and mechanical, immune, vascular, and primary cartilage derangements.

Radiological evidence of an osteoarthritic joint is present in 50 percent of the population and almost 100 percent of those over 50 years of age. However, histological and biochemical changes in osteoarthritic cartilage are only qualitatively, not quantitatively, similar to those of aging cartilage. For example, femoral heads, removed after femoral neck fractures in the elderly, have coverage by macroscopically healthy cartilage as opposed to the obviously abnormal cartilage of osteoarthritic femoral heads. Also, crystal deposits (hydroxyapatite, pyrophosphate, or even cholesterol) have been identified in the cartilage, menisci, and synovium of osteoarthritic joints, but the prevalence of these crystal deposits correlates more closely with age than with osteoarthritis. Thus, osteoarthritis and aging cannot be directly correlated.

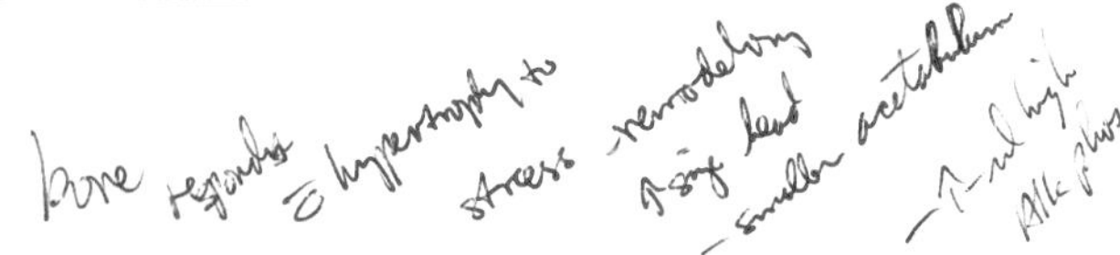

Loading is necessary for normal joint function, but abnormally increased loading, such as in posttraumatic or congenital incongruity, leads to osteoarthritis. The energy of repeated normal *loading* is absorbed by cartilage and subchondral trabecular bone. In human and animal specimens, microfractures leading to sclerosis and stiffness of subchondral bone have been identified in early osteoarthritis. Experimentally, it has been shown that increased stiffness of subchondral bone increases cartilage wear. Some researchers believe that the resultant subchondral stiffness creates increased stresses in the cartilage causing the chondrocytes to release an enzyme which destroys the matrix (a combined biomechanical and biochemical theory). This could explain incongruous, but not congruous, osteoarthritis. One study of 438 osteoarthritic hips showed that subchondral cysts that were part of the osteoarthritis process preceded the subchondral bone sclerosis and, by actually compressing the bone, led to bone necrosis adjacent to the cysts. This finding opposes the theory of subchondral microfracture as the primary event in osteoarthritis.

An altered local immune process has been suggested as part of the etiology of primary osteoarthritis. Lending credence to this theory is a recent report in which immune complexes were identified in the cartilage of 60 percent of 85 patients considered to have primary osteoarthritis. In contrast, similar findings were present in only 16 percent of thirty-two patients with secondary osteoarthritis and in only 3 percent of nonarthritic joints studied.

Some have identified a *primary defect* in the cartilage whereby the *chondrocytes*, damaged by any of various factors, fail to produce protease inhibitors, leading to loss of matrix and vascular invasion.

In conclusion there are several possible mechanisms to account for the cartilage destruction of osteoarthritis. In an attempt at repair, chondrocytes become more immature and hyperactive. They proliferate and produce more matrix. But, if the insult is too great or too prolonged, chondrocytes are unable to repair the damage and osteoarthritis results.

Rheumatoid Arthritis

For many years rheumatoid arthritis, a disease of unknown etiology, was considered to be simply a proliferative synovitis, typified by pannus formation and joint destruction. Now it is recognized that there are complex interactions among many pathogenic mechanisms in rheumatoid arthritis.

Immune mechanisms are implicated in the pathogenesis of rheumatoid arthritis. It is postulated that the immune response involving both T and B lymphocytes is triggered possibly by an infectious agent in a genetically susceptible individual (associated with HLA-DR4 antigens). The ensuing complex inflammatory response is associated with the presence of autoantibodies (e.g., rheumatoid factor, RF), synovial proliferation and pannus formation, recruitment of inflammatory cells (e.g., neutrophils), and the degradation of cartilage.

Findings of low complement levels in serum and synovial fluid support a role for immune complexes in the pathogenesis of rheumatoid arthritis. Rheumatoid factor, usually IgM with associated IgG, is one type of immune complex found in rheumatoid arthritis.

Other autoantibodies have been found recently in rheumatoid arthritis. These include antibodies directed mainly against type II collagen.

Inflammatory Arthritis Associated with Infectious Agents

Experimental arthritis has been induced by intraperitoneal injection of bacterial cell walls. Several experiments suggest that bacteria or bacterial components play a role in the initiation of the immune mechanisms which result in rheumatoid arthritis.

Mycoplasmas differ from other bacteria by their hereditary inability to form a cell wall. These microorganisms can cause various forms of spontaneous or experimental arthritis in animals and birds. The implication of mycoplasmas as an etiological factor is difficult because of the frequency of contamination of cell cultures by mycoplasmas that could have existed in the cultures prior to their inoculation with clinical specimens.

Many viral infections are accompanied by joint inflammation. However, viral induced arthritis is transient. Some studies in experimental arthritis suggest different theories on the role of a virus or viral subunits in the complex immune responses. Specific lesions in mice born after injection of the pregnant mother with homogenized rheumatoid synovial membrane and lesions in chick embryos after similar infection of embryonated eggs suggest the possibility of infection. The presence of a "slow" viral infection also has been suggested. These viruses are difficult to isolate, and there is no current evidence of their involvement in rheumatoid arthritis.

Lyme disease initially was recognized as a form of epidemic arthritis in a restricted geographic area. This oligoarticular inflammatory arthritis, most commonly involving the knees, is due to an organism transmitted by the *Ixodes dammini* tick. Synovectomy is beneficial in patients that progress to a chronic inflammatory state.

Treatment of Arthritis

Nonoperative The natural course of *osteoarthritis* is very slow. Thus, even with the use of arthrography, arthroscopy, intraosseous pressure monitoring, and scans, orthopaedic surgeons usually see patients years after the onset of the disease.

Nonsurgical treatment, including rest, physiotherapy, orthotics, local steroids, and nonsteroid anti-inflammatory drugs, can neither arrest nor cure the disease but may provide significant symptomatic relief. Repeated local steroid injections at short intervals may accelerate cartilage destruction.

The response to nonoperative treatment is variable and unpredictable because it is not specific. Many other therapeutic approaches have been tried (chondrocyte growth and glycosaminoglycan synthesis stimulation, substitution therapy with a sulfated glycosaminoglycan analogue, chondrocyte enzyme inhibitors, hyaluronic acid, and vitamin C) but have not been effective.

Recent laboratory work has shown that after creation of full-thickness cartilage defects in animals, continual passive motion results in better hyaline cartilage repair than either immobilization or active motion. In animals with septic arthritis, the same results occurred. Patient trials are currently underway to determine the clinical role of the findings.

In *rheumatoid* arthritis, immunosuppressive drugs are used. But, because T lymphocytes can inhibit the immunological process by their regulation of the B lymphocytes, some immunostimulators, such as transfer factor and levamisole, have been used successfully.

The pharmacological management of rheumatoid arthritis should be tailored to meet the needs of the patient. The drugs available can be considered in first, second, and third line categories. The first category consists of the nonsteroidal anti-inflammatory agents. (Table I). The goals are to select the agent that is most beneficial to the patient and to avoid polypharmacy. Individual patient response to the different drug classes varies. Because it is not possible to predict which drug class will be most beneficial in a particular patient, a commonly used plan is prescribe a sequence of one drug from each class to be taken individually during a succession of 2-week intervals. It is necessary to be certain that a therapeutic dose is being given. The patient should be monitored for clinical response as well as side effects, such as gastrointestinal distress, skin rash, and central nervous system distress (e.g., headaches). The drug providing the best response can then be selected for long-term use. Such a program should effectively control symptoms in 70 to 80 percent of patients with rheumatoid arthritis. This is also an appropriate method for selection of the optimum drug therapy for a patient with osteoarthritis.

The second and third line drugs may exert a fundamental effect upon the rheumatoid disease process but are potentially very toxic. These drugs are indicated for the 15 to 20 percent of rheumatoid arthritis patients with progressive disease. The second line drugs are known as remittive agents and include gold, penicillamine, and the antimalarials. As they may be toxic to blood, kidneys, skin, and eyes, meticulous monitoring is necessary.

Finally, the third line drugs may be considered for approximately 5 percent of rheumatoid arthritis patients that are not controlled with first and second line drugs. The third line drugs include continual systemic corticosteroids, ACTH, and cytotoxic drugs. They are highly toxic, and their long-term use is discouraged.

Table I

Classes of Nonsteroidal Anti-Inflammatory Agents

I. Salicylates
- acetylsalicylic
- trisalicylate magnesium choline
- salsalate
- diflunisal

II. Pyrazoles
- phenylbutazone
- apazone
- oxyphenbutazone

III. Indoles
- indomethacin
- sulindac
- tolmetin
- zomepirac

IV. Arylalkanoic acids (propionic acid derivatives)
- ibuprofen
- naproxen
- fenoprofen
- flurbiprofen
- ketoprofen

V. Oxicame
- piroxicam

VI. Fenamates
- mefenamic acid

(Courtesy of Daniel Stechschulte, M.D., Kansas City, Kansas)

TREATMENT

INCONGRUOUS JOINT DISEASE	CONGRUOUS JOINT DISEASE
HEAVY DEMAND (young, active, heavy, obese...)	
REALIGNMENT (pelvic, femoral, tibial Osteotomies) ± DEBRIDEMENT; BIOLOGICAL REPLACEMENT – ?	DECOMPRESSION – ? (tenotomies, forage); DEBRIDEMENT – ?; EXCISION (i.e. Girdlestone, patellectomy); BIOLOGICAL REPLACEMENT – ?; ARTHRODESIS
LOW DEMAND (old, inactive, light worker, skinny...)	
REALIGNMENT; PROSTHETIC REPLACEMENT	PROSTHETIC REPLACEMENT

Figure 5: Surgery of the arthritic joint. Left column lists the spectrum of procedures for incongruous joint disease, and the right column for congruous joint disease, depending upon whether the patient is categorized as heavy or low demand.

Surgery General indications and alternatives are shown in Figure 5. For more details, refer to the appropriate anatomical section.

Synovectomy Inflammation decrease and pain relief are the major benefits of synovectomy. However, it is doubtful whether a permanent cure is achieved. Regeneration of the synovium occurs, and, due to residual immune complexes in the cartilage, synovitis develops and eventually a rheumatoid synovium is reformed.

Synovectomy, chemical or surgical, is mainly useful in patients with severe prolonged synovitis and pain refractory to medical management. Specific criteria vary somewhat from joint to joint. For instance, in the knee, synovectomy is effective only when carried out in the early radiographic stages, whereas in the elbow it may be effective in late radiographic stages. Laser synovectomy is still experimental.

Debridement Joint debridement is indicated in osteoarthritis in combination with surgical realignment (i.e., osteotomy) but rarely as a single procedure. It is used for removal of loose bodies, osteophytes that block movement, and significantly torn menisci. Debridement is done to decrease symptoms and improve function. Arthroscopic debridement has been a useful procedure in some patients. It may be combined with osteotomy, avoiding the necessity of opening the joint.

Arthroscopic debridement, carried out as a single procedure, may provide some short-term benefits, but there is no hard data to suggest that this surgery provides good long-term results.

Excision Arthroplasty This has been shown to be of value for osteoarthritis of selected joints, such as the acromioclavicular, radiocapitate, first metacarpal, and patellofemoral.

Osteotomy A recent study of ninety-four varus knees revealed that if left untreated surgically, the varus and osteoarthritis progressed significantly over 10 years.

Thus, realignment of a joint is indicated in incongruous osteoarthritis when a portion of the joint is still healthy (as opposed to congruous disease when the entire articular surface is damaged). Osteotomy has been particularly useful in the hip (proximal femur or pelvis) and in the knee (proximal tibia and distal femur).

Osteotomy to realign a joint has several advantages. Decreasing the deformity lessens stretch on soft tissue (especially ligaments) and redistributes pressure over a larger, healthier articular surface. Bone division also lessens intraosseous pressure and divides nerve endings (likely a short-term effect). The healing process of the osteotomy allows subchondral microfractures to heal, cysts to disappear, and, perhaps, cartilage to regenerate.

An arthroscopic study of fifty-four knees that had previously undergone high tibial osteotomy revealed that if the deformity was overcorrected, ulcerated areas were capable of healing by fibrocartilage.

Arthrodesis Fusion of a major joint may be indicated when a joint has been completely destroyed in a young, active patient with no other joint involvement. To achieve a good arthrodesis after failure of an implant is difficult, and, therefore, new implants requiring less bone sacrifice are desirable.

Arthroplasty (Joint Replacement) Patients with advanced joint disease who are not suitable candidates for realignment or arthrodesis may be considered for replacement arthroplasty.

Implant Replacement Dramatic relief of pain and improvement of function are possible for a period of time depending upon the age, size, and demands of the patient as well as technical factors. The improvement of implant material, design, and careful attention to surgical technique has improved the long-term results in hip and knee replacement in the elderly patient. The younger, more active patient still presents a problem in terms of long durability.

One long-range follow-up series of total hip replacement patients showed a radiographic loosening rate of 30.5 percent at 5 years and 41.2 percent at 10 years. However, not all these joints were symptomatic or required surgical treatment. Standard actuarial analyses

UNIPOLAR FRAGMENT ALLOGRAFT

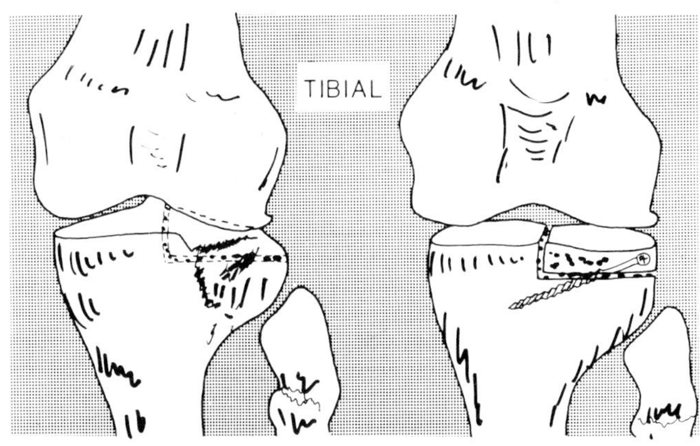

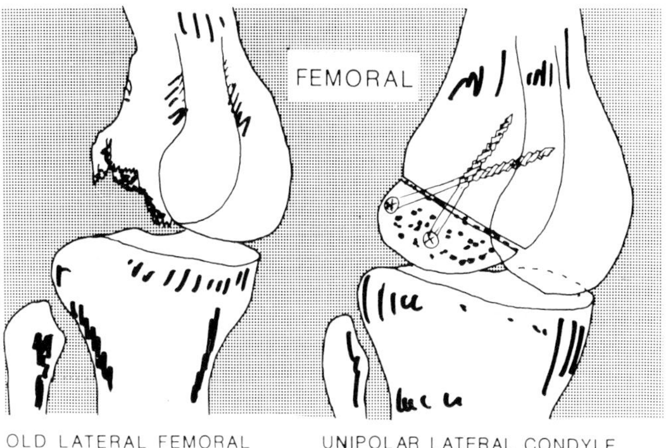

Figure 6: Schematic drawings of unipolar small fragment allograft.

BIPOLAR SMALL FRAGMENT ALLOGRAFT

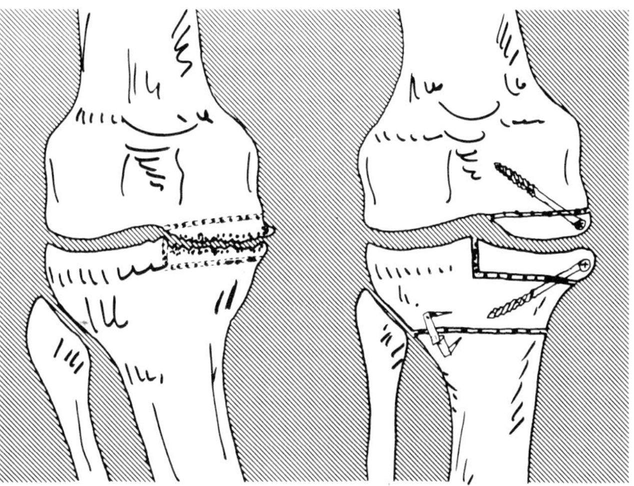

Figure 7: Schematic drawing of bipolar unicompartmental small fragment allograft.

demonstrated that 94 percent of the prostheses survived intact at 10 years. Average patient age in this series was 63.6 years. A recent study of total hip replacement in patients under the age of 30 years revealed good results at 1 year, but at 5 years 57 percent had significant loosening of one component (acetabular twice as frequently as femoral). Recently the results of knee replacement have paralleled those of the hip.

Because prosthetic joint replacements have a limited lifetime, the search for a biological alternative continues.

Biological Replacement As cartilage receives a significant part of its nutrition from synovial fluid, it has the potential to survive transplantation. Nonvascularized bone transplants are dead but retain structural integrity for a long time and eventually undergo host creeping substitution. Bone, collagen, proteoglycans, and chondrocytes are immunogenic; however, clinically, rejection does not appear to be as relevant as mechanical factors in determining the success of a graft.

Experimental: Rib perichondrial *autografts* produce cartilage that survives and demonstrates metabolic activity. When grafted into femoral condylar defects in rabbits (as an autograft), new cartilage formed filling the defect in 2 to 3 months, but slight degenerative changes occurred at 1 year.

Osteochondral *allografts* performed in animals have had early success but usually deteriorate with time. This deterioration may be partly due to the mechanical problems of animal experimentation. One experiment has demonstrated synovial reaction (both histological and biochemical) that has been offered as a cause for failure.

Factors that have been shown experimentally to improve the results of osteochondral allografts are: the use of immature cartilage; transplantation into nonarthritic (as opposed to papain-induced arthritic) joints; the use of fresh rather than stored grafts; the use of additives and tissue culture media if grafts are stored for short periods; and the use of cryopreservative agents (i.e., DMSO) and slow freezing in an attempt to preserve chondrocyte viability in deep frozen grafts.

Experiments have shown that osteochondral grafts that are stored for only 12 to 24 hours prior to grafting have the good qualities of live cartilage and dead bone (which has less immunogenicity than bone used immediately after harvesting).

Another approach to allografting has been the use of isolated chondrocytes in suspension or cultured chondroid tissue to fill articular defects. Chondrocytes can be stored in tissue culture for up to 3 months. This technique has some potential for pure cartilaginous defects without bone loss.

Clinical: Cartilage *autografts* have survived experimentally, but the practical usage is limited. They can be used for small lesions. Osteochondral grafts have been taken from the posterior aspect of the femoral condyles, the patella, and proximal fibula. Vascularized (pedicle) osteochondral autografts have been used around the knee and wrist. In plastic surgery, chondral and perichondrial grafts from the ear have been commonly used. The first successful reconstruction of an MP joint by a free rib perichondrial autograft was performed 10 years ago.

Cartilage *allografts* may be utilized as small or large fragment osteochondral grafts (Figs. 6 and 7).

Recent studies have shown that chondrocytes are antigenic but are at least partially protected from immunogenic cells and rejection by an intact matrix. As both fresh and deep frozen bone are immunogenic, there appears to be no advantage to freezing, a step that kills chondrocytes. For these reasons, most of these procedures

Figure 8: (A) Preoperative radiograph of a 54-year-old male with old lateral tibial plateau fracture. (B) Postoperative radiograph 5 years after allograft of lateral tibial plateau.

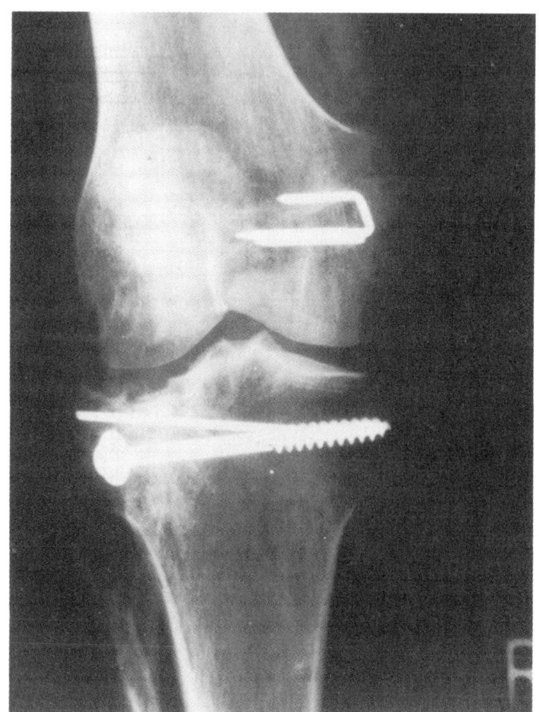

Figure 8-A

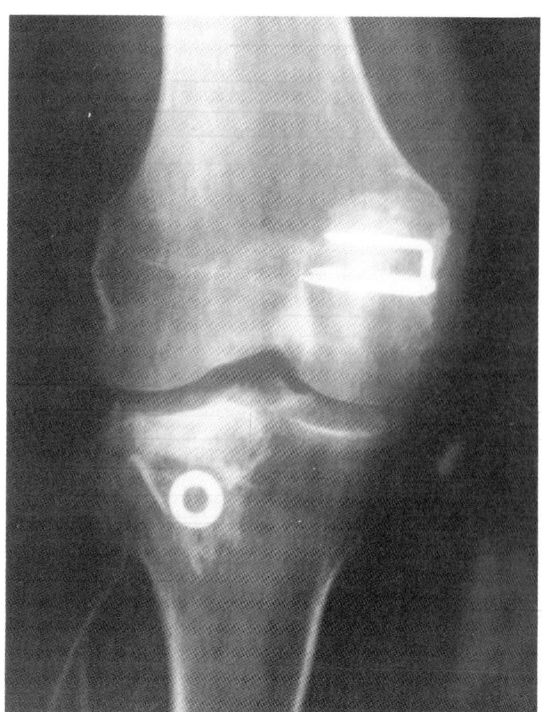

Figure 8-B

involve fresh, small osteochondral fragments.

Favorable results have been reported in the treatment of femoral head osteonecrosis and knee lesions, including old plateau fractures, osteonecrosis, and unicompartmental osteoarthritis. Best results were obtained when treating old plateau fractures and traumatic loss of bone and cartilage. Less predictable results were obtained in unicompartmental osteoarthritis, although twenty-four of thirty-seven patients did obtain an acceptable result (Figs. 8, 9, and 10). Tissue typing or blood grouping were not

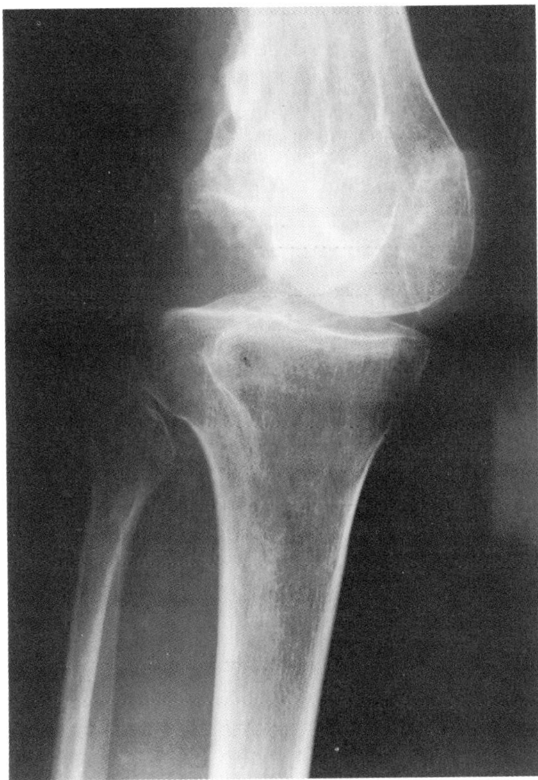

Figure 9-A

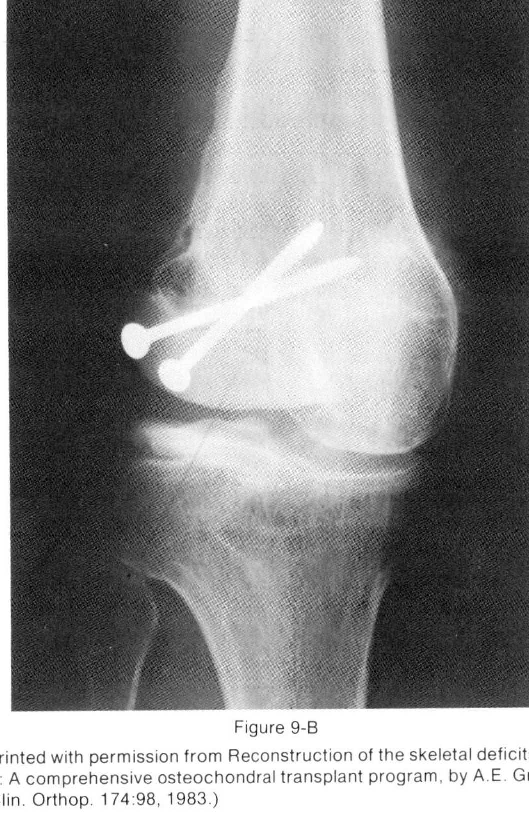

Figure 9-B

Figure 9: (A) Preoperative radiograph of a 17-year-old male with traumatic loss of lateral femoral condyle following an open fracture. (B) Postoperative radiograph 2½ years after allograft replacement of lateral femoral condyle. (Reprinted with permission from Reconstruction of the skeletal deficits at the knee: A comprehensive osteochondral transplant program, by A.E. Gross, et al., Clin. Orthop. 174:98, 1983.)

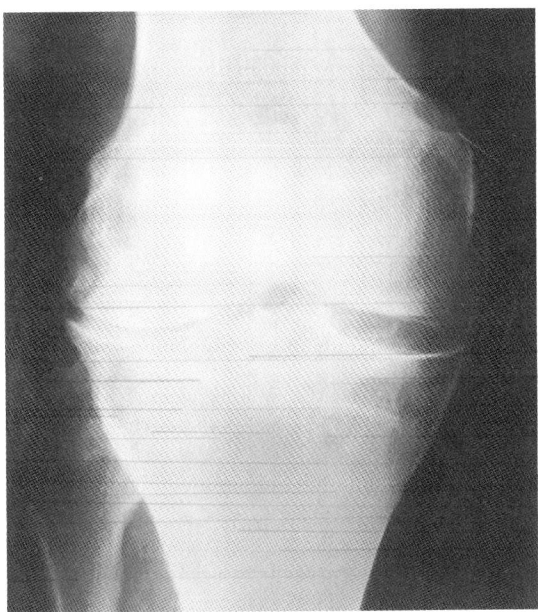

Figure 10-A

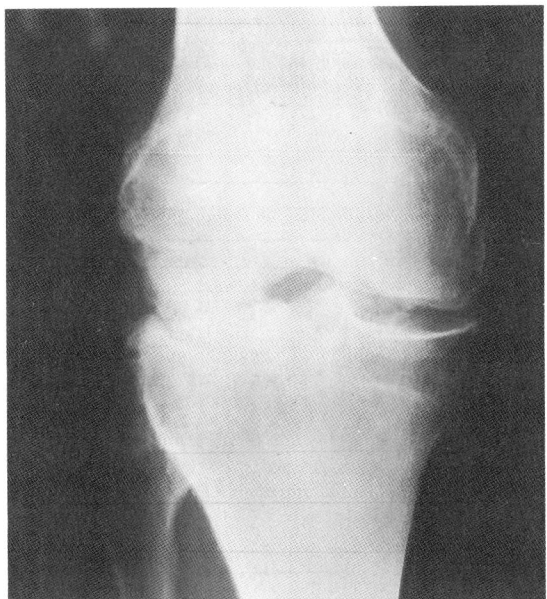

Figure 10-B

Figure 10: (A) Preoperative radiograph of a 52-year-old male with valgus deformity and severe osteoarthritis of lateral compartment. (B) Postoperative bipolar lateral compartment allograft at 40 months. The patient achieved a good clinical result. There has been loss of cartilage from both grafts but no bone compression or fragmentation thus allowing the knee to remain straight.

carried out as these factors had not been found to affect the clinical results.

One report of results with fresh small fragment osteochondral allografts in the treatment of femoral head osteonecrosis showed good results in all five patients with follow-up from 6 months to 2 years. These were vigorous patients under the age of 60.

In the young patient with severe unicompartmental osteoarthritis, osteotomy should be performed first, and if the patient is still symptomatic 1 year later, a bipolar osteochondral graft may be inserted into the decompressed compartment.

Recent advances in microvascular surgery have made it possible to reconstruct some bone deficits (after trauma or en bloc excision) with microvascularized fibulae providing live bone that heals like a fracture and requires no creeping substitution. For some large defects these microvascularized fibular autografts have been combined with allografts in an effort to reinforce the allograft.

ANNOTATED BIBLIOGRAPHY

General

Kelly, W.N.; Harris, E.D.; Ruddy, S.; and Sledge, C.B.: Textbook of Rheumatology. Philadelphia, W.B. Saunders, 1981.

This comprehensive text covers the data base of the field of rheumatology.

Normal Joint

Muir, H.: Proteoglycans: State of the art. Semin. Arthrit. Rheumat. (Supplement) 11:7-9, 1981.

Compressive stiffness of cartilage depends upon the content of hydrophilic proteoglycan macromolecules which are aggregated and therefore do not diffuse out when the collagen network is weakened. Enzymatic destruction of the aggregates allows proteoglycans to diffuse.

Radin, E.L.; Boyd, R.D.; Martin, R.B.; Goodwin, C.A.; and Brandt, K.D.: Relationship between bone and cartilage changes after impulsive loading. Orthop. Trans. 6:287, 1982.

The cartilage (^{35}S uptake) and subchondral bone (quantitative bone scanning) respond together to the effects of repetitive impulsive loads on joints in rabbits. This emphasizes the importance of the relationship between subchondral bone and cartilage in load bearing.

Osteoarthritis

Experimental

Altman, R.D.; Tenenbaum, J.; Pardo, V.; Blanco, L.N.; and Howell, D.S.: Morphological changes and swelling properties of osteoarthritic dog cartilage. Semin. Arthrit. Rheumat. (Supplement) 11:39-40, 1981.

In dogs with sectioned anterior cruciate ligaments, there is early disorganization of the perilacunar collagen allowing cartilage to swell due to imbibition of water by proteoglycans. Collagen breakdown could be mechanical or by collagenase and may be a factor in the pathogenesis of osteoarthritis.

Barrett, A.J.: Which proteinases degrade cartilage matrix? Semin. Arthrit. Rheumat. (Supplement) 11:52-56, 1981.

The glycosaminoglycan attachment region is vulnerable to proteolytic attack. The intramolecular cross-link which stabilizes collagen could be destroyed by a "cross-linkase," (i.e., elastase) thus weakening the collagen network and allowing cartilage to take up more water and swell.

Hulth, A.: Experimental osteoarthritis: A survey. Acta Orthop. Scand. 53:1-6, 1982.

Experimentally induced osteoarthritis (by immobilization, compression, partial resection, section of ligaments) results in hyperactivity of chondrocytes and increased matrix synthesis attempting repair prior to cartilage degradation. The definitive healing of cartilage comes from subchondral bone and marrow.

Radin, E.L.; Paul, I.L.; and Rose, R.M.: Current concepts of the etiology of idiopathic osteoarthrosis. Bull. Hosp. Joint Dis. 38:117-120, 1977.

An in vitro experiment in sheep demonstrated that cartilage wore out faster if the subchondral bone was stiffened by subchondral polymethyl methacrylate.

Human

Cooke, T.D.V.; Bennett, E.L.; and Ohno, O.: The deposition of immunoglobulins and complement in osteoarthritic cartilage. Internat. Orthop. 4:211-217, 1980.

In patients undergoing surgery for primary osteoarthritis, there was patchy deposition of immunoglobulins mainly IgA and complement in the cartilage of 60 percent of the patients, whereas in patients with secondary osteoarthritis the incidence was only 16 percent.

Howell, D.S., and Moskowitz, R.W.: Introduction: Symposium on osteoarthritis. A brief review of research and directions for future investigations. Arthrit. Rheumat. 20:96-103, 1977.

Osteoarthritis is caused by mechanical and biochemical factors. Abnormal forces cause microfractures leading to stiffness of subchondral bone. The resultant abnormal stress on the cartilage causes the chondrocytes to release enzymes which destroy the matrix. When attempts at repair (chondrocyte proliferation and production of proteoglycans) cannot keep up with destruction, osteoarthritis results.

Huskisson, E.C.; Dieppe, P.A.; Tucker, A.K.; and Cannell, L.B.: Another look at osteoarthritis. Ann. Rheumat. Dis. 38:423-428, 1979.

One hundred osteoarthritic patients have been compared with 100 rheumatoids. Based on the polyarticular distribution and evidence of inflammation, a metabolic abnormality of articular cartilage resulting in cartilage destruction, inflammation, and calcification is proposed as the etiology of osteoarthritis.

Pritzker, K.P.H.: Which comes first osteonecrosis or osteoarthritis? J. Rheumatol. 10:53-54, 1983.

The morphologic changes of osteoarthritis (cartilage edema, fissuring, chondrocyte proliferation) as well as the biosynthetic activity detected by $^{35}SO_4$ and ^{3}H-thymideine uptake are absent in osteonecrosis, and the cartilage above areas of osteonecrosis resembles resting cartilage. Focal superficial subchondral osteonecrosis is a common finding in advanced osteoarthritis but is different in pattern from that of primary osteonecrosis.

Pritzker, K.P.H.; Renlund, R.C.; and Cheng, P.T.: Synopsis: Which comes first crystals or osteoarthritis? A study of surgically removed femoral heads. J. Rheumatol. 10:38-39, 1983.

This study reviews 205 consecutive surgically removed femoral heads and found calcium pyrophosphate dihydrate (CPPD) crystals in cartilage in less than 2 percent (two of ninety-five) of specimens with osteoarthritis, whereas these crystals were found in 19 percent (sixteen of eighty-four) of femoral heads removed for fracture. Combined with the observation that the mean age of patients with CPPD crystal deposition was 18 years older than patients with morphologic changes of osteoarthritis, this indicates that CPPD arthropathy is a disease distinct from osteoarthritis and is associated with aging.

Solomon, L.: Patterns of osteoarthritis of the hip. J. Bone Joint Surg. 58B:176-183, 1976.

In a detailed study of 327 osteoarthritic patients, some predisposing abnormality was identified in 300. A classification was proposed: failure of normal cartilage due to abnormal loading, i.e., acetabular dysplasia; failure of damaged cartilage under normal loading, i.e., postinfection; and failure of normal cartilage under normal loading due to defective subchondral support, i.e., osteonecrosis.

Venn, M., and Maroudas, A.: Chemical composition and swelling of normal and osteoarthritic femoral head cartilage. Ann. Rheumat. Dis. 36:121-129 (Part I), 399-406 (Part II), 1977.

In osteoarthritis the damaged collagen network is no longer capable of opposing the swelling pressure of the proteoglycans, which are hydrophilic. Swelling could be induced in normal femoral heads by treating them with collagenase.

Rheumatoid Arthritis

Etiology

Person, D.A., and Sharp, J.T.: The etiology of rheumatoid arthritis. Bull. Rheumat. Dis. 27:888-893, 1977.

Immune mechanisms are deranged in this disease with the presence of immune complexes in synovial fluid and, at times, in serum. Cellular immune reactions also participate. The possibility that an infectious process may be an initiating event has been studied (bacteria, mycoplasmas, viruses). Research has failed to identify the causative organisms even though rheumatoid arthritis is suggested to be an infectious process by the clinical presentation and disease course.

Smith, C.A.: On a possible viral etiology of rheumatoid arthritis (Editorial). J. Rheumat. 6:113-115, 1979.

A possible viral etiology for rheumatoid arthritis deserves further investigation because the immunological findings are compatible and animal models of viral arthritis have been identified. Also there is evidence of specific lesions in mice born after injection of the pregnant mother with homogenized rheumatoid arthritis synovial membranes.

Wilkes, E., and Meek, E.S.: Rheumatoid arthritis: Review of searches for an infectious cause. Infection 7:125-128 (Part I), 192-197 (Part II), 1979.

A genetic predisposition is indicated. Immune complexes have been detected in the joint fluid in both seropositive and seronegative patients. There is still no evidence to confirm a bacterial or "slow virus" etiology. Mycoplasmas have been shown to cause arthritis in other species but thus far not in humans.

Treatment of Arthritis

Nonoperative

Gray, R.G.; Tenenbaum, J.; and Gottlieb, N.L.: Local corticosteroid injection treatment in rheumatic diseases. Semin. Arthrit. Rheumat. 10:231-254, 1981.

The occasional use of intra-articular steroids is useful in severe rheumatoid arthritis and osteoarthritis, but repeated injections at short intervals (weeks or months) may accelerate degeneration of articular cartilage, tendons, and ligaments as has been shown both experimentally and clinically.

Ilardi, C.F., and Sokoloff, L.: The pathology of osteoarthritis: Ten strategic questions for pharmacologic management. Sem. Arthrit. Rheumat. (Supplement) 11:3-7, 1981.

Future management of osteoarthritis will likely combine mechanical measures (i.e., continuous passive motion, realignment surgery) and biologic manipulation (i.e., stimulation of chondrocyte growth by somatomedin-like compounds, stimulation of glycosaminoglycan synthesis by compounds like Rumalon or substitute therapy with sulfated glycosaminoglycan analogues which competitively inhibit chondrolytic enzymes).

Salter, R.B.; Minster, R.R.; Clements, N.; Bell, R.S.; and Bogoch, E.R.: Continuous passive motion and the repair of full thickness articular cartilage defects: A one-year follow-up. Orthop. Trans. 6:266-267, 1982.

Continuous passive motion is more beneficial in the repair of full thickness articular cartilage defects in rabbits than regular cage activities or cast immobilization.

Surgery

Chandler, H.P.; Reineck, F.T.; Wixson, R.L.; and McCarthy, J.C.: Total hip replacement in patients younger than 30 years old: A five-year follow-up. J. Bone Joint Surg. 63A:1426-1434, 1981.

Twenty-nine patients with an average age of 23 years underwent total hip replacement and were followed up at 10 months and 5 years. At 10 months they scored well, but at 5 years over one-half had loosening of one component (acetabular loosening twice as frequently as femoral).

Fujisawa, Y.; Masuhara, K.; and Shiomi, S.: The effect of high tibial osteotomy on osteoarthritis of the knee. Orthop. Clin. North America 10:585-608, 1979.

Fifty-four knees were assessed by arthroscopic examination preoperatively and 4 months to 6 years postoperatively. When the osteotomy realigned the mechanical axis 30 to 40 percent lateral to the midpoint, repair of ulcerated areas by fibrous tissue or fibrocartilage occurred.

Hernborg, J.S., and Nilsson, B.E.: The natural course of untreated osteoarthritis of the knee. Clin. Orthop. 123:130-137, 1977.

Ninety-four osteoarthritic knee joints untreated surgically for 10 to 18 years became clinically worse with increasing varus deformity and instability. The prognosis was worse than in osteoarthritis of the hip.

Langlais, F.; Roure, J.L.; and Maquet, P.: Valgus osteotomy in severe osteoarthritis of the hip. J. Bone Joint Surg. 61B:424-431, 1979.

One hundred and fifty valgus osteotomies of the proximal femur performed for osteoarthritis were followed at 3 to 10 years. If joint congruity could be improved and the area of weight-bearing increased (particularly by using the cephalic medial osteophyte), good results were obtained in over 75 percent.

Scott, W.N.: Symposium on total knee arthroplasty (Foreword). Orthop. Clin. North America 13:1-249, 1981.

The surface replacement category, with the cruciate-retaining designs and the cruciate-sacrificing designs, now account of 85 percent of knee prostheses. The articulated (hinge) prostheses are applied in 15 percent only. Correct alignment is more important than in hip arthroplasty.

Biological Replacement: Experimental

Ashton, J.E., and Bentley, G.: Culture of articular chondrocytes as a method of storage: Assessment of maintenance of phenotype. J. Bone Joint Surg. 64B:384, 1982 (Abstract).

Banking of chondrocytes by freezing decreased their viability and capacity to repair when used as allografts. In vitro cultures of rabbit chondrocytes had a 70 percent survival at 6 weeks forming sheets of tissue and producing cartilage matrix. Similar techniques are being used for human articular cartilage grafts.

Bentley, G., and Greer, R.B., III: Homotransplantation of isolated epiphyseal and articular cartilage chondrocytes into joint surfaces of rabbits. Nature 230:385-388, 1971.

Isolated epiphyseal cells are superior to isolated articular cartilage cells when used as allografts to repair articular defects. At 8 weeks after transplantation, the defects were filled with cartilage indistinguishable from the surrounding cartilage.

DiNubile, N.A.; Jimenez, S.A.; Brighton, C.T.; Kaplan, F.; and Bashey, R.I.: Allotransplantation of preserved and fresh articular cartilage in an osteochondral plug model. Orthop. Trans. 4:203, 1980.

Osteochondral plug allografts were inserted fresh or after storage in tissue culture for 30 days in femoral condylar defects in rabbits. Histological and biochemical assessment at 6 and 12 months revealed the fresh grafts to be significantly better.

Green, W.T., Jr.: Articular cartilage repair: Behavior of rabbit chondrocytes during tissue culture and subsequent allografting. Clin. Orthop. 124:237-250, 1977.

Isolated chondrocytes when cultured, proliferated through many generations and produced a cartilage like matrix. Composite allografts of chondroid tissue in decalcified bone repaired large articular defects in 10 days.

Paccola, C.A.; Xavier, C.A.; and Goncalves, R.P: Fresh immature articular cartilage allografts: A study on the integration of chondral and osteochondral grafts both in normal and papain-treated knee joints of rabbits. Arch. Orthop. Trauma. Surg. 93:253-259, 1979.

Fresh immature chondral and osteochondral grafts were inserted into the knees of normal and arthritic (papain-induced) rabbits and studied macro- and microscopically and metabolically for 9 months. A significant percentage of the grafts achieved good results over 9 months, the best being the chondral grafts in the nonarthritic rabbits.

Rodrigo, J.J.; Thompson, E.; and Travis, C.: Frozen as compared to 4 degree preservation of avascular osteocartilaginous shell allografts in rats. Orthop. Trans. 4:201, 1980.

In a rat distal femur model, osteocartilaginous allografts preserved at 4 degrees centigrade for 12 to 24 hours after death showed live cartilage and dead or dying subchondral bone, with considerably lower antigenicity than the bone of fresh osteocartilaginous allografts.

Thomas, V.J.; Jimenez, S.A.; Brighton, C.T.; and Brown, N.: Sequential changes in the mechanical properties of in vitro stored articular cartilage. Transactions of the 28th Annual Orthop. Res. Soc. Meeting, p. 122, New Orleans, Louisiana, January 1982.

In vitro storage of articular cartilage in tissue culture media with additives (alpha-tocopherol, superoxide dismutase, and a mixture of protease inhibitors) improved chondrocyte viability and matrix preservation. This cartilage had superior mechanical properties, compared to cartilage stored in tissue culture media alone.

Tomford, W.W.; Fredericks, G.R.; and Mankin, H.J.: Cryopreservation of intact articular cartilage. Orthop. Trans. 6:269-270, 1982.

Chondrocyte viability of 50 percent was achieved by storage of intact bovine cartilage at minus 80 degrees centigrade with cryopreservative (DMSO) protection if the freezing rate was slowed to 3 hours between zero and -4 degrees centigrade.

Yablon, I.G., and Shirahama, T.: Acid hydrolase activity following allografting. Orthop. Trans. 6:244-245, 1982.

Fresh osteochondral allografts were inserted into the femoral condyles of dogs. The host synovium became hypercellular and invaded the allograft. Increased levels of acid phosphatase (an index of lysosomal activity) were found in host synovium.

Biological Replacement: Clinical

Engkvist, O., and Johansson, S.H.: Perichondrial arthroplasty: A clinical study in twenty-six patients. Scand. J. Plast. Reconstruct. Surg. 14:71-80, 1980.

Results of free autologous rib perichondrial autografts, mainly in the PIP and MP joints, were followed 3 to 41 months. Best results were in young rheumatoid patients. Twelve were for posttraumatic lesions, seven for osteoarthritic joints, five for rheumatoid joints, and two for congenital deformities. In bipolar joint surface transplants, an interposed silicone sheet was used. Thirteen patients were classified as excellent, three improved, and ten were not improved.

Gross, A.E.; McKee, N.H.; Pritzker, K.P.H.; and Langer, F.: Reconstruction of skeletal deficits at the knee. A comprehensive osteochondral transplant program. Clin. Orthop. 174:96-106, 1983.

From 1971 to 1982, 87 fresh, small fragment osteochondral grafts have been inserted for old plateau fractures (17 patients), osteonecrosis (26 patients), and osteoarthritis (37 patients) of the knee. Excellent results were obtained in young patients with old plateau fractures and traumatic loss of bone and cartilage. Biopsies have shown hyaline cartilage on the allografts as late as 8 years after transplantation.

Meyers, M.H.: The treatment of osteonecrosis of the hip with fresh osteochondral allografts and with the muscle pedicle graft technique. Clin. Orthop. 130:202-209, 1978.

Five vigorous young patients with osteonecrosis of the femoral head had partial replacement of the femoral head with fresh osteochondral allografts. Follow-up was from 6 months to 2 years with good clinical results in all five.

Salenius, P.; Holmström, T.; Koskinen, E.V.S.; and Alho, A.: Histological changes in clinical half joint allograft replacements. Acta Orthop. Scand. 53:295-299, 1982.

Biopsies of cartilage and bone were taken 10 weeks to 8 years after allotransplantation of nine deep frozen large osteochondral grafts inserted after en bloc excision of bone tumors around the knee. Rejection was not apparent. By 12 months substitution of live bone was well advanced subchondrally. Fibrocartilage was seen on the surface of the grafts at 12 months and chondrocytes at 18 months and some islands of hyaline cartilage at 7 years.

5 MUSCULOSKELETAL NEOPLASMS

The more commonly encountered primary tumors, metastatic carcinomas, and soft-tissue tumors are discussed. Recent advances in diagnosis and treatment are emphasized.

Primary Tumors

Osteosarcoma Except for myeloma, osteosarcoma is the most common primary sarcoma of bone. It accounts for 20 percent of all sarcomas. This tumor strikes children and usually occurs in the metaphyses of long bones, especially about the knee.

PATIENT EVALUATION: Diagnostic tests used are routine radiographs and laboratory studies, including calcium, phosphorus, and alkaline phosphatase determinations. It is believed that the osteoblastic form is more malignant than either the chondroblastic or fibroblastic types. Newer localizing studies that may be helpful include bone scans with technetium or gallium. Computed tomography has helped with bone localization and has aided in delineating soft tissue extension and in detecting pulmonary metastases at early stages.

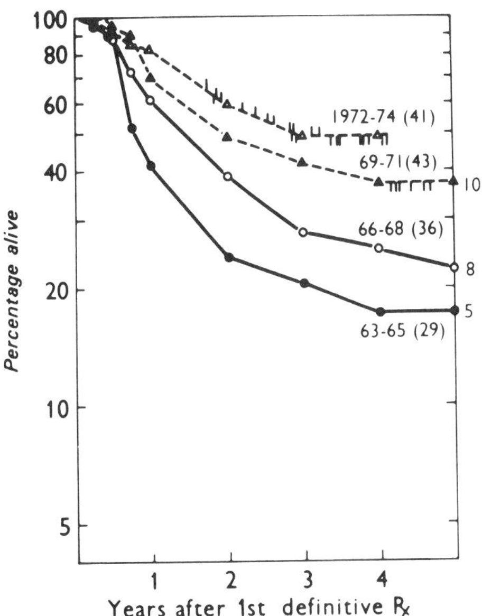

Figure 1: Actuarial estimates of percentages of patients still alive during first 5 years after initial definitive treatment for osteogenic sarcoma. Vertical marks along curves indicate time at which patient last known to be alive and withdrawn from survival analysis. Numbers along right margin indicate patients surviving at least 5 years, after which short time no deaths or metastases were observed. Total sample sizes in parentheses. (Reprinted with permission from Osteogenic sarcoma experience at the Mayo Clinic, 1963-1974, by Taylor, et al., Cancer Res. Ther. 6:257, 1978.)

A carefully selected *open biopsy* performed by a surgeon experienced in tumor surgery remains the principal means of obtaining a definitive tissue diagnosis. Parosteal osteosarcoma, located on the surface of long bone metaphyses, has an excellent survival rate and is an ideal tumor for a limb salvage procedure without need for adjunctive chemotherapy. Periosteal osteosarcoma also arises from the surface of bone but is chondrogenic and is considered more aggressive than the parosteal tumor but less so than the classic osteosarcoma. Telangiectatic osteosarcoma is the most malignant of all bone-forming tumors, and even with chemotherapy, patients with this unusual form rarely survive 5 years.

PROGNOSIS: Most historical studies of prognosis have cited a 20 to 25 percent 5-year survival rate for patients with osteosarcoma. A recent study indicates a 50 percent survival rate with amputation alone (Fig. 1) which suggests either a change in basic biology of the tumor or in host response to its growth. This creates controversy about evaluation studies of adjunctive chemotherapy so commonly used with surgical treatment. During the last decade, many complex chemotherapy programs have claimed survival rates varying from 50 to 93 percent. These studies, however, frequently did not include 5-year, disease-free figures. Only one important study has included randomized controls, and that study suggests that adjunctive chemotherapy has no significant effect upon the prognosis of osteosarcoma patients.

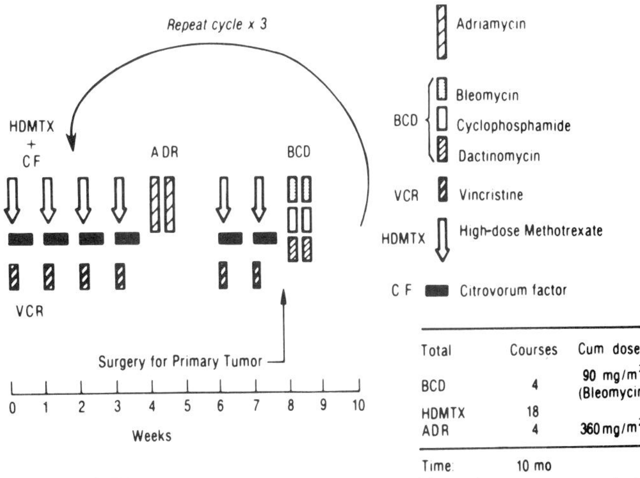

Total	Courses	Cum dose
BCD	4	90 mg/m² (Bleomycin)
HDMTX	18	
ADR	4	360 mg/m²
Time	10 mo	

Figure 2: T-7 preoperative chemotherapy protocol for osteosarcoma used at Memorial Sloan-Kettering Cancer Center, New York. (Reprinted with permission from Primary osteogenic sarcoma: The rationale for preoperative chemotherapy and delayed surgery, by G. Rosen, et al., Cancer 43:2163, 1979.)

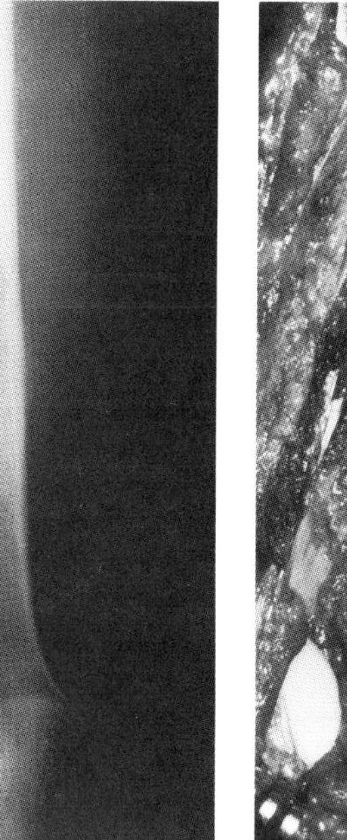

Figure 3-A

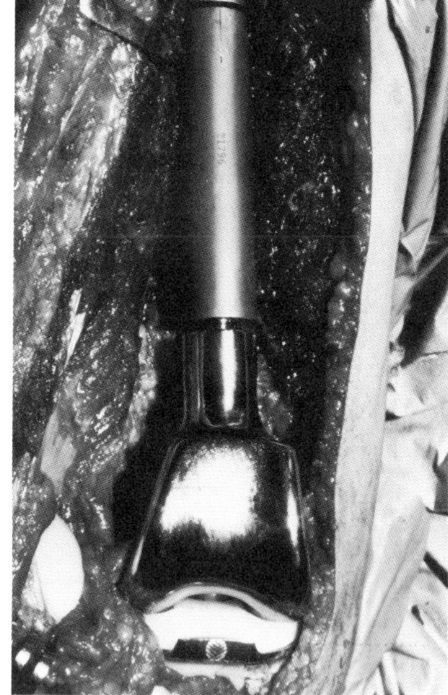

Figure 3-B

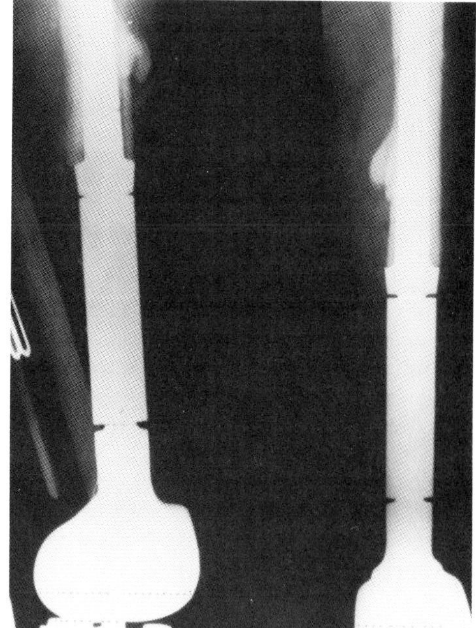

Figure 3-C

Figure 3: (A) Anteroposterior radiograph of osteosarcoma in distal femur of 20-year-old female patient. (B) Surgical photograph of a modular tumor resection endostem knee joint prosthesis inserted at surgical resection. (C) Postoperative radiograph.

TREATMENT: A recent study shows that approximately 70 percent of patients with sarcoma of any type have tumor cells circulating in their peripheral bloodstreams at the time of diagnosis. This suggests the presence of micrometastases throughout the body before treatment of the primary tumor is begun, an assumption upon which the rationale for chemotherapy is based.

The various *multidrug programs* characteristically include high-dosage methotrexate with citrovorum factor and Adriamycin. Bleomycin, cyclophosphamide, dactinomycin, and, more recently, cisplatin are also being used. The most encouraging recent protocol is the T-7 program (Fig. 2), which involves weekly pulses of chemotherapy for 2 months preoperatively and histologic observation of the effect on tumor death during surgery. Postoperatively, the program can be adjusted by stronger dosage or the addition of more toxic drugs such as cisplatin, which is used in the recently published T-10 program.

Immunotherapy may be a form of adjunctive therapy for osteosarcoma in the future. Investigators are currently searching for some form of vaccine that will stimulate the immune system to resist tumors, similar to the successful techniques employed in controlling bacterial and viral diseases. However, treatment attempts with tumor cell vaccines, BCG bacterial antigen, transfer factor, and human interferon have not as yet shown much promise and still must be considered experimental.

Surgical treatment is the mainstay in the management of osteosarcoma. Most authorities still recommend cross-bone amputation at about 7 to 8 cm proximal to the upper pole of the tumor. The surgeon must be aware of the rare occurrence of a skip metastasis high in the femur when considering a high thigh amputation. Technetium bone scans may help detect such lesions better than standard radiographs.

During the last ten years, a more aggressive approach has been taken toward treatment of *pulmonary metastases.* These lesions, which can be detected early using CT lung scans, are usually near the surface of the lung, allowing easy surgical resection. Many patients require multiple thoracotomies, which have improved survival times considerably. The longer a patient goes without a pulmonary metastasis, the better the prognosis.

Limb salvage procedures offer an attractive alternative to amputation. All these procedures include aggressive en bloc (or wide) local resection of the tumor which in most patients requires removal of the adjacent joint. With osteosarcoma for which adjunctive chemotherapy is used, the complication rate from infections and delayed bone healing is high.

There is a great deal of interest in the use of *custom prostheses* after tumor resection surgery. Figure 3 illustrates a lytic form of osteosarcoma in the distal femur of a 20-year-old female patient. This stage II-A (high-grade, intraosseous) lesion was resected by wide, local technique including a cuff of normal muscle and the entire knee joint. The defect was filled with a specially designed modular tumor resection knee joint prosthesis (availability subject to Food and Drug Administration regulations and patient specific prescription). Such a prosthesis can be adapted to any length of femoral or tibial resection at the operating table without the complexity of ordering a custom implant for a specific tumor patient. These new prosthetic implants must be considered experimental with limited long-term durability. Fatigue fractures through the intramedullary stems or repeated stem loosening, especially in young patients, are major concerns.

Ewing's Sarcoma Approximately 5 percent of primary bone sarcomas are Ewing's sarcoma, which mainly affects the pelvis and femur in children. The radiographic findings are nonspecific and may suggest osteomyelitis. Even the clinical evaluation may suggest infection since there can be low-grade fever, an elevated erythrocyte sedimentation rate, and anemia. During biopsy, purulent-appearing material may suggest a bone abscess. Thus, it is always advisable to send biopsy material to both pathology and bacteriology laboratories. Often, a touch preparation in the operating room can aid greatly in making an immediate diagnosis.

TREATMENT: As are most round cell lesions, Ewing's sarcoma is quite radiosensitive. For many years, 4,000 to 6,000 rads of irradiation without amputation was the suggested treatment for this tumor. Local control was achieved in 88 percent of patients, but only 5 to 10 percent survived. With the advent of multidrug chemotherapy combined with irradiation therapy and local surgery, the 5-year survival figures have reached about 50 percent. Because of this increased rate of long-term survival, a new group of late *complications* has arisen, including pathologic fracture through the irradiated bone. Figure 4 represents a typical lesion of the femur treated by combined irradiation and chemotherapy. After 4½ years, a pathologic fracture that progressed to nonunion occurred through the area of previous biopsy. This complication can result in amputation or, as in this patient, placement of a total femur into the thigh area.

Another complication arising because of long-term survival is a growing incidence of secondary irradiation sarcomas, such as osteosarcoma, which usually lead to amputation. In younger children, problems have resulted from growth plate irradiation damage and joint flexion contractures, so that severe discrepancies in leg length have occurred. For these reasons amputation followed by a multidrug program including such agents as cyclophosphamide, vincristine, dactinomycin, Methotrexate, and Adriamycin is recommended for lesions about or below the knee in children. Amputation rarely is indicated for upper extremity lesions.

Limb salvage may be considered in upper extremity lesions in older children or young adults. If the tumor tissue is not violated surgically, local irradiation is not needed. Postoperative chemotherapy is considered essential.

With large pelvic lesions, complete surgical resection is difficult because of adjacent vital structures. Therefore, consideration is urged of either preoperative chemotherapy to shrink the tumor before attempting removal or a debulking procedure when necessary, followed by combined local irradiation and continued chemotherapy.

Chondrosarcoma Representing 10 percent of primary bone tumors, chondrosarcomas typically occur in the trunk and limb girdles of young and middle-aged adults. A common example is a slow-growing tumor associated with minimal pain and a low incidence of pulmonary metastasis. The majority of these low-grade lesions have a good prognosis for survival if properly treated. High-grade chondrosarcomas are rare, rapidly growing tumors which present a myxomatous appearance grossly. These more aggressive sarcomas usually do not calcify. They metastasize early and are associated with a poor prognosis.

Low-grade chondrosarcomas will occasionally differentiate into high-grade sarcomas, such as malignant fibrous histiocytomas. This condition is associated with rapid growth and early metastasis with a resultant poor prognosis.

early bad sign

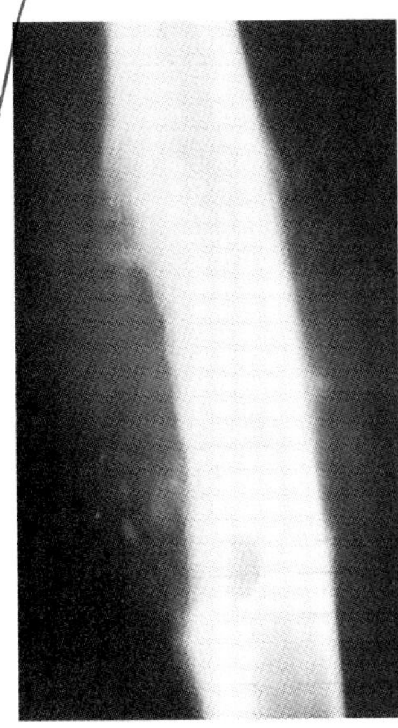

Figure 4-A

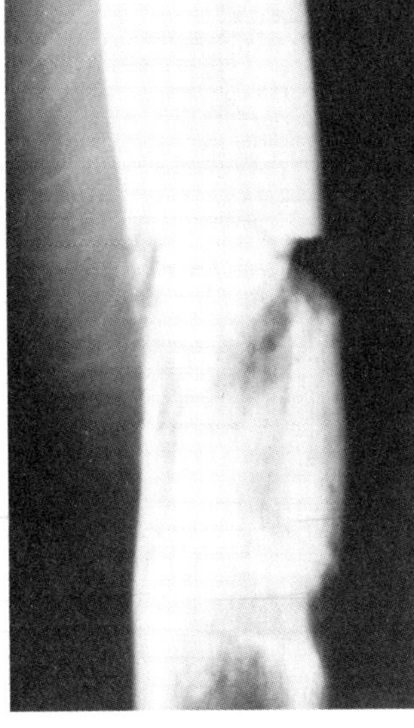

Figure 4-B

Figure 4: (A) Lateral radiograph of typical Ewing's sarcoma of femur in teenaged boy. (B) Anteroposterior radiograph 5 years later of pathologic fracture induced by irradiation therapy and biopsy stress riser.

TREATMENT: Chondrosarcomas are uniquely resistant to all forms of adjuvant therapy and, therefore, require wide local resection including a safe margin of surrounding normal tissue in most patients. Great care must be taken not to spill tumor cells into the surrounding tissue since this tumor may recur locally 20 years after resection.

Because of the low-grade nature of most chondrosarcomas, *limb salvage* procedures are well-suited to their management. Since no adjunctive chemotherapy or irradiation therapy follows limb salvage, the surgeon can rely more heavily on basic bone grafting such as excisional arthrodesis or allograft procedures using frozen cadaver bone. Imaginative combinations of allografts and synthetic implants such as long-stemmed endoprostheses can also be considered. Figure 5 shows a central primary low-grade chondrosarcoma arising from the supra-acetabular area of a 55-year-old woman. In the past, most surgeons would have elected a formidable hemipelvectomy procedure for this patient. A newer technique, the internal hemipelvectomy, is an optional limb-saving procedure that can provide adequately wide local resection of the entire tumor without cellular spillage. Replacement of the surgical defect with a pelvic allograft combined with a standard total hip prosthesis follows internal hemipelvectomy. These combined procedures are ideal for older patients because of the less complicated and more rapid postoperative rehabilitation programs associated with total joint replacement. For younger patients, particularly males, the more complex excisional arthrodesis procedures around the hip and knee might be best for the anticipated long, heavy use.

With a midshaft lesion, a viable alternative to amputation is wide-margin segmental resection of the tumor. This may be reconstructed utilizing either free fibular autogenous grafts or a deep frozen allograft supplemented with internal fixation. A more technically demanding procedure is the utilization of microsurgical techniques to insert a free fibular vascularized autograft into the surgical defect. This procedure may allow healing of a living graft

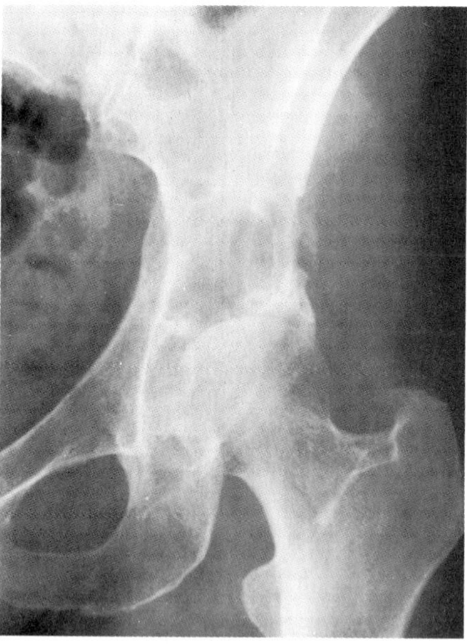

Figure 5-A

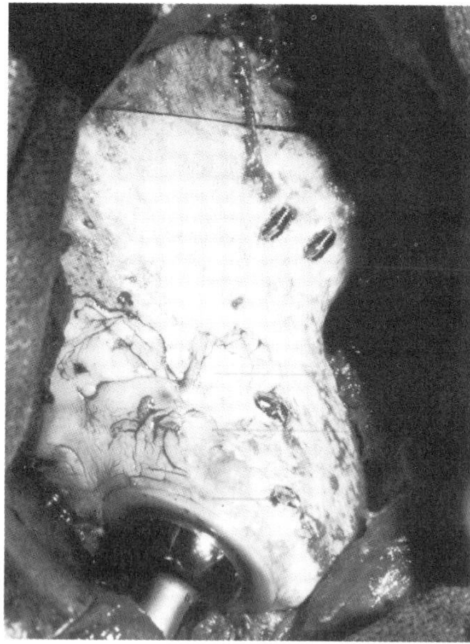

Figure 5-B

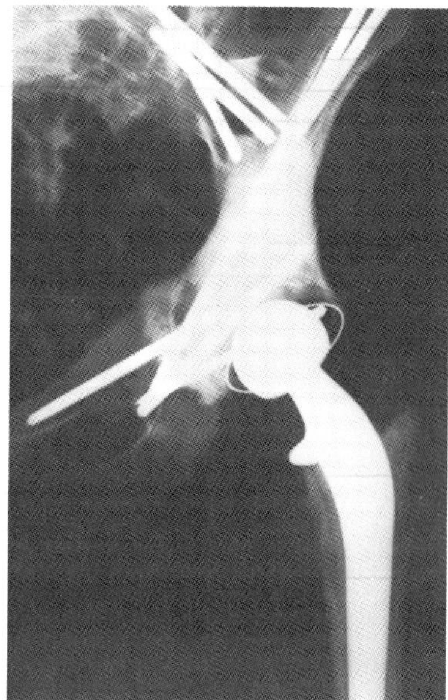

Figure 5-C

Figure 5: (A) Anteroposterior radiograph of primary chondrosarcoma in supra-acetabular area of 55-year-old female patient. (B) Surgical photography of combined pelvic allograft and total hip system after limb salvage internal hemipelvectomy. (C) Postoperative anteroposterior radiograph.

with greater potential for hypertrophy and perhaps less chance for delayed fatigue fracture, a frequent complication following nonviable allograft. Also, clinical trials with porous segmental metal implants are now in progress.

Giant Cell Tumor These tumors are usually benign lesions located in the epiphyseal-metaphyseal area of long bones in young adults and account for 20 percent of primary benign bone tumors. Approximately one-half occur about the knee joint. Care must be taken to distinguish the true giant cell tumor from the giant cell variants, including aneurysmal bone cyst, chondroblastoma, and osteoblastoma, which are usually pediatric lesions. In particular, the telangiectatic form of osteosarcoma must be differentiated because the many giant cells seen in this highly malignant sarcoma have an aneurysmal presentation. Giant cell tumors containing large numbers of giant cells have a better prognosis.

Treatment: As with chondrosarcomas, giant cell tumors do not respond well to adjunctive chemotherapy or irradiation therapy. The surgeon's responsibility is to remove the tumor completely and to preserve the best possible function. In the past, simple curettement resulted in an unacceptably high recurrence rate; now most surgeons use aggressive curettement followed by autogenous bone grafting as an initial approach. This yields a *local*

Figure 6: (A, B) Anteroposterior and lateral radiographs of typical benign giant cell tumor in distal femur. (C) Anteroposterior radiograph 9 years after aggressive curettement and packing with polymethyl methacrylate (PMMA).

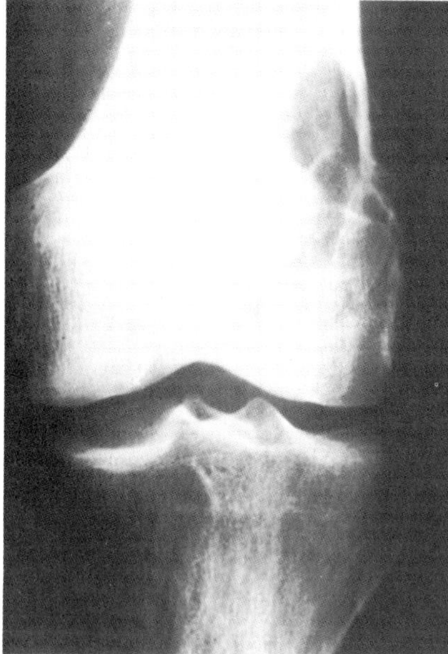

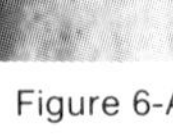

Figure 6-A

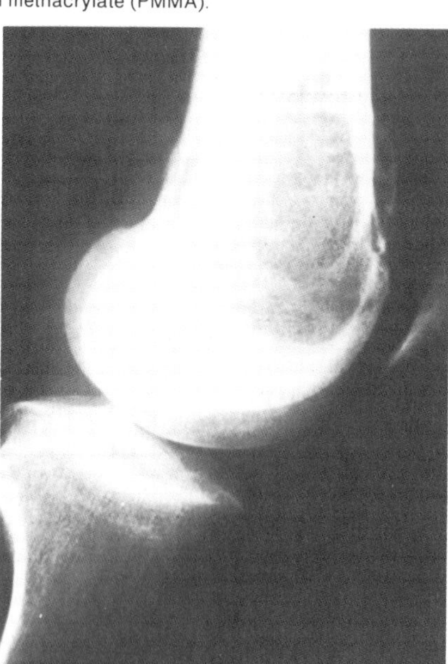

Figure 6-B

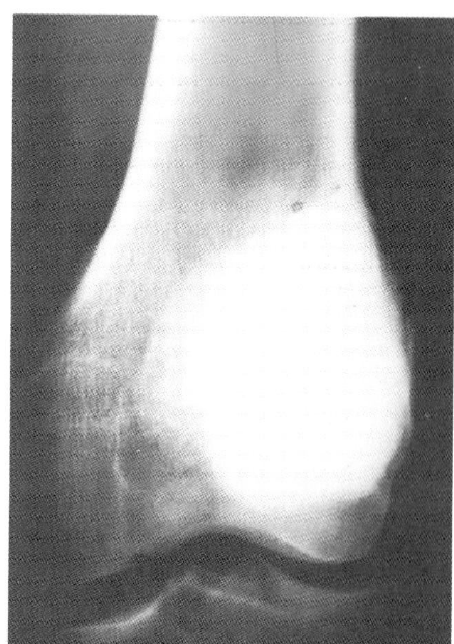

Figure 6-C

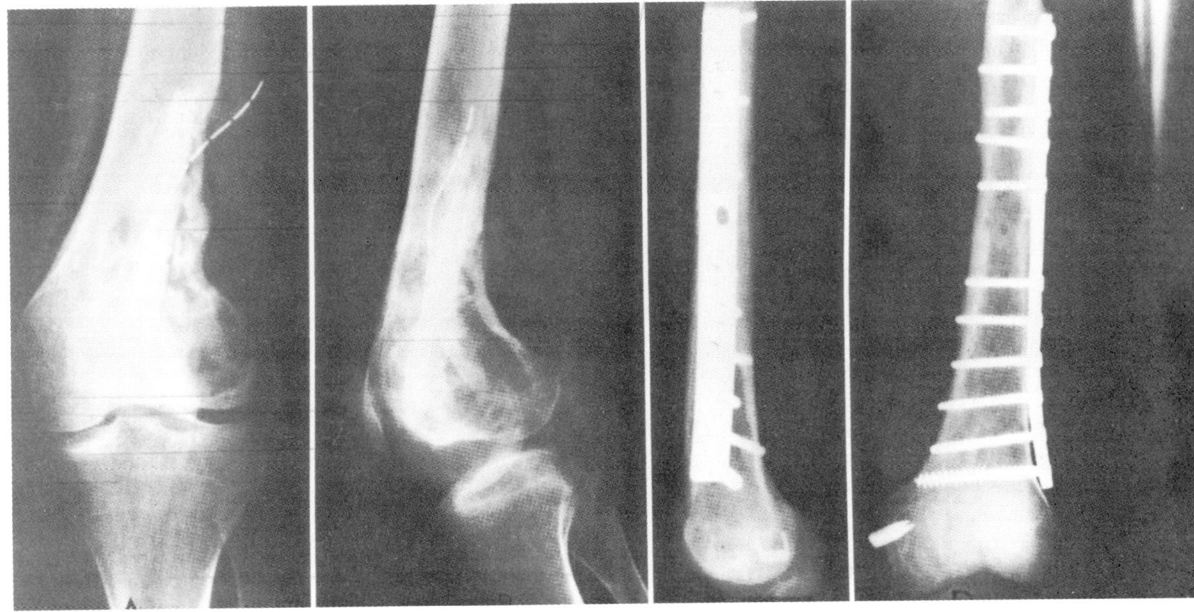

Figure 7-A Figure 7-B Figure 7-C Figure 7-D

Figure 7: (A, B) Anteroposterior and lateral radiographs in a 17-year-old patient 2 years after initial treatment and recurrence of giant cell tumor in distal femur just prior to allograft surgery in which distal femur with surrounding muscles and fascia was excised and replaced with allograft transplant. (C, D) Lateral and anteroposterior radiographs 5 years postoperatively showing good healing at anastomosis site and excellent preservation of joint space. (Reprinted with permission from Osteoarticular and intercalary allograft transplantation in the management of malignant tumors of bone, by H.J. Mankin, et al., Cancer 50:617, 1982.)

recurrence rate of about 50 percent in 5 years. Others have attempted to reduce this rate by using local phenol or liquid nitrogen following curettement to reduce the number of tumor cells remaining in the surgical site. Recurrence following this approach generally requires more aggressive wide local resection of the entire lesion and often involves partial resection of the adjacent joint. A still experimental approach to this initial surgical management consists of aggressive local curettement, followed by packing of the cavity with polymethyl methacrylate (PMMA). Figure 6 shows a typical giant cell tumor in the distal femur treated by this method which at 9 years follow-up had not recurred. The present recurrence rate using this technique is approximately 10 percent, which seems quite encouraging.

For recurrent cases or for larger lesions with extensive bone or joint involvement, more aggressive resection is required. As with chondrosarcomas, an excisional arthrodesis of the involved joint or perhaps an allograft replacement may be required (Fig. 7). Prosthetic implants can be used in young patients having a good prognosis for survival. However, the patient must be warned about the late complications of stem failure and PMMA loosening. The use of irradiation therapy for giant cell tumors is still controversial because a large percentage of malignant giant cell tumors have been induced by irradiation used to treat a preexisting benign lesion. But, in giant cell tumors of the sacrum or vertebrae where total surgical excision is technically difficult, irradiation therapy combined with an intralesional debulking procedure may be justified. New surgical techniques are being developed utilizing combined anteroposterior approaches for complete removal of a vertebral segment affected by a giant cell tumor.

Unicameral Bone Cyst Prior to 1974, this benign process in growing children was managed by a multitude of bone grafting procedures, yielding varying results dependent upon the size of the lesion, the age of the patient, and the aggressiveness of treatment. The recurrence rate ranged between 10 and 40 percent, varying with the magnitude of the operation.

During the past 8 years a simple nonoperative technique for the treatment of bone cysts in children has been described. Two large gauge needles are placed percutaneously into a cyst. Fluid is withdrawn from one needle as air enters the second needle. The air vent needle is then removed, and 80 to 200 mg of methylprednisolone acetate

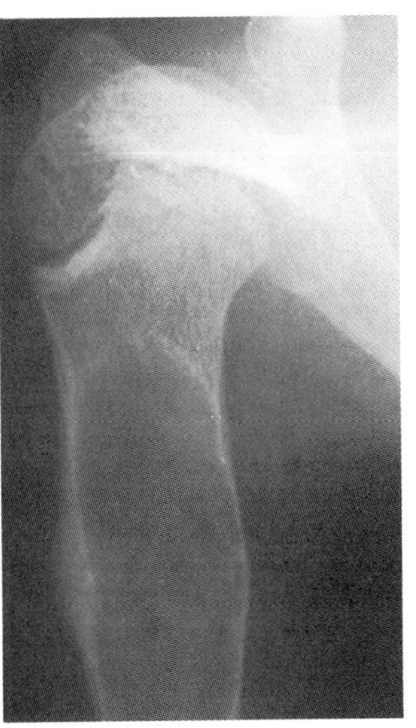

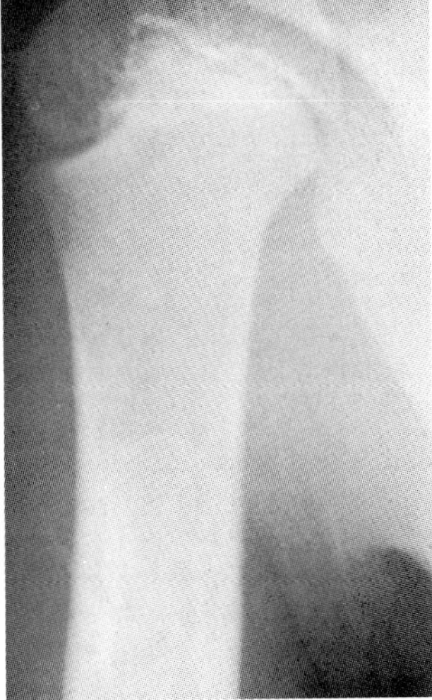

Figure 8-A Figure 8-B

Figure 8: (A) Anteroposterior radiograph of typical monoloculated solitary bone cyst in upper humerus of 8-year-old boy. (B) Anteroposterior radiograph more than 1 year after successful series of methylprednisolone acetate injections into cyst.

Figure 9-A

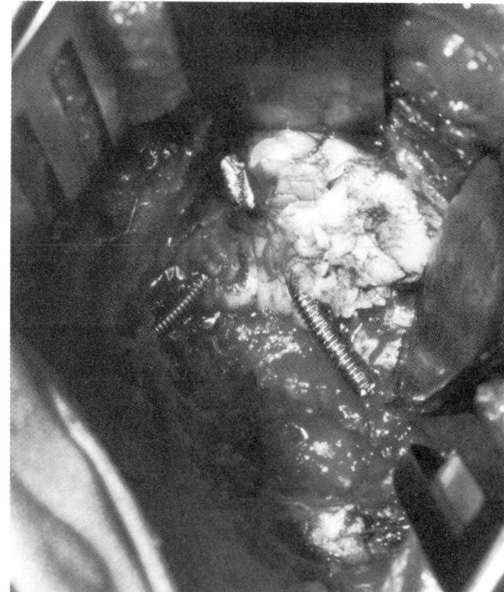

Figure 9-B

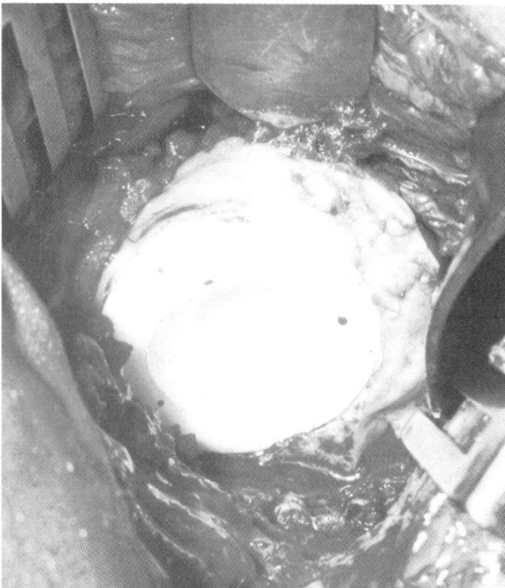

Figure 9-C

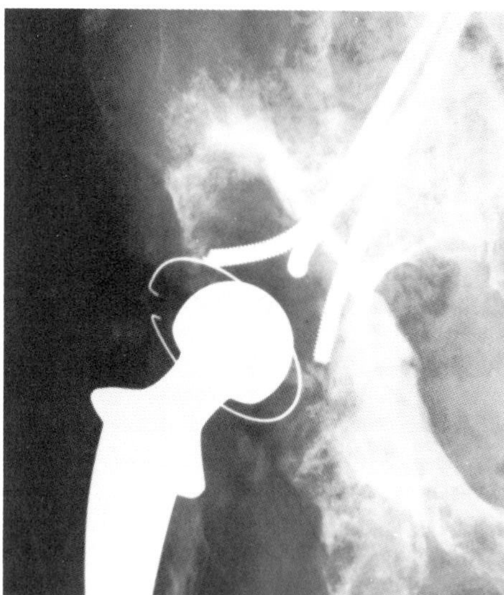

Figure 9-D

Figure 9: (A) Anteroposterior radiograph of elderly female patient with extensive lytic destruction of nearly the entire right half of pelvis secondary to metastatic breast cancer. (B) Surgical photograph after placement of three large Steinmann pins and PMMA up into solid bone at S1 joint level. (C) Surgical photograph of cup secured into position, with second batch of PMMA interphased over exposed bent foundation pins. (D) Anteroposterior radiograph more than 5 years postoperatively and after irradiation therapy.

is injected through the remaining needle. The injections are repeated every 2 months until the cyst is healed. The maximum number of injections needed to provide a satisfactory result is seven, with an average number of two to three. Good results were obtained in 80 percent of patients with minimal complications. The poorest results were in large multiloculated cysts and in children under 5 years of age. Figure 8 shows a typical monoloculated cyst in an 8-year-old child treated with two methylprednisolone acetate injections, following which the cyst healed completely.

Metastatic Carcinoma to Bone

Metastatic carcinoma to bone associated with pathologic fracture is a common problem. Nearly one-half of these lesions result from breast cancer, followed by cancer of the lung, prostate, kidney, thyroid, and other forms. The most common sites for pathologic fracture are the spine, humerus, and femur.

Micrometastases are very common in most high-grade tumors. The development of a clinical metastatic tumor apparently requires the production of tumor angiogenic factor, which attracts local vessel growth around the tumor to supply nutrients for its growth. In addition, recent studies suggest that metastatic carcinomas can produce prostaglandins that are responsible for osteolysis. Also, myeloma metastases can stimulate osteoclastic activity. Theoretically, prostaglandin inhibitors and diphosphonates might help prevent osteolysis in these situations.

Treatment: Hormonal therapy is the main form of treatment for breast and prostate cancer. Chemotherapy can be used for other carcinomas except thyroid and kidney, which do not respond well to chemotherapy.

Irradiation therapy is used to treat metastatic tumors either prophylactically or therapeutically starting 2 weeks after surgical treatment of a pathologic fracture. Irradiation is not indicated for asymptomatic lesions. Local control of the metastasis is quite successful, and the incidence of nonunion of pathologic fractures may be reduced by concentrating 2,200 rads in 4 days or a more conventional management program of 300 rads per day for 10 days.

If 50 percent of the cortical strength of a long bone is destroyed or if a lesion in long bone has a greater diameter than 2.5 cm, prophylactic nailing of the bone to prevent fracture is advisable. If a patient who has received irradiation therapy has pain on weight-bearing persisting beyond 1 month intramedullary fixation is indicated.

Surgical management of pathologic fractures about the hip requires various forms of internal fixation using adjunctive PMMA. For femoral neck fractures some surgeons prefer total hip systems to hemiarthroplasties because of the high incidence of occult acetabular lesions. For intertrochanteric lesions many surgeons still use telescoping hip nails with PMMA; but, long-stem total hip systems are also employed. For subtrochanteric fractures, the Zickel nail with PMMA or a long-stem total hip replacement is usually adequate. For femoral shaft lesions, strong intramedullary nails with PMMA work well. It is best to open the fracture site and debulk the tumor and necrotic bone before placing the nail and PMMA. Side plates for the femur are risky because of late fatigue fracture through the screwholes if the patient survives beyond 1 year.

With most metastases to the pelvis (including the acetabulum), irradiation therapy alone usually controls pain and allows continued ambulation. When pain persists or a pathologic fracture associated with severe bone deficiency occurs in the acetabular area, surgical reconstruction becomes a consideration. If justified on the basis of anticipated longevity, special steps can be taken to improve fixation (Fig. 9).

Metastases in the thoracic spine associated with cord compression now can be treated surgically. This condition can be approached anteriorly or posteriorly, utilizing PMMA and rods, depending upon the anatomic location and surgeon experience and preference. Prognosis is good for return of neurologic function if cord structure has remained partially intact, the rectal sphincter muscle is intact, and incomplete paraplegia has been gradual in onset. The poorest prognosis is associated with high thoracic lesions.

Paget's Disease

See Section 3, General: Bone Metabolism.

Soft-Tissue Sarcoma

Before launching a therapeutic program for a soft-tissue sarcoma, a careful diagnostic evaluation and staging process must occur. This evaluation usually involves an incisional biopsy (longitudinal incision), preferably by the surgeon who will perform the definitive resection. This biopsy material determines the biologic behavior of the tumor as either a low-grade lesion (stage I) or a high-grade lesion (stage II). If distant metastases are found in the lymph nodes or lung, the patient is considered to be in stage III. Next, the local anatomic extent of the tumor in relation to its fascial compartments is determined. If confined to one compartment, the tumor is stage A; if it violates a major fascial plane, it is stage B. Newer CT scanners are ideal for evaluating stage. Arteriograms may be required in certain patients, and isotope bone scans also may be helpful.

Following completion of this careful staging procedure, the tumor must be removed. For a low-grade intracompartmental (stage I-A) tumor, most authorities agree that wide local resection (as demonstrated by the dotted line in Fig. 10) is adequate. With a high-grade intracompartmental lesion (stage II-A), a more radical resection (as suggested by the dark line in Fig. 10) may be required to avoid local recurrence after surgery. Local control may be achieved in over 90 percent of patients with this approach. However, there is a pulmonary metastasis rate of between 40 and 50 percent regardless of the extent of the local surgery.

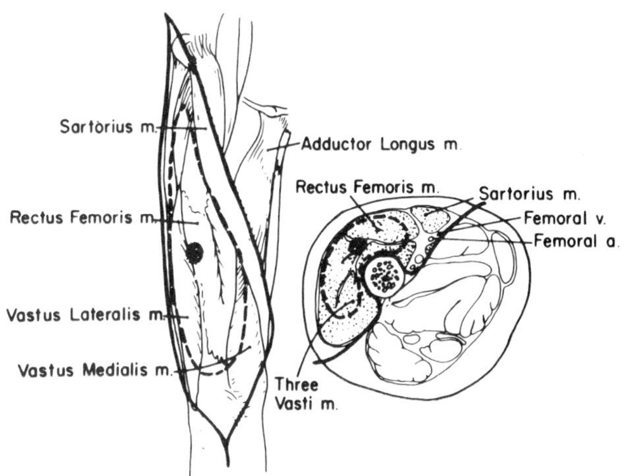

Figure 10: Longitudinal and transverse diagram of anterior compartment of thigh. Theoretical mass appears in midportion of vastus intermedius muscle. Dotted line indicates plane of dissection to achieve wide excision; solid line indicates radical resection. (Reprinted with permission from The effect of the anatomic setting on the results of surgical procedures for soft parts sarcoma of the thigh, by W.F. Enneking, et al., Cancer 47:1012, 1981.)

Another approach is adjunctive irradiation therapy after a more conservative wide local resection, leaving the patient with a more functional limb and still maintaining a 90 percent local control rate. The pulmonary metastasis problem is the same as with surgery alone.

Most stage III lesions in the lung should be resected aggressively and may require postthoracotomy chemotherapy.

ANNOTATED BIBLIOGRAPHY

Primary Bone Tumors

General

Fen, G., and Bufan, D.: Vascularized free fibula graft in bone tumors. Report of three cases. Chin. Med. J. (Engl.) 93:745-752, 1980.

The Chinese were among the first to adapt microvascular techniques to the management of neoplastic limb salvage procedures. This article outlines their technique in the management of three patients.

Kaiser, T.E.; Pritchard, D.J.; and Ritts, R.E., Jr.: The detection of tritiated thymidine labeled cells in the peripheral blood of sarcoma patients. Transactions of the 27th Annual Orthop. Res. Soc. Meeting, 6:127 [Abstract], Las Vegas, Nevada, February 24-26, 1981. Hyattsville, Maryland, Orthopaedic Research Society, 1981.

A study of the peripheral blood of sarcoma patients revealed 69 percent to have tumor cells. Those sarcoma patients with negative cell counts had no progression of their disease during the study period and 7 of 10 patients with circulating tumor cells who received chemotherapy had a decrease in cell count.

Mankin, H.J.; Doppelt, S.H.; Sullivan, T.R.; and Tomford, W.W.: Osteoarticular and intercalary allograft transplantation in the management of malignant tumors of bone. Cancer 50:613-630, 1982.

This is a review of 61 patients treated at Massachusetts General Hospital by limb salvage procedures involving the use of massive allografts, most of which included joint surfaces. The overall failure rate was 16.5 percent with a mean follow-up of 4½ years.

Mirra, J.M.; Gold, R.H.; and Marcove, R.C.: Bone Tumors. Diagnosis and Treatment. Philadelphia, J.B. Lippincott, 1980.

This textbook on bone tumors is clinically oriented toward the treating orthopaedic surgeon.

National Cancer Institute: Sarcomas of Soft Tissue and Bone in Childhood. *In* Proceedings of symposium held in Orlando, Florida, January 25-27, 1979. Washington, D.C., Government Printing Office, U.S. Dept. of Health and Human Services (NIH) Publication No. 81-2161 (National Cancer Institute Monograph No. 56), 1981.

This collection of papers presented at a 1979 symposium on sarcomas of soft tissue and bone in children includes the intergroup study reports on round cell tumors and osteosarcomas in children.

Pritchard, D.J.: Benign and Malignant Tumors of Bone. *In* Clinical Medicine, edited by J.A. Spittell, Jr., 4:1-19, New York, Harper & Row, 1981.

This review of the Mayo Clinic experience with benign and malignant tumors of bone includes the latest technique for diagnosis and management.

Schajowicz, F.: Tumors and Tumor-Like Lesions of Bone and Joints. New York, Springer-Verlag, 1981.

This text addresses tumor diagnosis from radiographic, gross, and microscopic materials.

Osteosarcoma

Eilber, F.R.: Adjuvant treatment of osteosarcoma. Surg. Clin. North America 61:1371-1378, 1981.

A review article on adjuvant chemotherapy and immunotherapy for osteosarcoma, includes surgical management of pulmonary metastases.

Goorin, A.M.; Frei, E., III; and Abelson, H.T.: Adjuvant chemotherapy for osteosarcoma: A decade of experience. Surg. Clin. North America 61:1379-1389, 1981.

This overview of the controversial subject of chemotherapy for osteosarcoma compares the experience of the Sidney Farber group with other groups in the United States during the past 10 years.

Rosen, G.; Caparros, B.; Huvos, A.G.; Kosloff, C.; Nirenberg, A.; Cacavio, A.; Marcove, R.C.; Lane, J.M.; Mehta, B.; and Urban, C.: Preoperative chemotherapy for osteogenic sarcoma: Selection of postoperative adjuvant chemotherapy based on the response of the primary tumor to preoperative chemotherapy. Cancer 49:1221-1230, 1982.

The Memorial Sloan-Kettering Cancer Center employed an aggressive five-drug preoperative (T-10) chemotherapy program that yielded a disease-free rate of 93 percent in a fifty-seven patient group followed for a median of 20 months.

Ewing's Sarcoma

Tepper, J.; Glaubiger, D.; Lichter, A.; Wackenhut, J.; and Glatstein, E.: Local control of Ewing's sarcoma of bone with radiotherapy and combination chemotherapy. Cancer 46:1969-1973, 1980.

This is a review of the National Cancer Institute's experience with adjuvant chemotherapy and irradiation therapy in ninety-four patients. Sites of primary lesion are divided into those with central, proximal, and distal lesions; 19, 33, and 57 percent of these patients, respectively, were alive.

Chondrosarcoma

Gitelis, S.; Bertoni, F.; Picci, P.; and Campanacci, M.: Chondrosarcoma of bone. The experience at the Istituto Ortopedico Rizzoli. J. Bone Joint Surg. 63A:1248-1257, 1981.

A review article on the surgical management of chondrosarcoma includes a critical review of the Italian experience with 125 patients. This article stresses the importance of adequate surgical resection and the significance of histologic grading.

Giant Cell Tumor

Sung, H.W.; Kuo, D.P.; Shu, W.P.; Chai, Y.B.; Liu, C.C.; and Li, S.M.: Giant-cell tumor of bone: Analysis of 208 cases in Chinese patients. J. Bone Joint Surg. 64A:755-761, 1982.

Surgical treatment of giant cell tumors by aggressive local resection and curettement followed by simple bone grafting without massive allografts or replacement prostheses resulted in a recurrence rate of 7 percent.

Unicameral Bone Cyst

Capanna, R.; Dal Monte, A.; Gitelis, S.; and Campanacci, M.: The natural history of unicameral bone cyst after steroid injection. Clin. Orthop. 166:204-211, 1982.

A recent review showed 80 percent good results in ninety patients from the simple injection of 80 to 200 mg of methylprednisolone acetate with an average two to three injections administered as an outpatient procedure.

Metastatic Disease to Bone

Levy, R.N.: Symposium on Metastatic disease of bone. Clin. Orthop. 169:15-114, 1982.

A collection of twelve recent articles addresses the clinical problems related to the surgical and adjuvant treatment of metastatic carcinoma to bone including exact techniques for surgical treatment of pathological fractures.

Soft-Tissue Sarcoma

Bolsen, B.: Soft tissue sarcoma of limbs: Better outlook. J. Am. Med. Assn. 246:2007-2008, 1981.

A review of the National Cancer Institute's experience with 107 patients having combined surgery, chemotherapy, and irradiation therapy shows a 3-year disease-free survival rate of 91 percent and a projected estimate of 80 percent at 5 years.

Das Gupta, T.K.; Patel, M.K.; Chaudhuri, P.K.; and Briele, H.A.: The role of chemotherapy as an adjuvant to surgery in the initial treatment of primary soft tissue sarcomas in adults. J. Surg. Oncol. 19:139-144, 1982.

This study comparing surgery alone with surgery and adjuvant chemotherapy indicates the disease-free rate in the 144 patients having surgery alone at 50 percent in contrast to 74 percent in the combined group having surgery with adjuvant chemotherapy.

Enneking, W.F.; Spanier, S.S.; and Malawer, M.M.: The effect of the anatomic setting on the results of surgical procedures for soft parts sarcoma of the thigh. Cancer 47:1005-1022, 1981.

This article presents an anatomic and biologic staging of soft-tissue tumors of the thigh prepared as a guide for the treating surgeon in planning surgery with the least chance of local recurrence.

Enzinger, F.M., and Weiss, S.W.: Soft Tissue Tumors. St. Louis, C.V. Mosby, 1983.

This text in the area of soft-tissue tumors reflecting the experience of the Armed Forces Institute of Pathology is illustrated with gross, microscopic, and electron microscopic material. The emphasis is on pathology and differential diagnosis with a brief discussion of treatment.

Leibel, S.A.; Tranbaugh, R.F.; Wara, W.M.; Beckstead, J.H.; Bovill, E.G., Jr.; and Phillips, T.L.: Soft tissue sarcomas of the extremities: Survival and patterns of failure with conservative surgery and postoperative irradiation compared to surgery alone. Cancer 50:1076-1083, 1982.

A comparative study of surgery alone in contrast to combined surgery and postoperative irradiation in a group of eighty-one patients shows a local control rate of 90 percent in the combined group.

6 INFECTION

Topics covered in this section include microbiology, antibiotics, perioperative prophylaxis, osteomyelitis, and infected total joint arthroplasty.

Microbiology

The microbiology of musculoskeletal sepsis, once chiefly concerned with staphylococci and streptococci, is now associated with a variety of microorganisms. The use of perioperative antibiotics alters the microbiology of infections, complicating elective surgical procedures. *Staphylococcus aureus* is the most frequently isolated causal organism in postoperative infections following elective surgical procedures performed without perioperative antibiotics. When perioperative antibiotics are administered, *Staphylococcus epidermidis* is the most frequently isolated causal organism. Anaerobic microorganisms are isolated from 25 percent of the postoperative infections associated with the use of perioperative antibiotics. Although gram-negative bacilli are recovered from 10 to 30 percent of infections complicating total hip arthroplasty, they are uncommon unless sinus tract drainage occurs. The rare infection in which gram-negative bacilli are the primary causal organisms is probably caused by hematogenous seeding of the hip from the genitourinary or gastrointestinal tract.

Anaerobic Infection Anaerobes now are isolated more frequently from musculoskeletal infections. The widespread use of antibiotics promotes an alteration of the flora of the gastrointestinal tract and skin. Normally, a symbiotic relationship between aerobic and anaerobic microorganisms restricts growth of the latter. Once the aerobic organisms are killed or reduced in number by antibiotics, the anaerobes tend to flourish.

Clostridial infections characterized the vast majority of anaerobic musculoskeletal infections in the past. Anaerobic gram-positive cocci, particularly members of the genus *Peptococcus*, are encountered increasingly in postoperative and posttraumatic infections of the musculoskeletal system. Anaerobic infections of the skeleton in patients with debilitating diseases are most frequently associated with isolation of members of the genus *Bacteroides*. A variety of anaerobes are recovered from deep tissue cultures of patients with osteomyelitis (Table I).

Anaerobic infections often occur in association with foreign bodies implanted during reconstructive procedures or utilized to stabilize fractures. There are few classic signs and symptoms of postoperative infections. Persistent pain may be the primary symptom. Febrile response and drainage are distinctly uncommon, and the peripheral white blood cell count is often normal while the sedimentation rate usually is elevated. Radiographic alterations can be diagnostic of an underlying septic problem (Fig. 1). Anaerobic gram-positive cocci, particularly *Peptococcus magnus*, are the most frequent causal organisms.

Table I

Anaerobes Isolated from Patients with Osteomyelitis

	Number of isolates	(%)	Number from cultures yielding only anaerobes*
Peptococcus magnus	17	(18.4)	2
Peptococcus prevotii	11	(11.9)	2
Peptococcus asaccharalyticus	6	(6.5)	—
Peptococcus varibilis	2	(2.2)	—
Peptococcus species	2	(2.2)	—
Peptostreptococcus species	16	(17.4)	2
Veillonella alcalescens	1	(1.0)	—
Bacteroides fragilis group	10	(10.9)	—
Bacteroides melaninogenicus	6	(6.5)	—
Bacteroides species	1	(1.0)	—
Fusobacterium naviforme	1	(1.0)	—
Fusobacterium nucleatum	1	(1.0)	1
Clostridium species	7	(7.6)	2
Propionibacterium acnes	8	(8.7)	3
Eubacterium lentum	3	(3.3)	1

*In mixed or pure anaerobic cultures

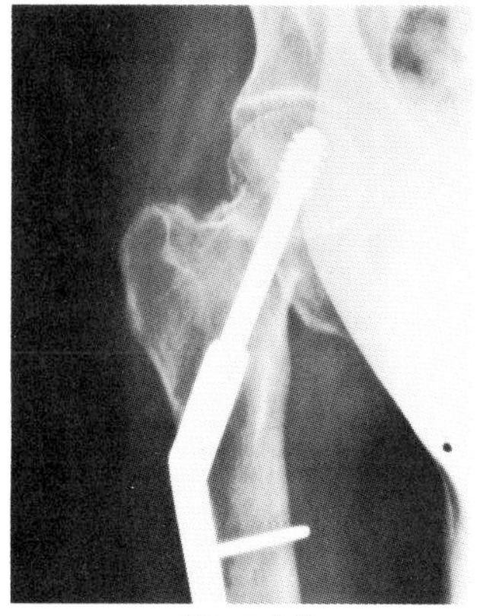
Figure 1-A

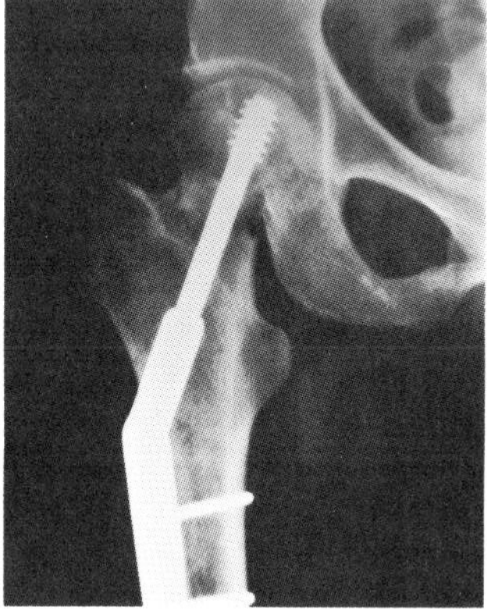
Figure 1-B

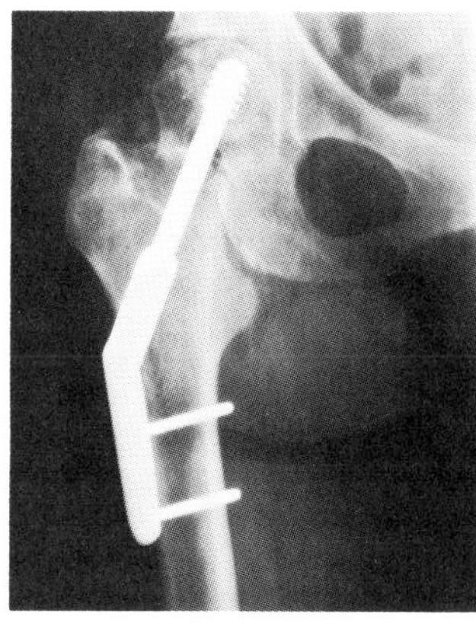
Figure 1-C

Figure 1: Narrowing of the hip joint associated with anaerobic septic arthritis of the hip. (A) Appearance of the hip immediately after open reduction and internal fixation of the hip. (B) Narrowing of the joint space and subchondral erosions 2 months after surgery. (C) Loss of the joint space and nonunion of the fracture 6 months after surgery. *P. acnes* was isolated in pure culture from tissue specimens obtained during resection arthroplasty.

Although anaerobic isolates from tissue cultures of bones and joints that also contain aerobic isolates may be contaminants, recent information suggests they have an important clinical role in the infectious process. Osteomyelitis caused by mixed aerobic-anaerobic organisms has resisted treatment more than osteomyelitis associated with either pure aerobic or anaerobic isolates. When selecting antimicrobial therapy for musculoskeletal sepsis, agents specific for anaerobic organisms require more time for identification. This usually necessitates the addition of a penicillin or clindamycin to the therapeutic agents specific for the aerobic isolates. *Bacteroides fragilis* is an exception. Once universally susceptible to ampicillin and clindamycin, resistant strains of *B. fragilis* now have emerged. Susceptibility testing of these isolates must be performed to identify those strains which produce beta-lactamase and must be treated with alternative therapeutic agents (e.g., metronidazole, chloramphenicol, or cefoxitin).

Toxic Shock Syndrome Toxic shock syndrome in menstruating women recently has become an established clinical entity. This syndrome is characterized by fever, profound multisystem dysfunction, desquamative erythroderma, and minimal infection or colonization with *S. aureus* occurring in previously healthy persons. It has not been widely recognized that the syndrome could result from staphylococcal infections at a wide variety of sites in persons of any age and of either sex.

The Center for Disease Control (CDC) reported the syndrome in thirteen patients following elective surgery. Three of the thirteen procedures were musculoskeletal in nature: spinal fusion, rotator cuff repair, and lumbar sympathectomy. There was a generalized toxic reaction with multisystem involvement and absence of overt wound infection among these patients. Four of the thirteen were male and four of the nine females were postmenopausal. Although no specific treatment has proved effective in resolving the altered microcirculation in the syndrome, drainage and irrigation of the surgical wound accompanied by a systemic antistaphylococcal antibiotic seems appropriate.

The etiology of toxic shock syndrome is not fully known. It seems to be a new disease associated with a new phage type strain of *S. aureus.* Three toxins and two other previously unidentified proteins have been extracted from staphylococcal isolates recovered from patients with this syndrome. One of these, enterotoxin F, elicits a limited antibody response in patients with the syndrome, whereas most "control patients" demonstrate elevated antibody titers. This indicates a selective susceptibility of toxic shock syndrome patients to this protein.

Resistant Microorganisms Resistant microorganisms, common in systemic and urinary tract infections, are being encountered in patients with musculoskeletal sepsis. *S. epidermidis* resistant to penicillin and semisynthetic penicillinase-resistant penicillins (oxacillin, nafcillin, or methicillin) accounts for 20 to 25 percent of clinical isolates of this organism. Clinicians should consider methicillin-resistant strains of *S. epidermidis* to be resistant to cephalosporins. Vancomycin is the agent of choice. Methicillin-resistant isolates of *Staphylococcus aureus* remain distinctly uncommon in musculoskeletal sepsis in North America.

Cefamandole, a second generation cephalosporin, has been advertised as the drug of choice in the therapeutic dilemma arising from the appearance of ampicillin-resistant *Haemophilus influenzae* type B. However, recent laboratory and clinical experience has documented the hydrolysis of cefamandole by certain concentrations and types of β-lactamases and incomplete lysis by certain strains of *H. influenzae.* Chloramphenicol with its effective bactericidal activity and favorable pharmacokinetic properties remains an alternative agent. Moxalactam, a third generation cephalosporin, is highly active against *H. influenzae* and does not carry the serious toxic side effects of chloramphenicol.

Tolerance, a new form of resistance, has been identified in patients with musculoskeletal and other forms of sepsis with isolates of *S. aureus* and *S. epidermidis.* This form of bacterial resistance differs from traditional types. The usual test indicates the isolate of either *S. aureus* or *S. epidermidis* to be susceptible to routine antibiotics. However, when the minimal bactericidal concentration (MBC) is determined, the organism exhibits resistance, i.e., an extraordinarily high MBC. When a patient with musculoskeletal sepsis caused by an apparent isolate of *S. aureus* or *S. epidermidis* fails to respond to specific parenteral therapy, the minimal bactericidal concentration should be determined.

Antibiotics

Antimicrobial agents are essential in the treatment of patients with musculoskeletal injury or disease. In fact, antibiotics in many hospitals are administered as primary or adjunctive therapy more often to patients with musculoskeletal disease than to any other group. The rapid proliferation of antibiotics and conflicting information in the literature have made the selection of antimicrobial agents for the prevention or treatment of musculoskeletal sepsis a formidable challenge.

Indications Antibiotics are prescribed for patients with musculoskeletal disease or injury in three clinical situations: the prevention of postoperative sepsis; the treatment of an incipient infection; and the treatment of an established infection. Rapid technological advancements in the past decade have permitted the orthopaedic surgeon to restore function dramatically to a diseased joint, extremity, or spine. However, most of these sophisticated surgical procedures necessitate the insertion of large metallic and/or acrylic implants. Numerous laboratory and clinical studies have documented the efficacy of administering prophylactic antibiotics to patients having musculoskeletal surgery that creates a residual dead space, results in hematoma formation, or requires implantation of large foreign bodies. Thus, a large portion of these procedures require the administration of prophylactic antibiotics.

Open injuries and fractures following vehicle and industrial accidents are common and difficult problems since most, if not all, are contaminated. Surgical debridement and administration of antibiotics are considered standard treatment. Some physicians may consider usage of antibiotics prophylactic, but it is, in fact, treatment of an incipient infection.

Although efforts in the past two decades have reduced the incidence of deep sepsis significantly following musculoskeletal surgery, the absolute number of postoperative infections actually has increased. This apparent discrepancy is explained by the larger number of patients having surgical treatment. Improved surgical modalities enable the orthopaedic surgeon to salvage traumatized and tumorous limbs formerly amputated. Additionally, the dramatic restoration of function with total joint arthroplasty has encouraged patients with arthritic afflictions to seek surgical treatment.

Even though the incidence of postoperative sepsis is low, the infections complicating these surgical procedures tend to be recalcitrant and polymicrobic with the isolation of multiple drug-resistant causal microorganisms. The rapid proliferation of antibiotics has generated divergent opinion as to the clinical role of the individual agents. The cephalosporin group of antibiotics, once considered a homogeneous group of agents with a similar in vitro spectrum of activity, has developed into a diverse group of agents with varying spectrums of in vitro antibacterial activity and pharmacokinetic properties. Even though clinical experience has begun to define the clinical indications for various cephalosporins, the newer second and third generation agents may be administered inappropriately.

The aminoglycoside group of agents has not expanded as rapidly as the cephalosporin group, but considerable information concerning the nephrotoxic and ototoxic side effects has emerged. Patients with osteomyelitis or other types of musculoskeletal sepsis who require prolonged antibiotic therapy are at greater risk to develop either of these toxic complications. Aminoglycosides cannot be administered indiscriminantly. When clinically indicated, their use necessitates monitoring of serum peak and trough levels at least weekly, serum creatinine every other day, and urinalysis weekly. A rising serum trough level, frequently the initial indicator of renal function alteration, necessitates adjustment of dosage and/or dosage interval. Careful questioning of the patient for the onset of tinnitus or dizziness is important, and weekly caloric functions can provide invaluable objective information to avoid ototoxicity. Weekly audiograms are recommended to detect loss of auditory acuity.

Pseudomembranous entercolitis is a feared complication of antimicrobial therapy. Although initially believed related to specific agents (e.g., clindamycin), careful screening has established an association with a wide spectrum of antimicrobials. The parenteral administration of antimicrobials disrupts the symbiotic microbial relationships of the gastrointestinal tract promoting the growth of *Clostridium difficile*. This organism produces a cytotoxin and an enterotoxin, both important in the development of colitis. When a patient receiving antibiotics develops diarrhea, the antibiotic should be discontinued and a stool specimen and serum sample obtained for culture and fluorescent antibody to *C. difficile*, respectively. Vancomycin is the drug of choice to eliminate *C. difficile* and prevent irreversible changes in the colon. orally

A wide variety of other adverse reactions have been associated with antimicrobial therapy (Table II). Neuro-

Table II

Serious Adverse Effects of Antimicrobial Agents

Nephrotoxic	*Ototoxic*
gentamicin	vestibular
tobramycin	streptomycin
amikacin	gentamicin
vancomycin	tobramycin
cephaloridine	amikacin
tetracycline	minocycline
methicillin	auditory
amphotericin B	neomycin
polymyxin	vancomycin
	erythromycin
Hepatotoxic	*Hemolytic anemia*
oxacillin	penicillins
erythromycin	cephalosporins
tetracycline	sulfonamides
isoniazid	
Hematoxic	*Bleeding Diathesis*
chloramphenicol	carbenicillin
flucytosine	moxalactam

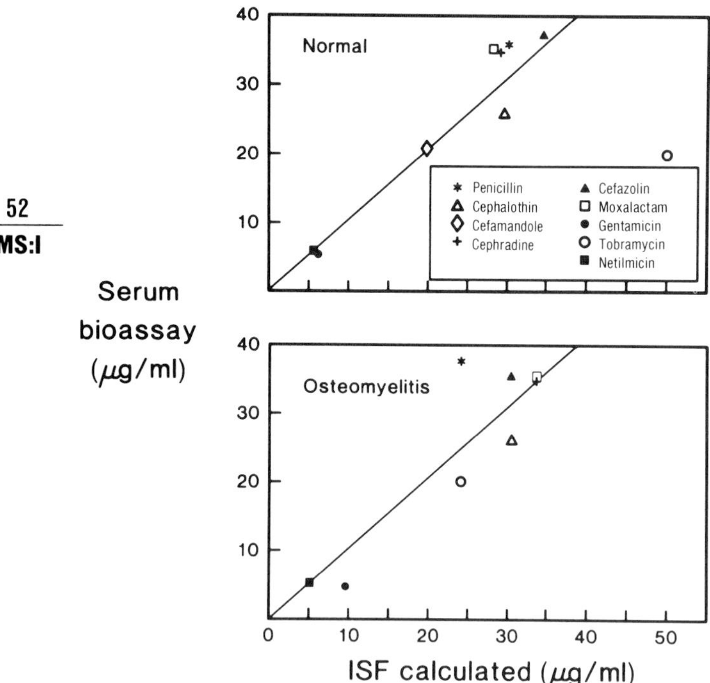

Figure 2: Comparison of the mean serum concentrations (determined with bioassay) with mean interstitial fluid concentrations (calculated) of the nine antibiotics studied in normal and osteomyelitic cortical bone. Except for tobramycin, there is a close correlation. The dose of tobramycin administered was inordinately high and quite possibly led to concentration in one or more of the fluid spaces. The serum level reflects the interstitial fluid concentration of each antibiotic. Each data point represents the mean of five experiments.

muscular blockade can be encountered with aminoglycoside therapy. Staining and deformity of the teeth are possible side effects with tetracycline therapy from the fourth month in utero through 8 years of age.

Assay There are conflicting reports concerning the ability of various antimicrobial agents to penetrate normal or infected osseous tissue. These disagreements reflect the difficulty of dealing with osseous tissue. A needle or probe cannot simply be inserted into cortical bone to extract an aliquot of interstitial or cellular fluid for analysis in the microbiology laboratory. Samples of whole or crushed bone usually are assayed biologically for antimicrobial concentrations. The variations in data generated reflect problems with methodology. In general, these bioassays of bone provide qualitative rather than quantitative data.

Bioassay of antibiotics in noninfected human osseous tissue unfortunately has led some investigators to recommend the superiority of one agent over others. This technique also has initiated the concept of a "blood-bone" barrier analogous to the "blood-brain" barrier to explain the recalcitrant nature of musculoskeletal infections to modern antimicrobial therapy. This hypothesis assumes the osseous capillary system prevents passage of antibiotics into the interstitial fluid space of normal or infected osseous tissue.

To circumvent the discrepancies of bioassay techniques of osseous tissue, a new method has evolved. Although not applicable to humans, it does provide a more fundamental understanding of antibiotic movement in osseous tissue. An isotope assay using physiological techniques (triple-tracer indicator dilution and volume of distribution studies) can define the ability of various antibiotics to cross the capillary membrane and their distribution in the various fluid spaces of normal and osteomyelitic bone in the research laboratory.

Recent research endeavors have addressed the ability of antibiotics to enter the fluid spaces of bone. Antibiotics were found to readily traverse the capillary membrane of normal and osteomyelitic bone. A strong correlation was found between the concentrations of antibiotics in the interstitial fluid space of both types of bone and the serum concentration (Fig. 2). All agents studied to date attained bactericidal concentrations in the interstitial fluid space in normal and osteomyelitic bone. These data refute the hypothesis of a capillary barrier to the passage of antimicrobials in osseous tissue. Furthermore, they suggest that the serum concentration under steady state conditions accurately reflects the osseous interstitial fluid concentration.

The clinical application of these findings suggests that it is unnecessary to consider the bone penetration of antibiotics, at least for the β-lactam and aminoglycoside groups, in the selection of an agent. The in vitro susceptibility data, allergic history, potential for toxicity, and cost are the important parameters in selecting an antimicrobial agent. Although of interest, bone bioassay data provide incomplete information and should not be the basis for the selection of an antimicrobial agent.

This information simplifies the selection of antimicrobial agents. This is particularly important when assessing the clinical role of the newer cephalosporins (Table III).

Cephalosporins *First generation* cephalosporins include

Table III

Bacterial Spectrum of Cephalosporins

Generation I	*Adequate for prophylaxis against:*
Cephalothin	S. aureus
Cephapirin	S. epidermidis
Cephradine	streptococci (not enterococcus)
Cefazolin	enteric GNB[1] (most clinically important)
	Anaerobes (except B. fragilis)
Generation II, III	*Same activity as Generation I* but less active against staphylococci *with activity against:*
Cefamandole	more enteric GNB H. influenzae
Cefoxitin	more enteric GNB some B. fragilis
Cefotaxime	more enteric GNB (many multiple drug-resistant GNB) some B. fragilis H. influenzae
Moxalactam	more enteric GNB (many multiple drug-resistant GNB) some P. aeruginosa some B. fragilis H. influenzae

[1] Enteric gram-negative bacilli. Enterobacteriaceae: e.g., E. coli, K. pneumoniae.

cephalothin, cephapirin, cephradine, and cefazolin. The pharmacokinetics of cephalothin, cephapirin, and cephradine are essentially the same (Table IV). Cefazolin has a significantly higher serum peak and half-life than the others, and thus its lower dosage and less frequent interval of administration make it less expensive to use. There is no difference in the spectrum of activity among the first generation cephalosporins. They are active against streptococci (except enterococcus) and *Staphylococcus aureus*, including penicillinase-producing strains. Methicillin-resistant *Staphylococcus aureus* may not respond, however. Some *Staphylococcus epidermidis* strains may be resistant to cephalosporins, but in general 90 to 95 percent are sensitive at an MIC (Minimum Inhibitory Concentration) of 4.0 μg/ml. Although not the agent of choice, these cephalosporins are active against most anaerobes except those, such as *Bacteroides fragilis*, that are β-lactamase producers. First generation cephalosporins are active against many commonly encountered gram-negative bacilli. The majority of strains of *Escherichia coli, Klebsiella pneumoniae*, and *Proteus mirabilis* are sensitive. These agents are usually ineffective in the treatment of infections caused by enterococcus, Enterobacter, Serratia, Pseudomonas species, indole-positive proteii, or *Bacteroides fragilis*.

The main adverse effects of first generation cephalosporins (and, in fact, second and third generation derivatives) are various hypersensitivity reactions. These include maculopapular rash, urticaria, eosinophilia, drug fever, serum sickness, angioedema, and anaphylaxis. Occasionally encountered are bone marrow suppression, transient hepatic abnormalities, or renal dysfunction. All cephalosporins are relatively nontoxic.

Second generation cephalosporins include cefamandole, cefoxitin, and cefotaxime. There are no major differences in pharmacokinetics within this group except for a somewhat longer half-life of cefamandole. The only advantage of these over the first generation is their increased activity against gram-negative bacilli. However, this greater coverage is offset by lessened activity against staphylococci. The gram-negative spectrum of *cefamandole* includes those organisms sensitive to cephalothin and many Enterobacter, most indole-positive proteii, and *Haemophilus influenzae*. *Cefoxitin* is active against many *Serratia marcescens*, most indole-positive proteii, and many *Bacteroides fragilis*. It is much more active against multiple drug-resistant enteric gram-negative strains than any other member of this group.

All second generation cephalosporins are advantageous in the treatment of gram-negative infections when causative organisms are resistant to first generation cephalosporins. However, *Pseudomonas aeruginosa* and many Enterobacteriaceae are resistant to the second generation cephalosporins. When they are effective (based on in vitro susceptibility testing), they certainly are preferable to aminoglycosides because of lesser toxicity. But, they should not be used frequently or routinely because resistant organisms will emerge. Their high cost is also a consideration.

Third generation cephalosporins, such as moxalactam and cefaperazone, have activity similar to first and second generation drugs but also are active against *P. aeruginosa*. They are less active than first generation cephalosporins against gram-positive cocci. Moxalactam has a gram-negative spectrum similar to all previously available cephalosporins which includes *H. influenzae*, indole-positive proteus, Enterobacter species, Serratia species, and many strains of *B. fragilis*. It is active against some, but not all, *P. aeruginosa*. It is also often active against multiple drug-resistant gram-negative bacilli.

Table IV

Pharmacodynamics of Cephalosporins Suitable for Prophylactic Use[1]

	I.V.	1 hour peak (μg/ml)	½ life (min)
Cephalothin	2 gm	25[2]	40[3]
Cephapirin	2 gm	<32[4]	36
Cephradine	2 gm	<32[4]	36
Cefazolin	1 gm	74	84

[1] Manufacturers published data
[2] Range of 10-40 μg/ml
[3] Range of 30-50 min.
[4] Peak at 30 min. is 32

The relatively long half-life of moxalactam allows the drug to be administered every 8 hours. In addition to the adverse reactions common to all cephalosporins, moxalactam has caused serious bleeding due to prolonged prothrombin time, and a disulfiram-like reaction has been reported after ingestion of alcohol. Superinfections with enterococci (Group D Streptococcus), occurring with an unusual frequency in the treatment of patients with osteomyelitis, are always resistant to moxalactam. Since it is inactive against most strains of *S. epidermidis* isolated from tissue specimens in patients with musculoskeletal sepsis, its application is precluded as a prophylactic agent. Use of moxalactam should be limited to prevent emergence of resistant bacteria. Again high cost is a factor. It may have a role in empiric treatment of polymicrobic infections and certainly is useful in an otherwise resistant infection.

In general, first generation cephalosporins always should be used for infections with sensitive organisms (Table III). This group is also appropriate for prophylactic use. Second and third generation cephalosporins should be used only for organisms resistant to first generation cephalosporins. They are preferable to more toxic antibiotics such as aminoglycosides. First generation drugs are more effective against gram-positive cocci whereas more recent derivatives have increased gram-negative activity.

Prevention of Postoperative Sepsis

Because of the devastating effects of septic complications of operative procedures on the musculoskeletal system, considerable interest has been generated over the past decade in their prevention.

Unidirectional Airflow Systems The introduction of unidirectional airflow systems in surgical theaters has generated considerable controversy within both the orthopaedic and general surgical communities. Numerous uncontrolled studies suggest that this ventilation of the operating room could reduce dramatically the incidence of postoperative sepsis. A multicenter, randomized prospective study over a 7-year period including 8,055 total hip or knee arthroplasties has provided data to support the hypothesis that a significant proportion of infections

occurring after elective surgery are caused by airborne bacteria. When all groups in the study were considered together, the analysis showed deep sepsis after 63 of 4,133 procedures (1.5 percent) performed in a conventional operating room (control group) and after 23 of 3,922 operations (0.6 percent) in the unidirectional airflow facilities ($P<0.001$). When a body-exhaust suit or isolator was worn, the reduction of sepsis was even greater. The use of conventional pattern gowns made of a small pore size
54 textile (as used in a body exhaust suit) did not lead to a
MS:I reduction of airborne bacterial contamination or a reduction in the incidence of sepsis. These data provide strong evidence for the use of ultraclean air (unidirectional airflow facilities) and of whole body exhaust suits by the surgical team.

Prophylactic Antibiotics Although this same study was not designed to address the effects of prophylactic antibiotics, the data generated suggest a substantial benefit from their administration: a fourfold reduction in the incidence of deep sepsis in patients receiving antibiotics.

The efficacy of prophylactic antibiotics during total hip arthroplasty has been addressed in a prospective, double-blind, randomized, placebo-controlled trial performed on 2,137 arthroplasties in nine centers throughout France over a 3-year period. Cefazolin administered just before surgery and continued for 5 days significantly reduced the number of hip infections from 3.3 percent (placebo) to 0.9 percent (cefazolin). The incidence of postoperative sepsis was not reduced statistically when cefazolin was administered prophylactically to patients whose surgeries were performed in ultraclean operating rooms. This contrasted with its prophylactic administration to patients whose surgeries were performed in conventional operating rooms. These data strongly support the administration of prophylactic antibiotics during total hip arthroplasty, especially when performed in a conventional operating room. The sample size of patients whose surgeries were performed in ultraclean operating rooms was too small to evaluate fully the impact of prophylactic antibiotics during total hip arthroplasty.

Several questions regarding the administration of prophylactic antibiotics during total joint arthroplasty remain: timing, duration, and type of antibiotic. The necessity of antibiotics prior to hematoma formation has been established. However, antibiotics have been prescribed as early as the day prior to surgery and as late as the time of wound closure. The ideal time varies with the surgical problem: in a patient without previous surgery on the joint, antibiotic dosage should be initiated at the beginning of the surgical procedure. When a patient has had previous surgery on the involved joint, the administration of antibiotics should be delayed until after deep tissue specimens have been obtained for aerobic and anaerobic culture and before implanting the polymethyl methacrylate.

Antibiotic usage has been continued for variable periods of time following surgery. There are no known advantages to administering antibiotics for a week following surgery, and there may be some distinct disadvantages. If the primary purpose of prophylactic antibiotics is to protect the open wound from infection, one dose in the operating room might be sufficient. For additional safety, dosage could be continued until the wound is sealed. With closed suction drainage, contamination of the wound about the drain sites is theoretically possible. Thus, antibiotics could be continued until the drains are removed at 24 to 36 hours following surgery and then discontinued.

The criteria for selection of a prophylactic agent for a patient having total joint arthroplasty are that it should be active against the most likely causal organism(s), achieve bactericidal concentration in osseous tissue, have attractive kinetic properties, and be safe. Additionally, if all other factors are equal, the cost of the agent should be considered. *S. epidermidis* and *S. aureus* are the most common causal organisms isolated from infected total joints. The semisynthetic penicillinase-resistant penicillins and the first generation cephalosporins are the two groups of antimicrobials (both β-lactam agents) that meet the preceding criteria. As previously noted, the β-lactam group of agents is able to traverse the capillary membrane of normal and infected osseous tissue to achieve bactericidal concentrations in the interstitial fluid space. The kinetic properties of these two groups of antibiotics have considerable variation. Cefazolin has the longest half-life of the first generation cephalosporins. Its half-life of 1.4 hours permits administration every 8 hours. This contrasts with other members of this group that require administration every 4 to 6 hours. The semisynthetic penicillinase-penicillins also require administration every 4 to 6 hours. Cefazolin achieves the highest serum levels following intravenous administration of all of the other agents in these two groups. Only cephaloridine and methicillin have excessive toxicity among the agents in both groups. Thus, cefazolin appears to be the ideal agent for prophylactic administration to patients having total joint arthroplasty.

Although some surgeons have administered and recommended agents in the second and third generations of cephalosporins as prophylactic agents, the in vitro activity spectrum of these agents provides for poor activity against the anticipated causal organisms. Thus, they should not be used as prophylactic agents. Cefamandole may be an exception to this observation. Its in vitro spectrum against gram-positive organisms is similar to that of the first generation cephalosporins. Additionally, it provides significant in vitro activity against a wide range of gram-negative bacteria. However, its pharmacokinetic parameters are not as attractive as those of cefazolin. Furthermore, gram-negative bacilli isolated from infected total joint arthroplasties are almost always secondary invaders once sinus tract drainage or subsequent surgical intervention has occurred. Finally, the cost of cefamandole is significantly greater than that of cefazolin.

Open Fractures and Joint Injuries The administration of antibiotics to patients with open fractures and joint injuries is not truly prophylactic but should be considered treatment of incipient infection. Several prospective studies demonstrate that the incidence of sepsis following treatment of open fractures can be reduced by antibiotics. However, there is a penalty associated with the administration of antibiotics to this group of patients. When patients receive no antibiotic therapy, 70 percent of the infections are associated with the isolation of *S. aureus*. When a first or second generation cephalosporin is used, the number of infections is reduced significantly, but 70 percent of the patients who develop an infection have gram-negative bacilli isolated. Thus, fewer infections occur, but they are more difficult to treat. An antibiotic program more selective in the identification of the patient to be treated and the agent to be administered could help prevent the more devastating gram-negative bacillary infections. Quantitative microbiologic techniques may provide an objective method upon which to base decisions regarding antibiotic therapy. Quantitative microbiology includes a quantitative Gram stain and culture. Following debridement of the open wound a 1 cm^3 tissue specimen is submitted to the microbiology laboratory. For the immediate quantitative smear (Gram stain), 0.01 ml of an undiluted homogenate is transferred onto a clean glass microscopic slide and spread in an area not exceeding 15 mm in diameter. After drying for 15 minutes at 75 degrees centigrade, it is Gram stained. The entire smear is examined microscopically at 1,000X. The presence of a single organism in any field indicates a positive smear, suggesting a high probability of infection. Since the results of the quantitative Gram stain can be available within 30 to 40 minutes, it can be used in the selection of an antibiotic. If a gram-positive organism is identified, a first generation cephalosporin can be administered. If a gram-negative organism is identified, an aminoglycoside can be administered. If the Gram stain reveals both gram-positive and gram-negative organisms, both agents should be used.

The remainder of the tissue homogenate can be serially diluted in nutrient broth for a quantitative culture. Twenty-four hours later the results are available. Cultures containing ten organisms per gram of tissue have a high probability of becoming infected.

The accuracy of quantitative microbiologic techniques following traumatic injuries of the upper extremity has been reported to be 84 percent for Gram stain and 89 percent for culture. When positive, the quantitative Gram stain provides objective information for the selection of an appropriate antibiotic.

Osteomyelitis

Chronic Osteomyelitis The cornerstone of surgical treatment of chronic osteomyelitis, a dreaded disease that is difficult to treat even with the new and more active antibiotics, remains a thorough debridement. This is most difficult in chronically infected bone. Recurrent sepsis is frequent following curettage and "bone scraping" procedures. Radical localized surgical resection of infected and marginally vascularized tissue is necessary to prevent recurrent sepsis.

Orthopaedic surgeons once held a pessimistic attitude toward chronic osteomyelitis that has now been partially allayed by improved surgical procedures that permit reconstruction following radical debridement.

Surgical reconstruction: Three procedures have become invaluable in surgical reconstruction of defects following radical debridement: localized muscle flap, cancellous bone grafting, and free tissue transfer. When bony continuity is retained and the primary problem is residual dead space, a local muscle flap can provide obliteration of the dead space with healthy vascularized tissue. The procedure requires an intimate knowledge of the neurovascular supply of the muscle to be transposed or the muscle becomes necrotic with an increased risk of recurrent sepsis. Recent experience with this technique proved successful in forty of forty-two patients followed for a minimum of 2 years after surgical debridement. The local muscle flap usually was performed within 7 days of sequestrectomy and saucerization. Although a single muscle can be mobilized to fill the residual defect in most patients, more than one muscle can be utilized in large defects.

When the residual defect is in anatomical areas not amenable to a local muscle flap (e.g., the distal third of the tibia or the dorsum of the foot), a cancellous bone graft can be applied after the exposed bony surfaces have become covered with healthy granulation tissue (Papineau procedure). Following debridement of the involved area, wet to dry dressings are applied to the exposed bony surfaces three to four times daily. Most residual cavities will be covered with healthy granulation tissue in 2 to 4 weeks. This technique also is utilized when the structural integrity of the osseous structures has been compromised by surgical debridement. Even though the treatment program can be prolonged with this technique, the patient need not be hospitalized while awaiting granulation to cover the exposed bony surfaces.

When a localized resection of the involved osseous structures or the soft tissue involvement precludes utilization of a local muscle flap, a free tissue transfer with microsurgical vascular anastomosis can permit reconstruction. The free tissue transfer can be composed of soft tissues, muscle with or without overlying skin or omentum, or a composite flap of bone, muscle, and skin (Fig. 3). This technique requires coordination of a team of physicians: the infectious disease expert, the treating surgeon, and a microvascular surgeon. It has permitted salvage of extremities that only a few years ago would have required amputation.

Another addition to the treatment of osteomyelitis is the introduction of electrically generated silver ions. This technique is based on the broad spectrum of bactericidal activity of silver ions in vitro. Preliminary evaluation shows success in thirteen of fifteen patients treated.

Some unusual forms of osteomyelitis have been encountered with the widespread use of drugs in society: heroin users are particularly prone to gram-negative bacillary infections in unusual anatomical sites. Heroin-related osteomyelitis and septic arthritis occur in a younger (and, generally, healthier) population. The most frequent causal organism is *Pseudomonas aeruginosa.* The clinical findings are sparse with localized tenderness the most common. The sedimentation rate and total serum globulins are usually elevated. Scintigraphy is a useful diagnostic tool for detecting osteomyelitis prior to radiographic alterations.

Four to 6 weeks of parenteral antimicrobial therapy has been empirically recommended for the treatment of chronic osteomyelitis. The prolonged hospitalization associated with this therapeutic regimen can be decreased by allowing the patient's continued antibiotic therapy with a heparin lock at home. If potentially toxic agents (e.g., aminoglycosides) are being administered, the patient needs to return for serum creatinines and peak and trough levels on a regular basis as an outpatient.

Acute Hematogenous Osteomyelitis The management of acute hematogenous osteomyelitis is improved with early diagnosis. Scintigraphy with the sequential use of technetium (99Tcm-MDP) and gallium (67GA-citrate)

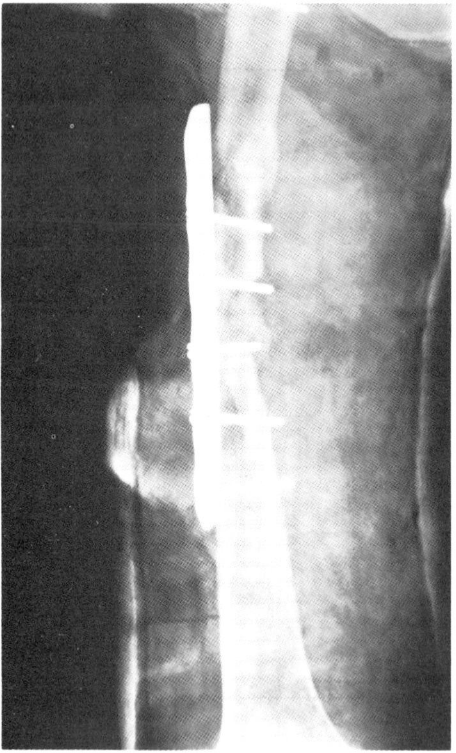

Figure 3-A

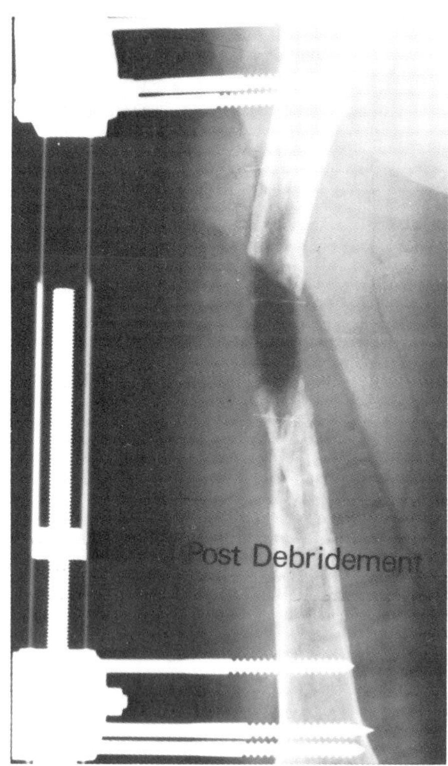

Figure 3-B

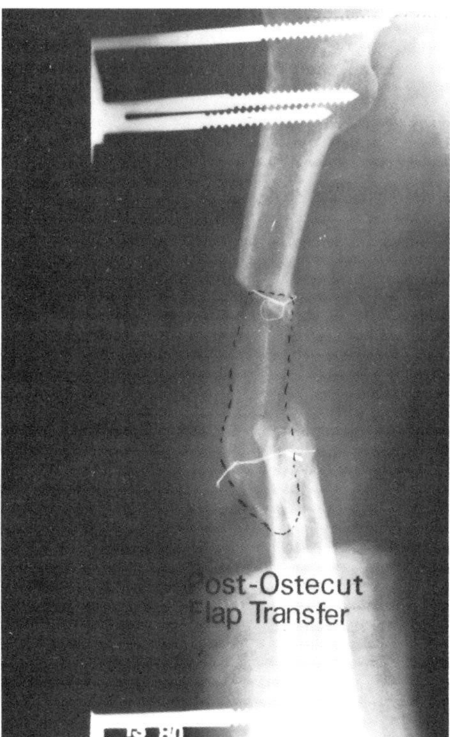

Figure 3-C

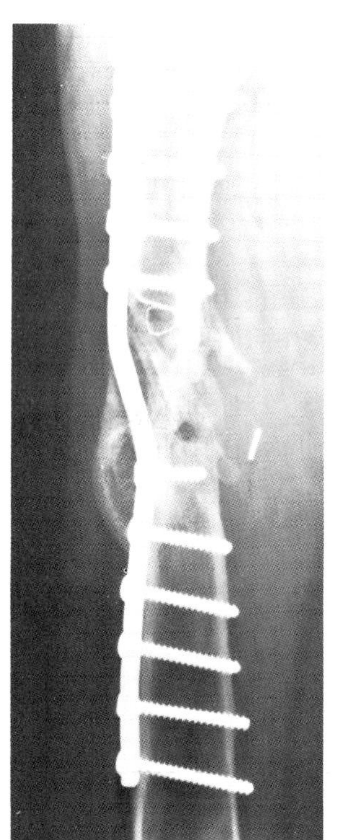

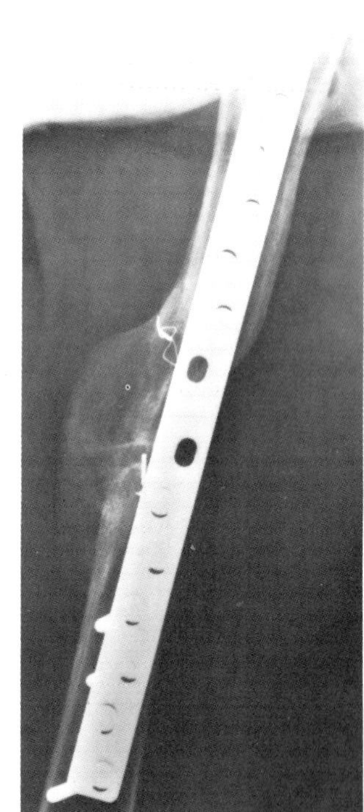

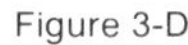

Figure 3-D

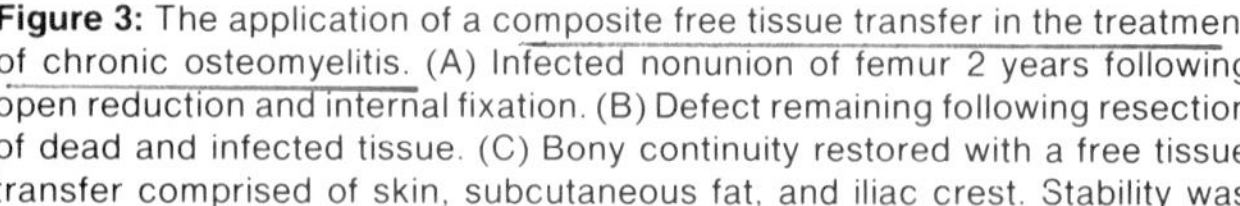

Figure 3: The application of a composite free tissue transfer in the treatment of chronic osteomyelitis. (A) Infected nonunion of femur 2 years following open reduction and internal fixation. (B) Defect remaining following resection of dead and infected tissue. (C) Bony continuity restored with a free tissue transfer comprised of skin, subcutaneous fat, and iliac crest. Stability was maintained with Wagner apparatus. (D) Two years following debridement, the patient is free of sepsis with united femur and legs of equal length. The plate and additional cancellous bone grafts were applied 6 months following the free tissue transfer.

has aided the nuclear radiologist's ability to differentiate trauma from acute osteomyelitis. Once the diagnosis of acute hematogenous osteomyelitis is made, prolonged parenteral therapy, difficult in the pediatric age group, may no longer be necessary. Short-term parenteral therapy of 2 to 5 days followed by oral therapy in a controlled environment has been effective in one study. Oral therapy necessitates a cooperative patient and family, as well as frequent serum assays to assure serum bactericidal titers of at least 1:8, i.e., the serum level of the antibiotic is 8 times greater than that necessary to kill the causal organism.

Infected Total Joint Arthroplasty

The adverse effects of monomeric polymethyl methacrylate on the cardiovascular system have been publicized, but it also appears there is an additional adverse effect on the ability of leukocytes to migrate, phagocytize, and kill *S. epidermidis, S. aureus,* and *Escherichia coli.* Surprisingly, *S. epidermidis* and *S. aureus* can survive in the presence of monomeric polymethyl methacrylate in concentrations ranging from 0.00 to 1.25 percent. The growth of *E. coli* is unaffected until the concentration of polymethyl methacrylate approaches 1.25 percent, when killing occurs. Although the clinical implication is unclear, it would appear that the monomeric polymethyl methacrylate released during the curing process may have an adverse effect on the local host defense mechanism.

Late hematogenous seeding of loose total joint arthroplasties has occurred with increasing frequency as this particular clinical condition has become more common. Metal salts and fragments of high density polyethylene and polymethyl methacrylate from failed arthroplasties are capable of inhibiting neutrophil chemotaxis. Thus, the local host defense mechanisms are affected adversely by the presence of a loose total joint arthroplasty. This, of course, should make such an arthroplasty more susceptible to infection.

The management of an infected total joint arthroplasty remains controversial. Successful salvage of a functional arthroplasty with parenteral antibiotics alone or when combined with surgical debridement is uncommon. The acutely infected hematoma in the immediate postoperative period is an exception and may be managed successfully by this means. According to some, a one-stage exchange arthroplasty with conventional polymethyl methacrylate without added antibiotics and parenteral antibiotics has been effective in patients with low-grade (subacute) infections from which highly susceptible organisms have been isolated. When this information merges with European experience with one-stage exchange arthroplasty, it would appear that patients with pure gram-positive infections sensitive to gentamicin are ideal candidates for a one-stage exchange arthroplasty.

Patients with gram-negative or mixed gram-positive and gram-negative infections are best treated by a thorough debridement and possibly by delayed reconstruction 3 to 12 months later. A two-stage exchange arthroplasty has been successful in 90 percent of 111 patients. Patients with early reimplantation and mixed gram-positive and gram-negative infections appear to have an increased incidence of recurrent infection. Retained cement during resection arthroplasty also predisposes the patient to recurrent sepsis (see Section 33, Pelvis Hip, and Femur: Reconstruction).

In some patients reimplantation is not advisable because of the high failure rate as a result of certain organisms and/or compromise of local tissue conditions. (See Section 13, General: Polymethyl Methacrylate, for the use of antibiotic impregnated cement for treatment of infected total joint replacements, which is not yet released for general use by the United States Food and Drug Administration.)

ANNOTATED BIBLIOGRAPHY

Microbiology

Bartlett, P.; Reingold, A.L.; Graham, D.R.; Dan, B.B.; Selinger, D.S.; Tank, G.W.; and Wichterman, K.A.: Toxic shock syndrome associated with surgical wound infections. J. Am. Med. Assn. 247:1448-1451, 1982.

Toxic shock syndrome is not limited to tampon use during menses. Thirteen patients developed toxic shock syndrome following surgical procedures. Three of the thirteen had musculoskeletal procedures. Postoperative toxic shock occurs in males, postmenopausal females, nonmenstruating and menstruating females. Characteristic features include fever, profound multisystem dysfunction, a desquamative erythroderma, and minimal infection with *Staphylococcus aureus* occurring in a previously healthy person.

Marks, M.I.: Antibiotic therapy of serious *haemophilus* infections—A continuing problem. J. Pediat. 98:910-912, 1981.

Effective and safe chemotherapy for Haemophilus infections of the musculoskeletal system has become complex with the isolation of ampicillin and cefamandole-resistant isolates. Cefamandole should not be used for the treatment of serious *H. influenzae* infections. Chloramphenicol or moxalactam appear to be the agents of choice.

Antibiotics

Eliopoulos, G.M., and Moellering, R.C., Jr.: Principles of antibiotic therapy. Med. Clin. of North America 66:3-15, 1982.

Effective antimicrobial therapy depends on identification of the infecting microbial pathogen. Proper selection of a specific agent with known pharmacokinetic properties, utilization of methods for monitoring antimicrobial drug levels, and a greater appreciation of the relevance of certain laboratory phenomena which make chemotherapy safe are the parameters to be considered in selecting an agent.

Fitzgerald, R.H., Jr.: Orthopaedic sepsis in osteomyelitis: Antimicrobial therapy for the musculoskeletal system. *In* AAOS Instructional Course Lectures 31:1-9, 1982.

Antibiotics, both β-lactam and aminoglycoside groups, are capable of crossing the capillary membrane and achieving bactericidal concentrations in the I.S.F. equivalent to those in the serum in normal and osteomyelitic bone. Antibiotic concentrations in bone determined with bone bioassay provide qualitative data that can be misleading as to the ability of a particular agent to penetrate osseous tissue.

Tetzlaff, T.R.; McCracken, G.H., Jr.; and Nelson, J.D.: Oral antibiotic therapy for skeletal infections of children: II. Therapy of osteomyelitis and arthritis. J. Pediat. 92:485-490, 1978.

Twenty-nine of thirty patients with acute hematogenous infections treated with a brief initial period of parenteral therapy followed by oral therapy were cured of the infectious process. Oral therapy in a controlled environment to assure a peak serum bactericidal titer of at least 1:8 appears to be safe and effective.

Prevention of Postoperative Sepsis

Cooney, W.P., III; Fitzgerald, R.H., Jr.; Dobyns, J.H.; and Washington, J.A., II: Quantitative wound cultures in upper extremity trauma. J. Trauma 22:112-117, 1982.

Quantitative microbiologic techniques, quantitative Gram stain and culture of tissue specimens immediately following debridement are accurate predictors of septic complications or primary wound healing in 89 percent of sixty-four traumatic wounds to the hand and forearm studied in a prospective fashion. Quantitative microbiologic techniques can be helpful in determining the method of wound management and the administration of antimicrobial therapy to traumatic wounds.

Hill, C.; Mazas, F.; Flamant, R.; and Evrard, J.: Prophylactic cefazolin versus placebo in total hip replacement. Lancet 1:795-797, 1981.

A statistically significant reduction in the postoperative wound infection rate following total hip arthroplasty occurred with prophylactic administration of cefazolin (beginning just before surgery and continuing for 5 days) in this double-blind, randomized, controlled study of 2,137 patients undergoing total hip replacement. Postoperative infections were less common when the procedure was performed in an unidirectional airflow environment, and the benefits of prophylactic antibiotics were restricted to patients undergoing surgery in conventional operating rooms.

Lidwell, O.M.; Lowbury, E.J.; Whyte, W.; Blowers, R.; Stanley, S.J.; and Lowe, D.: Effective ultraclean air in operating rooms on deep sepsis in the joint after total hip or knee replacement: A randomized study. British Med. J. 285:10-14, 1982.

In a prospective randomized study of 8,055 total hip and total knee replacement procedures, the incidence of postoperative wound infection was reduced by one-half with unidirectional airflow systems. When whole body exhaust ventilated suits were also utilized, the incidence of postoperative sepsis was one-fourth of that found after operations performed in conventional operating rooms. These reductions in the incidence of postoperative wound infection were statistically significant ($P<0.001$).

Osteomyelitis

Becker, R.O., and Spadaro, J.A.: Treatment of orthopaedic infections with electrically generated silver ions. J. Bone Joint Surg. 60A:871-881, 1978.

Electrically generated silver ions were effective in the treatment of twelve of fifteen patients with chronic osteomyelitis or pyarthrosis following wound debridement. One patient with an infected nonunion experienced eradication of the infection and union of the fracture. Two partial failures and one complete were associated with this technique.

Ger, R.: Muscle transposition for treatment and prevention of chronic posttraumatic osteomyelitis of the tibia. J. Bone Joint Surg. 59A:784-791, 1977.

Local muscle transposition and delayed skin grafting were successfully utilized in thirty-seven of forty-three patients with chronic osteomyelitis. This effective technique for the elimination of residual dead space following debridement provides healthy tissue to tissue partially compromised of vascularity. It aids rapid wound closure and healing of osteomyelitic defects.

Horoszowski, H.; Ganel, A.; Kamhin, M.; Zaltzman, S.; and Farine, I.: Sequential use of technetium 99m MDP and gallium 67 citrate imaging in the evaluation of painful total hip replacement. British J. Radiol. 53:1169-1173, 1980.

The use of Tc-phosphate compounds and Ga-citrate is recommended for the differentiation between mechanical loosening of a prosthesis and loosening of a prosthesis secondary to infection. The authors found this technique effective in the evaluation of fourteen patients with painful total hip arthroplasties.

May, J.W., Jr.; Gallico, G.G., III; and Lukash, F.N.: Microvascular transfer of free tissue for closure of bone wounds of the distal lower extremity. New England J. Med. 306:253-257, 1982.

The loss of soft tissue and the residual dead space following sequestrectomy and saucerization of osteomyelitic focus can be managed with the microvascular transfer of vascularized soft tissues. This free tissue transfer technique was effective in the treatment of eighteen patients with chronic infection and four patients with extensive traumatic injuries with short-term follow-up.

Roca, R.P., and Yoshikawa, T.T.: Primary skeletal infections in heroin users: A clinical characterization, diagnosis and therapy. Clin. Orthop. 144:238-248, 1979.

Heroin-related osteomyelitis and septic arthritis occur in a younger and generally healthier population. The causal organism is frequently a gram-negative bacillus. Sparse clinical findings with an elevated sedimentation rate and total serum globulin are common. Scintigraphy can be helpful in the diagnosis.

Septimus, E.J., and Musher, D.M.: Osteomyelitis: Recent clinical and laboratory aspects. Orthop. Clin. North America 10:347-359, 1979.

Effective treatment of osteomyelitis necessitates identification of the causal organism and the determination of the minimal inhibitory concentration and minimal bactericidal concentrations of antibiotics that would be likely to be used. Only in this manner can resistant and tolerant strains of offending pathogens be identified.

Sudmann, E.: Treatment of chronic osteomyelitis by free grafts of cancellous autologous bone tissue. Acta Orthop. Scand. 50:145-150, 1979.

Surgical debridement and grafting of the defect with cancellous and cortical cancellous bone in a one-stage procedure was effective in the treatment of twelve of thirteen patients with chronic osteomyelitis. This modification of the Papineau procedure (usually associated with a delayed cancellous bone grafting of the resulting defect) further substantiates the importance of obliteration of the residual dead space following sequestrectomy and saucerization of osteomyelitic fossae.

Waldvogel, F.A., and Vasey, H.: Osteomyelitis: The past decade. New England J. Med. 303:360-369, 1980.

A review of the literature detailing various bacterial and causal etiologies of musculoskeletal sepsis is described. Current concepts on laboratory evaluation of the patient with musculoskeletal sepsis are detailed. Recommendations for the selection and monitoring of antimicrobial agents are reviewed.

Infected Total Joint Arthroplasty

Cracchiolo, A.: The effects of metal salts and joint implant debris on neutrophil chemotaxis. Orthop. Trans. 6:265, 1982.

Neutrophil chemotaxis is reduced by exposure to metal salts and synovial fluid containing debridement from a failed total joint replacement. This altered leukocyte function documents a local form of depressed host resistance in the presence of a failed or loose total joint arthroplasty.

Fitzgerald, R.H., Jr.: Indirect exchange of the infected hip implant. Orthop. Trans. 5:372, 1981.

Delayed reconstruction of the infected hip arthroplasty, a resection arthroplasty followed by reconstruction with total hip arthroplasty at a subsequent date, was effective in alleviating the infection and providing a painfree functional arthroplasty in 90 percent of the patients 2 to 11 years following reconstruction.

Petty, W.: The effect of methylmethacrylate on bacterial phagocytosis and killing by human polymorphonuclear leukocytes. J. Bone Joint Surg. 60A:752-757, 1978.

The ability of leukocytes to phagocytize and kill strains of *Staphylococcus epidermidis, Staphylococcus aureus,* and *Escherichia coli* were impaired by monomeric polymethyl methacrylate. The ability of leukocytes to kill was affected to a greater degree than their ability to phagocytize.

7 TRAUMA: SPECIAL PEDIATRIC CONSIDERATIONS

In this section partial growth plate arrest and its treatment, as well as the general aspects of trauma resulting from child abuse are discussed.

The pathophysiological effects of multisystem trauma, as well as patient management following such injury is discussed in Section 10: Nonneuromusculoskeletal Systems and Section 31: Pelvis and Acetabulum: Trauma. Discussion of trauma to particular musculoskeletal anatomic areas is found in the specific anatomical sections.

Partial Growth Plate Arrest and Its Treatment

Introduction Premature partial arrest of an epiphyseal growth plate (physis) produces angular and length growth abnormalities of the involved bone. The arrest is produced when a bridge of bone forms from metaphysis to epiphysis, thereby crossing the physis. This continuity of bone has become known as a bone bridge or a bone bar and tethers growth. As the remaining physis grows, angular deformity occurs (Fig. 1). The size and location of the bar determine the clinical deformity.

Bone bars may result after any injury or insult to physeal cells. Anatomic differences between the various physes are important in the production of bone bars. These differences include size of the physis, rate of growth, and contour of the physis, i.e., whether the physis lies on one plane or is irregular. The age of the patient at physeal injury is the primary factor that determines the extent of subsequent deformity. Injury of the physis of a 14- or 15-year-old girl or a 16- or 17-year-old boy is of little consequence because these individuals have so little growth remaining that deformity is not likely to become clinically apparent. Any bone bar in an infant or young child, however, is a significant problem with wide-ranging clinical effects. Clinical follow-up until maturity is necessary in these children.

Evaluation History, physical examination, and routine radiographs will localize the involved physis. There should be careful evaluation of the relationship of the growth arrest line, physis, and joint surface (Fig. 1B). Radiographic bone age determination is necessary to assess the amount of remaining growth.

Tomograms determine both the configuration and area of bar involvement and, perhaps more important, the configuration and area of the remaining normal physis. Thin cuts (1 mm) taken every 3 mm in both the anteroposterior and lateral planes are used to construct both the area and configuration of the bar on a piece of paper. This may be referred to as a "map" of the bar. This aids in determining if the bar is resectable and, if so, the surgical approach.

Lengths of the involved and uninvolved extremities should be documented radiographically. Scanography is the preferred method because the distance can be measured directly on the film, the measurement is not affected by the thickness of the extremity, there is no magnifica-

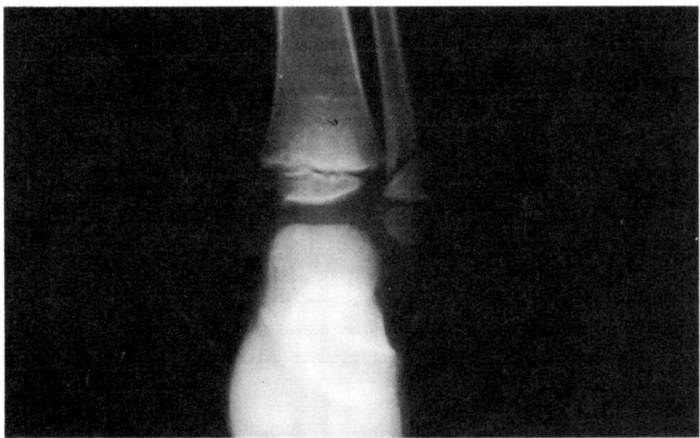

Figure 1-A

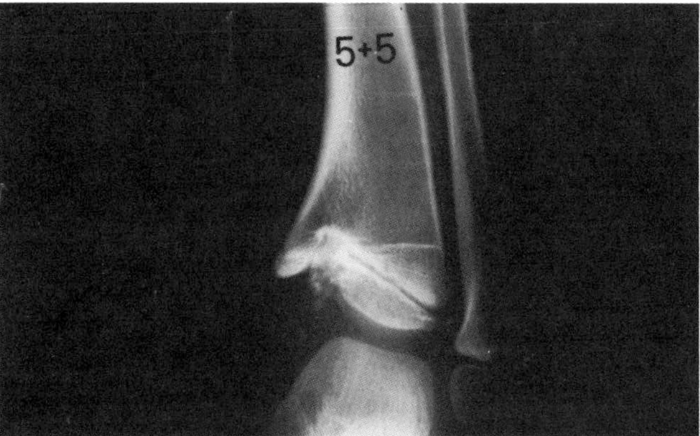

Figure 1-B

Figure 1: Three-year, 7-month-old boy fell from a tree. (A) Distal tibial physeal Salter-Harris type IV injury with proximal displacement. This was treated by cast immobilization without reduction. (B) Same child 22 months later (age 5 years, 5 months). Note physeal bar medially, growth arrest line perpendicular to longitudinal axis of the tibia, asymmetric growth of remaining normal physis producing 45 degree varus angulation of the physis, and adaptive contouring of the lateral edge of the tibial epiphysis allowing the ankle varus to be less than the physeal varus. The medial malleolus is present but not yet ossified. (Reprinted with permission from Operative correction of post-fracture arrest of the epiphyseal plate, by H.A. Peterson, J. Bone Joint Surg. 62A:1018, 1980.)

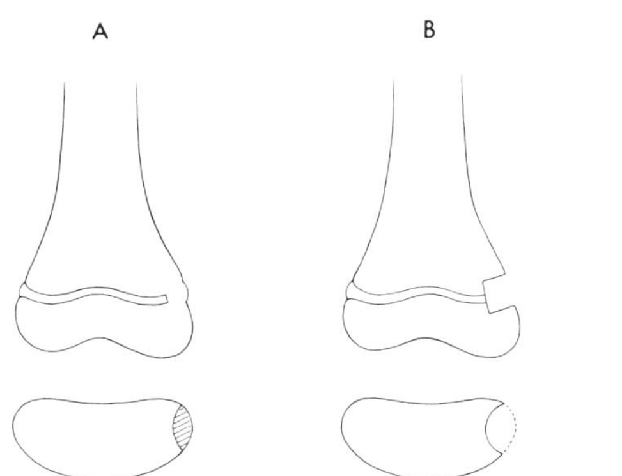

Figure 2: Peripheral bar: above, anteroposterior view; below, transverse section through physis. (A) With map of bar composed from tomograms. (B) Bar excised by direct approach.

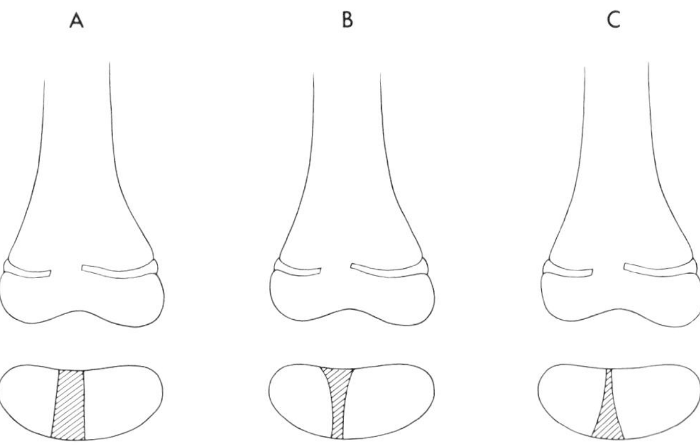

Figure 3: Elongated bar extending from anterior to posterior surfaces. Although these three bars have the same appearance on the anteroposterior view (above), they have different contours and areas on the transverse sections (below). To achieve complete bar removal with retention of as much normal physis as possible, the bar in (C) would be optimally approached anteriorly, that in (B) posteriorly.

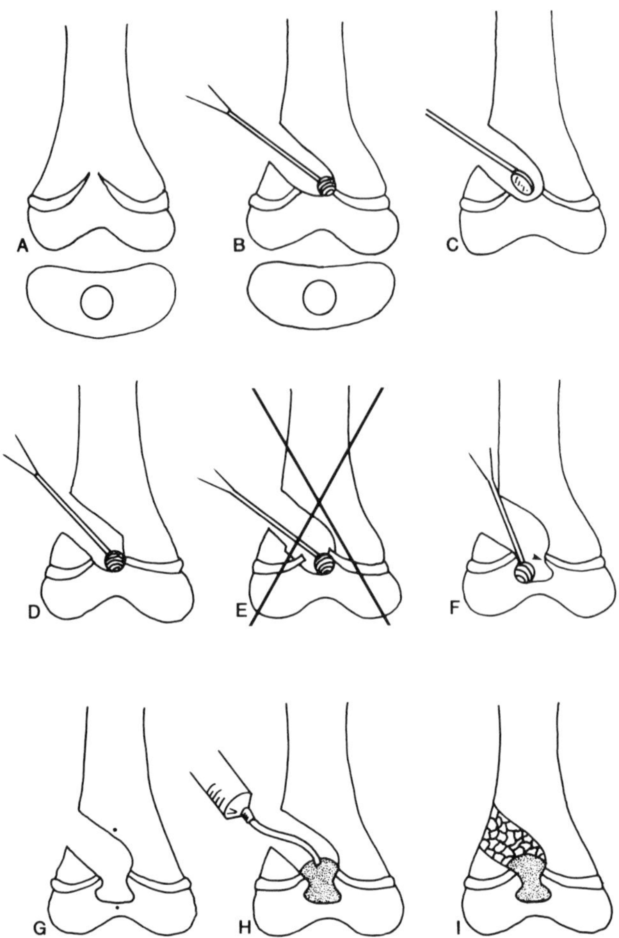

Figure 4: Central bar. (A) Bar in center with growth peripherally results in "tenting" or "cupping" of the physis. (B) Excision of central bar through window in metaphysis. (C) Visualization of entire physis with dental mirror. (D) As normal physis is exposed the adjacent metaphyseal bone surface should be smooth to help prevent the plug from staying with the metaphysis. (E) Undermining bone away from the physis should be avoided since the protruding physis would be deprived of its blood supply and prevented from growing inward over the plug as the epiphysis grows distally. (F) Bone in the epiphysis is undermined in an attempt to allow the plug to stay with the epiphysis. If this is done, a small rim of epiphyseal bone should be preserved to maintain viability of the physis (arrow). (G) Placement of markers in cancellous bone of metaphysis and epiphysis away from the interposition plug and longitudinally oriented to each other. (H) Using a syringe and catheter, insert only enough Cranioplast to bridge all physeal surfaces. (I) Remainder of defect filled with bone grafts.

tion, technical error can be easily detected (if the child moves during the examination, the image on the film will be wavy and the examination should be repeated), and the true measurements can be compared with previous and future scanograms in longitudinal studies.

Treatment Premature partial closure of the physis may be managed in many ways. If the patient is a teenager approaching maturity and little growth remains in the involved physis, no treatment may be necessary.

If the patient is young with significant growth remaining, a combination of many modalities may be used: (1) shoe lift; (2) arrest of the remaining growth of the injured physis; (3) arrest of the remaining growth of the physis of the adjacent bone (a forearm and lower leg); (4) arrest of the remaining growth of the corresponding physis or physes of the contralateral bone or bones; (5) open or closed wedge osteotomy to correct angular deformity; (6) bone lengthening (femur or tibia) or bone shortening (femur only); and (7) excision of the physeal bar.

All these preceding treatment options have been used in the management of physeal bars. But, when successful, excision of the bar avoids the use of the other modalities with their potential morbidities. If it is used and is unsuccessful, the other options may be used.

Excision of Physeal Bars

Technique The objectives of surgical excision of a bone bar are to remove the bar completely and preserve as much of the normal remaining physis as possible. This may be difficult if the bar is irregular or if there are multiple or satellite bars.

Peripherally located bars should be approached directly (Fig. 2). Any periosteum overlying the bar should be excised. Under direct visualization the bar can be removed from inside-out until normal physis can be seen on all sides of the cavity. The bone bar may be removed by using an osteotome, curet, and rongeur but is most precisely removed with a small, motorized burr. This allows excellent visualization of the physis and removal of as little normal physis as necessary to assure complete removal. It also facilitates contouring of the cavity in the epiphysis. The heat from the burr has no apparent deleterious effect upon the viability of the remaining physis.

Bars that extend completely across the physis (common after type IV fractures) require careful evaluation of the tomographic maps to determine surgical approach and to ensure complete removal of the bar (Fig. 3).

Centrally located bars that have normal physis peripherally and an intact perichondrial ring of Ranvier should not be approached from the periphery so that an attempt is made to save these structures (Fig. 4A). These bars should be approached through the metaphysis. This requires removing a window of cortical bone and a fair amount of cancellous metaphyseal bone before the physeal bar can be reached (Fig. 4B). After removing the entire bar, the normal physis must be visualized circumferentially in the cavity. This may be aided by the use of a small (5-mm diameter) dental mirror (Fig. 4C).

The sides of the cavity should be flat and smooth (Fig. 4D). Undermining the metaphyseal and epiphyseal bone from the physis deprives that portion of the physis of its blood supply and more of the physis would have to be removed than necessary (Fig. 4E). The contour of the cavity may be important. Bar reformation is less likely when the interposition material (plug) remains in the epiphysis than when the epiphysis grows away from it. Perhaps the easiest technique is to enlarge the cavity in the epiphysis like one-half of a button, maintaining a rim of bone next to the physis for vascular nourishment (Fig. 4F).

The only way to accurately measure subsequent growth of the involved physis is to place metal markers in the metaphysis and epiphysis (Fig. 4G). Without these markers, overgrowth of the physis at the other end of the bone may falsely enhance the result. These markers (one-half of a silver clip is commonly used) should be placed in cancellous bone, not in contact with the cavity, because they might become attached to a solid interposition material, or if fat is used, they might migrate into the cavity. The markers should be in the same longitudinal plane, proximal and distal to the defect.

The cavity should be filled with an interposition material to prevent hematoma and bone bar reformation (Fig. 4H). Fat, bone wax and fat, Gelfoam and sheet Silastic, Silastic elastomer, and methyl methacrylate have been used in humans. The approach hole is then filled with bone grafts (Fig. 4I). There are not enough patients followed to maturity in these studies to determine the superiority of one interposition material over the others. A recent study on rabbits has shown that bar reformation is prompt and predictable when no interposition material is used and that cartilage as an interposition material is superior to fat. Finding sufficient, suitable autogenous cartilage may be difficult in human patients. Another recent study on rabbits suggests that bar reformation following bar excision may be inhibited by the use of indomethacin given orally without the use of an interposition material.

An important feature of technique involves the effect of the size and shape of the interposition plug on the growth of the remaining physis. Presumably, as the epiphysis and its retained interposition material advance, the edges of the physis in contact with the plug grow inward over the plug. This has never been proved because biopsy of the growing epiphysis is not indicated. Thus, it is important to have the metaphyseal portion of the plug as small, smooth, and regular in outline as possible. A large metaphyseal portion of plug predisposes the epiphysis to grow away from the plug and should be avoided.

Mild angular deformity secondary to peripheral bars often corrects spontaneously with growth after excision of the bar. Angular deformities greater than 20 degrees will probably not correct spontaneously and usually require osteotomy. This may be performed at the same time as bar excision or later.

Postoperative joint motion may be begun immediately if solid interposition materials (e.g., Silastic or methyl methacrylate) are inserted. If a concomitant osteotomy is not done, a cast or other immobilization is unnecessary. Weight-bearing is encouraged on the day of operation or as soon as operative discomfort subsides. Cast immobilization to prevent fracture is recommended if a soft interposition material (e.g., fat, bone wax, Gelfoam) is used.

Follow-up Follow-up must be continued until maturity. Reestablished physeal growth may cease at any time. Recurrent bar formation has been successfully treated by reexcision of the bar. If a bar reforms near maturity or if the entire physis ceases growing on the injured side earlier than its contralateral counterpart (a fairly frequent finding), physeal arrest on the normal contralateral side may be considered. A typical patient is presented in Figure 5. A satisfactory result was achieved in this patient despite the fact that the interposition plug stayed in the metaphysis.

General Trauma Due to Child Abuse

Since the term "battered child syndrome" was introduced by Kempe in 1962, there has been a growing awareness that many traumatic injuries suffered by children are not accidental in origin. The orthopaedic surgeon is frequently involved in the management of these patients because of trauma to the musculoskeletal system.

It is important to recognize the signs of nonaccidental trauma to make a proper diagnosis. The patient and the patient's family can then be referred to other appropriate services to attempt management of the underlying cause or causes of the abuse. In addition, there may be an obligation to report the case to authorities outside of the treatment facility.

Recognition of these patients in order to initiate appropriate treatment and measures to avoid repetition of the trauma is not always simple. However, there are some characteristics of such patients, which may indicate the nonaccidental origin of the injury: (1) vague history which does not correlate with physical findings; (2) unrelated injuries indicating multiple impacts; (3) skin lesions and burn injuries in locations not normally associated with infantile accidents; (4) multiple injuries and evidence of previously healed and partially healed injuries in the same location (Fig. 6); (5) fractures of the long bones, ribs, and skull where other suspicious signs are present; (6) spiral or oblique fractures, especially in the lower limbs and in nonambulatory children (Fig. 7); (7) lesions involving the ribs posteriorly; (8) metaphyseal corner fractures and lower extremity fractures in nonambulators; and (9) bilaterality of acute fractures and epiphyseal fractures. If radiographs are normal in instances of suspected trauma, radionuclide bone scan may help in establishing the diagnosis (Fig. 8).

Proper treatment of the musculoskeletal injury serves

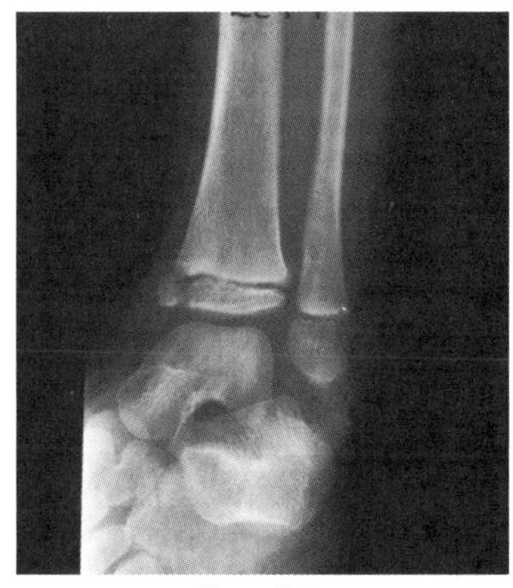

Figure 5-A

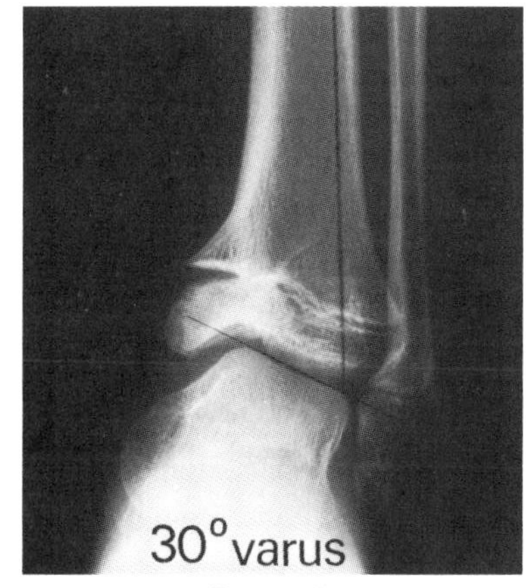

Figure 5-B

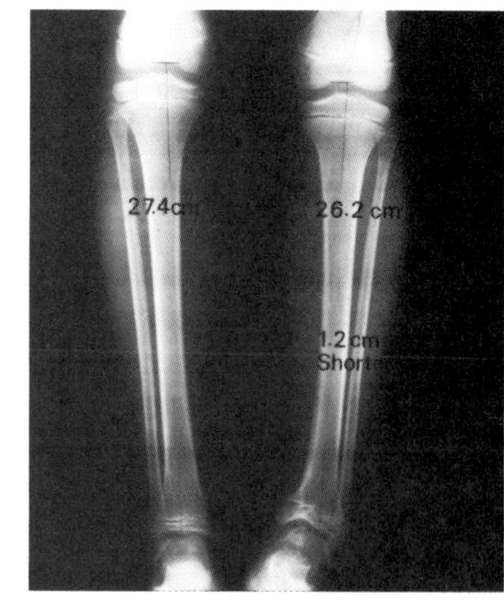

Figure 5-C

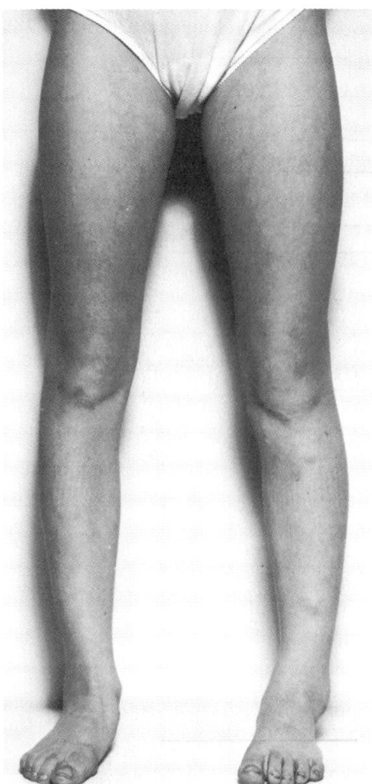

Figure 5-D

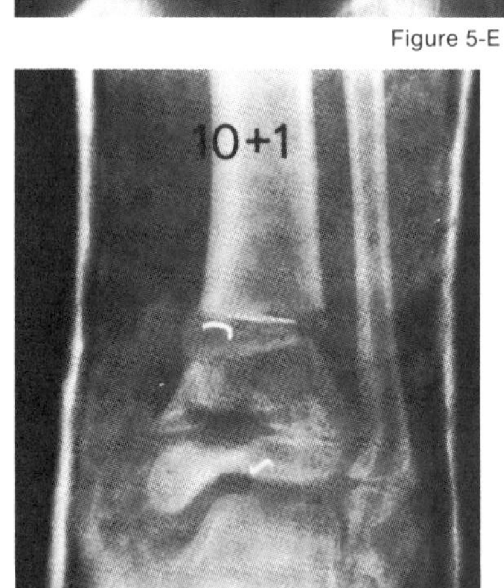

Figure 5-E

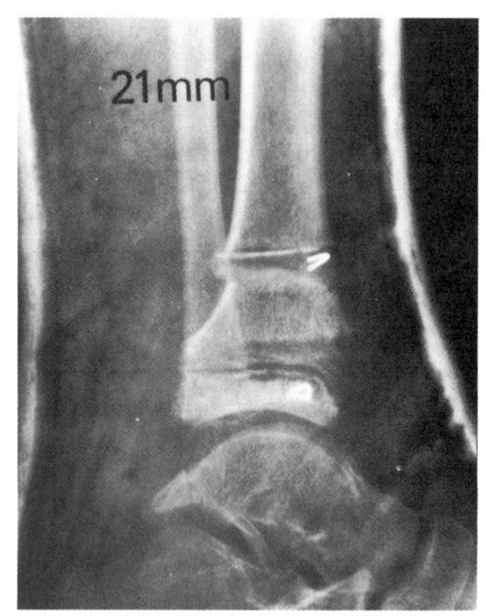

Figure 5-F

Figure 5-G

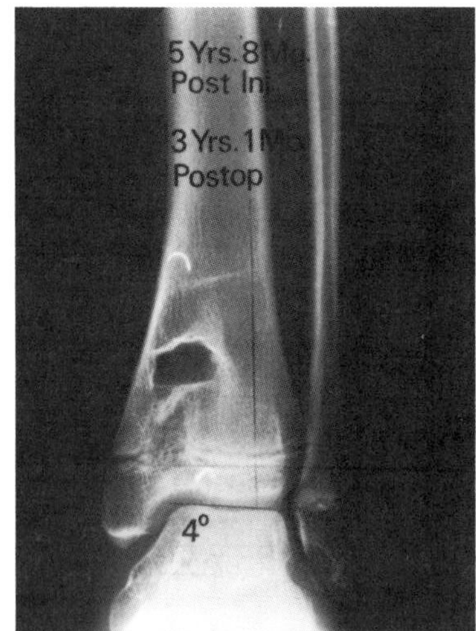

Figure 5-H

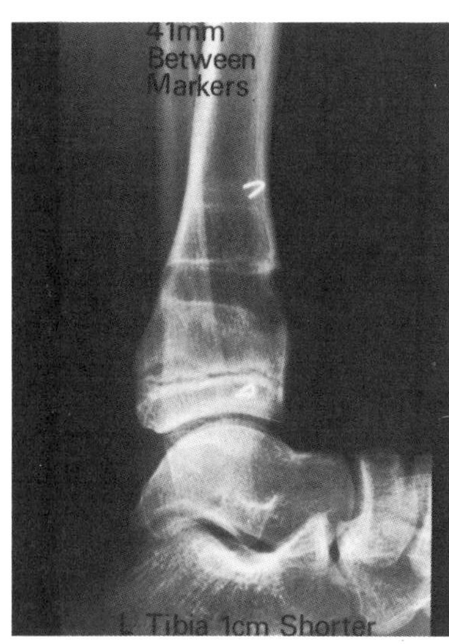

Figure 5-I

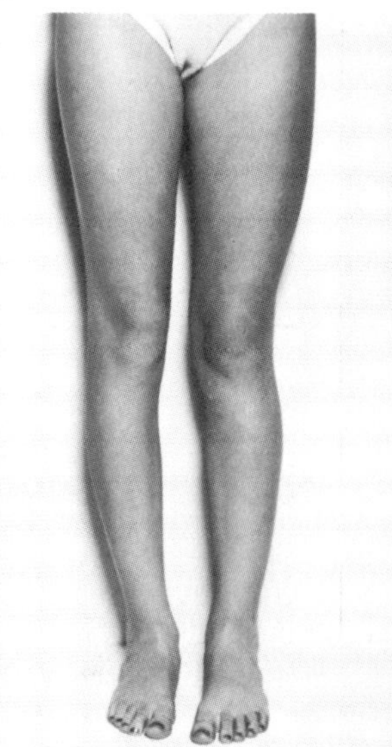

Figure 5-J

Figure 5: Girl (7 years, 4 months) sustained a mildly displaced Salter-Harris type IV fracture of the distal left tibia. After subsequent bar formation and excision, the plug stayed with the metaphysis. (A) Fracture of medial malleolus at age 7 years, 4 months, treated by cast 6 weeks. (B) Bar formation with 30 degrees ankle valgus 2 years, 6 months later, age 10 years, 1 month. (C) Scanogram at age 10 years, 1 month, shows left tibia 12 mm shorter than right. (D) Clinical appearance age 10 years, 1 month. Note left ankle varus. (E) Tomograms show elongated bar from anterior to posterior (See Fig. 3). (F, G) Bar excision by tunnel technique from periphery to periphery at age 10 years, 1 month. Distal tibial open wedge osteotomy, held open with autogenous iliac crest bone, corrected 20 degrees of the 30 degrees varus angulation. The metalmarkers (vascular silver clips) are 21 mm apart. A cast was used because of the osteotomy. (H, I) Three years, 2 months postoperatively (age 13 years, 3 months) the plug stayed in the metaphysis, the metal markers are 41 mm apart, and the varus has diminished from 10 degrees to 4 degrees (the contralateral normal ankle also measured 4 degrees varus). (J) Clinical appearance at age 13 years, 4 months. Scanograms showed the left tibia to be 10 mm shorter than the right. (Figures 5-B, F, G, H, and I reprinted with permission from Salter-Harris type-IV injuries of the distal tibial epiphyseal growth plate, with emphasis on those involving the medial malleolus, by J.R. Cass, et al., J. Bone Joint Surg. 65A:1068, 1069, 1983.)

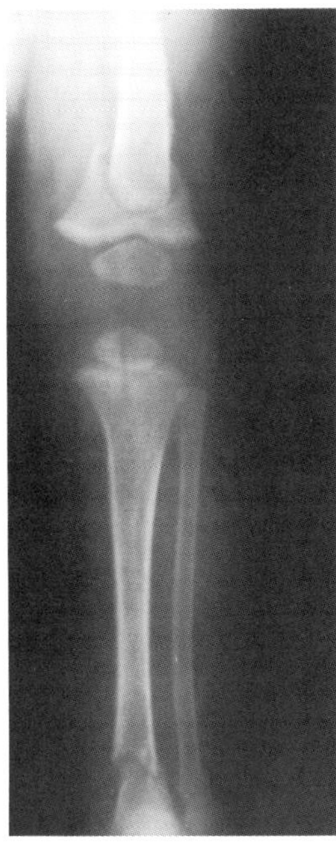

Figure 6: Anteroposterior radiograph of 7-month-old child showing an old fracture of the distal femur with periosteal new bone formation. Note the recent fracture of the distal end of the tibia.

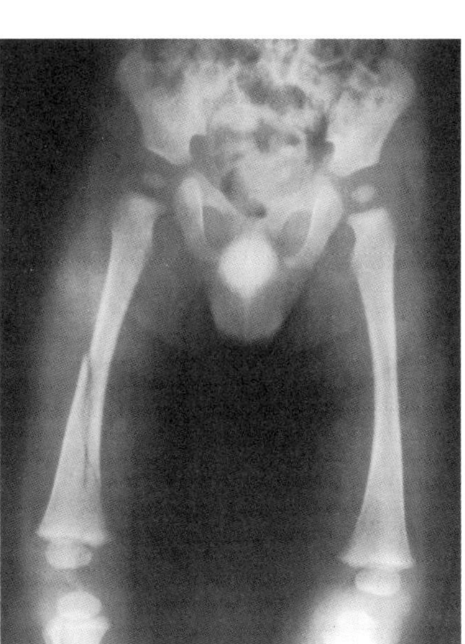

Figure 7: Radiograph of a child 8 months of age with a recent spiral fracture of the right femur. A fall from the crib was given as the history, but further investigation documented child abuse.

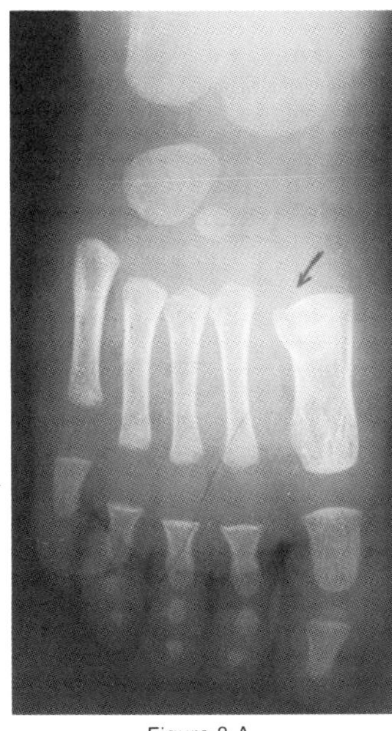

Figure 8-A

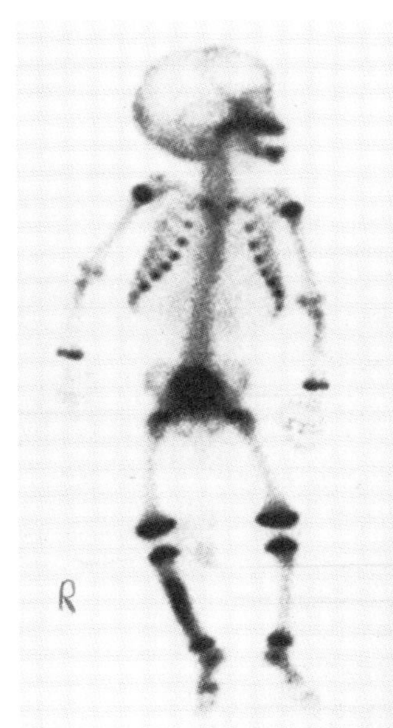

Figure 8-B

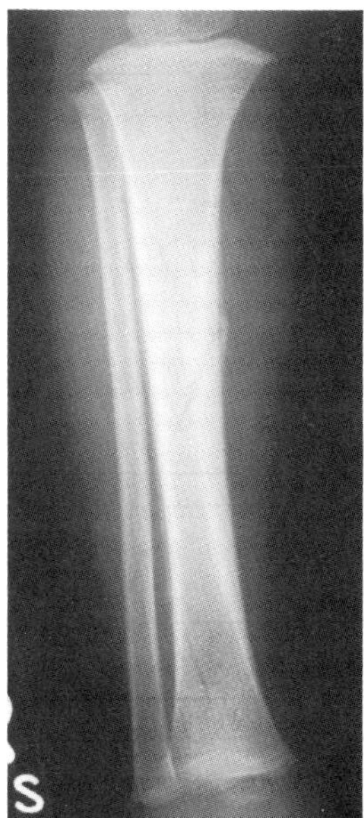

Figure 8-C

Figure 8: (A) Radiograph of the right foot shows a fracture of the base of the first metatarsal. (B) Technetium 99 bone scan shows increased uptake of the right foot as well as the right tibia. (C) Radiograph of the right tibia was then obtained which showed an old fracture of the midshaft of the tibia.

only part of the needs of these patients. Efforts should be made to alleviate the causes of the trauma as well.

ANNOTATED BIBLIOGRAPHY

Partial Growth Plate Arrest and its Treatment

Bright, R.W.: Partial growth arrest: Identification, classification, and results of treatment. Orthop. Trans. 6:65-66, 1982.

One hundred patients with physeal bar formation were treated by bar excision using Silastic as the interposition material. Radiographic evidence of renewed longitudinal growth was seen in 81 percent of patients.

Klassen, R.A., and Peterson, H.A.: Excision of physeal bars: The Mayo Clinic experience, 1968-1978. Orthop. Trans. 6:65, 1982.

Thirty-six patients with physeal bar formation were treated by bar excision using methyl methacrylate without barium as the interposition material. Growth of the operated physes equaled 94 percent (average) of the normal unoperated physis. Some growth occurred in all patients.

Langenskiöld, A.: Surgical treatment of partial closure of the growth plate. J. Pediat. Orthop. 1:3-11, 1981.

Thirty-eight patients with physeal bar formation were treated by bar excision using autogenous fat as the interposition material. Thirty-one showed resumption of growth and prevention or correction of deformity.

Lennox, D.W.; Goldner, R.D.; and Sussman, M.D.: Cartilage as an interposition material to prevent transphyseal bone bridge formation: An experimental model. J. Pediat. Orthop. 3:207-210, 1983.

A portion of physis, epiphysis, and metaphysis was removed from the periphery of the distal femur in three groups of rabbits. When no interposition material was inserted, bar formation was prompt. Cartilage as an interposition material was superior to fat.

Peterson, H.A.: Operative correction of post-fracture arrest of the epiphyseal plate: Case report with 10-year follow-up. J. Bone Joint Surg. 62A:1018-1020, 1980.

A tibia grew 16.7 cm (94 percent of the normal contralateral tibia) following excision of a distal tibial bar in 1968 in a boy 5 years old, followed 10 years. Sheet Silastic and Gelfoam were used as interposition materials.

Sudmann, E.; Husby, O.S.; and Bang, G.: Inhibition of partial closure of epiphyseal plate in rabbits by indomethacin. Acta Orthop. Scand. 53:507-511, 1982.

Bar reformation following bar excision without the use of an interposition material in rabbits appeared to be inhibited by the use of indomethacin given orally.

Vickers, D.W.: Premature incomplete fusion of the growth plate: Causes and treatment by resection (physolysis) in 15 cases. Australian New Zealand J. Surg. 50:393-401, 1980.

Fifteen patients with physeal bar formation were treated by bar excision and insertion of bone wax and fat in fourteen and methyl methacrylate in one. Some growth occurred in all. Methyl methacrylate is preferred in large defects prone to postoperative fracture.

General Trauma Due to Child Abuse

Akbarnia, B.; Torg, J.S.; Kirkpatrick, J.; and Sussman, S.: Manifestations of the battered-child syndrome. J. Bone Joint Surg. 56A:1159-1166, 1974.

Of 217 children admitted, one-third required orthopaedic management. This article describes the prevalence of the syndrome, orthopaedic and nonorthopaedic manifestations, and the legal responsibilities of the orthopaedic surgeon.

Bittner, S., and Newberger, E.: Pediatric understanding of child abuse and neglect. Pediat. in Review 2:197-207, 1981.

This review of child abuse includes social aspects and the management of victims of child abuse.

Galleno, H., and Oppenheim, W.L.: The battered child syndrome revisited. Clin. Orthop. 162:11-19, 1982.

This review of sixty-six children stresses the importance of the specific nature of the fracture (such as bilaterality or corner fractures) rather than the old adage of "three fractures in different stages of healing."

Haase, G.; Ortiz, V.; Sfakianakis, G.; and Morse, T.: The value of radionuclide bone scanning in the early recognition of deliberate child abuse. Trauma 20:873-875, 1980.

In forty-four children with histories of trauma, who had negative or positive radiographs for fractures, both bone scan and skeletal survey were done. None with negative radiographs and bone scans later developed radiologic evidence of a fracture.

Helfer, R.; Slovis, T.; and Black, M.: Injuries resulting when small children fall out of bed. Pediatrics 60:533-535, 1977.

Of 246 children less than 5 years of age who fell out of bed, there were three skull fractures, three clavicle fractures, and one humerus fracture. None were seriously injured.

Kempe, C.H.; Silverman, F.N.; Steele, B.F.; Droegenmueller, W.; and Silver, H.K.: The battered-child syndrome. J. Am. Med. Assn. 181:17-24, 1962.

This is the original description of the syndrome and describes the physical abuse as a possible cause of skeletal and nonskeletal injuries causing permanent damage or death.

McClelland, C.Q., and Heiple, K.G.: Fractures in the first year of life: A diagnostic dilemma. Am. J. Dis. Child. 136:26-29, 1982.

Thirty-four patients with 55 fractures were studied. Fifty-six percent were found to be a result of child abuse.

8 AMPUTATIONS AND PROSTHETICS

The major reason for limb amputation continues to be the elimination of disease or a functionally useless part. When amputation is performed, however, a new problem is introduced, and it is of the utmost importance that it be minimized insofar as technically possible. In this sense, amputation also must be considered a reconstructive procedure, and the extent of functional rehabilitation of the amputee is directly proportional to the surgeon's ability to create the best possible functional end organ. It is generally agreed that amputations should be performed at the lowest possible level consistent with tissue viability and the elimination of the disease process. In particular, every attempt should be made to save the knee and the elbow since they are key functional joints in the lower and upper limbs, respectively. The principle of myoplastic closure is now universally accepted as providing superior, functional amputation stumps. Surgeons who perform amputations should be familiar with the types of prosthetic replacements available and the rehabilitation needs of the amputee.

General Considerations

Children The major reasons for amputation in children are congenital limb deficiency, trauma, and tumor.

Congenital limb deficiencies may be transverse, longitudinal, and/or intercalary and frequently are multimembral. Conversion surgery by reamputation to produce a more functional stump rarely is indicated in the upper limb but may be necessary in many lower limb deficiencies, such as proximal femoral focal deficiency (PFFD) and congenital absence of the fibula or tibia. In such instances, disarticulation is preferred over transdiaphyseal amputation due to the problem of bony overgrowth in children. Prosthetic rehabilitation of the congenitally limb deficient child begins at the age of standing for lower limb deficiencies and at the age of sitting for upper limb deficiencies. The application of electrically powered or myoelectrically powered prostheses for congenital upper limb deficiencies, and, in particular, for the child with bilateral amputations is becoming more widespread because of technological advances.

In traumatic amputations, every effort should be made to save the distalmost epiphysis in order to preserve as much limb length as possible at maturity and to prevent bony overgrowth. The use of Silastic and polyethylene caps to prevent this overgrowth frequently has been complicated by extrusion of the material. A biological method of stump capping utilizing osteochondral graft over the terminal portion of the diaphysis now appears to be a better solution to this problem. The graft material may be taken from a portion of the ablated extremity.

In children undergoing amputation for tumor, prosthetic fitting should not be withheld as the early use of an artificial limb considerably minimizes the psychological consequences of this amputation.

Adults The most common cause of amputation in the adult population of the industrially developed world is peripheral vascular disease. In underdeveloped countries trauma remains a leading cause. In amputees suffering from peripheral vascular disease, maximal preservation of stump length, early prosthetic fitting, and a well-organized rehabilitation program are the major factors leading to successful rehabilitation outcomes.

In patients with severely traumatized extremities, it is important to assess the need for amputation at an early date since attempts to save a limb that should be amputated may be followed by excessive morbidity and even death.

Amputation as a primary treatment for malignant tumors of extremities is becoming less common with the advent of effective chemotherapy and improved surgical techniques for limb salvage.

Considerations in Vascular Disease

The incidence of major amputation for vascular disease in Sweden recently has been found to be 0.3 per 1000 persons over 40 years of age (with a 2:1 ratio of males to females). This rate increases exponentially with age.

In principle, arterial reconstruction should be the primary consideration in all patients with severe ischemia of the lower limb. Improved techniques such as prebypass arteriography, sequential reconstruction of tandem lesions, and the use of new materials including human umbilical vein and polytetrafluoroethylene (PTFE) grafts have resulted in improved limb salvage. Revascularization techniques now commonly result in a 50 percent patency rate at 5 years, although results are somewhat better after femoral-popliteal bypass than in bypasses to the tibial and peroneal arteries. Autogenous saphenous vein remains the material of choice for bypass surgery, but when not available, PTFE grafts have shown encouraging results. Controversy still exists as to whether revascularization procedures jeopardize a below-knee amputation, but some centers report that the incidence of below-knee amputation following such procedures is not affected.

Selection of Amputation Level In recent years, many methods have been devised to quantitate the healing potentials of the possible sites of amputation in dysvascular limbs. Although these procedures can be both helpful in selecting an amputation site and, in fact, predictive of successful healing, patients should not be denied a lower level of amputation purely on the basis of a single predictor due to the high false negative rate. Such studies should be combined with clinical judgment and the presence or absence of skin bleeding at the time of amputation to maximize the preservation of limb length. There are several techniques currently utilized for prediction of amputation healing.

Doppler ultrasound is the most available objective measurement of limb blood flow. Pressures obtained in the calf and ankle may be related to the brachial pressure to obtain an ischemic index. However, no demonstrable relationship between calf-arm pressure index and the degree of healing in below-knee amputations in diabetic or nondiabetic patients has been found.

Xenon 133 skin clearance has been used to successfully predict the level of healing in dysvascular patients. In one study, forty-three of forty-five patients with flow rates exceeding 2.4 ml/min/100 g of tissue healed primarily.

Segmental transcutaneous Po_2 measurements have been used to predict healing of below-knee amputations in thirty-seven patients with uniform healing occurring in patients with Po_2 values of 40 ml or more. However, seventeen of nineteen patients with values of more than 0 but less than 40 ml of mercury had delayed healing at the below-knee level as well.

Skin perfusion pressure has been measured preoperatively as the external pressure required to stop isotope washout using the radioactive isotope antipyrine mixed with histamine. This appears to be a reasonably reliable predictor of wound healing.

Preoperative fluorescein angiography likewise has been reported to be of predictive value for the assessment of skin viability and the determination of amputation level in patients with peripheral vascular disease.

Prognosis Although the incidence of reamputation in vascular disease has been reported as high as 18 percent after 6 months when delay in wound healing is encountered, the healed amputation secondary to vascular disease has a very low incidence of reamputation. Repeat angiographic studies should be performed in healed amputation stumps that present with evidence of gangrene since many of these limbs may be salvaged by vascular reconstruction. The risk of contralateral amputation is always present with an incidence of 11.9 percent within 1 year, 17.8 percent after 2 years, 27 percent after 3 years, and 44 percent after 4 years.

The prognosis for successful healing of a below-knee amputation in peripheral vascular disease is consistently reported at between 80 and 90 percent. Factors adversely affecting healing at the below-knee level include absence of the femoral pulses associated with cellulitis as opposed to those patients without cellulitis and an absent femoral pulse in which healing occurs in 85 percent. Hemoglobin levels are inversely proportional to success rates in patients with diabetes and cellulitis, and elevated white blood counts adversely affect healing in nondiabetic patients without cellulitis.

Operative mortality for above-knee amputation is in the range of 15 percent, prinicipally due to the extent of systemic disease, and an additional 26 percent mortality rate has been reported during a 2-year follow-up period in such patients as a result of related circulatory disorders. Below-knee amputation mortality rates in the dysvascular patient are approximately 2 percent. Successful prosthetic rehabilitation can be anticipated in below-knee amputees provided that such patients were ambulatory preoperatively. Successful prosthetic rehabilitation of the above-knee patient with peripheral vascular disease commonly occurs in only 50 to 60 percent as a result of the increased energy expenditure needed for walking.

Surgical and Prosthetic Management

Upper Limb Upper limb amputations constitute only 15 percent of all major limb amputations but are associated with more functional limitations and more profound psychological disturbances than lower limb amputations. Adequate prosthetic substitution has been more difficult in the upper limb than in the lower limb since the qualities of sensory feedback and manipulation within the grasp cannot be adequately substituted for by prosthetic replacement. Prosthetic rejection is common in upper limb amputees and is directly proportional to the amount of limb loss. Unilateral shoulder disarticulation and forequarter amputees uniformly reject their prostheses, preferring to function as one-handed individuals.

Controversy still exists regarding the merits of conventional prosthetic substitution versus the newer myoelectric designs. In general, conventional body-powered cable-driven prostheses are reliable and durable, provide a certain amount of sensory feedback through the harnessing mechanism, and require low maintenance and repair. They are also uncosmetic, provide weak grasp, and are relatively inconvenient because of the harnessing system. Myoelectric prostheses, on the other hand, are cosmetic and frequently self-suspending, provide excellent grip strength, and provide proportional control signaled by the patient's own muscular activity. But, they are extremely expensive, less durable, and frequently heavier. They also require maintenance and repair more often, and this is usually difficult to obtain.

As an alternative to a functional upper limb prosthesis, a cosmetic nonfunctional or aesthetic prosthesis may be utilized in proximal amputations and in partial hand amputations. Such prostheses particularly are indicated in females and have a high rate of acceptance.

With advances in microsurgical techniques, primary amputation and prosthetic replacement of the upper limb must be weighed against the degree of potential function from reimplantation of the severed part. Reimplantation is especially indicated in distal amputations with a short period of anoxia and relatively minimal tissue damage.

Research The principal areas of research in upper extremity prosthetics have been the development of externally powered components, myoelectric control systems, and sensory feedback designs. Although pneumatically controlled components have been used in the past, recent emphasis has been on the development of electrical components for prehension, wrist rotation, and elbow flexion and extension. Such electrically powered components are controlled either by electric switch or by an amplified myoelectric signal detected by transcutaneous electrodes within the prosthetic socket. Implanted electrodes over motorpoints through a percutaneous skin connection have also been developed on a research basis. To the extent possible, muscle control sites are selected to correspond to the patient's natural motor activity in operating the prosthesis, i.e., finger extensors control opening of the prosthetic hand and finger flexors control closing of the prosthetic hand. Myoelectric prostheses are commercially available for the below-elbow amputee as well as the above-elbow amputee, but higher amputations generally require custom fabrication of prostheses in research laboratories.

Sensory feedback mechanisms to indicate the power of prehension as well as some position sense are under clinical investigation at several centers with promising results. However, they are not yet available in commercially manufactured prostheses.

Also under investigation is the concept of myoelectrically controlled individual prosthetic digital movements.

Levels

FOREQUARTER AND SHOULDER DISARTICULATION: These mutilating amputation levels are fortunately necessary only rarely, either for tumor or extensive trauma. There is no satisfactory body-powered prosthesis available for this level of amputation, and nearly all patients will reject such an approach. Clinical investigation of myoelectrically controlled, externally powered prostheses is ongoing at several centers utilizing residual shoulder and trunk musculature to activate electric elbows and hands. Although partially successful, these sophisticated devices require considerable maintenance and are subject to frequent breakdown. Therefore, the fittings are often unsatisfactory from the patient's view.

Since a suitable functional prosthesis for this level of amputation does not yet exist, most prosthetic efforts have been directed toward a cosmetic substitute. Such devices may be endoskeletal in nature with a soft cosmetic cover and aesthetic hand with passive positioning of the elbow. With forequarter amputees, a simple soft plastic mold may be fashioned to fill out the shoulder as an alternative to a full-arm cosmetic prosthesis.

ABOVE ELBOW: Above-elbow amputations proximal to the deltoid insertion must be fitted as shoulder disarticulation amputees since there is no available motor to the amputation stump. In such instances an attempt should be made to reattach the deltoid to the distal portion of the humerus, if possible, so as to provide shoulder motion capable of controlling an above-elbow prosthesis. This should be performed as a myoplasty or myodesis, suturing the deltoid over the end of the humerus to the soft tissues or bone on the medial side. Myoplastic closure is recommended for any above-elbow amputation to preserve the functional activity of the biceps and triceps musculature. Above-elbow amputees may be fitted with conventionally body-powered prostheses, with myoelectrically controlled elbows and cable-controlled prehension, or with myoelectrically controlled prehension utilizing biceps and triceps with cable control for elbow flexion.

In the management of brachial plexus injuries above-elbow amputation may be elected depending upon the patient's desires. The necessity for shoulder arthrodesis combined with above-elbow amputation recently has been questioned in that the best return to gainful employment and prosthetic wearing habits were achieved with early above-elbow amputation alone in one clinical series.

BELOW ELBOW: The below-elbow level of amputation is an acceptably functional level, and prosthetic rehabilitation is achieved in 70 to 80 percent of such patients even with conventional body-powered techniques. Myoplastic closure of the below-elbow amputation stump should be performed to enhance proprioceptive feedback from the muscle spindle organs and to facilitate the use of myoelectric prostheses, if prescribed. The amputation should be performed as distal as possible to preserve effective pronation and supination which can be partially transmitted to the prosthesis if the amputation is in the distal one-third of the forearm.

In clinical practice the self-suspending myoelectric below-elbow prosthesis has achieved a great degree of acceptability which has been limited by the durability of the device and the cosmetic glove in work situations, as well as the frequent unavailability of servicing.

If a body-powered conventional below-elbow prosthesis is prescribed, most patients prefer having an interchangeable hook and hand since there are distinct advantages to both devices.

KRUKENBERG'S AMPUTATION: Krukenberg's kineplastic operation may be performed as a secondary procedure in below-elbow amputees who retain at least one-half of their forearm length. The operation transforms the below-elbow amputation stump into radial and ulnar pincers capable of strong prehension and excellent manipulative ability due to retained sensation on the "fingers" of the forearm. The operation is indicated particularly for the blind bilateral below-elbow amputee on either one or both sides. Such amputees can become completely independent in their daily activities due to the retained sensory ability of the amputation stumps, as well as the quality of the grasping mechanism. It may also be indicated, at least unilaterally, in the bilateral below-elbow amputee who has retained vision as it preserves sensory feedback at least unilaterally. The operation rarely is indicated in unilateral below-elbow amputees who have preserved sensory feedback in the remaining hand. Although the operation produces a superior functional below-elbow stump, its primary disadvantage is its rather grotesque appearance which many patients will not accept.

WRIST DISARTICULATION: This amputation level is to be preferred over below-elbow amputation when possible because a greater degree of pronation and supination is retained for prosthetic use and a self-suspending prosthesis can be utilized. The unsatisfactory hand which compares unfavorably with a prosthesis in function, comfort, and appearance may be better amputated at the wrist disarticulation level. Such a decision must be made jointly by the surgeon and the patient. Contributory factors include severe tissue loss, pain, appearance, functional requirements, and the patient's body image. In fifteen patients electing hand amputation for various combinations of these factors, eleven were fitted with a prosthesis at the time of operation and three within 3 weeks. All patients expressed satisfaction with their decision, and twelve were successful users of the prosthesis.

AMPUTATIONS WITHIN THE HAND: The incidence of these amputations has been reduced by the advent of microsurgical reimplantation techniques. However, there are still many patients for whom replantation of parts of the hand is either not feasible or results in failure. There is currently no satisfactory functional partial hand prosthesis, and restoration of prehension if unsatisfactory is best accomplished through reconstructive techniques, such as toe to hand transfer. In the complete absence of any prehensile ability, the partial-hand amputee may be best served by a cosmetic fitting for aesthetic purposes.

Bilateral upper limb amputee: Bilateral subtotal hand amputees with intact wrist joints do not need prosthetic fittings that interfere with the sensory capabilities of the remaining portion of the hand.

Wrist disarticulation and long below-elbow stumps, if not treated by the Krukenberg procedure, should be fitted by conventional prosthetic replacement and hooks as terminal devices, although hands may be utilized interchangeably for certain social activities.

Bilateral below-elbow amputees may be fitted with bilateral myoelectric prostheses, but it is generally preferable to supply the patient with at least one unilateral conventional prosthesis which gives the option of using the hook for certain activities. Most bilateral amputees, however, prefer bilateral hooks as terminal devices rather than hands since they are more versatile. Bilateral above-elbow amputees also perform better with bilateral conventional fittings utilizing hooks as terminal devices as well as wrist flexion units.

Lower Limb As in the upper limb, every effort should be made to perform amputation as low as possible. The higher the amputation, the more energy is expended in walking. This is a particular consideration in the dysvascular amputee who will frequently lose the other limb as well. The degree of energy expenditure required in walking with prostheses for a bilateral amputee with knee disarticulation, or higher, amputation will preclude prosthetic rehabilitation in the dysvascular amputee. On the other hand, bilateral below-knee amputees are nearly always rehabilitated to an ambulatory status provided they are ambulatory just prior to their second amputation.

Myoplastic closure should be performed in all lower limb amputations as this technique improves the circulatory physiology of the stump and enhances proprioceptive feedback.

Prosthetic rehabilitation of the elderly above-knee amputee and the young amputee with a hip disarticulation or hemipelvectomy level has been greatly improved by the development of endoskeletal prostheses. These are much lighter than the conventional exoskeletal prostheses of plastic laminate. In the endoskeletal design, a soft foam cover is applied over a rigid tubular weight-bearing assembly. Such prostheses are also much more cosmetic in appearance and may be indicated for the younger female patient with an above-knee amputation. However, very active young people are still fitted with the heavier exoskeletal design due to its superior durability.

It has been well demonstrated that prosthetic rehabilitation of the amputee is vastly enhanced by the concept of an amputee center utilizing a multidisciplinary approach to create a comprehensive program of care. This has resulted in a greatly improved healing rate, as well as a superior prosthetic rehabilitation rate.

Research Experimental research in rabbits has shown that diaphyseal amputation commonly results in proximal arteriovenous shunting whereas disarticulation or transdiaphyseal amputation with myoplastic closure prevents arteriovenous shunts and improves circulation to the distal stump.

Recent clinical investigation utilizing a sensory feedback mechanism from the shank of the prosthesis to a radiofrequency coupled implant on the sciatic nerve has improved the functional ability of thirteen patients so treated. Included were five hip disarticulation amputees, seven above-knee amputees, and one bilateral below-knee amputee. Improved ability to function in the dark, to walk up and down stairs, and to use ramps was noted in nearly all patients. If the implantation is performed at the time of amputation, a marked decrease in postoperative pain was also noted.

Levels

Hemicorpectomy: This mutilating procedure may be indicated as a last resort for life-threatening disease. It also may be used in rare instances to provide increased function in neurologically impaired patients who have severe and intractable pressure sores about the buttocks and pelvis.

Hemipelvectomy: This operation is generally performed as a life-saving procedure in patients with malignancies and yields a 35 percent 5-year survival in such patients. The standard posterior flap for closure is not always available in these patients, depending upon the resection dictated by the disease process, and a long anterior thigh flap and rectus abdominus myocutaneous flap have been described. With this procedure any soft-tissue defect resulting from hemipelvectomy can be safely closed primarily when the posterior flap is not available.

Postoperatively, comfort is enhanced by the application of a rigid dressing to contain the abdominal contents, and prosthetic fitting is feasible in the majority of patients with the newer endoskeletal designs.

Hip disarticulation: Hip disarticulation patients may also experience a high degree of successful prosthetic rehabilitation utilizing the lighter endoskeletal design prostheses. Although the gait of such a patient is slower than when utilizing crutches and no prosthesis, the energy requirements are considerably decreased due to the light weight of the prosthetic design. If preservation of the femoral head and trochanteric areas will not compromise the reason for amputation, retention of these portions of the proximal femur is beneficial in providing more stability within the socket of the prosthetic appliance.

Above knee: In amputations above the knee, the surgeon should strive to provide the longest possible segment to minimize energy expenditure in walking with the prosthesis. Myoplastic closure also facilitates control of the limb since both the quadriceps and hamstring muscles cross the hip joint.

The physiological, as well as psychological, aspects of rehabilitation are enhanced by early, temporary prosthetic fitting, which is generally performed 10 to 14 days following amputation. This technique has been applied with success in children as well as adults.

Prosthetic rehabilitation in the older patient is enhanced by the use of endoskeletal designs and stance phase control knee mechanisms which may be mechanical or hydraulic in nature. In the younger amputee, however, swing phase control knee mechanisms are preferable due to the fact that the cadence of gait is more variable. Also, there is less necessity for a stance phase control due to the superior balance, coordination, and strength of these younger individuals. New mechanisms now available provide both swing and stance control and give superior performance, particularly in the younger individual.

Knee disarticulation: Disarticulation through the knee is preferred over above-knee amputation when technically feasible. Its advantages include superior end bearing, improved prosthetic control, and the ability to utilize a self-suspending socket. When knee disarticulation is performed, the patellar tendon and hamstring tendons should be sutured over the end of the femur or to the cruciate ligaments to provide increased stump strength and proprioception. The patella should be preserved in its normal position.

Reliable and functional internal knee mechanisms are now available for the knee disarticulation amputee.

Below knee: Below-knee amputation remains the level of choice in the dysvascular patient when a more distal amputation cannot be performed. Most elderly and blind patients who were previously ambulatory can successfully be rehabilitated with a below-knee prosthesis.

The use of myocutaneous flaps and myoplastic closure is recommended in the dysvascular patient. Since the anterior flap is generally less well vascularized, either the long posterior flap or medial and lateral flaps are preferred, although short anterior and posterior flaps may also be indicated in certain patients. In posttraumatic amputations which are left open, healing may occur by secondary intention, split-thickness skin grafting, or revision and secondary closure. Split-thickness skin grafts generally hold up well when mature (even on the distal portion of the stump) and are not a contraindication to prosthetic use.

A rigid dressing is recommended postoperatively, and, if possible, the patient should be fitted 10 to 14 days following amputation with a temporary prosthesis. Utilization of early, temporary prosthetic fitting in combination with a newly described removable rigid dressing applied when the prosthesis is not in use greatly facilitate rehabilitation of the below-knee amputation patient.

Permanent prosthetic fitting is most frequently accomplished utilizing a standard exoskeletal design with supracondylar suspension. The endoskeletal design may be used for the very short, below-knee amputee, but distal to this level, reduction in prosthetic weight is not significant enough to sacrifice the added durability of the exoskeletal design.

Syme and foot: The Syme level of amputation has distinct advantages over the below-knee amputation because of its weight-bearing characteristics. It has application in children, adults, and dysvascular patients with diabetes who retain a posterior tibial pulse. It may be performed as a single-stage procedure or as a two-stage procedure if infection is present. The chief disadvantage of the Syme prosthesis is that it is cosmetically poor, but it is self-suspending and provides superior function to the below-knee level. The Syme level is also generally preferable to amputation through Chopart's joint due to subsequent deformity of the hindfoot and prosthetic fitting problems encountered at this level.

The transmetatarsal and Lisfranc amputations within the foot are superior to Syme amputation and require no prosthesis other than a special shoe insert and soft shoe modification to create a rigid forefoot lever arm. Partial foot amputations involving excision of one or more rays also produce a satisfactory functional limb without need for a prosthesis, but in diabetic patients with loss of sensation the increased pressures on the remaining ray or rays may result in ulceration and lead to further amputation.

In children the Boyd amputation in which the os calcis is arthrodesed to the distal tibial epiphysis has been shown to be superior to the Syme amputation. Better length is preserved, heel pad migration is minimized, and socket suspension is enhanced. Also, in children an analysis of partial foot amputations has revealed that midfoot amputations, including the Chopart level, have been superior to the Syme amputation, providing that the hindfoot is balanced and no equinus deformity has developed.

Complications

Pain Phantom pain occurs in nearly all amputees but generally is transient or intermittent and mild. Persistent and intolerable phantom pain is rare but is one of the most dreaded complications of amputation surgery. To date, no uniformly successful treatment has been devised, but the recent use of electrical stimulation has been beneficial in some patients, thus avoiding major neurological operations.

Pain secondary to neuroma formation has been treated successfully by proximal nerve ligation rather than resection of the neuroma which leads to further neuroma formation. Histological examination of nerve fascicles following nerve ligation confirms the fact that no significant neuroma formation occurs following this procedure.

Wound Healing Wound healing problems are frequent in dysvascular amputees. Careful tissue handling and accurate apposition of the skin edges with fine sutures or the use of tape closure may minimize these problems. Although delayed wound healing results in a longer period of rehabilitation, most wound healing problems can be managed without resorting to a signficantly higher level of amputation.

Fracture Fractures occurring in the residual limb of an amputee should be managed by nonoperative means with the exception of unstable intertrochanteric fractures and displaced fractures of the femoral neck. In a review of eighty-five lower limb amputees with ninety subsequent fractures of the residual limb, no indication was found for reamputation through the fracture site. Before fracture, all amputees used their prostheses, and after healing of the fracture, 97 percent of the patients with amputation below the knee and 82 percent of those with amputation above the knee resumed the use of a prosthesis.

Late Complications Late complications of amputation include arthritic changes in the lumbar spine and the remaining limb as well as circulatory problems. Compared to other injured veterans in World War II, patients undergoing extremity amputation had a mortality 1.4 times that of patients with other injuries. This increased mortality was due to ischemic heart disease, other disease of the cardiovascular system, suicide by poisoning, alcoholic cirrhosis, and pancreatitis.

ANNOTATED BIBLIOGRAPHY

General Consideration

Children

Marquardt, E.: The multiple limb-deficient child: Special surgical procedures. *In* Atlas of Limb Prosthetics: Surgical and Prosthetic Principles, p. 601. St. Louis, C.V. Mosby, 1981.

The surgical procedure of stump capping with osteochondral graft as applied to congenital and traumatic amputations in children is described.

Richardson, E.G., and Rambach, B.E.: Proximal femoral focal deficiency: A clinical appraisal. Southern Med. J. 72:166-173, 1979.

The surgical and prosthetic management of children with unilateral proximal femoral focal deficiencies are described.

Shaperman, J., and Sumida, C.T.: Recent advances in research in prosthetics for children. Clin. Orthop. 148:26-33, 1980.

This is an overview of advances in upper limb prosthetics for children, including body power designs as well as externally powered components.

Adults

Brotman, S.; Browner, B.D.; and Cowley, R.A.: Proper timing of amputation for open fractures of the lower extremities. Am. Surg. 48:484-486, 1982.

Considerations in the appropriate timing for amputating lower extremities with open fractures and major soft-tissue damage are outlined. Limb salvage through vascular repair and external fixation is frequently unjustified and may result in sepsis and death.

Considerations in Vascular Disease

Dardik, H.; Ibrahim, I.M.; Jarrah, M.; Sussman, B.; and Dardik, I.: Synchronous aortofemoral or iliofemoral bypass with revascularization of the lower extremity. Surg. Gynec. Ob. 149:676-680, 1979.

Synchronous correction of tandem lesions involving the aortoiliac and femoropopliteal segments should be considered for limb salvage, particularly in the presence of focal gangrene. In thirty-eight patients graft patency was 76 percent. Indications for the procedure are specified.

Evans, L.E.; Webster, M.W.; Brooks, D.H.; and Bahnson, H.T.: Expanded polytetrafluoroethylene femoropopliteal grafts: 48 month follow-up. Surgery 89:16-22, 1981.

Ninety-eight PTFE grafts were used for femoropopliteal reconstruction in eighty-one patients for specific indications including claudication, rest pain, and ischemic pregangrene. Overall cumulative patency rate was 75 percent at 6 months and 48 percent at 4 years.

Flanigan, D.P.; Williams, L.R.; Keifer, T.; Schuler, J.J.; and Behrend, A.J.: Prebypass operative arteriography. Surgery 92:627-633, 1982.

Operative arteriograms were performed in thirty-three patients and found to be beneficial in 91 percent of them. In 66 percent bypass was performed to vessels that were not visualized preoperatively, and major amputation was avoided in 86 percent of patients.

Klimach, O., and Charlesworth, D.: Femorotibial bypass for limb salvage using human umbilical vein. British J. Surg. 70:1-3, 1983.

Of forty-nine patients with pregangrene in whom human umbilical vein bypass worked longer than 2 months, only seven eventually required amputation in contrast to thirty-two of a group of thirty-nine similar patients in whom the bypass failed earlier.

Samson, R.H.; Gupta, S.K.; Scher, L.A.; and Veith, F.J.: Level of amputation after failure of limb salvage procedures. Surg. Gynec. Obstet. 154:56-58, 1982.

Failure of forty-five bypasses to arteries distal to the popliteal resulted in fourteen above-knee amputations. Following twenty-eight unsuccessful femoropopliteal bypasses only two patients needed above-knee amputation.

Selection of Amputation Level

Burgess, E.M.; Matsen, F.A.; Wyss, C.R.; and Simmons, C.W.: Segmental transcutaneous measurements of Po_2 in patients requiring below-the-knee amputation for peripheral vascular insufficiency. J. Bone Joint Surg. 64A:378-382, 1982.

Fifteen patients with below-knee transcutaneous Po_2 values of 40 mm or more had no delay in healing while seventeen of nineteen patients with values of more than 0 but less than 40 mm of mercury had delay of healing at the below-knee level.

Cederberg, P.A.; Pritchard, D.J.; and Joyce, J.W.: Doppler-determined segmental pressures and wound-healing in amputations for vascular disease. J. Bone Joint Surg. 65A:363-365, 1983.

In 102 diabetic and nondiabetic patients with severe vascular disease no demonstrable relationship between calf pressure or calf arm pressure index and the degree of healing of below-knee amputations was found.

Holstein, P.: Level selection in leg amputation for arterial occlusive disease: A comparison of clinical evaluation and skin perfusion pressure. Acta Orthop. Scand. 53:821-831, 1982.

In 102 leg amputations for arterial occlusion it was concluded that ischemia at the below-knee level could not be ruled out by clinical assessment alone and that preoperative determination of the skin perfusion pressure can be used in determining the healing potential in below-knee amputations.

Moore, W.S.; Henry, R.E.; Malone, J.M.; Daly, M.J.; Patton, D.; and Childers, S.J.: Prospective use of Xenon Xe 133 clearance for amputation level selection. Arch. Surg. 116:86-88, 1981.

In forty-five lower limb amputations, healing occurred in all patients with skin flow rates exceeding 2.4 ml/min/100 g of tissue, with two exceptions.

Tanzer, T.L., and Horne, J.G.: The assessment of skin viability using fluorescein angiography prior to amputation. J. Bone Joint Surg. 64A:880-882, 1982.

Fluorescein angiography is shown to be a simple, safe, and useful preoperative bedside technique for the assessment of skin viability and the determination of amputation level in patients with peripheral vascular disease.

Prognosis

Ebskov, B., and Josephsen, P.: Incidence of reamputation and death after gangrene of the lower extremity. Prosthet. Orthot. Internat. 4:77-80, 1980.

The risks of reamputation and loss of the second limb based upon 2,029 amputations from the Danish Amputation Registry since 1972 are described.

Kacy, S.S.; Wolma, F.J.; and Flye, M.W.: Factors affecting the results of below knee amputation in patients with and without diabetes. Surg. Gynec. Obstet. 155:513-518, 1982.

Factors, including cellulitis, hematocrit, cytosis, and use of drains, that affect the success of below-knee amputation in patients with vascular disease are identified.

Huston, C.C.; Bivins, B.A.; Ernst, C.B.; and Griffen, W.O., Jr.: Morbid implications of above-knee amputations: Report of a series and review of the literature. Arch. Surg. 115:165-167, 1980.

The operative mortality for above-knee amputation in vascular patients was 15 percent in a review of 100 patients with an additional 26 percent mortality during a 2-year follow-up.

Surgical and Prosthetic Management

Upper Limb

Research

Herberts, P.; Almström, C.; and Caine, K.: Clinical application study of multifunctional prosthetic hands. J. Bone Joint Surg. 60B:552-560, 1978.

The experimental clinical application of a prosthetic control system utilizing as many as six prosthetic movements is described.

Levels

Above elbow:

Rorabeck, C.H.: The management of the flail upper extremity in brachial plexus injuries. J. Trauma 20:491-493, 1980.

Three different treatment approaches were used in twenty-three patients with complete brachial plexus injuries. Return to gainful employment and prosthetic wearing habits were best achieved with early above-elbow amputation without shoulder arthrodesis.

BELOW ELBOW:

Northmore-Ball, M.D.; Heger, H.; and Hunter, G.A.: The below-elbow myo-electric prosthesis: A comparison of the Otto Bock myo-electric prosthesis with the hook and functional hand. J. Bone Joint Surg. 62B:363-367, 1980.

Forty-three patients who possessed both myoelectric prostheses and standard prostheses were evaluated in terms of use. There was a high rate of acceptance for the myoelectric arm, but acceptance would be increased if greater attention were paid to the durability of the device.

KRUKENBERG'S AMPUTATION:

Tubiana, R.: Krukenberg's operation. Orthop. Clin. North America 12:819-826, 1981.

Indications and contraindications to Krukenberg's amputation are described as well as the operative technique and results experienced.

WRIST DISARTICULATION:

Brown, P.W.: Sacrifice of the unsatisfactory hand. J. Hand Surg. 4:417-423, 1979.

Criteria for amputating the unsatisfactory hand are enumerated, and the decision-making process is discussed based upon fifteen patients who elected amputation. All patients were satisfied with their decision, and twelve were successful users of prostheses.

Lower Limb

Research

Clippinger, F.W.; Seaber, A.V.; McElhaney, J.H.; Harrelson, J.M.; and Maxwell, G.M.: Afferent sensory feedback for lower extremity prosthesis. Clin. Orthop. 169:202-206, 1982.

Sensory feedback has been used in thirteen patients whose sciatic nerves were stimulated by implantable electrodes receiving impulses from the prosthetic shank. Benefits are reduced pain and improved ability to function in the dark and when walking up and down stairs.

Hansen-Leth, C., and Karle, A.: Intracardial arteriographic study on vascular changes in amputated rabbits. Acta Orthop. Scand. 49:457-463, 1978.

Improved vascularization was found in myoplastic amputations and disarticulations as compared with transdiaphyseal amputations in experimental rabbits using angiographic technique.

Levels

HEMIPELVECTOMY:

Temple, W.J.; Mnaymneh, W.; and Ketcham, A.S.: The total thigh and rectus abdominis myocutaneous flap for closure of extensive hemipelvectomy defects. Cancer 50:2524-2528, 1982.

A new method for hemipelvectomy utilizing a thigh flap and rectus abdominus myocutaneous flap as applied to unusual pelvic and thigh tumors is described.

BELOW KNEE:

Wu, Y.; Keagy, R.D.; Krick, H.J.; Stratigos, J.S.; and Betts, H.B.: An innovative removable rigid dressing technique for below-the-knee amputation. J. Bone Joint Surg. 61A:724-729, 1979.

The technique of fabrication and utilization of a removable rigid dressing in the early postoperative period to enhance stump shrinkage is described.

SYME AND FOOT:

Greene, W.B., and Cary, J.M.: Partial foot amputations in children: A comparison of the several types with the Syme amputation. J. Bone Joint Surg. 64A:438-443, 1982.

Partial amputation is divided into three groups: Group I (six patients) with metatarsal ray or transmetatarsal amputation; Group 2 (five patients) with Lisfranc transtarsal or Chopart amputations without equinus contracture; and Group 3 (three patients) with Chopart amputation and equinus contracture. Compared to a Syme amputation group, function was clearly better in patients in Group I, and worse in Group 3.

Blum, C.E., and Kalamchi, A.: Boyd amputations in children. Clin. Orthop. 165:138-143, 1982.

Arthrodesis of the os calcis to the distal tibial epiphysis in forty-two patients is described as being superior to the Syme amputation in weight-bearing characteristics, prevention of heel pad migration, and prosthetic suspension.

Complications

Battista, A.F.; Cravioto, H.M.; and Budzilovich, G.N.: Painful neuroma: Changes produced in peripheral nerve after fascicle ligation. Neurosurgery 9:589-600, 1981.

Sixteen months after resection of the painful neuroma and classical ligation of the proximal nerve segments, no significant neuroma formation was found in the region of the ligation.

Bowker, J.H.; Rills, B.M.; Ledbetter, C.A.; Hunter, G.A.; and Holliday, P.: Fractures in lower limbs with prior amputation: A study of ninety cases. J. Bone Joint Surg. 63A:915-920, 1981.

In a review of eighty-five lower limb amputees with ninety subsequent fractures of the residual limb, most were managed by nonoperative methods. After healing of the fracture, 97 percent of below-knee amputees and 82 percent of above-knee amputees resumed the use of their prostheses.

Louis, D.S.; Hunter, L.Y.; and Keating, T.M.: Painful neuromas in long below-elbow amputees. Arch. Surg. 115:742-744, 1980.

Seven patients did not wear their prostheses because of neuromas in the amputation stumps. Proximal ligation of the median, radial, or ulnar nerve allowed prosthetic use in every patient.

Hrubec, Z., and Ryer, R.A.: Report to the Veteran's Administration Department of Medicine and Surgery on service-connected traumatic limb amputations and subsequent mortality from cardiovascular disease and other causes of death. Bull. Prosthet. Res. 16:29-53, 1979.

This is a comparative study of 36-year mortality in veterans who underwent limb amputations, disfiguration without loss of body part, and those who lost a portion of the hand or foot. Those with limb amputations had a mortality 1.4 and 1.3 times the other groups, respectively.

9 NEUROMUSCULAR DISORDERS AND GAIT

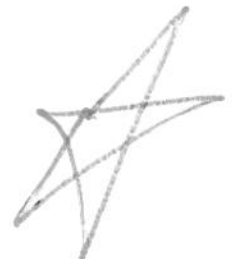

Topics considered in this section include cerebral palsy, muscle disease, spinal cord injury, and stroke. Since gait analysis has become a valuable tool for evaluating these patients and formulating operative plans, a discussion of gait precedes the separate clinical portions.

Gait

Mechanics Normal gait is a complex of postures and muscle activities producing propulsion at minimal energy expense (Fig. 1). Swing phase has been divided into initial, mid-, and terminal thirds (Fig. 2). Throughout swing, the pelvis rotates forward; the hip flexes to 30 degrees; the knee flexes 60 degrees initially and extends terminally; and the ankle plantar flexes 10 degrees initially and becomes neutral terminally. The hip flexors are the main motors advancing the limb in the first two-thirds of swing. The ankle dorsiflexors assure clearance in the final two-thirds of swing. The hamstrings decelerate the thigh in the terminal one-third of swing.

Stance phase is now considered a five-phase activity, involving contact, loading response, mid-stance, terminal stance, and pre-swing (Fig. 3). Throughout stance the pelvis gradually rotates backward and the hip extends. The knee is extended and the ankle is neutral (or slightly plantar flexed) at initial contact; however, during loading, the knee flexes 15 degrees while the ankle plantar flexes 15 degrees. This is an energy-conserving mechanism. By mid-stance the knee is extended and the ankle is neutral again. At pre-swing, the knee flexes 35 degrees and the ankle plantar flexes 20 degrees. In these last phases of stance, the toes, which have been neutral, dorsiflex at the metatarsophalangeal joints. Throughout the first phase of stance, the hamstrings and ankle dorsiflexors remain active. The quadriceps and gluteal muscles become active during loading and throughout early mid-stance to maintain hip and knee stability. In mid-stance, the triceps surae becomes active to control tibial advancement.

Pathological and developmental gait have been analyzed by observational analysis, optical systems, gait electromyography, electrogoniometry, force plate analysis, and oxygen consumption studies. Observational analysis requires an astutely trained eye, but it remains an important method. More precise documentation, however, can be made using optical or electrical systems. The more sophisticated of these systems involve diode reflectors and a computer analyzing scheme to translate key points into stick figures. Electrogoniometry measures three-dimensional joint motion by the use of potentiometers mounted adjacent to the joint.

Force plates, used to analyze direction and magnitude of forces expended during gait, can be utilized to compute gait efficiency. Another recent method of measuring gait efficiency is oxygen consumption.

Gait electromyography can be used to evaluate the temporal sequence of muscle activities in the gait cycle. Currently, there are three limitations to electromyography. The first is that since surface systems are unreliable, small wires must be introduced into the muscle to give good clinical output. Second, stretch reaction of the muscles may be misinterpreted as overactivity. However, if the observer notes the posture of the leg, this pitfall can be avoided. For instance, if a spastic foot is fixed in varus, the electromyogram may show continual activity of the stretched peroneals, but it is obviously illogical to believe that peroneal activity causes the varus. The third limitation is that electromyography is qualitative and not quantitative, indicating when but not how strongly the muscles are active. Despite these disadvantages, gait studies have proved to be valuable aids in preoperative planning for cerebrospastic patients.

Gait or stride analyzers are commercially available to measure the parameters of gait velocity, stride length, and cadence. Increased walking velocity increases stride length and cadence but decreases double stance time. Joint motion is little affected by velocity as demonstrated in these studies.

Development Studies in normal children under 2 years of age demonstrate greater external rotation and flexion at the hip, greater knee flexion, and greater ankle dorsiflexion during stance than normal adults. After 2 years of age angular motions are similar in the two groups. Reciprocal arm motion and heel strike usually are established by 18 months of age. Mature gait (as defined by duration of single limb stance, walking velocity, cadence, step length, and rotation of pelvis) is related to increased relative leg length and balance, and it develops after the age of 3 years.

Cerebral Palsy

Gait Analysis Gait analysis in cerebral palsy has shown that triceps surae action is an important determinant of knee position. Overactivity of the triceps surae can create knee recurvatum in stance phase. This may be controlled by an ankle-foot orthosis to maintain the ankle in neutral position. If the orthosis is not well tolerated, triceps surae lengthening may be necessary. Experimental, temporary paralysis of these muscles in normal individuals can lead to loss of knee stability due to loss of forward tibial restraint. Thus, triceps surae paralysis explains the knee

NORMAL GAIT

	SWING 40%			STANCE 60%				
	INITIAL SWING	MID-SWING	TERMINAL SWING	INITIAL CONTACT	LOADING RESPONSE	MID-STANCE	TERMINAL STANCE	PRE-SWING
TRUNK	ERECT NEUTRAL	ERECT NEUTRAL	ERECT NEUTRAL	ERECT NEUTRAL	ERECT NEUTRAL	ERECT NEUTRAL	ERECT NEUTRAL	ERECT NEUTRAL
PELVIS	LEVEL: BACKWARD ROTATION 5°	LEVEL: NEUTRAL ROTATION	LEVEL: FORWARD ROTATION 5°	LEVEL: MAINTAINS FORWARD ROTATION	LEVEL: LESS FORWARD ROTATION	LEVEL: NEUTRAL ROTATION	LEVEL: BACKWARD ROTATION 5°	LEVEL: BACKWARD ROTATION 5°
HIP	FLEXION 20° NEUTRAL ROTATION ABDUCTION ADDUCTION	FLEXION 20°-30° NEUTRAL ROTATION ABDUCTION ADDUCTION	FLEXION 30° NEUTRAL ROTATION ABDUCTION ADDUCTION	FLEXION 30° NEUTRAL ROTATION ABDUCTION ADDUCTION	FLEXION 30° NEUTRAL ROTATION ABDUCTION ADDUCTION	EXTENDING TO NEUTRAL NEUTRAL ROTATION ABDUCTION ADDUCTION	APPARENT HYPEREXT 10° NEUTRAL ROTATION ABDUCTION ADDUCTION	NEUTRAL EXTENSION NEUTRAL ROTATION ABDUCTION ADDUCTION
KNEE	FLEXION 60°	FROM 60° TO 30° FLEXION	EXTENSION TO 0°	FULL EXTENSION	FLEXION 15°	EXTENDING TO NEUTRAL	FULL EXTENSION	FLEXION 35°
ANKLE	PLANTAR FLEXION 10°	NEUTRAL	NEUTRAL	NEUTRAL HEEL FIRST	PLANTAR FLEXION 15°	FROM PLANTAR FLEXION TO 10° DORSIFLEXION	NEUTRAL WITH TIBIA STABLE AND HEEL OFF PRIOR TO INITIAL CONTACT OPPOSITE FOOT	PLANTAR FLEXION 20°
TOES	NEUTRAL	NEUTRAL	NEUTRAL	NEUTRAL	NEUTRAL	NEUTRAL	NEUTRAL IP EXTENDED MP	NEUTRAL IP EXTENDED MP

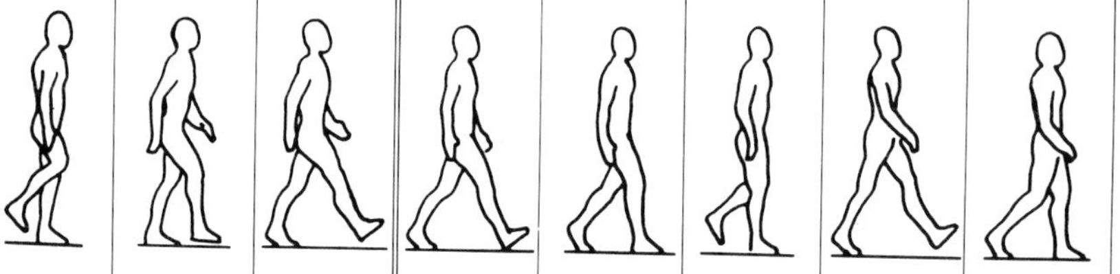

Figure 1: Normal gait.

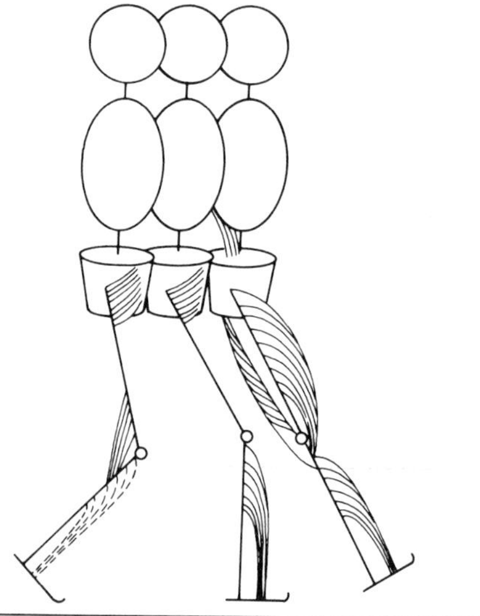

Figure 2: Swing phase of gait.

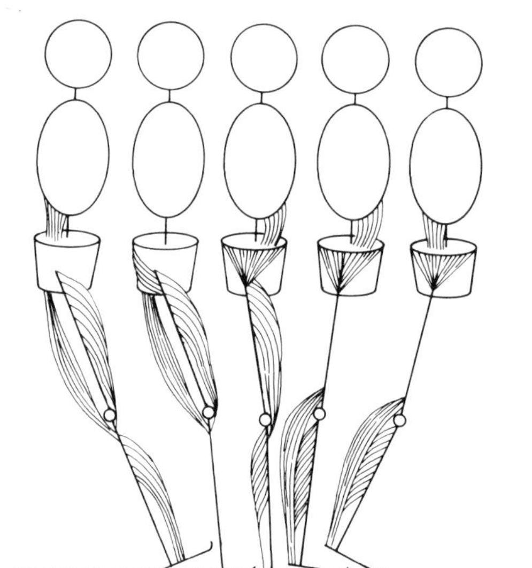

Figure 3: Stance phase of gait.

crouch that may develop in a cerebral palsy child with overcorrected equinus. The brain-damaged adult frequently has knee recurvatum which can be shown by gait electromyography to be related to overactivity of one or more of the quadriceps muscles. Individual release of the quadriceps may correct, or at least improve, the stiff knee gait.

Clinical Problems Cerebral palsy children are classified as hemiplegic (mostly one-sided neural deficit), diplegic (mostly both lower extremity involvement), or totally involved (new designation for quadriplegic). They may be spastic disorders, motion disorders (athetosis, ataxia, dyskinesia), or mixed problems. Ambulation can be expected in those with hemiplegia but rarely is accomplished in those with total involvement. Diplegic patients may ambulate if they have developed balance reaction and reciprocation by 3 years of age. Patients with spastic deformities are most amenable to treatment with orthopaedic surgical procedures and orthoses. Patients with motion disorders have unpredictable surgical and orthotic results.

Knee and foot positions in the cerebral palsy patient are developmental during the first 3 years of life and are subject to spontaneous change with plasters, bracing, and therapy. There is also a danger of overcorrection in dynamic (nonfixed) deformities of the ankle and knee in these first 3 years. Thus, surgery about the knee and ankle is discouraged, but hip surgery may be essential during these years to keep motion and prevent dislocation.

In ambulatory children 3 to 6 years of age, gait can be improved by appropriate tendon lengthenings and selected tendon transfers. Adducted, flexed hips may require adductor, psoas, or other flexor tendon lengthening; plantar flexed ankle deformity may require gastrocnemius or Achilles lengthening; varus feet may require posterior tibial or anterior tibial surgery. After hip and ankle deformities are corrected, hamstring lengthening or transfers may be required in patients with flexed or internally rotated knees. Gait studies can aid the clinician in selecting single or multiple procedures where clinical doubt might exist.

In older children, residual deformities may require bony procedures such as osteotomies of subluxated or rotated femurs and hindfoot stabilizations.

Myelodysplasia

Early closure of the myelodysplastic defect and more efficient shunting for hydrocephalus have resulted in both improved survival rates and neurological function for many of these children. Computed tomographic monitoring for hydrocephalus has proved effective over the last few years. Progressive neurological change also may be due to spinal cord lipomas, cervical hydromyelia, diastematomyelia, Arnold-Chiari deformity, and adherent scars that act as filum terminale tethers during growth.

The ability of myelomeningocele patients to ambulate correlates with the level of neurologic lesion (long-term functional walking is generally not possible with neurologic deficits higher than L3, i.e., less than fair [3+] quadriceps strength), age, obesity, contractures, and control of hydrocephalus. A unilateral dislocated hip, pelvic obliquity, and/or spinal deformity interferes with sitting posture and may result in pressure sores. Deformed insensate feet, even in nonambulators, may also result in pressure areas and local infection.

Muscle Disease

Diagnosis of muscular dystrophy requires a thorough family history, serum creatinine phosphokinase (CPK) determination, diagnostic electromyography, and muscle biopsy. By these means, the most common progressive muscular dystrophy may be separated from the rarer muscular dystrophies and the spinal muscular atrophies, which have a better prognosis. The gait of the muscular dystrophy child first becomes abnormal at the stage of development of lumbar lordosis, which is the result of increased anterior pelvic tilt secondary to gluteus maximus weakness. Gait studies of the leg muscles in these children demonstrate multiple out-of-phase muscle groups attempting to compensate for muscular imbalance. Achilles lengthenings and posterior tibial tendon transfers may improve gait by balancing the ankle forces, although there is no change in muscle activity detectable by gait electromyography. Treatment of progressive hip flexion-abduction contractures requires release of the iliotibial band. Progressive disability also can be delayed in these children by spinal fusions. Spinal muscular atrophy in children varies in its rate of progression. The key factor in evaluation remains serial muscle testing.

Contracture secondary to muscle weakness is the chief cause of disability. Fasciculations of the tongue and developmental scoliosis are important prognostic signs.

Head Injury

The child or adult who suffers a brain injury from trauma frequently has fractures, dislocations, or peripheral neuropathies that may go undetected. Therefore, cervical spine, chest, pelvic, and occasional thoracolumbar radiographs should be considered at the time of admission.

Spinal-Injured Patients

Spinal-injured patients with complete neurologic lesions are not improved by laminectomy, even when the condition is caused by gunshot. Patients with incomplete lesions due to gunshot injury have greater than a 70 percent probability of some improvement with or without laminectomy. Also, instability may be an unfortunate result of extensive laminectomy. Child and adult patients with complete thoracic-level paraplegia rarely ambulate even after intensive therapy. Those who do ambulate tend to stop within the first 5 years after injury. Functional ambulation implies that disabled persons rise from chairs independently, move to other areas to fulfill their own needs, and then sit without assistance. In contrast, exercise ambulators are patients who, if placed in an upright posture, can make forward progress in walkers or parallel bars. The oxygen consumption of paraplegic exercise ambulators has been found to be two to three times normal for a given distance covered. The same paraplegic patient when using a wheelchair may cover distances at speeds approaching normal walking with oxygen consumption similar to normal ambulators.

There are several different recognizable patterns of incomplete spinal cord injury (Table I). The prognosis is variable and depends upon the portion of the cord

76
N

Table I

Incomplete Spinal Cord Injuries and Their Prognoses for Recovery

Syndrome	Salient Features	Prognosis
Brown-Séquard (functional hemi-section)	Motor loss one side, pain and temperature loss opposite side	Good
Central cord syndrome	Usually cervical; all sensory motor functions involved, with greatest involvement at level of lesions; greater sparing distally	Variable; spasticity and poor hand function
Anterior cord syndrome	Complete or partial loss of pain, temperature and motor function; touch and position sense spared	Poor for motor recovery unless pain sensation spared
Posterior cord syndrome	Normal pain; temperature and motor loss; absent touch and position sense	Extremely rare
Concussion	Complete or partial loss momentary with rapid recovery	Normal within 48 hours

(Reprinted with permission from Spinal Cord Injuries, by R.W. Hussey, in Orthopedic Rehabilitation, p. 214. Edited by V.L. Nickel. New York, Churchill Livingstone, 1982.)

involved and the extent of injury.

The greatest problems in the spinal cord injured patient are pressure sores and urologic infections. Pressure-relieving inserts for wheelchairs and beds have been helpful. Plastic surgical flaps for skin closure and intermittent catheterization are newer management approaches for these problems.

Stroke Patients

After a period of initial flaccidity, there is a gradual increase in tone in the flexors and adductors of the lower limbs. Hyperactive tendon reflexes follow and, if spasticity is severe, may be associated with clonus. If muscle tone does not appear within 6 weeks, the prognosis for motor recovery is poor. Voluntary movement usually begins with hip flexion. Motor recovery generally follows a proximal to distal recovery pattern. Two types of voluntary motion have been defined. Pattern motion is the first to recover and consists of mass flexion or mass extension of the hip, knee, and ankle. Selective motor recovery (the ability to precisely control individual muscles and joints independent of activity of other muscles and joints) depends upon the extent of the cerebral cortical damage.

Walking To walk independently, the hemiplegic requires: (1) adequate balance to stand independently; (2) hip flexion to advance the limb; and (3) normal strength in the uninvolved side. If the patient meets these criteria and has retained acceptable cognition, ambulation can be restored in most patients by prescription of an appropriate orthotic aid and assistive devices.

Orthopaedic care of the stroke patient still involves control of limb deformities. Open phenol blocks of motor nerves to muscles with progressively increasing tone may avoid contractures, especially when performed in the first months after a stroke. After this period, lengthening or transfer of tendons may control dynamic deformities. Gait studies can aid the clinician in the selection of specific procedures. The role of functional electrical stimulation currently is being studied and may provide an excellent treatment modality in the future.

Hip Scissoring due to overactive adduction is the most common problem with the hip that can be corrected by surgery. Care should be taken not to release all adductors or perform anterior obturator neurectomy in patients whose adductor muscles are the sole means of limb advancement. Typically, these patients walk sideways so that adduction advances the limb in the line of progression. A patient who has a scissoring gait but walks directly forward also has functioning hip flexors, detectable by palpation and electromyography.

Knee Inappropriate quadriceps activity in the terminal stance and early swing phases of gait prevents adequate knee flexion in some patients. To compensate, the patient must hike the pelvis or circumduct the leg to clear the foot in the swing phase. Electromyographic studies have shown that abnormal activity in the different components of the quadriceps mechanism is often restricted to the rectus femoris and vastus intermedius. If these isolated portions of the quadriceps are tenotomized, knee flexion will improve. However, if spasticity in the other portion of the quadriceps is noted during terminal stance and initial swing phases, release of the rectus femoris and vastus intermedius will likely not improve knee flexion, particularly if both the vastus lateralis and vastus medialis are active at this time. Release of all four components is not indicated since some extensor function must be preserved to stabilize the knee in stance.

Knee flexion deformity in ambulatory hemiplegic patients increases the demand on the quadriceps and may lead to knee instability. This deformity is most often due to overactivity (spasticity) of the hamstring tendons with or without associated myostatic contracture, rather than primarily the result of quadriceps paresis. Although a long-leg orthosis may be used temporarily as a training aid to provide knee stabilization, this device is difficult for the stroke patient to put on and wear and is, therefore, contraindicated for permanent usage. Hamstring tendon release eliminates the dynamic component of the deformity. Residual joint deformity can be corrected by postoperative serial casting. Dynamic electromyograms enable more precise identification of the muscles responsible for knee flexion deformity and enable selective release.

Ankle-Foot Surgical correction of *equinus* most often is indicated when the foot cannot be maintained in the neutral position (with the heel in firm contact with the sole of the shoe) by a well-fitted orthosis which was selected to maintain the ankle in a neutral position. Despite a wide variety of methods designed to weaken the triceps surae, none are believed to be more effective than Achilles tendon lengthening (TAL) in adult patients. Posterior tibial nerve block with a local anesthetic can be a valuable tool in patient assessment. It demonstrates preoperatively the potential benefits of a TAL if the deformity is due to increased muscle tone. The potential exists for the patient to be ambulating brace-free postoperatively if, after a local anesthetic block, the patient is able to dorsiflex the ankle to neutral. However, most hemiplegic patients lack sufficient active dorsiflexion following posterior tibial nerve block and/or TAL and will require some permanent orthotic support to hold the foot in neutral.

Increased ankle dorsiflexion following heel cord tenotomy increases tension on the long toe flexor and frequently leads to painful excessive toe flexion. Therefore, if there is active toe flexion during the stance phase of gait, the extrinsic long toe flexors may be divided prophylactically at the time of TAL.

Electromyographic studies performed in stroke patients with equinus indicate that the triceps surae fire abnormally in most patients prior to heel contact as a part of mass firing of all extensors of the hip, knee, and ankle. Anterior tibialis firing often is delayed in the initial swing phase. Consequently, even following heel cord lengthening, persistent firing of the triceps surae prior to heel contact may result in inadequate dorsiflexion in the late swing phase, even if the anterior tibialis is active. This requires orthotic management to hold the foot in neutral.

Surgical correction of *varus* is indicated to correct a deformity that cannot be corrected by a well-fitted orthosis or to enable the patient to walk without an orthosis.

The tendons of the anterior tibialis, posterior tibialis, flexor hallucis longus, flexor digitorum longus, and gastrosoleus pass medial to the axis of the subtalar joint and, therefore, may potentially cause a varus deformity. The anterior tibialis is nearly always the key muscle responsible for varus, and in most patients this can be confirmed by visual examination and palpation while the subject walks. The split anterior tibialis transfer procedure changes the anterior tibialis from an inverting to an everting force.

Toe flexion deformity is usually due to both long and short toe flexor activity and is responsible for excessive toe flexion causing pain. Treatment consists of dividing the long and short flexors via transverse incisions over the volar aspect of each toe.

ANNOTATED BIBLIOGRAPHY

Gait

Beck, R.J.; Andriacchi, T.P.; Kuo, K.N.; Fermier, R.W.; and Galante, J.O.: Changes in the gait patterns of growing children. J. Bone Joint Surg. 63A:1452-1457, 1981.

The gait patterns, including time and distance measurements and ground reaction forces, of fifty-one normal children were studied. An increase in height was found to be the major factor in determining the changes in gait patterns with age.

Norlin, R.; Odenrick, P.; and Sandlund, B.: Development of gait in the normal child. J. Pediat. Orthop. 1:261-266, 1981.

Velocity, stride length, cadence, and the temporal phases of the stride of 230 normal children were studied. Parameters changed with age, and the changes were most pronounced up to 8 and 10 years of age.

Sutherland, D.H.; Cooper, L.; and Daniel, D.: The role of the ankle plantar flexors in normal walking. J. Bone Joint Surg. 62A:354-363, 1980.

Gait studies demonstrated that the ankle plantar flexion muscles contribute to knee and ankle stability by restraining forward rotation of the tibia on the talus during stance.

Sutherland, D.H.; Olshen, R.; Cooper, L.; and Woo, S.L.: The development of mature gait. J. Bone Joint Surg. 62A:336-353, 1980.

Normative data on 186 children, ages 1 through 7 years, demonstrated increased knee and ankle dorsiflexion under the age of 2 years. Thereafter, cadence decreased, while velocity and step length increased.

Cerebral Palsy

Csongradi, J.; Bleck, E.; and Ford, W.F.: Gait electromyography in normal and spastic children, with special reference to quadriceps femoris and hamstring muscles. Devel. Med. Child Neurol. 21:738-748, 1979.

The average child with spastic cerebral palsy was found to have a shorter stance phase than normal. However, the cadence, while more variable, was nearly the same as normal. The spastic muscles typically exhibited prolonged phasic activity or a dysphasic pattern. Most of the patients with spastic hamstrings also had spastic quadriceps.

Hoffer, M.M., and Koffman, M.: Cerebral palsy: The first three years. Clin. Orthop. 151:222-227, 1980.

Surgical procedures in the first 3 years of life are usually limited to the adductor releases about the hip. Stretching and plaster splints about the ankle and knee, followed by ankle-foot orthoses, are frequently effective in correction of deformity.

Simon, S.R.; Deutsch, S.D.; Nuzzo, R.M.; Mansour, M.J.; Jackson, J.L.; Koskinen, M.; and Rosenthal, R.K.: Genu recurvatum in spastic cerebral palsy. Report on findings by gait analysis. J. Bone Joint Surg. 60A:882-894, 1978.

Gait patterns of fifteen children demonstrated the calf muscle and tibial movement relationships causing recurvatum. This was corrected by ankle-foot orthoses in some.

Sutherland, D.H.: Gait analysis in cerebral palsy. Devel. Med. Child Neurol. 20:807-813, 1978.

A review article of all recent cerebral palsy gait studies showed electromyograms obtained during walking are of great value in planning treatment.

Waters, R.L.; Garland, D.E.; Perry, J.; Habig, T.; and Slabaugh, P.: Stiff-legged gait in hemiplegia: Surgical correction. J. Bone Joint Surg. 61A:927-933, 1979.

Selective tenotomy of one or two heads of the quadriceps based on electromyographic criteria improved knee flexion in hemiplegic patients who walked with a unilateral stiff-legged gait.

Muscle Disease

Benady, S.G.: Spinal muscular atrophy in children: Review of 50 cases. Devel. Med. Child Neurol. 20:746-757, 1978.

An early age of onset and the presence of tongue fasciculation carry a poor prognosis for disability. Scoliosis appears early in children with the more severe forms. Contractures are the main cause of progressive disability.

Evans, G.A.; Drennan, J.C.; and Russman, B.S.: Functional classification and orthopaedic management of spinal muscular atrophy. J. Bone Joint Surg. 63B:516-522, 1981.

The subdivision of patients into four groups, based on the maximal physical function, correlates well with the severity of deformity of the limbs and spine.

Melkonian, G.J.; Cristofaro, R.L.; Perry, J.; and Hsu, J.D.: Dynamic gait electromyography study in Duchenne muscular dystrophy (DMD) patients. Foot and Ankle 1:78-83, 1980.

In patients with weakened leg muscles, multiple muscle groups fire out-of-phase in an attempt to overcome the action of the stronger muscles, thus stabilizing the limb for ambulation.

Siegel, I.M.: The management of muscular dystrophy: A clinical review. Muscle Nerve 1:453-460, 1978.

Progressive disability can be delayed by surgical release of lower extremity contracture, repair of foot and ankle deformity, and correction of scoliosis.

Sutherland, D.H.; Olshen, R.; Cooper, L.; Wyatt, M.; Leach, J.; Mubarak, S.; and Schultz, P.: The pathomechanics of gait in Duchenne muscular dystrophy. Devel. Med. Child Neurol. 23:3-22, 1981.

The earliest postural change in gait of patients with this disease is increased lumbar lordosis secondary to gluteus maximus weakness. Insufficiency of this muscle causes anterior pelvic tilt, restricted hip extension, and maintenance of the line of floor reaction force in front of the knee.

Head Injury

Garland, D.E., and Bailey, S.: Undetected injuries in head injured adults. Clin. Orthop. 155:162-165, 1981.

Of 254 adults admitted over a period of 2 years to the Head Trauma Service, twenty-nine (11 percent) had ten previously undiagnosed fractures and/or dislocations and twenty-nine had previously undetected peripheral neuropathies.

Spinal-Injured Patients

Cerny, K.; Waters, R.; Hislop, H.; and Perry, J.: Walking and wheelchair energetics in persons with paraplegia. Phys. Ther. 60:1133-1139, 1980.

The energetics of walking with orthoses and wheelchair propulsion at free velocity were tested. Walking was significantly more difficult for paraplegics to perform than wheelchair propulsion.

Mikelberg, R., and Reid, S.: Spinal cord lesions and lower extremity bracing: An overview and follow-up study. Paraplegia 19:379-385, 1981.

Sixty people tended to use their orthoses at home only for standing and exercise.

Nickel, V.L.: Orthopedic Rehabilitation. New York, Churchill Livingstone, 1982.

A review of all phases of orthopaedic rehabilitation. This stresses a disease-oriented approach involving the orthopaedic surgeons directly with the allied health team.

Stauffer, E.S.; Hoffer, M.M.; and Nickel, V.L.: Ambulation in thoracic paraplegia. J. Bone Joint Surg. 60A:823-824, 1978.

Complete paraplegic children and adults rarely ambulate functionally even after intense therapy. After 5 years those that did ambulate cease to do so.

Stauffer, E.S.; Wood, R.W.; and Kelly, E.G.: Gunshot wounds of the spine: The effects of laminectomy. J. Bone Joint Surg. 61A:389-392, 1979.

In a review of 185 patients, laminectomy did not improve any complete lesion. Seventy-one percent of patients with incomplete lesions treated by laminectomy and 76 percent of patients with incomplete unoperated lesions improved. Thus, laminectomy did not affect prognosis for neurological recovery.

Stroke Patients

Frazier, J.K.; Waters, R.L.; and Garland, D.: Electromyographic analysis of equinovarus before and after surgical correction. *In* Proceedings of the 26th Annual Orthop. Res. Soc. Meeting, p. 284, Atlanta, Georgia, February 5-7, 1980.

Dynamic walking electromyograms on twenty-five patients hemiplegic from stroke, head trauma, or brain tumor with equinus or equinovarus deformities were done before and at least 6 months after surgery. Conclusions were: (1) premature and prolonged firing of the triceps surae were present in most patients; (2) muscle firing pattern did not change as a result of surgery; (3) tibialis anterior was a major contributor to varus deformity; (4) split anterior tibialis tendon transfer to the third cuneiform and cuboid redirected excessive varus pull creating a corrective valgus force; and (5) if active in swing phase, the flexor hallicus longus was satisfactory for transfer to assist ankle dorsiflexion.

10 CIRCULATORY, RESPIRATORY, HEMATOPOIETIC, GASTROINTESTINAL, GENITOURINARY, AND INTEGUMENTARY SYSTEMS

Topics in this section include diagnosis, prevention, and treatment of thromboembolism disease; osteonecrosis; fat embolism; adult respiratory distress syndrome; hemophilia; hemorrhagic shock; and skin ulcers.

Circulatory, Respiratory, and Hematopoietic Systems

Thromboembolism Thromboembolism is the most prevalent complication after lower extremity surgery in adults, and pulmonary embolism is the most common fatal complication following lower extremity trauma or surgery. Thrombophlebitis occurs in 40 to 60 percent of patients over the age of 40 undergoing surgery about the hip or knee, and the incidence is similar following tibia and femur fractures. Fewer thrombi occur in the calves of patients on whom tourniquets are used probably because there is increased systemic fibrinolytic activity following tourniquet release. The incidence of thromboembolic disease following spine fusion is much less than that following lower extremity surgery. More likely in extensive operations which involve longer fusions and increased blood loss, this complication tends to be encountered in the proximal venous system, usually in the left iliac vein which is more vulnerable to stasis when a patient is prone.

EVALUATION: Patients at risk for thromboembolic disease may be evaluated by physical examination, phlebography, radioactive scanning, outflow obstruction measurement, and thermography. Sole reliance on other findings such as complaints of pain, swelling, tenderness, Homan's sign, fever, and leukocytosis leads to marked underdiagnosis of thromboembolic disease. Only 5 to 30 percent of thrombophlebitis will be detected by physical examination alone. Furthermore, approximately 50 percent of patients suspected of having thrombophlebitis have negative findings on the laboratory evaluations described above.

Phlebography is the most exact evaluation technique for diagnosing thrombophlebitis. Its disadvantages include pain, inability to be repeated frequently, and resultant complications (such as thrombophlebitis and allergic reaction to the dye which occurs in approximately 1 in 5,000 patients). Despite disadvantages, phlebography is accurate in the calf and femoral veins and approximately 70 percent reliable in the iliac veins. Because of this accuracy, it is the test by which other evaluation methods are measured and is especially valuable in clinical research involving thromboembolic disease.

Radioactive fibrinogen (I125) is 90 percent accurate in detecting thrombophlebitis in the absence of recent trauma or operation in the area being evaluated. Any such area will normally reveal increased uptake when scanned. For example, this examination is not helpful in the proximal thigh following hip surgery. The significant advantages of this scan include little patient discomfort and the ability to repeat as desired.

Measurements of outflow obstruction include pneumatic plethysmography, cuff-impedence phlebography, and Doppler ultrasound techniques. These methods are most accurate for thrombi in major veins and are less so in the presence of small vein thrombi because of the insignificant difference in outflow. These tests are not as exact as either venography or radioactive fibrinogen scanning. Thermographic techniques have been tested on a small scale and may have future application but currently are limited to experimental use.

Another method under investigation is a *coagulolysis assay* that measures coagulation and fibrinolysis processes by the products in the serum. These methods show some promise but will require considerable technique improvement and documentation before consideration for routine clinical use.

Arterial oxygenation evaluation has been suggested as a screening test for pulmonary embolism. Used alone it is unreliable, and if pulmonary embolism is suspected clinically, the patient should have a *ventilation and perfusion scan*. If questions still remain, *pulmonary angiography* may be necessary. These objective tests also may be necessary with suspected recurrent pulmonary embolus. Vena caval interruption may become necessary in patients on adequate anticoagulation therapy.

Prophylactic Treatment of Thromboembolic Disease Methods recommended for prevention of thromboembolic disease include: physical or mechanical measures; anticoagulants, including heparin and Coumadin; and antithrombotic drugs.

The ideal treatment, of course, would be a highly effective method associated with little or no potential complications. Present anticoagulant drugs remain the most effective prophylactic methods, but their use carries a risk of bleeding complications. *Sodium warfarin* and *dextran-70* are most useful in reducing the occurrence of serious thromboembolic disease.

Heparin in low dose is effective in thoracic, abdominal, and pelvic surgical procedures, but evaluation of its effectiveness following lower extremity surgery and trauma has produced contradictory results. The action mechanism of low-dose heparin probably is an increased rate at which antithrombin-3 inhibits activated factor X and thrombin. In a major surgical procedure (such as total hip arthroplasty) or after major trauma the coagulation system activation may be so intense that thrombin generation exceeds its inhibitory rate, even in the presence of small amounts of heparin. Thrombin generation also releases platelet factor IV which has anti-heparin activity.

Somewhat higher doses of heparin than recommended after abdominal procedures have been used for the prevention of thromboembolic disease in the lower extremity. A small device known as a coagulometer was used in one group of patients to assess the state of the coagulation system and, thus, the heparin dose. Using this technique, heparin in relatively low dosage was effective in preventing thromboembolic disease following surgery for hip fractures. An additional finding was that most patients exhibited a state of significant hypercoagulability at 5 to 7 days following surgery; thus, heparin was continued well beyond this time. Many low-dose heparin regimes are discontinued at 5 to 7 days or at the time of patient mobilization. Though incidence of bleeding complications in general surgical procedures administering low-dose heparin has been minimal or nonexistent, most patients with lower extremity orthopaedic surgical procedures experience an increased likelihood of bleeding complications.

A potentially serious complication with heparin use for antithromboembolism prophylaxis is the paradoxical effect of arterial embolism. Clinically apparent arterial embolisms may occur 7 to 15 days after the onset of heparin administration. Heparin-induced thrombocytopenia often results in a platelet count of less than 100,000 and perhaps as low as 30,000. Most patients who develop clinically apparent embolisms have premonitory symptoms involving the gastrointestinal tract and musculoskeletal system for 1 to 2 days prior to major embolus. The most common embolization site is the aortic bifurcation with occurrences possible in other major arteries, including the iliac and femoral. The emboli consist of platelet-rich fibrin with a few red blood cells which may be caused by aggregation of platelets due to prolonged administration of heparin. It has also been suggested that an anti-heparin antibody may become active, leading to platelet aggregation. Major embolism occurring during heparin therapy carries a 60 percent mortality rate. The treatment recommended is immediate surgery for embolus removal and discontinuation of heparin therapy.

The antithrombotic action of *aspirin* is related to its inhibition of the prostaglandins, thromboxane (a potent stimulus to platelet aggregation), and prostacyclin (a vasodilator and inhibitor of platelet aggregation synthesized by human endothelial cells). Aspirin blocks the activity of prostaglandin cyclo-oxygenase by irreversible acetylation, thus preventing the formation of active prostaglandins. By this inhibition, aspirin has both a thrombotic and antithrombotic effect. In low dosage (no more than 600 mg b.i.d.) the platelet prostaglandin may be affected more than that produced by human endothelial cells, resulting in a net antithrombotic effect. An excessive dose of aspirin (ten times that required for an antithrombotic effect) may reduce its effectiveness or even increase thrombosis. In general, low-dose aspirin is useful in reducing the incidence of both thrombophlebitis and pulmonary embolism. At least one study found a significant difference in the effectiveness between males and females, with aspirin prophylactically useful only in males. However, this is controversial since another study shows effectiveness in females, though not as great as in males. There has been no evidence of increased bleeding complications with aspirin. With the exception of fractures about the hip, the effectiveness of aspirin has not been evaluated in lower extremity trauma.

Hydroxychloroquine and *sulfinpyrazone*, two drugs with antithrombotic activity, have been suggested for prophylactic use in thromboembolic disease. The results of their administration in orthopaedic surgery have been somewhat controversial with less evidence for the effectiveness of sulfinpyrazone than for hydroxychloroquine.

Numerous investigations of various combinations of anticoagulant and antithrombotic medications have yielded no evidence that a drug combination is more effective than the use of one agent—and in many instances the use of combination therapy has resulted in increased complications, particularly bleeding.

Physical and *mechanical* means of prevention of thromboembolic disease include early mobilization of patients after surgery or trauma, the use of antithromboembolism stockings, and the early initiation of muscle exercises with lower extremity motion. More sophisticated mechanical means investigated include passive motion applied during the operation and use of mechanical compression devices surgically and postsurgically to improve venous outflow from the lower extremities. None of these methods effectively prevents or reduces the incidence of thromboembolic disease when used alone. Investigation of these methods should continue since they have the advantage of a low complication rate.

Osteonecrosis Death of bone tissue may occur anywhere in the skeleton. When necrosis of bone occurs in limited areas of the diaphysis or metaphysis, the skeleton continues to perform its support function. Unless a radiograph is taken for another reason, these infarcts go unnoticed. A possible, but rare, long-term complication of bone infarct may be transformation to a malignant fibrous tumor. Only when necrotic bone no longer performs its support function, usually adjacent to a joint surface, do symptoms occur.

ETIOLOGY: The cause of osteonecrosis following a specific episode of trauma is the loss of blood supply for a time sufficient to result in cellular death. The etiology of nontraumatic osteonecrosis is less clear. Compromise of blood supply to bone tissue may be present, but there may be other factors. Steroid administration may be involved in the pathogenesis of osteonecrosis following renal transplantation as well as in other diseases, but it is difficult to correlate the steroid dosage with the occurrence of osteonecrosis. Older patients who have a low serum phosphorus have evidence of significant bone disease and experience delay in renal function normalization following the procedure are more likely to develop osteonecrosis following renal transplantation. An additional complication found in one large series of patients following this procedure was a 26 percent incidence of fractures, which included the pelvis more commonly than the long bones. All fractures healed without complication, usually following closed methods of treatment.

Steroid intake results in an increase in serum cholesterol, fatty metamorphosis of the liver, and occurrence of

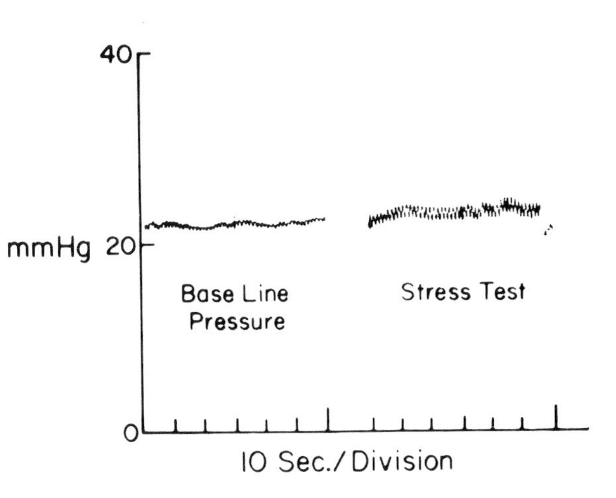

Figure 1-A

Figure 1-B

Figure 1: Intraosseous pressure and stress test measured in the proximal femoral metaphysis. (A) Normal pressure and stress test. (B) Slightly increased baseline pressure and substantially increased stress test in a patient with Stage I alcoholism-associated osteonecrosis. (Reprinted with permission from Alcoholism associated ischemic necrosis, by Hungerford, et al., Clin. Orthop. 130:144-153, 1978.)

fat emboli in small vessels. In addition, there is an increase of approximately 25 percent in the marrow fat cell volume and of 15 percent in the total volume of the marrow compartment due to osteoporosis. An increased cell volume greater than the marrow compartment space volume may cause heightened pressure and damage to the vascular sinusoidal elements. Similar changes may occur with heavy alcohol intake.

Elevated vascular pressure and delayed emptying of radiopaque dye from the intraosseous space are found in patients who have osteonecrosis associated with alcohol intake (Figs. 1, 2, and 3). The mechanism of development of osteonecrosis in patients presenting with severe pressure changes is probably multifactorial, involving ischemia due to intravascular and extravascular nitrogen bubbles, fibrin thrombi, platelet aggregation, clumping of formed elements of blood (mainly erythrocytes with lipids), and blood flow changes. It is suggested that emboli may not be a cause of osteonecrosis in metabolic disorders. Instead, it is proposed that the bone cells are unhealthy because of metabolic disorders and toxic substances, such as alcohol and steroids, may be enough additional insult to cause cell death, eventually resulting in osteonecrosis.

There are no significant alterations in the biochemical and metabolic parameters of cartilage overlying necrotic bone in either traumatic or nontraumatic forms of osteonecrosis. Secondary changes due to mechanical factors and similar to those in osteoarthritis eventually occur in cartilage.

In patients who present with unilateral symptomatic osteonecrosis, a search for similar skeletal lesions at other sites is warranted (particularly in a contralateral hip) since some forms of treatment are effective only if performed before osteochondral collapse and significant symptoms develop. If a patient is symptomatic and no radiographic changes are noted, a radioactive bone scan may be helpful. Tomography may demonstrate the "crescent sign" or transchondral fracture earlier than plain radiographs.

TREATMENT: The treatment for osteonecrosis depends upon etiology, stage of involvement (Table I), symptoms, and location. The most common site of osteonecrosis requiring surgical treatment is the femoral head. If post-traumatic, or a form of nontraumatic, osteonecrosis is diagnosed before an osteochondral fracture or collapse occurs, a fibular bone graft may retard those developments and prevent symptomatic osteonecrosis. Once osteochondral fracture and collapse occur in the femoral head, most patients require major reconstructive surgery such as arthroplasty or arthrodesis. Successful early results have been reported with the transtrochanteric anterior rotational osteotomy of the femoral head by one author. Patients with osteonecrosis associated with alcoholism may benefit from decompression of the femoral head and neck by drilling. Patients who demonstrate no osteochondral fracture prior to this procedure have no further progression following decompression. Those with a crescent sign or osteochondral fracture have shown temporary symptomatic improvement but continue to have progressive destruction on radiographs. Osteonecrosis of the femoral condyle may heal if detected early and protected by nonweight-bearing, appropriate immobilization, or realignment osteotomy. Individuals who develop osteone-

Table I
Stages of Osteonecrosis

Stage I	Normal x-ray, diagnosis based on histologic changes of ischemic necrosis.
Stage II	X-ray changes are present but may not be typical for ischemic necrosis. No osteochondral fracture.
Stage III	Characteristic changes of ischemic necrosis with wedge-shaped increased density and mottled osteoporosis. A subchondral lucent line is visible, and the head is no longer spherical.
Stage IV	Marked changes in the femoral head with secondary degenerative changes in the hip joint.

Classification of ischemic necrosis of Arlet and Ficat.

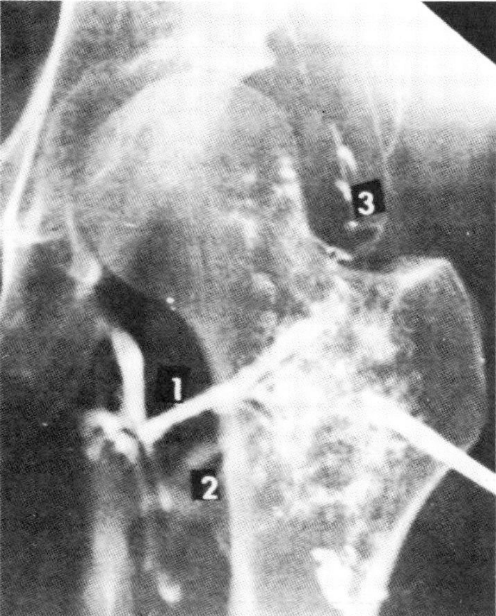

Figure 2-A

Figure 2-B

Figure 2: Normal intraosseous venogram of the proximal femur. (A) The venogram demonstrates: (1) liminocapsular veins; (2) circumflex femoral veins; and (3) gluteal veins. (B) Five minutes after injection most of the Renografin has cleared the bone. (Reprinted with permission from Alcoholism associated ischemic necrosis of the femoral head, by D.S. Hungerford, et al., Clin. Orthop. 130:144-153, 1978.)

crosis at this site following renal transplantation occasionally may heal their osteonecrotic segment without sequelae. Those patients progressing to osteochondral fracture and collapse may require realignment osteotomy, removal of loose bodies, arthrodesis, or prosthetic reconstruction.

Both posttraumatic and nontraumatic osteonecrosis of the talus may require major surgical reconstruction. Osteonecrosis of the humeral head not associated with a major traumatic episode should be treated with activity limitation to reduce the forces across the shoulder joint and passive or assisted exercises to maintain motion. Healing may occur without surgical intervention. Even with moderate deformity many patients will continue to function well. Those who develop severe symptoms can be treated successfully with prosthetic replacement usually not requiring resurfacing of the glenoid. Osteonecrosis in itself is not painful, and symptoms are the result of attempted biological repair of necrotic bone. Methods which prevent the reparative process in experimental animals may allow continued function of skeletal support without development of symptoms. Such therapeutic techniques involve the chemical fixation of bone to prevent repair or the removal of necrotic bone and replacement with a nonliving plastic. Another procedure still considered experimental is the replacement of the subchondral bone and articular cartilage with human allografts. These techniques currently are being studied and may have future application in the treatment of osteonecrosis.

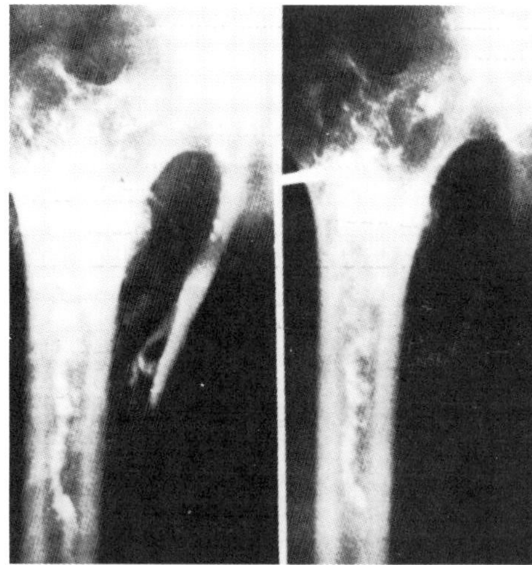

Figure 3: Intraosseous venogram of the proximal femur in a patient with Stage I alcoholism associated osteonecrosis. Poor filling of the main drainage veins (left). Delayed venous emptying of the proximal femur (right). (Reprinted with permission from Alcoholism associated ischemic necrosis of the femoral head, by D.S. Hungerford, et al., Clin. Orthop. 130:144-153, 1978.)

Fat Embolism Syndrome Fat embolism syndrome is a clinical symptom complex consisting of tachypnea, tachycardia, fever, mental status change, and petechiae. It occurs much more commonly in young adults than in any other age group and is quite rare in children, only occurring in about 0.05 percent with femur fractures. Its incidence correlates positively with the number of long bones fractured, open fractures, and fractures caused by vehicular accidents.

It was believed that fat embolism syndrome was caused by the alteration of pulmonary function brought on directly by fat emboli from the fractured bone. Whereas fat emboli are found in the lungs of patients sustaining fractures and other major musculoskeletal trauma, there is now evidence that fat emboli are metabolized into free fatty acids which have a toxic action on the lung parenchyma and produce respiratory distress and chemical pneumonitis. There is a strong stimulus to platelet aggregation by thromboplastin released from damaged tissue. Thromboplastin causes disseminated intravascular coagulation and a disturbance of the colloidal stability of plasma lipids, allowing the formation of additional intravascular fat particles. Both platelets and erythrocytes adhere to fat particles resulting in emboli that consist of fat macroglobules, platelets, and erythrocytes which lodge in the lungs resulting in further release of free fatty acids. Finally, hypovolemia and poor oxygenation have an important role in development of the clinical manifestations of fat embolism syndrome.

TREATMENT: Maintenance of normal blood volume and proper oxygenation are important in preventing these clinical manifestations. Treatment includes blood volume replacement, cardiotonic drugs, and respiratory support. Thirty to 40 percent oxygen delivered by mask is adequate in many patients, but some will require positive pressure breathing. In addition to supportive measures, alcohol or steroids have been recommended. Patients who have a blood alcohol level of less than 0.02 g per 100,000 are more likely to develop clinical fat embolism syndrome than are patients with higher blood alcohol levels. On this basis, alcohol has been recommended as a treatment for this syndrome, but results are inconclusive. In experimental animal studies, methylprednisolone suppresses many abnormalities that occur during this syndrome. Steroids inhibit platelet aggregation, platelet factor III availability, and serotonin release; stabilize the release of tissue thromboplastin from injured tissues; and result in an increase in lung surfactant. Atelectasis, inflammation, and alveolar membrane thickening are reduced with methylprednisolone administration. There is also increased cardiac output, increased pulmonary vasodilatation, and decreased pulmonary shunt. Glucose administration partially ameliorates the decrease in Pa_{O_2} following trauma but does not prevent occurrence of the syndrome. Most evidence suggests that patients with clinical fat embolism syndrome should be treated by cardiorespiratory support, but in resistant cases or in the presence of multiple fractures, methylprednisolone treatment may be considered.

A similar syndrome has been reported following total hip arthroplasty and femoral prosthetic placement in which methyl methacrylate is used. Less commonly, the syndrome may occur following total knee replacement, usually with a long-stem prosthesis (although it has been reported following implantation of a total condylar prosthesis).

Adult Respiratory Distress Syndrome This condition occurs following trauma and is similar to fat embolism syndrome in symptomatology and pathogenesis. The occurring tachypnea, dyspnea, and hypoxemia are resistant to routine methods of oxygen administration. Patients also exhibit restlessness, anxiety, cough with significant pulmonary secretions, and often an expiratory wheeze. In later stages of the disease an almost complete consolidation in the lung fields may occur. The mortality rate of adult respiratory distress syndrome, even with modern forms of treatment, is 25 to 59 percent, which is higher than that seen with fat embolism syndrome. The incidence of the syndrome reportedly is approximately 2 percent of all patients sustaining severe trauma.

The etiology is probably multifactorial. Fluid overload, lung emboli, aspiration of gastric contents, shock, and particulate matter (such as platelet aggregates and fibrin thrombi passing through standard blood filters and lodging in the pulmonary capillaries) have been suggested as etiologic factors. Recent investigations indicate the presence of leukoagglutinants in transfused blood that may be responsible for this syndrome. Finally, there is experimental evidence that cerebral hypoxia or injury will cause some changes consistent with respiratory distress syndrome.

Mechanical ventilation may be successful treatment, but if the Pa_{O_2} cannot be raised to 70 mm of mercury with an FI_{O_2} of 0.5, positive end expiratory pressure is necessary. In addition to respiratory support, these patients require adequate volume and blood replacement as well as the use of cardiotonic drugs, if necessary to maintain cardiac function.

Hemophilia Hemophilia is a genetically inherited group of bleeding disorders characterized by deficiency or absence of specific coagulation factors, most commonly VIII. The degree of deficiency and, thus, the degree of coagulation defect determine the severity of the clinical problems. Patients with marked deficiency (less than 1 percent) exhibit coagulation deficiency and bleeding episodes at very early ages and may develop characteristic radiographic joint findings by the age of 5 years.

TREATMENT: Hospital treatment of patients with severe hemophilia has been reduced substantially in recent years by home treatment programs. The home administration of factor VIII allows earlier treatment of bleeding complications (such as hemarthrosis), reduces cost of treatment, and probably improves social development.

Severe hemophiliac arthropathy generally is correlated with the severity and frequency of bleeding into the joint. Though both mechanical and chemical means are responsible for damage to joints, enzymatic processes appear to be the primary cause of cartilage matrix degradation. In addition to hemophiliac arthropathy, there may be other serious musculoskeletal complications. Bleeding within closed compartments may cause neuropathy and muscle contracture. Patients who present with hemophilia and symptoms and signs suggestive of compartment syndrome should have immediate replacement therapy to achieve a level adequate for surgery. If increased compartment pressure is confirmed, fasciotomy should be performed. Repeated bleeding into muscles may cause an expanding pseudotumor which may be life-threatening. Excision is sometimes necessary.

Patients with hemophilia commonly suffer fractures as a result of osteoporosis, joint stiffness, and muscle weakness. Most fractures can be treated nonoperatively. Circular casts should not be applied initially. Instead, the fracture should be splinted, and the patient treated with replacement therapy until all bleeding is under control. A factor level of 30 percent or more should be maintained for 2 to 7 days, depending upon the severity of the fracture.

In patients with synovitis and recurrent hemarthroses but with preservation of joint (cartilage) space, synovectomy may decrease pain and prevent recurrent bleeds. Release of contractures may result in substantial functional improvement in patients with joint contractures resulting from bleeding into muscle and/or compartment syndromes. Patients with severe hemophiliac arthropathy may be treated successfully with total joint replacement. Caution must be exercised in patients with such arthropathy because they probably have some increased risk of infection due to the frequent necessity for intravenous replacement therapy throughout their expected long life spans.

Patients with lesser forms of hemophilia or other coagulation defects may present with musculoskeletal disorders requiring surgery. If these coagulation deficiencies are unrecognized, catastrophic postoperative bleeding may result. The most effective means of avoidance is an adequate history. Many drugs (such as aspirin and other anti-inflammatory agents) may increase the bleeding tendency by decreasing coagulation efficiency. All patients undergoing surgery should be asked about previous bleeding tendency, particularly in connection with dental extraction or tonsillectomy. If there is any question of coagulation defect based on history, the most appropriate evaluation is assay for specific coagulation factors. If coagulation defects are found, the patient should receive adequate replacement therapy of cryoprecipitate or factor concentrate pre- and postoperatively.

Inhibiting antibodies to replacement factors occurs in 4 to 20 percent of patients with classic hemophilia but is much less common in patients with mild to moderate forms. Such inhibiting antibodies contraindicate surgery except for the most life-threatening problems. If surgery is necessary for a life- or limb-threatening situation in a hemophiliac with inhibiting antibodies, activated factors are available, but there is considerable controversy about the safety of their use.

Sickle Cell Anemia Patients with sickle cell anemia tend to have associated musculoskeletal problems, including osteonecrosis, sickle cell arthropathy, and sickle cell dactylitis. Osteonecrosis in the femoral head is commonly associated with sickle cell disease but is believed to occur rarely in patients with sickle cell traits. Arthropathy is common and usually manifests itself as a transient noninflammatory effusion which normally does not lead to severe joint destruction. Some patients develop chronic destructive synovitis resulting in articular cartilage damage and severe joint destruction. Various surgical reconstructions may be necessary in patients who develop severe joint dysfunction due to osteonecrosis or sickle cell arthropathy. There is no higher complication rate in sickle cell disease patients with tourniquet usage for orthopaedic procedures than in any other patients. Patients with this disease who undergo a major operation (such as total hip arthroplasty) are more likely to develop such complications as infection and pulmonary problems. These problems may be minimized by adequate transfusion, adequate hydration, and avoidance of hypoxia and acidosis.

Dactylitis often is an early manifestation of sickle cell disease and may be the presenting complaint that leads to diagnosis. It occurs at about 18 months of age, and the initial diagnosis is often in error. Mistaken diagnoses may include osteomyelitis, rheumatoid arthritis, meningitis, and leukemia. Dactylitis is a self-limiting problem that lasts a few days to a few weeks. The radiographic features initially are soft tissue swelling, but within 1 to 2 weeks radiographs will reveal subperiosteal bone formation in a rectangular shape along the phalanges and cortical thinning and irregular medullary densities in the involved bone. The radiographic changes usually disappear after several months.

Platelet Deficiencies Patients who present with congenital musculoskeletal defects, such as radial clubhand, commonly have an associated platelet deficiency. A significant advance in their treatment is the transfusion of platelets from tissue-matched donors. If pooled platelets from random donors are used, patients become refractory to treatment after several weeks and may exhibit signs of clinical rejection, including bleeding, fever, chills, and headache. Tissue-matched donor platelets are more effective, and fewer donor packs are required than when random-donor platelets are used.

Hemorrhagic Shock Vigorous ventilatory and circulatory supports are essentials of early resuscitation of patients in shock. Blood replacement and crystalloid administration form the most important treatment for hypovolemic shock. The effectiveness of synthetic oxygen-carrying blood replacement products for replacement in patients who have sustained blood loss is being evaluated experimentally. However, their place in treatment of patients who sustain traumatic or surgical blood loss is yet to be determined.

After initial resuscitation, the orthopaedist often is faced with treatment of multiple fractures, which may be associated with significant hemorrhage. Hemorrhage remains the most common cause of death following pelvic fractures. Methods recommended for control of hemorrhage from these fractures include direct surgical approach for ligation of vessels, ligation of the internal iliac vessels, use of the G-suit, external fixation of the fracture, skeletal traction, massive fluid and blood replacement, and therapeutic embolization of bleeding vessels. Patients who present with pelvic fractures also may have intra-abdominal injury that should receive priority. An injured viscus should be treated surgically. However, the retroperitoneal space should not be opened as it is usually impossible to control the bleeding vessels by direct surgical treatment. The G-suit is effective because of compression and tamponade of the bleeding sites and immobilization of the fractures.

A technique used increasingly in recent years for severe pelvic bleeding following both trauma and surgical procedures is diagnostic angiography followed by therapeutic embolization of bleeding sites with an autologous clot of gelatin sponge (Fig. 4). Stabilization of the pelvic fracture should be accomplished as soon as possible either by pelvic slings, traction, or external and/or internal fixation.

Anesthesia Hypotensive anesthesia during major hip and spinal surgery is a proven, effective technique for reducing intraoperative and total blood loss and for shortening operative time.

Intravenous regional anesthesia is becoming more common for reduction of fractures and major surgery in the upper extremity (and at times in the lower extremity). It may be utilized for procedures distal to the elbow joint in patients who otherwise would require general or regional block anesthesia. Major potential complications associated with this technique include sensitivity to the drug, cardiac and neural reactions, and tourniquet pain. Patients who have excessive cortical stimulation following release of the tourniquet may experience lightheadedness, agitation, and confusion. On rare occasions, muscle twitching and convulsions follow these symptoms. Rapid

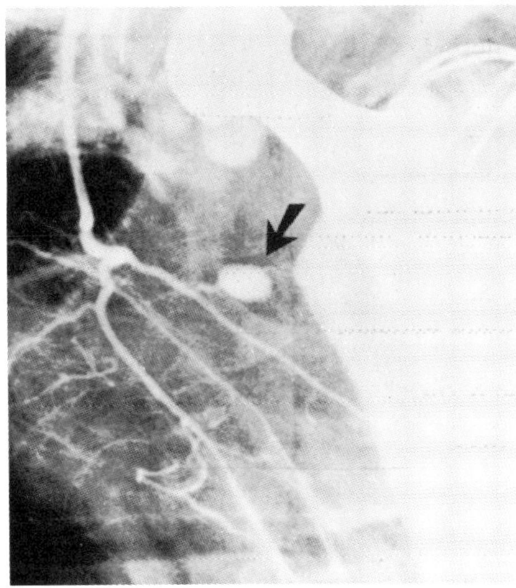

Figure 4-A

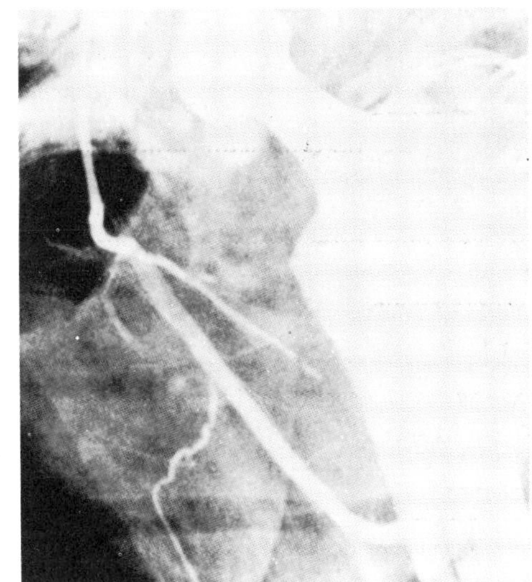

Figure 4-B

Figure 4: Transcatheter embolization for the control of wound hemorrhage following hip surgery. (A) Arteriogram shows extravasation from the medial femoral circumflex artery (arrow). (B) Repeat arteriogram after embolization shows no extravasation. Bleeding had stopped. (Reprinted with permission from Transcatheter embolization for the control of wound hemorrhage following surgery, by Stock, et al., J. Bone Joint Surg. 62A:1000-1003, 1980.)

release of the anesthetic agent may result in cardiac arrest and shock due to depression of respiration and cardiovascular centers in the medulla oblongata. Patients with severe reactions must be treated with respiratory support, fluid administration, anticonvulsants, and vasopressor agents. Reactions can be reduced or eliminated by delaying release of the tourniquet until 1 hour following drug administration. If release is necessary sooner, it should be done gradually.

Patients with osteogenesis imperfecta who require musculoskeletal surgical procedures present a difficult problem in anesthetic management. The anesthesiologist must be aware of their fragile bones and teeth. These patients often have large heads, large tongues, short necks, and thoracic deformities that make intubation difficult. They are also prone to hyperthermia which usually is nonmalignant. Since fasciculations associated with succinylcholine may lead to fractures, a nondepolarizing muscle relaxant (such as d-tubocurarine or pancuronium bromide) is recommended to avoid these muscle contractions.

Malignant Hyperthermia This autosomal dominant abnormality of muscle physiology may be triggered by many stimuli, including stress and various anesthetic agents. Patients with this condition are particularly prone to musculoskeletal abnormalities, including myopathy, recurrent dislocations, scoliosis, and kyphosis. The agents halothane and succinylcholine most commonly are implicated in stimulation of a hyperthermic reaction, the first signs of which are rapidly rising temperature and tachycardia. Sinus tachycardia may lead to ventricular tachycardia, fibrillation, and death. The core body temperature may rise as rapidly as 2 degrees centigrade per 5-minute period and reach 47 degrees centigrade. The pathogenesis of malignant hyperthermia involves a calcium transport abnormality which results in recurrent sarcomeric contraction and muscle rigidity, leading to increases in metabolic rate, temperature, CO_2, and oxygen use with resultant cyanosis. Myoglobinuria may occur and lead to renal failure. The mortality rate, which is directly related to the severity of the fever, is high.

Patient evaluation: Serum levels of creatinine phosphokinase may be elevated in some patients susceptible to malignant hyperthermia, but this is not a consistently reliable screening test. An accurate family and personal history is the best method. The report of a serious illness or death following stress of any type, including surgery, is a key diagnostic indication. Patients may have large muscle mass with a history of cramping, exercise intolerance in hot weather, and acrocyanosis associated with stress.

Management: Careful intraoperative monitoring is important. Any rise of temperature of 1 degree centigrade or more, even from the subnormal, requires investigation. If malignant hyperthermia is suspected intraoperatively, the surgical procedure should be terminated as rapidly as possible, muscle relaxants and anesthetic agents should be discontinued, and the patient hyperventilated with oxygen. Dantrolene sodium acts as an inhibitor of calcium release from the sarcotubular system. It should be administered intravenously in an initial dose of 1.5 mg (1-3 mg) per kilogram body weight, followed by incremental doses of 1 mg per kilogram body weight (up to a total dose of 10 mg per kilogram) until a clinical response is seen. Sodium bicarbonate is used to manage acidosis. Mannitol and furosemide may be needed to maintain urine output. Administration of glucose is helpful in reducing the serum potassium level. Procainamide is an effective treatment for arrhythmias. Cooling of the patient with ice bath and/or fans is essential. The use of iced intravenous fluids is also helpful. Cooling methods may be discontinued when the patient's temperature falls to 38 degrees centigrade. Patients who recover from malignant hyperthermia will have severe muscle pain and swelling. Most will experience muscle soreness and weakness with any significant activity for many months.

Dantrolene sodium in a dose of 1 to 1.5 mg per kilogram given orally 12 and 4 hours prior to surgery may be effective in preventing this syndrome.

Gastrointestinal System

Patients suffering severe trauma or undergoing major surgery are susceptible to significant gastrointestinal complications with hemorrhage the most common serious problem. Patients with gastric hemorrhage postoperatively should be evaluated by endoscopy and/or angiography. Bleeding is usually from a vessel supplied by the left gastric artery and can be controlled in most patients with vasopressin infusion into this artery. Another effective nonoperative method for control involves administration of antacid by a nasogastric tube on an hourly basis to maintain the stomach pH at 7.0. The administration of cimetidine also may be helpful. If antacid is given as a prophylaxis in high-risk patients, development of bleeding ulcers is reduced substantially by maintaining the stomach pH at 3.5 or greater. Surgery for gastrointestinal hemorrhage in patients who have already had major surgery or suffered severe trauma carries a high mortality rate and should be used only as a last resort.

Experimental studies have revealed that there is a marked slowing in the emptying of stomach contents following trauma related more to the time of development of severe pain, edema, and shock than to the time of injury. Nembutal sedation significantly slows the emptying of stomach contents both before and after trauma. Casting or splinting of an injured extremity substantially reverses delayed emptying time.

Genitourinary System

Urinary tract infections are the most common nosocomial infections, ranging in incidence from 5.4 to 8.6 percent of all hospitalized patients. Use of antibiotics and catheterization are both important associated factors. In a large group of males requiring catheterization following total hip arthroplasty, the deep infection rate of the arthroplasty was 6.2 percent. If a male requires catheterization following total hip arthroplasty, there is a 30 percent chance that he will require prostatectomy, which in one series had a mortality rate of incidence of 8.6 percent. Male patients who complain of urinary tract symptoms should have urologic evaluation and treatment prior to total joint replacement.

Patients presenting urinary tract infections should have them cleared prior to elective surgery, particularly that involving orthopaedic implants. Traditional treatment for urinary tract infections is the administration of antibiotics, based on appropriate sensitivity studies, for 10 to 14 days. Recent evidence suggests that in females with no evidence of urinary tract abnormalities, urinary tract infections can be cleared with a 3-day treatment that seems as effective as the 10-day course. Preliminary investigation also suggests that even shorter courses of antibiotic therapy may be equally as effective.

Most surgeons utilize perioperative antibiotics when implanting prostheses. There is evidence that prolonged administration of prophylactic antibiotics may be harmful in that the bacterial flora of the urinary tract is significantly changed. If an antistaphylococcal agent is used, there is often overgrowth of gram-negative organisms, especially pseudomonas. Since there is no evidence that prolonged "prophylactic" antibiotics are more beneficial than short-term, their administration probably should not exceed 48 to 72 hours.

Skin

Skin Ulcers In patients with various medical problems that are linked with decreased sensation whether due to peripheral neuropathy associated with diabetes or traumatic neural injury, skin ulcers are a frequent problem. Improved education of patients with sensory deficits reduces the occurrence of pressure ulcers. When they do develop, the ulcers are usually small and clean, can be excised, and the wound closed primarily. Antiembolism stockings may contribute to the development of heel ulcers in patients with spinal cord injury and should be used with great caution or not at all.

TREATMENT: When skin ulceration develops which does not heal or cannot be closed primarily, various techniques are available for treatment. Because skin on the sole of the foot is specialized and often subject to great stress, it is particularly troublesome. Split thickness skin grafts from distant areas may be used but sometimes develop complications, such as hyperkeratotic areas on their border. In traumatic problems as well as others, split thickness skin grafts 0.5 mm thick, harvested from the medial non-weight-bearing area of the foot, have achieved success in covering deficient skin areas in the weight-bearing areas of the foot. In patients with decreased sensation as a cause of skin defect, innervated flaps have been utilized. The lateral calcaneal artery skin flap as well as a full-thickness island graft based on the sural nerve have been used effectively to provide sensate skin on the plantar surface of the foot and the posterior aspect of the heel. Intercostal neurovascular island flaps have been used with favorable results in paraplegic patients having severe resistant ulcers in the lower trunk.

Muscle transposition, or transfer, for coverage of traumatic defects have been successful, particularly in the lower leg. The gluteus maximus muscle may be utilized for rotation flaps to cover resistant ulcers in the sacral and ischial regions. Bone excision has also been performed in areas of resistant ulcer. Partial or total calcanectomies have been useful in nondiabetics and occasionally in diabetics. There is some functional disability with such a procedure, but function is nearly always better than that obtained with a lower limb prosthesis. Ischiectomy may be necessary for severely resistant ischial ulcers, but significant morbidity may result. If ischiectomy is performed unilaterally, pressure is transferred to the contralateral side and may result in the formation of another ischial ulcer. When bilateral ischiectomies are performed, pressure is transferred to the perineal area, and occasionally this may lead to severe ulceration with urethral and rectal fistulae. These latter complications are particularly probable in patients with dislocated hips or resection arthroplasty of the hip.

The most significant advance in skin defect coverage in the last decade has been the use of free flaps with microvascular anastomosis. Free flaps consist of single free tissue transfers which may involve skin, bone, muscle, nerve, and intestine. Compound flaps consist of various combinations, e.g., osteocutaneous, musculocutaneous, neurovascular, and whole body portions such as toe to hand transfer. Free flaps may be used when a direct flap is not possible or is very difficult. When a tube pedicle flap may be necessary or when more conventional flaps or transpositions have failed, free flaps also may be indicated. There are several donor areas that leave little cosmetic or functional deficit. A major advantage of free flaps is that they can be accomplished in one stage with the corresponding disadvantage that the operation is difficult and prolonged.

ANNOTATED BIBLIOGRAPHY

Circulatory, Respiratory, and Hematopoietic Systems

Thromboembolism

DeLee, J.C., and Rockwood, C.A., Jr.: Current concepts review. The use of aspirin in thromboembolic disease. J. Bone Joint Surg. 62A:149-152, 1980.

Aspirin in low dose (600 to 1200 mg per day) is effective in reducing thromboembolic disease in men over the age of 40 following total hip arthroplasty.

Dorr, L.D.; Sakimura, I.; and Mohler, J.G.: Pulmonary emboli following total hip arthroplasty: Incidence study. J. Bone Joint Surg. 61A:1083-1087, 1979.

Pulmonary embolism, diagnosed by the development of new perfusion defects without associated ventilatory defects and confirmed by pulmonary angiography, occurs in 6 percent of patients undergoing major orthopaedic surgery. Arterial oxygen Pa_{O_2} may not be a good indicator of pulmonary embolism following major hip surgery.

Fahmy, N.R., and Patel, D.G.: Hemostatic changes and postoperative deep-vein thrombosis associated with use of a pneumatic tourniquet. J. Bone Joint Surg. 63A:461-465, 1981.

Lower extremity tourniquet use increases fibrinolytic activity and in this small series of patients reduced the likelihood of thrombophlebitis.

Moskovitz, P.A.; Ellenberg, S.S.; Feffer, H.L.; Kenmore, P.I.; Neviaser, R.J.; Rubin, B.E.; and Varma, V.M.: Low-dose heparin for prevention of venous thromboembolism in total hip arthroplasty and surgical repair of hip fractures. J. Bone Joint Surg. 60A:1065-1070, 1978.

Patients were given 70 U.S.P. units of heparin per kilogram every 8 hours for 7 days. Heparin was moderately effective in the prevention of thromboembolism following total hip arthroplasty and ineffective following surgery for hip fractures. There were significant bleeding complications and increased transfusion requirements for those patients receiving heparin.

Osteonecrosis

Chryssanthou, C.: Dysbaric osteonecrosis: Etiological and pathogenetic concepts. Clin. Orthop. 130:94-106, 1978.

Dysbaric osteonecrosis appears to be independent of decompression sickness and the incidence is influenced by the number of exposures, degree of compression, decompression rate, obesity, and possibly the rate of compression. The etiology is multifactorial.

Elmstedt, E., and Svahn, T.: Skeletal complications following renal transplantation. Acta Orthop. Scand. 53:279-286, 1981.

Overall incidence of osteonecrosis in renal transplantation patients is 11 percent. Fractures are also common (26 percent). All fractures healed without complications.

Glimcher, M.J., and Kenzora, J.E.: The biology of osteonecrosis of the human femoral head and its clinical implications. Clin. Orthop. 138:284-286, 139:283-312, and 140:273-312, 1979.

Osteonecrosis is probably a disease of multifactorial etiology. A newly suggested approach to treatment involves prevention of the repair process since it appears that symptoms relate to the presence of this process.

Hungerford, D.S., and Zizic, T.M.: Alcoholism associated ischemic necrosis of the femoral head. Clin. Orthop. 130:144-153, 1978.

Osteonecrosis in alcoholic patients is associated with increased intraosseous pressure in the proximal femur. Core decompression of the femoral head and neck may be beneficial in prevention of disease progression if the procedure is performed prior to osteochondral collapse.

Sugioka, Y.; Katsuki, I.; and Hotokebuchi, T.: Transtrochanteric rotational osteotomy of the femoral head for the treatment of osteonecrosis. Clin. Orthop. 169:115-126, 1982.

Excellent results are obtained in 98 (77 percent) of 128 hips followed 2 to 9 years postoperatively. Results are related to extent of head avascularity.

Fat Embolism Syndrome

Pollak, R., and Myers, R.A.M.: Early diagnosis of the fat embolism syndrome. J. Trauma 18:121-123, 1978.

Patients with the highest risk for fat embolism syndrome are males less than 30 years of age who demonstrate hypoxemia early following fractures to the long bones of the lower extremities.

Stoltenberg, J.J., and Gustilo, R.B.: The use of methylprednisolone and hypertonic glucose in the prophylaxis of fat embolism syndrome. Clin. Orthop. 143:211-221, 1979.

Methylprednisolone may reduce severity of respiratory problems in fat embolism syndrome by reducing endothelial damage occurring in the lung. Fat embolism syndrome is closely related to respiratory insufficiency syndrome.

Adult Respiratory Distress Syndrome

Amato, J.J.; Rhinelander, H.F.; and Cleveland, R.J.: Posttraumatic adult respiratory distress syndrome. Orthop. Clin. North America 9:693-713, 1978.

Adult respiratory distress syndrome is an often fatal complication of severe trauma which involves complete respiratory failure. Adequate treatment depends on careful monitoring and sophisticated respiratory support.

Hemophilia

Blood Coagulation. *In* Clinical Hematology, edited by M.M. Wintrobe, pp. 405-452. Philadelphia, Lea and Febiger, 1981.

A discussion of the components and mechanism of coagulation is presented. Treatment of coagulation deficiencies depends on accurate diagnosis and an understanding of the coagulation system.

Boardman, K.P., and English, P.: Fractures and dislocations in hemophilia. Clin. Orthop. 148:221-232, 1980.

Most fractures can be treated closed, but full cast should not be applied until the danger of continued hemorrhage is past. Open reduction and internal fixation can be performed with adequate replacement therapy.

McCollough, N.C., III; Enis, J.E.; Lovitt, J.; Lian, E.C.; Niemann, K.N.W.; and Loughlin, E.C., Jr.: Synovectomy or total replacement of the knee in hemophilia. J. Bone Joint Surg. 61A:69-75, 1979.

No patients experienced recurrent bleeding episodes following synovectomy. Total knee arthroplasty, although successful in most patients, has a high complication rate.

Spear, C.V.; Mason, J.A.; Williamson, S.R.; Neff, R.S.; Comeaux, L.J., Jr.; and Gwathmey, F.W.: Undiagnosed bleeding states and medical treatment. Clin. Orthop. 134:249-260, 1978.

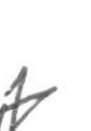

Surgery on patients with undiagnosed bleeding states may have disastrous consequences. An appropriate history is the most important factor for avoiding this. A history of substantial bleeding following tonsillectomy or dental extraction must not be ignored.

Sickle Cell Anemia

Schenkar, D.L.; Roeckel, I.E.; Bailey, H.L.; and Brower, T.D.: Thrombocytopenia and its management in the surgical patients needing multiple reconstructive procedures. Am. J. Surg. 133:572-574, 1977.

Platelets harvested from tissue-matched donors are more effective and result in fewer complications than platelets from random donors for patients with thrombocytopenia requiring surgery.

Stein, R.E., and Urbaniak, J.: Use of the tourniquet during surgery in patients with sickle cell hemoglobinopathies. Clin. Orthop. 151:231-233, 1980.

Tourniquet use for both upper and lower extremity surgery does not increase the complication rate in patients with sickle cell disease.

Hemorrhagic Shock

Flint, L.M., Jr.; Brown, A.; Richardson, J.D.; and Polk, H.C.: Definitive control of bleeding from severe pelvic fractures. Ann. Surg. 189:709-716, 1979.

The use of a G-suit is effective in patients with severe hemorrhage following pelvic fractures. Its effectiveness depends on compression and tamponade of bleeding vessels and immobilization of fractures.

Matalon, T.S.; Athanasoulis, C.A.; Margolies, M.N.; Waltman, A.C.; Novelline, R.A.; Greenfield, A.J.; and Miller, S.E.: Hemorrhage with pelvic fractures: Efficacy of transcatheter embolization. Am. J. Roentgenol. 133:859-864, 1979.

Diagnostic angiography and therapeutic transcatheter occlusion of bleeding vessels utilizing clot of gelatin sponge are found effective in eighteen patients angiographically and seventeen patients clinically in controlling severe hemorrhage following pelvic fracture. Transfusion requirements are markedly reduced.

Stock, J.R.; Athanasoulis, C.A.; Harris, W.H.; Waltman, A.C.; Novelline, R.A.; and Greenfield, A.J.: Transcatheter embolization for the control of wound hemorrhage following hip surgery. J. Bone Joint Surg. 62A:1000-1003, 1980.

Techniques similar to those used for bleeding following pelvic fractures are used for continued hemorrhage after hip surgery. Autologous clot or surgical gelatin is effective in stopping hemorrhage.

Anesthesia

Haas, L.M., and Lendeen, F.H.: Improved intravenous regional anesthesia for surgery of the hand, wrist, and forearm. The second wrap technique. J. Hand Surg. 3:194-195, 1978.

The hand and forearm are wrapped a second time with an elastic bandage after instillation of local anesthetic, and the second tourniquet is inflated. The technique allows better distribution of the anesthetic agent with decreased tourniquet pain and a drier operative field.

Jardon, O.M.; Wingard, D.W.; Barak, A.J.; and Connolly, J.F.: Malignant hyperthermia. A potentially fatal syndrome in orthopaedic patients. J. Bone Joint Surg. 61A:1064-1070, 1979.

The most important factor in recognizing the potential of malignant hyperthermia is a positive family history or past medical history of sudden death or serious illness following stress of any type. Dantrolene sodium is effective in preventing development of the syndrome.

Katz, J., and Aidinis, S.J.: Current concepts review. Complications of spinal and epidural anesthesia. J. Bone Joint Surg. 62A: 1219-1222, 1980.

The mortality rate is much reduced in patients having spinal, rather than general, anesthesia. Complications from spinal anesthesia include total spinal anesthesia, headache, backache, bladder dysfunction, and neural deficit. Major complications are rare.

Libman, R.H.: Anesthetic considerations for the patient with osteogenesis imperfecta. Clin. Orthop. 159:123-125, 1981.

Special precautions must be taken when patients with osteogenesis imperfecta require anesthesia; these include careful padding and positioning, avoidance of agents that cause muscle fasciculations, and monitoring.

Vazeery, A.K., and Lunde, O.: Controlled hypotension in hip joint surgery. An assessment of surgical hemorrhage during sodium nitroprusside infusion. Acta Orthop. Scand. 50:433-441, 1979.

Both intraoperative and total blood loss are substantially reduced by use of sodium nitroprusside infusion to maintain the mean arterial blood pressure in the range of 60 to 70.

Gastrointestinal System

Curtis, L.E.: Management of postoperative gastrointestinal bleeding. Orthop. Clin. North America 9:791-797, 1978.

Gastrointestinal hemorrhage is a common complication following major surgery or trauma. Nonoperative treatment is most effective, usually with vasopressin infusion into the left gastric artery or antacid treatment.

Genitourinary System

Fair, W.R.; Crane, D.B.; Peterson, L.J.; Dahmer, C.; Tague, B.; and Amos, W.: Three day treatment of urinary tract infections. J. Urol. 123:717-721, 1980.

A 3-day course of antibiotics is as effective in the treatment of urinary tract infections in females without genitourinary abnormalities as a 10-day course of antibiotics.

Wroblewski, B.M., and del Sel, H.J.: Urethral instrumentation and deep sepsis in total hip replacement. Clin. Orthop. 146:209-212, 1980.

The incidence of deep sepsis and mortality is significantly increased in patients who undergo total hip replacement and require catheterization and/or prostatectomy.

Skin

Crandall, R.C., and Wagner, F.W.: Partial and total calcanectomy: A review of 31 consecutive cases over a ten-year period. J. Bone Joint Surg. 63A:152-155, 1981.

Patients without diabetes who had ulcers refractory to treatment obtained excellent results following calcanectomy. Failure rate was high in diabetics, but the procedure may still be useful for active diabetic patients with adequate blood flow.

Daniel, R.K., and May, J.W., Jr.: Free flaps: An overview. Clin. Orthop. 133:122-131, 1978.

The advantages of free flaps include improved function, cosmesis, and attainment of adequate tissue coverage in a one-stage procedure. Normal vessel to normal vessel anastomosis with the use of vein graft, if necessary, is required for success.

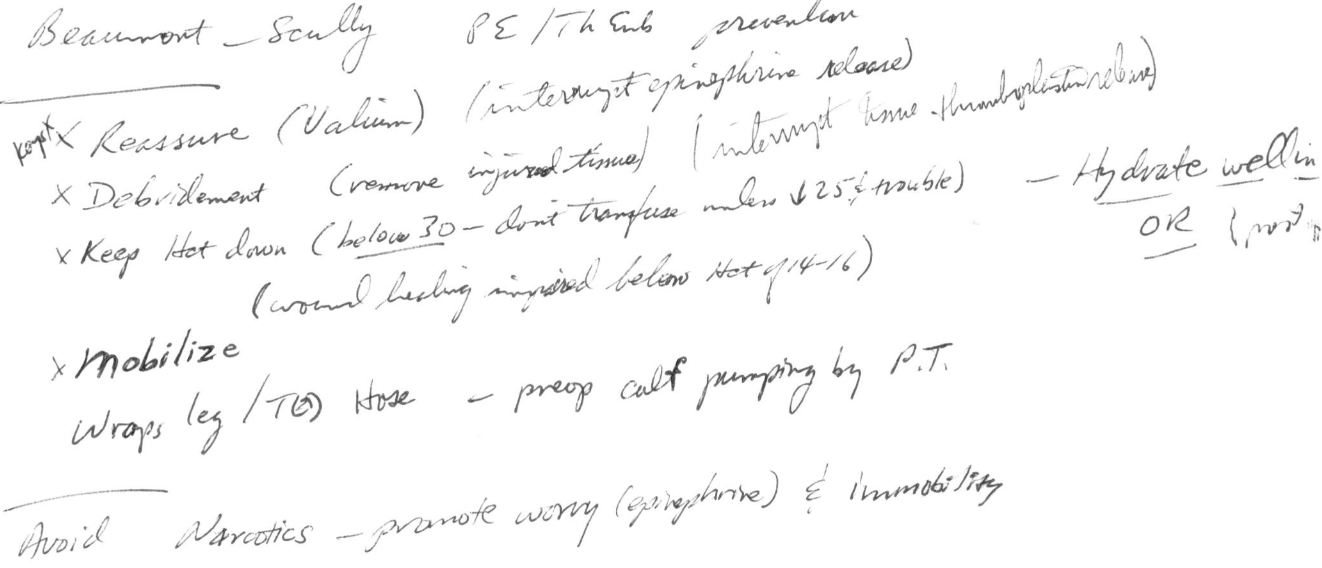

11 METALS USED IN ORTHOPAEDIC SURGERY

This section discusses metallic and some newer porous materials used for orthopaedic implants.

Introduction

Orthopaedic surgery has advanced considerably during the last 15 years. Foremost in this change is the extensive use of implanted devices for reconstruction of skeletal structures. It is now commonplace for the orthopaedic surgeon to use metallic alloys, polymers, and, in certain environments, ceramics for joint replacement. The implantation of prosthetic devices imposes severe requirements on the biomaterials used. The issue of biocompatibility is important. Interactions between implanted materials and surrounding tissues can translate into biological hazards to the living organism and into mechanical failure of the device. In many instances, the implanted device is required to function without failure for the life of the patient. This is an extraordinary engineering requirement since the lifetime of a prosthesis in many patients may exceed 30 to 50 years.

Metallic Materials

Metallic materials have certain properties that make them ideal for load-bearing applications. They can achieve very high strength under severe conditions, such as aggressive environments, maximum-load excursions, fluctuating loads, and the presence of flaws. These materials have a certain capacity to undergo irreversible, or plastic, deformation under load (ductility). This property is used extensively in manufacturing to produce complex shapes, and it also confers resistance to fracture. A variety of manufacturing processes are possible with metallic materials. The biocompatibility of metallic materials is related directly to their corrosion resistance. There are several families of metallic alloys fulfilling the demand of tissue tolerance required for human application.

Metals rarely are used in pure elemental form since they do not possess all the properties required for service and manufacturing. Other elements, usually more than two, are added to form metallic alloys. To fit given applications and requirements (such as strength and corrosion resistance), special alloying conditions are used. Four metallic alloys are used extensively in orthopaedic devices today: iron-chromium-nickel (stainless steel), cobalt-chrome, titanium, and cobalt-nickel-chromium-molybdenum (Table I).

Stainless Steel There are at least fifty alloys and grades of alloys identified as commercial stainless steels. Only the austenitic grades, the iron-chromium-nickel alloys, are used as biomaterials in orthopaedic surgery. Unalloyed iron, carbon steels, and alloyed carbon steels cannot be used because they corrode in oxygenated saline solutions. Despite their very good corrosion resistance, stainless steels are subject to several other types of corrosion processes, including crevice, pitting, intergranular, and stress corrosion. These processes can lead to the release of metallic ions into the surrounding tissue with undesirable biological consequences and, in addition, can profoundly degrade the mechanical strength of the alloy.

The stainless steels designated as ASTM F-55-56 (316, 316L) are used extensively when stainless steel is the material of choice. The following composition of alloying elements is present in type A: 17/20 percent Cr, 10/14 percent Ni, 2/4 percent Mo, 0.08 percent C (maximum), 2 percent Mn (maximum), and 0.75 percent Si (maximum). Alloying with chromium generates a protective, self-regenerating oxide film which resists perforation, has a high degree of electrical resistivity, and, thus, provides a major protection against corrosion. The nickel imparts more corrosion resistance and outstanding fabricability. The molybdenum addition provides exceptional resistance to pitting corrosion. The manganese and silicon additions are limited and serve to control problems in manufacturing. The presence of carbon is undesirable. Under certain conditions, the carbon segregates from the major elements of the alloy, taking with it a substantial

Table I
Metallic Alloys Used in Prostheses

	Yield Strength ($X10^2$MPa)	Fatigue Strength ($X10^2$MPa)	Elastic Modulus ($X10^5$MPa)
Annealed 316 Stainless Steel	2.07	1.52	1.93
Cold Worked 316 Stainless Steel	6.90	2.90	1.93
Cast Co-Cr-Mo Alloy	5.18	2.55	2.21
Forged Co-Cr-Mo Alloy	8.98	7.59	2.21
Hot Isostatic Pressed Co-Cr-Mo-Alloy	8.40	7.65	2.21
Titanium Alloy (Ti6A14V)	8.63	5.52	1.10
Hot Forged MP35N Alloy	9.65	6.21	2.28
Cold Worked MP35N Alloy	15.88	8.98	2.28

amount of chromium forming chromium carbide precipitates. Local depletion of chromium deprives those zones of corrosion resistance, and since the carbides form most frequently at the alloy crystal interfaces, the resultant corrosion occurs selectively in the intercrystalline paths. This steel is called "sensitized" and has the potential of failing dramatically after a moderate exposure to a corrosive medium. As a precaution there is a special high grade of F-55-56 stainless steel designated as type B (316L) with a guaranteed maximum of only .03 percent carbon.

All metallic materials are subjected to *fatigue fracture* under conditions of fluctuating load, such as might be expected in a femoral stem during gait. Fatigue fracture begins with small crack-like flaws within the material that grow with each stress fluctuation until a critical magnitude of crack size is reached and ends with total failure of the part. These crack-like flaws can be generated by inclusions within the material. To increase resistance to fatigue failure, 316L steel is available in a special grade with smaller and more widely spaced inclusions. This grade, designated as AISI 316LVM and identified as ASTM F-138, is produced by a special vacuum-melting procedure, which produces a cleaner metal.

All stainless steels are prone to *crevice corrosion.* When two parts of a stainless steel device (such as plate and screw) are fitted close together, the fluid in the intervening gap is lower in dissolved oxygen than elsewhere. This establishes a so-called oxygen concentration cell with a voltage capable of overcoming the passive film character intrinsic to the steel, thus allowing local corrosion to proceed more rapidly. This phenomenon commonly is seen in plates and screws retrieved from patients. Crevice corrosion is not expected in a monolithic device, such as a femoral stem.

The 316 stainless steels are capable of substantial yield strengths achieved by plastic deformation at room temperature, with a range between 260 MPa and 896 MPa. Although there are obvious advantages to using cold drawn 316LVM in highly stressed applications, it cannot be utilized in every instance because the larger diameter bars required for manufacturing purposes are not available in the higher strength material due to limitations in existing cold drawing equipment.

Following forming and machining operations and prior to use as a finished implant, stainless steel as well as other metallic alloy devices are exposed to a *passivation process.* This involves immersion of the finished part in a strong nitric acid solution for 10 to 30 minutes. The solution not only dissolves imbedded iron particles resulting from machine operations but also generates a thin, transparent, but dense oxide film on the surface of the alloy. This process is important in enhancing the corrosion resistance of the alloy.

Cobalt-Chromium-Molybdenum Alloy (ASTM F-75) The specifications for this alloy require 27 to 30 percent Cr, 5 to 7 percent Mo, 0.35 percent C (maximum), and Co for the balance. For many years this material was used primarily as a *casting alloy.* Faced with the need for a higher strength material, manufacturers have used two additional fabrication techniques, hot isostatic pressing (HIP) and forging, to obtain materials with superior strength characteristics.

As with stainless steels, the chromium content of this alloy generates a highly resistive passive film which contributes substantially to corrosion resistance. The cast alloy has a minimum yield strength of 517 MPa, which makes it stronger than 316LVM but at the lower end of the cold worked band of available yield strengths for stainless steel.

Although the mechanical properties of the cast alloy are adequate for most orthopaedic applications, they are not sufficient for high stress requirements. The casting procedure imposes some variables in the microstructural features of the material that may alter its mechanical properties and affect its fatigue life. As the molten alloy hardens during the freezing process, the distribution of carbides within the alloy can change (i.e., they can be segregated in the form of continuous bands) and add a measure of relative brittleness to the material. Also associated with the freezing process is a volume change as the material transforms from the liquid to the solid state. This shrinkage process can result in voids trapped between the growing alloy crystals. Voids also can form by the expulsion of gases during the freezing process. These voids must be regarded as precursors of microcracks that affect the fatigue life of the alloy, as well as allowable stresses in fatigue. When the alloy is produced void-free or the voids are closed, as with *HIP* or *forging,* ductility and fatigue resistance of the alloy are improved measurably.

There is a strong relationship between grain size and strength. The alloy crystals of the cast material are 5 to 15 mm in diameter, whereas much smaller crystals in the order of .01 mm can be obtained either by the HIP or the forging process. The yield strength of the HIP product is 896 MPa and 517 MPa for the cast material.

In the *HIP process* the liquid alloy is atomized to powder. Loose powder is consolidated to a void-free solid, resulting in a part reasonably close in shape to the ultimate device. The preformed part is finished by machining and polishing. The resulting structure has a very fine alloy crystal size and very fine uniform dispersion of carbide particles.

In the *forging process* the stems are forged from bar stock produced with specific composition and properties. Various operations then are performed to obtain the finished prosthesis.

The F-75 alloy has superior *corrosion resistance* to the F-138 stainless steel, particularly in crevice corrosion. There is an extensive, decades-long history of biocompatibility in human implantation. The availability of the high strength varieties and their superior corrosion resistance and biocompatibility make them an excellent choice for high-stress applications such as the femoral stem of a total hip prosthesis.

Cobalt-Chromium-Tungsten-Nickel Alloy (ASTM F-90) This alloy is composed of 19/21 percent Cr, 14/16 percent W, 9/11 percent Ni, and 0.05/0.15 percent C. It is very different from the F-75 alloy with which it is often confused. This alloy can be hot forged and cold drawn and is not used in the cast form. Yield strengths range from 690 MPa for the soft condition to as much as 6,090 MPa for severely cold drawn wire. In clinical practice it is used to make wire and internal fixation devices (e.g., plates, intramedullary rods, and screws).

Unalloyed Titanium (ASTM F-67) Titanium and its

alloys are of particular interest for biomedical application due to their outstanding biocompatibility. In general, their corrosion resistance significantly exceeds that of the stainless steels and the cobalt-chromium alloys. In saline solutions near neutral pH, the corrosion rate is extremely small, and there is no evidence of pitting, intergranular, or crevice corrosion. Data from in vivo animal experimental models and from human sources indicate truly superior biocompatibility.

So-called unalloyed titanium actually is alloyed by the level of oxygen dissolved into the metal. In large amounts, oxygen embrittles titanium and its alloys. However, in small, regulated amounts it helps control the yield strength of the materials. ASTM F-67 is a specification for oxygen providing 345 MPa of yield strength in grade III and 485 MPa of minimum yield strength in grade IV. Other elements in unalloyed titanium include N 0.07 percent (maximum), C 0.15 percent (maximum), H 0.015 percent (maximum), and Fe 0.35 percent (maximum). Any excess of these elements may degrade the performance of the basic material. Unalloyed titanium is not used extensively in orthopaedic surgery today. It is available in various configurations, such as plain wire for manufacturing purposes. It would appear to be the material of choice for a porous layer in a titanium-based, cementless total joint device.

Ti6A14V Titanium Alloy (ASTM F-136) ASTM F-136 specifies a content of 5.5/6.5 percent Al, 3.5/4.5 percent V, 0.25 percent Fe (maximum), 0.05 percent N (maximum), 0.08 percent C (maximum), 0.0125 percent H (maximum), and other 0.1 percent (maximum 0.4 percent total). Developed by the aircraft industry as one of a number of high strength titanium alloys, this particular formulation has the capability for as much as 1,110 MPa of yield strength. As used in biomedical applications in the annealed form, yield strength is 896 MPa with a substantial degree of ductility. High strength levels that are obtainable by heat treatment have not been used for biomedical applications. The ASTM F-136 specification limits the oxygen to an especially low level of 0.13 percent maximum. This is also known in the industry as the ELI grade (extra low interstitial). Limiting the level of oxygen improves the mechanical properties of the material, particularly increasing its fatigue life.

One interesting feature of titanium and its alloys is the low modulus of elasticity of 100 gigaPa as compared to 200 gigaPa for the cobalt-chrome alloys. This feature leads to their use in plates for internal fixation of fractures. Some have found that the lower stiffness of these plates may decrease the severity of bone stress shielding which results in cortical osteoporosis under these devices. Controversy still exists regarding its advantages over more rigid metals for femoral stem manufacturing.

Some investigators have reported that titanium alloy wears when articulating with ultrahigh molecular weight polyethylene (UHMWPE) during in vitro wear testing. It appears this problem relates to the mechanical stability of the passive film covering the surface of the alloy. On a carefully polished surface, the film is highly passive but mechanically weak. When the passive film is developed through a specific process to a thickness that is mechanically much stronger, its wear ceases, and the polyethylene wear is similar to that seen when stainless steel or cast cobalt-chrome articulate against it.

MP35N, Cobalt-Nickel-Chromium-Molybdenum-Titanium (ASTM F-562-78) MP35N is one of several alloys of the multiphase family. It has a nominal composition of 35 percent Co, 35 percent Ni, 20 percent Cr, and 10 percent Mo. The carbon content is controlled to 0.035 percent (maximum). An addition of 0.65 to 1 percent titanium ensures that the carbon is fixed as titanium carbide so that precipitation of the chromium carbide and sensitization (as with stainless steel) does not occur. The alloy is vacuum melted and cast to ingot so that the nonmetallic inclusion contents are very low. The material is hot forged to preliminary formed parts which provides for a very fine grade of material that consequently is strengthened by cold deformation. Two manufacturers use this alloy for femoral stem applications. The reported yield strength for one of the manufacturers is 965 MPa and 1,929 MPa for the other. Fatigue resistance is also outstanding. In the United States femoral stems are marketed with a cast and polished F-75 head which is welded onto the neck, and in Europe a polished alumina head is press fitted on. This is done because of the difficulty of polishing the hard MP35N femoral head surfaces.

The alloy has excellent corrosion resistance and biocompatibility. In vitro and in vivo studies indicate that the resistant passive films on the surface of the alloy are sufficiently stable and can be coupled with cast F-75 or with titanium alloys without hazard of accelerated corrosion. Its main application currently lies in the area of femoral stems where high strength and high fatigue resistance are required. Because of the lack of long-term biological experience, it probably should not be used in a porous configuration where the surface areas are very large and different biocompatibility problems may arise.

Metal Failure in Clinical Practice Failure of an implanted device always constitutes a dramatic event. In devices used for internal fixation, fractures occur because the implants are not designed to replace the weight-bearing function of the underlying bony skeleton. Although material defects occasionally may play a causative role, more often technique problems, delayed or nonunion of the fracture, and excessive, early weight-bearing may be the responsible factors. Prosthetic devices, on the other hand, are meant to bear weight.

Recognition that *fractures* of the *femoral stem* can occur as a long-term complication of total hip surgery has led to the use of new metallic alloys and the development and application of many improved surgical techniques.

Failures have been reported in a variety of prosthetic designs and have occurred in stems manufactured from all of the conventional metallic materials, including forged, cast, and cold worked 316L stainless steel, cast cobalt-chromium alloy of both European and American origins, and, recently, forged cobalt-chrome alloy. The incidence of this complication varies from 0.23 to 11 percent as reported in different studies. The device used, the material from which the prosthesis is made, the surgeon, and the patient population are some of the variables involved.

The most frequent location of the fractures has been in the middle one-third of the stem. High body weight, body habitus, high level of activity, limitation of motion of the hip, and bilateral hip disease have been associated with an increased incidence of fracture. Several radiographic

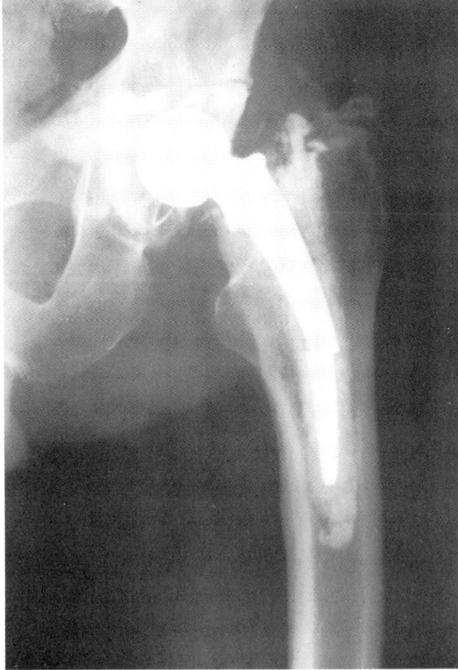

Figure 1: Femoral stem fracture.

findings are present with varying frequency, including loosening of the stem, lack of support at the level of the calcar femorale, and varus position of the stem (Fig. 1). Analytical and experimental studies have indicated that these clinical and radiographic findings have one common denominator: they tend to produce a high level of stress in the femoral stem.

The appearances of the fracture surfaces have been studied by direct observation, conventional stereoptic microscopy, and scanning electron microscopy. In every patient in whom some part of the original fracture surface was undisturbed, the characteristic features of fatigue fractures have been identified. These include a series of parallel or concentric striations that are uniquely characteristic of fatigue fractures (Fig. 2). Several investigators have indicated that the origin of the fracture often appears to be localized to the anterolateral corner of the prosthesis and, in addition, the prosthetic stem seems to have been twisted along its longitudinal axis. These findings would result from the combination of the longitudinal and posteriorly directed loads that act on the femoral head during gait, probably the most important mechanism in the generation of femoral stem fractures.

Metallographic analysis done on polished cross-sections have indicated the presence of *microstructural defects* in almost every instance. Most investigators have reported defects of this type but have differed in the interpretation of their significance. Quite likely, the presence of these defects in the vicinity of the fracture associates them with the mechanism of failure because of the specific nature of fatigue fractures and their control by local defects.

The most common defect identified in annealed 316 stainless steel is the presence of coarse crystals which very often occur near the surface of the prosthesis (Fig. 3). This phenomenon could result from a combination of the forging and subsequent annealing procedures that are utilized in manufacturing. Experimental studies on the

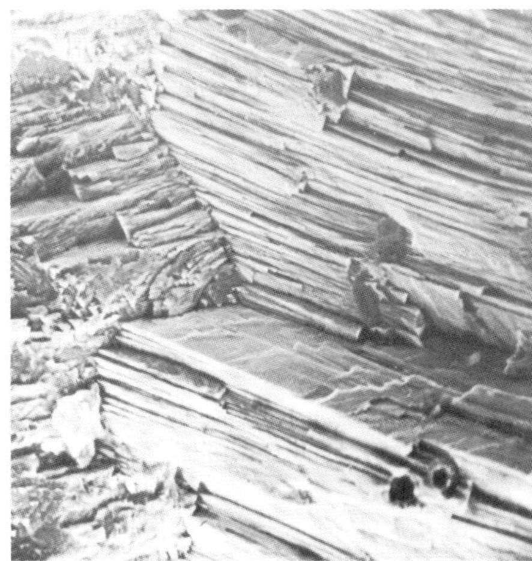

Figure 2: Scanning electron microscopic appearance of a fatigue fracture surface.

fatigue strength of this alloy have indicated a direct relationship to grain size: the smaller the grain, the higher the fatigue strength. Other abnormalities encountered in annealed 316 stainless steel include large inclusion populations and inclusion stringers, which can have a deleterious effect on the fatigue life of the alloy.

The most common defects reported in cast cobalt-chromium alloys have been related to microporosity of the shrinkage or gas expulsion (Fig. 4). Other defects found in cobalt-chromium alloys include nonmetallic inclusions, undissolved master alloy, and abnormal carbide segregation.

All these defects can cause a significant decrease in the fatigue resistance of the alloys. Many prosthetic devices manufactured from these materials may contain some microstructural defects. Only a very few of these, however, actually fail early by fatigue. This implies that the early failure probably results from the combination of a microstructural defect with a relatively large local stress (e.g., that generated by a heavy, active individual with an improperly oriented and/or improperly cemented femoral stem).

The details of correct use of surgical and cementing techniques are important in the *prevention* of stem failure

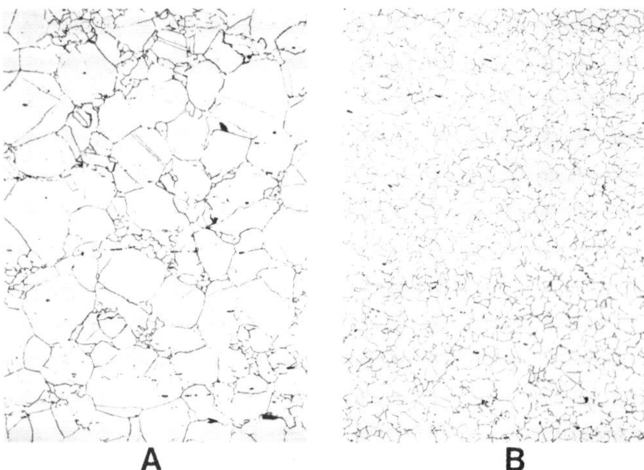

Figure 3: Abnormal large grain, structure in 316 annealed stainless steel. (A) Large grains in the surface. (B) Small grain structure in the center.

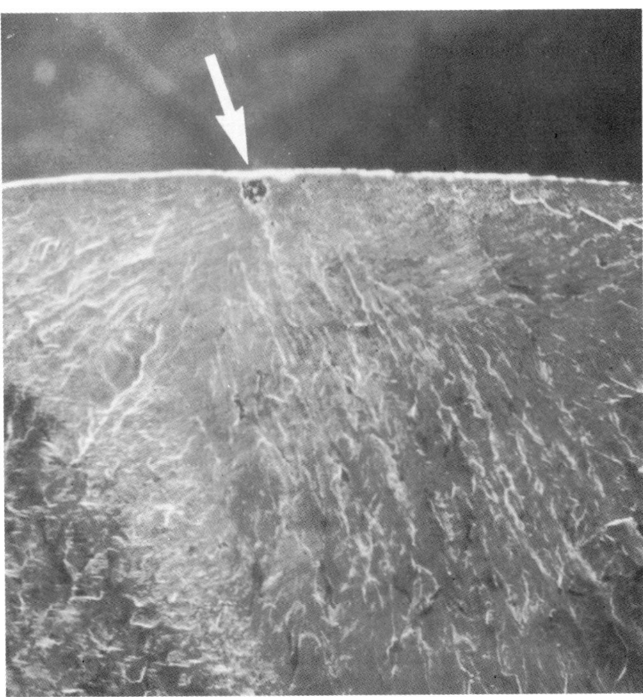

Figure 4: Porosity at the fracture surface in a cast cobalt-chromium failed device.

as is the incorporation of improvements in current designs of femoral stems. In addition, the choice of metallic alloys is critical. It constitutes the justification for the use of newer high strength alloys in orthopaedic surgery, including Ti6A14V, the cobalt-chromium-molybdenum alloy using the HIP or the forging process in manufacturing, and the MP35N alloy. All these materials have outstanding yield and fatigue strength characteristics, and their use in femoral stems constitutes an important advance in current hip replacement surgery.

Choice of Metallic Alloys for Femoral Stems There is considerable controversy concerning titanium rather than other high strength alloys as the material of choice for a femoral stem. The basic issue is the difference in the modulus of elasticity that makes a prosthesis manufactured from titanium more flexible than one made from more rigid metals.

Some believe that the compressive stress in the cement immediately adjacent to the proximal stem is a critical consideration in evaluating the overall efficacy of a stem design. Through the use of finite element analysis techniques, investigators have concluded that with a collarless prosthesis an increase in component flexibility (e.g., one made with titanium) would result in higher stresses in the cement about the proximal stem and lower stresses in the cement about the distal tip. They also reported increased loading of the proximal medial femoral cortex using the titanium component. However, this increase was relatively small when compared to physiologic loading. They found that if calcar contact could be achieved and maintained in a prosthesis with a collar, an increase in proximal femoral loading would be present and significantly higher with a titanium prosthesis than with a more rigid component. However, proximal cement stresses still would be higher with a titanium prosthesis. Also, the cement trapped beneath the collar would be subjected to very high stresses with the likelihood of failure, resulting in a collar that would not function as expected. These investigators concluded that the use of titanium stems in most patients would result in an increase in the proximal compressive stress in the acrylic cement and, thus, the likelihood of loosening.

Using a similar technique, another study reached similar experimental results but drew different conclusions. Finite element studies, verified by a laboratory experiment, disclosed some increases in proximal cement stresses for the titanium stem, but the stresses on the cement at the distal tip of the prosthesis were higher with a cobalt-chrome device. The investigators believed that the critical region was the distal area and that the use of a titanium stem would result in increased longitudinal proximal bone compression and lower cement stresses at the distal tip, thus making it the material of choice for the stem.

The three issues between these two groups are whether the critical region for cement stress is at the calcar or at the distal tip of the stem, whether strain levels in the bone at the calcar are the critical factor in resorption and loosening, and whether a collar can function to load the bone at the calcar. Although not all these issues can be answered currently, there is an important factor that must be considered in the evaluation of results from finite element studies. These studies assume a perfect bond between the cement and the prosthetic device. But, a perfect bond does not exist, and bond failure appears to occur at relatively low loads, drastically changing the mechanical environment. For a given stem, the differences in cement and bone stress that are predicted from changing stem properties can be much less than the differences that are predicted from bond failure.

In one study where bond failure was included in the experimental design, no significant differences in stem, cement, bone stress, or bond failure regions were predicted when stem properties were changed from steel to titanium. In addition to the choice of material and its relation to stem stiffness, there are other factors of major importance, including geometry of the stem cross-section, thickness of the cement mantle, and effects of stem position.

Porous Materials

The most serious clinical problem in total joint replacement today is failure of fixation. This remains true even if technical shortcomings are eliminated. An alternative approach to cement for the fixation of prosthetic devices is the use of porous materials that allow bone ingrowth into their porous structure. A variety of materials currently are undergoing laboratory and clinical evaluation for this application. Metals, polymers, and ceramics in porous forms have been considered. Metallic porous materials may offer the most promising alternative.

Porous materials usually are used as a surface layer which is bonded onto a central load-bearing stem to form a composite prosthetic device. Metallic porous materials have been manufactured by several techniques which include powder metallurgy, fiber metallurgy, and flame-spraying techniques used with titanium and cobalt-chrome alloys. All these techniques involve a sintering operation required to bond the porous layer to the solid portion of the prosthetic device. The temperature and time

94
MET

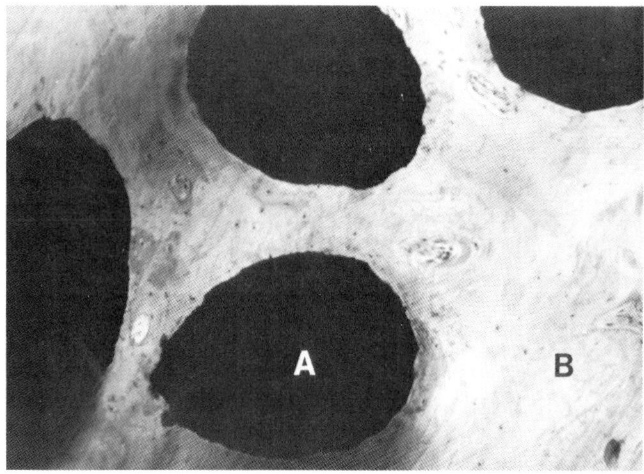

Figure 5: Bone ingrowth in fiber titanium composite 8 years following implantation in an adult baboon. (A) Titanium fiber. (B) Bone. Note the close apposition of bone to the titanium fiber.

of sintering, as well as the surrounding atmosphere, generally control the mechanical properties of the resulting materials. The effect of sintering is particularly important on the structure and properties of the solid alloy. Grain growth and a general degradation of mechanical properties occur as a result of its exposure to high temperatures. With cobalt-chrome alloys, the final product has properties that are similar to those of cast cobalt-chrome alloy but not in the range of the new high strength varieties of this material. With titanium, degradation does occur, but careful control of the sintering conditions can result in minor changes. The important issue in the design and use of these devices is that consideration must be given to the mechanical properties of the solid metal alloys to avoid potential stem fractures.

In powder metallurgy techniques, particles of metal are coated onto the central solid stems using a binder or a mold assembly and are sintered. Points of contact between particles and the solid become metallurgical bonds, and the composite acquires structural strength. The size and shape of the particles and their degree of compaction determine the eventual diameter of the pores and interconnecting channels. Fiber metallurgy techniques have been used with unalloyed titanium fibers. The fibers are cut to a short length, kinked, and consolidated by compaction in dyes. The sintering process is used to bond the fibers to each other and to the central solid stem. Flame-spraying techniques have not been used for cementless fixation. One manufacturer uses this technique to produce porous coated prostheses to enhance cement bonding.

The *histological events* surrounding the phenomenon of bone ingrowth into a porous material are very similar to those that occur during fracture healing and have been studied in experimental animals. In the initial stages following implantation, blood cellular elements can be identified within the porous spaces. This is followed by ingrowth of young connective tissue, and within 10 days after implantation, bone ingrowth can be identified in the periphery of the implant. This ingrowth progresses rapidly thereafter with values of 1,500 μ reported at 3 weeks and 2,600 μ at 6 weeks. The characteristics of the ingrowing bone have been described as that of immature bony trabeculae in the early stages following implantation. These trabeculae undergo a process of maturation, become thicker, and develop haversian systems. Considerable remodeling occurs in the bone present within the implant and in that surrounding it in response to the stresses applied during weight-bearing. Long-term histological studies (up to 7 years) in titanium fiber composites have indicated excellent biocompatibility with the presence of healthy living bone in close contact with titanium surfaces (Fig. 5).

Intimate contact and *adequate immobilization* are important prerequisites for bone ingrowth. Intimate contact is relative because close apposition is required over a significant surface of the implant but not throughout. Experimental animal models have indicated that, particularly in the intramedullary cavity of the femur, bone bridges significant gaps, fills in spaces, and grows into the porous material. Immobilization is important since fibrous tissue ingrowth occurs under conditions of implant motion.

Pore size is an important variable. In general, bone formation in experimental animals has not been observed when the pore size is smaller than 30μ. Materials with pore sizes between 175 and 450 μ have exhibited the best characteristics for bone ingrowth and related interfacial shear strengths.

Several investigators have performed mechanical tests to determine the shear strength of the porous metal-bone interface. Values of up to 14.5 to 15.8 MPa have been reported when using push-out tests. There is some controversy about the effect of pore size. It appears that interfacial shear strengths do not increase indefinitely with increasing pore size. Recent studies indicate a lower interfacial shear strength of cobalt-chromium specimens with a pore size range of 400 to 800 μ than in specimens with a pore size range from 50 to 400 μ after implantation times between 8 and 12 weeks.

Some have explored the use of electrical stimulation and hydroxyapatite impregnation as a method of enhancing bone ingrowth with porous titanium implants and have measured significant increases in the maximum shear stress. Using hydroxyapatite, a significant increase in the interfacial shear strength has been shown between 2 and 4 weeks after implantation. However, at 12 weeks no difference existed between the impregnated and nonimpregnated specimens. The study indicated that the effect of impregnation is to induce bone enhancement only in the very early stages after implantation. This method may prove to be a useful tool to facilitate early biological fixation of a prosthesis in clinical applications.

Some have used porous metallic materials in *animal models* to evaluate their effectiveness. Successful fixation by bone ingrowth in dogs has been reported in both hip surface and total replacements, including femoral and acetabular components using cobalt-chrome beads, titanium beads, and titanium fiber composites. Successful fixations of long bone segmental replacements, total knees, and patellar replacements also have been reported. These studies have confirmed that meticulous surgical preparation of the bony surfaces is required to obtain intimate contact between the device and the surrounding bone over a significant area of the device. Failures of fixation generally could be traced to technical shortcomings. These studies have shown that although the process of initial bone ingrowth is important in allowing the incorporation of the device and its fixation, the process of active bone remodeling occurring thereafter is essential for the long-term maintenance of that fixation. It probably is related to the patterns of stress transfer although the relationship between stress and resulting bone remodeling is not clearly understood.

One serious concern regarding the use of porous ingrowth fixation is the development of secondary osteoporosis in the surrounding femoral cortex. This has been well demonstrated in animals following femoral head surface, segmental long bone, and total knee replacements. The design of prosthetic devices incorporating porous material for bone ingrowth must consider the need for stress transfer from the prosthetic device to the surrounding bone to prevent extensive bone resorption.

The mechanical properties of the porous layer may play a significant role in the resulting remodeling process. The influence of modulus of the porous composite has not been investigated.

One important consideration in the use of metallic porous material relates to the large surface areas present and the potential for significant metal ion migration into the surrounding tissues. Biocompatibility and corrosion resistance of the base alloys are important considerations, and there exists considerable controversy about the relative advantages of titanium over cobalt-chrome alloy. Titanium migration has been studied following long-term implantation of titanium fiber composites used for the fixation of long bone replacements in adult baboons. Concentrations up to six times larger than the control were detected in the urine and the lungs. Although toxic effects from the metal ion migration have not been shown, the presence of these large surface areas and the concomitant increase in metal ion release indicate that further study is necessary. Stainless steel with its known propensity for crevice corrosion is not a suitable candidate for use in this application.

Successful *clinical experiences* have been reported in cementless fixation of total hip and total knee prostheses. Total hip prostheses manufactured with an irregular surface have been used extensively in Europe. Satisfactory results with femoral and acetabular fixation have been reported in over 95 percent of the 1,500 patients operated upon between 1975 and 1981 using a cobalt-chrome prosthesis coated with one layer of large cobalt-chrome beads. In the United States, porous cobalt-chrome manufactured with powder metallurgy techniques has been used successfully to fix femoral stems without cement in some patients.

A success rate of over 90 percent has been reported in the cementless fixation of forty-six total knee prostheses followed up to 75 months. A double layer of sintered cobalt-chrome beads with an average pore size of 425 μ was used.

There are several clinical studies in progress evaluating the efficacy of total hip and total knee prostheses using cobalt-chrome and titanium porous composites. Results of these clinical experiments will help to determine objectively the actual indications for the use of these devices and their proper place in reconstructive joint surgery.

Biocompatibility

In the study of materials for prospective applications as implants in the human body, the issue of biocompatibility is critical. Biocompatibility denotes absolute tolerance of the material by the host in which it has been implanted. In its assessment, it is important to think in terms of the implant, the presence of the metal ions, chemical moieties that leave the implant by corrosion degradation or mechanical wear, local tissue surrounding the implant, and remote tissues and organs of the host. Interactions between the implant and its product of degradation with the tissues of the host locally and systemically and the magnitude of the responses elicited determine the biocompatibility of the material.

Assessment requires an evaluation of each of the factors involved. In addition, the eventual application of the proposed material must be considered.

The standard recommended practices for the assessment of biocompatibility developed by the ASTM F-4 Committee on Medical and Surgical Materials and Devices take a number of variables into account and provide the basis for a uniform system of evaluation using standard histological techniques.

In addition, the use of histochemical techniques has been proposed to allow for a numerical quantitation of tissue response. Acid phosphatase and amino peptidase determinations have been used as an index of lysosome hydrolytic activity. This activity would result from toxic effects of the material on tissue macrophages and subsequent release of lysosomal enzymes.

In vitro evaluation techniques, such as cell and organ cultures, offer the possibility of quantitating the different elements of a bioassay system. Toxicity can be evaluated by determinations of growth rates, cell counts, or morphological changes of the cells. Activities of the different enzymes can be measured accurately and reflect cell damage. Concentration of soluble products from the material tested can be evaluated in tissue culture media. These techniques can be extremely useful as a screening method and also provide information on the fundamental mechanisms of implant toxicity. The more subtle responses that are observed with very inert materials, such as corrosion-resistant metals after prolonged implantation times, may be more difficult to assess. The final evaluation of a material depends upon the results of long-term in vivo evaluation studies.

The corrosion resistance of the metallic materials currently used in orthopaedic surgery accounts for their inert behavior in animal tissues. However, metal ions from a metallic prosthetic device are released into the tissues and bloodstream usually by wear and/or corrosion.

Spectrochemical analyses to determine the concentration of metallic dissolution products in the tissue surrounding metal implants in the paravertebral muscles of rabbits have shown increased concentrations when compared to controls. These analyses of the various organs have indicated that the spleen has the greatest tendency to store metals, followed by the lungs, liver, and kidneys. Cobalt and nickel particularly tend to be found in these organs.

A correlation between the histological appearance as determined by the thickness of the fibrous encapsulating membrane and concentration of the metallic constituent elements in the surrounding tissue has been described. The exception appears to be titanium, which is extremely well tolerated despite high tissue concentrations.

It has been suggested that slow release of metal ions by

corrosion of a surgical metal implant could lead to an increase in the systemic burden of each of the metals in a surgical alloy. The predicted values for chromium and nickel were high and of concern because of their known toxic effects, particularly since they have been associated with specific serum proteins.

96 MET

Regarding the potential systemic effects of metal ion release, little clear evidence exists directly establishing the causal relationship between observed clinical manifestations of implant failure and metal ion release. Evidence indicating that metal ion release may be a problem has been found in only two categories of system effects: immunological effects and carcinogenicity.

One possible effect of the release of metallic constituents is the development of *tissue sensitivity.* Metal ions behave as haptens, which, when complexed with serum proteins, can trigger an immune response. Clinical evidence is, at best, inconclusive. Several studies have found a very high incidence of metal sensitivity in patients with unexplained loosening of total joint prostheses. Sensitivity to cobalt was seen most commonly and less frequently to chromium and nickel. Histological studies in these patients disclosed extensive tissue necrosis, marked proliferation of macrophages and giant cells with intracellular metal containing particles, and obliterative vascular changes. Others found no relation between the occurrence of loosening and hypersensitivity. It has been suggested that the widely varying results are caused by improper testing procedures. The use of other techniques besides skin tests, such as leukocyte inhibition factor (LIF) or migratory inhibition factor (MIF with macrophages), have been shown to be more indicative of metal sensitivity in patients. However, they have not been related as yet to clinical implant failure.

The evidence concerning *tumorigenesis* as a result of the clinical implantation of metallic devices is limited. Data on the potential carcinogenic activity of implanted materials comes from animal studies. There is a latent period that precedes the development of a tumor in response to the introduction of an implant. This latent period is related to the life of the animal species under study. Most experimental work has been done in rodents, which are prone to develop tumors and exhibit latent periods that can be as short as 5 months. These studies have indicated that not only is the chemical reactivity of an implanted material important but also its physical characteristics, geometry, and surface texture. Plain films induced far more tumors than perforated films, fabrics, or powders. It appears that the difference in tumorigenicity is related to the development of a fibrous capsule and the ability for the implant to be encapsulated entirely. Certain compounds containing beryllium, cadmium, chromium, cobalt, iron, lead, nickel, selenium, zinc, and titanium appear to be carcinogenic in experimental animals, as do many plastics. However, there have been only a few animal studies of the carcinogenic hazards of the metallic alloys and plastics commonly used for orthopaedic surgical implants. Sarcomas in rats have been induced when experimentally produced cobalt-chromium-molybdenum wear products from total joint replacement prostheses were implanted in muscles, but other studies found no such relationship. There is a need for further careful investigation into the possible hazards of such wear products. Experimental observations strongly suggest that polyethylene wear particles are not carcinogenic in animals.

The behavior of metallic alloys used in orthopaedic surgery has been evaluated, and in solid form these materials do not appear to constitute a carcinogenic hazard. In powder form, more tumors at the implant site have been found with MP35N and cobalt-chrome alloys. The effect of implantation of these same materials in porous form is not known.

There have been rare clinical reports of tumor formation following the use of implants in humans and, in the veterinary literature, in dogs. The orthopaedic literature reports three patients with implant site tumors. One was a sarcoma and the second a hemangioendothelioma, both occurring after internal fixation for a fractured tibia. The third was a Ewing's sarcoma following internal fixation for a fractured humerus occurring 30 years after the initial implantation. These clinical studies disclosed corrosion in the metal implants which may have contributed directly to the development of a neoplastic response. There are isolated reports of tumor formation following the use of polymers in nonorthopaedic applications. These reports have indicated that tumors occur only after considerable periods of time. On the basis of animal experiments, induction periods for tumor formation in man could be well over 20 years, and if so, the potential for carcinogenicity of many implanted materials may have not been realized as yet. Careful clinical follow-up and continuing research in the field are essential to clarify such hazards of implant materials in man.

ANNOTATED BIBLIOGRAPHY

Metallic Materials

Black, J.: Biological performance of materials. *In* Fundamentals of Biocompatibility. New York, Marcel Dekker, 1981.

The text summarizes interrelations between material properties, structure, and related biocompatibility problems as used in orthopaedic applications.

Mears, D.C.: Materials and Orthopaedic Surgery. Baltimore, Williams & Wilkins, 1979.

Structure, mechanical properties, corrosion, biocompatibility, and applications of biomaterials in orthopaedic surgery are presented.

Uhthoff, H.K.; Bardos, D.I.; and Liskova-Kiar, M.: The advantages of titanium alloy over stainless steel plates for the internal fixation of fractures. J. Bone Joint Surg. 63B:427-434, 1981.

Experimental femoral fractures were internally fixed with stainless steel or less rigid titanium plates. The titanium-plated femora exhibited equal fracture stability and less bone resorption due to reduced stress shielding.

Metal Failure in Clinical Practice

Galante, J.O.: Current concepts review. Causes of fractures of the femoral component in total hip replacement. J. Bone Joint Surg. 62A:670-673, 1980.

Fractures of the femoral stem occur as a combination of factors that include metallurgical defects, loosening, abnormal position or lack of support at the femoral calcar, patient-related factors (e.g., level of activity and weight), and prosthetic design. Prevention should be directed at each issue.

Choice of Metallic Alloys For Femoral Stems

Crowninshield, R.D.; Brand, R.A.; Johnston, R.C.; and Pedersen, D.R.: An analysis of collar function and the use of titanium in femoral prostheses. Clin. Orthop. 158:270-277, 1981.

Femoral components made from titanium produce more flexible stems. In a collarless prosthesis, higher stresses result in the cement about the proximal stem. Loading of the proximal medial femoral cortex is increased, but it is small compared to physiologic loading. If the result of prosthesis collar function is to increase proximal medial femoral stresses, titanium prostheses offer advantages over more rigid devices. If collar function is designed to reduce proximal cement stresses, a more rigid device is the choice.

Hampton, S.J.; Andriacchi, T.P.; Draganich, L.F.; and Galante, J.O.: Stresses following stem cement bond failure in femoral total hip implants. Orthop. Trans. 5:284, 1981.

Analytical stress analysis models were used to simulate stem cement bond failure. Stresses that were four to five times greater than under conditions of perfect bonding were predicted under conditions of bond failure.

Lewis, J.; Kramer, G.; Wixson, R.L.; and Askew, M.J.: Calcar loading by titanium total hip stems. Orthop. Trans. 5:245, 1981.

Using three-dimensional finite element models and strain-gauged femora, the stresses in cement on bone were studied using a cobalt-chromium and a titanium femoral component. Increased proximal radial cortical bone stresses were obtained with the titanium stem. The highest polymethyl methacrylate stresses occurred at the stem tip with the cobalt-chromium stems.

Porous Materials

Bobyn, J.D.; Cameron, H.U.; Abdulla, D.; Pilliar, R.M.; and Weatherly, G.C.: Biologic fixation and bone modeling with an unconstrained canine total knee prosthesis. Clin. Orthop. 166:301-312, 1982.

Total knee replacements with porous coated condylar type femoral components were performed on canine subjects. The femoral component became firmly fixed by bony ingrowth, but significant remodeling occurred with resorption of the anterior femoral cortex and hypertrophy of the bone surrounding the prosthetic stem.

Bobyn, J.D.; Pilliar, R.M.; Cameron, H.U.; and Weatherly, G.C.: The optimum pore size for the fixation of porous-surfaced metal implants by the ingrowth of bone. Clin. Orthop. 150:263-270, 1980.

Pore size of 50 to 400 μ provided the strongest and most rapid fixation when porous coated implants were placed in canine femora.

Bobyn, J.D.; Pilliar, R.M.; Cameron, H.U.; and Weatherly, G.C.: Osteogenic phenomena across endosteal bone-implant spaces with porous surfaced intramedullary implants. Acta Orthop. Scand. 52:145-153, 1981.

Porous coated rods of varying diameters were inserted into canine femora. All implants, regardless of size, induced osteogenesis. However, there generally was a direct relationship between the proximity of the implant to the endosteal surface and the rate of bone formation.

Chen, P.Q.; Turner, T.M.; Ronnigen, H.; Galante, J.; Urban, R.; and Rostoker, W.: A canine cementless total hip prosthesis model. Clin. Orthop. 176:24-33, 1983.

A canine total hip replacement model was used with porous titanium fiber composites for fixation. Fixation by bony ingrowth and progressive remodeling of the bone surrounding the prosthetic device were obvious. The pattern of bone remodeling was believed to be important due to its implications on design and long-term viability of the fixation system.

Ducheyne, P.; Hench, L.L.; Kagan, A., II; Martens, M.; Bursens, H.; and Mulier, J.C.: Effect of hydroxyapatite impregnation on skeletal bonding of porous coated implants. J. Biomed. Mater. Res. 14:225-237, 1980.

Fiber metal implants coated with hydroxyapatite showed substantially greater amounts of bony ingrowth than did untreated controls at 2 and 4 weeks postimplantation. This enhancement phenomenon was documented by mechanical testing, microscopic, and microprobe analyses.

Engh, C.A.: Hip arthroplasty with a Moore prosthesis with porous coating: A five year study. Clin. Orthop. 176:52-66, 1983.

Twenty-six patients had total hip replacements using a femoral component coated with sintered cast cobalt-chrome spheres. Average pore size was 100 μ. At 2- to 5-year follow-up, the experience was comparable to that in a cemented total hip replacement population. There was no radiological evidence of osteoporosis.

Harris, W.H.; White, R.E., Jr.; McCarthy, J.C.; Walker, P.S.; and Weinberg, E.H.: Bony ingrowth fixation of the acetabular component in canine hip joint arthroplasty. Clin. Orthop. 176:7-11, 1983.

A hemispherical acetabular prosthesis coated with a cobalt-chrome porous composite and initially fixed by screws was evaluated in five mature dogs. Extensive bone ingrowth covering an average of 53 percent of the porous surface of the implant was observed.

Hedley, A.K.; Clark, I.C.; Kozinn, S.C.; Coster, I.; Gruen, T.; and Amstutz, H.C.: Porous ingrowth fixation of the femoral component in a canine surface replacement of the hip. Clin. Orthop. 163:300-311, 1982.

Porous coated canine surface hip prostheses were found to be securely fixed via bony ingrowth. Stress shielding with bony resorption and fibrous membrane formation at the bone implant interface occurred when porous fixation pins were added to the implants.

Hungerford, D.S., and Kenna, R.V.: Preliminary experience with a total knee prosthesis with porous coating used without cement. Clin. Orthop. 176:95-107, 1983.

These are the preliminary results of a cobalt-chrome alloy, porous coated, total knee prosthesis implanted without cement in forty-six knees. No interface failures were seen in forty-one patients followed from 4 to 25 months. Intimate contact between bone and prosthesis was maintained for up to 2 years.

Lord, G., and Bancel, P.: The madreporic cementless total hip arthroplasty. Clin. Orthop. 176:67-76, 1983.

In 235 cementless arthroplasties with a minimum follow-up of 5 years, 196 (83.4 percent) were rated as excellent or good. In 175 femora, no radiological changes were present, and in fifty-four of those (22.9 percent) definite evidence of bony ingrowth on the radiographs was observed. Radiolucent lines were present in seven femora. The acetabular experience was similar. In revisions of loosened cemented total hip replacements, satisfactory results at 2 years were maintained in 75 percent of the patients.

Park, J.B.; Salman, N.N.; Kenner, G.H.; and Von Recum, A.F.: Preliminary studies on the effects of direct current on the bone-porous implant interfaces. Ann. Biomed. Eng. 8:93-101, 1980.

Porous polymethyl methacrylate and cobalt-chrome-molybdenum cylinders were implanted in canine femora and stimulated with direct electric current. The stimulated implants exhibited a faster rate of bony ingrowth and increased interfacial shear strengths when compared to nonstimulated controls.

Spector, M.; Harmon, S.L.; and Kreutner, A.: Characteristics of tissue growth into Proplast and porous polyethylene implants in bone. J. Biomed. Mater. Res. 13:677-692, 1979.

Ingrowth of fibrous tissues, rather than bone, into Proplast rods implanted into canine femora was found to be due to the material's small interconnecting pore size (50 to 75 μ). In addition, no structural continuity was found between the fibrous tissue within the pores and the surrounding bone. Porous polyethylene (pore size 400 μ) and Proplast teased to increase the pore size both inhibited osseous ingrowth.

Biocompatibility

Heath, J.C.; Freeman, M.A.E.; and Swanson, S.A.V.: Carcinogenic properties of wear particles from protheses made in cobalt chromium-alloy. Lancet 1:564-566, 1971.

Sarcomas were observed in rats at sites of intramuscular injection of cobalt-chrome-molybdenum particles suspended in horse serum.

Meachim, G.; Pedley, R.B.; and Williams, D.F.: A study of sarcogenicity associated with Co-Cr-Mo particles implanted in animal muscle. J. Biomed. Mater. Res. 16:407-416, 1982.

Co-Cr-Mo particles in the ranges of 100 to 250 μm and 0.5 to 50 μm were implanted in adult female rats and guinea pigs. No malignant neoplasms developed at the test or control operation sites.

Memoli, V.A.; Woodman, J.L.; Urban, R.M.; and Galante, J.O.: Malignant neoplasms associated with orthopaedic implants materials. Orthop. Trans. 6:264, 1982.

Preliminary results indicate that animals with nickel-containing metal implants may be at greater risk for increased development of malignancy including sarcomas and lymphoreticular neoplasms.

Merritt, K., and Brown, S.A.: Metal sensitivity reactions to orthopaedic implants. Internat. J. Dermatol. 20:89-94, 1981.

Metal sensitivity, an infrequent orthopaedic complication, results from haptenization of metal salts to body proteins. Nickel and cobalt are most commonly implicated. Systemic and/or local (i.e., loosening) reactions may occur. Suspected individuals may be identified by lymphocyte migration inhibition testing.

Rae, T.: The toxicity of metals used in orthopaedic prostheses: An experimental study using cultured human synovial fibroblasts. J. Bone Joint Surg. 63B:435-440, 1981.

Tissue cultures of human synovial fibroblasts were grown in media containing various metals used in orthopaedic implants. Cytotoxicity and morphologic changes were produced by several metals. However, the only comparable clinical situation in which experimental metal concentrations could be reached was with cobalt-chrome-molybdenum articulating with itself.

12 POLYETHYLENE IN TOTAL JOINT REPLACEMENT

Subjects in this section include a description of the structure of the polyethylenes, in vitro and in vivo wear rates, and factors affecting wear rates.

The Material

The term *polyethylene* refers to plastics formed from polymerization of ethylene, $CH_2=CH_2$, to produce polymers with the general formula $(CH_2)_n$ or, more accurately, $(CH_2CH_2)_n$. The possibilities for structural variation on molecules formed by this simple repeating unit for different molecular weight, crystallinity, branching, cross-linking, etc., are so numerous and dramatic with such a wide range of attainable properties that the term *polyethylene* truly refers to a subclass of materials. The earliest type of polyethylene was made by reacting ethylene at high (20,000-30,000 pounds per square inch) pressure and temperatures of 200-400 degrees centigrade with oxygen as catalyst. Such material is referred to as "conventional" or *low density* polyethylene. Much polyethylene is produced now by newer, low-pressure techniques using aluminum-titanium (Ziegler) catalysts. This is called "linear" polyethylene due to the linearity of its molecules, in contrast to the branched molecules produced by high-pressure processes. The linear polymers can be used to make *high density* polyethylene by means of the higher degree of crystallinity attained with the regularly shaped molecules. Typically there is no great difference in molecular weight between the low-density and high-density varieties, e.g., 100,000-500,000. However, if the low-pressure process is used to make extremely long molecules, i.e., *ultrahigh molecular weight polyethylene* (UHMWPE), the result is different and quite remarkable. This material, with a molecular weight between 1 and 10 million, is less crystalline and less dense than high-density polyethylene and has exceptional mechanical properties. It is extremely tough (a 0.357 magnum bullet fired from 25 feet bounces back from a 1-inch thick slab of UHMWPE) and is remarkably wear resistant. The material is used in very demanding applications (e.g., ore chutes in mining equipment) and is by far the most successful material used in total joint replacements. It far outperforms the various acrylics, fluorocarbons, polyacetals, polyamides, and polyesters which have been used for such purposes.

Measurement of Wear

In Vivo The first measurement of polyethylene wear was performed in vivo by radiography. The observed wear rates for the Charnley total hip prosthesis were 0-0.45 mm per year, with an average of 0.15 mm per year. That is to say, the femoral component advances into the acetabular component at such rates. A careful analysis of the limitations of the radiographic method has been made. It should be noted that this method yields at best a dimensional measurement, and the "wear" thus calculated is a sum of the actual wear plus any other dimension change, e.g., creep or plastic deformation, which may occur in vivo. Inevitably, therefore, the in vivo measurements disagree markedly with early laboratory measurements predicting wear rates about an order of magnitude lower. The implication is that creep is a significant component of radiographic "wear."

In Vitro Early wear measurements in vitro were numerous and highly variable. Specimen geometries tested included pin-on-flat, annulus-on-flat, and journal bearings, whereas lubricants tested ranged from synovial fluid,

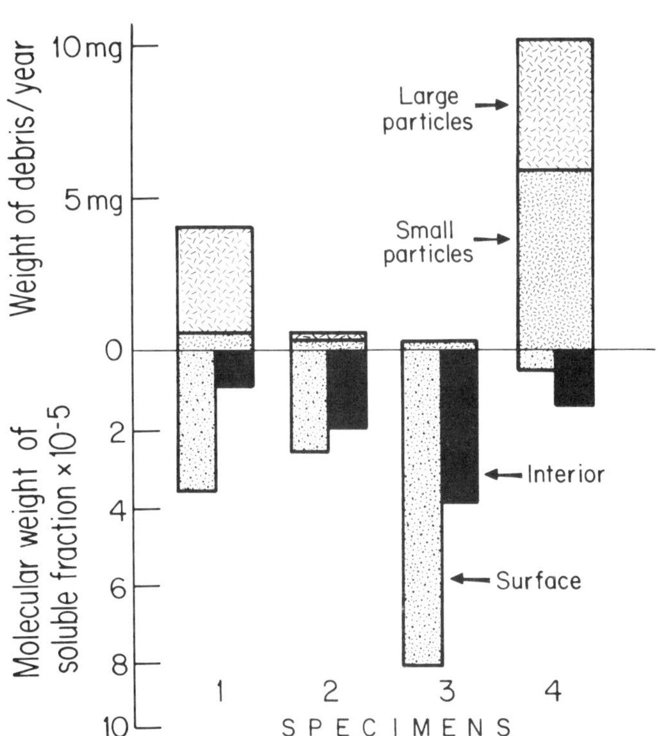

Figure 1: True wear rate vs. molecular weight of soluble fraction at articular surface and interior for four different Charnley-Mueller acetabular components. Molecular cross-linkage caused by radiation sterilization renders part of polyethylene insoluble; note the appearance of large debris particles with high wear rates. (Reprinted with permission from On the true wear rate of ultra high-molecular-weight polyethylene in the total hip prosthesis, by R.M. Rose, et al., J. Bone Joint Surg. 62A:547, 1980.)

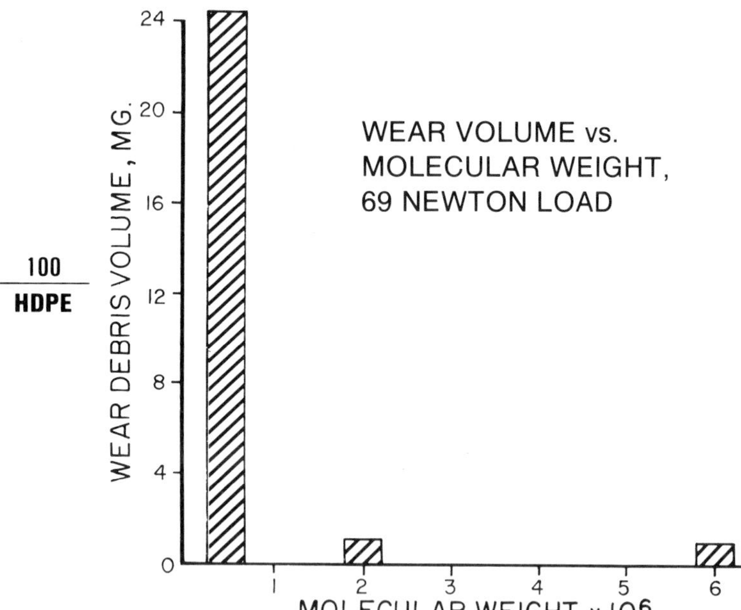

Figure 2: Dependence of wear on molecular weight of polyethylene resin used to make specimens. (Reprinted with permission from Exploratory investigations on the structure dependence of the wear resistance of polyethylene, by R.M. Rose, et al., Wear 77:89, 1982.)

plasma, saline solutions, to mineral oil. The wide variability of test conditions would preclude any essential agreement even if the material itself were consistent. Substantial understanding of the general wear behavior of ultrahigh molecular weight polyethylene has been achieved. Static and dynamic tests show that creep is a substantial component of the dimensional changes observed in the acetabular component of the total hip prosthesis. Thus, there is reason to expect disagreement between the clinical (radiographic) and in vitro measurements from the various wear machines. For that matter, the in vitro measurements also will vary among themselves. Some investigators of wear in vitro attempt to measure wear by weight loss, only to find their specimens gaining weight. The weight gain is, in fact, caused by radiation sterilization; one consequence of the radiation damage is oxidative degradation of the polyethylene molecule. The carbonyl groups created by the degradation are hydrophilic and lead to continuous water absorption.

Present Status: Wear

There is no satisfactory method for direct measurement in vivo of the true wear rate. To infer in vivo wear rates from in vitro measurement, four requirements must, at minimum, be met: (1) the most accurate possible method, biomechanically and chemically, of total joint simulation; (2) an accurate method for measurement of dimensional changes in acetabular cups (and other polyethylene components as well, if possible); (3) a quantitative method for the recovery and evaluation of wear debris; and (4) reliable experimental characterization of the structure of the polyethylene.

The combination of (1) to (3) should permit the separation of true wear and creep under clinically realistic conditions. Requirement (4) is absolutely necessary since the wear rate is known to be sensitive to the structure of the polyethylene, and at the least it must be known whether or not the materials in the in vitro specimens are comparable to clinical material. The results of subsequent experiments which met these requirements are striking (Fig. 1). The implications are that: (1) at least for prostheses available in 1975-1980, there was considerable variability of molecular structures between the products as manufactured; (2) there was a corresponding variation of true wear rate by a factor of 30-40 and that the lowest molecular weights were associated with the highest wear rates; and (3) the type of wear was different for the high- and low-wear rates. We now know that the high-wear rates are characterized by the generation of large (typically 1/2 to 1 mm) particles of polyethylene debris and crater formation in the articular surface of the prosthesis. Low-wear rates are associated with very smooth articular surfaces and fine, fibrous debris.

Wear and Molecular Weight The extreme sensitivity of wear rate to molecular weight is demonstrated independently by wear tests on polyethylene where molecular weight is varied by molding specimens from resins with different molecular weights (Fig. 2). Again, there is a difference in wear rate of more than an order of magnitude. It is apparent then that the term *polyethylene* is generic and refers to a subclass of materials, which, although they have similar, nominal chemical compositions, may have very dissimilar structures and, therefore, different properties.

Hip simulator experiments indicate that proper control of the molecular weight of the acetabular component should reduce wear considerably in total hip prostheses of the metal-HDPE type. However, this is definitely not true for knee prostheses in which the shape conformity between tibial and femoral components is relatively low. In such prostheses, the contact stresses are high compared to the hip prostheses, and much higher

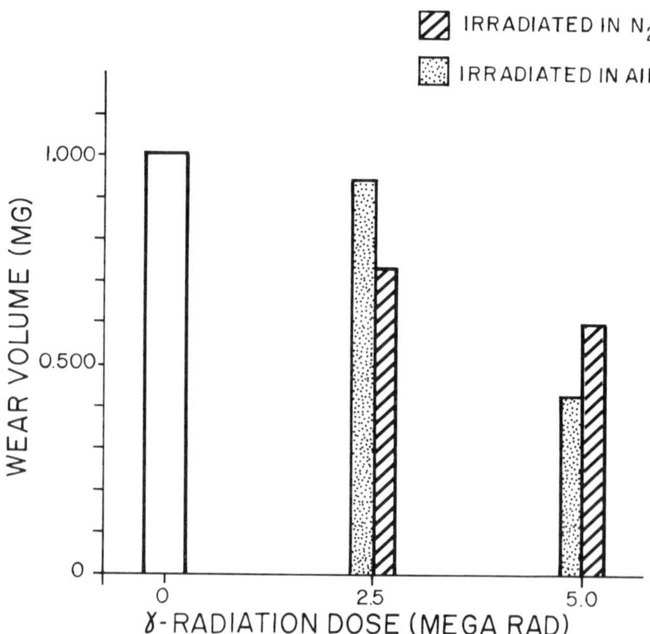

Figure 3: Dependence of wear rate on sterilizing (gamma ray) dose. (Reprinted with permission from Exploratory investigations on the structure dependence of the wear resistance of polyethylene, by R.M. Rose, et. al., Wear 77:89, 1982.)

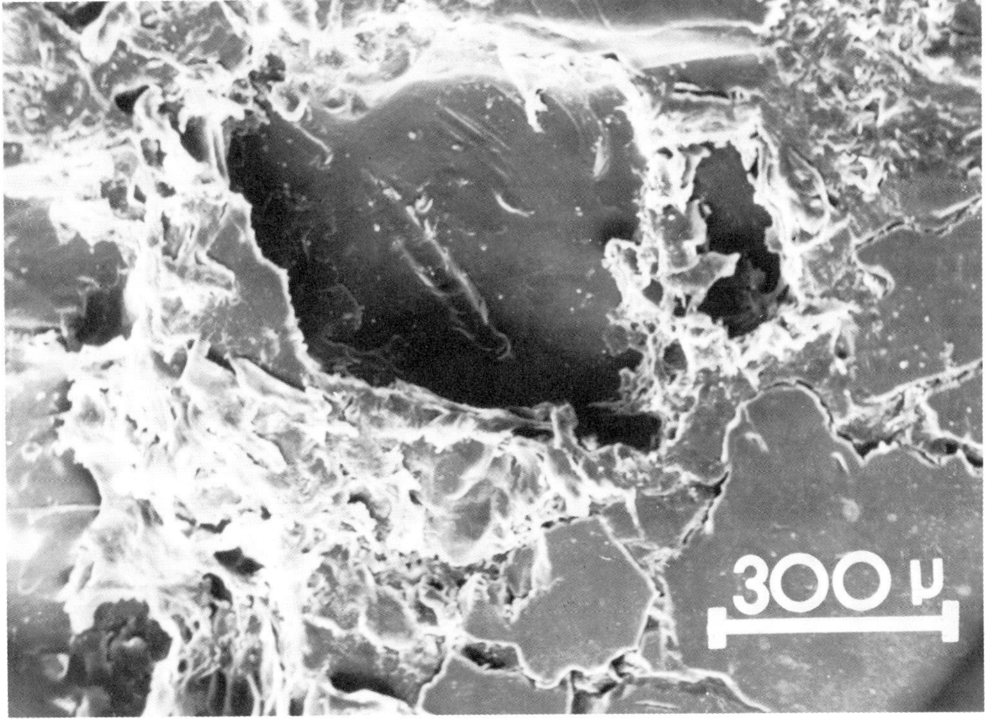

Figure 4: Damage by acrylic debris in a clinical retrieval. Departure of an embedded fragment leaves a polyhedral crater. Still embedded fragments are also visible.

wear rates may be expected according to recent measurements of the dependence of wear rate on contact stress. Whether wear rates in total knee replacements are indeed high and whether such wear rates are controllable by suitable choice of polyethylene microstructure and molecular structure remain to be seen.

Composite materials with carbon fibers incorporated in the polyethylene have been developed to improve wear and deformation characteristics of the bearing surface of total joint prostheses. Clinical trials of these composites are under way (see Section 11, General: Metals Used in Orthopaedic Surgery).

Wear and Manufacture of the Plastic Component Even when the basic resin granules are well characterized, differences in molding conditions will introduce variability in crystallinity (and, therefore, density of the plastic), molecular degradation by oxidation and mechanical deformation, voids due to incomplete fusion of the granules of resin, etc. Finally, there are marked structural changes due to radiation sterilization, particularly degradation and cross-linking.

Radiation Sterilization Whether the polyethylene is sterilized by gamma rays or high-energy electrons, the structural changes are essentially the same. Molecules are fragmented by high-energy collisions, and the scission process propagates, leaving many free radical fragments. Some react to form a cross-linked polymer; some remain, ultimately to oxidize, the first step in the environmental degradation of this material. Recent research results indicate that the short-term consequences of radiation sterilization are slight. The long-term consequences are still a matter of concern. Dosage is also important. As Figure 3 shows, the wear may decrease for dosages up to five MRAD (the accepted sterilizing dose is 2.5 MRAD). Some investigators find increases in wear rate at 5 to 10 MRAD. Thus, the issue of resterilization by radiation is now controversial.

Acrylic Cement Debris It is generally assumed that particles of acrylic cement caught between the articular surfaces cause substantial abrasion of the polyethylene. Although this idea has yet to be critically tested, some clinical retrievals illustrate how the surface of the polyethylene is disrupted by acrylic cement debris (Fig. 4). The craters tend to be polyhedral, reflecting the shapes of the hard, brittle acrylic particles that are embedded in the softer, extremely ductile polyethylene before breaking up and departing for other locations. Whether or not substantial true wear (i.e., actual release of polyethylene debris into the surrounding tissues) is caused by loose acrylic cement debris has not been proved. On the other hand, it is known that substantial true wear can occur in the absence of acrylic debris.

ANNOTATED BIBLIOGRAPHY

General Reference

Walker, P.S.: Human Joints and Their Artificial Replacements. Springfield, Charles C Thomas, 1977.

This is an introduction to basic concepts of biomechanics, materials, lubrication, friction and wear, fixation, and history.

The Material

Schwartz, S.S., and Goodman, S.H.: Plastics, Materials and Processes. New York, Van Nostrand-Reinhold, 1982.

This is a reference to the structure, properties, and processing of plastics and composites.

Measurement of Wear

In Vivo

Atkinson, J.R.; Dowling, J.M.; and Cicek, R.Z.: Materials for internal prosthesis: The present position and possible future developments. Biomaterials 1:89-99, 1980.

This paper shows that most of the "wear" observed by in vivo radiography (see following) is, in fact, creep or plastic deformation of the acetabular component.

Charnley, J., and Cupic, Z.: The nine and ten year results of the low friction arthroplasty of the hip. Clin. Orthop. 95:9-25, 1973.

The paper describes 9- to 10-year clinical follow-ups on the early Charnley total hip replacements, including the first attempt at in vivo wear measurement using radiography and wire "markers" in the acetabular component.

Charnley, J., and Halley, D.K.: Rate of wear in total hip replacement. Clin. Orthop. 112:170-179, 1975.

An improved approach to the in vivo radiographic measurement (see preceding) correlates apparent wear to time, weight, activity, and age.

Clarke, I.C.; Black, K.; Rennie, C.; and Amstutz, H.C.: Can wear in total hip arthroplasties be assessed from radiographs? Clin. Orthop. 121:126-142, 1976.

This is an analysis of the experimental limitation of "wear" (i.e., dimensional change) measurements on the acetabular component by radiography.

In Vitro

Clarke, I.C.: Wear of artificial joint materials IV: Hip joint simulator studies. Engineering in Medicine 10:189-198, 1981.

This comparative review of simulator studies of wear in total hip replacements follows earlier reviews on wear screening.

Dumbleton, J.H., and Shen, C.: The wear behavior of ultrahigh molecular weight polyethylene. Wear 37:279-289, 1976.

An early exploration of wear in UHMWPE measures wear as a function of pressure.

Present Status: Wear

Rose, R.M.; Nusbaum, H.J.; Schneider, H.; Ries, M.; Paul, I.; Crugnola, A.; Simon, S.R.; and Radin, E.L.: On the true wear rate of ultra high-molecular-weight polyethylene in the total hip prosthesis. J. Bone Joint Surg. 62A:537-549, 1980.

This paper addresses in vitro wear behavior of different polyethylene acetabular components related to molecular structure. Low wear is associated with high molecular weight polyethylene and high wear with low molecular weight polyethylene at the implant surface. Clinical radiographic evaluations of wear are more an indication of dimensional change due to creep or plastic flow than of true wear.

Radiation Sterilization

Nusbaum, H.J., and Rose, R.M.: The effects of radiation sterilization on the properties of ultrahigh molecular weight polyethylene. J. Biomed. Mater. Res. 13:557-576, 1979.

This article describes the structure and properties of the plastic and the effects on radiation on same.

Acrylic Cement Debris

Rose, R.M.; Crugnola, A.; Ries, M.; Cimino, W.R.; Paul, I.; and Radin, E.L.: On the origins of high in vivo wear rates in polyethylene components of total joint prostheses. Clin. Orthop. 145:277-286, 1979.

This evaluation of the nature and causes of wear in retrieved hip and knee joint replacements examines the role of acrylic debris.

13 POLYMETHYL METHACRYLATE

Subjects considered in this section include mechanical properties, bone-cement interface, adverse cardiac physiology, antibiotic impregnated cement, and adjunctive applications.

Mechanical Properties The mechanical behavior of polymethyl methacrylate has been implicated in a high percentage of failed total hip and knee arthroplasties. The surgical team controls a number of variables potentially critical in the mechanical behavior of the acrylic cement. Use of a slow beating frequency while mixing the monomer with the polymer and limiting the mixing time to 90 seconds can maximize the ultimate compressive strength of the polymerized acrylic. Rapid beating while mixing decreases this strength by 10 percent, and mixing for 2½ minutes leads to an 11 percent reduction.

The viscosity of the acrylic cement increases slowly at first and then more rapidly after mixing. Early insertion of the acrylic cement while the viscosity is low prevents laminations which significantly weaken the polymerized cement mass. Cement specimens formed 7½ minutes after initiation of mixing exhibit a 43 percent reduction in the ultimate compression strength as compared to specimens formed after mixing for a total of 2½ minutes. Since the acrylic mass is not controllable in the surgeon's hands during the early states of mixing, it is necessary to handle the cement in an injection device. This technique also permits pressurization which can enhance both the ultimate compressive and tensile strengths by 30 percent depending upon the amount of pressure applied. The application of two atmospheres for even 15 seconds upon insertion of the dough can increase the ultimate compressive strength by 11 percent.

Other variables influencing the mechanical behavior of the acrylic cement in the operating room are only partially controllable by the surgeon. These variables include blood and tissue inclusions, stress risers, physical constraints, and cement thickness. The inclusion of blood within the cement mass can have a dramatic detrimental influence on the mechanical behavior of cement with reductions up to 77 percent in tensile strength and 69 percent in shear strength. Although it is rarely possible to eliminate blood totally from bony surfaces during total hip arthroplasty, the degree of bloody contamination can be minimized with use of hypotensive anesthesia, instillation of an epinephrine solution, jet lavage of the bone surface, and/or use of suction prior to insertion of the acrylic dough.

Acrylic cement is brittle and exhibits a limited plastic deformation prior to failure. Exposure of polymerized cement to stress risers leads to mechanical failure at lower levels. Thus, prosthetic devices should not have sharp edges or corners.

Bone cement does not immediately reach a state of equilibrium with reference to its physical properties following polymerization. Polymethyl methacrylate polymerized at 37 degrees centigrade achieves 90 percent of its strength in 4 hours and ultimate strength at 24 hours.

Creation of mechanical constraints for polymerized bone cement may be one of the most important variables during clinical application. The mechanical behavior of constrained cement is not only enhanced in the research laboratory but also in recent clinical studies the advantages of plugging the femoral canal to constrain the cement are documented. When this technique is combined with early insertion (a lower viscous state) and pressurization, the incidence of lucent zones at the bone-cement interface has been reduced significantly.

There are several variables influencing the mechanical behavior of bone cement over which the surgeon has no control, including environmental temperature, moisture content, strain rate, and the effect of aging.

When mixing the monomer with the polymer in the operating room, the acrylic is exposed to the ambient room temperature. When the acrylic mass is transferred to the surgeon's hands and inserted into the bony cavity or surface, it is exposed to an environmental temperature approaching 37 degrees centigrade. The ultimate compressive strength of cement that polymerizes at 37 degrees centigrade is reduced by 10 percent (Fig. 1).

Polymerized acrylic cement exposed to a moist environment gradually increases in weight due to absorption of

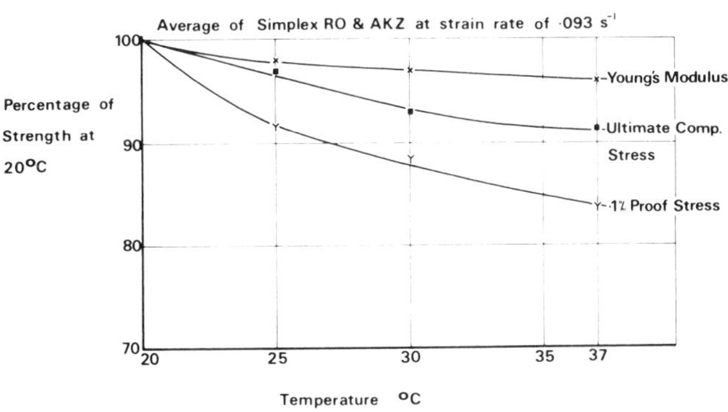

Figure 1: Relationship of environmental temperature to mechanical properties of cement. (Reprinted with permission from Some clinically relevant variables affecting the mechanical behavior of bone cement, by A.J. Lee, et al., Arch. Orthop. Trauma Surg. 92:1-18, 1978.)

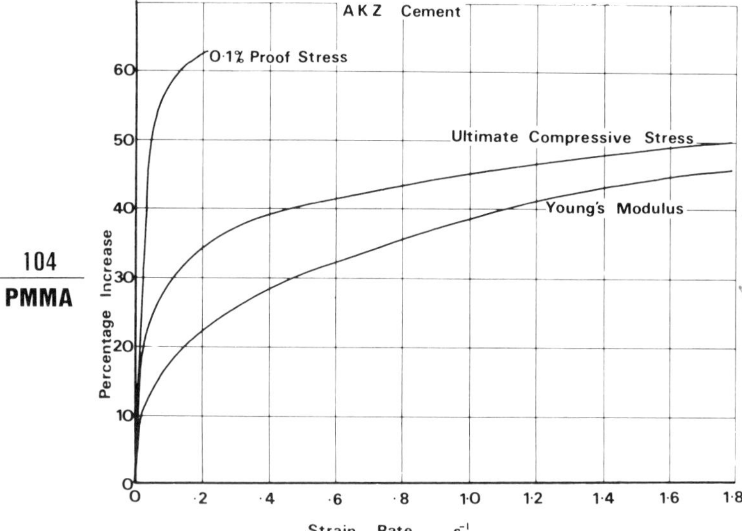

Figure 2: Relationship of strain rate to mechanical properties of cement. (Reprinted with permission from Some clinically relevant variables affecting the mechanical behavior of bone cement, by A.J. Lee, et al., Arch. Orthop. Trauma Surg. 92:1-18, 1978.)

fluid. The equilibrium moisture content leads generally to a 3 percent reduction in ultimate compressive strength in comparison with dry specimens.

Polymers, including acrylic bone cement, are viscoelastic and thus are stiffer and stronger at high strain rates than at low (Fig. 2).

The effects of aging on polymerized acrylic cement are controversial. Acrylic cement aged in bovine serum at 37 degrees centigrade for up to 2 years apparently does not deteriorate in static properties or in compression fatigue behavior. However, acrylic cement placed in a soft-tissue envelope in the paraspinal muscles of an animal demonstrates a nonsignificant trend toward increasing strength in the first 12 months. However, a significant drop in fracture stress as determined by 3-point bending is noted in the period between 12 and 26 months. Acrylic cement specimens machined from cement specimens obtained following total hip arthroplasty up to 7½ years following implantation have not mechanically deteriorated. This suggests that acrylic cement which is stressed does not deteriorate with aging.

The improved mechanical behavior of polymethyl methacrylate when handled early in a lower viscous state led to the development of low viscosity polymethyl methacrylate. However, the mechanical behavior of low viscosity cement required reinforcement with carbon fibers which decreased crack velocity of the acrylic mass by one order of magnitude and increased the tensile fracture strength by 20 percent. The presence of the carbon fibers adversely affected the flow behavior of the acrylic cement. Thus, the improvement of the mechanical behavior of low viscosity cement with carbon fibers has been offset by impaired flow characteristics.

Bioactive glass ceramic particles have been added to polymethyl methacrylate to improve the strength of the bone-cement interface. There is less local tissue necrosis with this bioactivated cement. The integrated glass ceramic particles frequently are surrounded on all free surfaces by bony ingrowth with integration into the trabecular system. An intermediate connective tissue has not formed at the contact surfaces during animal investigations. The viscosity of this material is high and the handling properties are poor. This particular composite of polymethyl methacrylate is not currently applicable for use in humans.

Bone-Cement Interface The radiolucent lines forming at the bone-cement interface of total joint arthroplasties have been a disconcerting phenomenon. Histologically, the tissue forming at the bone-cement interface is laced with macrophages. The stromal cells have an orientation similar to synovium with palisades of cells lining the cement surface. In tissue culture, these cells reveal growth unique to normal and rheumatoid synovium and secrete large amounts of prostaglandin E_2 and collagenase. These two agents are capable of resorbing bone. The secretion of prostaglandin E_2 and collagenase is enhanced when these cells are exposed to a peripheral blood factor known to be elaborated by macrophages.

Macrophages are precursors of osteoclasts. Thus, the macrophage may play a critical role in the development of the radiolucent zones (Fig. 3). The stimuli which activates macrophages and maintains the deleterious activity remains an enigma. It is also not known whether this biochemical phenomenon is a cause of clinical loosening at the cement-bone interface or whether it occurs only after loosening takes place.

Effects on Cardiac Physiology The significant advances in prosthetic joint surgery made possible by polymethyl methacrylate have been offset by the occasional cardiovas-

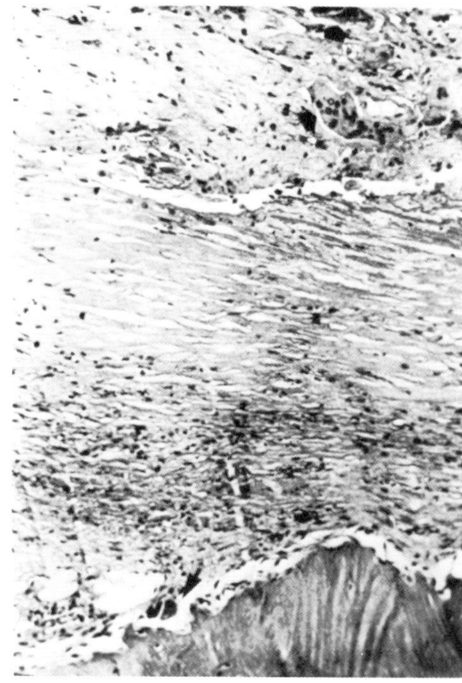

Figure 3: Photomicrograph of the tissue between bone and polymethyl methacrylate, PMMA, (Zone 1) showing two distinct regions. The upper region contains numerous macrophages and giant cells containing PMMA and HDP debris (broad arrows). The lower region is less cellular fibrous tissue. Note osteoclastic resorption of bone (small arrow). Hematoxylin-eosin x 50. (Reprinted with permission from Observations upon the interface between bone and polymethylmethacrylate cement, by M.A.R. Freeman, et al., J. Bone Joint Surg. 64B:491, 1982.)

cular collapse or irreversible cardiac arrest associated with its surgical use. Clinicians feared that the monomeric form of polymethyl methacrylate released into the circulation system might be cardiotoxic. Subsequent experience demonstrates that monomeric polymethyl methacrylate is metabolized to methacrylic acid. It has been impossible to define a quantitative correlation between the maximum concentrations of either methyl methacrylate or methacrylic acid and reduction in arterial blood pressure. The onset of hypotension (usually 30 to 75 seconds following the insertion of acrylic cement) always precedes the appearance of methyl methacrylate and methacrylic acid in the serum.

In patients who develop cardiac collapse, fat emboli and other marrow contents are consistently identified in the pulmonary system during postmortem examinations. A transient elevation of intramedullary pressure is correlated with the insertion of polymethyl methacrylate and the femoral component into the femoral canal during total hip arthroplasty. Some clinicians suggest that elevated intramedullary pressures might precipitate fat embolization, and pressures ranging from 290 to 900 mm of mercury have been documented during insertion of the femoral component. Radioactive albumin placed within the femoral canal before the insertion of the acrylic cement or the prosthetic component appears in the lung 10 to 120 seconds after cementing. Thus, it seems that the cardiovascular changes result from embolization of fat and marrow contents which precipitate aggregation of platelets and fibrin consequent to the release of tissue thromboplastin products into the pulmonary circulation.

Methacrylic acid is the coenzyme A ester which is a normal intermediate in the catabolism of valine. This and other recently developed biochemical information indicate that methyl methacrylate released during the curing process is metabolized via the tricarboxylic acid cycle to carbon dioxide.

Antibiotic Impregnated Cement Recently there has been considerable interest in the use of antibiotic impregnated

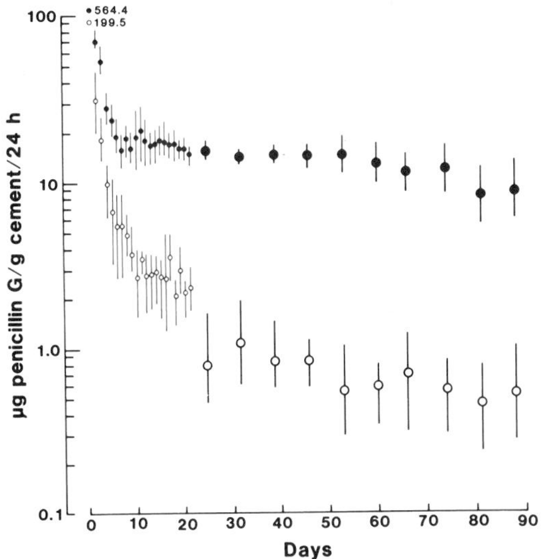

Figure 4: In vitro elution of penicillin from Simplex P (O) and Palacos (●) acrylic cement. (Reprinted with permission from The depot administration of penicillin G and gentamicin in acrylic bone cement, by Hoff, et al., J. Bone Joint Surg. 63A:800, 1981.)

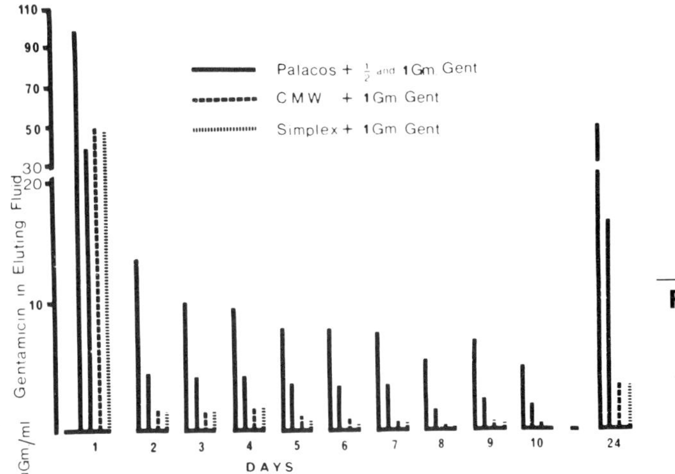

Figure 5: Concentrations of gentamicin eluted from blocks of gentamicin-loaded acrylic cements. Comparison of Palacos R containing 1.0 g and 0.5 g per 40-gram powdered polymer before curing, with CMW and Simplex containing 1.0 g. (Reprinted with permission from Antibiotic-loaded acrylic cement, by R.A. Elson, et al., J. Bone Joint Surg., 59B:201, 1977.)

polymethyl methacrylate. If 1 g of powdered antibiotic is thoroughly mixed with the polymer, the average reduction in the ultimate compressive strength does not exceed 4 percent.

The elution of antibiotics from the polymethyl methacrylate varies with the type of acrylic cement. Antibiotics elute from Palacos acrylic cement better than any other commercially available cement (Figs. 4 and 5). Although heat stable gentamicin was initially believed the agent of choice, more recent data would suggest that a variety of agents, including β-lactams, leach in bactericidal concentrations (Figs. 6 and 7).

The application of this technique in the treatment of the infected hip implant has proved remarkably successful over the last decade in Europe where eradication of infection was reported in 77 percent of 583 patients with an infected hip implant treated with a one-stage exchange arthroplasty. The magnitude of this procedure in patients with an infected hip implant is underscored by a mortality rate of 2.7 percent. Careful analysis of the causal organisms of the infected arthroplasties treated with a one-stage exchange arthroplasty utilizing gentamicin-impregnated acrylic cement suggests that this technique should be limited in scope rather than applied to all patients with infected implants (Table I). The technique was most effective in the treatment of infections from which *Propionibacterium acnes* (anaerobic Corynebacterium) and Peptococcus species were isolated. The actual role played by gentamicin in the treatment of infections with causal organisms against which gentamicin has no activity must be questioned. Meticulous surgical debridement of the involved area and nuances of the symbiotic relationships of aerobic-anaerobic microorganisms may be responsible for the success of this technique. Furthermore, extremely high local concentrations of gentamicin may be bactericidal to organisms normally resistant to the usual physiological concentrations of gentamicin.

Less spectacular results associated with the application of this technique to the treatment of an arthroplasty infected with gram-negative bacillary organisms appears to indicate a limitation of the technique. These patients

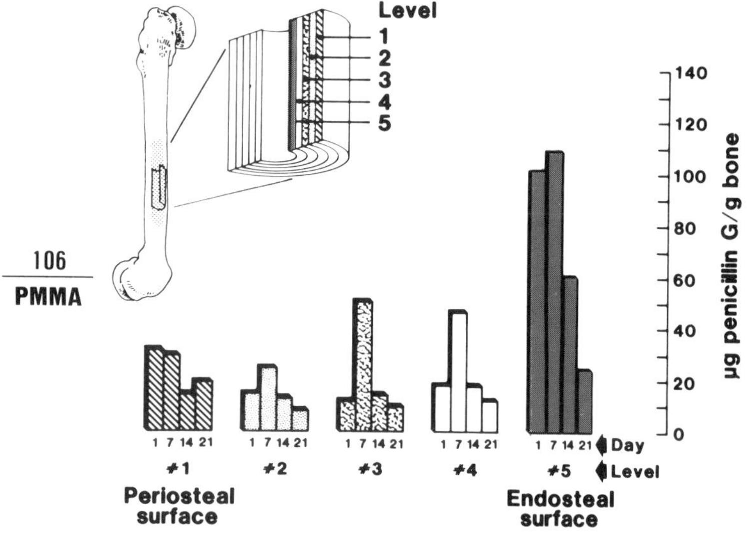

Figure 6: Osseous concentrations of penicillin between the first and twenty-first days following implantation of penicillin-impregnated Palacos acrylic cement in canine femora. (Reprinted with permission from The depot administration of penicillin G and gentamicin in acrylic bone cement, by Hoff, et al., J. Bone Joint Surg. 63A:802, 1981.)

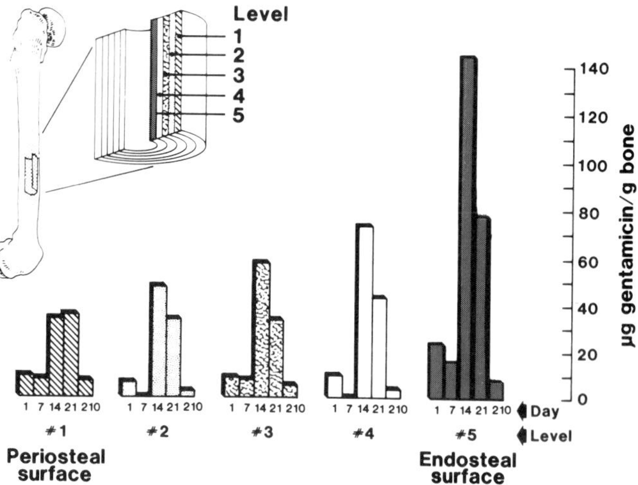

Figure 7: Osseous concentrations of gentamicin between the first and twenty-first days and at 210 days following the implantation of gentamicin-impregnated Palacos acrylic cement in canine femora. (Reprinted with permission from The depot administration of penicillin G and gentamicin in acrylic bone cement, by Hoff, et al., J. Bone Joint Surg. 63A:802, 1981.)

probably are served better by a resection arthroplasty and delayed reconstruction rather than a one-stage exchange arthroplasty.

Application of the depot administration of antibiotics in polymethyl methacrylate to the treatment of osteomyelitis is less successful. Some investigators have initiated the use of the depot administration of antibiotics in patients with osteomyelitis with two basic alterations: temporary implantation and increased surface area. Permanent implantation of polymethyl methacrylate into an osteomyelitic cavity conflicts with the principles of treatment of osseous infections. Since the elution of antibiotics from polymethyl methacrylate is related to surface area, alteration of the shape of the acrylic mass could be crucial. Introduction of preformed beads of polymerized acrylic cement impregnated with gentamicin connected on a wire permits removal of the foreign body and an enhanced elution of gentamicin into the local tissues (Fig. 8).

Implantation of gentamicin-impregnated acrylic beads into the defect following debridement of an osteomyelitic cavity is as efficacious as conventional treatment. The chains of acrylic beads must be removed manually between the tenth and fourteenth days. If removal is delayed, surgical excision becomes necessary. Although to date the depot administration of gentamicin from acrylic beads has been combined with parenteral antimicrobial therapy, future clinical studies relying solely on the depot form of antimicrobial may prove equally as effective.

Adjunctive Applications Although the adjunctive use of polymethyl methacrylate to stabilize pathological fractures of diaphyseal bones has become routine, implantation of polymethyl methacrylate about the cervical spine has been limited because of the exothermic reaction during the curing process. Bone-cement interfacial temperatures of 60 to 65 degrees centigrade during total knee arthroplasty and of 80 to 90 degrees during total hip

Table I

Causal Organisms in a Series of Infected Total Hip Arthroplasties Treated with One-stage Exchange Arthroplasty

	Total Bacterial incidence	Good results after first exchange: Number	Good results after first exchange: Percent
Corynebacterium (anaerobic)	64	54	84
Peptococcus group (anaerobic)	74	56	75
Staphylococcus aureus	274	197	71
Escherichia coli	28	17	60
Streptococcus group D	38	20	52
Klebsiella group	15	8	53
Proteus	33	16	48
Pseudomonas group	69	31	44
Sterile	80	71	88

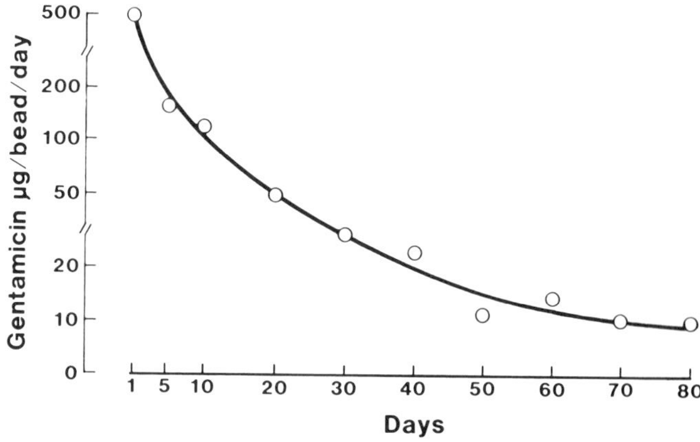

Figure 8: A graph showing the rate of release of gentamicin from PMMA beads in vitro (µg/bead/day). (Reprinted with permission from The release of gentamicin from polymethylmethacrylate beads, by H. Wahlig, et al., J. Bone Joint Surg. 60B:271, 1978.)

arthroplasty have been reported. These are of sufficient magnitude to cause degradation of protein. The adverse effects of such temperatures on the cerebrospinal fluid and spinal cord can be avoided by precooling the soft tissues and bone, placing the cement on the dorsal aspect of the intact lamina, and applying precooled Gelfoam over exposed dura. Thus, acrylic cement and wire fixation of pathological fractures of the cervical spine can be performed safely to allow early mobilization of patients with limited life expectations.

When attempting to reinforce polymethyl methacrylate with carbon fiber, stainless steel wire, or perforated metal sheet, only the perforated metal sheet provides sufficient shear strength at its interface with methyl methacrylate.

ANNOTATED BIBLIOGRAPHY

Mechanical Properties

Hennig, W.; Blencke, B.A.; Brömer, H.; Deutscher, K.K.; Gross, A.; and Ege, W.: Investigations with bioactivated polymethyl methacrylates. J. Biomed. Mater. Res. 13:89-99, 1979.

Addition of glass ceramic particles to polymethyl methacrylate can lead to a tight and durable bond between acrylic and newly formed osseous tissue. An intermediate connective tissue does not form at the contact surface.

Lee, A.J.; Ling, R.S.; and Vangala, S.S.: Some clinically relevant variables affecting the mechanical behavior of bone cement. Arch. Orthop. Trauma Surg. 92:1-18, 1978.

The authors delineate the results of a carefully performed mechanical study of polymethyl methacrylate. Their studies have pertinent application to the handling properties of polymethyl methacrylate in the operating room indicating that containment of the cement, early insertion, and pressurization will lead to enhanced mechanical fixation.

Peterson, L.J.; Pennel, B.M.; McKinney, R.V., Jr.; Klawitter, J.J.; and Weinstein, A.M.: Clinical, radiographical, and histological evaluation of porous rooted polymethyl methacrylate dental implants. J. Dental Res. 58:489-496, 1979.

Porous coated methyl methacrylate (50 and 170 micron pores) dental implants exhibit bony ingrowth and stabilization for up to 3 years following implantation. A PMMA plastic implant was bioacceptable without eliciting a foreign body response.

Rostoker, W.; Lereim, P.; and Galante, J.O.: Effect of an in vivo environment on the strength of bone cement. J. Biomed. Mater. Res. 13:365-370, 1979.

A nonsignificant trend toward increasing strength can be observed during the first 12 months following curing. However, a significant drop in strength between 12 and 26 months was documented.

Bone-Cement Interface

Freeman, M.A.R.; Bradley, G.W.; and Revell, P.A.: Observations upon the interface between bone and polymethyl methacrylate cement. J. Bone Joint Surg. 64B:489-493, 1982.

Macrophages are inherently attracted by PMMA and may explain the presence of radiolucent lines at the bone-cement interface. Since macrophages are osteoclast precursors, bone resorption at the bone-cement interface can occur easily.

Wahlig, H.; Dingeldein, E.; Bergmann, R.; and Reuss, K.: The release of gentamicin from polymethyl methacrylate beads: An experimental and pharmacokinetic study. J. Bone Joint Surg. 60B:270-275, 1978.

Gentamicin-impregnated Palacos R beads released gentamicin in bactericidal concentrations over a several-month period. Application of this technique to an osteomyelitic model in a dog proved to be efficacious.

Effects on Cardiac Physiology

Crout, D.H.G.; Corkill, J.A.; James, M.L.; and Ling, R.S.M.: Methacrylate metabolism in man. Clin. Orthop. 141:90-95, 1979.

Methyl methacrylate in the human body is rapidly hydrolyzed to methacrylic acid which is coenzyme A, a normal intermediate in the catabolism of valine. Methacrylic acid subsequently exerts a catabolic direct influence on cardiovascular function.

Antibiotic Impregnated Cement

Buchholz, H.W.; Elson, R.A.; Engelbrecht, E.; Lodenkämper, H.; Röttger, J.; and Siegal, A.: Management of deep infection of total hip replacement. J. Bone Joint Surg. 63B:342-353, 1981.

A one-stage exchange arthroplasty utilizing gentamicin-impregnated Palacos R bone cement was successful in the treatment of 77 percent of 583 patients with infected total hip arthroplasties. The technique was most effective in the treatment of patients in whom tissue cultures were negative or *Propionibacterium acnes*, Peptococcus species, or *S. aureus* were isolated. It was effective in only one-half of patients with gram-negative infections.

Hedström, S.; Lidgren, L.; Törholm, C.; and Önnerfält, R.: Antibiotic containing bone cement beads in the treatment of deep muscle and skeletal infections. Acta Orthop. Scand. 51:863-869, 1980.

Beads of polymethyl methacrylate impregnated with gentamicin provide for an increased surface area for the elution of gentamicin in higher doses. The temporary implantation of gentamicin-impregnated Palacos R beads was effective in twenty-one of twenty-three patients as compared to twenty-one of twenty-five patients treated with conventional techniques.

Adjunctive Applications

Wang, G.-J.; Reger, S.I.; McLaughlin, R.E.; Stamp, W.G.; and Albin, D.: The safety of cement fixation in the cervical spine: Studies of a rabbit model. Clin. Orthop. 139:276-282, 1979.

Precooling of the soft tissues in bone rather than acrylic cement or monomer provides adequate protection for the central nervous system when PMMA is utilized for stabilization of the cervical spine with neoplastic disease.

14 SHOULDER AND HUMERUS: PEDIATRIC

These afflictions are arranged in the following categories: embryology and growth, congenital and developmental, infection, trauma, neuromuscular, and arthritis.

Embryology and Growth

Development of the shoulder girdle proceeds rapidly during the first 8 weeks in utero. Abnormalities in development can result in absence, malformation, or duplication of parts. The cephalad tip of the scapula migrates from the fifth cervical to the fifth thoracic level, beginning in the fifth week and is essentially complete by the eighth week. Failure of descent results in congenital elevation of the scapula.

The proximal end of the humerus ossifies from three centers. The humeral head ossification center appears between the fourth and sixth months and unites with the epiphyses of the greater and lesser tuberosities between the seventh and fourteenth years. The head of the humerus fuses with the shaft at approximately 19 years.

The ossification center for the body of the scapula is present at birth. That of the coracoid unites with the body of the scapula by the fifteenth year. The acromion arises from two centers of ossification that are united by the twenty-second year.

The clavicle has two cartilaginous centers, one medially for the inner two-thirds and one for the lateral one-third. Failure of coalescence of these two centers may be a cause of congenital pseudarthrosis of the clavicle.

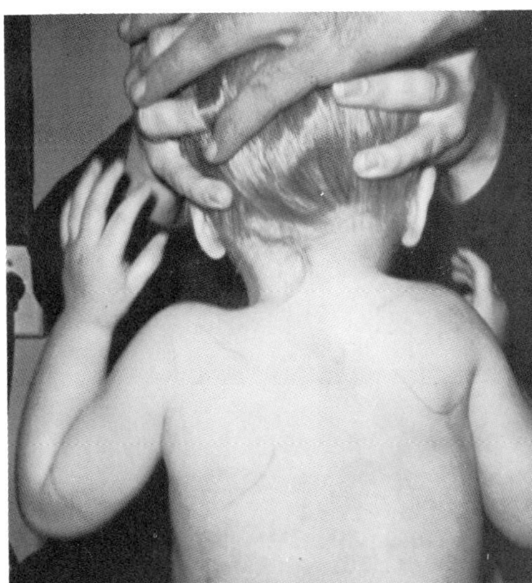

Figure 1: Sprengel's scapula with elevation of the right shoulder in a 2 year old. Hypoplasia and rotation are evident. (Reprinted with permission from Congenital and developmental defects of the shoulder, by S.M.K. Chung and M.M. Nissenbaum, Orthop. Clin. North America 6:381-392, 1975.)

Table I

Congenital and Developmental Defects of the Shoulder

I. Congenital anomalies of the shoulder
  A. Anomalies of the scapula
    1. Sprengel's deformity
    2. Bipartite acromion
    3. Glenoid dysplasia
  B. Anomalies of the clavicle
    1. Segmental defects of the clavicle
    2. Congenital coracoclavicular bar (synostosis)
    3. Cleidocranial dysostosis
    4. Congenital pseudarthrosis
    5. Congenital neural foramina
  C. Anomalies of the humerus
    1. Humerus varus
    2. Congenital retroversion
    3. Bicipital groove aberrations
    4. Aplasia of head of humerus
  D. Anomalies of the glenohumeral articulation
    1. Congenital dislocations
    2. Epiphyseal separation
II. Congenital anomalies of the soft tissues of the shoulder—the musculature
  A. Congenital fibrotic bands of the deltoid
  B. Anomalies of muscular origins and insertions
III. Developmental anomalies of the shoulder
  A. Paralytic dislocations
  B. Secondary contractures of the deltoid
  C. Posttraumatic pseudarthrosis of the clavicle

(Reprinted with permission from Congenital and developmental defects of the shoulder, by S.M.K. Chung and M.M. Nissenbaum, Orthop. Clin. North America 6:382, 1975.)

Table I lists a number of the congenital and developmental defects of the shoulder. Some represent normal and asymptomatic variations in anatomy rather than true deformities.

Congenital and Developmental

Sprengel's Deformity Although the deformity was described earlier, in 1891 Sprengel theorized that this condition was caused by failure of the scapula to descend from its origin as a cervical appendage. This is the most common congenital anomaly of the shoulder and has a high incidence of associated skeletal and soft-tissue anomalies including scoliosis, cervical ribs, anomalies of rib and vertebral segmentation, torticollis, clavicular

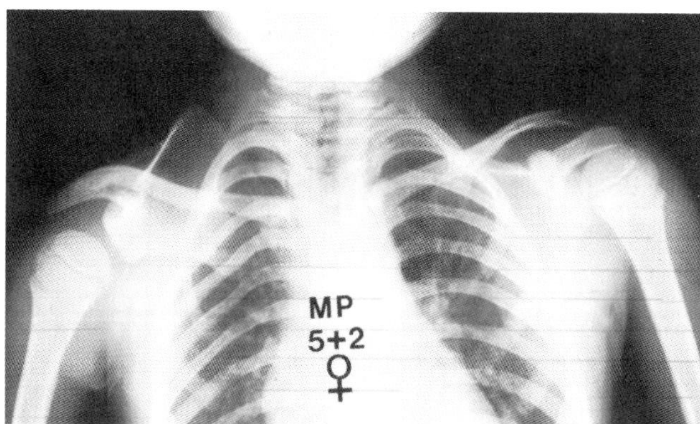

Figure 2: Radiograph of older child with Sprengel's showing typical radiographic findings of elevation, significant rotation, decreased length of medial border, and inferior direction of glenoid. Acromion is prolonged.

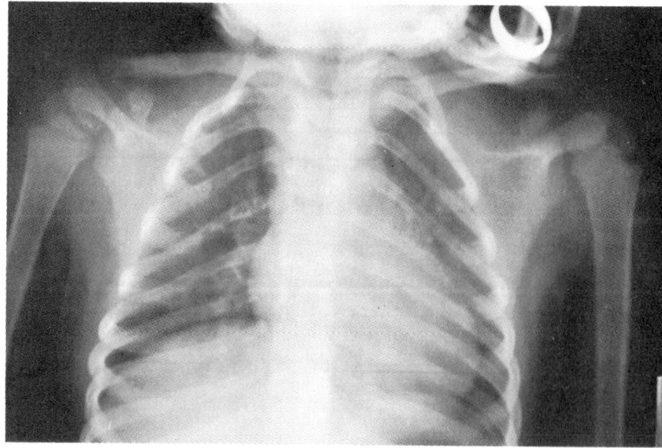

Figure 3: Postoperative radiograph following relocation of right scapula with good position and reformed right clavicle with good curve over first rib after morcellation.

anomalies, renal abnormalities, and muscular hypoplasia of the pectoralis major, rhomboids, serratus anterior, latissimus dorsi, and, most commonly, the trapezius muscle (Fig. 1).

The affected scapula is elevated and hypoplastic, giving the appearance of an equilateral triangle. The superomedial angle may be prolonged which accentuates the true malrotation. Inferior tilt of the glenoid of varying degrees may be seen on radiographs (Fig. 2).

An attachment between the scapula and vertebral column consisting of bone, fibrous tissue, or cartilage may be present in 30 percent or more of patients. This can severely limit scapulocostal motion, but glenohumeral motion is affected less. Abduction should be greater than 90 degrees if no omovertebral bone is present. Computed tomography may be useful for identification of the location and the nature of the omovertebral communication. A true omovertebral bone may be palpable when present.

Because the entire shoulder girdle (including the clavicle) is elevated, there is no stimulus for the clavicle to form an accommodating curve to the neurovascular structures and the first rib. The resulting straight clavicle can cause thoracic outlet compression following surgical displacement of the elevated scapula, and this must be considered during the performance of any surgery in the area.

Although advocated in the past, early passive stretching and active exercises have not been found to alter the natural course of the deformity. Surgery is indicated in those children with significant functional and cosmetic abnormalities. The usual age for such procedures is between 3 and 7 years. The Putti, Schrock, Ober, and Green procedures utilize detachment of the scapular insertions of the muscles prior to caudal relocation of the scapula. The Woodward procedure involves resection of the supraspinous portion of the scapula with detachment of the vertebral origins of the muscles. Relocation and derotation of the scapula are performed with suturing of the detached muscles further caudally on the vertebral spinous processes. Further temporary fixation of the relocated scapula may be achieved by suturing the inferior pole of the scapula to a rib and the medial border to a vertebral spinous process using large absorbable suture material so that the superior border of the scapula is at an equal level to the normal opposite side.

Because of the occasional complication of neurovascular compression by the straight clavicle scissoring over the first rib, morcellation (Robinson procedure) or osteotomy of the clavicle will allow it to mold about the thoracic outlet and avoid compression (Fig. 3).

When a deformity is not severe, or in patients over the age of 8 years, simple excision of the superior angle of the scapula and any omovertebral communication can give improved function and cosmesis.

Congenital Pseudarthrosis of the Clavicle Although there have been a few reports of autosomal dominant transmission with other associated anomalies, most cases of pseudarthrosis of the clavicle are nonfamilial. Congenital pseudarthrosis of the clavicle is not associated with birth trauma. Almost all reported cases involve the right clavicle. Failure of union between the medial and lateral ossification centers of the clavicle has been blamed for this entity. It causes very little early functional disability.

Clinically, a painless, nontender bony mass is usually noted at birth with increasing deformity evident with age. True birth fractures, on the other hand, will cause pseudoparalysis, pain on passive motion, and progressive callus formation on radiographs. In true pseudarthrosis there is

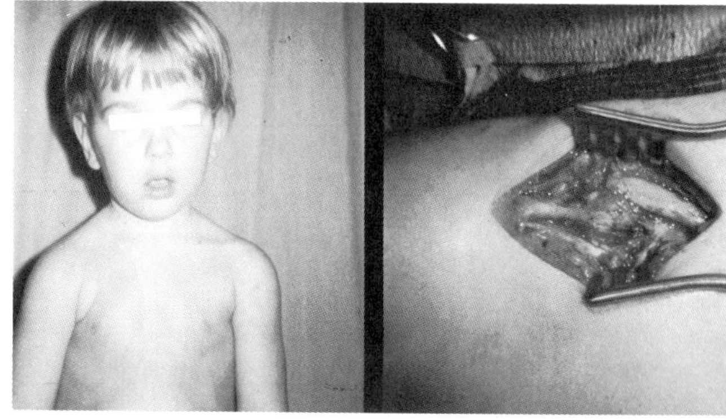

Figure 4-A Figure 4-B

Figure 4: Congenital pseudarthrosis of the right clavicle in a 4 year old. Clinical photograph demonstrates droop of the right shoulder with asymmetry of the anterior axillary folds. Intraoperative photograph shows overlapping and fibrous nonunion. (Reprinted with permission from Congenital and developmental defect of the shoulder, by S.M.K. Chung and M.M. Nissenbaum, Orthop. Clin. North America 6:381-392, 1975.)

Figure 5-A

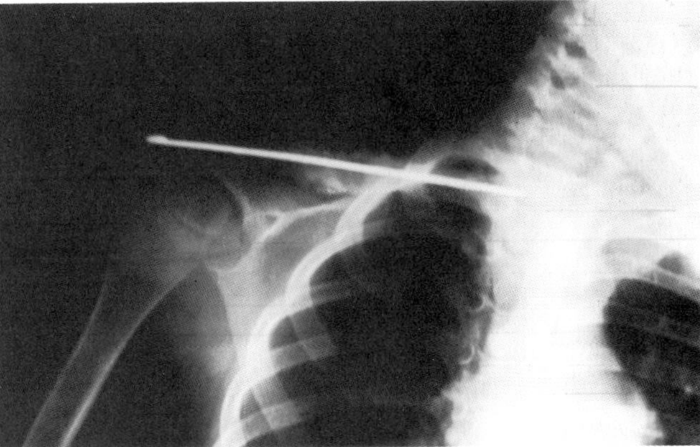

Figure 5-B

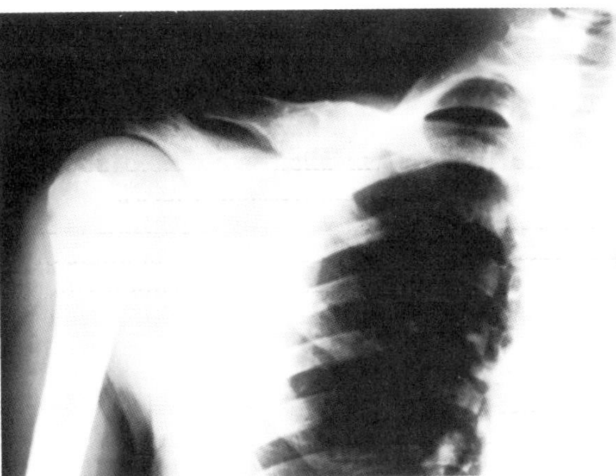

Figure 5-C

Figure 5: (A-C) Preoperative, early postoperative, and final radiographs of congenital nonunion of the clavicle demonstrating results from iliac crest bone grafting with Steinmann pin fixation.

no reactive bone, and bone ends are usually rounded, without the classic "sucked candy" appearance seen in congenital pseudarthrosis of the tibia and neurofibromatosis (Fig. 4). However, little or no discomfort or functional impairment occur.

With subsequent growth, increased asymmetry of the shoulder, winging of the scapula, and abnormal mobility of the fragments are found.

Surgery may not be necessary but can be considered for patients in whom the cosmetic deformity is unacceptable and those with significant functional symptoms. Appropriate surgical treatment, if indicated, is cancellous bone grafting with stable internal fixation (Fig. 5). External electrical stimulation cannot be used because of difficulties in positioning electrodes. Internal stimulation (Brighton technique) has been reported to achieve union, but the complication rate, including pin breakage and pin tract irritation, remains relatively high.

Congenital and Iatrogenic Fibrotic Bands of the Deltoid Replacement of a portion of the deltoid muscle by a short, fibrous band can cause abduction contracture of the shoulder. This deformity is characterized by elevation and winging of the scapula when the arm is adducted and disappearance of the scapular deformity when the arms are raised above horizontal. The shoulders are asymmetrical (Fig. 6A). The fibrous bands may often be palpated. Radiographs demonstrate elevation and rotation of the involved scapula, and remodeling of the humeral head in the older child may occur (Fig. 7). Surgical resection of the band restores good motion (Fig. 6B).

Another cause of deltoid contracture in children is multiple intramuscular injections. These are often bilateral, and the patients are unable to adduct the shoulders sufficiently to approximate the forearms. Intramuscular tetracycline in children may cause this fibrosis. As in a congenital band, excision of the scar gives good results.

Infection

There is debate regarding medical versus surgical treatment of acute osteomyelitis in children (see Section 6, General: Infection). Because the clavicle is an unusual site for acute osteomyelitis, diagnosis is often delayed and identification of offending organisms frequently requires open biopsy.

Surgical treatment of the septic shoulder in children still requires formal arthrotomy, complete irrigation, and drainage with drilling of the proximal humeral metaphysis if osteomyelitis is suspected. Diaphysectomy can be performed provided the periosteal sleeve is preserved and closed.

Trauma

Clavicular Fractures The clavicle is subjected to all medially directed forces exerted on the upper limb and is the most frequently fractured bone in children. Displacement of the fracture is caused by the cephalad pull of the sternocleidomastoid muscle and caudal depression of the lateral fragment by the attachments of the pectoralis major and the trapezius muscles and the weight of the limb.

Fracture at birth causes pseudoparalysis with decrease in the observed voluntary motion of the limb. Reflexes remain intact, unlike brachial plexus paralysis. Treatment is gentle strapping in the infant. In children, a soft figure-of-eight dressing is appropriate. Following healing, small bumps will remodel with growth. Older children may require a plaster figure-of-eight dressing for maintenance of reduction.

Epiphyseal Fractures The highest incidence of fractures of the proximal humeral epiphysis occurs between the ages of 11 and 15 years with males outnumbering females three to one. However, these fractures also can occur in the course of a traumatic delivery. The findings in infants include pseudoparalysis. In the older child there is localized swelling, the arm appears shortened, and there may be a prominence in the anterior axillary fold.

Reduction should be performed on any fracture angulated greater than 20 to 40 degrees, dependent upon the age and remodeling potential. Remodeling may not be complete, particularly in patients older than 12 or 13 years of age. Rarely, interposition of the biceps tendon or capsule prevents closed reduction, a situation more common in adults.

Diagnosis of epiphyseal fractures of the proximal humerus, humeral head, and scapular fractures can be aided with the use of anterior oblique radiographs of the shoulder.

Acromioclavicular Separations These injuries rarely occur in children. Usually children tend to fracture the distal end of the clavicle rather than suffer acromioclavicular separations.

These lesions include simple sprains (type I) and subluxation (type II) which are treated in children and teenagers with simple strapping and sling immobilization. Often, chronic dislocations of the acromioclavicular joint (type III) are not significantly symptomatic in children and may not require formal surgical procedures. However, when symptomatic, a variety of procedures have been proposed. Stabilization either with ligamentous reconstruction, prosthetic substitution for the coracoclavicular ligaments, or transfer of the coracoacromial ligament into the lateral end of the clavicle appears to give satisfactory results, according to the recent literature.

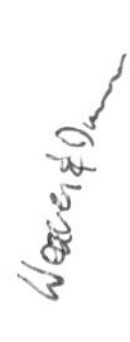

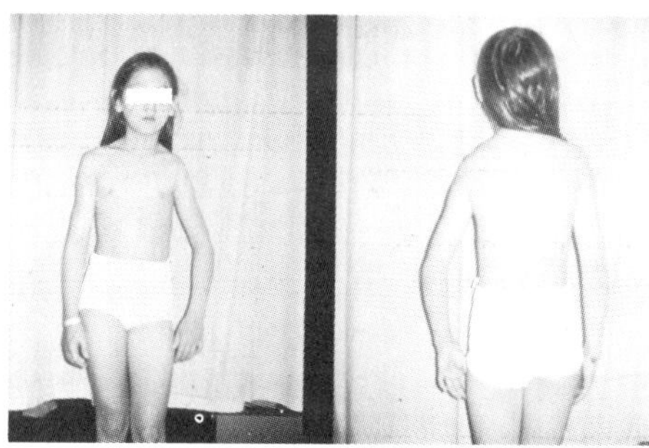

Figure 6-A

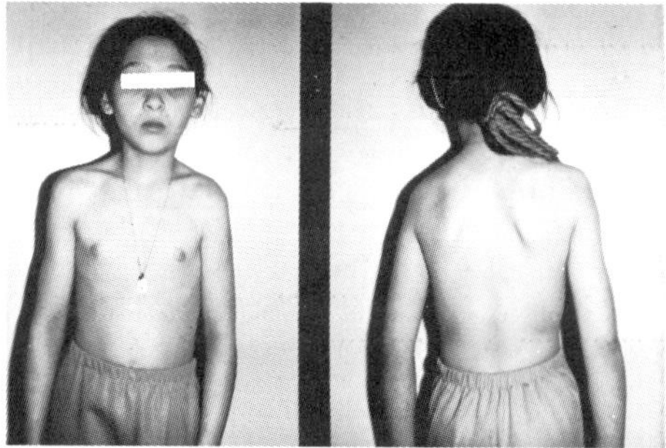

Figure 6-B

Figure 6: (A) Ten year old with congenital fibrotic band of the left deltoid with inability to adduct. Scapular prominence also present. (B) Following excision, full adduction is possible. (Reprinted with permission from Congenital and developmental defects of the shoulder, by S.M.K. Chung and M.M. Nissenbaum, Orthop. Clin. North America 6:381-392, 1975.)

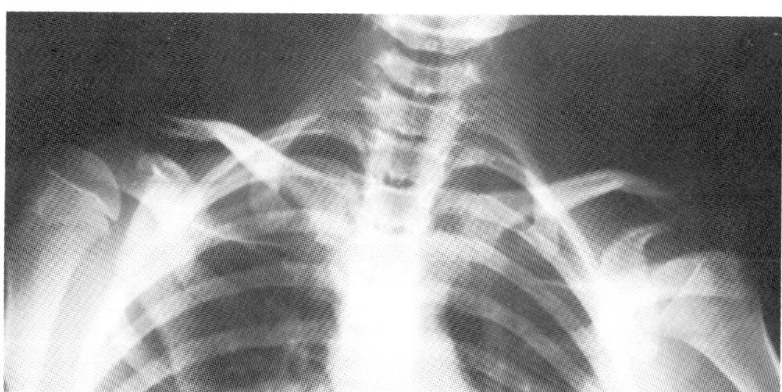

Figure 7: Radiograph of patient with congenital fibrotic band of deltoid in humeral head. (Reprinted with permission from Congenital and developmental defects of the shoulder, by S.M.K. Chung and M.M. Nissenbaum, Orthop. Clin. North America, 6:381-392, 1975.)

Neuromuscular

Obstetrical Paralysis With the improvement in obstetrical techniques in the past 20 years, the incidence of obstetrical paralysis producing trauma to the brachial plexus has decreased significantly. The primary cause of these injuries is traumatic manipulation during delivery, usually due to large fetal size and undiagnosed cephalopelvic disproportion. Factors include breech position, overuse of sedation resulting in maternal relaxation requiring increased instrumentation, and hypotonia in a large infant.

Nerve lesions cover the range from slight stretching (neurapraxia) with early recovery to complete rupture (neurotmesis) and no recovery.

Most commonly involved are the fifth and sixth cervical roots (Erb's palsy) with weakness in the deltoid, biceps, brachialis, supinator, supraspinatus, infraspinatus, and subscapularis (Fig. 8A).

Total plexus involvement is the second most common injury (Fig. 8B). The extremity is usually limp with loss of tendon reflexes, loss of the Moro reflex, Horner's syndrome from involvement of the cervical sympathetic nerves, and diaphragmatic paralysis from phrenic nerve injury. Along with parascapular paralysis, these suggest a poor prognosis because of root involvement.

Radiographs of the neck and both upper extremities should be taken since accompanying bone and joint injuries can be present. Fractures through the proximal humeral epiphysis may be difficult to diagnose since it is not ossified at birth. With upper or total plexus involvement, fixed internal rotation and adduction deformities of the shoulder become evident and, in time, secondary bony changes, including elongation and hooking of the coracoid and acromion, are noted on radiographs. The scapula shows hypoplastic development, and chest radiographs may show unilateral elevation and loss of motion of the diaphragm.

Damage to the seventh and eighth cervical roots (Klumpke's paralysis) results in weakness of wrist and finger flexors and hand intrinsics. Sensation is usually intact except in total plexus involvement.

Differential diagnosis includes pseudoparalysis from fractures or osteomyelitis in the clavicle, humerus, or forearm. Arthrogryposis and congenital bone deformities, such as humerus varus or congenital dislocation of the shoulder also should be considered.

Electromyography may be useful to document recovery

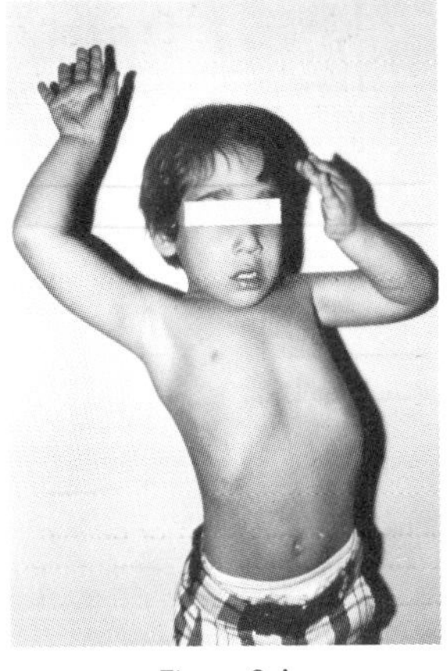

Figure 8-A

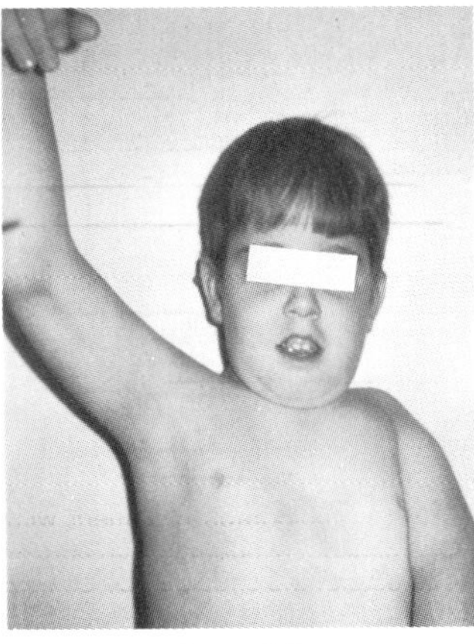

Figure 8-B

Figure 8: (A) Decreased abduction and external rotation of the left arm with normal hand in patient with Erb's palsy. (B) Obese child of diabetic mother with complete left arm paralysis and deltoid atrophy. (Reprinted with permission from Obstetrical paralysis, by S.M.K. Chung and M.M. Nissenbaum, Orthop. Clin. North America 6:396, 1975.)

and also to identify muscles available for tendon transfers in the older cooperative child. Myelography is not particularly useful in view of its morbidity and the fact that the appearance of traumatic meningoceles may not truly indicate root avulsion.

Initial therapy through the first 18 to 24 months of life is directed at preventing fixed deformities while watching for neurologic recovery. The mainstay of treatment for the first 24 months remains gentle range of motion, formal physical therapy as necessary, and intermittent static splinting. However, prolonged splinting in abduction may result in contracture.

Previous attempts at early surgical exploration of the brachial plexus met with failure but are again being revived utilizing newer microsurgical techniques. Some encouraging results in selected patients are being reported. However, additional experience is necessary to evaluate whether this previously discarded approach merits further attention.

In the past, surgical reconstructive procedures emphasized release of fixed contractures and bypassing muscle weakness by using humeral osteotomy to place the arm in a more advantageous position, especially when the hand was functional. Osteotomy continues to have a role in the shoulder joint which is unstable or dislocated. Otherwise, the procedure of choice is the modified L'Episcopo procedure. This involves release of the short head of the biceps and coracobrachialis from the coracoid process; a Z-lengthening of the tendinous portion of the pectoralis major on the humerus; division of the subscapularis; release of the latissimus dorsi and teres major at their insertions on the humerus; transfer of the latissimus dorsi and teres major tendons into the posterior surface of the humerus to act as external rotators; repair of the lengthened subscapularis and pectoralis major; and return of the coracobrachialis and biceps to the coracoid.

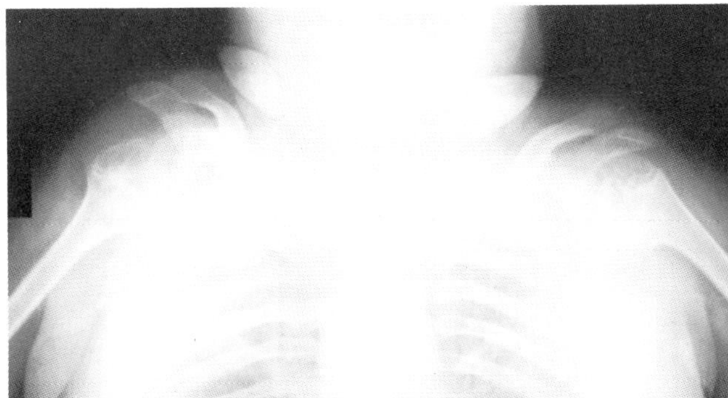

Figure 9: Shoulders in juvenile rheumatoid arthritis with widening and deformity of the humeral heads with cyst formation adjacent to growth plate. Widened joint space noted in right shoulder.

Juvenile Rheumatoid Arthritis

Approximately 5 percent of patients with juvenile rheumatoid arthritis will demonstrate progressive and severe joint involvement. Among these, shoulder destruction is quite rare. When it occurs, initial radiographic features include deformity of the greater tuberosity with progression to cyst formation and erosions (Fig. 9). Eventually, flattening of the medial portion of the humeral head can occur, and, with continued involvement over a period of several years, subluxation occurs. A report of patients with Charcot-like changes has been presented.

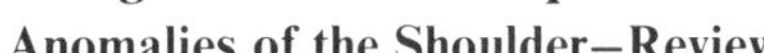

ANNOTATED BIBLIOGRAPHY

Congenital and Developmental

Congenital Anomalies of the Shoulder–Review

Samilson, R.L.: Congenital and developmental anomalies of the shoulder girdle. Orthop. Clin. North America 11:219-231, 1980.

This review of embryology, growth, and phylogenetic changes of the shoulder girdle includes classification and examples of scapular, clavicular, and proximal humeral anomalies.

Sprengel's Deformity

Braun, R.M.: Iatrogenic compression of the thoracic outlet. Johns Hopkins Med. J. 145:94-97, 1979.

Compression of the brachial plexus secondary to operative correction of Sprengel's deformity can occur. The anatomy of the costoclavicular area and the mechanism of injury with scissoring of neurovascular structures are described.

Carson, W.G.; Lovell, W.W.; and Whitesides, T.E., Jr.: Congenital elevation of the scapula. Surgical correction by the Woodward procedure. J. Bone Joint Surg. 63A:1199-1207, 1981.

Eleven patients following the Woodward procedure for Sprengel's deformity are reviewed, including range of motion and scapular lowering. Correction of rotational deformity is stressed.

Klisic, P.; Filipovic, M.; Uzelac, O.; and Milinkovic, Z.: Relocation of congenitally elevated scapula. J. Pediat. Orthop. 1:43-45, 1981.

Soft tissue release of scapula combined with extraperiosteal "greenstick" fracture of clavicle to prevent brachial plexus compression follows relocation of the scapula, which is stabilized with large absorbable sutures from the median and inferior angles to the fourth thoracic spinous process and the eighth rib respectively.

Wilkinson, J.A., and Campbell, D.: Scapular osteotomy for Sprengel's shoulder. J. Bone Joint Surg. 62B:486-490, 1980.

An alternative technique for treatment of Sprengel's deformity consisting of medial release and vertical displacement osteotomy of the scapula is described.

Congenital Pseudarthrosis of the Clavicle

Kohler, R.; Chappuis, J.P.; and Daudet, M.: Congenital pseudarthrosis of the clavicle. A report of seven cases. Chir. Pediat. 21:201-207, 1980.

Diagnostic findings are reviewed. The recommendation is surgery at age 3 to 5 years with resection of pseudarthrosis and bone grafting.

Ogden, J.A.; Conlogue, G.J.; and Bronson, M.L.: Radiology of postnatal skeletal development. III. The clavicle. Skeletal Radiol. 4:196-203, 1979.

Cadaver clavicles from birth to 14 years are reviewed in detail. Ossification centers, curve patterns, sternoclavicular joint anatomy, and the radiographic aspect of development are discussed.

Quinlan, W.R.; Brady, P.G.; and Regan, B.F.: Congenital pseudarthrosis of the clavicle. Acta Orthop. Scand. 51:489-492, 1980.

The right-sided predominance of congenital pseudarthrosis of the clavicle is emphasized in this review of the differential diagnosis between birth trauma, cleidocranial dysostosis, and congenital pseudarthrosis.

Toledo, L.C., and MacEwen, G.D.: Severe complications of surgical treatment of congenital pseudarthrosis of the clavicle. Clin. Orthop. 139:64-67, 1979.

A brachial plexus neurapraxia occurred after bone grafting for congenital pseudarthrosis of the clavicle. Although rapid improvement followed removal of internal fixation, the pseudarthrosis healed with angulation.

Infection

Donovan, R.M., and Shah, K.J.: Unusual sites of acute osteomyelitis in childhood. Clin. Radiol. 33:222-230, 1982.

Usual sites of osteomyelitis in children are femur, tibia, and humerus. In unusual sites, such as the clavicle, clinical and radiographic findings may not be specific or conclusive. Early biopsy may be necessary.

Morrey, B.F.; Bianco, A.J.; and Rhoades, K.H.: Hematogenous osteomyelitis at uncommon sites in children. Mayo Clin. Proc. 53:707-713, 1978.

When osteomyelitis presents at uncommon sites (such as the pelvis, clavicle, or calcaneus), diagnosis may be delayed. Drainage is recommended in abscess formation.

Schmidt, D.; Mubarak, S.; and Gelberman, R.: Septic shoulders in children. J. Pediat. Orthop. 1:67-72, 1981.

The standard surgical treatment of septic shoulders in children, consisting of arthrotomy, full drainage of all recesses, and drilling of the proximal humeral metaphysis, is again advocated.

Trauma

Shoulder

Cohen, A.W., and Otto, S.R.: Obstetric clavicular fractures: A three year analysis. J. Rep. Med. 25:119-122, 1980.

Statistical evaluation of fractures show correlation with birth weight, physician experience, and mid-forceps delivery. One of fifteen showed brachial plexus paralysis.

Cumming, W.A.: Neonatal skeletal fractures. Birth trauma or child abuse? J. Can. Assoc. Radiol. 30:30-33, 1979.

Usual sites of birth fractures are clavicle, humerus, or femur. Fractures at other sites or absence of calcification at fracture site after 11 days posttrauma suggest possible child abuse.

DeSmet, A.A.: Anterior oblique projection in radiography of the traumatized shoulder. Am. J. Roentgenol. 134:515-518, 1980.

Anterior oblique projection can be useful in shoulder trauma, particularly in humeral head and scapular fractures.

Eidman, D.K.; Siff, S.J.; and Tullos, H.S.: Acromioclavicular lesions in children. Am. J. Sports Med. 9:150-154, 1981.

A review is presented of surgical options in twenty-five children between 5 and 16 years with complete acromioclavicular separations undergoing surgical repair.

Gregg, J.R.; Labosky, D.; Harty, M.; Lotke, P.; Ecker, M.; DiStefano, V.; and Das, M.: Serratus anterior paralysis in the young athlete. J. Bone Joint Surg. 61A:825-832, 1979.

Ten patients with isolated serratus anterior paralysis from traction injury to the long thoracic nerve are treated by range of motion exercises and observation. All recover with no residual scapular winging within 9 months.

Rauschning, W.; Nordesjö, L.O.; Nordgren, B.; Sahlstedt, B.; and Wigren, A.: Resection arthroplasty for repair of complete acromioclavicular separations. Arch. Orthop. Trauma Surg. 97:161-164, 1980.

Resection of the distal end of the clavicle combined with transfer of the coracoacromial ligament into the medullary cavity give excellent results and allow return to heavy work and competitive sports. Stress radiographs show good stability.

Deltoid Contracture (Iatrogenic)

Shanmugasundaram, T.K.: Post-injection of fibrosis of skeletal muscle: A clinical problem. A personal series of 169 cases. Internat. Orthop. 4:31-37, 1980.

This large series of iatrogenic fibrosis of deltoid, quadriceps, and gluteal muscles was caused from multiple IM injections. In deltoid fibrosis, the patients are unable to approximate forearms. Tetracycline consistently causes fibrosis. Myotomy gives good results.

Neuromuscular Disease

Eng, G.D.; Koch, B.; and Smokvina, M.: Brachial plexus palsy in neonates and children. Arch. Phys. Med. Rehabil. 59:458-464, 1978.

This study with careful follow-up describes the importance of prevention of contractures and exercise of functional muscles. It stresses preoperative EMGs to select muscle for transfer to be combined with rotational osteotomy of the humerus.

Solonen, K.A.; Telaranta, T.; and Ryöppy, S.: Early reconstructions of birth injuries of the brachial plexus. J. Pediat. Orthop. 1:367-370, 1981.

Three patients with brachial plexus paralysis at birth had nerve grafting before 3 months. Followed for 2 years, they report return of deltoid, biceps, and external rotators.

Rheumatoid Arthritis

Dabrowski, W.; Fonseka, N.; Ansell, B.M.; Liyanage, I.S.; and Arden, G.P.: Shoulder problems in juvenile chronic polyarthritis. Scand. J. Rheumat. 8:49-53, 1979.

Progressive involvement of shoulders in JRA begins with deformity of greater tuberosity, may cause cyst formation and erosions, and progresses to flattening of the medial humeral head. Subluxation often occurs but only after 7 years of involvement.

Rothschild, B.M., and Hanissian, A.S.: Severe generalized (Charcot-like) joint destruction in juvenile rheumatoid arthritis. Clin. Orthop. 155:75-80, 1981.

Although only 5 percent of patients with juvenile rheumatoid arthritis demonstrate severe joint involvement, shoulder destruction is rare. Two patients with Charcot-like changes are presented.

Miscellaneous

Pediatric Prosthetics

Shaperman, J., and Sumida, C.T.: Recent advances in research in prosthetics for children. Clin. Orthop. 148:26-33, 1980.

A review of children's prosthetics includes new powering systems for standard devices and entirely new components. Also described are attempts at providing extended physiologic proprioception.

Surgical Approaches

Bouyala, J.M.; Chrestian, P.; Jacquemeir, M.; Ramaherison, P.: Axillary approach in surgery of the shoulder and proximal extremity of the humerus in children. Chir. Pediat. 21:287-288, 1980.

Good access to the proximal humerus is possible through an axillary approach with excellent cosmetic scars, often a problem in shoulder surgery using other approaches.

Kline, D.G.; Kott, J.; Barnes, G.; and Bryant, L.: Exploration of selected brachial plexus lesions by the posterior subscapular approach. J. Neurosurg. 49:872-880, 1978.

Posterior subscapular approach with resection of the first rib gives access to roots and trunks of the brachial plexus in complicated thoracic outlet syndromes or in patients with previous anterior scarring from either surgery or radiation.

15 SHOULDER AND HUMERUS: TRAUMA

Subjects considered in this section include the traumatic aspects of rotator cuff lesions and shoulder instability.

Brachial Plexus Injuries

Injuries to the brachial plexus pose a formidable problem both to the patient and the surgeon. Recent data suggest an increased optimism for the results of selective operative intervention. A gratifying surgical solution is based on a thorough understanding of the anatomy of the brachial plexus as well as the pathophysiology of injury and repair of the neurologic system.

Injuries to the plexus can be broadly divided into open and closed. Open injuries are usually produced by a sharp object, such as glass or a knife. More extensive damage can be created by missiles such as bullets. Management of the plexus deficit should be based on the overall condition of the patient. Complicating factors may be present which include such associated life- or limb-threatening problems as vascular or chest injury. If there are no severe associated injuries, lacerations of the brachial plexus can be explored and a direct repair undertaken on an elective basis. In those plexus injuries arising from gunshot wounds, it is permissible to delay exploration until spontaneous recovery of any lesion from neuropraxia or axonotmesis has occurred. In open injuries in adults the best prognosis is with the repair of the upper or intermediate trunks and their branches. Improved results can also be anticipated in younger individuals.

Closed or traction injuries are more difficult to reconstruct. They can be divided into supra- and infraclavicular lesions with the supraclavicular further subdivided into preganglionic (root avulsion) and postganglionic injuries. This classification correlates with prognosis. The preganglionic lesions have a poor prognosis and are not amenable to surgical intervention. The postganglionic lesions, however, can be reconstructed in some patients. Clinical, electromyographic, and myelographic evaluation are helpful in establishing the location of the avulsion injury in relation to the ganglion. EMG and myelography should be delayed for 1 month following injury to give the most accurate assessment. Some helpful, but not absolute, physical findings to distinguish preganglionic lesions include a Horner's syndrome, winging of the scapula, a flail arm, and a normal axon response. These findings are not present in the postganglionic injury. In addition, EMG findings confirm abnormalities in the paravertebral muscle activity, and myelography shows traumatic pseudomeningoceles which obliterate all root detail for the preganglionic lesion. Indications for surgical intervention include no evidence of recovery by 3 months following injury and some portion of the plexus believed to be intact at the preganglionic level.

Infraclavicular plexus injuries can result from fractures or dislocations about the shoulder which damage the nerves either by direct local compression or by traction. As a general rule, these injuries can be managed nonoperatively. If, however, there is a combined supraclavicular and infraclavicular injury, the overall management is determined by the more proximal lesions.

Shoulder

Recent interest in shoulder disorders has enhanced understanding of the basic nature and treatment of problems commonly seen about the shoulder joint. Two general problems are receiving the most attention: (1) lesions of the tendons of the rotator cuff, including inflammatory processes, as well as tears; and (2) shoulder instability, including recurrent anterior dislocations, transient anterior subluxations, and multidirectional instability. Although fractures, fracture-dislocations, acromioclavicular injuries, and adhesive capsulitis are problems that arise, their discussion in the recent orthopaedic literature is far less than that of these two problems.

Disorders of the Rotator Cuff and Biceps Tendon Tendons of the rotator cuff and biceps are subjected to chronic, repetitive mechanical irritation from impingement on the coracoacromial ligament, the anteroinferior surface of the acromion, and the undersurface of the acromioclavicular joint. Although the subacromial bursa is interposed between the acromial arch and the underlying tendons, it may not provide sufficient protection from long-term wear and tear on the underlying tendons. In addition, the hypovascular area of the supraspinatus tendon just proximal to its insertion into the greater tuberosity contributes to early rotator cuff tendon degeneration. In younger patients (under 40 years), the effects of this repeated trauma are manifested as acute or chronic inflammatory tendinitis. In older patients with fraying and degeneration of the tendons, there often is tearing or rupture of the cuff tendons. This spectrum of disorders of the subacromial space has been termed *impingement syndrome, supraspinatus syndrome,* or *painful arc syndrome.*

In the younger patient, there is usually evidence of an inflammatory process in the rotator cuff tendons. Frequent causes of such tendinitis include overuse syndromes due to throwing activities, racket sports with overhead motions, and swimming. The most frequent complaint is pain associated with activity that is improved by rest and does not interfere with sleep.

Physical examination seldom reveals any evidence of atrophy. Motion is usually normal or, if restricted, limited by discomfort rather than by capsular contracture. It is important to determine on examination that there is no significant weakness in external rotation or initiation of abduction.

Pain can be localized to the rotator cuff by three maneuvers. One is done by stabilizing the scapula and abducting the internally rotated humerus against the acromial arch. Another, often termed the biceps resistance test, is performed while the patient maintains the extremity in shoulder forward flexion of 90 degrees, elbow extension, and forearm supination. When positive, downward pressure applied to the anterior surface of the distal humerus produces pain. A third test is the impingement sign, in which shoulder pain is produced by hyperflexion of the humerus. There may also be tenderness about the cuff or the biceps, and the acromioclavicular joint frequently is tender or prominent. A plain radiograph does not provide significant clues to the diagnosis.

TREATMENT: Initial therapy consists of at least temporary avoidance of the causative activity. After a period of rest and anti-inflammatory agents, a program of local heat and gentle stretching exercises may be helpful. Occasionally, injection of the subacromial space with local anesthetic and steroid is indicated. After the acute episode subsides, the patient may resume previous activities gradually but on each occasion should apply heat to the shoulder and do stretching exercises beforehand and apply ice to the joint afterward.

Most patients respond to this nonoperative approach. Generally, a regimen of 6 months or more of nonoperative treatment is advised prior to consideration of any surgery. On the unusual occasion when a nonoperative therapeutic program fails, arthrography may be valuable to rule out rotator cuff rupture.

The role of the biceps tendon in this syndrome remains controversial. Some investigators believe that the biceps rarely plays an important role in the painful arc syndrome, and others believe the changes in the biceps are part of the spectrum of this disease process.

Those who believe that the problem usually lies with the tendons of the rotator cuff recommend resection of the coracoacromial ligament, often with an anteroinferior acromioplasty. Others have drawn attention to the role of the acromioclavicular joint and suggest that acromioclavicular arthroplasty should be considered as a component of the subacromial decompression. If the biceps is involved by the disease, a tenodesis of the biceps in the groove, with resection of the intra-articular component of the tendon, can be considered.

Rotator Cuff Tears Tears of the rotator cuff occur more commonly in older patients (over 40 years of age) because of the attritional effects of wear and tear on the cuff tendons through repeated irritation by the acromial arch. Traumatic tears can occur with a fall on the outstretched arm (with no fracture or dislocation of the shoulder), with anterior dislocation of the shoulder (with or without a displaced fracture of the greater tuberosity), and with a fracture of the acromion or the greater tuberosity. Axillary views are necessary to determine the degree of displacement of a tuberosity fracture since the tendons of the cuff pull the fracture into external rotation and posterior displacement. Any greater tuberosity fracture that is retracted under the acromion represents a tear of the rotator cuff insertion. This usually requires open reduction and internal fixation with repair of the rotator cuff to restore good function.

In the patient with a rotator cuff tear without associated fracture, the initial *physical examination* may demonstrate inability to abduct the arm. The drop arm test of passively placing the arm in 90 degrees abduction and asking the patient to maintain it may be positive. If the arm drops to the side, a complete tear of the rotator cuff is suggested. The patient likewise may show marked weakness in external rotation, localized tenderness over the cuff, and significant pain with palm-down abduction. In the later stages, when the tear becomes chronic, active abduction may improve but remain weak. Many such patients may show nearly normal motion, a fact that confuses many examiners and frequently results in misdiagnosis. The presence or absence of a drop-arm test neither establishes nor excludes a diagnosis of rotator cuff tear. In the late stages, weakness in external rotation and abduction can be determined through physical examination. Pain with palm-down abduction also localizes the lesion to the rotator cuff. A consistent feature of chronic tears of the rotator cuff is pain at night. Chronic attritional tears are common but often missed because the patient demonstrates good motion.

Plain radiographic assessment may be unrevealing, but there may be cystic changes, small areas of erosion, and sclerosis noticeable just medial to the greater tuberosity at the area of insertion of the supraspinatus tendon. With a massive or chronic tear, superior subluxation of the humeral head is a significant finding (Fig. 1). An acromiohumeral interval of less than 6 mm also is highly suggestive of a tear. An arthrogram is necessary to establish the diagnosis of rotator cuff tear in a patient without a displaced fracture of the greater tuberosity. The presence of dye simultaneously in the glenohumeral joint and the subacromial or subdeltoid bursa is diagnostic of a tear in the rotator cuff since this anatomic communication does not exist in the normal shoulder (Fig. 2).

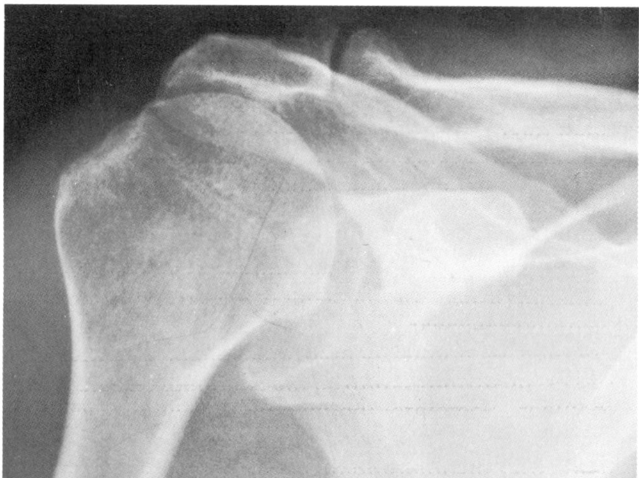

Figure 1: Superior migration of the humeral head in relation to the inferior margin of the glenoid is highly suggestive of a rotator cuff tear. (Reprinted with permission from Tears of the rotator cuff, by R.J. Neviaser, Orthop. Clin. North America 11:298, 1980.)

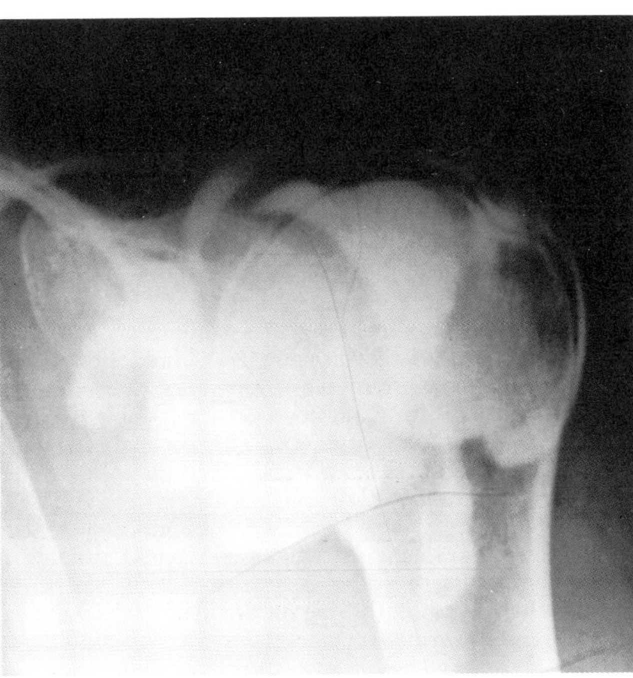

Figure 2: Arthrographic finding of dye in the glenohumeral joint and the subdeltoid bursa simultaneously is diagnostic of a tear of the rotator cuff.

TREATMENT: For the acute stage patient with inability to abduct and externally rotate the arm after injury, the local anesthetic injection test can be done. The subacromial space is injected with 5 to 10 ml of 1 percent lidocaine, and after several minutes the patient is asked to abduct the arm. The local anesthetic diminishes the pain and sometimes permits the patient to raise the arm. Nevertheless, the arm should be maintained in a sling, and the patient should be examined frequently the first 2 weeks. If there is improvement in pain and ability to raise the arm, nonoperative therapy can be continued. If there is little improvement after 2 weeks, an arthrogram should confirm the diagnosis and the repair considered. Statistics support the contention that repair of an acute tear within the first 3 weeks results in significantly better overall function than later reconstruction.

In the patient with a chronic tear, the primary indication for surgical repair is pain. The likelihood of restoring abduction is less predictable than relief of pain, and operative intervention solely to restore motion should be undertaken with complete understanding by the patient and physician that success is questionable.

For the patient whose pain is intolerable, several *operative approaches* are available. The anterior or anterosuperior approach with a deltoid-splitting incision now is recommended. The deltoid muscle is reflected from the superior aspect of the lateral end of the clavicle, the acromioclavicular joint, and the anterior acromion. Restoration of normal deltoid attachment is critical to the success of any procedure on the tendinous structures of the shoulder. Therefore, the method of deltoid elevation or detachment and subsequent repair is extremely important. After the appropriate exposure beneath the deltoid, the coracoacromial ligament is excised, and an anteroinferior acromioplasty is performed. There is no longer any indication for a lateral or complete acromionectomy. These procedures can result in postoperative deltoid detachment, which causes inability to abduct the shoulder because of distal retraction of the origin of the deltoid.

Due to the role of the acromioclavicular joint in the painful arc syndrome, an acromioclavicular arthroplasty often is performed. This may contribute to pain relief and increases exposure of the rotator cuff. The subdeltoid bursa is incised, reflected, and retained for closure later unless severely scarred or diseased. The friable, scarred, or necrotic edges of cuff tears should be resected to healthy tissue. Generally, extensive resection is unnecessary. Stay sutures are used to apply traction to the edges of the cuff, and the tendons are brought lateralward with blunt mobilization. Every effort should be made to reinsert the tendons into their original anatomic site. A variety of techniques can be used for direct repair, but all include tendon-to-bone suture.

If the defect is too large to close by direct repair, several options have been described. A satisfactory procedure for pain relief is inserting the tendon edges to whatever point they reach in the humeral head, as described by McLaughlin in 1944. Alternatives presented in the literature include an interposition of free biceps tendon graft, a transfer of the subscapularis alone or in conjunction with the teres minor, an interpositional freeze-dried cadaver rotator cuff graft, or weaving fascia lata into the defect or using it as an interpositional graft.

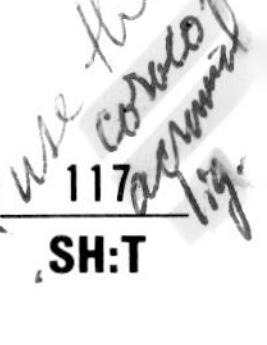

Postoperative care is directed toward rehabilitation of the rotator cuff. Within the first week, guarded passive exercises of the involved shoulder may be started within the limits of the repair. This usually involves passive forward flexion and passive external rotation. The degree of mobility permissible can be determined at the time of surgery by moving the shoulder after the repair to see when the repair comes under stress. That point constitutes the limit of passive mobility. These passive exercises are continued for the first 3 to 6 weeks, and then an increase in exercises is permitted, emphasizing abduction, forward flexion, and external and internal rotation of the shoulder under the supervision of a physical therapist. For those patients with special procedures, such as a freeze-dried rotator cuff graft, the biceps graft, or tendon transfers, active exercises are not instituted until 6 weeks after surgery, but passive exercises are continued in the interim. The patient's arm should be protected at night and between exercise periods with a sling and swathe. Maximum functional improvement cannot be expected in less than 6 months.

Instability Emphasis recently has centered on four problems: recurrent anterior dislocation, recurrent anterior subluxation, involuntary multidirectional instability, and chronic unreduced dislocation.

Recurrent Anterior Dislocation and Subluxation It has been suggested that in anterior instability there is a spectrum of disorders with similar underlying pathophysiology. These have been classified as type I, subluxation without prior dislocation; type II, recurrent dislocation with interval subluxation; and type III, recurrent dislocation without interval subluxation. Patients with recurrent anterior subluxation can also be divided into those who have experienced a major traumatic event or those whose problems have occurred without trauma. Whether the dislocation can be produced voluntarily or occurs nonvoluntarily can also be considered.

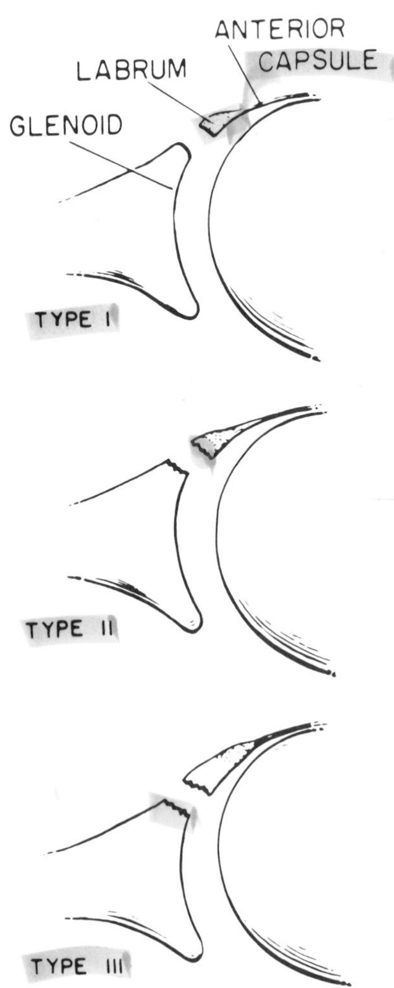

Figure 3: Classification of the severity of Bankart lesions on the basis of damage to the anterior glenoid rim. (Reprinted with permission from Recurrent transient subluxation of the shoulder, by C.R. Rowe, et al., J. Bone Joint Surg. 63A:868, 1981.)

Recent literature implicates the Bankart lesion as a prominent feature of the pathologic anatomy. The most commonly includes avulsion of the capsule and cartilaginous labrum from the anterior portion of the glenoid rim. Less commonly the capsule and labrum avulse a small piece of glenoid rim (Fig. 3). Some variation of the Bankart lesion is found in up to 65 percent of patients. Less frequently capsular tearing or redundancy alone is responsible for the recurrent subluxation.

A new concept in the pathologic anatomy of recurrent anterior dislocation and subluxation is the presence of a defect in the musculotendinous cuff and capsule superiorly in the interval between the supraspinatus and subscapularis (Fig. 4). This has not been previously recorded, and whether it is a normal finding or has a role as a causative factor in recurrent anterior instability is not well defined.

The history is usually characteristic. The patient often is involved in athletic activities and is unable to use the arm in the overhead position with any force. The arm is described as "going dead" when throwing hard or serving a tennis ball. It is important to recognize that a patient may have sustained an injury with the arm in the abducted, extended, and externally rotated position but that such an injury is not requisite. The problem also may arise from repetitive forceful use of the arm in this position. With the onset of the paralyzing numb or "dead" feeling in the arm, the patient may lose control of the extremity and may drop any object being held or readied for throwing. Although the pain subsides quickly when the subluxation is reduced, a sense of soreness persists for several hours.

Physical examination is valuable in establishing the diagnosis. There is often a positive apprehension test (Fig. 5). This is performed by placing the arm in abduction, external rotation, and extension. With the examiner's thumb placed posteriorly on the humeral head, force is directed anteriorly while the arm is increasingly externally rotated and extended. The patient will suddenly become apprehensive and complain of pain in the shoulder. Occasionally, the humeral head can be palpably subluxated anteriorly. Some patients may have a history of being loose-jointed.

Some have advised utilizing a true axillary radiograph or modified axillary radiograph (the so-called "West Point view") to establish the presence or absence of a defect in the anterior surface of the glenoid. This view is obtained by placing the patient prone on the x-ray table with the shoulder built up approximately 7 to 8 cm from the table by bolsters. The arm is abducted to 90 degrees and rotated so that the forearm is resting over the edge of the table and the hand is pointing toward the floor. The patient's head is turned away from the affected shoulder, and the x-ray tube is directed into the axilla at an angle 25 degrees downward from the horizontal and 25 degrees medial from the longitudinal plane of the body. The central ray of the x-ray beam enters posteriorly approximately 12 to 14 cm inferior and 3 to 4 cm medial to the acromial edge. The

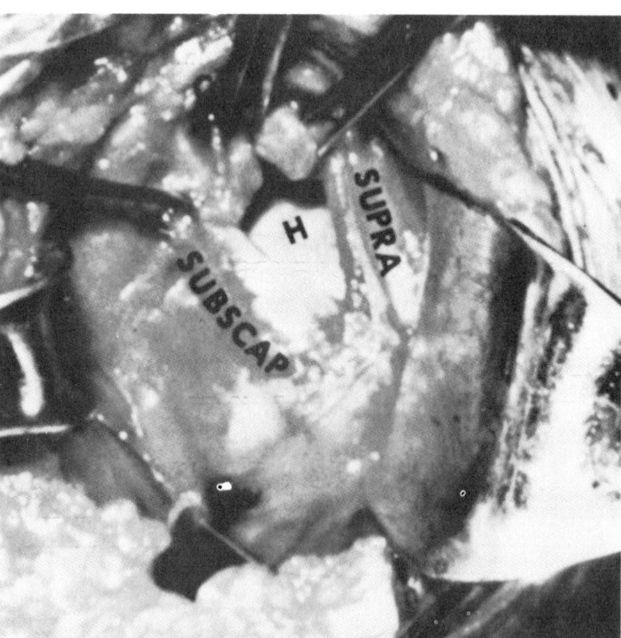

Figure 4: A large opening in the shoulder capsule between the superior and inferior glenohumeral ligaments into the subscapular bursa is seen between the subscapularis and supraspinatus tendons. This opening leads into the left shoulder joint. The floor of the subacromial bursa has been removed to expose the opening, which would have gone unnoticed had the coracoid process not been osteotomized and traction applied to the arm. SUBSCAP = subscapularis; SUPRA = supraspinatus; C = coracoid process; H = humeral head. The large retractor is on the deltoid muscle. (Reprinted with permission from Recurrent transient subluxation of the shoulder, by C.R. Rowe, et al., J. Bone Joint Surg. 63A:868, 1981.)

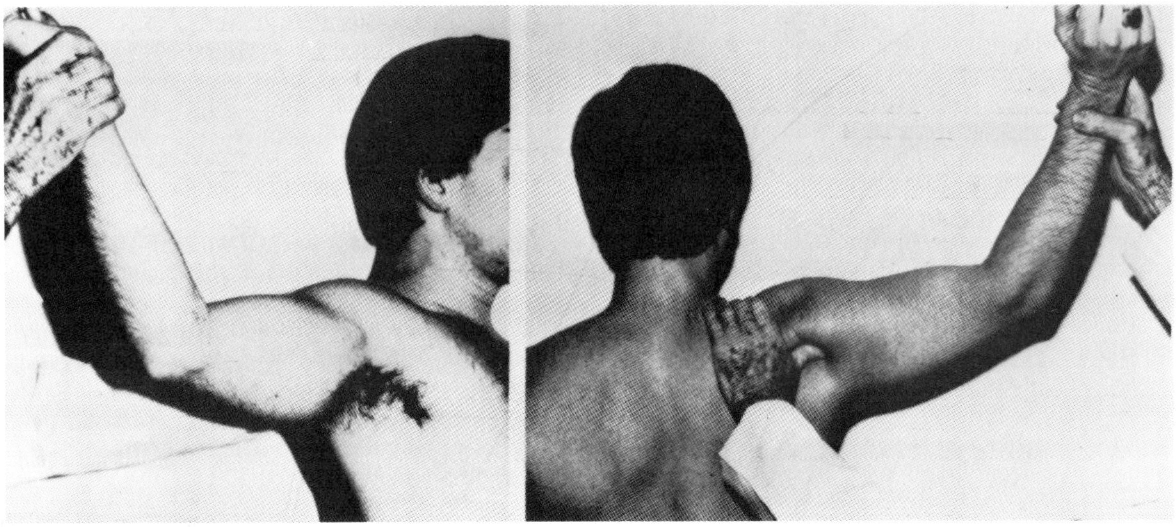

Figure 5-A

Figure 5-B

Figure 5: (A,B) Apprehension test. The arm is rotated externally in a position of abduction while anteriorly directed pressure is applied to the posterior aspect of the humeral head. This maneuver produces sudden pain and weakness in the arm if there is anterior subluxation of the shoulder. (Reprinted with permission from Recurrent transient subluxation of the shoulder, by C.R. Rowe, et al., J. Bone Joint Surg. 63A:865, 1981.)

beam travels in a cephalic-posteroanterior direction tangential to the rim of the glenoid. The plate is placed above the shoulder perpendicular to the x-ray beam.

Other diagnostic tests, such as arthrotomography and arthroscopy, have some usefulness but their role is not clearly defined. In particularly difficult diagnostic situations, the patient can be examined under anesthesia with or without the aid of fluoroscopic control.

TREATMENT: Voluntary subluxation should be ruled out since many patients with this problem have emotional disorders of varying degrees. There may also be an element of secondary gain with voluntary subluxation which is absent in those with involuntary subluxations. For those with involuntary subluxation, physical therapy emphasizing muscle strengthening, especially the internal rotators and abductors, is important to assure the patient that every effort at nonoperative treatment has been undertaken. Occasionally, such an exercise program, combined with an adjustment in the style of throwing or swinging a racket, may solve the problem.

For patients not aided by this approach, surgical reconstruction of the anterior supporting structures of the shoulder can be recommended. Although a number of procedures, including the Putti-Platt and Bristow, are being used to correct recurrent anterior instability, recent emphasis has been on the efficacy of the Bankart (Fig. 6) or modified Bankart technique (Fig. 7). One advantage of these procedures is restoration of the anteroinferior gle-

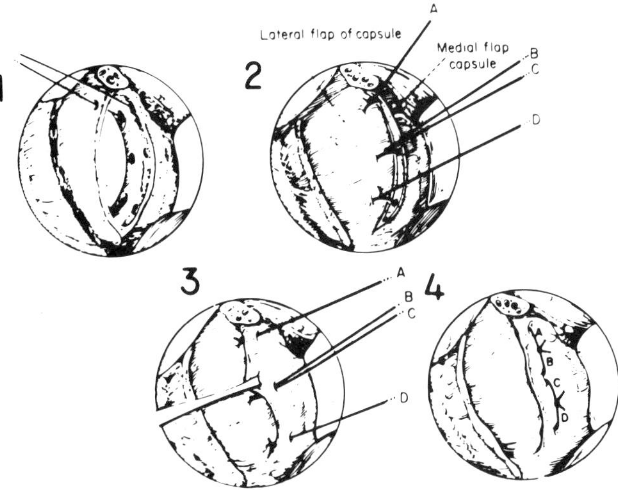

Figure 6: The standard Bankart procedure is used when the capsule and labrum are avulsed from the glenoid rim. (1) Three drill holes are made in the anterior glenoid rim. (2) Three sutures are used to reattach the lateral flap of the capsule to bone. (3) Once the sutures are tied, four of the six ends of the tied sutures are passed through the medial flap of the capsule as shown, and (4) are tied to one another as indicated to form a double-layered reinforcement at the site of repair. (Reprinted with permission from Recurrent transient subluxation of the shoulder, by C.R. Rowe, et al., J. Bone Joint Surg. 63A:866, 1981.)

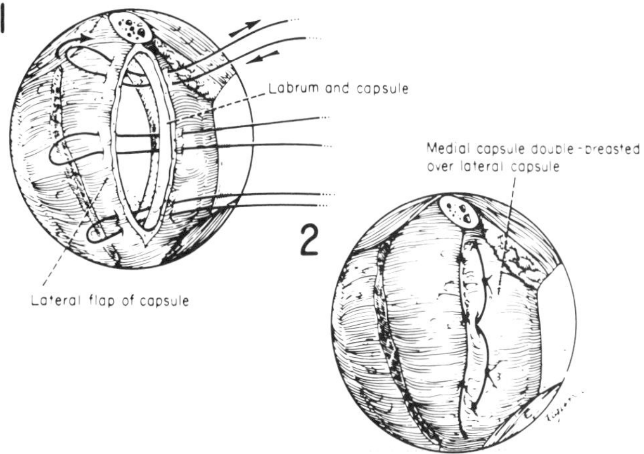

Figure 7: Anterior shoulder capsulorrhaphy is performed when a Bankart lesion is not present. Since the capsule and labrum are not avulsed from the glenoid, they are used to anchor the sutures at the rim of the glenoid when reefing the anterior and inferior parts of the capsule. (1) The sutures are passed through the medial flap of the capsule deep to the labrum, through the lateral flap of the capsule and back under the labrum and through the capsule, where they are tied. (2) Four of the six ends of the sutures then are tied to one another as in the Bankart procedure, and the free margin of the medial flap is sutured to the underlying lateral flap with interrupted sutures to produce a double-layered reinforcement as indicated. (Reprinted with permission from Recurrent transient subluxation of the shoulder, by C.R. Rowe, et al., J. Bone Joint Surg. 63A:866, 1981.)

noid labrum, which is an extension of the inferior glenohumeral ligament. Since this is a basic pathologic entity, this operation may attack the lesion itself. Another advantage is the minimal loss of external rotation following the Bankart. If a rotator cuff defect is discovered in the interval between the subscapularis and supraspinatus, it is repaired. Demonstration of this lesion is accomplished by placing traction inferiorly on the shoulder while sliding a finger along the lateral aspect of the base of the coracoid process to palpate the cuff. Although the role of the tendinous defect in the production of an anterior dislocation has not been clearly established, it has been suggested that this represents congenital absence of the middle glenohumeral ligament, allowing increased anterior mobility.

Involuntary Multidirectional Instability The pathological anatomy has been found to be redundancy of the ligaments and inferior part of the capsule of the glenohumeral joint.

The history in these patients is somewhat different from those with anterior subluxation. Many report having discomfort or fatigue when carrying heavy loads that apply an inferior or downward force on the upper extremity. They also may describe an inability to throw, swim, or work with the arm overhead. There may be a variable history of injury, with some patients reporting only a mild injury and others a severe one. They are generally athletically active. Many mistakenly are diagnosed as having subluxated or dislocated in one direction only. These patients give a history of uncontrollable or involuntary inferior subluxation or dislocation in addition to anterior and/or posterior instability. This can be demonstrated clinically on physical examination by either applying traction inferiorly on the arm or asking the patient to hold heavy weights in both arms with the shoulders relaxed (Fig. 8A).

Stress radiographs taken in this position demonstrate further inferior subluxation of the humerus in relation to the glenoid on the involved side as opposed to the uninvolved side (Fig. 8B). Generalized hyperlaxity of other joints is present in a significant number of these patients.

TREATMENT: Initially this consists of changing the form of use of the shoulder and doing strengthening exercises. The latter should be directed at improving the strength and tone of the rotator cuff and deltoid. But if such a program is unsuccessful over an extended period of time, surgical intervention may be considered. It should be emphasized that patients who have voluntary multidirectional subluxation often have emotional disorders and should not be operated upon.

Surgical treatment is directed toward tightening the inferior capsular laxity. The incision may be either anterior or posterior, depending upon the associated direction of instability. Preoperatively this often can be determined clinically, but a reassessment of the shoulder under

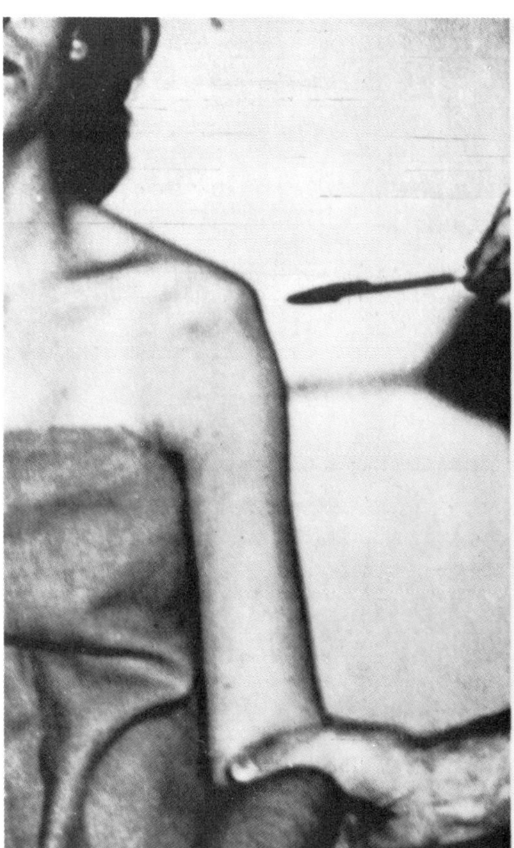

Figure 8-A

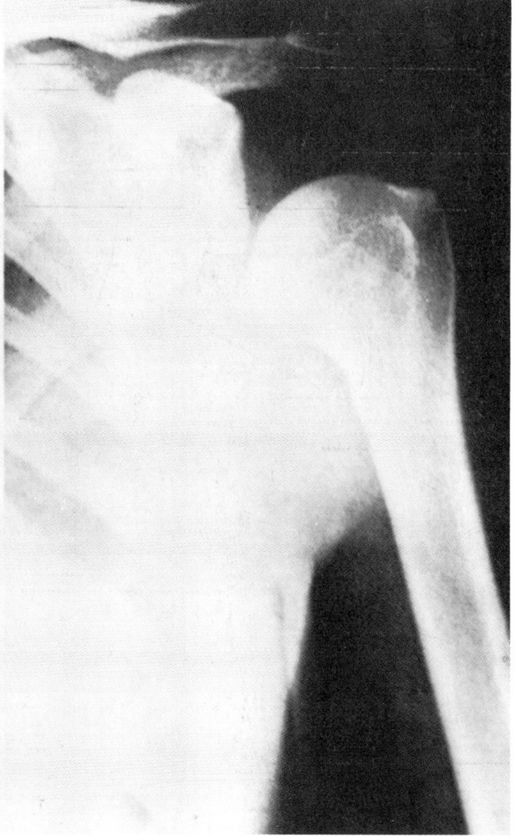

Figure 8-B

Figure 8: (A) A 30-year-old woman with symptomatic inferior and multidirectional instability. Inferior subluxation is produced by downward traction on the arm. (B) Traction radiograph of the same shoulder showing marked inferior subluxation. (Reprinted with permission from Inferior capsular shift for involuntary inferior and multidirectional instability of the shoulder: A preliminary report, by C.S. Neer, II, et al., J. Bone Joint Surg. 62A:898, 1980.)

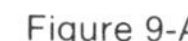

Figure 9-A

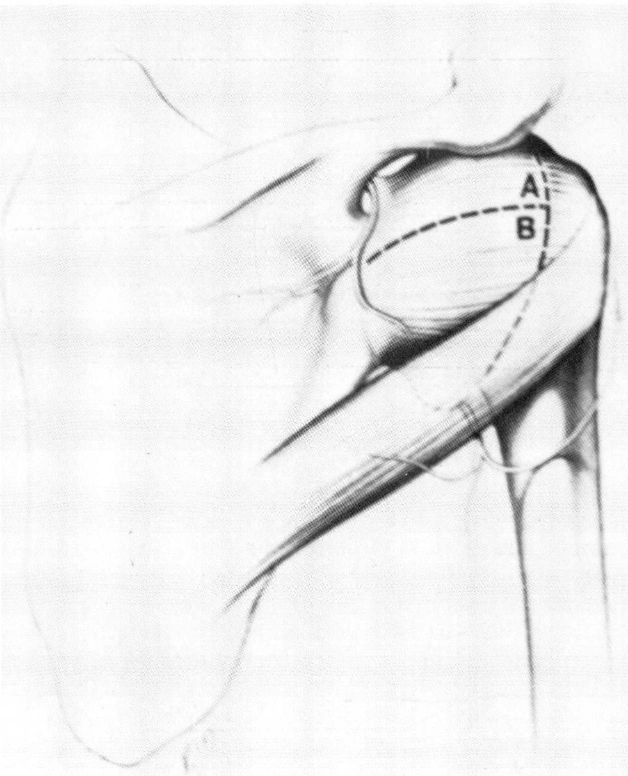

Figure 9-B

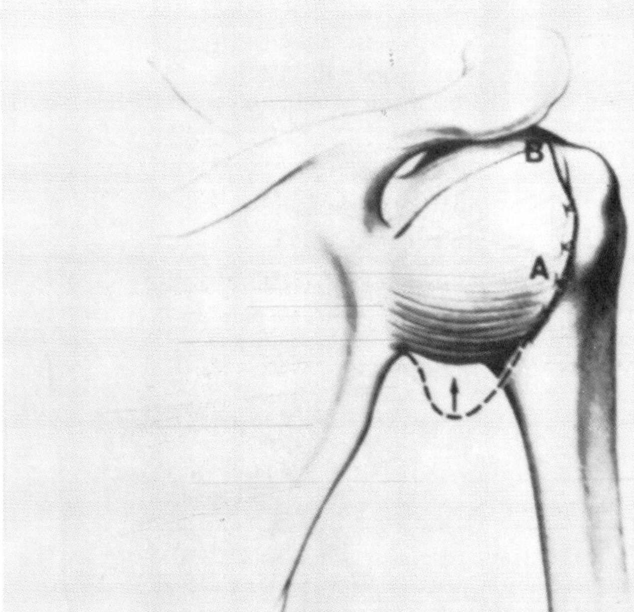

Figure 9-C

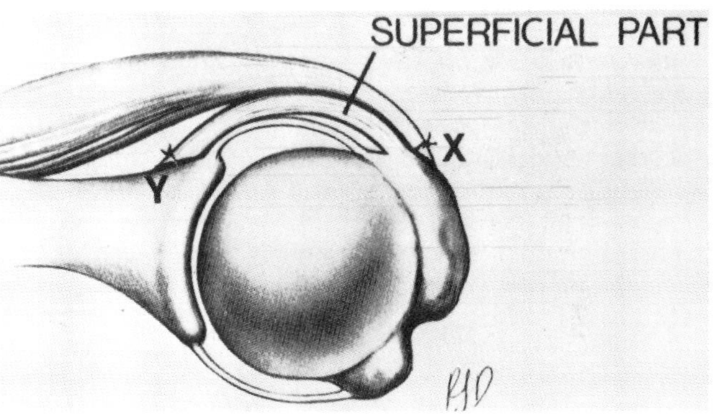

Figure 9-D

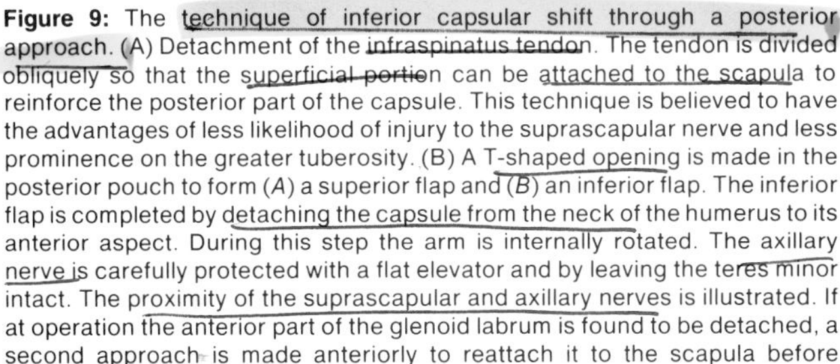

Figure 9: The technique of inferior capsular shift through a posterior approach. (A) Detachment of the infraspinatus tendon. The tendon is divided obliquely so that the superficial portion can be attached to the scapula to reinforce the posterior part of the capsule. This technique is believed to have the advantages of less likelihood of injury to the suprascapular nerve and less prominence on the greater tuberosity. (B) A T-shaped opening is made in the posterior pouch to form (*A*) a superior flap and (*B*) an inferior flap. The inferior flap is completed by detaching the capsule from the neck of the humerus to its anterior aspect. During this step the arm is internally rotated. The axillary nerve is carefully protected with a flat elevator and by leaving the teres minor intact. The proximity of the suprascapular and axillary nerves is illustrated. If at operation the anterior part of the glenoid labrum is found to be detached, a second approach is made anteriorly to reattach it to the scapula before proceeding with the inferior capsular shift. (C) Relocation of the flaps. After a shallow slot has been made in the neck of the humerus, the arm is held in moderate external rotation and extension as the flaps are reattached. The superior flap (*B*) is then pulled downward and reattached. The inferior flap (*A*) is then pulled backward and upward over it, reducing the redundancy of the capsule anteriorly, inferiorly, and posteriorly and reinforcing it posteriorly. (D) Reinforcement of the capsular flaps. The superficial part of the infraspinatus tendon (*Y*) is brought down and sutured against raw bone on the scapular neck. The deep portion of the infraspinatus tendon (*X*) is sutured over this so that it will remain a strong external rotator. (Reprinted with permission from Inferior capsular shift for involuntary inferior and multidirectional instability of the shoulder: A preliminary report, by C.S. Neer, II, et al., J. Bone Joint Surg. 62A:902-903, 1980.)

anesthesia is helpful in determining the directions of subluxation. It is rather easy to confuse reducing a subluxation with producing one on clinical examination.

If the primary directions of instability are posterior and inferior, a posterior approach is utilized. An incision is made over the posterior aspect of the acromion, and the deltoid is detached on the posterior lateral aspect of the acromion and spine of the scapula. The infraspinatus is detached, leaving a deep layer attached to the capsule for further reinforcement (Fig. 9A). A T-shaped opening is made in the capsule posteriorly (Fig. 9B), and a superior capsular flap developed. An inferior capsular flap is made subsequently, with care taken to prevent injury to the axillary nerve. The joint is distracted, and an inspection of the anterior rim of the glenoid is made. If a Bankart lesion is found, a separate anterior approach is made to repair it. If not, the posterior portion of the capsule is drawn backward to eliminate the inferior pouch and reduce any anterior capsular laxity. A slot is made at the junction of the inferior aspect of the humeral articular cartilage with the humeral shaft so the capsular flap will approximate to cancellous bone while the arm is held in slight extension and moderate external rotation. Traction is applied to the inferior flap to determine how far it can be advanced to eliminate the anterior and inferior instability. Once this has been determined, the superior flap is sutured in position first, and the longer inferior flap is imbricated over the superior one (Fig. 9C). The infraspinatus is then reattached (Fig. 9D), and the deltoid closed.

For those patients with primarily anterior and inferior instability, an anterior axillary incision is used. The standard approach to the anterior surface of the joint is accomplished. The subscapularis is split, leaving the deep portion attached to the anterior capsule to provide further reinforcement (Fig. 10A). The capsule is opened in T-shaped fashion (Fig. 10B), and a superior and inferior flap developed (Fig. 10C). Care must be taken to protect the axillary nerve. The interior of the joint is inspected, and posterior instability is tested both with and without traction anteriorly on the inferior flap. This allows for an adequate estimate of the new location of the inferior flap to reduce posterior and inferior instability. A similar shallow cancellous groove is made on the humeral neck. In this approach the inferior flap is sutured first, and the superior flap imbricated over it (Fig. 10C). The arm must be held in slight flexion and in 10 degrees of external rotation while the capsular flaps are being sutured. The subscapularis is reattached to its normal location. Postoperative care includes immobilization in a splint or cast for 5 to 6 weeks, followed by heat and gentle exercises. The objective is to recover motion gradually rather than rapidly. Return to athletic activities is slow, and strenuous sports are avoided for at least 9 months and until muscle strength is normal on manual testing.

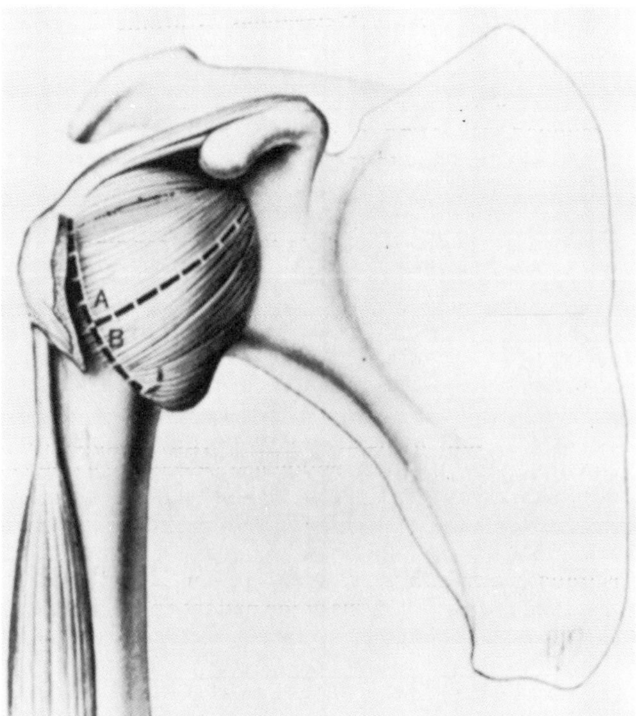

Figure 10-B

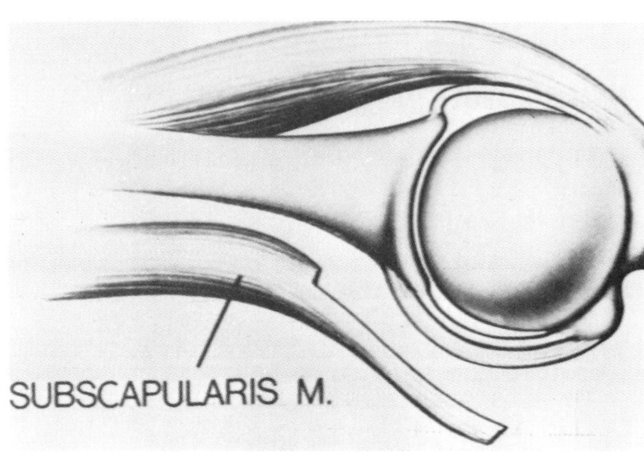

Figure 10-A

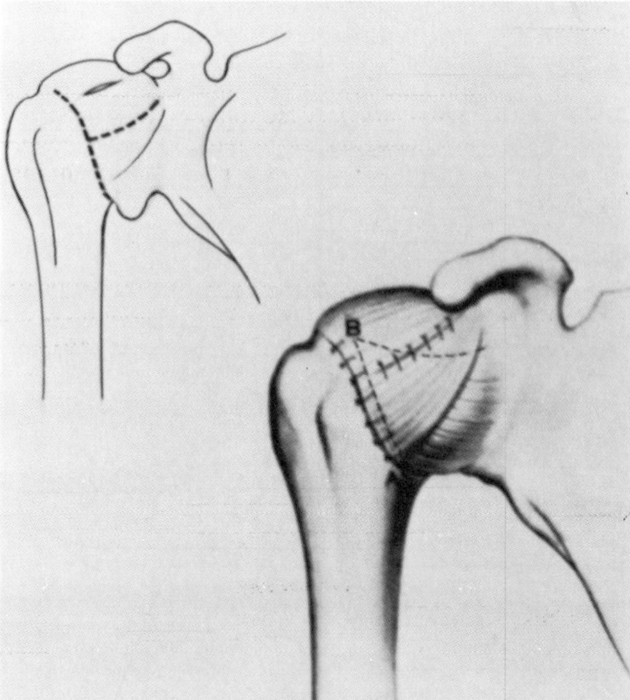

Figure 10-C

Figure 10: The technique of inferior capsular shift through an anterior approach. (A) Reinforcement of the capsular flaps. Approximately 50 percent of the thickness of the subscapularis tendon is left attached to reinforce the capsule. (B) Capsular incisions. The opening between the superior and middle glenohumeral ligaments (which is almost constant) is closed with nonabsorbable sutures. A T-shaped opening is made by incising longitudinally between the middle and inferior glenohumeral ligaments and detaching the capsule and ligaments from the neck of the humerus anteriorly, inferiorly, and to the posterior part of the neck. (C) Relocating the flaps. The arm is held in slight flexion and 10 degrees of external rotation on the arm board. The inferior flap (*B*) is relocated first. It is pulled forward to tighten the posterior part of the capsule until posterior subluxation no longer occurs, and it is pulled upward until the inferior capsular pouch is eliminated. The flap then is sutured to the stump of subscapularis tendon and to the part of the capsule remaining on the humerus to hold it against the slot. The surplus portion of the flap is usually folded over to further reinforce the capsule. The superior flap (*A*), which contains the middle glenohumeral ligament, is brought down over the inferior flap so that it suspends the humerus and reinforces anteriorly as well. Note the sutures used to close the cleft between the middle and inferior glenohumeral ligaments prior to making the capsular incision. Finally, the subscapularis tendon is brought to its normal position and secured with nonabsorbable sutures so that it will remain a strong internal rotator. (Adapted with permission from Inferior capsular shift for involuntary inferior and multidirectional instability of the shoulder: A preliminary report, by C.S. Neer, II, et al., J. Bone Joint Surg. 62A:901, 1980.)

Chronic Unreduced Dislocations Chronic unreduced dislocations of the shoulder are more frequent than previously appreciated. A recent survey of over 200 orthopaedic surgeons in New England indicated that the likelihood of seeing a chronic unreduced dislocation increases directly with the length of time in practice. This survey also indicated that the most frequently encountered type of chronic unreduced dislocation is an anterior dislocation which contradicts the long-standing opinion that the posterior dislocation is more commonly missed.

Five treatment options are available: (1) no treatment; (2) manipulation and closed reduction; (3) open reduction; (4) prosthetic replacement; and (5) humeral head resection and reattachment of the rotator cuff.

No treatment need be offered if the patient's lifestyle or activities of daily living are not sufficiently disabled by the chronic dislocation. This option was selected in 42 percent of the patients in a recent study. When evaluated over a long period, these patients have a significantly poorer rating than those treated by other means. Closed reduction is fraught with danger. It should be considered only after assessing the overall status of the patient and the extremity as well as the radiographic appearance. There is a significant risk of producing an associated fracture. Open reduction is the most commonly utilized procedure. The anterior approach is useful for anterior and posterior dislocations, but a utilitarian, superior approach with detachment of the deltoid from the anterior, lateral, and posterior aspects of the acromion has been suggested. Prosthetic replacement is justified when there is extensive, severe posttraumatic arthritis. Simple humeral head resection with reattachment of the rotator cuff is an alternative to consider; however, open reduction with humeral head retention or replacement is preferable to humeral head resection.

Transfer of the subscapularis, either with or without a piece of the lesser tuberosity, should be utilized in those patients in whom chronic posterior dislocation appears to be unstable after open reduction, and in whom there is an anterior humeral impression fracture. Postoperative care includes maintaining the arm either anterior or posterior to the coronal plane of the body, depending upon the original direction of the dislocation. This approach has eliminated the need for transarticular pin fixation to prevent redislocation. Gentle active motion, again in the appropriate plane, can be initiated shortly after surgery. The overall results are better than previously suspected.

Humerus

Fractures In 1979 Neer classified fractures of the proximal humerus according to displacement of the major anatomic segments, a classification similar to Codman's earlier description. The recommendations arising from the conclusions of that study have not changed. Two-part fractures can be treated successfully by closed means, but if unacceptable displacement of the fragments cannot be reduced, open reduction is indicated. This is especially true of displaced fractures of the greater tuberosity (more than 5 to 10 mm of residual displacement) because they represent a tear of the rotator cuff.

Displaced three-part fractures or fracture-dislocations require open treatment with meticulous care taken to achieve anatomic reduction and secure fixation. Secure fixation may be achieved by cancellous screws and/or tension band techniques. The displaced four-part fractures or fracture-dislocations may be treated by a humeral head prosthetic replacement with repositioning of the tuberosities and cuff repair. In young patients primary repair may be attempted even though the success rate is very low.

Humeral shaft fractures with radial nerve palsy continue to present a therapeutic dilemma. Currently, recommendations for treatment emphasize that most, if not all, radial nerve palsies associated with these fractures recover spontaneously within 3 months. Operative exploration of the nerve in a closed injury should be delayed until recovery is not evident at 3 months. In an open humeral shaft fracture with radial nerve palsy, exploration of the nerve is justified especially if the nerve is directly in the operative field at the time of debridement. It should be noted, however, that most radial nerve injuries associated with humeral shaft fractures are contusion or traction palsies and not lacerations.

Recent experience with functional bracing for humeral shaft fractures has shown that the rate of union is high. There is also less associated morbidity in terms of regaining shoulder and elbow function. A limitation of functional bracing is a persistent varus deformity that the brace does not always correct. Treatment includes passive exercises and a collar and cuff for the first 3 weeks while wearing the brace. The collar and cuff then can be discontinued in most patients.

ANNOTATED BIBLIOGRAPHY

Brachial Plexus Injuries

Hoffer, M.M.; Braum, R.; Hsu, J.; Mitani, M.; and Temes, K.: Functional recovery and orthopedic management of brachial plexus palsies. J. Am. Med. Assn. 246:2467-2470, 1982.

Functional recovery in 133 patients with brachial plexus palsy (45 birth, 18 childhood trauma, and 70 adult trauma) was best predicted by serial clinical examination. For patients with complete recovery and those with substantial recovery, the latest onset of return of function was 3 months and 5 to 6 months respectively.

Kline, D.G., and Judice, D.J.: Operative management of selected brachial plexus lesion. J. Neurosurg. 58:631-649, 1983.

Treatment recommendations based on a 12-year operative experience with 171 consecutive patients are made. Delayed exploration is recommended unless the injury is one of sharp transection of neural elements.

Leffert, R.D.: Brachial plexus. *In* Operative Hand Surgery, edited by D.P. Green, pp. 1091-1108. New York, Churchill Livingstone, 1982.

An extensive review of the current status of management of brachial plexus injuries with operative details about reconstructive techniques.

Narakas, A.: Brachial plexus surgery. Orthop. Clin. North America 12:303-323, 1981.

Experience with 800 patients with brachial plexus injuries concluded that gratifying results can be obtained with injuries to C-5, 6, and 7, but not those involving C-8 and T-1. Lesions that involve the plexus origin of such nerves as the suprascapular, the axillary, the musculocutaneous, radial and to some degree the median are amenable to surgical intervention. The ulnar nerve results have been disappointing.

Rorabeck, C.H., and Harris, W.R.: Factors affecting the prognosis of brachial plexus injuries. J. Bone Joint Surg. 64B:404-407, 1981.

In 131 patients (134 injuries) the best recovery was observed in those with isolated injuries to the upper trunk and the poorest prognosis in those with complete injury of the plexus.

Shoulder

Disorders of the Rotator Cuff and Biceps Tendon

Cofield, R.H.: Subscapular muscle transposition for repair of chronic rotator cuff tears. Surg., Gynec. Obstet. 154:667-672, 1982.

Twenty-two of twenty-six patients achieved pain relief and abduction of 120 degrees or greater following transfer of the subscapularis into a large defect in the supraspinatus and infraspinatus. It should not be used in smaller tears where direct closure is possible.

Cofield, R.H.: Tears of rotator cuff. *In* AAOS Instructional Course Lectures, XXX:258-273. St. Louis, C.V. Mosby, 1981.

This is a review of the incidence, physical and radiographic findings, and treatment options. Statistical documentation is presented to support repairing acute tears within the first 3 weeks after injury.

Neer, C.S., II, and Marberry, T.A.: On the disadvantages of radical acromionectomy. J. Bone Joint Surg. 63A:416-419, 1981.

Thirty patients who had radical (80 percent) or complete (100 percent) acromionectomy had poor results. The loss of the lever arm of the deltoid and distal retraction of its origin resulted in marked weakness and an unaesthetic appearance of the shoulder.

Neviaser, R.J.: Symposium on disorders of the shoulder. Orthop. Clin. North America 11:185-373, 1980.

The current status of the broad spectrum of shoulder disorders is presented. Topics include rotator cuff tears, tendinitis, fractures, dislocations, and adhesive capsulitis.

Neviaser, R.J., and Neviaser, T.J.: Lesions of musculotendinous cuff of shoulder: Diagnosis and management. Part A: Tears of rotator cuff. *In* AAOS Instructional Course Lectures, XXX:239-250. St. Louis, C.V. Mosby, 1981.

The mechanism of production of cuff tears is categorized, diagnostic criteria are outlined, and surgical indications are defined. The techniques for repairs of massive tears are described.

Neviaser, R.J., and Neviaser, T.J.: Transfer of the subcapularis and teres minor for massive defects of the rotator cuff. *In* Shoulder Surgery, edited by J.I. Bayley and L. Kessel, pp. 60-69. New York, Springer-Verlag, 1982.

Seventeen patients underwent transfer of the subscapularis and teres minor for otherwise irreparable massive, chronic tears of the rotator cuff. Only two failures occurred, and twelve patients could abduct more than 90 degrees without pain. Three patients had pain relief but persistent loss of abduction due to deltoid detachment from previous surgeries.

Neviaser, T.J., and Neviaser, R.J.: Lesions of musculotendinous cuff of shoulder: Diagnosis and management. Part B: Lesions of the long head of biceps tendon. *In* AAOS Instructional Course Lectures, XXX:250-257. St Louis, C.V. Mosby, 1981.

The anatomic basis and pathomechanics of the painful arc syndrome with biceps tenosynovitis are outlined. Measures for establishing the diagnosis and treatment rationale are presented. In the unusual instance where operative intervention is required, the four-part operative approach is described.

Neviaser, T.J.; Neviaser, R.J.; Neviaser, J.S.; and Neviaser, J.S.: The four-in-one arthroplasty for the painful arc syndrome. Clin. Orthop. 163:107-112, 1982.

The painful arc syndrome is described, and an anatomic and pathologic basis for its development outlined. The four-part surgical approach is discussed and recommended for the unusual patient in whom nonoperative means fail. Sixty-one of sixty-two patients followed from 2 to 6 years achieved pain relief and returned to their normal activities.

Instability

Hill, J.A.; Lombardo, S.J.; Kerlan, R.K.; Jobe, F.W.; Carter, V.S.; Shields, C.L., Jr.; Collins, H.R.; and Yocum, L.A.: The modification Bristow-Helfet procedure for recurrent anterior shoulder subluxations and dislocations. Am. J. Sports Med. 9:283-287, 1981.

Although 89 percent of 107 patients were satisfied, only six of forty-one with dominant shoulder surgery could throw in the same manner as before. Five of twenty-four patients (21 percent) with a diagnosis of recurrent anterior subluxation remained symptomatic.

Leach, R.E.; Corbett, M.; Schepsis, A.; and Stockel, J.: Results of a modified Putti-Platt operation for recurrent shoulder dislocations and subluxations. Clin. Orthop. 164:20-25, 1982.

Seventy-seven of seventy-eight repairs were successful, allowing all patients to return to athletic activities. Limitation of external rotation varied between 12 to 19 degrees at 90 degrees abduction but was not a functional disability.

Protzman, R.R.: Anterior instability of the shoulder. J. Bone Joint Surg. 62A:909-918, 1980.

Classification of anterior instability into three types is established. A Bankart or modified Bankart procedure was successful in eliminating anterior instability in these patients.

Rowe, C.R., and Zarins, B.: Recurrent transient subluxation of the shoulder. J. Bone Joint Surg. 63A:863-872, 1981.

Transient subluxation of the shoulder may cause the dead arm syndrome. A positive apprehension test is strongly supportive of the clinical suspicion. Bankart or modified Bankart anterior repair was successful in eliminating the cause of the dead arm syndrome.

Involuntary Multidirectional Instability

Neer, C.S., II, and Foster, C.R.: Inferior capsular shift for involuntary inferior and multidirectional instability of the shoulder: A preliminary report. J. Bone Joint Surg. 62A:897-908, 1980.

Thirty-six patients with involuntary inferior and multidirectional instability underwent evaluation. Inferior capsular laxity was found in all patients. Capsular reefing anteriorly or posteriorly, associated with tightening of the inferior capsule, was successful in reducing involuntary instability.

Chronic Unreduced Dislocations

Rowe, C.R., and Zarins, B.: Chronic unreduced dislocations of the shoulder. J. Bone Joint Surg. 64A:494-505, 1982.

Unreduced dislocations of longer than 3 weeks were found to be more frequently anterior than posterior. Open reduction gave results which were better than previously appreciated. Surgical options are outlined.

Humerus

Balfour, G.W.; Mooney, V.; and Ashby, M.E.: Diaphyseal fractures of the humerus treated with a ready-made fracture brace. J. Bone Joint Surg. 64A:11-13, 1982.

Diaphyseal fractures of the shaft of the humerus were treated with a polyethylene brace which allowed passive motion to the elbow and pendulum exercises to the shoulder. Seventy-four patients were treated, but only forty-two reviewed at follow-up. The major complication was persistent varus deformity of the humerus which was present in a majority of patients and could not be controlled by the brace.

Pollock, F.H.; Drake, D.; Bovill, E.G.; Day, L.; and Trafton, P.G.: Treatment of radial neuropathy associated with fractures of the humerus. J. Bone Joint Surg. 63A:239-243, 1981.

Eight percent of patients with radial neuropathy associated with humeral shaft fracture required exploration of the nerve because no return was present after 3½ to 4 months. These patients showed good recovery after delayed operation. Closed treatment for 3½ to 4 months after injury is recommended.

16 SHOULDER AND HUMERUS: RECONSTRUCTION

Topics discussed in this section include diagnostic techniques, acromiohumeral reconstruction, acromioclavicular joint reconstruction, and total shoulder replacement arthroplasty.

Diagnostic Techniques and Arthroscopy Due to its soft tissue and osseous complexity, the diseased shoulder frequently presents a confusing clinical picture. Sole reliance upon conventional radiographs may not yield a definition of the structural disorder; in fact, these radiographs tend to understate the problems. The newer techniques of arthrography, arthrotomography, bursography, arthroscopy, computed tomography, and ultrasound are helping clarify this difficult diagnostic area. In addition, nuclear magnetic resonance shows promise as a diagnostic tool.

Shoulder arthrography is useful in the diagnosis of rotator cuff tears, adhesive capsulitis, recurrent dislocation, loose osseous bodies, biceps tendon lesions, synovitis, and arthritis. Arthrographic techniques include single-contrast procedures (positive contrast material or air) and double-contrast procedures (positive contrast material and air). Although more difficult to perform and interpret than the single-contrast procedure, the double-contrast technique may yield more information, particularly about labral and rotator cuff injuries. Rotator cuff tears are characterized by extravasation of the dye into the subacromial or subdeltoid bursa. Normal and abnormal arthrographic anatomy and findings are illustrated in Figure 1.

Normally, the glenohumeral joint holds 25 to 30 ml of contrast solution, but in patients with adhesive capsulitis this is markedly reduced. The subscapular recess, axillary pouch, and bicipital tendon sheath are contracted and thus fill to a lesser degree. Distension and manipulation with arthrography may be beneficial to patients with adhesive capsulitis since afterward some report an improved range of motion.

In patients with recurrent dislocation, the Hill-Sach's defect, the Bankart lesion, or a loss of demarcation between the subscapular and axillary recesses may be shown by arthrography. Intra-articular osseous loose bodies also may be demonstrated. Biceps tendon abnormalities are more difficult to define, but dislocation and rupture of the tendon as well as tenosynovitis may be noted. Abnormalities of the synovial membrane may be defined by the presence of an irregularity, a corrugated appearance, or a nodular filling defect instead of the unfurrowed, uniform distribution of contrast material seen in the normal synovium. Such changes are indicative of inflammatory synovitis, septic arthritis, or rheumatoid arthritis. Arthrography of the acromioclavicular joint may assist in the evaluation of the severity of an acromioclavicular dislocation and in differentiation of incomplete and complete ruptures.

Arthrotomography (a radiographic technique designed to assist in outlining the glenoid labrum, the articular surfaces, and the capsular attachments in the shoulder joint) may help in evaluating patients with shoulder instability or unexplained shoulder pain.

Subacromial bursography has been used to assess chronic impingement syndromes in athletes. The subacromial bursa normally accepts 5 to 10 ml of contrast material, but in a chronically diseased bursa, only a few milliliters of material may be injected. Thus, a normal bursogram would tend to exclude chronic impingement syndrome with fibrosis.

The indications for arthroscopy are not clearly defined. It may be useful in diagnosing rotator cuff tears, synovitis, biceps tendon lesions, loose osseous bodies, adhesive capsulitis, and glenoid labrum tears. Unlike arthrography, arthroscopy provides direct visualization of intra-articular anatomy. Some surgery through the arthroscope is possible: labral lesions may be removed; chondroplastic shaving and synovectomy are possible, as is removal of loose osseous bodies; and lesions of the rotator cuff, biceps tendon, or synovium and adhesive capsulitis also may be amenable to such surgery. The general distension and manipulation occurring during arthroscopic diagnostic procedures may help patients with adhesive capsulitis.

Although arthroscopy for the shoulder may be performed under local anesthesia, general anesthesia is used more commonly. The patient is positioned laterally; light traction on the arm in 45 degrees of abduction is helpful. Entry is usually posterior and inferior to the acromion; an additional entry anteriorly may be helpful. Use of a three cannula technique allows the inflow scope and surgical instruments to be exchanged among the cannulas. Generally, the joint is distended with saline through a long, 18-gauge needle before the instruments are inserted.

Computed tomography will play an increasing role in the accurate delineation of subtle pathologic lesions of the shoulder. Its use may be combined with that of arthrography. Certainly, subtle lesions of the bony and soft-tissue structures will be more easily defined than by any other presently available diagnostic procedure.

Ultrasonography, with improvement, may be of diagnostic value in demonstrating soft-tissue lesions about the shoulder joint. Increased sonographic resolutions beyond 0.2 mm and computer-enhanced color sonography may

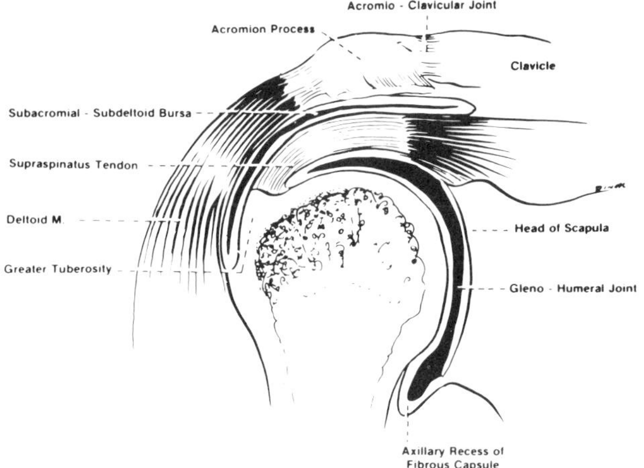

Figure 1-A

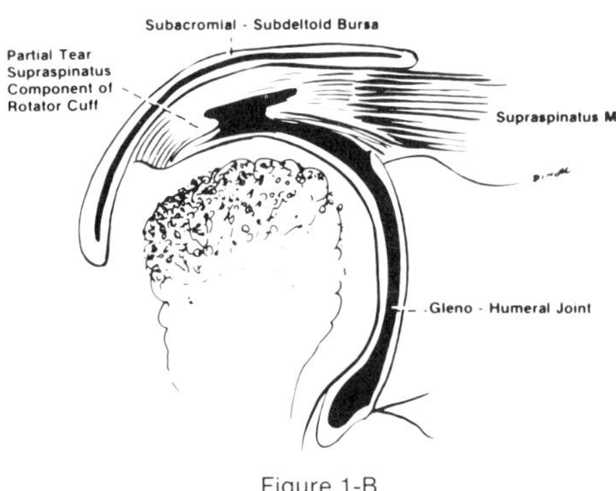

Figure 1-B

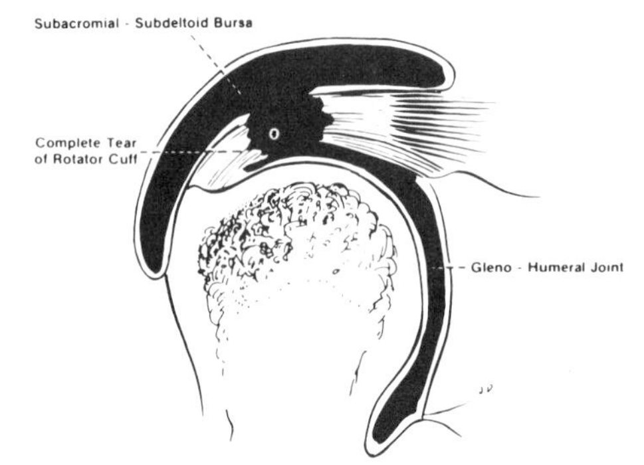

Figure 1-C

Figure 1: (A) Drawing of coronal section through middle of shoulder joint with normal anatomy. (B) Partial thickness tear of undersurface of rotator cuff. During arthrography, dye enters the tear but not the subacromial subdeltoid bursa. (C) Complete tear of rotator cuff. Dye fills both the glenohumeral joint space and the subacromial subdeltoid bursa. (Reprinted with permission from Arthrography of the shoulder joint: State of the art, by R.M. Tirman, et al., CRC Crit. Rev. Diag. Imaging 17:19-76, 1981.)

provide additional information about lesions, such as rotator cuff tears and tendon injuries about the shoulder as well as periarticular and intra-articular fluid collections.

Acromiohumeral Disease and Reconstruction

Subacromial Syndromes The subacromial space is an extra-articular area of limited confines and complex structures. It is spanned by an arch which from anterior to posterior aspect consists of a portion of the coracoid process, the coracoacromial ligament, and the acromion (Fig. 2). Tenting from its lateral border are the broad origin and expanse of the deltoid musculature. The subacromial or subdeltoid bursa is just underneath and acts as a cushioning and gliding mechanism. Beneath the subacromial bursa are the structures of the rotator cuff and capsule, which cover the humeral head. From medial to lateral are the subscapularis and its insertion, the bicipital groove and transverse ligament, and the biceps tendon and sheath with overlying ligaments. Superior and posterior are the structures of the remainder of the rotator cuff: the supraspinatus, infraspinatus, and teres minor muscles.

The subacromial space increases and decreases in size as the arm is abducted in a variety of degrees of rotation and anterior and posterior positioning. Throughout the complex arc of motion, the scapula, or the roof of the arch, does not keep pace with the movements of the proximal humerus, and impingement occurs. If the structures involved become overused, inflamed, traumatized, or worn with age, pain and inhibition of function occur. Later changes include degenerative and traumatic destruction of the elements of the cuff and arch. Overuse, aging, and/or impingement cause the painful arc syndrome, also called the supraspinatus syndrome or the rotator cuff impingement syndrome. This syndrome may include any or all of the following: subacromial bursitis, rotator cuff attrition and inflammation, biceps tendinitis, dorsal luxation of the humeral head, adhesive capsulitis, synovitis, and formation of subacromial osteophytes.

There are generally three groups of patients involved: the young athlete with frequent high-speed, high-load oscillations and overuse at the extremes of motion and power; the middle-aged patient with sporadic overhead strain; and the older patient with chronic degeneration secondary to accumulated wear and tear of aging tissues.

Most overhead motion in man occurs with the shoulder in the anterior, internally rotated position. As the arm is elevated without external rotation, the eventual lag in scapular motion relative to humeral motion causes impingement between the osseous humeral structures and the fibro-osseous coracoacromial structures. This traps and compresses the subacromial bursa and the rotator cuff. Hypertrophy or inflammation with overuse further diminishes the space available and aggravates the impingement compression. Some primates with extensive overhead activities form a layer of fibrocartilage over the supraspinatus tendon and tuberosity. This layer serves as a smooth protective buffer and glide plate to protect the musculotendinous structures.

In the simple overuse group, there is inflammation of the subacromial bursa, the tendons of the rotator cuff, the biceps, or any combination of these changes as well as inflammation of the capsule of the shoulder. In older people with chronic degeneration, the pathologic process includes attritional changes, chronic inflammation, and thickening of the tendinous structures, as well as destructive and osteophytic changes in the bony surfaces of the acromion and the proximal humerus. Extension of the disease may include total rupture of the rotator cuff and degenerative changes in the glenohumeral and coracoacromial joint. Neer has defined three stages of the syndrome: stage I, seen in the athletic or young person, consisting of edema, hemorrhage, and inflammation; stage II, consisting of fibrosis and tendinitis; and stage III, consisting of tendon degeneration, bony changes, and ruptured tendons. The degree of involvement tends to worsen with aging. Athletes particularly prone to develop stage I disease are those involved in sports requiring frequent overhead use of the arms to the extreme limitations of range, e.g., swimmers, tennis players, pitchers, and quarterbacks.

In the athlete and the middle-aged worker, the intermittent age and stress group, the initial treatment should include diminution of the inflammation with rest, ice packs, anti-inflammatory agents, occasional steroid injections, and, sometimes, ultrasound. After the inflammatory phase has subsided, shoulder strengthening exercises should be initiated to improve function and diminish impingement. In patients in whom nonoperative treatment has failed, excision of the coracoacromial ligament and anterior acromioplasty may be indicated.

Surgical intervention in stage I and II patients rarely is needed unless an acute rotator cuff tear, the most acute form of this syndrome, is present (see Section 15, Shoulder and Humerus: Trauma, regarding repair of rotator cuff tears). Although radical acromionectomy was performed in patients with refractory chronic disease, there is now a consensus that partial anterior acromionectomy is a better form of treatment. The basis for this procedure and the excision of the coracoacromial ligament is that most of the impingement occurs in the anterior arc of movement. Thus, the involved structures are usually the coracoacromial ligament and the underside of the anterior acromion where decrease in space, degenerative loss of convexity, and osteophytic formation are frequent. The disadvantage of radical acromionectomy was that it often resulted in secondary loss of deltoid function.

Subacromial disease and rotator cuff injuries in particular present a continuum of progressive disease severity. These injuries may be partial thickness (on the undersurface), incomplete (involving only a portion, e.g., the supraspinatus), or complete. They are more frequent in patients over 40 years of age. The cause may be acute trauma or degeneration of tendon tissue. They occasionally may occur as the result of massive trauma in younger patients. Clinical manifestations vary from minimal discomfort in the elderly group to severe pain, weakness, and loss of shoulder function following acute ruptures.

When indicated, partial anterior acromionectomy may be combined with repair of the rotator cuff, removal of osteophytes from the bicipital groove and the undersurface of the acromion, excision of the coracoacromial ligament, and subperiosteal excision of the outer centimeter of the clavicle. The rationale for excision of the coracoacromial ligament in conjunction with partial anterior acromionectomy is that most impingement occurs in the anterior one-third of the coracoacromial arch during hyperabduction of the arm. A proximal, anterior, or an anterolateral deltoid-splitting approach are the incisions of choice. Disruption of the deltoid origin should be kept to a minimum during this procedure.

Lesions of the Long Head of the Biceps Lesions of the long head of the biceps may be difficult to diagnose and may occur in conjunction with rotator cuff impingement syndrome or glenohumeral instability. If biceps tendinitis is a secondary part of impingement syndrome, it is the impingement syndrome that requires treatment. If the biceps tendon is involved, biceps tenodesis may be effective. Therefore, at the time of operation, when biceps

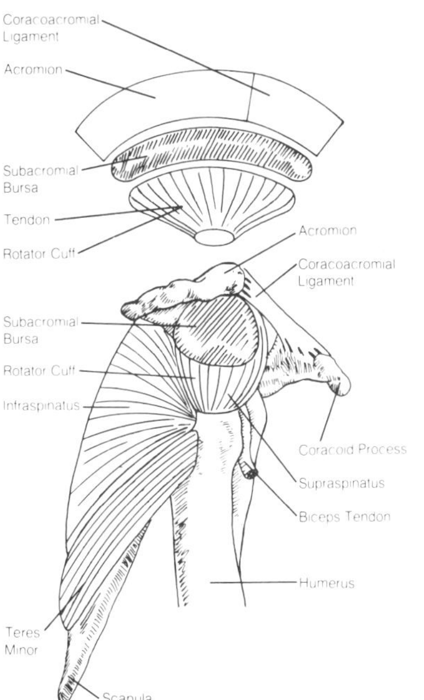

Figure 2: Drawing of the structures arching across the subacromial space. The arch consists of the acromion (posterior two-thirds) and the coracoacromial ligament (anterior one-third). (Reprinted with permission from Rotator cuff impingement syndrome in sports, by M.E. Brunet, et al., Phys. Sportsmed. (McGraw-Hill publication) 10:188, 1982.)

disease is suspected and tenodesis is contemplated, the coracoacromial arch and the contents of the coracoacromial space should be reviewed for possible primary or secondary disease.

Acromioclavicular Joint Reconstruction Injuries to the acromioclavicular joint are categorized in three grades. Grade I injuries result in tearing of a few fibers of the acromioclavicular ligament and joint capsule. The acromioclavicular joint is stable, and pain is minimal. There is no joint laxity since the ligaments remain intact. In grade II injuries, there is disruption of the capsule and acromioclavicular ligament. The coracoclavicular ligament remains intact, but there may be subluxation of the acromioclavicular joint. This is best demonstrated on stress radiographs. Grade III lesions result in disruption of the acromioclavicular as well as the coracoclavicular ligament and the capsule of the joint; the acromioclavicular joint is dislocated and the clavicle is displaced superiorly.

Nonoperative management of acromioclavicular separation consists of mild analgesics and immobilization with a sling (the Kenny-Howard or one of its derivatives) to pull the clavicle down and the acromion up, followed by early range of motion exercises of the shoulder and resumption of activities in accord with patient comfort.

Methods of operative treatment include transarticular fixation, fixation of the clavicle to the coracoid, distal clavicle resection with substitution of a Dacron graft for the torn coracoclavicular ligament, and coracoacromial ligament transfers. Transarticular fixation of the joint with a small Steinmann pin or Kirschner wires was used in the past but has been largely discontinued because of the hazards of pin breakage, loosening, and migration. These problems can be minimized by using a single pin, such as that designed by Simmons, since it is stable enough to inhibit breakage if removed early and has a head that

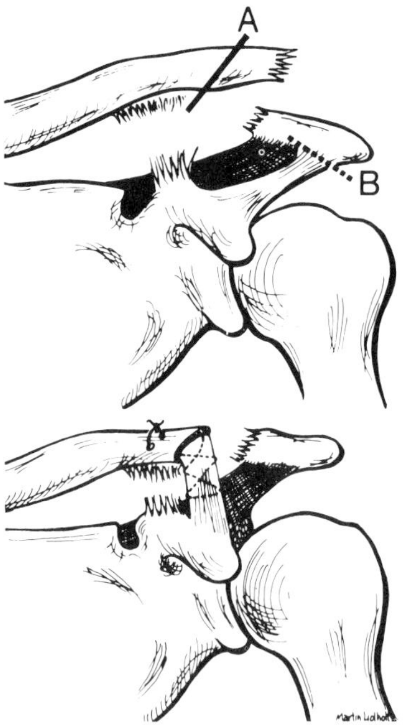

Figure 3: Lateral end of the clavicle is resected obliquely along line (A), and the coracoacromial ligament is detached along line (B) and anchored in the medullary cavity of the proximal clavicle. (Reprinted with permission from Resection arthroplasty for repair of complete acromioclavicular separations, by W. Rauschning, et al., Arch. Orthop. Trauma Surg. 97:161-164, 1980.)

prevents its migration and facilitates its extraction.

The Weaver-Dunn technique, the oblique resection of the lateral end of the clavicle and transfer of the coracoacromial ligament into the medullary cavity of the clavicle, is another option (Fig. 3). This procedure addresses the problem of insufficient suspension from the shoulder by the clavicle with secondary deformity and muscle weakness. Transposition of the coracoacromial ligament stabilizes the remaining lateral end of the clavicle during arm movements.

A relatively new operative procedure utilizes a Dacron graft as a substitute for the coracoclavicular ligament (Fig. 4). In late repairs the distal end of the clavicle is resected as well. Potentially undesirable effects of this operation are probable enhanced risk of infection with implantation of a foreign body, possibility of malpositioning the Dacron loop, and resorption of the bone along the superior border of the distal clavicle. Its potential advantages are retention of the coracoacromial ligament, ease of performance, and theoretical fibroblastic infiltration that may occur with the potential for reconstituting the disrupted coracoclavicular ligament.

Total Shoulder Replacement Arthroplasty The first artificial shoulder joint was inserted 90 years ago by Péan of France. However, it was Neer who initiated the modern era of shoulder arthroplasty when he inserted the first proximal humeral replacement prosthesis in 1952. During the subsequent 30 years, its use has been expanded to include painful and chronic glenohumeral incongruities with major involvement of the humeral head and four-part humeral neck and comminuted head fractures. With development of the total shoulder joint prosthesis, indications have further expanded to include resurfacing of the diseased glenoid in conditions such as rheumatoid, degenerative, and posttraumatic arthritis.

Biomechanical Considerations An important design consideration in a total shoulder replacement is that if there is a conforming curve on the glenoid component of any degree (i.e., one curved surface against another), some degree of constraint is present. Constraint is the force imposed to restrict the motion of a mechanical body to a particular mode. However minimal the constraint may be, some degree of shear and compressive force is transferred to the glenoid component. Even with an "unconstrained" device, compressive forces may be transferred into varying loads on the glenoid components as their points of articulation move from the center. Even a theoretically flat, frictionless glenoid surface is loaded by compression as the vectors and instant center shift in abduction, and flexion, extension, and off-center rocking movements stress the glenoid anchorage.

Biomechanical studies reveal that the humerus is on the verge of subluxating upward whenever the glenohumeral joint is in neutral rotation up to 60 degrees of abduction. Therefore, in the absence of a rotator cuff, particularly the supraspinatus part, some instability is expected. At 90 degrees of abduction, resultant forces on the glenoid reach a maximum of 0.89 times body weight. Shearing components on the face of the glenoid are maximal at 60 degrees of abduction and equal 0.42 times body weight. Therefore, even the less constrained glenoid resurfacing components are stressed to some extent as compression and shear interact. With a diseased rotator cuff, the humeral head instant center shifts, allowing compression and shear to act as stressing vectors on the scapular anchorage. Thus, clinical studies covering more than 2 or 3 years are necessary to determine the true rate of glenoid loosening, even for the relatively unconstrained type of prosthesis. It is obvious that surgical and cementing techniques are of utmost importance in achieving fixation to the limits of the design.

Prostheses Total shoulder joint replacement devices can be categorized into two types: the constrained and the relatively unconstrained. It is generally agreed that if constrained prosthetic devices are used, they should be reserved for the most grossly unstable shoulders with unreconstructable rotator cuffs and significant soft-tissue

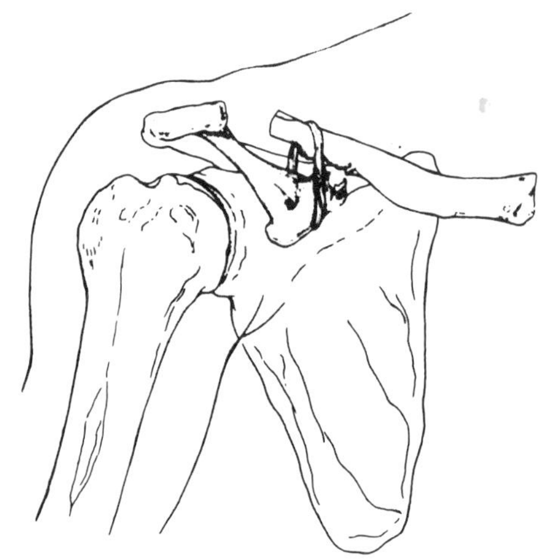

Figure 4: Dacron loop substitution for the coracoclavicular ligament. (Reprinted with permission from Treatment of acromioclavicular separations: A retrospective study, by J.P. Park, et al., Am. J. Sports Med. 8:251-256, 1980.)

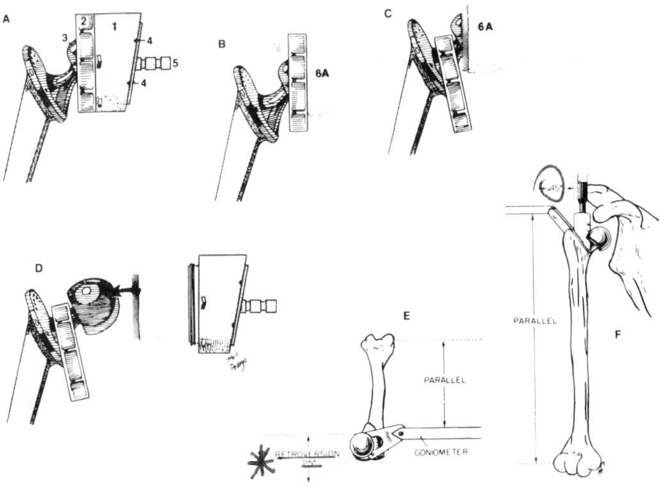

Figure 5: Post constrained total shoulder prosthesis. (A) Assembled prosthesis. (B) Metal glenoid cup has been removed. (C) Metal locking ring has been slipped down over humeral neck to show polyethylene peripheral lip. (D) Steps in assembly. Metal locking ring is placed on neck, polyethylene pieces are placed around head, head is placed into metal glenoid cup to be held in place by tightening metal locking ring. (E) and (F) Details of insertion. (Reprinted with permission from Total shoulder replacement with a constrained prosthesis, by M. Post, et al., J. Bone Joint Surg. 62A:327-335, 1980.)

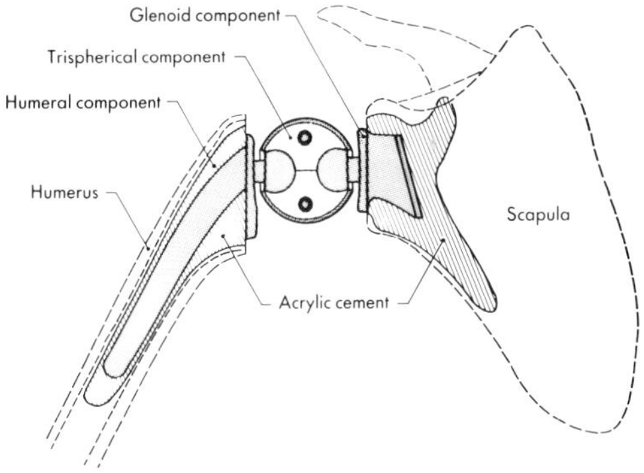

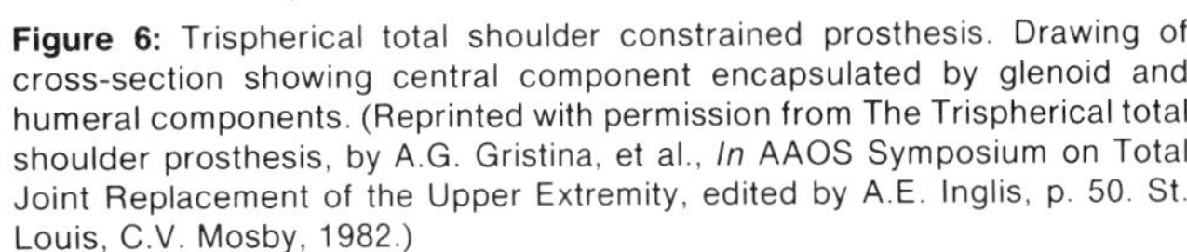

Figure 6: Trispherical total shoulder constrained prosthesis. Drawing of cross-section showing central component encapsulated by glenoid and humeral components. (Reprinted with permission from The Trispherical total shoulder prosthesis, by A.G. Gristina, et al., *In* AAOS Symposium on Total Joint Replacement of the Upper Extremity, edited by A.E. Inglis, p. 50. St. Louis, C.V. Mosby, 1982.)

and osseous defects. Figures 5 and 6 illustrate the Post and Trispherical types of constrained shoulders. The unconstrained category of shoulder prostheses includes the Neer II (Fig. 7), the Monospherical (Fig. 8), and the UCLA (Fig. 9).

Indications The indications for total shoulder replacement are significant unrelenting pain with associated loss of motion in rheumatoid, degenerative, or posttraumatic arthritic disease. Neoplastic disease with proximal humeral or glenoid destruction also may be an indication. The primary indication in all patients must be severe pain due to incongruity of the humeral head and glenoid. Loss of motion is a secondary indication as gain of motion is highly variable and unpredictable. Stiffness alone is not an indication for a total joint replacement. In patients with acute fractures or osteonecrosis, and in younger patients, humeral head replacement alone is best. Contraindications to total shoulder replacement include infection and extensive paralysis. Neer points out that the two indications (subgroups of the above) that are the most difficult to assess are prosthetic revisions and arthropathy after rotator cuff tear.

Technique Surgical approaches for total shoulder replacement vary. The extended deltopectoral approach is useful. The incision extends from the outer one-third of the clavicle over the coracoid process and curves into the deltopectoral groove. The deltopectoral interval is used without detachment of the proximal deltoid or the conjoined tendon. With adequate elongation of the incision and retraction of the arm and proximal humerus, the capsule can be entered through the subscapularis for full exposure of the humeral head and glenoid. In patients with severe rheumatoid arthritis, internal rotation contracture requires careful dissection and release of adherent capsule and synovium; the axillary artery and nerve must be protected.

Critical features of the surgical technique include: (1) careful curettement of the scapular recess for removal of cancellous bone while preserving the subchondral cortical bone of the glenoid face and the use of aqueous lavage, drying, and cement gun injection techniques to obtain optimal cement penetration and maximal fixation, particularly in the glenoid; (2) preservation or maintenance of adequate humeral length for appropriate stability, capsular tension, and abductor function; and (3) adequate and stable reconstruction of the capsule and rotator cuff for maximum function, humeral head stability, and synergistic motion of the rotator cuff-deltoid complex.

Postoperatively, adequate immobilization and carefully supervised rehabilitation should be planned according to the particular prosthetic design and to the soft-tissue limitations and surgical requirements of the patient.

Results Preliminary results indicate that there is good pain relief following total shoulder replacement. Near normal function also may be achieved in a patient whose shoulder musculature is not severely damaged or can be rehabilitated. But, in the more seriously involved shoulder with significant soft-tissue disease, range of motion is much more limited.

Possible complications of total shoulder replacement include subluxation and dislocation, loosening of the

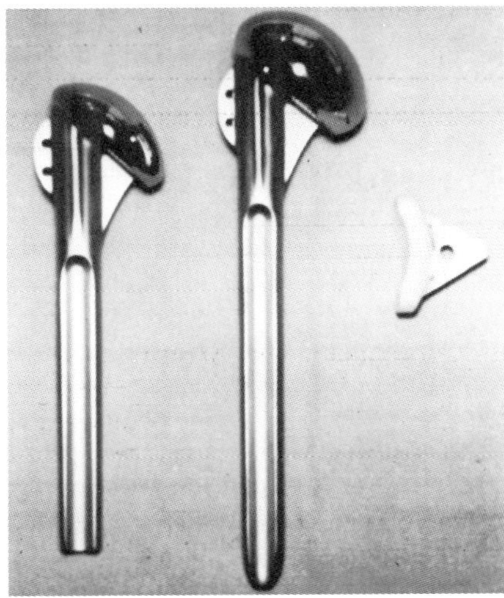

Figure 7: Neer II unconstrained total shoulder prosthesis. Different sized heads and humeral shafts are used. Glenoid component (polyethylene) has keel which is placed within the scapula. (Reprinted with permission from Total joint arthroplasty: The shoulder, by R.H. Cofield, Mayo Clin. Proc. 54:500-506, 1979.)

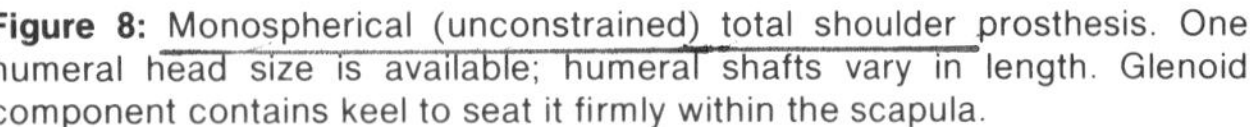

Figure 8: Monospherical (unconstrained) total shoulder prosthesis. One humeral head size is available; humeral shafts vary in length. Glenoid component contains keel to seat it firmly within the scapula.

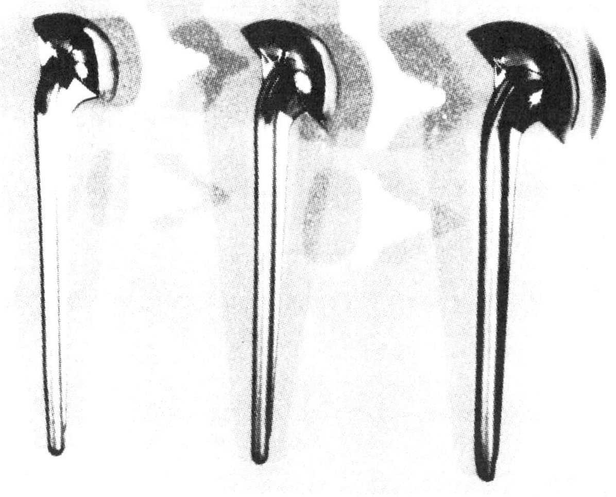

Figure 9: UCLA unconstrained total shoulder prosthesis. Glenoid component can be either standard or hooded. The latter is used where the rotator cuff is nonfunctional or absent. Three humeral head and humeral neck sizes are available. (Reprinted with permission from UCLA anatomic total shoulder arthroplasty, by H.C. Amstutz, et al., Clin. Orthop. 155:7-20, 1981.)

prosthetic device (especially the glenoid component), and axillary and musculocutaneous nerve injury. Failure of the glenoid component due to loosening may be salvaged by recementing a scapular component or by simple removal of that component, retention of the humeral prosthesis, reconstruction of the capsule, and debridement of the glenoid region. A lucent zone at the glenoid bone-cement interface may not be a sign of clinical loosening since it has been seen in 30 percent or more of patients after several years follow-up. The infection rate has been minimal, and there has been no significant incidence of pulmonary emboli.

Conclusions Total shoulder replacement cannot be equated with total hip replacement. In total hip replacement, the basic joint structure is that of simple static congruity and architectural stability (i.e., motion restricted to a particular mode). In total shoulder replacement, the result is highly dependent upon the integrity or the reconstructability of the muscles, tendons, and capsule. Stability and function of the unconstrained implant are a result of the interrelationship of critical factors such as humeral length and humeral and glenoid version, appropriate deltoid tension, and rotator cuff integrity. If these are not present and preserved, they must be reconstructed.

Total shoulder replacement currently must be considered a relatively new procedure with few follow-ups exceeding 36 months. The results (especially from Neer's extensive series) indicate some optimism for the durability of this procedure. But, until long-term results can be assessed, the indications for total shoulder replacement and selection of patients must be strict. The surgical technique is demanding and precise.

Continuing improvement in unconstrained prosthetics appears to be leading toward their use in most patients and may obviate the need for constrained types. But, long-term results may show that the stability of the minimally constrained prosthesis needs improvement. Cement insertion techniques must be improved for more dependable long-term fixation. Fixation by bony ingrowth for both the humeral and glenoid components may be ideal.

Other Reconstructive Procedures of the Shoulder

Debridement and Synovectomy In posttraumatic or degenerative disease of the shoulder, limited areas of deformity and osteophyte formation (especially anteriorly and inferiorly on the humeral head) occasionally can be excised and combined with soft-tissue debridement and capsuloplasty to achieve significant pain decrease and a concomitant increase in motion. Best results occur when the major articular surfaces are not involved. In specific circumstances (such as massive infection or tumor nonamenable to placement of a prosthesis), resection of the humeral head may be required. Synovectomy is a worthwhile consideration, especially early in rheumatoid disease before significant articular, capsular, and rotator cuff destruction have occurred. At the same time, anterior capsular release and lengthening of the subscapularis may be required for a fixed internal rotation contracture. Concomitant rotator cuff restructuring, biceps tenodesis, coracoacromial synovectomy, and anterior acromial excision also may be indicated. Arthroscopic chondroplastic shaving and synovial debridement may prove useful in at least temporarily relieving symptoms.

Arthrodesis of the Shoulder Arthrodesis of the shoulder is a reasonably reliable and effective procedure in appropriately chosen patients with the residual of infection, paralysis, or arthritis. As total joint replacement techniques in the shoulder improve, it is likely that more patients will select joint replacement. But, there will be some (particularly those with paralysis or postseptic disorders) for whom an arthrodesis is preferable. Over the past 20 years, fusion has been used in rheumatoid arthritis as well as sepsis and paralysis.

Techniques of arthrodesis vary, but a useful and commonly applied procedure consists of apposition of the humeral head to the glenoid and acromion by multiple compression-type screw fixation (Fig. 10). There is controversy over the position of fusion. Currently less abduction is recommended than the 45 degrees suggested in the past. This is combined with 20 to 30 degrees of forward flexion and internal rotation. Bilateral arthrodesis may be performed with good results in carefully selected patients. Fusion may be achieved in 80 to 90 percent of patients with one procedure. Possible postoperative complications are some residual pain (approximately 25 percent of patients) due to internal fixation devices or suboptimal position of the scapula, subsequent fractures of the more rigid extremity, pseudarthrosis, and infection. Some form of postsurgical immobilization and splinting is required for 9 to 12 weeks. Scapulothoracic motion may increase following fusion.

Double Osteotomy Double osteotomy of the shoulder has been reported to be efficacious in relieving the pain of arthritis. The success of the procedure is believed to be due to relief of pain from subchondral hyperemia and intraosseous hypertension; the increase in range of motion is entirely due to the decrease in pain, which allows glenohumeral motion and scapulothoracic compensation. The reported experience is small, and nonunion may occur.

Muscle Flap Reconstruction Massive trauma-induced cutaneous defects about the shoulder may be repaired by muscle flap reconstruction. Delineation of vascular territories of the pectoralis and latissimus muscle and the overlying skin used to form myocutaneous flaps allows single procedure correction of defects previously requiring staged procedures. Such flaps provide durable coverage of damaged bone and joint structures and are particularly useful for problems secondary to radiation damage and major limb avulsion defects. They may be used as skin-graft-covered muscular flaps. For anterior shoulder defects, the pectoralis muscle may be used; for more posterior and superior defects, the latissimus dorsi flap is more reliable and versatile.

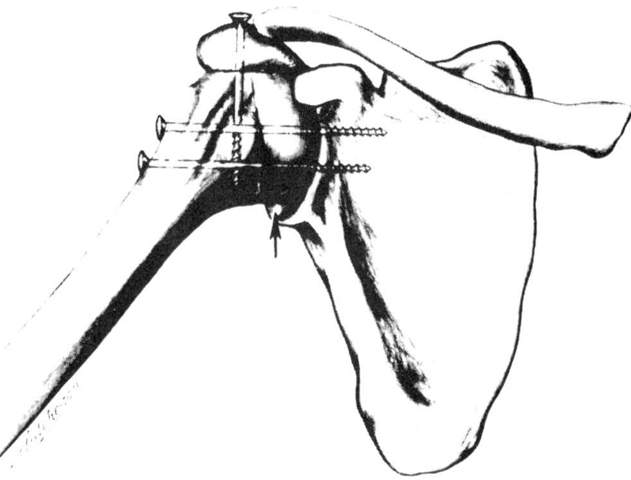

Figure 10: Operative technique for obtaining arthrodesis of the shoulder. Humeral head is apposed to the glenoid and acromion with screws. If glenohumeral contact is compromised by upward subluxation (arrow), the acromion is cracked where it joins the scapular spine and displaced downward, hinging through the acromioclavicular joint. (Reprinted with permission from Glenohumeral arthrodesis: Operative and long-term functional results, by R.H. Cofield, et al., J. Bone Joint Surg. 61A:668-677, 1979.)

ANNOTATED BIBLIOGRAPHY

Diagnostic Techniques and Arthroscopy

Caspari, R.B.: Shoulder arthroscopy: A review of the present state of the art. Contemp. Orthop. 4:523-531, 1982.

Arthroscopy through a posterior approach provides better visualization of shoulder structures than most surgical exposures. Rotator cuff tears and the mechanism of subluxating the shoulder can be identified. Synovectomy as well as removal of loose bodies is possible.

El-Khoury, G.Y.; Albright, J.P.; Abu Yousef, M.M.; Montgomery, W.J.; and Tuck, S.L.: Arthrotomography of the glenoid labrum. Radiology 131:333-337, 1979.

In eight unstable shoulders, arthrotomography correctly identified surgically confirmed lesions of the glenoid labrum and failed to show an abnormality in one shoulder that was normal at operation. The technique is described.

Johnson, L.L.: Arthroscopy of the shoulder. Orthop. Clin. North America 11:197-204, 1980.

Shoulder arthroscopy affords an opportunity for better understanding of the anatomy and pathophysiology of the joint and may prove particularly useful in the diagnosis of occult subluxation of the shoulder joint, loose bodies, and entrapment of the biceps tendon.

McGlynn, F.J.; El-Khoury, G.; and Albright, J.P.: Arthrotomography of the glenoid labrum in shoulder instability. J. Bone Joint Surg. 64A:506-518, 1982.

Arthrotomographically, twenty-five of twenty-eight patients with painful subluxation had abnormal glenoid labra. Two with voluntary subluxation and seven with pain but no prior instability had normal labra. The correlation between arthrotomograms and labral lesions was excellent.

Tirman, R.M.; Nelson, C.L.; and Tirman, W.S.: Arthrography of the shoulder joint: State of the art. CRC Crit. Rev. Diag. Imaging 17:19-76, 1981.

Arthrography (either single- or double-contrast) often helps to diagnose disease with nonspecific symptoms: rotator cuff tear, adhesive capsulitis, recurrent dislocation, biceps tendon lesions, arthritis, and synovitis. The combination of arthrography with air and subsequent computed tomography may prove to be of even greater value.

Acromiohumeral Disease and Reconstruction

Subacromial Syndromes

Ha'eri, G.B.: Ruptures of the rotator cuff. Canadian Med. Assn. J. 123:620-627, 1980.

Arthroscopy, arthrography, and other special techniques have increased the frequency of ruptured rotator cuff diagnosis. Nonoperative and surgical treatments of these ruptures are discussed, as is the importance of physiotherapy.

Hawkins, R.J., and Kennedy, J.C.: Impingement syndrome in athletes. Am. J. Sports Med. 8:151-158, 1980.

Impingement against the anterior edge of the acromion and the coracoacromial ligament irritates the avascular region of the supraspinatus and biceps tendons, which may lead to rotator cuff degeneration and tearing (impingement syndrome).

Neer, C.S., II, and Marberry, T.A.: On the disadvantages of radical acromionectomy. J. Bone Joint Surg. 63A:416-419, 1981.

A study of thirty unsuccessful radical acromionectomies (80 to 100 percent removed) indicated that the procedure weakens the deltoid by removing its lever arm and encouraging retraction of its middle section, which adheres to the rotator cuff and/or humerus.

Watson, M.: The refractory painful arc syndrome. J. Bone Joint Surg. 60B:544-546, 1978.

Excising the outer end of the clavicle and dividing the coracoacromial ligament through a deltoid approach relieved night pain in twenty-three patients with severe refractory painful arc syndrome. Six still had mild movement pain.

Lesions of the Long Head of the Biceps

Dines, D.; Warren, R.F.; and Inglis, A.E.: Surgical treatment of lesions of the long head of the biceps. Clin. Orthop. 164:165-171, 1982.

Thirty percent of biceps tenodesis procedures for biceps tendinitis or instability failed over 7 years, primarily due to misdiagnosis or failure to release the coracoacromial ligament. Biceps tendinitis secondary to impingement cannot be corrected by tenodesis.

Acromioclavicular Joint Reconstruction

Park, J.P.; Arnold, J.A.; Coker, T.P.; Harris, W.D.; and Becker, D.A.: Treatment of acromioclavicular separations: A retrospective study. Am. J. Sports Med. 8:251-256, 1980.

An H-beam double-Velour Dacron graft was substituted for double-loop wire in clavicle-to-coracoid process fixation of thirty-nine type III shoulder separations. The distal clavicle was usually resected. Long-term results were good.

Rauschning, W.; Nordesjö, L.O.; Nordgren, B.; Sahlstedt, B.; and Wigren, A.: Resection arthroplasty for repair of complete acromioclavicular separations. Arch. Orthop. Trauma Surg. 97:161-164, 1980.

For type III shoulder separations, obliquely resectioning the lateral clavicular end and transferring the coracoacromial ligament into the clavicular medullary canal provided good cosmesis and nearly normal function in seventeen patients.

Total Shoulder Replacement Arthroplasty

Amstutz, H.C.; Sew Hoy, A.L.; and Clarke, I.C.: UCLA anatomic total shoulder arthroplasty. Clin. Orthop. 155:7-20, 1981.

Among eleven patients with UCLA total shoulder endoprostheses, nine were painfree at 1½ to 3½ years, and five with good rotator cuffs had near normal function and full range of motion.

Cofield, R.H.: Total joint arthroplasty: The shoulder. Mayo Clin. Proc. 54:500-506, 1979.

This survey of seventy-five patients having total shoulder arthroplasty with the Neer prosthesis covers patient selection, technique, postoperative management, complications, and long-term results. An unconstrained device is usually adequate.

Gristina, A.G., and Webb, L.X.: Proximal Humeral and Monospherical Glenoid Replacement: Surgical Technique, pp. 1-6. Rutherford, N.J., Howmedica, Inc., 1982.

The step-by-step technique of total shoulder replacement with a Monospherical endoprosthesis is illustrated. Care must be taken to reconstruct any deficiency in the capsule and rotator cuff.

Gristina, A.G., and Webb, L.X.: The Trispherical total shoulder replacement. *In* Shoulder Surgery, edited by J.I. Bayley and L. Kessel, pp. 153-157. New York, Springer-Verlag, 1982.

The Trispherical total shoulder prosthesis, useful where the rotator cuff is deficient, comprises a scapular component, a humeral component, and a central sphere. The three-bar linkage allows greater than anatomical range of motion. Relief of pain and improvement in function in twenty patients with this endoprosthesis have been good.

Lettin, A.W.F.; Copeland, S.A.; and Scales, J.T.: The Stanmore total shoulder replacement. J. Bone Joint Surg. 64B:47-51, 1982.

Among fifty patients, nine had the Stanmore endoprosthesis removed (one infection, one dislocation, nine loosenings) and one died. All but four of the rest had some relief of pain, and all had functional improvement.

Lugli, T.: Artificial shoulder joint by Péan (1893): The facts of an exceptional intervention and the prosthetic method. Clin. Orthop. 133:215-218, 1978.

In 1893, Péan, a French surgeon, implanted a platinum and rubber total shoulder endoprosthesis in a patient with tuberculous shoulder joint. The total shoulder prosthesis was functional but was removed 2 years later because of infection.

Neer, C.S., II; Watson, K.C.; and Stanton, F.J.: Recent experience in total shoulder replacement. J. Bone Joint Surg. 64A:319-337, 1982.

No clinical loosening occurred in 194 unconstrained total shoulder replacements followed for 2 to 8½ years, although a halo at the glenoid bone-cement interface developed in 30 percent. Postoperative stability depended upon height and version of components; nine sizes of humeral components and five different glenoid components were used. Neither loss of bone nor deficient rotator cuff was a contraindication. Postoperative function depended upon meticulous reconstruction and rehabilitation of the rotator cuff and deltoid muscles. Eighty-six percent of patients had good to excellent results; twelve of twenty-four complications required reoperation.

Poppen, N.K., and Walker, P.S.: Forces at the glenohumeral joint in abduction. Clin. Orthop. 135:165-170, 1980.

Electromyographic and geometric data were used to assess forces in the glenohumeral joint during abduction. The force of a muscle appears proportional to its area times integrated electromyographic signal. Forces across the glenohumeral joint were 0.89 times body weight at 90 degrees abduction.

Post, M.; Haskell, S.S.; and Jablon, M.: Total shoulder replacement with a constrained prosthesis. J. Bone Joint Surg. 62A:327-335, 1980.

Indications for use of a constrained total shoulder were intact glenoid rim and scapular neck, strong serratus anterior and trapezius muscles, no severe soft-tissue contracture, and a strong deltoid muscle.

Other Reconstructive Procedures of the Shoulder

Benjamin, A.; Hirschowitz, D.; and Arden, G.P.: The treatment of arthritis of the shoulder joint by double osteotomy. Internat. Orthop. (SICOT) 3:211-216, 1979.

Double osteotomy without displacement of the scapular and humeral necks was done in sixteen painful, arthritic shoulders. One patient had nonunion, one delayed union, and one 20 degrees less abduction. Pain was relieved in thirteen patients.

Cofield, R.H., and Briggs, B.T.: Glenohumeral arthrodesis: Operative and long-term functional results. J. Bone Joint Surg. 61A:668-677, 1979.

Internal fixation and fusion of seventy-one shoulders for intractable pain was successful in 75 percent of patients (average follow-up of 9.5 years). Pain requiring removal of the fixation device developed in seventeen shoulders. Ten shoulders fractured, and one became infected.

Copeland, S.A., and Howard, R.C.: Thoracoscapular fusion for facioscapulohumeral dystrophy. J. Bone Joint Surg. 60B:547-551, 1978.

The thoracoscapular muscle paresis resulting from fascioscapulohumeral dystrophy was treated in eleven shoulders by fusion of the scapula to the ribs with tibial grafts. Improvement in stability, function, and cosmesis was maintained over long periods.

Cruess, R.L.: Rheumatoid arthritis of the shoulder. Orthop. Clin. North America 11:333-342, 1980.

This review covers clinical findings, radiographic changes, and management of rheumatoid arthritis of the shoulder, emphasizing the value of early synovectomy and the favorable results with Neer humeral head prosthetic replacement.

Rybka, V.; Raunio, P.; and Vainio, K.: Arthrodesis of the shoulder in rheumatoid arthritis: A review of 41 cases. J. Bone Joint Surg. 61B:155-158, 1979.

Internal fixation arthrodesis combined with external splinting for approximately 9 weeks provided good to excellent results in 68 percent of forty-one shoulders with advanced destruction due to rheumatoid arthritis.

Muscle Flap Reconstruction

Dowden, R.V., and McCraw, J.B.: Muscle flap reconstruction of shoulder defects. J. Hand Surg. 5:382-390, 1980.

The development of muscle and myocutaneous flaps enables a single procedure correction of soft-tissue defects in the shoulder area, especially difficult ones with irradiation damage or exposed, infected bone.

17 ELBOW AND FOREARM: PEDIATRIC

Subjects discussed in this section include normal development, congenital and developmental problems, arthritis, neuromuscular diseases, tumors, and osteochondrosis dissecans.

Normal Development

At birth children normally have a 30 degree flexion contracture of the elbow which resolves by 3 months of age.

The epiphyses of the elbow develop throughout growth and can lead to confusion in the interpretation of the radiographic appearances at different ages. The capitellum, the first epiphyseal center of the elbow to ossify, is always visible before the age of 2 years and sometimes by the age of 6 months. Fusion of the capitellum usually is complete by 14 years of age. It frequently fuses to the trochlea and the lateral epicondyle before uniting with the humerus. The normal position of the capitellum may be misinterpreted because the ossification center is situated anteriorly, it is often tilted downward during development, and its physis tends to be wider posteriorly than anteriorly.

Several lines can be drawn on the true lateral radiograph which are helpful in assessing the capitellum.

The coronoid line, drawn through the coronoid fossa and continued downward, should just touch or project slightly anterior to the developing capitellum (Fig. 1A). This can be helpful in assessing anterior and posterior displacements of the capitellum.

The humeral shaft line is a straight line drawn parallel to the anterior shaft of the humerus, just touching the anterior surface of the humerus where the coronoid line arises (Fig. 1B). This line should project through the posterior half of the developing capitellum. Most of the ossified epiphysis normally lies between the coronoid and the humeral shaft lines (Fig. 1C).

The radiocapitellar line bisects the proximal end of the radial shaft and should always pass through the capitellum on all radiographic views. It confirms the position of articulation between the radial head and the capitellum. If the line fails to pass through the capitellum, it indicates dislocation of the radial head. However, before the epiphysis of the radial head ossifies, it may appear (in the anteroposterior view) that the radius is pointing laterally and there is abnormal angulation of the radial neck. This is the normal appearance in an elbow with nonossification of the radial head. A lateral radiograph reliably demonstrates the alignment of these structures.

The medial epicondylar ossification center appears at an average age of 4 years. Multicentric ossification may occur although it is quite uncommon. It is the last of the six epiphyses to unite with the humeral shaft, and, therefore,

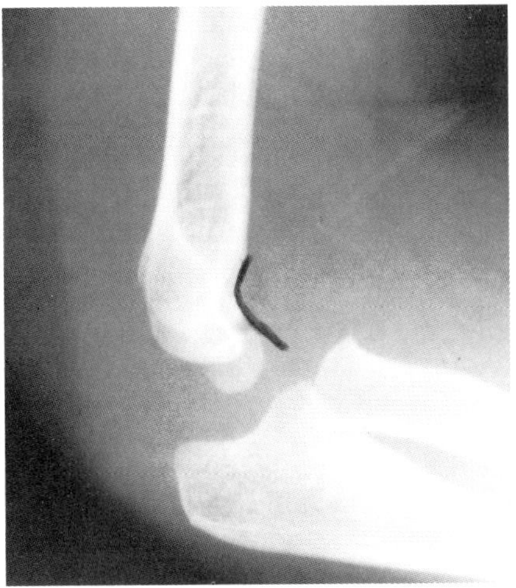

Figure 1-A

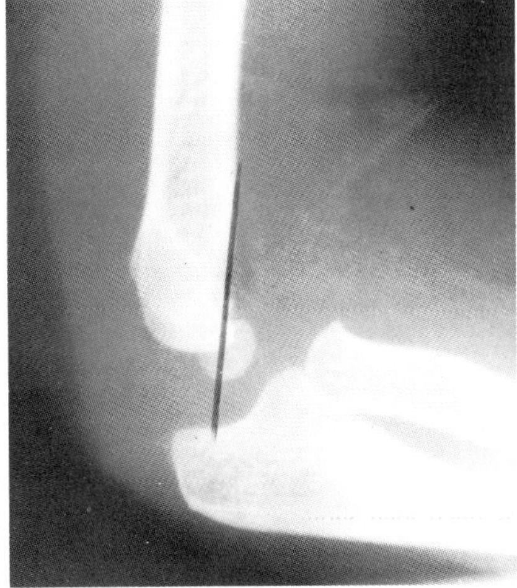

Figure 1-B

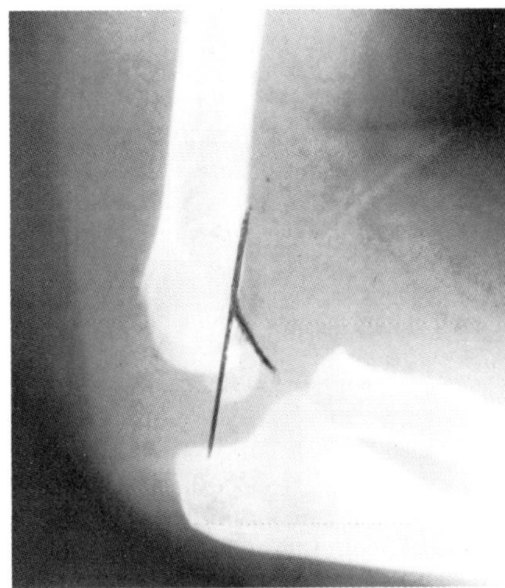

Figure 1-C

Figure 1: (A) Two dense curved lines at end of the humerus form a teardrop; the coronoid anteriorly and the olecranon line posteriorly. The coronoid line is drawn along the anterior shaft of the humerus, over the coronoid, and is continued downward. It should just touch or project slightly anterior to the developing capitellum. (B) The humeral shaft line is drawn on the anterior border of the humerus. Continued distally, it normally projects through the posterior half of the developing capitellum. (C) The coronoid and humeral shaft lines drawn on the same radiograph. These two lines describe an angle within which most of the ossified portion of the capitellum normally lies.

closure indicates that maturation of the elbow joint is complete. In addition, just before ossification, a sharp, straight sclerotic border develops on the metaphyseal surface of the distal end of the humerus. The epiphysis of the medial epicondyle normally lies posterior to the distal end of the humerus, and it may appear to be quite a distance from the humeral epiphysis. A slight off-center oblique radiograph may accentuate its normal posterior position and mimic separation. The medial epicondyle does not take part in the articulation of the elbow joint and, thus, may not be associated with a positive fat pad sign if it is injured. It does, however, contribute to the longitudinal growth of the humerus.

Congenital and Developmental

Amputations Children rarely are born with congenital amputations of the wrist, forearm, or elbow. When this does occur, the ideal rehabilitation includes restoration of strong prehension and good sensation. Prehension can be restored satisfactorily with a prosthetic fitting, but the lack of tactile feedback makes artificial limbs less than ideal. If a prosthesis is to be utilized in children with an absent distal hand or forearm, they should be fitted with a smooth plastic prosthesis when they are 6 to 12 months of age so that they can use both limbs for grasping large objects, crawling, and standing. A plastic hook is added to the prosthesis at 18 to 20 months of age, and the child is taught to use the prosthesis for grasp with a cable-controlled shoulder harness. Later a sturdier hook with stronger elastic bands or a hand is added to the end of the prosthesis. It is important that children learn to use their artificial limbs very early to pattern their development.

Children with bilateral upper limb aplasia develop tremendous skill and dexterity with their feet which they use for their daily needs. However, as they get older, social pressure prohibits them from using their feet in public or at work. Recent developments in the construction of hydraulic or electro-powered prostheses triggered by shoulder motion have been helpful. The hook or the hand at the end of these prostheses can exert relatively strong grasp without a tremendous amount of shoulder motion. Myoelectric prostheses are activated by amplified electrical impulses from "contracting muscles." Sensory feedback can be obtained from some artificial limbs by placing a pressure-sensitive transducer in the prosthetic hook. An induction-powered radio receiver is implanted into the median nerve in the upper arm. When the pressure increases on the hook, the voltage transmitted from the transducer is increased, and the patient experiences a progressively increasing stimulus in the median nerve. Although this sensory feedback mechanism is attractive, its practical application has been limited.

Children born with aplasia of the hand at the level of the distal radius can acquire a sensible prehensile limb by surgical separation of the radius from the ulna at the distal two-thirds of the forearm, creating a grasping forearm. This is particularly useful in children with bilateral amputations and is recommended in those who are blind. It is important in creating these Krukenberg stumps to maintain tactile sensation over the distal ends of the stump. Usually a 6- to 12-cm opening can be created depending upon the size of the forearm. The muscle belly of the pronator teres limits the depths of the division proximally. When the forearm pronates, the radius and ulna adduct and can grasp and hold up to 10 kg. When the forearm supinates, the radius and ulna diverge up to 45 degrees. The main advantage of the procedure is the preservation of normal sensibility and proprioception in a useful limb. The forearm becomes functional and is helpful in dressing, eating, and toilet activities. With a bilateral hand amputee, a prosthetic fitting is recommended on the contralateral side. There is concern that the stump, although functional, is unattractive and will be hidden and rejected by the child. It has been noted that in children with bilateral aplasia the Krukenberg stump became the dominant hand, and these children showed no desire to wear an artificial limb over it. This stump should be created in children before the second year of life when prehension is rapidly developing.

Radial Aplasia (Radial Clubhand) Intercalary aplasia, typically on the radial side of the limb, presents a spectrum of deformity ranging from hypoplasia of the thumb to partial or total aplasia of the radial side of the arm and hand. In children with partial or total absence of the radius, the muscles of the lateral side of the forearm displace the unsupported hand into pronation, flexion, and radial deviation until the carpal bones lie on the lateral side of the ulna. Usually the ulna is bowed and grows to only 60 percent of its normal length. The thumb is hypoplastic in 80 percent of patients with radial aplasia, and the elbow may be stiff in extension. Abnormalities are not limited to the osseous structures and include dysplasia or aplasia of the musculotendinous units, neurovascular structures, and other soft-tissue components along the radial border of the upper limb.

Despite numerous proposed theories, the cause of radial aplasia remains unknown. It is believed that some event occurs during the fourth to sixth weeks of gestation when the mesenchymal and cartilaginous analogues of the extremities are recognizable. Other anomalies associated with radial aplasia include thrombocytopenia with absent radius syndrome (TAR syndrome), cardiac defects (Holt-Oram syndrome), craniosynostosis (Baller-Gerold syndrome), Fanconi's syndrome, and the VATER association (which consists of abnormalities of the vertebral or vascular system, imperforate anus, tracheoesophageal fistula, and radial limb or renal system).

The coincidental finding of radial aplasia with amegakaryocytic thrombocytopenia (TAR syndrome) is recognizable in the neonate with bilateral radial aplasia, petechiae, melanotic stools, and obvious rectal bleeding. The TAR syndrome is believed to be an autosomal recessive disorder. By utilizing fetal radiography, it can be diagnosed correctly between 16 and 20 gestational weeks in mothers with the responsible gene. In these children, early and continued hematopoietic support may be necessary for the first year of life during which platelet function is suboptimal. Spontaneous improvement in thrombogenesis usually occurs after 12 months of age, and the prognosis is excellent. It is of interest that although the radius is frequently absent in the TAR syndrome, the thumb, even though it may be hypoplastic, is seldom missing entirely.

The TAR syndrome must be differentiated from macrocytic anemia with pancytopenia, which may be associated with radial dysplasia (Fanconi's syndrome). The latter usually occurs at 3 to 5 years of age and has a poor prognosis.

TREATMENT: Treatment is begun at birth with stretching and plaster casts applied to gradually stretch the soft-tissue contractures of the lateral side of the forearm and to position the hand parallel to the ulna. Centralization of the hand at the end of the ulna has proved to be satisfactory in correcting the deformity and providing a stable carpoulnar pseudarthrosis. This procedure is performed in the first year of life by excising the central area of the carpal bones and fitting the ulna into the defect. The hand is held in the corrected position with a Steinmann pin for at least 1 year. A radial approach to the hand is used with release of the soft-tissue contractures and lengthening of the tight muscles on the radial side of the arm. However, some have preferred a transverse ulnar approach which allows the operation to be performed in an area where there are nearly normal anatomic structures and where soft-tissue stabilization procedures and excision of excessive skin and soft tissue on the ulnar side of the wrist can be accomplished. This results in a cosmetically pleasing closure and may contribute to ulnar stability of the wrist. The ulnar approach allows stabilization of the carpoulnar pseudarthrosis by advancement of the extensor carpi ulnaris tendon, proximal transfer of the hypothenar musculature, and ulnar capsular reefing. If the ulna is severely bowed, it may be straightened by an osteotomy at its apex 6 weeks following centralization.

Active elbow flexion to at least 60 degrees is a prerequisite for the procedure. The elbow may be stiff at birth but becomes more mobile during the first year of life. If elbow motion does not develop, the centralized hand cannot reach the face or head. Forearm flexion usually can be achieved by surgical release of the posterior elbow ligaments and transfer of the triceps tendon anteriorly.

There are four functional advantages of a stable carpoulnar pseudarthrosis: provision of a stable hand-forearm articulation, improvement of the mechanical effects of finger flexors by reducing the power wasted in further radial deviation, increase in the effective length of the upper extremity distal to the elbow, and facilitation of thumb reconstruction or pollicization after displacement of the hand from its close proximity to the radial side of the forearm. Following relocation of the hand, its position can be stabilized by tendon transfers to the ulnar side of the hand. An aligned hand supported by the ulna is strong, functional, and relatively aesthetic.

Free transfer of the proximal fibula with its epiphysis to the radial side of the forearm has been disappointing in the radial clubhand patient. Recently, composite transfer of the proximal fibula utilizing microsurgical vascular anastomoses has been accomplished to support the carpus. It is uncertain whether this will result in fibular growth that parallels that of the ulna and whether the joint between the fibula and carpal bones will permit satisfactory wrist motion.

A shortened forearm in a child, secondary to a radial clubhand, can be lengthened by osteotomy and gradual distraction of the ulna. As much as 3 cm in length have been achieved by this method.

Attempts have been made to scientifically evaluate the results of centralization arthroplasty. Pre- and postoperative hand-forearm angles were measured by evaluating the angle between the longitudinal axis of the long finger metacarpal and the longitudinal axis of the distal ulna on the anteroposterior radiograph (Fig. 2). Furthermore, the hand-forearm position on the anteroposterior radiograph was measured to establish the position of the hand relative to the distal ulna (Fig. 3). Postoperative change in the ulnar direction is considered an improvement in position of the hand. It was found that the hand-forearm position more accurately reflects the major objective of the centralization arthroplasty: to reposition the hand on the distal ulna.

The thumb in these children can be hypoplastic or missing. If hypoplastic, but potentially functional, an opponensplasty utilizing the abductor digiti minimi mus-

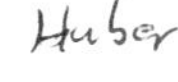

Figure 2-A

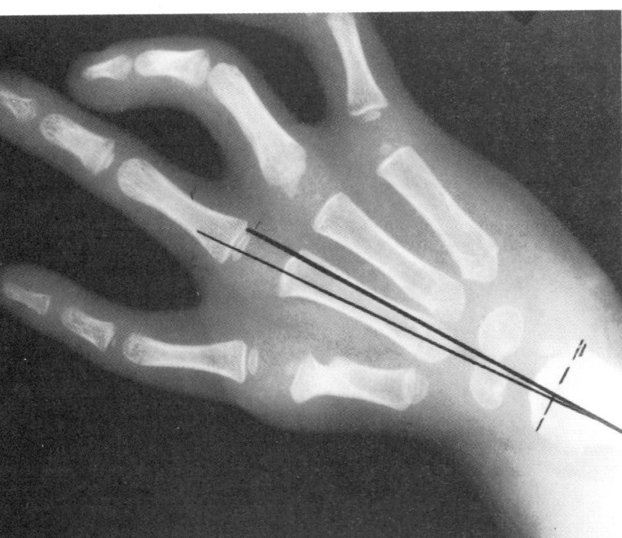

Figure 2-B

Figure 2: (A, B) Hand-forearm angle measured on the anteroposterior radiograph preoperative and postoperative centralization. This shows the acute angle of the intersection between the longitudinal axis of the long finger metacarpal and the longitudinal axis of the distal ulna. It is important to note that the angulation of the ulna is not included in its longitudinal line. To standardize a technique of determining the longitudinal axis of the ulna, a line is drawn across the face of the distal ulnar epiphyseal plate. A line drawn perpendicular to the midpoint of the epiphyseal plate is designated as the longitudinal axis of the distal ulna. The angle at which this line intersects with a second line drawn through the midshaft of the long finger metacarpal is recorded as a hand-forearm angle.

cle may be helpful. If absent, pollicization can be accomplished prior to opponensplasty.

Ulnar Aplasia Ulnar deficiency is among the least common types of congenital aplasia and is not the postaxial counterpart of radial aplasia. The deformity usually occurs sporadically, and there is no known related chromosomal abnormality. Although radial deficiency frequently is accompanied by cardiac, gastrointestinal, and hematopoietic problems, the abnormalities associated with ulnar aplasia usually involve only the musculoskeletal system. These include contralateral hand defects, scoliosis, proximal focal femoral deficiency, microcephaly and micrognathia, facial agenesis, short palate, deformed external ears, and hypospadias.

Like radial aplasia, ulnar aplasia represents a spectrum of dysplasia ranging from total absence to hypoplasia at either the proximal or distal end of the bone. Ulnar aplasia is usually partial, and the proximal ulnar epiphysis is present. One in three patients is bilateral, and most children with ulnar aplasia have failure of formation of one or more digits on the involved side.

Ulnar deviation of the carpus is usually mild and often does not progress beyond 20 degrees. Resection of the ulnar analogue should be reserved for those patients in whom there is progressive ulnar deviation of the hand or subluxation of the radial head. Major deformities usually are found at the elbow and may include instability due to deficiency of the ulna and the interosseous membrane, radiohumeral or ulnohumeral synostosis, or dislocation and proximal migration of the radius. No correlation has been found between severity of the ulnar deficiency, the elbow deformity, or the severity of the ulnar deviation at the radiocarpal joint. In some patients, the proximal third of the ulna articulates normally with the distal humerus, and the radial head is dislocated anteriorly, which reduces elbow flexion. In these patients a stable and mobile elbow and wrist can be achieved by creating a one-bone forearm. Forearm rotation is lost, but a one-bone forearm improves the function and appearance of the limb.

Twenty percent of patients with ulnar aplasia have no elbow joint. Osteotomy through the ulnohumeral ankylosis can be done to place the forearm in an improved functional position. Arthroplasty of the elbow in patients with a congenital synostosis is not advisable because neither stability nor satisfactory motion can be expected. Free joint transfers have been successful in laboratory animals, but the procedure has not been performed for congenital synostosis of the elbow and appears to have little likelihood of success.

Radioulnar Synostosis Proximal radioulnar synostosis results from failure of the developing cartilaginous precursors of the forearm to separate. There is a familial predisposition for radioulnar synostosis believed to be transmitted by a dominant phenotype with variable expression. Chromosomal abnormalities have been reported in some patients with bilateral radial synostosis.

Radioulnar synostosis is bilateral in 60 percent of patients and frequently is associated with other muscular abnormalities. Disability associated with this disorder is caused by severe pronation of the forearm. The hand positioned in pronation gets little help by substitute motion of the shoulder to place it in functional supination.

TREATMENT: There have been a number of ingenious operations devised to separate the synostosis and to permit active forearm rotation. Included are the insertion of a plastic membrane between the bones following release of the synostosis or insertion of a bone cap or specially constructed metallic swivel joint at the site of the synostosis. In addition, tendon transfers have been proposed to

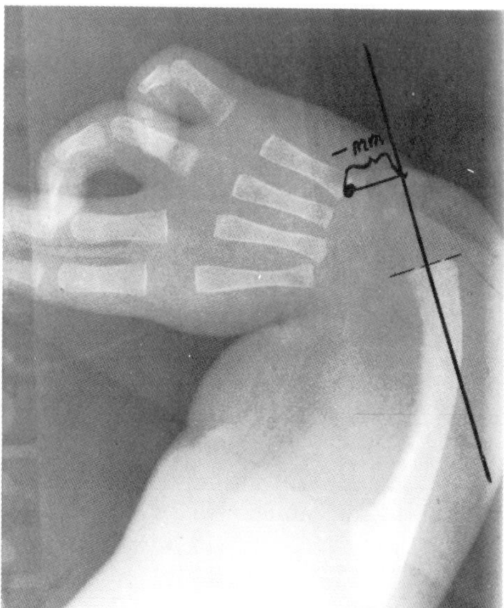

Figure 3-A

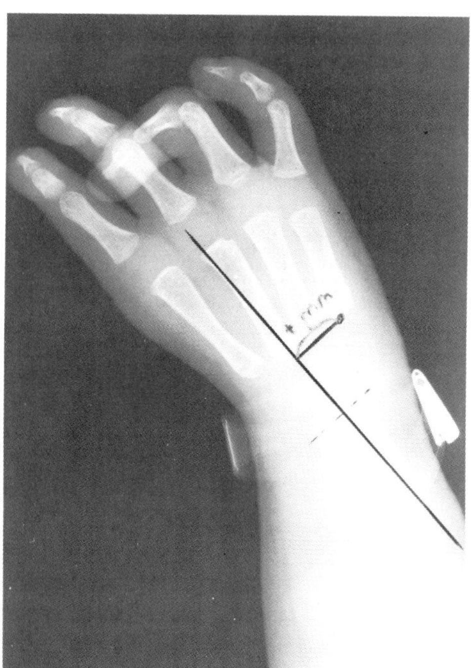

Figure 3-B

Figure 3: (A, B) Hand-forearm position measured on the anteroposterior radiograph preoperative and postoperative centralization. Hand-forearm position is measured by first drawing the longitudinal axis of the ulna as described in Figure 2. The second line is drawn from the proximal pole of the little finger metacarpal perpendicular to the longitudinal axis of the distal ulna, and the distance between the two is measured. (A) If the proximal pole is located radial to the axis of the distal ulna, it is recorded negatively in millimeters. (B) If the proximal pole of the little finger metacarpal is ulnar to the axis of the distal ulna, it is recorded positively in millimeters.

provide active rotation. Results of these procedures have been inconsistent, and frequently new bone rebridges the gap between the bones. Tendon transfers have not been effective in providing rotation.

Osteotomy through the synostosis is the preferred method of correcting deformity. With unilateral synostosis, osteotomy is not indicated unless the position of pronation is extreme. The desired position should be 10 to 20 degrees of supination. A hand in the forward working position of mild supination and a flexed elbow can obtain a degree of functional pronation by controlled amounts of internal rotation, flexion, and abduction at the shoulder.

In patients with bilateral radioulnar synostosis, it is recommended that the nondominant hand (that not used for writing) should be rotated to a position of 20 to 35 degrees of supination. If one hand is in supination, the other can remain in considerable pronation. If the other arm also is to be osteotomized, it should be placed in 30 to 45 degrees of pronation. In general, it has been noted that once the nondominant arm is rotated into supination, the other arm is usually in an appropriate position and does not have to be rotated.

The osteotomy should be done through the distal end of the fusion mass since it heals rapidly and is technically easy to position. Osteotomy through both bones at various levels in the forearm has presented difficulties with angulation and nonunion. It is important that the forearm be rotated in the direction that provides functional lengthening of the nerves of the forearm. Tightening of the pronator teres may occur during rotation and cause nerve or vascular dysfunction. If this happens or if there is any vascular difficulty, the pronator teres should be lengthened by sliding it proximally. It is probably preferable to rotate the arm in early childhood since it will provide a maximal range of motion during the growing period. Increased flexibility usually will develop at the wrist and shoulder in these children.

Madelung's Deformity Madelung's deformity manifests itself during late childhood or adolescence. It occurs bilaterally twice as often as it does unilaterally. It is inherited as an autosomal dominant trait and is more common in females than males by a four to one margin.

Radiographic changes, in contrast to clinical deformity, usually begin to appear at 2 years of age. The ulnar and volar half of the distal radial epiphysis does not grow as rapidly as the remaining portion, resulting in a radius whose ulnar half is shorter than the radial half. This shorter portion of the radial epiphysis receives its vascular supply from the anterior and posterior interosseous pedicles, which has prompted speculation that the etiology of the deformity may be caused by injury or atrophy of these vessels.

With time, the carpal articular surface of the radius slants ulnarly (up to 80 degrees) and volarly (up to 60 degrees), and the carpus and hand shift into flexion and ulnar deviation. The ulna remains in its usual position resulting in a dorsal prominence. The proximal end of the radius usually is normal but occasionally may be deformed. Some consider Madelung's deformity a local manifestation of a systemic disorder termed *dyschondrosteosis,* a variant of mesomelic dwarfism. Madelung's deformity also may be associated with multiple enchondromatosis, Turner's gonadal dysgenesis, Hurler's syndrome, and Morquio's syndrome.

The deformity commonly presents in girls 6 to 13 years of age with the insidious onset of pain and progressive deformity of the wrist. It limits extension and radial deviation of the wrist and supination of the forearm. The deformity progresses with growth until maturity at which time it is usually painful.

TREATMENT: This is directed primarily toward alleviation of pain and restoration of the function lost as a result of the deformity. Many patients with Madelung's deformity do not require any treatment. Surgery may be indicated to correct the deformity and improve range of motion following epiphyseal closure. The preferred method is a closing wedge osteotomy of the distal radius which is based dorsally and radially, fashioned to correct both volar and ulnar angulation. A limited resection of the distal ulna also is accomplished by the Darrach method in adults or the Milch cuff method in skeletally immature patients. This usually results in improved dorsiflexion and supination of the wrist and hand.

Congenital Pseudarthrosis of the Forearm Few patients with congenital pseudarthrosis of the forearm due to neurofibromatosis have been reported in the literature. The pseudarthrosis may involve either the radius or the ulna separately or, even more uncommonly, both. It may present as a nonhealing fracture, similar to the tibia and invariably is associated with generalized neurofibromatosis.

Treatment is directed toward gaining union of the bones of the forearm. Several investigators have reported difficulty in obtaining union of the pseudarthrosis by bone grafting and internal fixation in children. They subsequently have suggested that bone grafting the pseudarthrosis may be more successful in older children and recommend that the arm be supported in an orthosis until the child is mature, when bone grafting is accomplished. Others have used free transfer of the vascularized fibula to obtain union after resecting the pseudarthrosis. They have achieved union, but a normal arm has not been obtained.

It has been noted that in patients with pseudarthrosis of the ulna normal growth of the radius may cause increased pressure on the lower humeral epiphysis. This impairs development of the capitellum and part of the trochlea, making the radiohumeral joint unstable. Bowing of the radius and eventual dislocation of the radial head may occur. In order to maintain the normal length of the ulna, early excision of the pseudarthrosis has been recommended. This is believed to remove the restraining effect of the ulna on the radius, allow normal development of the lower end of the humerus, and prevent dislocation of the radial head.

Arthritis

Hemophilia The elbow joint may be commonly involved in patients with hemophilia. Free blood within the joint is an irritant and may cause an inflammatory response with synovial hypertrophy resulting in recurrent hemorrhage into the joint. It also appears to cause enzymatic destruction of articular cartilage.

TREATMENT: Acute treatment involves the infusion of factor VIII concentrate as soon as there is any indication of bleeding into the joint. This is supplemented by application of ice and appropriate splinting to decrease the intensity of the response and physical therapy to regain motion following the bleed.

Synovectomy is recommended in the early stages before advanced arthropathy has occurred to reduce the frequency of hemarthrosis. The usual indication for synovectomy is recurrent bleeding into the joint which is uncontrolled by hematologic management. Results of elbow synovectomy (in contrast to knee synovectomy) have been encouraging in that bleeding episodes have decreased from an average of twenty-five to three per year in a recent study. Complications of hemorrhage in the early postoperative period despite adequate factor VIII replacement and infection occur in approximately 25 percent of patients. Most elbow joints lose 25 to 30 degrees of mobility following synovectomy, but this does not cause a functional disability. Most patients reported the operation worthwhile. Recently, "medical synovectomy" using radioactive gold has been reported to decrease the incidence of bleeding and reverse early arthropathy. This may hold promise in the future, but further studies are necessary.

When elbow synovectomy should be done is still controversial. Some have found that reduction in bleeding frequency delays progression of chronic elbow arthropathy and recommend early synovectomy. Others believe it is not indicated until medical management has proved unsuccessful. It would seem that synovectomy plays a useful role in the treatment of recurrent hemarthroses of the elbow that do not respond to clotting factor treatment.

Neuromuscular Disorders

Arthrogryposis Multiplex Congenita This disorder is characterized by congenital failure of development of skeletal muscles, joint contractures, and deformities with associated absence of function. The degree of involvement is variable. Typical upper extremity deformity includes bilateral adduction and internal rotation of the shoulders, bilateral extension contractures of the elbows, pronation of the forearms, and palmar flexion and ulnar deviation of the wrists. Hand function may be comparatively good despite fixed elbow extension and wrist deformities.

Two elbow motions are necessary in children with arthrogryposis: elbow flexion for self-feeding, preferably with one hand; and elbow extension for toilet care, the use of a long arm crutch, and the required pushoffs when rising from a chair. In these patients, perineal care, ambulation, and pushoffs are achieved most easily with the elbow in extension, and eating is accomplished with the elbow in flexion. It is not always possible to achieve adequate flexion and extension in the same upper extremity, and, therefore, procedures to restore elbow flexion should be accomplished in only one extremity. Function of the child's elbow and shoulder should be considered together because correction of the elbow is dependent upon the position and mobility of the shoulder.

Treatment: Active flexion of the elbow can be gained by anterior transfer of the triceps brachii, pectoralis major muscle transfer, or Steindler flexorplasty. The indication for surgical procedures should be based upon the severity of involvement, the muscle or muscles available for transfer, and which muscles are strong enough for transfer. Prerequisites for any of these transfers include passive elbow flexion to a right angle prior to introduction of an active elbow flexor. Extension contracture of the elbow can be corrected by posterior and lateral capsulotomy of the joint combined with elongation of the triceps muscle. Improved flexion has been achieved most often by pectoralis major transfer since this muscle is usually available and strong. Anterior transfer of the triceps has not always been successful in these children. Steindler flexorplasty is successful in children with satisfactory muscles available for transfer, but this is not often the case. Properly selected, these procedures greatly improve the ability of these severely involved children to flex their elbows.

Poliomyelitis

Paralysis of the biceps brachii and brachialis with resultant loss of active elbow flexion often resulted from poliomyelitis. Proximal and lateral transfer of the medial epicondyle (Steindler flexorplasty as modified by Mayer and Green) became a standard transfer for this deficit, and satisfactory long-term results continue to be reported. The prerequisites are a functional hand, forearm flexor power sufficient to justify transfer, and a lack of need for full elbow extension for transfer or ambulation. The procedure may be used for patients meeting these criteria as a result of cerebral palsy, brachial plexus palsy, and arthrogryposis multiplex congenita.

Cerebral Palsy

Flexion Contracture Children with cerebral palsy may have elbow flexor spasticity which causes the limb to assume a position of elbow flexion. This posturing may be constant, or it may occur with voluntary activity. Involuntary dynamic flexion at the elbow eventually may result in a secondary flexion contracture which interferes with use of the limb by eliminating reach and functional activities of the hand.

Emotion or positionally induced hypertonia often exaggerate the elbow flexion deformity. This flexion attitude during activity is cosmetically disabling, particularly in adolescents. Unfortunately, there is no medication effective in controlling this deformity. The use of orthoses and exercise most often results in only minor or temporary improvement.

Pessimism concerning the results of surgery on the upper extremity in patients with spasticity due to cerebral palsy generally has been justified. However, most have attempted to improve function of the hand by operations directed at the wrist and fingers, not at the elbow and forearm. Functional use of the hand depends to a large extent upon a functional elbow. It must be recognized that although some improvement in function and appearance may be realistic for these patients, normalcy can rarely, if ever, be achieved.

The elbow flexors can be lengthened to decrease the elbow flexor predominance and allow the triceps to regain balance and power. The procedure consists of complete excision of the lacertus fibrosus, Z-lengthening of the biceps tendon, and release of the brachialis aponeurosis (Fig. 4). A flexion contracture of 45 degrees or more is one indication for surgery. Children with a flexion contracture of the elbow and a pronation contracture of the forearm may dislocate the radial head, and this may be another indication for the procedure. Reasonable intelligence in a child who has not completely rejected the extremity is one prerequisite for elbow release. The procedure usually results in decreasing the flexion contracture by 30 degrees

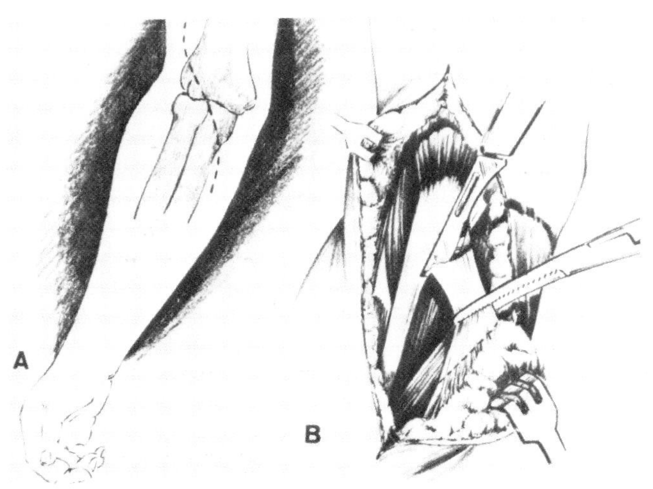

Figure 4: Sequential steps of lengthening the elbow flexors in children with cerebral palsy. (A) Initial incision. (B) Exposure and excision of the lacertus fibrosus. (C) Z-lengthening of the biceps tendon. (D) Incision of the aponeurotic fascia covering the biceps brachialis tendon at several levels. (Reprinted with permission from Lengthening of the elbow flexors in cerebral palsy, by M.A. Mital, J. Bone Joint Surg. 61A:516, 1979.)

or more without loss of the preoperative flexor range so that all children can get their hands to their mouths postoperatively. Most patients believe that the major benefit from this procedure may be improvement in cosmesis. The appearance of the extremity should not be underestimated and may be as important as improvement of function, particularly in the adolescent child with normal or near normal intelligence. In addition, patients who utilize crutches for upright balance benefit from reduction of the flexion deformity.

Pronation Contracture This also occurs in children with flexion contractures of the forearm. They lack the ability to supinate and, therefore, cannot turn doorknobs, receive change, and use a key. It has been reported that a pronation contracture can be treated by changing the insertion of the pronator teres and, therefore, changing it into a supinator. This is accomplished by rerouting the pronator teres from the anterior aspect of the radius around laterally and posteriorly and reinserting it into its original position. Preoperative patient selection is very important. Prerequisites include satisfactory sensation to light touch and pinprick, as well as good stereognosis. Forty-five degrees of passive supination of the forearm is desirable but not required. It is recommended that the operation be performed between the ages of 6 and 10 years, so that the child can develop the use of the extremity to its optimal degree and prior to the development of a pronator teres contracture. One report noted improvement of active supination by 50 percent and good to excellent results were reported in 82 percent of the patients by one author, but others have not been able to duplicate these results with this procedure.

Tumors

There are no tumors that have a specific predilection for the elbow or forearm. The tumors which present in childhood may occur in this area and usually simulate other disease processes.

An intra-articular *osteoid-osteoma* of the distal humerus may simulate synovitis and may cause an erroneous diagnosis of an inflammatory arthritic process. A juxta-articular osteoid-osteoma of the distal humerus may present with subperiosteal new bone formation on the adjacent radius and ulna as well as on the humerus. *Infantile cortical hyperostosis* may present in the humerus or radius and mimic pulled elbow or Erb's palsy. This process usually presents under 5 months of age with a sudden onset of soft-tissue swelling, fever, irritability, high white blood cell count, and increased sedimentation rate, all characteristic of an inflammatory response. Differential diagnosis of this process includes osteomyelitis, vitamin A deficiency, scurvy, congenital syphilis, and bone tissue repair. Typically, the diagnosis of infantile cortical hyperostosis is made as the bony changes become apparent or there is involvement of the mandible which is diagnostic of the condition. This should be considered when dealing with a disease process which has an inflammatory nature but does not appear to respond in the usual fashion.

Multiple hereditary exostoses commonly occur bilaterally at the elbow and forearm. Exostoses of the distal radius (80 percent) and ulna (85 percent) are frequently involved. The distal end of the ulna is always more seriously affected than the radius. Over one-half of the patients with multiple radial exostoses have severe deformity of the forearm, and one-third have restriction of either pronation or supination (Fig. 5). Either pronation or supination usually is restricted with free movement in the other direction. Exostoses are less common in the elbow, occurring in 5 percent of the distal humerus, 38 percent of the proximal radius, and 37 percent of the proximal ulna. Dislocation of the radial head occurs in approximately 20 to 25 percent of elbows (Fig. 6).

No deformity, once identified, has improved with growth. Deformity of the upper extremity can be treated surgically by excision of the dislocated radial head at skeletal maturity or by osteotomy of the radius to increase rotation. Excision of a distal osteochondroma from the radius to increase rotation is sometimes effective, but the results may be inconsistent.

Ewing's sarcoma rarely occurs in the radius and the ulna. Traditional treatment includes amputation, radiation therapy, and chemotherapy. Recently, moderate radiotherapy (5,000 rads) and adjunct chemotherapy have been used and have improved forearm function, but the 5-year survival rate has been dismal.

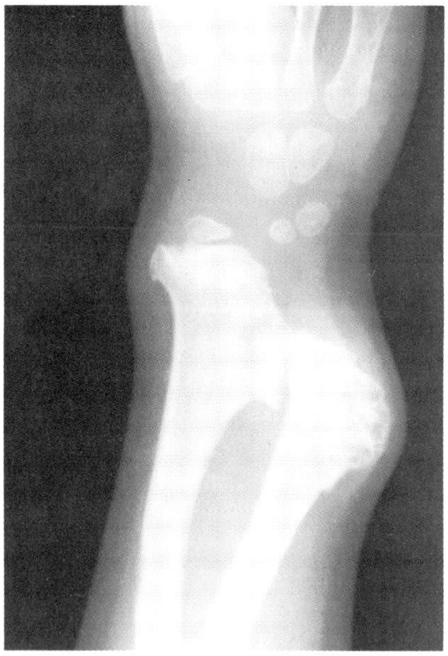

Figure 5: Severe deformity of the distal radius and ulna in a child with hereditary multiple exostoses. The exostoses are present in both the ulna and the radius. Note that there is considerable obliquity of the distal radial epiphysis and the ulna is shortened.

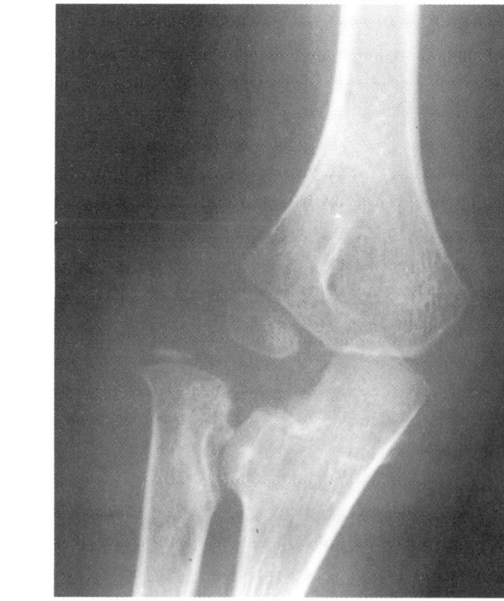

Figure 6: Elbow radiograph in a child with hereditary multiple exostoses shows exostosis of the proximal ulna and dislocation of the radial head.

Miscellaneous

Osteochondrosis Dissecans This term is preferred over osteochondritis dissecans since there is no evidence that the lesion is inflammatory, as was originally proposed. The elbow is an uncommon site for osteochondrosis dissecans. There are two concepts of its pathogenesis: reaction to repeated trauma of the radial head against the capitellum, and spontaneous, focal osteonecrosis of the capitellum. Trauma has been identified as a factor in the etiology in 50 percent of the patients, but it is unclear whether it causes the lesion or is the precipitating factor. Repetitive throwing motions are frequently associated with osteochondrosis dissecans of the elbow. The final stage of throwing is associated with a progressive extension of the elbow and pronation of the forearm which may result in compression and shearing at the radiohumeral joint. However, although trauma may lead to osteochondral fragment formation in some individuals, the possibility of focal osteonecrosis in constitutionally vulnerable individuals cannot be excluded as an etiology.

Osteochondrosis dissecans usually causes pain and restricted range of motion of the elbow. Locking may occur if a free fragment is present in the joint. It is most commonly found in boys in early adolescence (skeletal age of 13 years for boys and 11 years for girls). A radiograph demonstrates a characteristic crescent-shaped area of radiolucency in the anterolateral aspect of the capitellum. The lesion is best localized by anteroposterior, lateral, and tangential views of the elbow. The osteochondral fragment may be in situ, incompletely detached, or completely detached and free within the joint. Prognosis and treatment varies depending upon the age of patient and the stage of the lesion, (in situ, incompletely detached, or free fragment). In early adolescence, when the epiphysis is still open, the prognosis for healing is excellent. Treatment consists of modification of activity, particularly if baseball pitching is responsible. A resting splint may be necessary to relieve the symptoms.

Young adults who are beginning skeletal maturation (skeletal age of 14 years for boys and 12 years for girls) until approximately age 20 do not heal the lesions as readily. They are ideal candidates for arthrotomy, drilling, and possible bone graft to the affected area, particularly if the fragment is partially attached. This usually prevents the fragment from becoming a loose body with progressive articular degeneration and articular incongruity. The preoperative state of the overlying cartilage can be assessed arthroscopically.

ANNOTATED BIBLIOGRAPHY

Normal Development

Hoffer, M.M.: Joint motion limitation in newborns. Clin. Orthop. 148:94-96, 1980.

Newborn infants and children undergo changes in tone and joint motion with growth and development. Fifty neonates were examined in the first days of life and then followed up for 1 year. Elbow extension was limited by 30 degrees in many newborn children, but this limitation completely disappeared by the 3-month examination.

Silberstein, M.J.; Brodeur, A.E.; and Graviss, E.R.: Some vagaries of the capitellum. J. Bone Joint Surg. 61A:244-247, 1979.

The capitellum is the first epiphyseal center of the distal humerus to ossify and is subject to misinterpretation because the ossification center is situated anteriorly tilted downward and its physis tends to be wider posteriorly than anteriorly. Radiographic development is traced to fusion. The author discusses the use of the humeral shaft line and the coronoid line to interpret the position of the capitellum.

Silberstein, M.J.; Brodeur, A.E.; Graviss, E.R.; and Luisiri, A.: Some vagaries of the medial epicondyle. J. Bone Joint Surg. 63A:524-528, 1981.

These authors outline the radiographic development of the medial epicondyle of the humerus and discuss why it may be prone to misinterpretation radiographically.

Silberstein, M.J.; Brodeur, A.E.; Graviss, E.R.; and Luisiri, A.: Some vagaries of the olecranon. J. Bone Joint Surg. 63A:722-725, 1981.

This article details the features of the olecranon through its maturation and discusses why it may be prone to misinterpretation radiographically.

Congenital and Developmental

Amputations

Swanson, A.B., and Swanson, G.D.G.: The Krukenberg procedure in the juvenile amputee. Clin. Orthop. 148:55-61, 1980.

This paper outlines the indication and the operative procedure used in constructing the Krukenberg stump in patients with unilateral or bilateral loss of the hand. Improved prehension and sensibility have appeared to have improved their quality of life. The Krukenberg stump was accepted cosmetically by all children in this series.

Radial Aplasia (Radial Clubhand)

Dell, P.C., and Sheppard, J.E.: Thrombocytopenia, absent radius syndrome: Report of two siblings and review of the hematologic and genetic features. Clin. Orthop. 162:129-134, 1982.

The paper discusses two patients with thrombocytopenia and radial dysplasia (TAR syndrome). Combined hematologic and orthopaedic management is recommended in these children who usually resolve their thrombocytopenia by 1 year of age.

Feingold, M.; Sklower, S.L.; Willner, J.P.; Desnick, R.H.; and Cohen, M.M.: Cranial synostosis–radial aplasia: The Baller-Gerold syndrome. Am. J. Dis. Child. 133:1279-1280, 1979.

This report describes two patients with Baller-Gerold syndrome and points out it is probably transmitted by autosomal recessive inheritance. The authors distinguish this syndrome from the TAR syndrome, the Holt-Oram syndrome, and Fanconi's syndrome.

Luthy, D.A.; Hall, J.G.; and Graham, C.B.: Prenatal diagnosis of thrombocytopenia with absent radii. Clin. Genet. 15:495-499, 1979.

Six pregnant women with a fetus at risk for thrombocytopenia with absent radius (TAR syndrome) between 16 and 20 menstrual weeks were studied utilizing fetal radiography. Two affected and four unaffected fetuses were correctly identified with this technique which can provide reliable prenatal diagnosis in pregnancies at risk.

Manske, P.R., and McCarroll, H.R., Jr.: Abductor digiti minimi opponensplasty in congenital radial dysplasia. J. Hand Surg. 3:552-559, 1978.

The abductor digiti minimi opponensplasty was utilized in patients with radial aplasia and isolated thenar aplasia, thenar muscle aplasia with other radial abnormalities, and in patients with weakness of opposition after pollicization. Satisfactory results were obtained in twenty of twenty-one transfers.

Manske, P.R.; McCarroll, H.R.; and Swanson, K.: Centralization of the radial club hand: An ulnar surgical approach. J. Hand Surg. 6:423-433, 1981.

Centralization arthroplasty by a transverse ulnar approach was used to correct the radial clubhand deformity in twenty-two hands. The results were evaluated at an average of 34 months postoperatively by clinical exam and measurement of the hand-forearm angle and hand-forearm position. Stable carpoulnar pseudarthroses were established in twenty of twenty-one extremities.

Roberts, A.; Wickstrom, J.; and McKay, D.: Congenital absence of the radius. Southern Med. J. 73:702-706, 1980.

This article reviews the Shreveport Children's Hospital experience in eighteen children with twenty-seven congenitally absent radii. The authors found the prognosis for hand function in patients treated nonoperatively to be poor, but the majority of patients had good function following centralization.

Weber, T.R.; Smith, W.; and Grosfeld, J.L.: Surgical experience in infants with VATER association. J. Pediat. Surg. 15:849-854, 1980.

The surgical experience in thirty infants with the VATER association of multiple congenital abnormalities is described. The authors suggest the infants can be managed by a multisystem approach with well-planned operative therapy. Satisfactory growth and development takes place in most of these infants with few long-term complications.

Ulnar Aplasia

Broudy, A.S., and Smith, R.J.: Deformities of the hand and wrist with ulnar deficiency. J. Hand Surg. 4:304-315, 1979.

The authors reviewed twenty-six upper limbs in twenty patients with ulnar deficiency. They described the various deformities of the hand and elbow associated with this syndrome, as well as their method of treatment and its results.

Radioulnar Synostosis

Danielsson, L.G.: Iatrogenic pronator syndrome: Case report. Scand. J. Plast. Reconstr. Surg. 14:201-203, 1981.

Complete loss of motor and sensory function in the median nerve following rotational osteotomy for radioulnar synostosis is reported. The author recommends lengthening of the pronator teres at the time of surgery to avoid this complication.

Green, W.T., and Mital, M.A.: Congenital radio-ulnar synostosis: Surgery treatment. J. Bone Joint Surg. 61A:738-743, 1979.

Fourteen patients with congenital radioulnar synostosis, followed 10 to 25 years after a transverse supination osteotomy through the conjoint mass of the radius and the ulna, are discussed. The results of osteotomy through the synostosis were good and excellent in twelve children. In patients not rated excellent, it would have been preferable to rotate them further into supination.

Madelung's Deformity

Dawe, C.; Wynne-Davies, R.; and Fulford, G.E.: Clinical variation in dyschondrosteosis: A report on 13 individuals in 8 families. J. Bone Joint Surg. 64B:377-381, 1982.

Madelung's deformity associated with dyschondrosteosis is described as are the other deformities associated with dyschondrosteosis. It is recommended that patients with dyschondrosteosis be kept under observation during their growth period.

Congenital Pseudarthrosis of the Forearm

Ali, M.S., and Hooper, G.: Congenital pseudarthrosis of the ulna due to neurofibromatosis. J. Bone Joint Surg. 64B:600-602, 1982.

This paper draws attention to the effect on the elbow in two patients with isolated pseudarthrosis of the ulna due to neurofibromatosis. The authors theorize a tethering effect of the ulna which results in distortion of the capitellum and part of the trochlea, bowing of the radius, and proximal dislocation of the radial head.

Allieu, Y.; Gomis, R.; Yoshimura, M.; Dimeglio, A.; and Bonnel, F.: Congenital pseudarthrosis of the forearm: Two cases treated by revascularized fibular grafts. J. Hand Surg. 6:475-481, 1981.

The authors report two patients with congenital pseudarthrosis of the forearm, treated with a vascularized fibular graft. Union was achieved in both patients, but the arms are not normal and the ultimate outcome is unknown.

Manske, P.R.: Forearm pseudarthrosis–neurofibromatosis: Case report. Clin. Orthop. 139:125-127, 1979.

A 3½-year-old girl with pseudarthrosis of the radius and ulna secondary to neurofibromatosis is reported. The author recommends that surgical attempts to achieve union of a forearm pseudarthrosis associated with neurofibromatosis be postponed until the child reaches skeletal maturity.

Arthritis

Hemophilia

Ahlberg, A., and Pettersson, H.: Synoviorthesis with radioactive gold in hemophiliacs: Clinical and radiographic follow-up. Acta Orthop. Scand. 50:513-517, 1979.

The authors report that intra-articular injection of radioactive gold decreased the frequency of bleeding and reversed the progression of arthropathy if accomplished early in the disease process. They speculate that the reduction in bleeding frequency delays the progression of chronic arthropathy in affected joints.

Kay, L.; Stainsby, D.; Buzzard, B.; Fearns, M.; Hamilton, P.J.; Owen, P.; and Jones, P.: The role of synovectomy in the management of recurrent haemarthroses in haemophilia. British J. Haematol. 49:53-60, 1981.

The article presents eighteen patients with severe hemophilia A, who underwent synovectomy of twelve elbows. Recurrent bleeding was decreased from twenty-four to three episodes per year. Patient acceptance was good, despite an average loss of 28 degrees of mobility and a complication rate of 25 percent.

Neuromuscular Disorders

Arthrogryposis Multiplex Congenita

Doyle, J.R.; James, P.M.; Larsen, L.J.; and Ashley, R.K.: Restoration of elbow flexion in arthrogryposis multiplex congenita. J. Hand Surg. 5:149-152, 1980.

The authors compared the results of four procedures to improve elbow flexion including seven patients with pectoralis transfer, seven patients with anterior transfer of the triceps, and two patients with Steindler flexorplasty. They report that pectoralis transfer was the most effective procedure in improving elbow flexion in children with arthrogryposis.

Poliomyelitis

Dutton, R.O., and Dawson, E.G.: Elbow flexorplasty: An analysis of long-term results. J. Bone Joint Surg. 63A:1064-1069, 1981.

In twenty-five patients (twenty-five elbows) with elbow flexor paralysis secondary to poliomyelitis (twenty-two), birth palsy (two), and arthrogryposis multiplex congenita (one), excellent and good results were reported in twenty elbows with a definite improvement in all but one. The average postoperative arc of flexion was 95 degrees—from 36 degrees lack of full extension to 131 degrees flexion.

Cerebral Palsy

Mital, M.A.: Lengthening of the elbow flexors in cerebral palsy. J. Bone Joint Surg. 61A:515-522, 1979.

The article reviews the results of surgical release at the elbow to decrease elbow flexion deformity in twenty-six children with cerebral palsy. The flexion deformity was decreased from 48 to 10 degrees with improvement in reach, two-handed activities, and use of the limb. A major benefit is improvement of cosmesis in the upper extremity.

Sakellarides, H.T.; Mital, M.A.; and Lenzi, W.D.: Treatment of pronation contractures of the forearm in cerebral palsy by changing the insertion of the pronator radii teres. J. Bone Joint Surg. 63A:645-652, 1981.

The authors present a new procedure for decreasing the pronation deformity of the forearm and enhancing supination function in patients with cerebral palsy. This is accomplished by rerouting the pronator teres which achieves good results in 82 percent, with an average gain of active supination of 46 degrees.

Tumors

Cronemeyer, R.L.; Kirchmer, N.A.; DeSmet, A.A.; and Neff, J.R.: Intra-articular osteoid-osteoma of the humerus simulating synovitis of the elbow: A case report. J. Bone Joint Surg. 63A:1172-1174, 1981.

Intra-articular osteoid-osteoma of the distal humerus is rare and may pose diagnostic difficulties by mimicking an inflammatory or arthritic process. The authors point out that juxta-articular osteoid-osteomas will cause periosteal new bone formation on adjacent bones, in this instance the radius and ulna.

Finsterbush, A., and Husseini, N.: Infantile cortical hyperostosis with unusual clinical manifestations. Clin. Orthop. 144:276-279, 1979.

Three patients with infantile cortical hyperostosis who presented with a picture of Erb's palsy, a pulled elbow, or torticollis are reported. The authors point out that infantile cortical hyperostosis may mimic a variety of other common conditions in early infancy.

Kliman, M.; Harwood, A.R.; Jenkin, R.D.; Cummings, B.J.; Langer, F.; Quirt, I.; and Fornasier, V.L.: Radical radiotherapy as primary treatment for Ewing's sarcoma distal to the elbow and knee. Clin. Orthop. 165:233-238, 1982.

The authors reviewed twenty-two patients with Ewing's sarcoma distal to the elbow and knee treated by moderate dose (5,000 rads) radiotherapy and, in some instances, adjuvant chemotherapy. The functional results following this protocol in the forearm tumors were good. Unfortunately, all patients expired within 3 years with this regimen.

Shapiro, F.; Simon, S.; and Glimcher, M.J.: Hereditary multiple exostoses. Anthropometric, roentgenographic, and clinical aspects. J. Bone Joint Surg. 61A:815-824, 1979.

The authors reviewed thirty-two patients with hereditary multiple exostoses. Sixty percent of the patients had moderate to severe involvement of the upper extremity, including dislocation of the radial head in 22 percent and moderate to severe rotational limitation in 33 percent of the forearms. Operative excision of the radial head at maturity and excision of exostosis of the distal radius improved forearm rotation in most patients.

Miscellaneous

Osteochondrosis Dissecans

Pappas, A.M.: Elbow problems associated with baseball during childhood and adolescence. Clin. Orthop. 164:30-41, 1982.

The elbow is the most frequent area of complaint in child and adolescent baseball players. The motions of throwing as well as the injuries which can occur to the medial, lateral, anterior, and posterior elbow joint are reviewed. Diagnosis and treatment are discussed.

Pappas, A.M.: Osteochondrosis dissecans. Clin. Orthop. 158:59-69, 1981.

This review presents the problems of osteochondrosis dissecans as related to the knee, ankle, hip, and elbow joints, in terms of its etiology, presenting symptoms, radiographic demonstration, and treatment.

18 ELBOW AND FOREARM: TRAUMA

This section considers injuries of adults and children.

Elbow

Anatomy The elbow joint is a complex of three joints that are held together by a combination of ligamentous structures. These structures are important to identify as they are the key to selecting the proper treatment regimen in the injured patient.

The lateral ligament is not a true collateral ligament. Rather than spanning the joint from lateral condyle to radius and ulna, it attaches to the annular ligament (Fig. 1B). The anconeus muscle functions as more of a lateral stabilizer (Fig. 1A).

On the medial side there is a well-developed collateral ligament, consisting of three basic components: an anterior oblique ligament, a posterior oblique ligament, and a small transverse ligament (Fig. 1C).

The posterior oblique ligament is absent in many primates and is not believed to be an essential stabilizer of the medial aspect of the elbow. The anterior oblique ligament is fundamentally the most important part of the medial collateral ligament. It is a thick band which runs from the undersurface of the medial epicondyle to a point on the medial aspect of the ulna just below the coronoid process. In extension, the most anterior fibers of the anterior oblique ligament become tight, and in flexion, the posterior fibers become taut. Therefore, the anterior oblique ligament functions throughout the range of motion of the elbow joint and, except at full extension, is responsible for the inherent stability of the entire joint through its range of motion. In full extension, even with all the medial collateral ligament disrupted, the olecranon process locks into the fossa stabilizing the joint to valgus stress.

Adult Fractures

Supracondylar Fractures Supracondylar fractures in adults are usually comminuted, forming the *T, Y, or M* configuration. In addition, unusually severe fragmentation as a treatment problem is becoming more common due to improved survival rates following high-speed vehicular injuries and falls from heights. Controversy continues concerning nonoperative versus surgical management.

Those advocating nonsurgical management of supracondylar fractures in adults condemn the surgical approach as leading to osteonecrosis after the extensive dissection necessary to obtain reduction. Additionally, increased adhesions often develop, limiting postoperative motion.

Conversely, others claim that surgical management lends more stability and correction of deformity. Some surgeons combine both methods of treatment by anatomically reducing the intra-articular portion of the fracture with a single screw or K-wire through a minimal

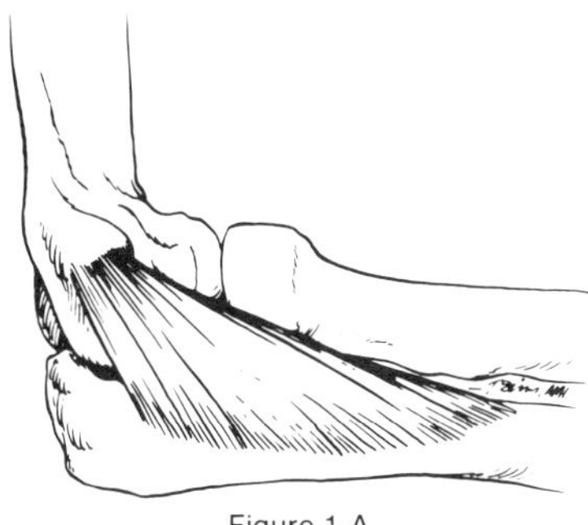

Figure 1-A

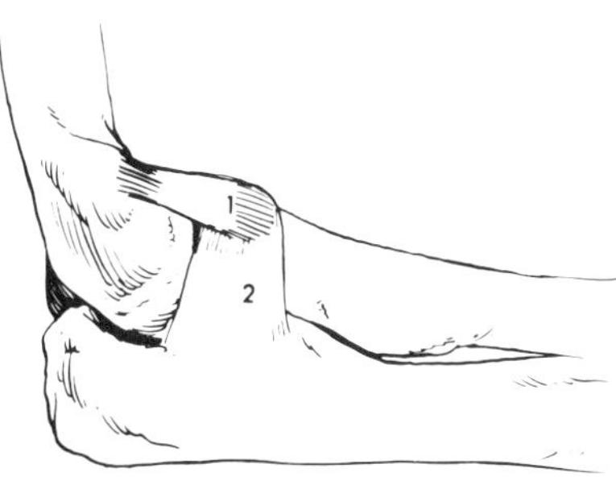

Figure 1-B

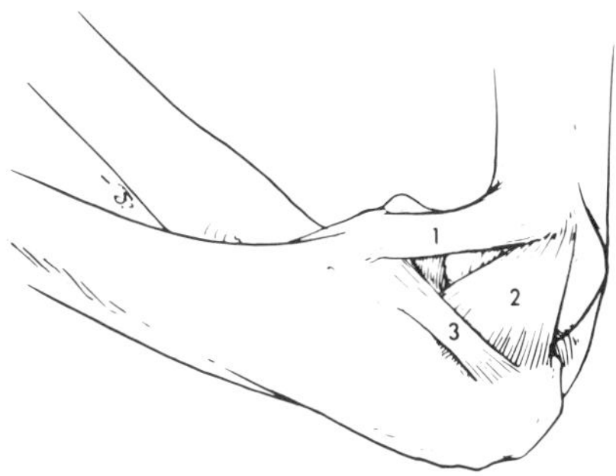

Figure 1-C

Figure 1: (A) Anconeus muscle. (B) Lateral ligaments: 1, Lateral collateral ligament; 2, Annular ligament. (C) Medial elbow ligaments: 1, Anterior oblique; 2, Posterior oblique; 3, Transverse oblique. (Reprinted with permission from Factors influencing elbow instability, by H.S. Tullos, et al., *In* AAOS Instructional Course Lectures, XXX:186, St. Louis, C.V. Mosby, 1981.)

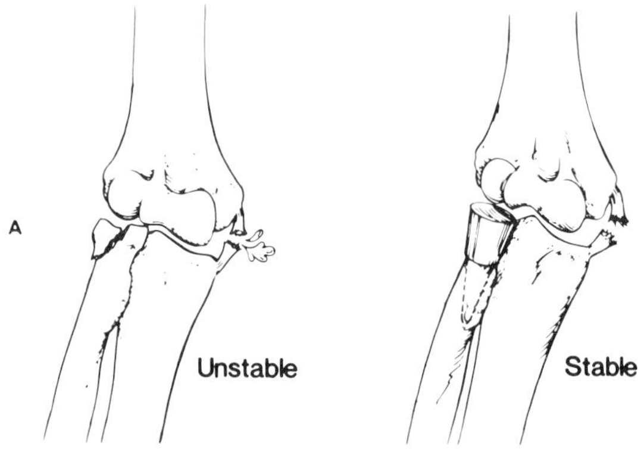

Figure 2: (A) Elbow is unstable with fracture of radial head and rupture of medial collateral ligament. (B) Elbow may be stabilized by repair of medial collateral ligament, replacement of radial head, or both. (Reprinted with permission from Factors influencing elbow instability, by H.S. Tullos, et al., AAOS Instructional Course Lectures XXX:195, St. Louis, C.V. Mosby, 1981.)

incision, while treating the remaining extra-articular fragments as a closed supracondylar fracture with immobilization for approximately 3 weeks. This treatment seems most appropriate for the adolescent.

In the elderly patient, severe comminution can be treated with a collar and cuff, combined with a well-padded plaster posterior splint. Active exercise begins 3 weeks after the injury.

Osteosynthesis may be achieved by screw and/or plate fixation. The advantage of this procedure is accurate reduction and very early active motion (2 to 5 days postfixation). However, extensive dissection is required for exposure. Neurovascular compromise and adhesions may be increased by the procedure. Finally, rigid internal fixation is difficult to achieve because of the complex anatomy of the distal humerus.

There seems to be a consensus favoring a nonoperative approach for the Riseborough and Radin types I, II, and IV fractures, whereas type III fractures are treated surgically. Ulnar nerve transposition is recommended in the treatment of type III fractures except in elderly patients for whom nonsurgical treatment is recommended.

An orthopaedist occasionally sees an undisplaced supracondylar fracture in the adult without involvement of the elbow joint. Treatment consists of a posterior splint for 3 weeks, followed by an active range of motion exercise program.

Olecranon Fractures Open reduction and internal fixation compose the currently recommended treatment for most olecranon fractures. However, the current literature stressing the importance of the anterior oblique ligament may influence selection of an appropriate operative procedure in the treatment of the fractured olecranon. If the fracture is proximal to the insertion of the anterior oblique ligament, the olecranon fragment can be removed safely without fear of creating an unstable elbow. The technique of fragment removal with triceps reattachment may prove to be the preferred treatment in severely comminuted fractures. Operative complications associated with wire and pin fixation, such as metal breakage, protrusion, and reduction resulting in incongruous joint surfaces, can thus be avoided. Additionally, secondary procedures for removal of fixation devices are not required.

Fractures distal to the coronoid process require open reduction and stable internal fixation. These fractures are

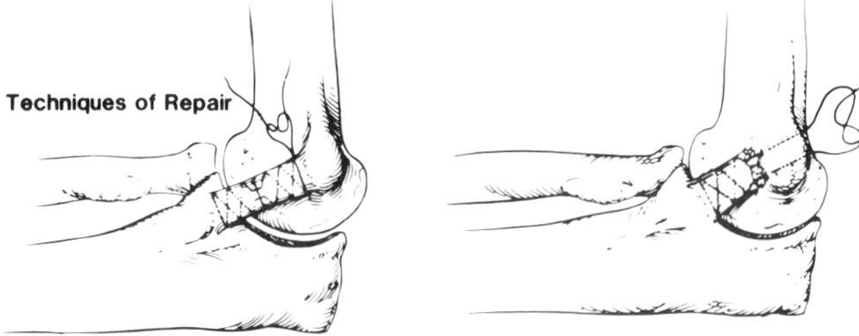

Figure 3: Techniques of repair and reattachment of medial collateral ligament. (Reprinted with permission from Factors influencing elbow instability, by H.S. Tullos, et al., AAOS Instructional Course Lectures XXX:196, St. Louis, C.V. Mosby, 1981.)

not intra-articular and should be treated as proximal third ulna fractures. Noncomminuted, nondisplaced fractures of the olecranon can be treated by immobilizing the patient in a posterior splint at 150 degrees of extension. Active motion is begun at 3 weeks after injury.

Elbow Dislocations Elbow dislocations always involve rupture, stretching, or avulsion of the ligamentous structures of the joint. In the unusual dislocation in which the radial head cannot be salvaged, an unstable condition may develop, and the use of a radial head prosthesis may be indicated (Fig. 2). Reconstruction of the anterior oblique ligament may be advisable if the lateral joint line is irreparably damaged because of an associated comminuted fracture of the capitellum. The use of intraoperative stress radiographs may help the surgeon select the proper procedure. When tested, the elbow should be flexed beyond 30 degrees to free the olecranon process from the constraint of the fossa. The most likely lesion of the anterior oblique ligament is avulsion from the medial epicondyle. End-to-end repair can be performed for a midportion tear (Fig. 3).

Elbow dislocations usually do well after a short period of immobilization (2 to 3 weeks) followed by active motion. Formal rehabilitation should stress active rather than assistive range of motion exercises to establish full range of motion to the joint. Stability is dependent upon an intact ligamentous structure, and, therefore, muscle strengthening exercise programs aimed at preventing further dislocation are not necessary.

Radial Head Fractures Many radial head fractures can be treated nonoperatively. Prognosis does not seem to be affected by the extent of depression, size of fragments, or degree of comminution. If radial head excision is to be done because of persistent pain or intra-articular bone impingement, at least one investigator has found poor results following a delay of more than 6 weeks before operation. The fact that distal radioulnar subluxation occurred did not appear to cause significant clinical symptoms. It now appears that Silastic radial head replacement in acute trauma of the elbow should be reserved for posterior dislocations combined with radial head (or capitellum) comminution. According to some the only indication for surgical treatment of an acute comminuted radial head fracture is a loose fragment in the joint. If there is one fragment and it is of adequate size, open reduction and internal fixation may be considered.

Rarely, a fracture of the radial head may be associated with a tear or complete avulsion of the triceps tendon. The clinical findings of diffuse swelling, tenderness, and ec-

Figure 4-A

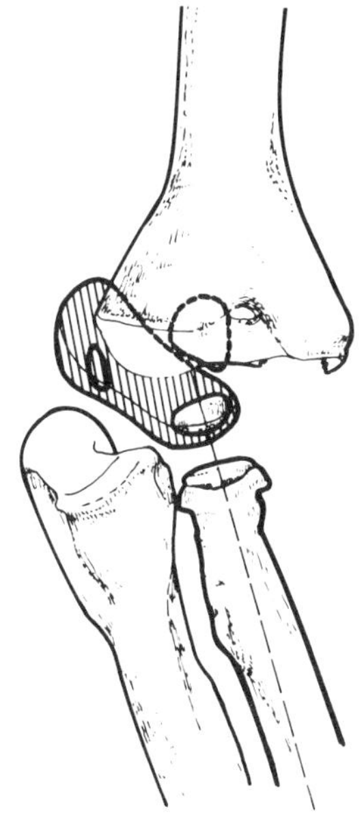

Figure 4-B

Figure 4: (A) Anteroposterior view of a type II Salter-Harris epiphyseal separation with medial displacement. It can easily be confused with a dislocated elbow. (B) Diagrammatic representation of the lesion. The ossified portion of the capitellum continues to articulate with the radius (a straight line drawn through the radius will transect the capitellum). The osseous metaphyseal segment lies posteriorly and is represented by stippled lines. It can be seen on the lateral view (Fig. 5A). The cartilaginous epiphysis is represented by the striped area. It does not appear on the radiograph since it has not yet calcified. The entire epiphysis has been displaced posteriorly and medially. (Reprinted with permission from Fracture separation of the lower humeral epiphysis with medial displacement, by S.S. Kaplan, et al., J. Bone Joint Surg. 53A:1105, 1971.)

chymosis along the posterior surface of the elbow, associated with a palpable gap in tendon continuity, confirm the diagnosis. The gap in the triceps tendon may be best demonstrated by asking the patient to extend the affected elbow against gravity. Care must be taken to check for this injury complex because fracture pain from the radial head may mask the clinical presentation of the ruptured tendon.

Children's Fractures

Supracondylar Fractures There is no unanimity of opinion regarding treatment of supracondylar fractures of the humerus. Many large series continue to show that closed reduction and plaster splint immobilization, incorporating collar and cuff, appear to be most efficacious. The use of Dunlap's traction results in an increased incidence of cubitus varus and increased cost of hospitalization. However, this type of treatment is still appropriate for patients with severe swelling, angulation, and late presentation (a few days). In those patients in whom adequate reduction cannot be maintained because of the increased swelling or intrinsic instability, percutaneous pinning appears to be the most appropriate method. Certainly, this is the preferred method when there are associated ipsilateral injuries of the shoulder and forearm. These fractures are true emergency situations. The quicker the reduction after injury, the more likely closed methods are to be successful. Furthermore, appropriate reduction techniques are important as remanipulation only causes further swelling and trauma to the intact periosteal sleeve. The use of interscalenus block or general anesthetic is necessary, and utilization of an image intensifier C-arm fluoroscopy unit aids in the reduction. Admission to the hospital for observation is indicated so that any neurovascular compromise may be detected early.

Closed reductions can be accomplished most easily if care is taken to secure the forearm in pronation when the medial condyle is reduced from its posterior position. The final position of pronation at the forearm should be secured with a plaster splint after the elbow is flexed to 90 degrees. This corrects the varus position and results in a more acceptable and secure reduction.

Open reduction is reserved for those patients with neurovascular compromise that does not resolve rapidly after reduction, severe displacement with suspected interposition of vessels, or unacceptable position.

Slight loss of the carrying angle or cubitus varus does not appear to cause functional disability but may result in a cosmetic deformity for which later osteotomy may be necessary.

Epiphyseal Separations at the Distal Humeral Epiphysis Epiphyseal separations of the lower humeral epiphysis with medial displacement (Figs. 4 and 5) may be confused with a dislocated elbow, a supracondylar fracture of the humerus, or a lateral condyle fracture (Fig. 6) in children less than 9 years of age. The importance of recognizing this fracture is that closed reduction is the treatment of choice. Open reduction has led to significant cubitus varus deformity and functional impairment usually due to inadequate reduction. Once closed reduction is accomplished, anatomic restoration is usually obtained and is stable. However, after reduction, two percutaneous Kirschner wires can be inserted from the lateral side for fixation. A posterior splint should be applied after the reduction, and the patient admitted to the hospital to allow neurovascular monitoring for 48 hours.

Medial Epicondylar Fractures Radiographic misinterpretation of the developing epiphysis of the medial epicondyle of the humerus may lead to improper diagnoses

Figure 5-A

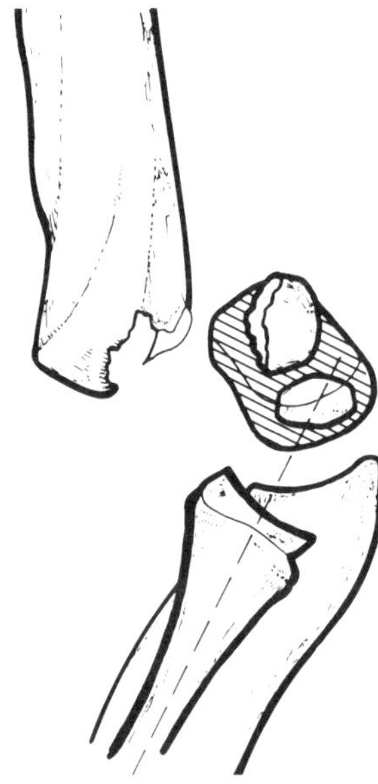

Figure 5-B

Figure 5: (A) Lateral view of a type II Salter-Harris epiphyseal separation of the distal end of the humerus. It can be easily confused with the supracondylar fracture of the elbow. Note that the fracture line appears to be running obliquely into the joint. (B) Diagrammatic representation of the lesion. Note that the entire cartilaginous epiphysis has been displaced posteriorly along with the ossified portion of the capitellum and portion of the metaphysis. (Reprinted with permission from Fracture separation of the lower humeral epiphysis with medial displacement, by S.S. Kaplan, et al., J. Bone Joint Surg. 53A:1106, 1971.)

and needless operative intervention. The medial epicondyle can confuse the surgeon in that it ossifies early and fuses late and is often involved in dislocations and avulsions of the elbow. As a general rule, operative intervention should be considered for medial epicondylar injuries when the fracture fragment is within the joint, dysfunction of the ulnar nerve is detected, or there is displacement of a large fragment to the joint level.

Medial Condylar Fractures Displaced fractures of the medial humeral condyle should be identified and treated by open reduction and internal fixation to avoid growth disturbance, articular incongruity, and functional disability. Because the trochlear epiphysis does not ossify before the age of 9 or 10 years, radiographic diagnosis of the fracture of the medial condyle is difficult to establish and may, in fact, be mistaken for avulsion of the medial epicondyle. Therefore, marked displacement of the medial epicondyle in a child whose trochlear epiphysis has not yet ossified often represents medial condyle displacement. Surgical intervention is justified. In an older child, displacement of the metaphyseal fragment is a reliable sign of an epiphyseal injury. This latter injury always is associated with a positive fat pad sign as it is intra-articu-

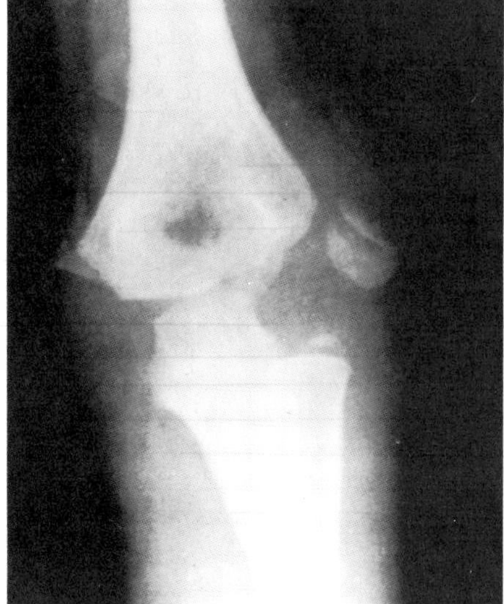

Figure 6-A

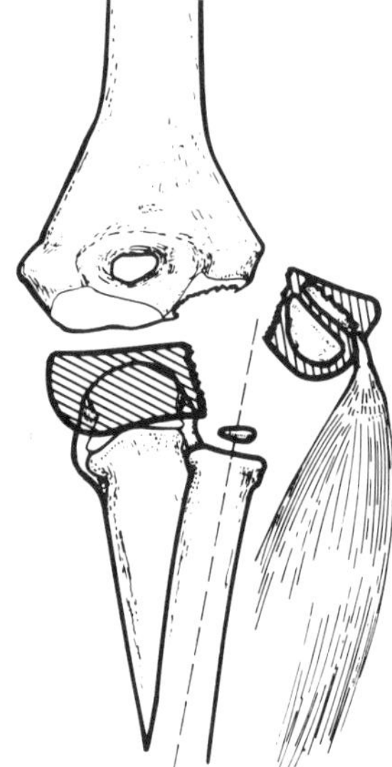

Figure 6-B

Figure 6: (A) Anteroposterior radiograph of a type IV Salter-Harris epiphyseal injury. Note that a straight line drawn through the radius does not transect the fractured condylar fragment. (B) Diagrammatic representation of the lesion. The fracture line is through the cartilaginous epiphysis into the joint. Note that the strong forearm extensor group of muscles distracts the fractured epicondylar fragment laterally and distally. (Reprinted with permission from Fracture separation of the lower humeral epiphysis with medial displacement, by S.S. Kaplan, et al., J. Bone Joint Surg. 53A:1107, 1971.)

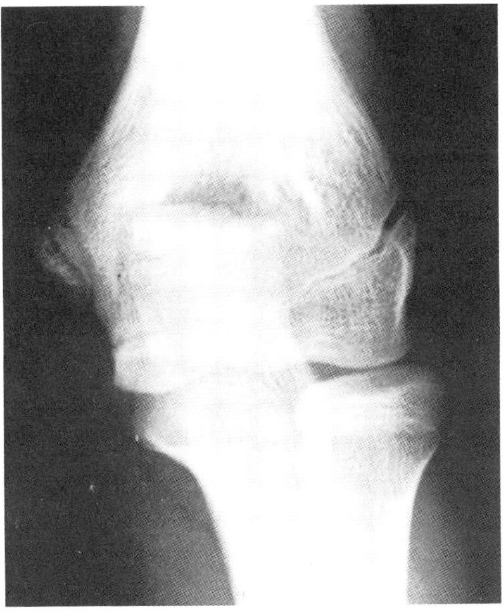

Figure 7: The distal part of the epiphysis of the lateral epicondyle usually fuses with the capitellum before the proximal part unites with the humerus. (Reprinted with permission from Some vagaries of the lateral epicondyle, by M.J. Silberstein, et al., J. Bone Joint Surg. 64A:445, 1982.)

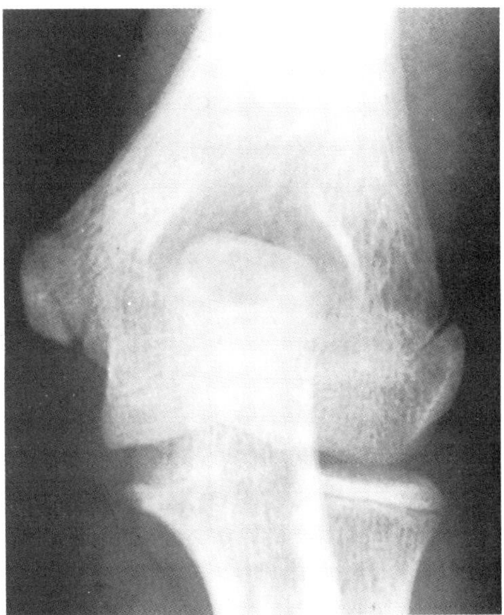

Figure 8: Once the distal part of the lateral epicondylar epiphysis has fused, the proximal part of the physis may closely resemble a fracture. The absence of elevated fat pads and associated soft-tissue swelling, in association with the faintly sclerotic margins of the physis should prevent misinterpretation. (Reprinted with permission from Some vagaries of the lateral epicondyle, by M.J. Silberstein, et al., J. Bone Joint Surg. 64A:445, 1982.)

lar, whereas a true epicondylar injury is extra-articular and not associated with a joint hemarthrosis. The use of two Kirschner wires to fix the medial condylar fracture is an effective way to prevent rotation of the fragment after reduction.

Lateral Epicondylar Fractures The lateral epicondyle also presents a diagnostic dilemma following trauma to the immature elbow. The distal part of the epiphysis fuses with the capitellum before the proximal part unites with the adjacent humerus. This frequently results in the physis appearing like a fracture (Figs. 7 and 8). Lack of a fat pad sign and associated soft-tissue swelling help prevent misinterpretation. A clinical exam should localize the tenderness directly to the epicondyle.

Olecranon Fractures Fractures of the olecranon in children are common. Nondisplaced fractures generally present no problem in treatment, but the diagnosis may be confusing, particularly when the physis of the olecranon extends distally into the joint, thus simulating a fracture (Fig. 9). This dilemma may be clarified by identifying the

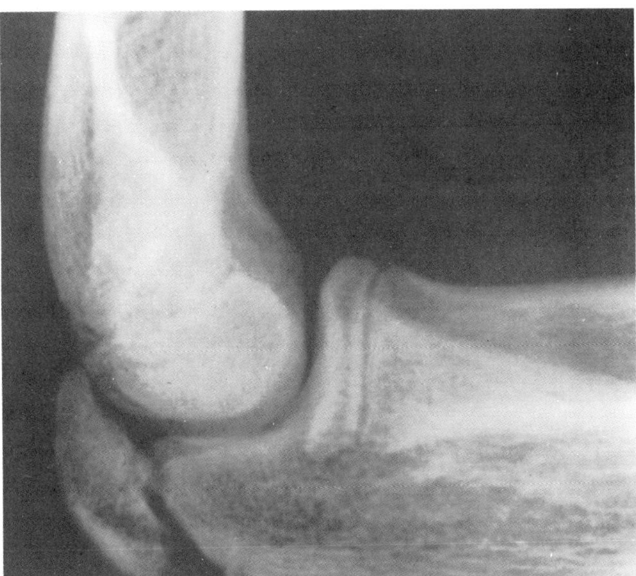

Figure 9: The olecranon physis has migrated distally and is entering the joint surface. Note its well-defined sclerotic margins, its wider posterior portion, and the absence of a positive fat pad sign. It should not be mistaken for a fracture line. (Reprinted with permission from Some vagaries of the olecranon, by M.J. Silberstein, et al., J. Bone Joint Surg. 63A:723, 1981.)

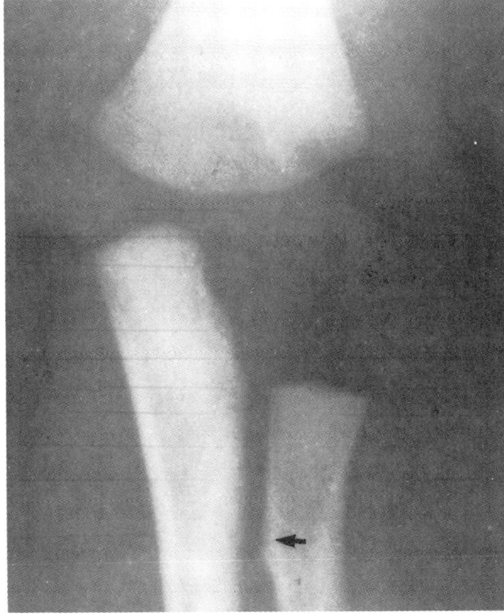

Figure 10: In an infant, the radial neck appears only slightly medially angulated on the anteroposterior radiograph. The radial tuberosity is small and just visible on the medial aspect of the proximal end of the radius at the point of maximum angulation (arrow). (Reprinted with permission from Some vagaries of the radial head and neck, by M.J. Silberstein, et al., J. Bone Joint Surg. 64A:1153, 1982.)

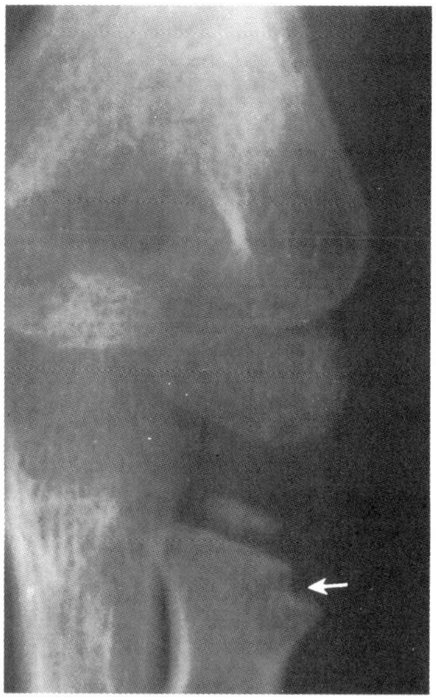

Figure 11: A notch may be found on the lateral aspect of the proximal radial metaphysis (arrow). This is a normal variant and not a compression fracture. (Reprinted with permission from Some vagaries of the radial head and neck, by M.J. Silberstein, et al., J. Bone Joint Surg. 64A:1154, 1982.)

sclerotic margins of the physis and noting that it is wider in its posterior portion. Additionally, the fat pad sign is negative. The clinical examination supports the suspicion of a normal physis on radiographs. In acute elbow fractures in children, return to normal function may take as long as 12 weeks, and passive motion should be avoided.

Radial Head and Neck Fractures The normal radiographic appearance of the radial head and neck may be misinterpreted as representing an injury. The radial neck in the infant is laterally displaced in the frontal plane and may mimic a dislocation of the radial head (Fig. 10). Also, the radial tuberosity is small, is barely visible on the medial aspect of the proximal end of the radius, and may mimic a fracture. Additionally, a notch may be found in older children on the lateral aspect of the proximal radial metaphysis. This is a variant of normal and not to be mistaken for a compression fracture (Fig. 11).

Fractures of the radial head and neck have the worst prognosis in older children. Best results are obtained if treatment is initiated early and if closed, rather than open, reduction is used. Significant impairment of pronation and supination after either closed or open reduction was observed in one series. Most authors have concluded that open reduction is required for only completely displaced fractures and for the occasional fracture that cannot be reduced to an acceptable angulatory position. The consensus is that acceptable angulation may be as high as 40 to 50 degrees. Internal fixation is not generally recommended.

Forearm

Adult Injuries

Radius and Ulna Fractures Most authors consider open reduction and internal fixation with compression plates the preferred treatment for fractures of both bones of the forearm. Early motion is important in the treatment regimen. Considerably less motion loss occurs when im-

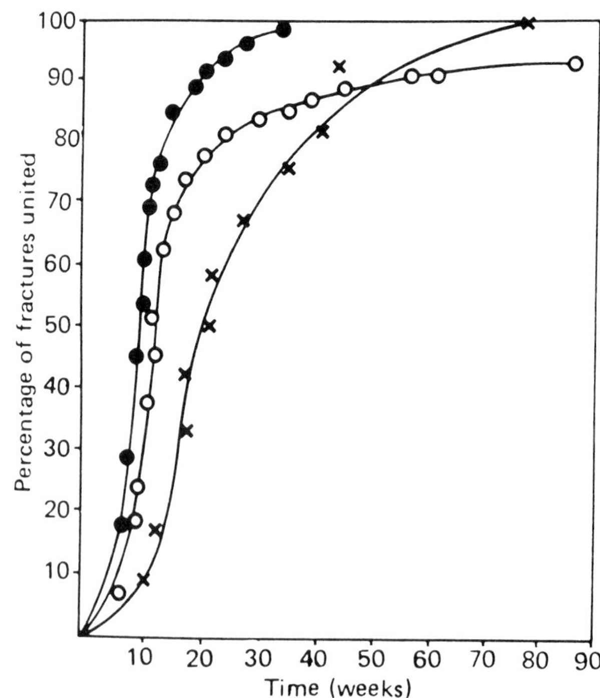

Figure 12: Cumulative percentage graph to show speed of union. Fractures in proximal third, X---X; fractures in middle third, 0---0; fractures in distal third, ●---●. (Reprinted with permission from The treatment of isolated fractures of the ulnar shaft in adults, by J.R. Corea, et al., Injury 12:367, 1980.)

mobilization is discontinued after the initial swelling has decreased, during the first 5 to 10 days postsurgery. On the other hand, early motion does not seem to significantly influence the results of single bone fractures as compared to cast immobilization. All series report increased loss of pronation and supination with open fractures. Additionally, care must be taken to correct completely any residual angulation. Experimental conditions have shown that midshaft fractures of the radius and ulna demonstrate loss in range of rotation when residual convergent angulation of 20 degrees or more exists. One series indicated that the frequency of union may be enhanced by delaying surgery for 1 to 3 weeks after fracture and by using primary bone grafting.

However, compression plating is not without complications. Implantation of plates and screws produces a temporary stress riser effect which appears again after removal. On the other hand, as long as a rigid plate remains in place, the bone will remain weak due to a stress shielding effect. Therefore, there appears to be a significant difference of opinion as to whether the plates should be removed. This requires a second operation, raises the possibility of sepsis, and produces a stress riser effect at the screw holes. There is general agreement that if the fixation is to be removed, it should not be removed for 18 to 24 months after implantation. Once removed, at least 6 weeks of limited activity is recommended.

Fractures of the Ulna Fractures of the middle and distal thirds of the ulna require internal fixation only if they are angulated greater than 15 degrees or are displaced more than one-quarter of the bone's diameter. These fractures may result in limitation of pronation and supination. In general, the use of a short cast or functional brace appears to be the treatment of choice for minimally angulated, minimally displaced ulna fractures (nightstick fracture). Union requires an average of 12.7 weeks (Fig. 12).

Monteggia and Galeazzi Fractures Most authors are in agreement that the Monteggia fracture in adults is best treated by open anatomical reduction and internal fixation of the ulna fracture and closed reduction of the radial head. Repair of the annular ligament is not necessary. In special instances, excision of the radial head, along with internal fixation of the ulna, gives good results in adults.

Operative intervention usually is indicated for isolated proximal third fractures of the ulna. If internal fixation is not used, instability of the radial head leading to a Monteggia's fracture-dislocation may result. Also, a disguised Monteggia's fracture-dislocation may occur in which a subluxated or dislocated radial head has reduced spontaneously.

The radial component of a Galeazzi fracture should be treated by open reduction and internal fixation. Cast immobilization in a long-arm cast with the forearm in supination is appropriate treatment for the distal radioulnar subluxation, although some might prefer percutaneous K-wire fixation.

Children's Forearm Fractures Studies are available indicating that malunited midshaft fractures of the radius and ulna in infants spontaneously correct with bone remodeling. However, limited rotation of the arm is noted in children with residual angular deformities of the proximal and mid-forearm of greater than 10 degrees. Under the age of 5 years, an angulation of 15 degrees is acceptable, provided the site of fracture is in the distal forearm. Between the ages of 6 and 10 years, remodeling is unlikely to correct deformity of 10 degrees or more. In children over the age of 10 years, angular deformity of greater than 20 degrees requires surgical intervention in the unlikely circumstance of failed closed reduction.

Refracture of the forearm in children occurs in about 13 percent of patients, generally following a greenstick fracture of one or both of the forearm bones. Duration of immobilization or residual axial deviation after healing appears to have no relationship to refracture. This suggests that mid-forearm greenstick fractures in children should be completed by manipulation during reduction to prevent refracturing.

Cyst-like cortical defects have been noted following greenstick fractures in children. These cysts are due to bony resorption within the excessive periosteal callus that occurs with healing of greenstick fractures. Cysts do not appear to cause refracture. They can be confused with fibrous cortical defects, eosinophilic granulomas, or interosseous ganglia.

Although experience with ipsilateral elbow and forearm injuries in children is small, several studies now indicate that open reduction and internal fixation of the supracondylar fracture and closed treatment of the forearm fracture give the best results.

General Problems Involving Elbow and Forearm

Compartment Syndromes The key to treating compartment syndromes involving the upper extremity is the clinical awareness that they can occur insidiously as well as rapidly. The results of an undiagnosed compartment syndrome can be devastating if treatment, in the form of fasciotomy, is not performed promptly. Unfortunately, the most frequent symptom is nonspecific pain. It is a mistake to wait for the development of paralysis as full function rarely returns after true paralysis has occurred. The most sensitive diagnostic test appears to be pain with passive motion of the fingers associated with reduced hand sensibility or paresthesias and loss of two-point discrimination. Once this occurs, fasciotomy must be done immediately.

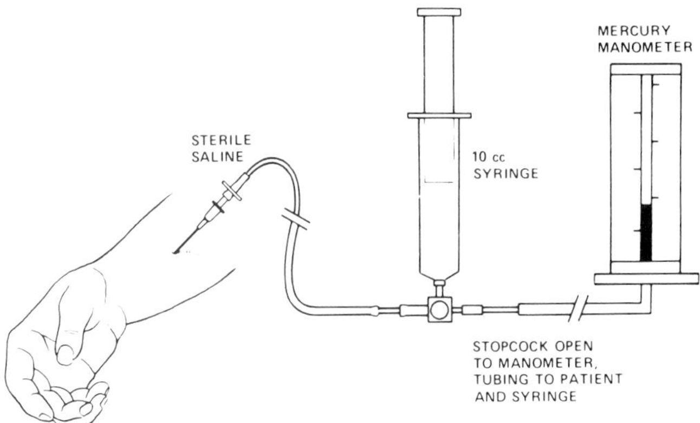

Figure 13: Diagram of the apparatus for measuring compartment pressure using equipment available on any hospital ward: standard intravenous tubing, an 18-gauge needle, a 10-cc syringe, a three-way stopcock, and a mercury manometer. (Reprinted with permission from Compartment syndromes of the forearm: Early recognition using tissue pressure measurements, by A.A. Halpern, et al., J. Hand Surg. 4:263, 1979.)

Measurement of intracompartmental pressures is helpful in documenting the diagnosis. Some investigators use the Wick catheter technique, but this may not be easily or readily available. An easier technique for pressure measurement utilizing equipment available on many hospital wards has been described and is illustrated (Fig. 13). The only error commonly encountered using this simple setup is that a stopcock must be used which connects all three portals simultaneously. The standard metal nondisposable three-way stopcock, available at some hospitals, is not sufficient. Most disposable stopcock systems allow for simultaneous connection so that the intracompartmental pressure can be transmitted to both plunger and manometer simultaneously. Most authors advise careful monitoring if initial pressures exceed 30 mm of mercury in the upper extremity.

When pressures exceed 40 mm of mercury and are accompanied by any neurovascular compromise, fasciotomy is advised. Fasciotomy should be done as an emergency procedure (Fig. 14 shows the incisions). The volar incision should be performed initially and pressures remeasured in the dorsal compartment. Occasionally, both compartments require decompression. It is important to decompress routinely the carpal tunnel at the wrist and the lacertus fibrosus at the elbow. Care must be taken to check the proximal edge of both the pronator teres and the flexor digitorum superficialis.

None of the investigators believe there is a direct correlation between the magnitude of the pressure elevations and the results from forearm decompression. Pressure determinations are most helpful in evaluating the comatose patient and patients with equivocal physical findings. Prompt action is the key to avoiding significant permanent functional damage.

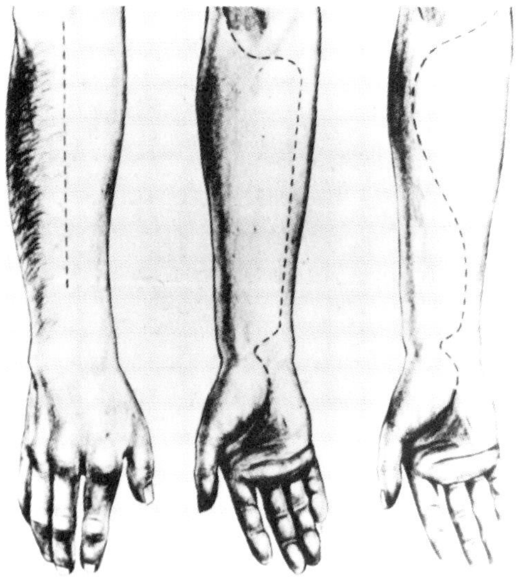

Dorsal Volar—Ulnar Volar

Figure 14: Dorsal and volar forearm incisions. (Adapted with permission from Compartment syndromes of the forearm: Diagnosis and treatment, by R.H. Gelberman, et al., Clin. Orthop. 161:259, 1981.)

Periarticular Heterotopic Ossification The elbow is the most common site of periarticular heterotopic ossification following head injury in an adult. The posterior aspect appears to be more commonly involved than the anterior. The elbow joints involved were not initially injured in the direct trauma, and spasticity was not always present in the involved joint. Resection of mature heterotopic bone generally restores satisfactory motion of the elbow.

Plaster Burns in the Upper Extremity When treating fractures of the elbow and forearm, plaster splints commonly are used because circumferential plaster dressings may cause neurovascular compromise. Studies now indicate that occasional burns from plaster splints can occur. These burns are more common in upper extremities. Recommendations for preventing plaster burns include avoiding water temperature higher than 24 degrees centigrade, limiting plaster splint thickness to eight plies or less, and allowing heat to dissipate by using proper ventilation. However, if a patient complains of severe burning sensation after application of a plaster splint dressing, the splint should be removed immediately to prevent second or third degree burns.

ANNOTATED BIBLIOGRAPHY

Elbow

Anatomy

Schwab, G.H.; Bennett, J.B.; Woods, G.W.; and Tullos, H.S.: Biomechanics of elbow instability: The role of the medial collateral ligament. Clin. Orthop. 146:42-52, 1980.

This article outlines the anatomy of the elbow ligaments and their clinical significance in relation to elbow fractures and/or dislocations. The role of the anterior oblique portion of the medial collateral ligament is stressed.

Adult Fractures

Supracondylar Fractures

Horne, G.: Supracondylar fractures of the humerus in adults. J. Trauma 20:71-74, 1980.

The article concludes that nonoperative rather than surgical management is indicated for all adult supracondylar fractures except the most simple types.

Riseborough, E.J., and Radin, E.L.: Intercondylar T fractures of the humerus in the adult: A comparison of operative and nonoperative treatment in 29 cases. J. Bone Joint Surg. 51A:130-141, 1969.

These fractures were classified into four types: I, no displacement; II, trochlear and capitellar fragments separated but not appreciably rotated; III, fragments separated and rotated; and IV, severe comminution of the articular surface and wide separation of the humeral condyles.

Thompson, D.M.: T-Shaped fractures of the elbow in adults. J. Bone Joint Surg. 64B:142, 1982. (Abstract)

This paper concludes that all complex adult elbow fractures, except those with significant rotatory deformity, should be treated nonsurgically. In the elderly, it is recommended that the nonsurgical approach be used even if rotatory components are present.

Wadsworth, T.G.: Adult trauma *In* The Elbow, pp. 210-216. New York, Churchill Livingstone, 1982.

The chapter dealing with supracondylar fractures in adults concludes that operative intervention is technically difficult and, in general, undesirable. Discussion is given to various forms of internal fixation.

Olecranon Fractures

Gartsman, G.M.; Sculco, T.P.; and Otis, J.C.: Operative treatment of olecranon fractures. J. Bone Joint Surg. 63A:718-721, 1981.

A comparison is made between excision of the olecranon and internal fixation. The study supports the rationale for excision of fragments of the olecranon with repair of the triceps tendon as the preferred method of treatment for fracture of the olecranon.

Elbow Dislocations

Hanson, C.T.; Jaslow, B.; Danoff, J.V.; and Alon, G.: Electromyographic response of elbow flexors to a changing, dislocating force. Arch. Phys. Med. Rehab. 62:631-634, 1981.

EMG studies were monitored during application of externally generated dislocating forces across the elbow joint. The article concludes that the practice of strengthening muscles as a means of protecting joint integrity did little to resist elbow joint dislocation with loads up to 18 newtons.

Radial Head Fractures

Farrar, E.L., III, and Lippert, F.G., III: Avulsion of the triceps tendon. Clin. Orthop. 161:242-246, 1981.

The article summarizes the clinical findings of the triceps tendon avulsion following deceleration stress to the upper extremity and its relation to radial head fractures. The importance of differentiating complete and partial tears while examining the active range of motion is stressed.

Levy, M.; Goldberg, I.; and Meir, I.: Fracture of the head of the radius with a tear or avulsion of the triceps tendon.: A new syndrome? J. Bone Joint Surg. 64B:70-72, 1982.

The article points out that this combination of injuries is a new, but rare, syndrome. Clinical awareness is important to its discovery.

Mackay, I.; Fitzgerald, B.; and Miller, J.H.: Silastic replacement of the head of the radius in trauma. J. Bone Joint Surg. 61B:494-497, 1979.

The article confirms that prosthetic replacement of the radial head is particularly effective after posterior dislocation of the elbow.

Miller, G.K.; Drennan, D.B.; and Maylahn, D.J.: Treatment of displaced segmental radial-head fractures. J. Bone Joint Surg. 63A:712-717, 1981.

This article reports a long-term follow-up on radial head fractures. Good results were achieved in most patients by nonoperative treatment. The only indication for surgery in the segmental radial head fracture was a loose fragment in the joint.

Morrey, B.V.; Askew, L.; and Chao, E.Y.: Silastic prosthetic replacement for the radial head. J. Bone Joint Surg. 63A:454-458, 1981.

The article reviews radial head prostheses inserted following acute fractures. Conclusions indicate that this type of prosthesis should not be used routinely.

Stephen, I.B.: Excision of the radial head for closed fracture. Acta Orthop. Scand. 52:409-412, 1981.

The article concludes that excision of the radial head for closed fractures does not appear to give rise to significant clinical disability and that radial head prosthetic replacement does not offer sufficient advantages to warrant its general use.

Children's Fractures

Supracondylar Fractures

Buhl, O., and Hellberg, S.: Displaced supracondylar fractures of the humerus in children. Acta Orthop. Scand. 53:67-71, 1982.

A large group of patients were reviewed. A discussion of results after closed reduction and plaster dressing technique versus percutaneous K-wire pinning and plaster is presented. Those treated with percutaneous K-wire pinning included the most severe fractures. Nevertheless, results equal those obtained by closed methods.

Dameron, T.B., Jr.: Transverse fractures of distal humerus in children. *In* AAOS Instructional Course Lectures. XXX:224-235. St. Louis, C.V. Mosby, 1981.

This instructional course lecture discusses the anatomy of the transverse fracture of the distal humerus in children. A discussion of management and complications resulting from this fracture is presented. The significance of pronation and supination is diagramatically explained.

Prietto, C.A.: Supracondylar fractures of the humerus. J. Bone Joint Surg. 61A:425-428, 1979.

The article compares results of treatment of supracondylar fractures using Dunlap's traction and those using percutaneous pinning. Range of motion in those treated with pin fixation was slightly better, and hospital costs were significantly less. Dunlap's traction was associated with an increased incidence of gunstock deformity.

Epiphyseal Separations at the Distal Humeral Epiphysis

Ariño, V.L.; Lluch, E.E.; Ramirez, A.M.; Ferrer, J.; Rodriguez, L.; and Baixauli, F.: Percutaneous fixation of supracondylar fractures of the humerus in children. J. Bone Joint Surg. 59A:914-916, 1977.

This article describes percutaneous fixation of supracondylar fractures of the humerus in children using two percutaneous Kirschner wires from the lateral aspect of the elbow. The article indicates that parallel or crossed Kirschner wires are acceptable fixation.

DeLee, J.C.; Wilkins, K.E.; Rogers, L.F.; and Rockwood, C.A.: Fracture separation of the distal humeral epiphysis. J. Bone Joint Surg. 62A:46-51, 1980.

A description of fracture separations of the distal humeral epiphysis is given. Displacement was posteromedially. Postinjury cubitus varus, which developed in three patients, was believed to be due to inadequate reduction and did not progress clinically.

Peiro, A.; Mut, T.; Aracil, J.; and Martos, F.: Fracture-separation of the lower humeral epiphysis in young children. Acta Orthop. Scand. 52:295-298, 1981.

A description of the Salter-Harris classification and its application to the radiographic diagnosis of the fracture is made. Good results were obtained with closed treatment if the lesion was correctly diagnosed.

Medial Epicondylar Fractures

Kiss, A., and Vincze, J.: Fractures of the medial humeral epicondyle in children. Magy Traumatol. Orthop. Helyreallito Sebesz 24:1-7, 1981.

A summary of an experience with medial epicondylar fractures is reported. Good results were obtained with closed reduction. Only three clinical events were considered to warrant surgical intervention.

Silberstein, M.J.; Brodeur, A.E.; Graviss, E.R.; and Luisiri, A.: Some vagaries of the medial epicondyle. J. Bone Joint Surg. 63A:524-528, 1981.

The normal radiographic appearance of the medial epicondyle in children is presented with clear pictures differentiating normal variations from trauma.

Medial Condylar Fractures

Fowles, J.V., and Kassab, M.T.: Displaced fractures of the medial humeral condyle in children. J. Bone Joint Surg. 62A:1159-1163, 1980.

This article emphasizes that early diagnosis and accurate reduction with internal fixation is important to avoid growth disturbances and functional disability.

Lateral Epicondylar Fractures

Silberstein, M.J.; Brodeur, A.E.; and Graviss, E.R.: Some vagaries of the lateral epicondyle. J. Bone Joint Surg. 64A:444-448, 1982.

Aids are given to assist in distinguishing between the radiographic appearance of normal ossification centers and fractures of the lateral epicondyle.

Olecranon Fractures

Matthews, J.G.: Fractures of the olecranon in children. Injury 12:207-212, 1980.

The article presents a series of children followed at least 3 years. Most fractured olecranons were associated with other injuries which complicated recovery. Treatment and complications are thoroughly discussed.

Silberstein, M.J.; Brodeur, A.E.; Graviss, E.R.; and Luisiri, A.: Some vagaries of the olecranon. J. Bone Joint Surg. 63A:722-725, 1981.

Misinterpretations of normal radiographic characteristics of a maturing olecranon are discussed. Features distinguishing a normal olecranon from fracture are illustrated.

Radial Head and Neck Fractures

Silberstein, M.J.; Brodeur, A.E.; and Graviss, E.R.: Some vagaries of the radial head and neck. J. Bone Joint Surg. 64A:1153-1157, 1982.

This article points out how the normal developing radial head and neck may be prone to misinterpretation following trauma. First, the radial neck of the infant is slightly medially angulated in the frontal projection, mimicking a dislocated radial head. Second, the early proximal radial epiphysis is wedge-shaped simulating an avulsion fracture of the radial head. Third, notches and clefts of the proximal metaphysis may resemble posttraumatic appearances. All these are actually normal variants in the infant and young child.

Tibone, J.E., and Stoltz, M.: Fractures of the radial head and neck in children. J. Bone Joint Surg. 63A:100-106, 1981.

Fractures of the proximal radial epiphysis had a worse prognosis in older children. Associated medial injuries were noted. Closed reduction gave satisfactory results.

Forearm

Adult Injuries

Radius and Ulna Fractures

Grace, T.G., and Eversmann, W.W.: Forearm fractures. J. Bone Joint Surg. 62A:433-438, 1980.

Patients with open fractures or with fractures of both bones of the forearm lost significantly more rotation of the forearm. A program of early active motion without immobilization increased range of motion of the forearm in patients with fractures of both bones of the forearm.

Matthews, L.S.; Kaufer, H.; Garver, D.F.; and Sonstegard, D.A.: The effect on supination-pronation of angular malalignment of fractures of both bones of the forearm. J. Bone Joint Surg. 64A:14-17, 1982.

The effects of residual angulation from simulated fractures of both bones of the forearm on the potential for range of rotation of the forearm and limitation of pronation and supination were studied. The study indicated loss in range of motion can be expected with residual angles of 20 degrees or more.

Teipner, W.A., and Mast, J.W.: Internal fixation of forearm diaphyseal fractures: Double plating versus single compression (tension band) plating—a comparative study. Orthop. Clin. North America 11:381-391, 1980.

Complications after removal of orthopaedic devices are presented. The article concludes that double- and single-compression plating ensure a high rate of union and an excellent functional result. The authors believe that internal fixation should not be removed as a routine procedure.

Fractures of the Ulna

Corea, J.R.; Brakenbury, P.H.; and Blakemore, M.E.: The treatment of isolated fractures of the ulnar shaft in adults. Injury 12:365-370, 1980.

Proximal third fractures of the ulnar shaft should be internally fixed, and fractures at the mid-third of the shaft, particularly near the junction with the distal third, are at risk of nonunion. Fractures that are displaced by more than one-quarter of the bone's diameter or angulated 15 degrees or more should be fixed. Most isolated fractures of the ulnar shaft, however, can be adequately treated by closed means.

Monteggia and Galeazzi Fractures

Reckling, F.W.: Unstable fracture-dislocations of the forearm (Monteggia and Galeazzi lesions). J. Bone Joint Surg. 64A:857-863, 1982.

This article discusses in detail the classification of the Monteggia fracture-dislocation. Additionally, the Galeazzi fracture is discussed with the recommendation that open reduction of the radius be performed. Contrary to Mikic's recommendation, this series showed that long-arm cast immobilization in full supination appears to give good results for the distal radioulnar subluxation component of the Galeazzi lesion.

Children's Forearm Fractures

Bhuller, G.S., and Hardy, A.E.: Ipsilateral elbow and forearm injuries in children. Australian New Zealand J. Surg. 51:65-68, 1981.

Serious complications following ipsilateral elbow and forearm injuries were low. Open reduction and internal fixation of the supracondylar fracture with closed treatment of the forearm gave the best results.

Daruwalla, J.S.: A study of radioulnar movements following fractures of the forearm in children. Clin. Orthop. 139:114-120, 1979.

The largest number of fractures occurred in the 6- to 10-year age group. Fractures united within 8 weeks. Angulatory deformity of more than 10 degrees in children above the age of 10 years failed to remodel adequately, particularly in the fractures in the proximal-half of the forearm.

Fuller, D.J., and McCullough, C.J.: Malunited fractures of the forearm in children. J. Bone Joint Surg. 64B:364-367, 1982.

The article concludes that malunion of the distal third of the radius and ulna will remodel satisfactorily provided the child is less than 14 years of age. However, gross malunion of the midshaft and ulna will spontaneously correct only in infancy. Little correction of deformity can be anticipated in diaphyseal fractures in children over the age of 8 years.

Gruber, R., and von Laer, L.R.: The etiology of refracture of the forearm in childhood. Akt. Traumatol. 9:251-259, 1979.

A large number of children who sustained a refracture of the forearm were studied. The incidence of refracture was 13 percent when the primary fracture was an incompletely broken greenstick fracture. Duration of immobilization and residual deviation had no relationship to refracture. The author recommends that greenstick fractures in the forearm be completed.

Pfister-Goedeke, L., and Braune, M.: Cyst-like defects following fractures in children. Pediat. Radiol. 11:83-86, 1981.

Cyst-like cortical defects appearing a few weeks after greenstick fractures in the undamaged part of the radius were noted in some children. Some of the lesions disappeared within 1 to 3 years postfracture. The authors believe that these are benign lesions and represent resorption cysts within the excessive periosteal reaction related to the subperiosteal hematoma accompanying these fractures.

General Problems Involving Elbow and Forearm

Compartment Syndromes

Gelberman, R.H.; Garfin, S.R.; Hergenroeder, P.T.; Mubarak, S.J.; and Menon, J.: Compartment syndromes of the forearm: Diagnosis and treatment. Clin. Orthop. 161:252-261, 1981.

The article describes incisions for release of forearm compartmental syndromes and stresses the physical findings related to compartment syndrome.

Halpern, A.A., and Nagel, D.A.: Compartment syndromes of the forearm: Early recognition using tissue pressure measurements. J. Hand Surg. 4:258-263, 1979.

The article describes Whitesides' method of measuring tissue pressures. The authors suggest that fasciotomy be performed when tissue pressures exceed 40 mm of mercury and are accompanied by neurovascular compromise.

Periarticular Heterotopic Ossification

Garland, D.E.; Blum, C.E.; and Waters, R.L.: Periarticular heterotopic ossification in head-injured adults. J. Bone Joint Surg. 62A:1143-1146, 1980.

The article indicates that heterotopic bone developed in head-injured patients at joints not involved in trauma. Sixteen percent of all joints underwent ankylosis, with the elbow being most frequently involved. Surgical excision of this heterotopic bone about the elbow led to satisfactory results.

Plaster Burns in the Upper Extremity

Kaplan, S.S.: Burns following application of plaster splint dressings. J. Bone Joint Surg. 63A:670-672, 1981.

This article stresses the fact that second and third degree burns occur more commonly after plaster splint application in the upper extremity. The cause is unknown and, fortunately, the occurrence is rare. The phenomenon is time-related. Removal of plaster splint dressings when the patient complains of serious burning pain will prevent the development of this complication.

Lavalette, R.; Pope, M.; and Dickstein, H.: Setting temperatures of plaster casts: The influence of technical variables. J. Bone Joint Surg. 64A:907-911, 1982.

The article points out that plaster casts can cause second and third degree burns if dip water temperature is greater than 24 degrees centigrade or if the thickness of the cast is greater than eight-ply. Burns occur when dissipation of heat from the cast is limited by pillows or wrapping.

19 ELBOW AND FOREARM: RECONSTRUCTION

Subjects covered in this section include elbow synovectomy and total replacement arthroplasty, radius and ulnar reconstruction with vascularized transfers, nerve compression syndromes, and tennis elbow.

Elbow Joint

Arthroscopy in a Gas Medium Arthroscopy, using saline and then carbon dioxide to inflate the joint, has demonstrated advantages. Small details are more visible with gas arthroscopy because liquid tends to disperse light more evenly, thus muting the contours. In a gas medium, a small elevation of cartilage leads to a shadow on the far side, therefore heightening the visual contrast. The procedure is particularly useful for small joints where synovial folds may float free in a liquid medium and obscure pathological details.

Surgical Approach to Anterior and Posterior Elbow Compartments Portions of the joint may be visualized by several different approaches. Recently a single radiodorsal approach has been described that allows excellent visualization of the ventral and dorsal portions simultaneously without detaching collateral ligaments or resecting the radial head. This approach is useful for synovectomy in the treatment of rheumatoid arthritis as well as joint debridement for osteoarthritis or osteochondromatosis. An extensive detachment of joint capsule for restoration of motion is possible.

There are several anatomical considerations affecting this new radiodorsal approach. Most synovial tissue is located anteriorly in a single space which is easily visible in flexion. On the ulnar side of the joint, the synovial space is reduced because of a dense ligament system covering the bone on all sides. On the radial side, the most important portion of the ligament system is the radioventrally located common extensor origin. Thus, surgical exposure includes detachment of the extensor carpi radialis brevis origin and penetration on the front of the elbow joint with the elbow relaxed and detachment of the anconeus with penetration on the dorsal margin of the extensor carpi ulnaris with the elbow extended to expose the posterior regions.

Osteochondritis Dissecans Osteochondritis dissecans of the elbow often is related to forceful or repetitive physical activity. Some patients have bilateral lesions in the capitellum, and a few have an additional focus on the articular surface of the ulna. A defect in the capitellum commonly is associated with loose bodies in the anterior joint or in the coronoid fossa. Some patients show early osteoarthritic changes. Patients complain of local pain, tenderness, locking, and loss of motion. All routine laboratory examinations are normal. If temporary immobilization and restriction of activities fail to relieve symptoms, loose bodies and fragments may be excised. At follow-up, many patients have some pain and tenderness, and only about one-half have normal joint motion. Radiologically some remodeling with gradual filling in of the defect generally occurs. Osteoarthritic changes and formation of new loose bodies are frequent, and a cubitus valgus deformity may develop due to growth disturbances. Although osteochondritis dissecans of the elbow and Panner's disease (osteochondrosis) may have similar clinical presentation, there is no osteochondral fracture fragment in the latter, and the disease generally is treated effectively by nonoperative measures. Nonsurgical treatment for osteochondritis dissecans is recommended, but surgery may be necessary if symptoms are caused by loose bodies.

Elbow Synovectomy Elbow synovectomy done for rheumatoid arthritis tends to improve range of motion. Patients generally have good or excellent relief of pain, and results are comparable with or without radial head excision. Preservation of the radial head probably improves elbow stability and precludes additional stress on the elbow medial collateral ligament and the distal radioulnar joint. Pain relief and preservation of existing motion are about the same whether the radial head is excised or replaced with a Silastic prosthesis. The Silastic radial head prosthesis probably confers additional stability to the elbow in advanced cases.

The indication for elbow synovectomy in hemophilia is continual or recurrent bleeding that is uncontrolled by medical management and causes major disability. Patients experience fewer hemarthroses postoperatively. This marked improvement is apparent in the immediate postoperative year and is maintained subsequently. Postoperatively bleeding may occur in some patients despite adequate hemostatic levels of factor VIII. Some patients lose motion postoperatively whereas others gain. Results for elbow synovectomy are significantly better than for similarly treated knees.

Excisional Arthroplasty of Elbow Excisional arthroplasty has been performed with some frequency. Various interpositional substances (including fascia lata, fat, muscle, dermis, acrylic, nylon, and homographs) have been used. Recently, excisional arthroplasty with interposition of Gelfoam has been reported for treatment of posttraumatic ankylosis, rheumatoid arthritis, osteoarthritis, and septic arthritis. Pain relief is good, and the average flexion-extension arc achieved is 80 degrees. However, lateral instability of from 10 to 40 degrees of varus-valgus motion can be expected. This instability is minimized by muscle contraction during functional activity and uncommonly prevents patients from returning to their previous employment. Best results are in young adults with recent ankylosis due to trauma. Patients with rheumatoid arthritis have difficulties because of muscle weakness and tendency for bone resorption.

Treatment of Chronic Elbow Instability Although rare, chronic dislocation or subluxation of the elbow causes persistent disability. Tendon transfer, anterior bone block, capsular and ligamentous reinforcements have been described but provide only limited success. An improved treatment includes reattachment of the brachialis and anterior elbow capsule to the coronoid with pull-through sutures in the ulna. Gentle motion is begun 2 weeks later. Patients generally regain useful range of motion. Forearm rotation is full and elbow stability is restored.

Elbow Arthrodesis Elbow arthrodesis is difficult to achieve, and reported failure rates with existing techniques have averaged 50 percent. Recently a new procedure has been reported. Patients with tuberculous arthritis of the elbow with a draining sinus received triple antibiotic therapy immediately preoperatively and for 3 months postoperatively. Highlights of the procedure are illustrated in Figure 1.

Transient nerve palsy may occur. There is minimal shortening of the limb, and the postoperative appearance is cosmetically acceptable. In addition to the high success rate, advantages of this procedure are that it requires no exogenous bone and that a complete joint debridement and synovectomy can be performed.

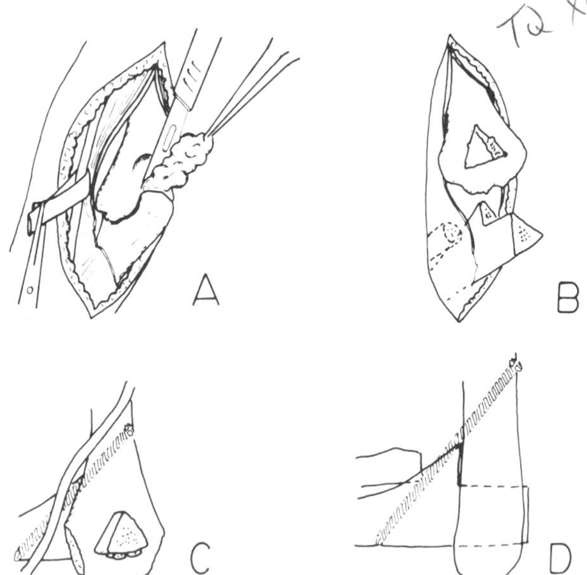

Figure 1: A new operative technique for elbow arthrodesis. (A) Isolation of the ulnar nerve, splitting, and release of the triceps tendon from the olecranon and posterior synovectomy. (B) Excision of the radial head and anterior synovectomy; shaping the olecranon and creation of the triangular hole through the distal end of the humerus. (C) Insertion of the olecranon through the hole in the distal end of the humerus, screw fixation, medial and lateral epicondylectomy, and anterior transposition of the ulnar nerve. The resulting bone chips are used to fill any gaps around the stump of the olecranon. (D) Lateral view of the completed fusion showing the fixation screw in place. (Reprinted with permission from A new technique of fusion for tuberculous arthritis of the elbow, by R.P. Arafiles, et al., J. Bone Joint Surg. 63A:1397, 1981.)

Total Elbow Replacement

DESIGN CONSIDERATION: Most activities of daily living are performed in a position of slight forearm pronation. These activities can be accomplished with 100 degrees of elbow flexion (from 30 to 130 degrees) and 100 degrees of forearm rotation (50 degrees each of pronation and supination). These minimum ranges should be sought following elbow reconstruction.

In the past, technical limitations produced conflicting results concerning elbow kinematics. Using different techniques, several groups now have shown that elbow motion occurs about a single axis which passes through the bottom of the trochlear sulcus and across the periphery of the capitellum. Joint surface motion is of a sliding type except at the extremes of flexion and extension where a rolling motion occurs. The carrying angle of the forearm remains constant throughout elbow flexion and extension. These results suggest a total elbow prosthesis should also be uniaxial with the axis of motion identical to that of the normal joint.

The shortcomings associated with the semiconstrained, hinged prosthesis are well known. Forces are transmitted across the hinge which produce tensile forces at the bone-cement interface. Rotatory forces are also transmitted, and certain designs have experienced axle failures. Conversely, the nonconstrained or resurfacing prostheses are less subject to loosening and breakage; however, they are less stable and can only be successfully implanted when adequate bone stock and good ligaments are present. In one experimental design, magnetic force holds the components together and maintains some constraint during motion. Stability is greater than nonhinged devices. Since the magnetic force is elastic, shocks or overloads are not transmitted directly to the bone-cement interface because of the temporary displacement of the component. The magnetic force thereafter acts to restore the initial configuration.

TECHNIQUES AND RESULTS: Even though experience with total elbow arthroplasty still lags behind the more commonly performed hip and knee procedures, several large series of elbow replacements with 3-year follow-ups are now available for study.

A new report has been published of sixty-nine nonconstrained capitellocondylar metal-to-plastic total elbow replacements for rheumatoid arthritis with an average follow-up of 3½ years. The metal humeral component and the polyethylene ulnar component required minimal bone removal (Fig. 2). Postoperatively, pain relief was good, flexion and pronation were improved, but there were no significant changes in extension or supination. Eighty-seven percent of patients had good or excellent results. Loosening, either clinically or radiographically, was uncommon. Complications occurred often, but only one patient had an absolute failure of treatment. The major problems were recurrent dislocations and ulnar nerve palsies, some of which were permanent. A modification of stem design allowed for an increased carrying angle. This modified stem, used in patients who have an increased

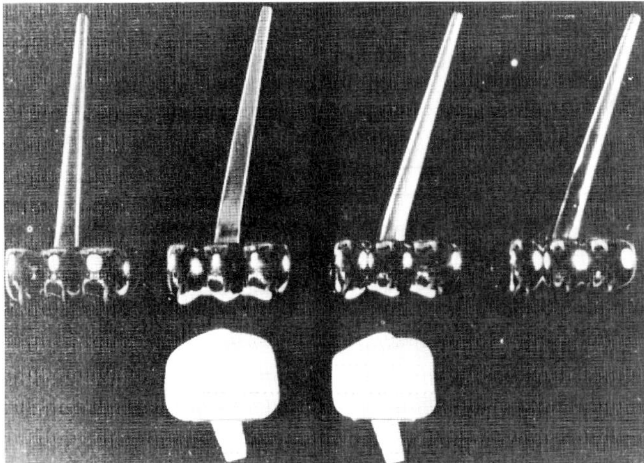

Figure 2: The metal-to-plastic capitellocondylar total elbow prosthesis. The metal humeral components have medullary fixation stems in 5, 10, 15, and 20 degrees of valgus angulation. The polyethylene ulnar component has two thicknesses. (Reprinted with permission from Capitellocondylar total elbow arthroplasty, by F.C. Ewald, et al., J. Bone Joint Surg. 62A:1260, 1980.)

carrying angle preoperatively, improved the ligamentous support, and problems of instability and dislocation were reduced. Several patients with ulnar nerve palsies subsequently were discovered to have an underlying peripheral neuropathy on the opposite side. A change of surgical exposure from a triceps-dividing approach to a lateral exposure with subperiosteal dissection of the common extensor origin eliminated further ulnar nerve complications. Fractures, wound infections, and delayed skin healing were other complications encountered.

Another report discussed thirty-six total elbow replacements done with either the semiconstrained Pritchard-Walker or the semiconstrained triaxial prosthesis, followed for an average of 3.7 years (Fig. 3). One-fourth of the patients had posttraumatic arthritis, and the remainder had rheumatoid arthritis. Those with rheumatoid arthritis improved markedly in all areas of clinical assessment with gain of motion measuring 60 degrees and concomitant gain in strength and function. Patients with juvenile rheumatoid arthritis gained somewhat less motion, and the posttraumatic group gained the least. There was an overall complication rate of 53 percent. Complications included postoperative wound hematoma, humerus fracture, symptomatic excess cement, deep wound infection, prosthesis failure, prosthetic loosening, ulnar palsy, triceps muscle rupture, and minor skin sloughs. Only five of the complications adversely affected the final results. Some believe that the less constrained triaxial designs lead to less loosening. Since this prosthesis was used late in the series, the follow-up is presently insufficient to prove this point. The best candidates for total elbow replacement appear to be patients with painful and disabling rheumatoid arthritis with significant radiographic changes.

Other studies of total elbow arthroplasty either with nonconstrained or semiconstrained prostheses parallel these results. Basically there appears to be less loosening with the nonconstrained prosthesis. Joint stability depends upon the integrity of the patient's connective tissue and preservation of adequate bone stock to support the resurfacing. Conversely, there are higher rates of loosening with the semiconstrained and constrained prostheses. However,

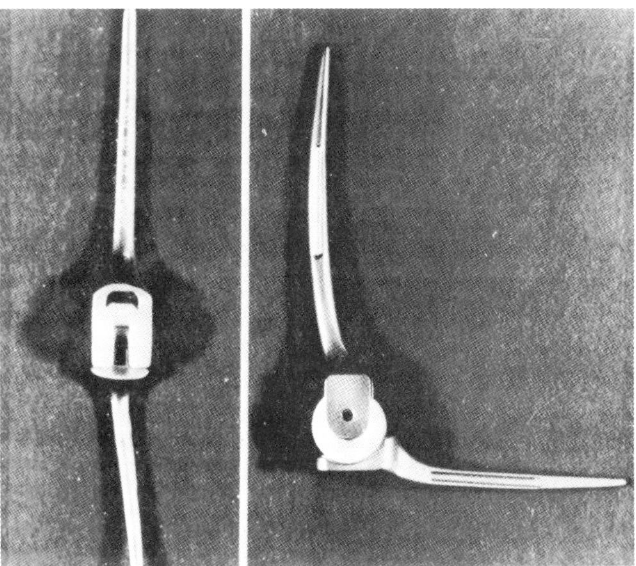

Figure 3: Second generation triaxial prosthesis. The articulation is via a polyethylene bearing which facilitates insertion. (Reprinted with permission from Total elbow replacement, by A.E. Inglis, et al., J. Bone Joint Surg. 62A:1254, 1980.)

these devices can be used in the presence of greater bony or ligamentous destruction. Complication rates are quite high in all series. It appears that with additional experience and improvement in techniques, complication rates are diminished. Great care must be taken during surgery to avoid fracture of the condyles of the humerus since loss of this bony support is difficult to overcome. Likewise, most surgeons now use a posterolateral approach with reflection of the triceps tendon and adjacent ulnar periosteum without entirely detaching them from the ulna. This technique has been reported to reduce the complications of ulnar nerve palsy, joint subluxation, and triceps rupture. Relief of pain is excellent in all series. Most series show increases in the flexion arc but no significant gain in extension.

Forearm

Radius and Ulna Reconstruction Loss of radial or ulnar length following massive trauma or tumor resection presents a difficult problem. When bone loss is less than 1 cm, shortening will not generally compromise function. With larger defects, shortening usually produces an unacceptable appearance and impaired limb function.

Methods of restoring normal length and gaining union of the affected bones include fibular interposition grafts, full-thickness iliac-crest grafts stabilized by intermedullary rods, dual onlay iliac-crest grafts stabilized by plate and screws, and radioulnar cross-unions. A method of stabilizing bone fragments with a plate and bridging the nonunion with a section of pure cancellous bone was described in 1956. Two recent papers report the technique and results using a tricortical iliac-crest graft with compression plating for segmental defects ranging from 1.2 to 4.5 cm in length. The secure internal fixation allows for early mobilization of adjacent joints (Fig. 4). Patients may have a significant restriction of forearm rotation related to the severity of the initial soft-tissue injury or to the presence of an infection following the initial injury. Average time to radiographic evidence of graft incorpora-

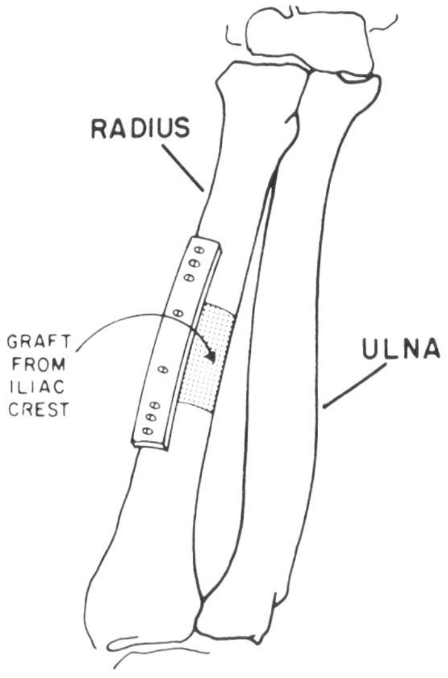

Figure 4: Tricortical iliac-crest graft has been internally fixed to the remaining normal bone using a plate and screws. A single mechanical unit thus is created, allowing early postoperative range of motion exercises. (Reprinted with permission from The management of segmental bone loss associated with forearm fractures, by T.G. Grace, et al., J. Bone Joint Surg. 62A:1151, 1980.)

tion was 13.5 weeks. Complications included flare-ups of previous infection, nonunion, and fracture at the end of the plate. Some recommend plate removal 18 to 24 months after placement with the patient cautiously avoiding excess stress on the extremity for an additional 6 months.

For reconstruction of the distal radius following resection of large benign tumors or low-grade malignant tumors, transfer of the proximal fibula has been advocated. Two recent studies report on a surgical technique designed to overcome previously encountered shortcomings (e.g., failure of the graft to heal to the proximal radius, fracture of the graft, wrist subluxation, and loss of forearm motion). This procedure has been used for low-grade chondrosarcomas, giant cell tumors, and hemangiomas. Return to useful hand function was achieved by 3 to 6 months postoperatively, and full graft incorporation appeared to be well-established by 1 year. Wrist motion was approximately 50 percent that of the uninvolved side. The patient should be advised about the possibility of a subsequent wrist replacement or arthrodesis because of eventual articular degeneration. This joint destruction may result from adverse mechanical stress, relative joint incongruity, or cartilage death because of alterations in synovial nutrition.

In an alternative approach a segment of ulna with its undisturbed blood supply is transferred into the radial defect. An ulno-lunate-scaphoid arthrodesis is performed distally and a radioulnar osteosynthesis proximally. Forearm rotation and intercarpal motion are preserved.

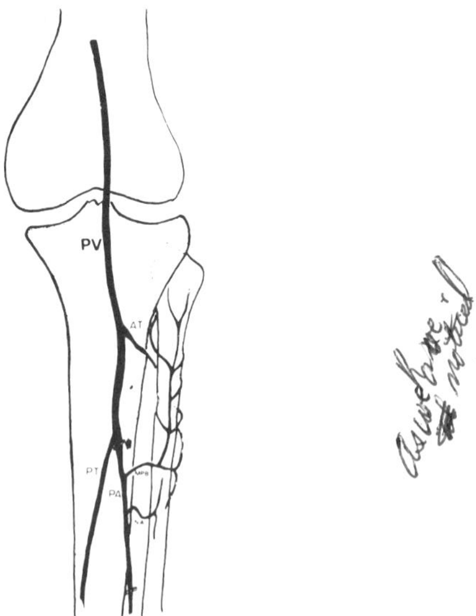

Figure 5: Schematic representation blood supply to the proximal one-half of the fibula. PV, popliteal artery; AT, anterior tibial artery; PT, posterior tibial artery; PA, peroneal artery (arrow indicates the level where peroneal artery was transected); NA, nutrient artery to fibula; MPB, muscular periosteal branches supplying the fibula. (Reprinted with permission from Free vascularised fibular transplant for replacement of the lower radius, by R.W.H. Pho, et al., J. Bone Joint Surg. 61B:362-365, 1979.)

Vascularized bone transfers: Living bone, transferred on its blood supply, has been used to reconstruct large defects in the radius and ulna. By transferring the graft with its blood supply, the bone junction between host bone and graft heals much like a fracture rather than gradually being incorporated by creeping substitution. Vascularized bone transfers primarily use the fibula but also may use rib and iliac crest. The main upper limb application is for radius reconstruction following excision of giant cell tumors. The transfers also have been used following trauma and after massive bone resection for other tumors or chronic osteomyelitis in the humerus and in the forearm bones.

The proximal one-half of the fibula receives its blood supply from the peroneal artery through a main nutrient artery and numerous segmental vessels (Fig. 5). The fibula is removed extraperiosteally on all surfaces with a cuff of flexor hallucis brevis remaining posteromedially. In this cuff of tissue lies the undisturbed peroneal artery and its venae comitans along with the feeder vessels to the fibula. The transferred segment of peroneal artery can be interposed into the radial artery in the forearm so that the blood passes proximally from the radial artery into peroneal artery segment and back into radial artery more distally. Anastomosis between the peroneal venae comitans and a forearm vein establishes venous return.

The advantage of vascularized over nonvascularized bone transfer is the ability to transfer large segments of bone without sacrificing viability and, therefore, allowing for a shorter immobilization with more rapid incorporation and hypertrophy of the graft. The disadvantages are prolonged operating time, difficulty of assessing vessel patency in the early postoperative period, and sacrifice of the peroneal artery in the leg. Preoperative arteriograms of the donor leg and recipient upper limb are valuable in assessing unsuspected vascular anomalies or injuries.

Neuromuscular

Nerve Compression Syndromes

Cubital Tunnel Syndrome Compression neuropathy of the ulnar nerve at the elbow was first described in 1878, and several etiologies have since been recognized. The first known cause was a paralysis of the ulnar nerve occurring many years after a fracture in the elbow area, particularly with the development of cubitus valgus deformity. Other lesions have been recognized including impingement by osteophytes, ganglia or tumors on the nerve, repetitive or acute trauma to the area, and various congenital anomalies. Prolonged elbow flexion or prolonged external pressure on the nerve during coma or general anesthesia frequently lead to ulnar nerve palsy. Additionally, the syndrome may develop from subluxation or dislocation of the ulnar nerve from behind the medial epicondyle. It is likely that the degree of compression, rather than its duration, causes the symptoms. Therefore, patients with a mild compression over a long period of time have a better prognosis than those with a high degree of compression for a short time. Tardy ulnar palsy following fracture in the elbow area has been seen as late as 60 years after injury. An anomalous muscle, the epitrochleoanconeus, spans transversely from the medial epicondyle to the olecranon and is believed to be an accessory elbow extensor. This muscle hypertrophies particularly among people performing repetitive forceful activities of the elbow and is implicated as an additional cause of cubital tunnel syndrome.

When examining a patient with ulnar nerve compression symptoms, the site or sites of compression must be defined carefully. Cubital tunnel syndrome may coexist with thoracic outlet syndrome or with a compression of the ulnar nerve in Guyon's canal at the wrist. Compression at these other sites can be evaluated by a thorough history and physical examination and confirmed by nerve conduction studies and electromyogram. Nerve compression at more than one level is additive and termed the *double crush syndrome*. Once pressure is relieved on the nerve at one level, the patient is frequently asymptomatic even though there may be residual physical and laboratory indicators for pressure at additional levels.

The appropriate method of treatment of cubital tunnel syndrome is controversial. The simplest surgical treatment is in situ decompression of the ulnar nerve. This procedure has the advantage of leaving the main nerve, its branches, and its vascular supply undisturbed while relieving any overlying compression on the convexity of the nerve at the flexed elbow. This decompression may be adequate treatment for patients with early and mild changes. Anterior subcutaneous transposition necessitates transection of some of the segmental blood supply to the nerve as well as a possible disturbance of the nerve branches to the elbow joint and to the flexor carpi ulnaris. The nerve is relieved on its concavity from pressure against the medial epicondyle. A noncompressing fascio-dermal sling to maintain the nerve anteriorly is useful particularly for symptoms of nerve subluxation during forceful extension activities, such as pitching baseballs.

An alternative surgical procedure to simple decompression or anterior subcutaneous transposition, originally described in 1950, is removal of the medial epicondyle (Fig. 6). Postoperative elbow mobilization can be rapid because of the wide fascial origin of flexor pronator muscles (in addition to the clearly defined origin on the medial epicondyle). The procedure has the advantage of decompressing the ulnar nerve on the concave side of its curve without mobilizing it and consequently jeopardizing its blood supply or nerve branches. Theoretical risk of later trauma to the vulnerable ulnar nerve over the medial aspect of the elbow has not been recognized as a real problem.

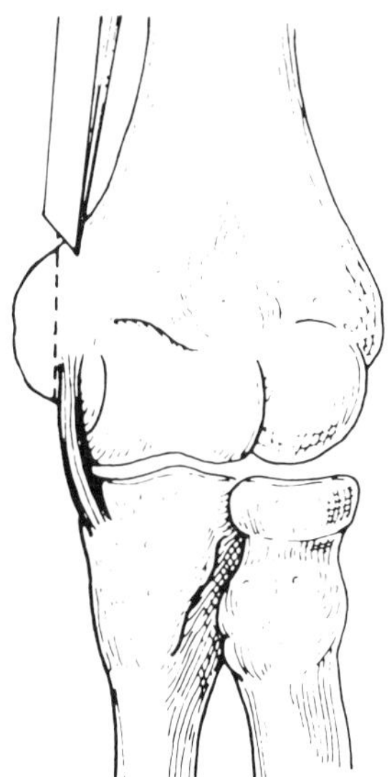

Figure 6: The medial epicondyle must be resected without disturbing the medial collateral ligament to avoid instability. (Reprinted with permission from Treatment of compression neuropathy of the ulnar nerve at the elbow by epicondylectomy and neurolysis, by A.I. Froimson, et al., J. Hand Surg. 5:394, 1980.)

The final surgical procedure for cubital tunnel syndrome is the anterior submuscular transposition. This procedure elevates the flexor pronator origin off the medial epicondyle. The ulnar nerve is mobilized for a considerable distance, necessitating some segmental devascularization as well as mobilization of its branch to the flexor carpi ulnaris. The ulnar nerve is transposed anteriorly and laterally to lie under the flexor pronator origin.

Results from these various procedures are difficult to compare, and no randomized, prospective studies have been done. It appears that all the procedures result in relief or significant improvement of symptoms in 75 to 85 percent of patients, providing they do not have an underlying peripheral neuropathy. Medial epicondylectomy seems to offer the best decompression of the ulnar nerve with the least surgical intervention and the least risk of jeopardizing its blood supply or branches.

Pronator Teres Syndrome The median nerve may be compressed by the pronator teres muscle belly in the proximal forearm. Although the resulting pronator teres syndrome has been recognized for some time, it remains a difficult diagnostic and therapeutic challenge.

Symptoms of median neuropathy localized to the forearm and hand are frequently caused by repetitive hand motions which demand forced forearm rotation. Nocturnal awakening, frequently encountered with carpal tunnel syndrome, is typically absent in patients with more proximal nerve compression. Symptom duration prior to treatment averages almost 2 years. Nonspecific symptoms and subtle physical findings may lead to an initial suspicion of functional neurosis or conversion hysteria. Some patients have undergone unsuccessful carpal tunnel release or ulnar nerve transposition prior to establishment of the proper diagnosis.

The outstanding positive physical findings of this syndrome are tenderness in the proximal part of the pronator teres, over the median nerve in the pronator teres, and over the median nerve in the antecubital space. Resisted

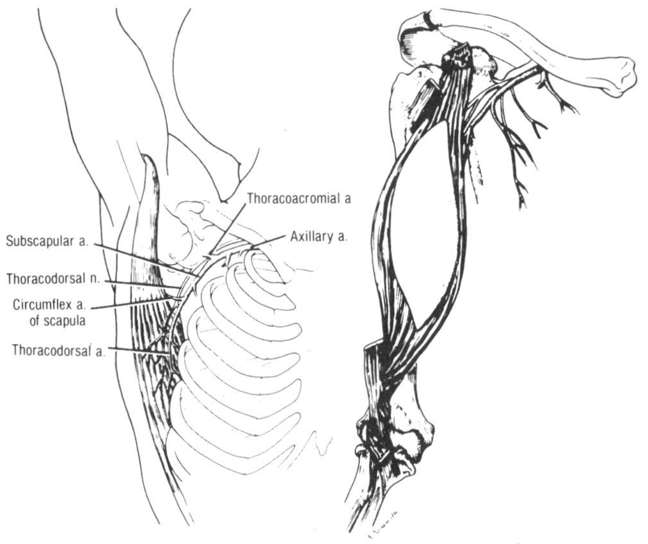

Figure 7-A Figure 7-B

Figure 7: (A) Anatomy of latissimus muscle. Note lengthy neurovascular pedicle entering on posterolateral surface. (B) Flap has been passed to anterior brachium. Proximal fixation to coracoid and distal fixation to biceps tendon are depicted. (Reprinted with permission from Latissimus dorsi musculocutaneous flap for elbow flexion, by P.J. Stern, et al., J. Hand Surg. 7:26, 27, 1982.)

pronation of the forearm frequently causes paresthesias in the median nerve distribution, and a positive Tinel's sign often is found at the proximal edge of the pronator teres. This sign is rarely positive at the wrist although patients may have a positive Phalen's sign.

Compression is located under one or more of the following structures: lacertus fibrosus, a tendinous band in the pronator teres, and a tendinous proximal arcade of the flexor digitorum superficialis. Compression by each of these can be elicited by specific muscle testing. The lacertus fibrosus draws tightly across the median nerve when the forearm is held in resisted supination and flexion. The pronator teres can be implicated when the arm is held in resisted pronation and flexion and then gradually extended while in the pronated position. Independent flexion of the middle finger flexor digitorum superficialis localizes the level of entrapment to the fibrous arcade of the flexor superficialis. Electrical studies show only mild and nonspecific changes in the median nerve function resulting in conduction velocities within a normal range. Normal electrical studies can neither exclude the diagnosis of pronator teres syndrome nor predict the surgical outcome. Electrical studies may distinguish other peripheral nerve disorders that present similar symptoms and may accurately locate the median nerve compression in a small percentage of patients. Clinical examination may suggest that a tight lacertus fibrosus indents the proximal portion of the pronator teres, a finding confirmed at surgery. The most frequent site of median nerve compression is in the substance of the pronator teres where a tendinous band, either in the superficial or deep portion of the pronator, presses against the nerve. In a similar percentage of patients, the fibrous arcade of the superficialis compresses the nerve slightly more distally. Symptoms usually resolve or diminish after release of the offending fascial band. Some patients who improve after fascial decompression in the proximal forearm have electromyographic evidence of carpal tunnel syndrome. Therefore, pronator teres syndrome may coexist with compression on the nerve at other levels, and these other disorders may improve after decompression of the median nerve proximally.

Posterior Interosseous Nerve Entrapment In addition to tennis elbow, pain on the lateral side of the elbow may be caused by entrapment of the posterior interosseous nerve by a fibrous band in the supinator muscle. The differential diagnosis may be difficult.

Of patients with posterior interosseous nerve entrapment, two-thirds have tenderness over the lateral epicondyle, and all have tenderness more distally over the site of entrapment. Pain is almost universally experienced with resisted supination of the forearm and frequently with resisted pronation. More than two-thirds of patients have pain with resisted extension of the middle finger. Most show a diminished grip strength on the affected side.

Surgery consists of decompressing the posterior interosseous nerve from under the proximal edge of the superficial supinator muscle. The edge of the superficial supinator is frequently fibrous at the intersection with the nerve. At surgery the nerve is commonly compressed by the supinator edge on passive forearm pronation. In some patients there is a visible indentation in the nerve with proximal enlargement. Postoperative pain relief occurs gradually.

Placement of a fat pad over the decompressed nerve to reduce scarring may improve the surgical outcome. The presence of a fibrous margin on the supinator muscle is associated with better results. The vast majority of patients with the supinator muscle compressing a seemingly normal nerve during passive pronation have good results. Only one-half of patients preoperatively show some decrease in conduction velocity. Results of surgery seem unrelated to the presence or absence of preoperative electrophysiological abnormalities. Of those having repeat electrical studies postoperatively, most show no definite changes, and a small percentage show either an increase or decrease in conduction velocity. From available data, approximately 5 percent of patients diagnosed with tennis elbow syndrome actually have posterior interosseous nerve entapment.

Painful Neuromas in Below-Elbow Amputees In long below-elbow amputees, painful scars of the nerves ordinarily supplying the hand may be disabling and preclude prosthetic use. Ligation of the median, radial, and ulnar nerves proximally in the forearm physiologically transposes the sensitive nerve endings under better muscle cover in the proximal forearm. These nerves provide no sensibility to the forearm, and, therefore, ligation does not diminish forearm sensibility. Proximal ligation of the major hand nerves during the original amputation or at an early elective time should aid in rapid rehabilitation and full prosthetic use.

Acquired Flexor Spasticity Acquired flexor spasticity in adults with internal rotation of the shoulder and flexion of the elbow, wrist, and fingers is a difficult problem. Surgical treatment for the shoulder, wrist, and hand has been well described. Treatment for the flexed elbow remains difficult.

TREATMENT: Phenol injection into the musculocuta-

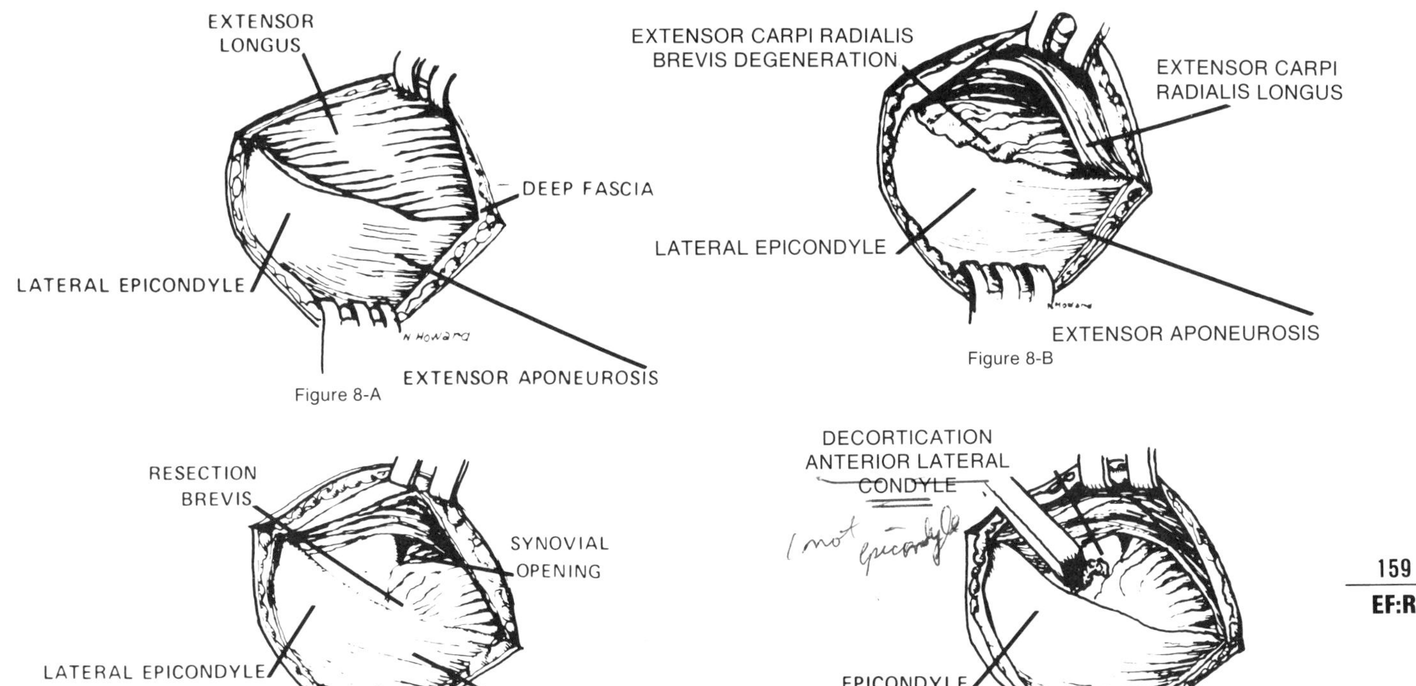

Figure 8: Surgical technique for the treatment of tennis elbow. (A) Deep structures are identified. (B) Retraction of the extensor carpi radialis longus anteriorly reveals the origin of the extensor carpi radialis brevis. Gross change is generally seen in the proximal three-quarters of the tendon. Note that the extensor aponeurosis and the lateral epicondyle are not disturbed. (C) Diseased tissue is resected. Generally three-quarters of the proximal part of the extensor brevis tendon is resected. The anterior edge of the underside of the extensor aponeurosis and the underside of the extensor longus are inspected as well, and all abnormal tissue is removed as indicated (although it is rare to release the extensor aponeurosis from its attachment to the epicondyle). A small opening is made in the synovial membrane to inspect the joint. An intra-articular lesion or an alternation in the orbicular ligament is rare. (D) Decortication or drilling of the anterior part of the lateral condyle is undertaken to enhance blood supply to the area. The lateral epicondyle is not disturbed. (Reprinted with permission from Tennis elbow by R.P. Nirschl, et al., J. Bone Joint Surg. 61A:836-837, 1979.)

neous nerve temporarily interrupts nerve conduction to the spastic elbow for 4 to 6 months. This is a useful procedure for the patient with a recently acquired spasticity interfering with function or leading to progressive contracture. Since the effects of the block are temporary, there is no functional loss if eventual central neurologic recovery occurs. If central recovery is incomplete and spasticity reappears 6 to 9 months following the phenol block, definite surgery can be performed.

Musculocutaneous neurectomy is recommended after 6 months in the stroke-injured patient and 1½ years in the adult head-injured patient. The goals of surgery are to increase the ability for self-care and to improve ambulation, personal hygiene, and appearance. Preoperatively, the brachial plexus block differentiates between muscle spasticity and myostatic contracture. If this shows a residual flexion contracture of 75 degrees or more, a muscle release at the elbow is planned in addition to the musculocutaneous neurectomy. Radiographs are obtained to ascertain the presence of any heterotopic bone at the elbow. If resection of this bone does not include resection of significant soft tissue at the elbow, a musculocutaneous neurectomy also is performed. This is done in the proximal arm where the musculocutaneous nerve is identified by a nerve stimulator between the coracobrachialis and the short head of the biceps. For elbows with more than 75 degrees fixed flexion contracture, the soft-tissue release includes sectioning of the biceps and brachialis muscles and occasionally the brachioradialis and anterior joint capsule. The average extension gain expected is 40 degrees. Surgery generally improves ability for self-care. Patients have not complained of impaired sensation in the distribution of the lateral cutaneous nerve of the forearm.

The brachioradialis must function preoperatively, or there will be no active elbow flexion, an undesirable outcome unless the procedure is performed for reasons of hygiene alone. Postoperatively, more severe contractures are treated with serial splinting and physical therapy to preserve the surgical correction.

Tendon Transfers for Restoration of Elbow Motion For brachial plexus injury or severe loss of soft tissue in the arm, refinement of available transfer techniques has improved restoration of elbow motion. With the recent interest in myocutaneous flaps, some have reported transfer of the latissimus dorsi with overlying skin for restoration of elbow flexion or extension and for coverage of large soft-tissue defects (Fig. 7). A refinement of the pectoralis major transfer to restore elbow flexion includes complete transfer of the pectoralis insertion from the humerus to the acromion with attachment of the pectoralis origin onto the biceps tendon at the radial tuberosity. Thus, the muscle is rotated approximately 90 degrees, and the more proximal attachment on the acromion not only places the muscle in a more advantageous position for strong elbow flexion but also improves stability of the

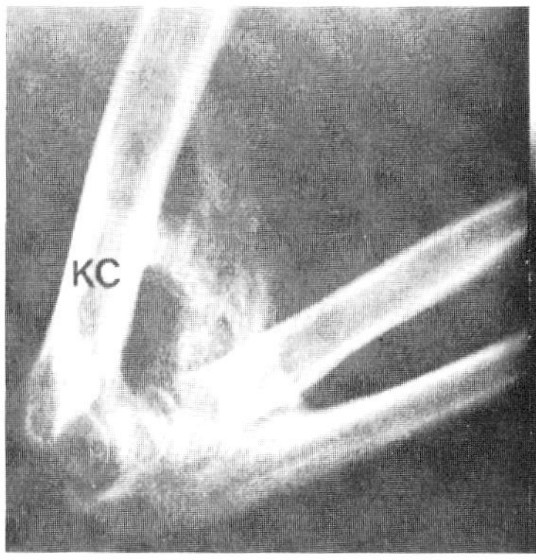

Figure 9: Preoperative and postoperative lateral radiographs of an elbow with complete ankylosis preoperatively. At follow-up 11 months after surgery, there are 100 degrees of flexion-extension and full supination-pronation. The joint space is well preserved, and there is no evidence of recurrence on the follow-up radiograph. (Reprinted with permission from The surgical treatment of heterotopic ossification at the elbow following long-term coma, by J.B. Roberts, et al., J. Bone Joint Surg. 61A:760, 1979.)

160
EF:R

glenohumeral joint. Care must be taken to avoid undue stretching of the neurovascular supply to the transferred muscle.

Miscellaneous

Tennis Elbow Considerable controversy has centered over the pathophysiology of this condition. Recent data suggest that the basic underlying lesion is a microscopic rupture and subsequent incomplete tendinous repair with immature tissue in the origin of the extensor carpi radialis brevis. One reason for failing to recognize this site of pathological change results from a lack of proper surgical visualization. The extensor carpi radialis longus must be retracted to expose the origin of the extensor brevis, which characteristically contains greyish, immature scar tissue that is edematous, shiny, and pliable. Microscopically, there is a characteristic invasion of fibroblasts and vascular granulation, described as angiofibroblastic hyperplasia. The extensor brevis origin may be found detached, indicating a disruption or tear of these tissues. Also, a portion of the extensor carpi radialis brevis originates from the underlying orbicular ligament, accounting for the pathological changes noted. Highlights of the operative technique are illustrated in Figure 8.

The elbow is immobilized for 10 days postoperatively, followed by gradual return to normal activities. The patient may begin to play tennis at 6 weeks following surgery. As for treatment of any pain syndrome, the patient's emotional outlook and stability is a factor deserving emphasis. Most patients with tennis elbow are highly motivated and vigorously follow the postoperative course of rehabilitation.

Fractional lengthening of the extensor carpi radialis brevis tendon above the wrist for treatment of lateral epicondylitis also provides excellent relief of symptoms. However, the procedure was not satisfactory for one patient who had previous and unsuccessful surgery in the elbow area for lateral epicondylitis.

Heterotopic Ossification Encouraging results following resection of heterotopic ossification at the elbow secondary to long-term coma has been reported (Fig. 9). When the mental state and motor control of the patient have improved to a degree that increased elbow function would facilitate self-care, feeding, or the use of ambulatory aids, surgical intervention should be considered. In this procedure, heterotopic bone is removed, but no effort is made to correct the soft-tissue contractures. A vigorous postoperative therapy program is instituted early to preserve and improve elbow motion. A functional excursion of the elbow is obtained immediately, and the range increases over the first 6 months postoperatively. The reason for postoperative recurrence of heterotopic ossification at the hip and not at the elbow is uncertain.

Forearm Rotation Contracture Forearm rotation contracture may be secondary to Volkmann's ischemia, fractures, chondrodysplasia, congenital radial head deformities, posterior dislocation of proximal radius, congenital synostosis, polio, Erb's palsy, spastic paralysis, and as a heritable disorder. In another group of patients, symptoms begin in early teenage years, and the contracture (pronation) progresses over the next 8 to 10 years until the patients seek surgical attention because of physical restrictions. These patients have no family history of congenital anomaly and do not recall specific acute trauma to the forearm. Typical findings include supination only to neutral and pronation to 45 degrees. Radiographs show only pronounced dorsal bowing of the distal ulna.

Correction obtained by surgery is maintained by a transverse Kirschner wire placed between the distal radius and ulna with the forearm in maximum supination (Fig. 10). When the pin is removed and mobilization is begun at 3 weeks, some loss of correction occurs although 10 to 50 degrees of supination generally can be maintained.

Tumors Although *nodular (pseudosarcomatous) fasciitis* occurs anywhere in the body except on the hands and feet, approximately 40 percent of the lesions occur on the forearm or arm. The lesion, characteristically present for

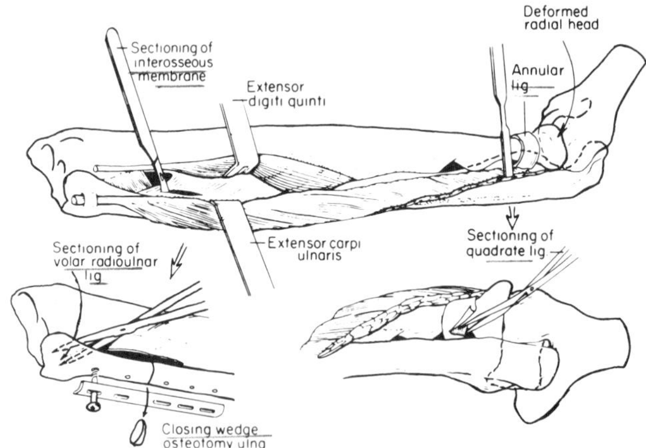

Figure 10: Surgical treatment of forearm rotation contracture. Top: Exposure of the interosseous membrane and distal radioulnar joint is achieved by an incision between the extensor carpi ulnaris and the extensor digiti quinti in the distal third of the forearm. Proximally, through the Boyd incision, the interosseous membrane is exposed by reflecting the extensor carpi ulnaris tendon extraperiosteally. This also allows exposure of the annular ligament and the radial head. Distally, the contracted volar portion of the distal radioulnar joint may be incised with scissors. Bottom right: The quadrate ligament may be incised by inserting a scissors between the two leaves of the annular ligament from the posterior approach. Bottom left: Excessive angular bowing of the distal end of the ulna can be corrected by wedge osteotomy and application of a compression plate. This releases tension on the interosseous membrane and capsule of the distal radioulnar joint to achieve greater supination. (Reprinted with permission from Rotatory contracture of the forearm, by J.M. Bert, et al., J. Bone Joint Surg. 62A:1166, 1980.)

only a short time prior to surgery, rarely exceeds 4 cm in size. Most are smaller than 2 cm. Even incompletely resected lesions may not recur. Histologically, the nodular fasciitis resembles reparative tissue, and it is possible that the lesion is an atypical form of granulation tissue brought about by minor trauma. Nodular fasciitis is a nonrecurrent lesion. Recurrence of a lesion originally diagnosed as nodular fasciitis should lead to a careful review of the pathological findings.

Several recent reports are reminders that tumors which generally are seen in the soft tissues may occasionally appear intra-articularly or interosseously. *Pigmented villonodular synovitis* occurs in the elbow and may mimic neoplasm. Epidermoid cysts are common in soft tissue. A patient with an epidermoid cyst in the distal ulna recalled a minor blunt injury approximately 10 years previously. The diagnosis was made histologically.

ANNOTATED BIBLIOGRAPHY

Elbow Joint

Surgical Approach

Gschwend, N.: Our operative approach to the elbow joint. Arch. Orthop. Trauma Surg. 98:143-146, 1981.

A single surgical incision on the lateral aspect of the elbow allows for extensive view into the anterior and posterior aspects of the elbow joint. This incision has proved valuable for rheumatoid synovectomy, posttraumatic capsulotomy, and loose body removal.

Osteochondritis Dissecans

Lindholm, T.S.; Österman, K.; and Vankka, E.: Osteochondritis dissecans of elbow, ankle and hip: A comparison survey. Clin. Orthop. 148:245-253, 1980.

Osteochondritis dissecans of the elbow occurs during adolescence and sometimes responds to rest. Occasionally loose body removal is indicated.

Elbow Synovectomy

Copeland, S.A., and Taylor, J.G.: Synovectomy of the elbow in rheumatoid arthritis: The place of excision of the head of the radius. J. Bone Joint Surg. 61B:69-73, 1979.

Twenty-seven of thirty patients undergoing elbow synovectomy for rheumatoid arthritis obtained pain relief, and twenty-one obtained increased motion. Approximately one-half had their radial heads preserved but with no difference in the overall result.

Kay, L.; Stainsby, D.; Buzzard, B.; Fearns, M.; Hamilton, P.J.; Owen, P.; and Jones, P.: The role of synovectomy in the management of recurrent haemarthroses in haemophilia. British J. Haematol. 49:53-60, 1981.

Eighteen hemophiliac patients with recurrent elbow hemarthroses resistant to medical management benefited from synovectomy. The effects of surgery on motion were variable; however, all experienced fewer hemarthroses postoperatively.

Low, W.G., and Evans, J.P.: Synovectomy of the elbow and excision of the radial head in rheumatoid arthritis. Southern Med. J. 73:707-709, 1980.

Elbow synovectomy in rheumatoid arthritis provided pain relief and increased range of motion even in the late stages of the disease.

Excision Arthroplasty of Elbow

Shahriaree, H.; Sajadi, K.; Silver, C.M.; and Sheikholeslamzadeh, S.: Excisional arthroplasty of the elbow. J. Bone Joint Surg. 61A:922-927, 1979.

A Gelfoam interpositional elbow arthroplasty was performed in thirty patients, most of whom had sustained injuries. Eighty percent were relieved of pain, and 90 percent were able to return to their jobs.

Elbow Arthrodesis

Arafiles, R.P.: A new technique of fusion for tuberculous arthritis of the elbow. J. Bone Joint Surg. 63A:1396-1400, 1981.

A new technique for elbow arthrodesis creates a mortise and tenon type of joint between the olecranon and distal humerus. All eleven patients operated on achieved union.

Total Elbow Replacement

Brumfield, R.H., Jr.; Volz, R.G.; and Green, J.F.: Total elbow arthroplasty: A clinical review of 30 cases employing the Mayo and AHSC prostheses. Clin. Orthop. 158:137-141, 1981.

Adequate bone structure is required for use of an unconstrained total elbow prosthesis. Disruption of bony architecture requires a semiconstrained or constrained prosthesis depending on degree of disorganization.

Ewald, F.C.; Scheinberg, R.D.; Poss, R.; Thomas, W.H.; Scott, R.D.; and Sledge, C.B.: Capitellocondylar total elbow arthroplasty. J. Bone Joint Surg. 62A:1259-1263, 1980.

Sixty-nine nonconstrained total elbow arthroplasties were followed 3.5 years. A high complication rate included only one loosening.

Inglis, A.E., and Pellicci, P.M.: Total elbow replacement. J. Bone Joint Surg. 62A:1252-1258, 1980.

Thirty-six total elbow replacements using a semiconstrained prosthesis were followed 3.7 years. Patients with posttraumatic arthritis and disability from a restricted motion benefited least.

Kudo, H.; Iwano, K.; and Watanabe, S.: Total replacement of the rheumatoid elbow with a hingeless prosthesis. J. Bone Joint Surg. 62A:277-285, 1980.

Twenty-four nonconstrained total elbow replacements for rheumatoid arthritis were followed for nearly 4 years. Pain relief was excellent, and the loosening rate was very low.

Morrey, B.F.; Askew, L.J.; An, K.N.; and Chao, E.Y.: A biomechanical study of normal functional elbow motion. J. Bone Joint Surg. 63A:872-877, 1981.

Most daily activities can be accomplished with elbow motion from 30 to 130 degrees and forearm rotation from 50 degrees of pronation to 50 degrees of supination.

Morrey, B.F.; Bryan, R.S.; Dobyns, J.H.; and Linscheid, R.L.: Total elbow arthroplasty: A five-year experience at the Mayo Clinic. J. Bone Joint Surg. 63A:1050-1063, 1981.

Eighty Mayo and Coonrad total elbow replacements followed at least 2 years gave excellent pain relief and some motion improvement but were associated with a high complication rate.

Forearm

Radius and Ulna Reconstruction

Grace, T.G., and Eversmann, W.W., Jr.: The management of segmental bone loss associated with forearm fractures. J. Bone Joint Surg. 62A:1150-1155, 1980.

Eighteen forearm bone fractures with segmental defects were treated with interposed corticocancellous iliac-bone grafts. The rare unsatisfactory outcome was associated with preoperative infection.

Mack, G.R.; Lichtman, D.M.; and MacDonald, R.I.: Fibular autografts for distal defects of the radius. J. Hand Surg. 4:576-583, 1979.

A nonvascularized fibular autograft was successful in all three patients in reconstruction of the distal radius following resection for tumor.

Shelton, W.R., and Sage, F.P.: Modified Nicoll-graft treatment of gap non-unions in the upper extremity. J. Bone Joint Surg. 63A:226-231, 1981.

Sixteen upper limb, long bone gap nonunions responded well to full-thickness iliac interposition graft and compression plating.

Weiland, A.J.; Kleinert, H.E.; Kutz, J.E.; and Daniel, R.K.: Free vascularized bone grafts in surgery of the upper extremity. J. Hand Surg. 4:129-144, 1979.

Vascularized fibular transfers were used in five patients with upper limb segmental bone loss reconstruction by transferring the fibula and its nutrient vessels to appropriate recipient vessels in the upper limb. The osteocytes survived, negating the need for graft incorporation by creeping substitution.

Neuromuscular

Cubital Tunnel Syndrome

Froimson, A.I., and Zahrawi, F.: Treatment of compression neuropathy of the ulnar nerve at the elbow by epicondylectomy and neurolysis. J. Hand Surg. 5:391-395, 1980.

Discomfort and pain subsided in all thirty patients undergoing medial epicondylectomy for cubital tunnel syndrome.

Leffert, R.D.: Anterior submuscular transposition of the ulnar nerves by the Learmonth technique. J. Hand Surg. 7:147-155, 1982.

The operative technique for submuscular transposition of the ulnar nerve in cubital tunnel syndrome is described. Patients with significant scarring or with severe preoperative pain fared less well postoperatively.

Pronator Teres Syndrome

Hartz, C.R.; Linscheid, R.L.; Gramse, R.R.; and Daube, J.R.: The pronator teres syndrome: Compressive neuropathy of the median nerve. J. Bone Joint Surg. 63A:885-890, 1981.

162 EF:R The cause of failure in five of thirty-six patients undergoing surgery for proximal median nerve compression was either inadequate decompression or misdiagnosis.

Johnson, R.K.; Spinner, M.; and Shrewsbury, M.M.: Median nerve entrapment syndrome in the proximal forearm. J. Hand Surg. 4:48-51, 1979.

Median nerve entrapment by various fibrous structures in the proximal forearm was successfully treated in sixty-seven of seventy-one patients by surgical decompression.

Posterior Interosseous Nerve Entrapment

Werner, C.: Lateral elbow pain and posterior interosseous nerve entrapment. Acta Orthop. Scand. 174:1-62, 1979. (Supplement)

A review of diagnosis and treatment of posterior interosseous nerve entrapment is presented and the findings are contrasted to those of tennis elbow.

Neuromas

Louis, D.S.; Hunter, L.Y.; and Keating, T.M.: Painful neuromas in long below-elbow amputees. Arch. Surg. 115:742-744, 1980.

Prosthetic use was permitted in seven long below-elbow amputees with painful neuromas following proximal ligation of median, radial, and ulnar nerves.

Acquired Flexor Spasticity

Garland, D.E.; Thompson, R.; and Waters, R.L.: Musculocutaneous neurectomy for spastic elbow flexion in non-functional upper extremities in adults. J. Bone Joint Surg. 62A:108-112, 1980.

Spastic elbow flexion can be reduced by musculocutaneous neurectomy in the proximal arm. Improved self-care, ambulation, personal hygiene, and appearance result.

Miscellaneous

Tennis Elbow

Nirschl, R.P., and Pettrone, F.A.: Tennis elbow: The surgical treatment of lateral epicondylitis. J. Bone Joint Surg. 61A:832-839, 1979.

Eighty-eight operative patients with tennis elbow consistently demonstrated immature fibroblastic and vascular infiltration of the extensor carpi radialis brevis origin. Excision of the identified lesion and repair of the origin provided an overall improvement rate of 98 percent.

Heterotopic Ossification

Roberts, J.B., and Pankratz, D.G.: The surgical treatment of heterotopic ossification at the elbow following long-term coma. J. Bone Joint Surg. 61A: 760-763, 1979.

Heterotopic ossification at the elbow following cerebral injury was surgically removed with satisfactory restoration of motion and without reformation of bone in all nine patients.

Forearm Rotation Contracture

Bert, J.M.; Linscheid, R.L.; and McElfresh, E.: Rotatory contracture of the forearm. J. Bone Joint Surg. 62A:1163-1168, 1980.

Idiopathic progressive loss of supination occurring during adolescence benefited from surgical sectioning of quadrate ligament, release of interosseous membrane, and corrective osteotomy of distal ulna.

20 WRIST AND HAND: PEDIATRIC

Subjects covered in this section include congenital deformity (syndactyly, thumb duplication, congenital constriction rings), trauma, replantation, cerebral palsy, and tumors.

Congenital Deformities

Classification A classification for congenital limb malformations has been adopted by the American Society for Surgery of the Hand, the International Federation of Societies for Surgery of the Hand, and the International Society of Prosthetics and Orthotics. This system, based upon certain patterns of embryological failure, groups similar abnormalities. The main categories of the classification are: (I) failure of formation; (II) failure of separation; (III) duplication; (IV) overgrowth; (V) undergrowth; (VI) congenital constriction band syndrome; and (VII) generalized skeletal abnormalities. This classification, which has replaced the confusing Latin and Greek terminology, is practical and easily applied. The deformities are considered here in the order of their frequency.

Failure of Separation (Syndactyly) Syndactyly, the most common congenital anomaly of the hand, appears in 1 per 2,500 births and often is associated with other congenital abnormalities of the extremities. It represents a failure of separation of the developing mesenchymal tissue that normally occurs between the fifth and eighth weeks in utero.

It is classified into complete or incomplete and simple or complex. Complete syndactyly involves webbing of the entire length of the fingers, including the tips, and incomplete syndactyly a partial webbing. The simple form has only soft tissue between the digits, and the complex has fusion of adjacent bones and joints. Syndactyly occurs most often between the long and ring fingers. The thumb index web space is affected least frequently.

TREATMENT: The timing of surgery is dependent upon the web space involved and the degree of complexity. If there is complete syndactyly between two digits of disparate length, the longer will eventually develop a flexion contracture and/or a lateral deviation deformity. For proper hand function development, early separation of the border digits is important. A less significant deformity is simple syndactyly between the long and ring fingers.

Of the several techniques described for release of syndactyly, the two most common are either dorsal and volar triangular flaps (Fig. 1) or separation of the fingers with Z-incisions and a wide dorsal rectangular flap (Fig. 2). Although the common digital nerves can be readily split proximally, the distal Y-division of the common digital artery limits the extent of proximal recession of the flaps in the web. It usually is unnecessary, however, to divide one of the proper digital arteries to create a deep enough web. Full-thickness skin grafts usually are used to cover defects after syndactyly release since they have less tendency to develop secondary contractures than split-thickness skin grafts. Longitudinal incisions to release syndactyly are also very prone to develop contractures.

Approximately 50 percent of patients with major associated hand anomalies require a second operative procedure to provide satisfactory results. Thirty percent with isolated syndactyly require further surgery for partial recurrence of the web, usually within 2 years. Patients with complex syndactyly and those treated before 18 months of age are more likely to require revision surgery. In those with complete complex syndactyly, functional results can be improved if separation of the bony elements is done early in life and further soft-tissue procedures are delayed until after the age of 18 months. Certain patients, particularly those with Apert's syndrome, may function satisfactorily with the creation of a three-fingered hand.

Duplication of the Thumb This fairly common congenital abnormality is almost always unilateral and sporadic in occurrence. When the duplication includes a triphalangeal thumb, it is frequently of autosomal dominant inheritance. There are a great many syndromes associated with duplication of the thumb; acrocephalosyndactyly is probably the most common. Syndactyly, brachydactyly, deafness, and facial abnormalities, including clefting, also may

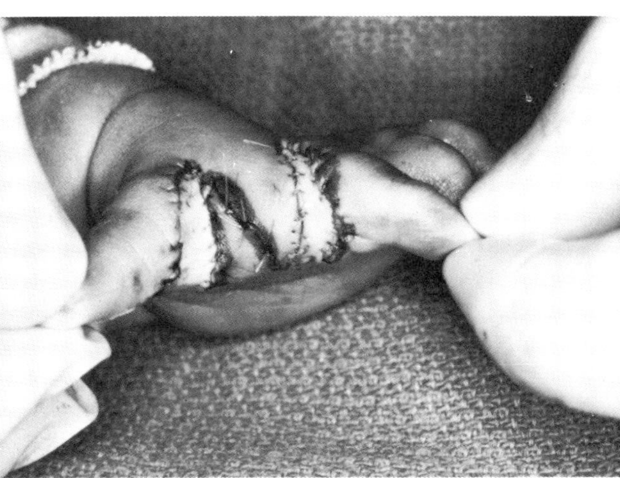

Figure 1: An incomplete simple syndactyly of the index-long web is released with dorsal and volar triangular flaps. The donor sites are covered with full-thickness skin grafts.

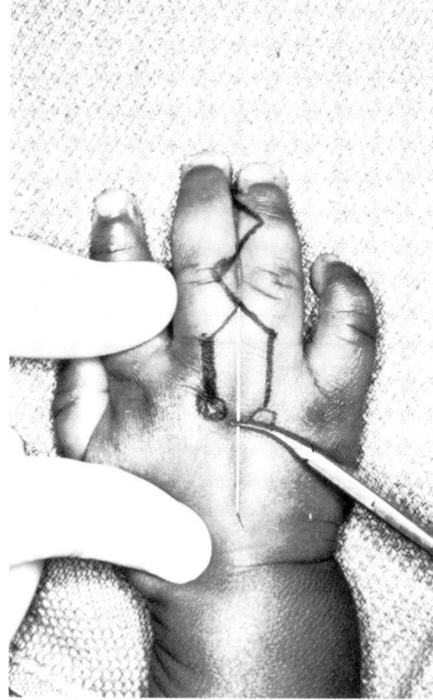

Figure 2-A

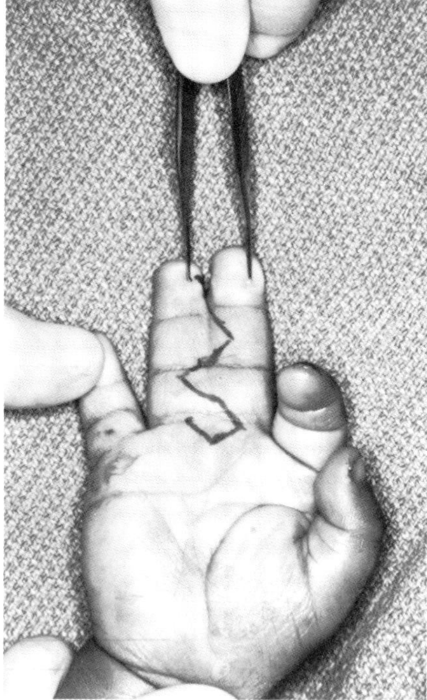

Figure 2-B

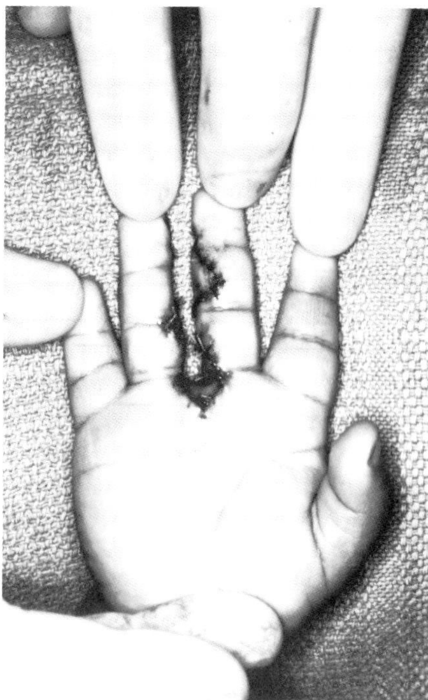

Figure 2-C

Figure 2: (A,B) A complete simple syndactyly of the long-ring web is to be released with Z-incisions and a dorsal flap to create a new web. (C) The newly created web with primary closure of all wounds. A skin graft is usually necessary.

occur. The preferred classification for duplication of the thumb is that of Wassel. The most common is type IV, the duplication of both proximal and distal phalanges. Type VII duplication involving triphalangism of one of the thumbs is the second most commonly encountered deformity.

Treatment: There are several important principles concerning ablation of one of the duplicated thumbs. In most patients, the radially duplicated thumb is smaller and functionally less well developed and is usually the one

Figure 3: (A,B) A severe angular deformity of the thumb occurred after simple ablation because of a longitudinal radial incision and failure to rebalance the flexor and extensor insertions into the distal phalanx.

removed. Careful placement of the suture line prevents a contracted linear scar along the radial side of the remaining digit (Fig. 3). Identification of the neurovascular bundles is mandatory to prevent injury to those supplying the remaining thumb. The extensor and flexor tendons may have anomalous insertions in the remaining thumb and should be corrected to prevent deforming forces. Reconstruction of the capsule and collateral ligaments about the metacarpophalangeal (MP) or interphalangeal (IP) joints and proper reinsertion of the thenar muscles, particularly the abductor pollicis brevis, are important to avoid weakness and a flail or unstable joint.

Several problems may develop in the treatment of this condition. Loss of interphalangeal joint motion occurs in 40 percent of patients, and lateral deviation of the MP or IP joints of over 10 degrees develops in 33 percent. Nail deformities are almost universal following the Bilhaut-

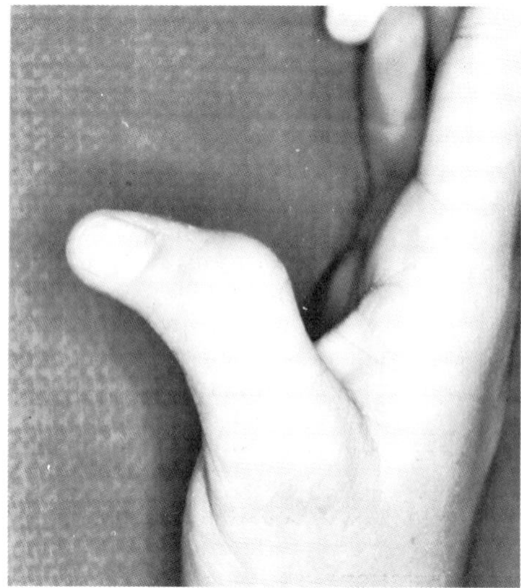

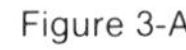

Figure 3-A

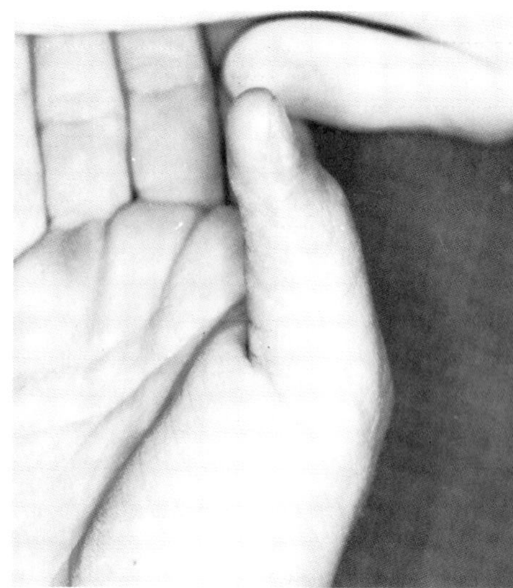

Figure 3-B

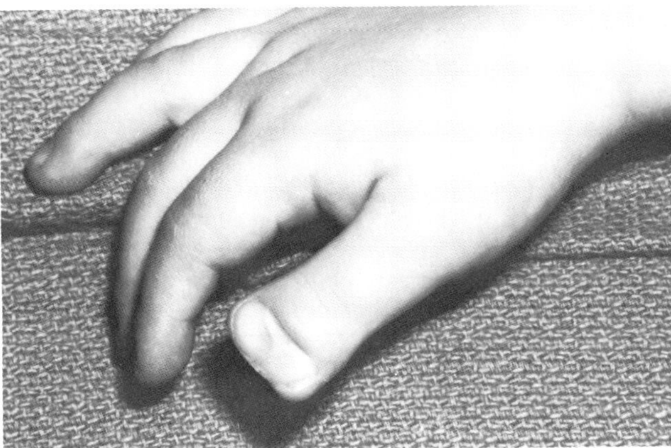

Figure 4-A

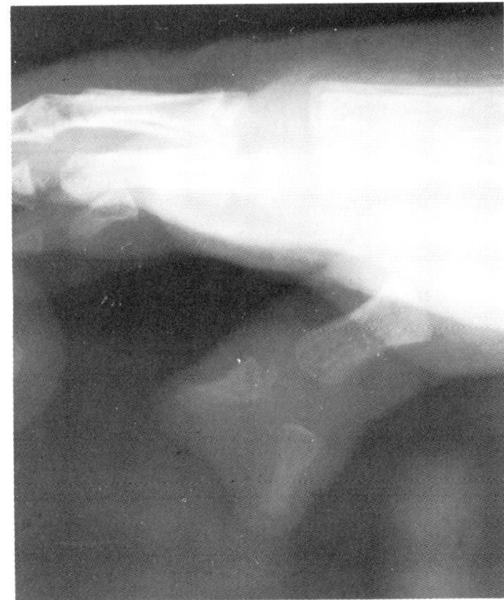

Figure 4-B

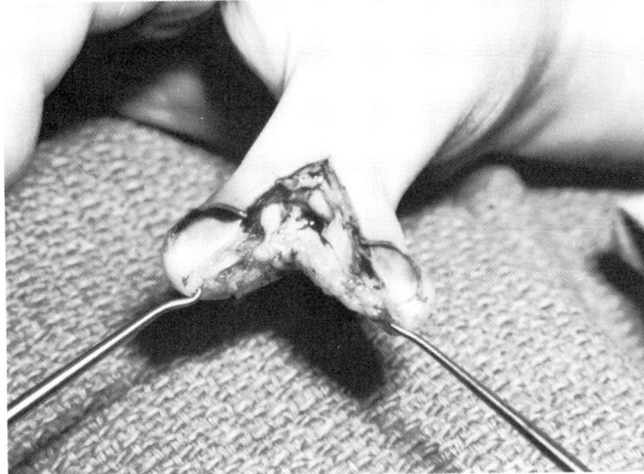

Figure 4-C

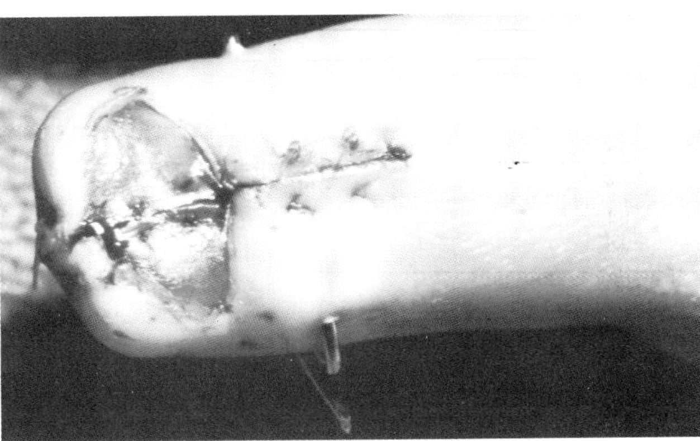

Figure 4-D

Figure 4: (A,B) A type II polydactyly of the thumb with duplication of the distal phalanx and fusion of the duplicated digits. (C,D) Wedge excision of the central portion of the duplication (Bilhaut-Cloquet). Nail deformity is common with this procedure.

Cloquet method involving wedge excision of a terminally duplicated thumb with repair of the nail bed (Fig. 4). Patients having this procedure also experience the most loss of motion at the interphalangeal joint. Other problems encountered may be deformity of the bones requiring late osteotomy, adduction contracture of the web space of the thumb necessitating Z-plasty and release, or lack of soft-tissue coverage of the thumb.

Duplication with triphalangism presents a more difficult surgical problem. In treating this particular polydactyly, the best results seem to be obtained by removing the triphalangeal digit rather than the biphalangeal thumb. A more acceptable appearance may result if the rudimentary thumb is transposed from the ulnar to the radial position. Occasionally pollicization of the triphalangeal thumb is the procedure of choice, depending upon the configuration of the duplicated thumbs.

Congenital Constriction Rings The exact etiology of congenital constriction ring syndrome is unknown. Streeter's theory of a defect in germ plasm development and Torpin's theory implicating early rupture of the amniotic membrane are the two discussed most frequently. Since there are many reports of deformed amputated limbs being delivered at birth and recently a thumb with a well-defined fibrous band in the constriction ring, it is believed that entrapment of the limbs within the amnion is the most likely cause.

Congenital constriction rings occur in 1 of 5,000 to 10,000 live births. Typically, there is no family history of constriction rings although there is a high incidence of familial foot anomalies. They are more common in first pregnancies, and there does not appear to be any relationship to drug ingestion, maternal illness during the first trimester, or oligo- or polyhydramnios. There is a common association with other developmental anomalies, deformity of the hand with syndactyly being the most common. Often foot deformities are encountered, and 25 percent of patients have a combination of syndactyly with constriction rings in the upper extremity and clubfoot deformity. The ring constrictions are most prevalent in the digits.

It is unusual to have a functional impairment due solely to constriction rings. Rings situated proximally in the limb have a greater tendency for compromise of circulatory function, and decreased capillary refill and edema is present in 70 percent of such patients. Peripheral cyanosis after prolonged exertion, dependency, or exposure to cold is present in 50 percent of proximal rings. Only 10 percent of patients with distal constriction rings demonstrate circulatory compromise. Alteration of neural function (particularly sensation) can occur and is associated with temperature gradients across the constriction ring. An

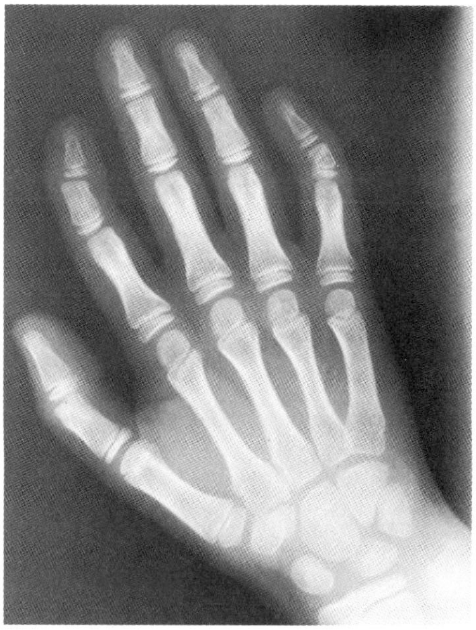

Figure 5: Clinodactyly of the index and small fingers. The middle phalanx of the small finger has a delta phalanx with the epiphysis extending along its radial margin. Function of this hand is excellent.

increase in ring depth with growth is found in almost 60 percent of patients.

TREATMENT: Several surgical techniques for constriction rings have been described, but staged excision and Z-plasty is the preferred method. This usually is a two-stage technique for distal rings, and either a two- or three-stage procedure for more proximally located rings.

In one series, 75 percent of patients so treated had no functional loss, no cosmetic deformity, no recurrence, and a decreased extent of edema and cyanosis. Another 20 percent experienced little or no functional loss with some mild cosmetic deformity or slight recurrence of the ring, but circulation improved. Staged Z-plasty remains the treatment of choice and should be considered when there is distal edema, cyanosis, or an increased depth of the constriction. In the absence of these complications, treatment can be delayed until the child is older.

Clinodactyly Clinodactyly, angular deviation of a digit in the radial-ulnar plane of greater than 10 degrees, is a physical sign which may have many etiologies. Often the deformity represents an autosomal dominant mode of inheritance not associated with any other congenital anomaly. It also may be due to trauma either from a fracture of the epiphyseal plate or frostbite with resultant irregularities in epiphyseal plate growth. It also may be associated with an assortment of chromosomal abnormalities including Down's, Klinefelter's and Turner's syndromes. Clinodactyly of the thumb, commonly associated with Apert's syndrome, may be severe.

Clinodactyly most often is seen in the small finger and consists of a short deformed middle phalanx. The epiphyseal plate of the middle phalanx may be abnormal, causing an asymmetrical longitudinal growth of the phalanx (Fig. 5). Less commonly, the proximal phalanx is affected.

Those patients requiring surgical correction should be carefully selected since most patients function quite satisfactorily without treatment. If severe angulation without a delta phalanx occurs, a closing-wedge osteotomy can be performed after skeletal maturity. When a delta phalanx is present, significant angular deformity may develop early in life and should be corrected then. The preferred treatment method is a reverse-wedge osteotomy in which a wedge of bone from the long side of the phalanx is inserted into the opposite side. This effectively breaks up the abnormal epiphyseal plate and prevents recurrence. A delta phalanx in a triphalangeal thumb without polydactyly should be excised early with ligamentous reconstruction and stabilization of the joint.

The long-term consequences of clinodactyly of a finger are unknown, but it is believed that there is no greater predisposition to degenerative arthritis.

Congenital Central Hand Deficiency Absence of the central digits of the hand is a relatively uncommon group of disorders primarily due to failure of longitudinal formation of central rays. The incidence ranges from 0.14 to 0.4 per 10,000 births. Although a predominant feature is failure of formation, many of these deformities also are associated with failure of separation in other portions of the hand and with hypoplasia of part or all of the hand.

A classification system based upon the number of rays involved has been proposed with group 0 being all bones present with some minor failure of differentiation and groups 1, 2, and 3 having 1, 2, or 3 rays involved, respectively. Of the two-thirds of patients having unilateral involvement, the vast majority are group 3 (i.e., three involved rays). The other one-third of patients have bilateral hand anomalies, and most also have a similar degree of bony involvement on each side. The long finger ray is the most frequently involved, with the index the next, and the ring finger ray the least. There is correspondingly more severe involvement in the order of long, index, and ring finger rays.

Many patients with bilateral central ray deficiencies of the hand also have them in the feet. Approximately one-third of all patients with these deficiencies have associated major musculoskeletal anomalies.

There are two types of patients with central hand deficiency. One presents with unilateral hand involvement, no foot involvement, a negative family history, and no transference to subsequent generations. This type probably represents a sporadic anomaly. The other has a strong family history of bilateral hand and foot involvement, probably representing an autosomal dominant trait with some variable expression.

TREATMENT: The primary goal of surgical management is a hand with good grasp and pinch. Cosmetic appearance is of less concern. The thumb and small finger rays are the major determinants of grasp, and efforts should be made to maximize their function. For group 1 hands, usually involving deficiency of the long finger ray, closure of the cleft with a skin flap to form a shallower web may be performed. The long finger metacarpal should be preserved in closing this defect if possible, because it tends to maintain a broader palm and preserve some hand strength. Also, a progressive gap between the index and ring fingers may develop in the adult years. There may be a problem in adult years if the central metacarpal is excised to close the cleft with a progressive gap between the index and ring fingers developing. Finally, patients

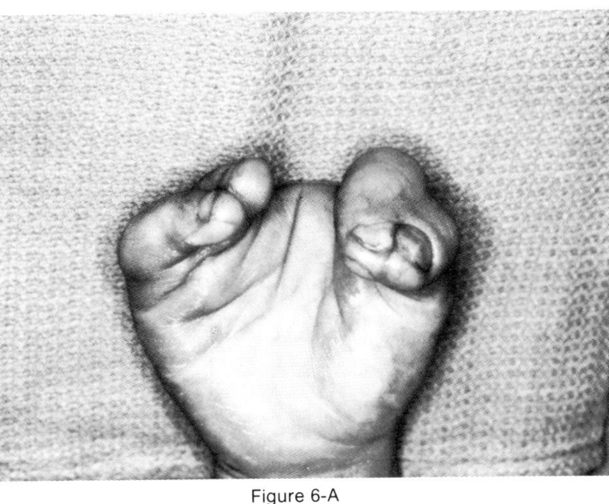

Figure 6-A

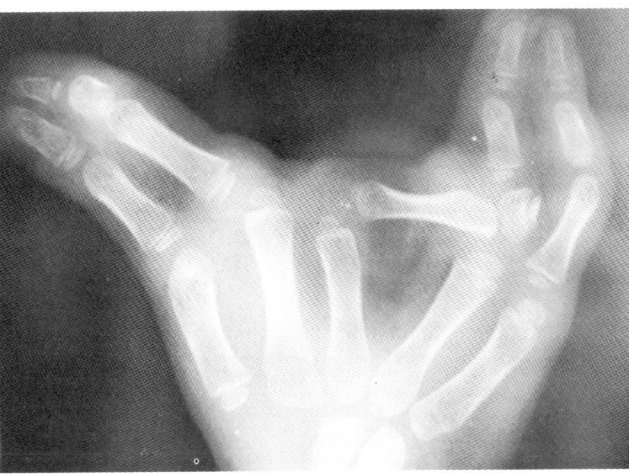

Figure 6-B

Figure 6: (A) An isolated central ray deficiency involving the middle finger with syndactyly of the first and fourth web spaces. This is the maximum opposition obtainable. (B) The radiograph demonstrates a transverse phalanx in the central portion of the hand.

with a closed cleft may have deepening of the web during the adolescent growth spurt.

Transverse phalanges in the central portion of the hand should be excised because they frequently block motion of adjacent digits and cause divergence of the remaining rays (Fig. 6). However, ligamentous instability and flexion contractures of the remaining joints following removal of these transverse bones may develop. In groups 2 and 3 preservation of the most structures possible with excision of central structures to widen the span of grasp is urged. Efforts should be directed toward maximizing thumb and small finger mobility, and any delta phalanges present should be treated with osteotomy to correct progressive deformities of the border digits.

Most patients with central hand deficiency function quite satisfactorily throughout life given the basic functions of grasp and pinch.

Reconstruction of Congenital Absence of the Fingers and Thumb Hand reconstruction with partial or complete failure of formation of the digits is a worthwhile endeavor. With the advent of several new surgical techniques, restoration of grasp and pinch is now possible with predictably good results.

The use of toe phalanges for reconstruction of hypoplastic digits with intact digital skin tubes is an established technique. Previously obtained by subperiosteal dissection, the potential for growth was limited. The use of toe phalanges with intact epiphyses obtained by extraperiosteal dissection results in considerably improved survival of the graft, presumably due to the improved revascularization through the intact periosteum. In one study of patients operated on between 6 and 18 months of age, 91 percent of the epiphyseal plates remained open, and approximately 90 percent of the predicted growth of those phalanges occurred. From 18 months to 5 years of age, the epiphyseal plates remained open in 67 percent of patients, and over 5 years of age 50 percent of the plates remained open. Of those with open epiphyseal plates in the latter two age groups, approximately 90 percent of the predicted growth occurred. The operation is relatively simple and provides a reasonably functional joint because of the preserved flexor and extensor tendon insertions often found in the soft tissues of these digital buds. Sensation is preserved on the tip of the reconstructed digit, and fine pinch can be restored.

Another technique involves lengthening of the remaining portions of the hand using a special distraction device (Fig. 7). Osteotomy and gradual distraction of the bone are performed for approximately 1 month. The elongation achieved varies between 2.5 and 3.8 cm, and spontaneous consolidation of the gap occurs with continued immobilization. This technique is especially applicable to the thumb provided most of the first metacarpal is present and there is good soft-tissue coverage over the stump (Fig. 8). The gradual distraction of 1.0 to 1.5 mm per day does not cause vascular compromise or neurologic loss in the reconstructed digit. Few complications are encountered using this technique so long as the pins do not loosen. Because an average treatment time is 4 months and considerable patient cooperation is required, careful patient selection is mandatory.

The ability to transfer tissues with an intact blood supply adds a new dimension to the reconstruction of the hand with absent fingers or thumb (Fig. 9). Generally, the second toe is chosen for transfer although successful

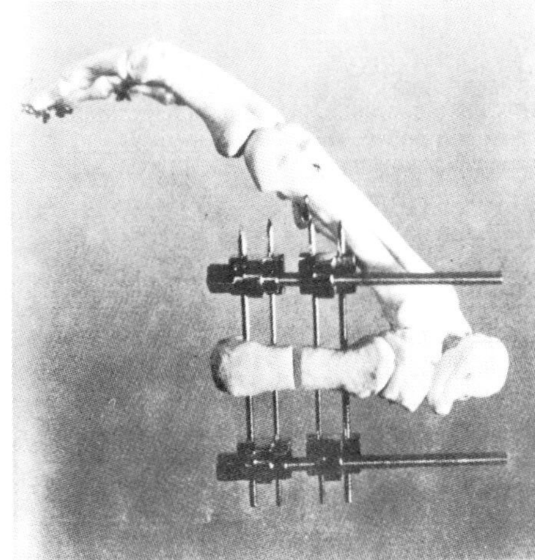

Figure 7: The distraction device used to lengthen the thumb metacarpal and site of osteotomy is shown. Secure pin fixation in both fragments is essential. (Reprinted with permission from Thumb reconstruction in children through metacarpal lengthening, by I.B. Matev, Plast. Reconstr. Surg. 64:665-669, 1979.)

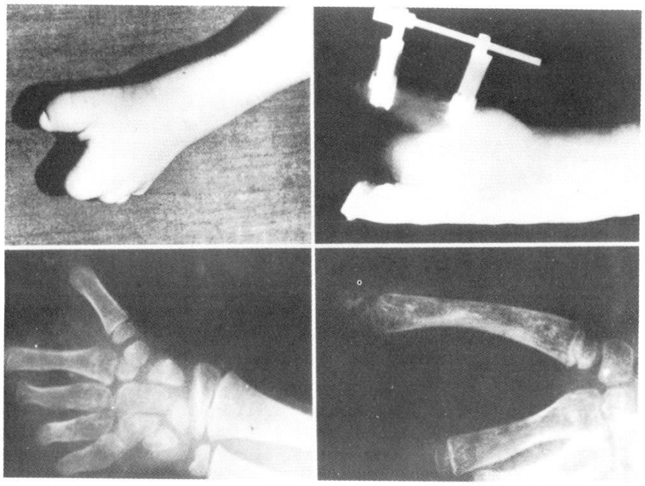

Figure 8: Congenital absence of the thumb (left, top, and bottom) is treated by the distraction method (right, top). Spontaneous consolidation of the metacarpal has occurred (right, bottom). (Reprinted with permission from Thumb reconstruction in children through metacarpal lengthening, by I.B. Matev, Plast. Reconstr. Surg. 64:665-669, 1979.)

one-stage transfer of the great toe for total congenital absence of the thumb is reported. Multiple-staged transfers to the same hand for loss of multiple digits can be performed to improve the overall cosmetic and functional appearance of the hand. With microvascular techniques, failure due to vascular thrombosis is infrequent. The youngest patient undergoing the procedure was 18 months of age with many under the age of 3 years. A consistent postoperative problem is lack of mobility of the transferred toe. There is commonly a flexion contracture of the toe, and the average active range of motion varies from 40 to 60 degrees. Secondary tenolysis procedures have not been very helpful. The overall function of the transferred toe is much better in the thumb position with intact thenar musculature and first metacarpal. Sensibility has been less than 10 mm two-point discrimination in most patients.

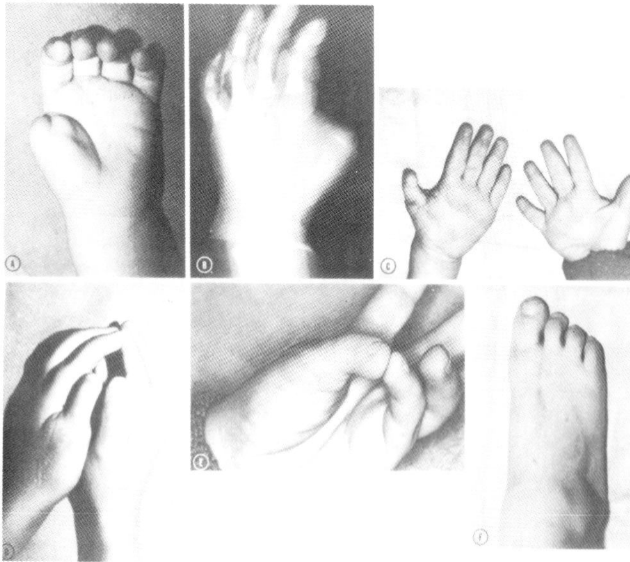

Figure 9: (A,B) Congenital absence of the thumb. (C,D,E) Treated with microvascular transfer of the second toe. Appearance and function are excellent. (F) The donor site of the foot is quite acceptable. (Reprinted with permission from Toe transfers for congenital hand defects, by A. Gilbert, J. Hand Surg. 7:118-124, 1982.)

Toe transfers appear to fare better when the digital loss is due to congenital constriction ring syndrome since there is normal architecture of the remaining portion of the hand. In digital aplasia there can be hypoplasia, aplasia, and deformities of the remaining vessels, tendons, and nerves in the hand. Patients with total aplasia of the digits where the transferred toe sits in an isolated fashion above the palm exhibit the worst functional results.

The aesthetic results of transfer are reasonably satisfactory provided there is careful patient selection. For complete absence of the thumb, pollicization of the index finger is the procedure of choice.

Trauma

Fingertip Injuries Loss of portions of the fingertip due to crushing injuries is common in childhood. The long finger is most frequently involved, followed by the index finger. There are several modalities for treatment of lost fingertips. Split-thickness skin grafting is the usual procedure. Many local flaps including Kutler's lateral flaps and the Atasoy-Kleinert volar advancement flap are used for transverse and dorsally oblique amputations. The need for more distant flap coverage is unusual. Wound healing by secondary intention with frequent dressing changes has become another accepted method of treatment. It is reported that although nonoperative treatment necessitates an additional 2 or 3 weeks for satisfactory healing, there is no need for general anesthesia or hospitalization. The procedure is also much more convenient. In one series, the cosmetic appearance of the fingertip, and, more importantly, the return of two-point discrimination was best with this method. In view of the considerable time and expense involved in more elaborate management of fingertip injuries in children, nonoperative treatment with dressing changes and healing by secondary intention would appear to be the procedure of choice.

Fractures Fractures of the phalanges are not always without problems. Distal phalanx fractures are the most common. Epiphyseal fractures are most frequently the Salter-Harris type II and are most prevalent among the 10 to 14 year old age group. Most of these fractures occur at the base of the proximal phalanx of the fingers and thumb. Remodeling of fractures of the base of the proximal phalanx in the dorsal-volar plane as well as in the lateral plane can be expected. Rotational deformities do not correct by remodeling. Fractures at the base of the middle phalanx tend to remodel better in the dorsal-volar plane; therefore, lateral angulation cannot be accepted.

An interesting childhood fracture is the longitudinal splitting fracture, usually caused by a crushing injury. It is often minimally displaced and does well with early mobilization.

Shaft fractures of the phalanx are the most difficult to manage, and in children the most common type is a transverse fracture through the neck of the phalanx. Since there is not an epiphysis at the distal end of the phalanx, the potential for remodeling is limited, and accurate anatomical reduction should be achieved.

Although fractures of the scaphoid are considered rare in children and adolescents, a series of 147 scaphoid fractures in a 14-year period has been reported. Almost all fractures were located in the distal one-third of the scaphoid, and approximately one-half of these were so-called avulsion fractures of the distal pole. This particular fracture seems unique to children. Fractures through the waist were less common and those of the proximal pole were extremely rare. All fractures united with plaster immobilization, usually a short arm thumb spica cast, for a period of 4 to 8 weeks. Three missed fractures healed with a period of immobilization from 7 to 16 weeks.

Diagnosis of avulsion fractures of the distal pole of the scaphoid may be difficult without oblique projections. These fractures, however, have no great clinical significance because of their rapid healing. Although nonunion is possible in children, the vast majority of fractures of the scaphoid appear to heal satisfactorily.

Replantation in Children Replantation of amputated parts in children is frequently successful and has been accomplished in patients as young as 13 months. Because of generally better return of sensibility and motion in children, the indications for replantation are less restrictive than in the adult. Isolated amputation of a finger, even proximal to the superficialis insertion, should be considered for replantation if the conditions of the wound and amputated part are suitable.

As expected, guillotine amputations and those with a limited crushing component tend to have a better rate of survival of the part (average 72 percent) as compared to avulsion injuries (average 62 percent). A few studies have noted a decreased success rate in children, and others have found no difference from adult patients. As with most highly technical procedures, the success rate increases with experience.

Most children with replantation can be expected to regain two-point discrimination of less than 10 mm. Range of motion may be normal, but some stiffness is usually present. Secondary procedures are often necessary and commonly are directed at reconstructing the flexor tendon system. Growth of the replanted part has been found to be normal or slightly delayed in most patients. There may be some delay or cessation of growth in the immediate area of the amputation site.

Replantation of major limbs can have potentially fatal metabolic consequences. Careful monitoring of the fluid and acid-base status of these patients is necessary, and preventive measures should include adequate transfusions and infusion of bicarbonate when appropriate.

Juvenile Rheumatoid Arthritis

The types of deformities and problems occurring in the hand of the child with juvenile rheumatoid arthritis (JRA) differ significantly from the adult with rheumatoid arthritis. Unlike adults in whom volar subluxation and dislocation and loss of extension of the metacarpophalangeal joints are often seen, children with JRA usually have loss of flexion and develop radial deviation. Volar subluxation and ulnar deviation are unusual. At the proximal interphalangeal joint, lack of flexion as a result of proliferative synovitis is the most common deformity. Distal interphalangeal joint involvement also is seen and is manifested by synovitis and a mild flexion contracture. Involvement of the wrist, with loss of extension being the most common deformity, occurs in approximately 25 percent of patients. Ankylosis of the joints of the wrist (particularly the carpometacarpal joints) is more frequent in the juvenile than the adult with rheumatoid arthritis.

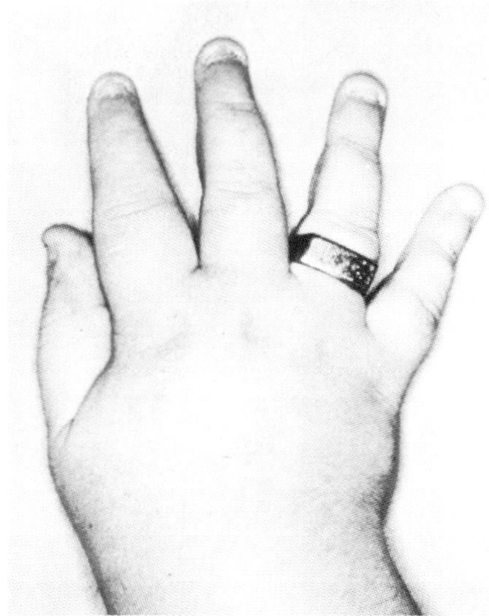

Figure 10: The hand in juvenile rheumatoid arthritis commonly has ulnar deviation of the wrist and radial deviation of the metacarpophalangeal joints. (Reprinted with permission from The hand in the child with juvenile rheumatoid arthritis, by W.M. Granberry, et al., J. Hand Surg. 5:105-113, 1980.)

Wrist ulnar deviation averaging 13 degrees is also seen. This may contribute to the radial deviation deformities at the metacarpophalangeal joints (Fig. 10). Ulnar shortening averaging 4 mm is also very common.

Surgical procedures are not often indicated for JRA. Although tenosynovitis occurs, tenosynovectomy is very infrequent except, occasionally, to correct triggering of the flexor tendons in the palm. Synovectomy does not seem to improve function and often leads to more stiffness. Severe loss of flexion at the joints, particularly the metacarpophalangeal, can be treated successfully with capsu-

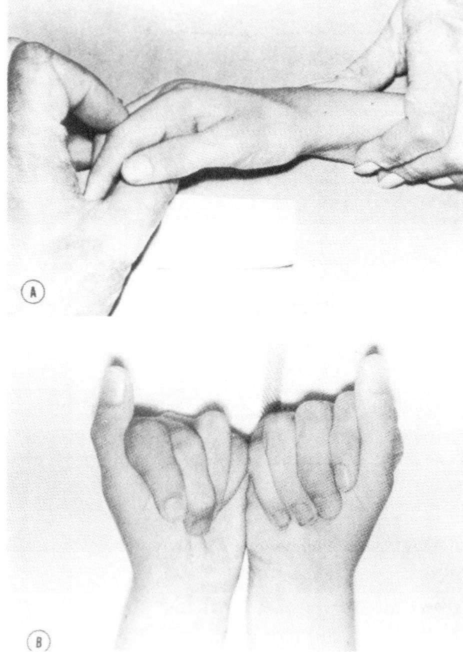

Figure 11: (A) Lack of flexion of the metacarpophalangeal joints is common in JRA. (B) Flexion can be restored by capsulotomies and collateral ligament releases. (Reprinted with permission from The hand in the child with juvenile rheumatoid arthritis, by W.M. Granberry, et al., J. Hand Surg. 5:105-113, 1980.)

Figure 12-A

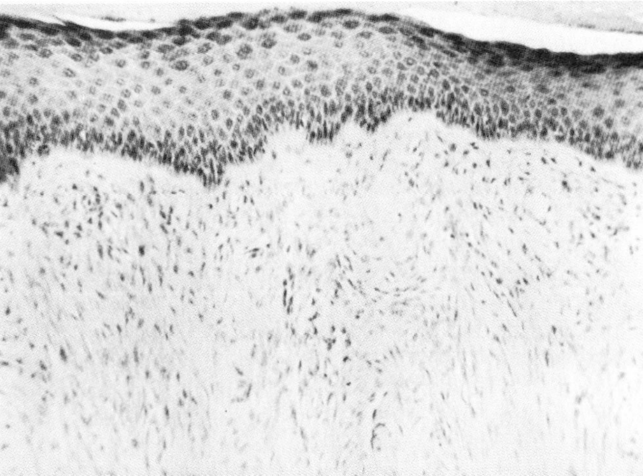

Figure 12-B

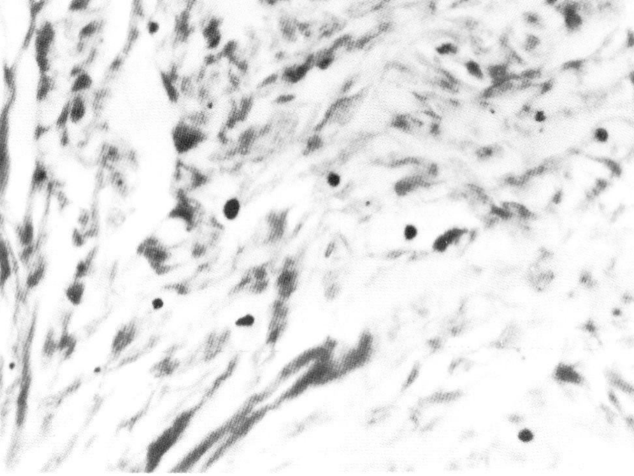

Figure 12-C

Figure 12: (A) Multiple recurring digital fibrous tumors of childhood are seen on the right hand. (B) Microscopic section (180X) demonstrates fusiform fibroblasts and collagen bundles forming the intradermal growths. (C) Intracytoplasmic inclusion bodies are diagnostic (600X). (Reprinted with permission from Recurring digital fibrous tumor of childhood, by R.J. Cosky, et al., Cutis 23:359-362, 1979.)

lotomy and collateral ligament release (Fig. 11).

The most typical combination of deformities in JRA is loss of wrist extension, ulnar deviation at the wrist, and loss of flexion at the MP and PIP joints. Careful follow-up of these patients for early detection of these problems and correction with splinting and therapy is encouraged.

Neuromuscular

Cerebral Palsy The varying degrees of spasticity, sensibility, and voluntary control in cerebral palsy make reconstructive surgery a complex undertaking. Several factors need to be carefully evaluated preoperatively in considering patients for surgery. Patients with the spastic type of cerebral palsy are most amenable to surgical correction. Patients with extrapyramidal or dystonic forms, including athetosis, are poor surgical candidates. A profound lack of mental ability, speech, vision, and hearing defects, as well as behavioral problems, may compromise the postoperative rehabilitation program and thus necessitate considerably simplified goals for surgery. Patients with hemiplegia seem to do much better than those with quadriplegia. Two common patterns of involvement in the hand are an imbalance of the flexors and extensors of the wrist and fingers and assorted degrees of adduction and flexion deformities of the thumb. These problems may all coexist to varying degrees. Successful correction of deformities in the hand is reported in patients as young as 18 months of age. Earlier surgical correction of many of these deformities, in addition to early therapy and splinting, should be considered.

Wrist and Finger Imbalance Imbalance of flexion and extension of the wrist and fingers can be categorized into three groups with group 1 having minimal flexion spasticity (usually the flexor carpi ulnaris, FCU) and the ability to extend the fingers completely with the wrist in neutral or less than 20 degrees of flexion. Group 2 patients are able to extend the fingers but only with more than 20 degrees of wrist flexion. Spasticity is located in the wrist and finger flexor muscles, and an important factor is whether or not the patient can extend the wrist actively with the fingers flexed. In group 3 there is severe spasticity of all flexor muscles with paralysis of the extensor muscles and inability to extend the fingers, even with maximal wrist flexion.

The choice of reconstructive procedures is dependent upon the severity of involvement. For group 1 patients, tenotomy of the FCU with partial release of the origin of the flexor pronator mass is sufficient. In group 2 patients, which are the most common, two procedures have been recommended to improve wrist and finger positioning. For relatively mild deformities, a transfer of either the FCU or the brachioradialis (BR) into the radial wrist extensors can provide satisfactory results. It is reported that transfer of the BR into the extensor carpi radialis brevis with tenotomy or lengthening of the FCU is the best combination of procedures. An alternative method recently has been reported and involves transfer of the FCU through the interosseous membrane into the extensor carpi radialis associated with an aponeurotic release of the medial epicondyle muscles. Long-term results are pending. In group 3 patients the goal should be to improve the basic positioning of the hand to enhance appearance and hygiene.

Thumb Deformities These can be classified into four types. Type I the most common deformity, is an isolated metacarpal adduction contracture, typically due to spasticity of the adductor pollicis and possibly the first dorsal interosseous. Secondary contracture of the skin of the first web can occur. Type II is metacarpal adduction and metacarpophalangeal (MP) flexion due to involvement of both the adductor pollicis and flexor pollicis brevis. Type

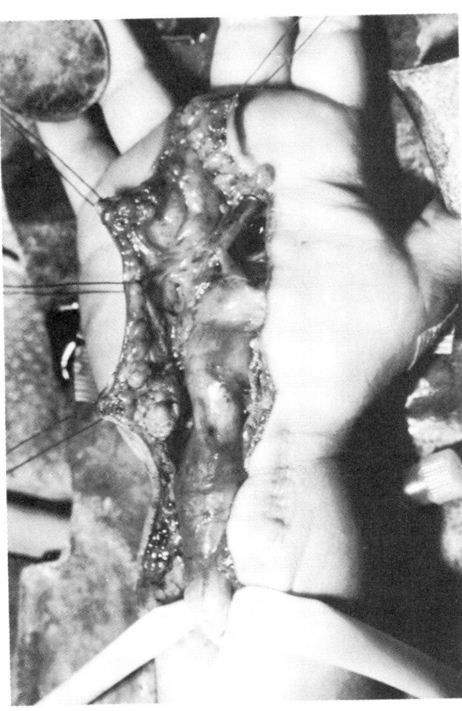

Figure 13: A lipofibromatous hamartoma of the median nerve and its terminal branches is seen in a 3-year-old female who presented with pain in the hand. The enlarged nerve is flattened in the carpal tunnel. Decompression relieved her symptoms.

III is metacarpal adduction and MP hyperextension or instability due to compensatory overactivity of the extensor pollicis longus. Type IV is metacarpal adduction and MP and IP flexion from spasticity of the flexor pollicis longus in addition to the adductor pollicis.

Reconstruction of thumb deformities needs to be carefully tailored to these multiple factors. Best results are obtained in those patients with good voluntary control and normal or near normal sensibility. Three steps to deformity correction involve release of contractures of skin and spastic muscles, augmentation of weak muscles, and joint stabilization.

Tumors

Recurrent Digital Fibrous Tumor Recurring digital fibrous tumor of childhood is benign, appears on the digits of the hands or feet and is characterized by one or more circumscribed reddish pink nodules (Fig. 12A). These tumors typically appear in the first year of life in both sexes.

The lesion histologically consists of whorls of spindle cells and fibrous tissue which may extend into the subcutaneous tissue (Fig. 12B). Characteristically, there are intracytoplasmic inclusion bodies 3 to 10 μ in diameter (Fig. 12C). Special staining techniques are usually necessary as the inclusion bodies are difficult to see with standard hematoxylin-eosin stains.

Treatment of this benign condition is nonoperative. If functional impairment develops, surgical excision may become necessary. Recurrence following excision is approximately 60 percent and may prove to be problematic. A few patients have undergone spontaneous remission, which indicates allowing a period of observation.

Lipofibromatous Hamartoma of the Median Nerve This rare, benign tumor usually involves the median nerve or its terminal branches in the palm but may develop in the ulnar nerve. It usually presents as a painless, enlarging soft-tissue mass in the palm or wrist. This tumor also is associated with macrodactyly. Presenting symptoms of pain and numbness are due to compression of the median nerve in the carpal tunnel (Fig. 13).

The tumor, confined to the epineural sheath, is usually yellow, firm, thick, and very difficult to dissect from the normal nerve fibers which it intimately surrounds. Due to its appearance early in life, it is probably developmental or congenital in origin. The tumor most appropriately is classified as a hamartoma because it is composed of normal cell types found in the peripheral nerve but in abnormal proportions. It should be distinguished from a lipoma which is a well-circumscribed mass, easily separable from the nerve.

Since the tumor is benign, a nonoperative approach to its management seems warranted. If suspected or when discovered during surgical exploration, the best procedure seems to be minimal biopsy and release of all overlying fascia and the transverse carpal ligament. Some patients experience diminution in tumor size following surgical decompression. Continued growth of the mass after carpal tunnel release has been very unusual. Some reports recommend microsurgical excision of the fat and fibrous tissue with preservation of the nerve, but this is a time-consuming procedure with considerable chance of neural function loss. Other reports suggest radical excision of all involved nerve, but considering the benign natural course, this seems more than necessary.

ANNOTATED BIBLIOGRAPHY

Congenital Deformities

Classification

Swanson, A.B.: A classification for congenital limb malformations. J. Hand Surg. 1:8-22, 1976.

A classification system, widely adopted throughout the world for categorizing congenital limb malformations, is described that is based upon recognizable patterns of embryological failure.

Syndactyly

Toledo, L.C., and Ger, E.: Evaluation of the operative treatment of syndactyly. J. Hand Surg. 4:556-564, 1979.

Sixty-one patients with 176 surgically treated webs are reported. Average follow-up is 14 years. Recurrence of web and contractures of fingers are usually associated with use of split-thickness skin grafts and straight incisions to release the web. Treatment before age 18 months and of complex syndactyly frequently requires subsequent operations.

Polydactyly

Miura, T.: Duplicated thumb. Plast. Reconstr. Surg. 69:470-479, 1982.

A review of seventy-seven hands with duplicated thumbs stresses the importance of proper incisional placement, ligament reconstruction, reinsertion of intrinsic muscles, preservation of neurovascular bundles, modification of extrinsic tendon insertions, and osteotomy when indicated at the time of thumb ablation.

Wood, V.E.: Polydactyly and the triphalangeal thumb. J. Hand Surg. 3:436-444, 1978.

A modification of Wassel's classification is proposed. Early treatment, preferably by excision of the radial digit, is emphasized. Multiple procedures, including ligament reconstruction, osteotomy, excision of delta phalanx, and first web widening are required.

Congenital Constriction Rings

Moses, J.M.; Flatt, A.E.; and Cooper, R.R.: Annular constricting bands. J. Bone Joint Surg. 61A:562-565, 1979.

Forty-five patients with average follow-up of 15.8 years are reported. Most were first pregnancies of young mothers. Other anomalies, usually of the hand, were common. Neural deficits (23 percent) and circulatory compromise (16 percent) were noted, usually with proximal limb bands. Staged excision and Z-plasty is the procedure of choice when surgery is indicated.

Clinodactyly

Burke, F., and Flatt, A.: Clinodactyly. A review of a series of cases. Hand 11:269-280, 1979.

Six of fifty patients needed surgery for functional and cosmetic problems. Early reverse wedge osteotomy for delta phalanges and late closing-wedge osteotomy for brachymesophalangism is preferred.

Congenital Central Hand Deficiency

Nutt, J.N., III, and Flatt, A.E.: Congenital central hand deficit. J. Hand Surg. 6:48-60, 1981.

A classification system is proposed. A sporadic anomaly with only hand involvement and a familial disorder with associated central foot deficits are seen. Surgical decisions are based upon the classification system. Hand function cannot be predicted from the anatomy present.

Congenital Absence of Digits

Gilbert, A.: Toe transfers for congenital hand defects. J. Hand Surg. 7:118-124, 1982.

Microvascular transfer of twenty-one second toes in seventeen patients without vascular failure is reported. Active motion is limited and function depends on mobility of the metacarpal remnant. Normal growth of the transfer is documented. Results are better in amniotic band amputations than in aplasia.

Goldberg, N.H., and Watson, H.K.: Composite toe (phalanx and epiphysis) transfers in the reconstruction of the aphalangic hand. J. Hand Surg. 7:454-459, 1982.

Toe phalanges with intact periosteum and without vascular supply are placed into soft-tissue pouches to reconstruct thirty-six digits. Ninety percent of normal growth is documented when open epiphyses are preserved (90 percent operated less than 18 months of age, 50 percent when 5 to 13 years).

Matev, I.B.: Thumb reconstruction in children through metacarpal lengthening. Plast. Reconstr. Surg. 64:665-669, 1979.

Seven patients between 10 and 14 years had thumb metacarpal lengthening of 2.5 to 3.8 cm. Spontaneous consolidation of the metacarpal is noted after 2 to 3 months' immobilization. The technique requires a nearly complete metacarpal and a cooperative patient for success.

Trauma

Fingertip Injuries

Das, S.K., and Brown, H.G.: Management of lost finger tips in children. Hand 10:16-27, 1978.

A comparison of split-thickness skin grafts, local digital flaps, and healing by secondary intention is made. While taking longer to heal by the nonoperative method, there is better cosmetic appearance, less nail deformity, improved sensibility, and more convenience to all involved.

Fractures

Barton, N.J.: Fractures of the phalanges of the hand in children. Hand 11:134-143, 1979.

Crush injuries produce a longitudinal splitting fracture unique to children. Epiphyseal fractures of the proximal phalanx are common and remodel in all planes except rotation. Fractures of the neck of the proximal and middle phalanges require anatomic reduction.

Vahvanen, V., and Westerlund, M.: Fracture of the carpal scaphoid in children: A clinical and roentgenological study of 108 cases. Acta Orthop. Scand. 51:909-913, 1980.

Distal pole fractures predominate, and an avulsion fracture of the distal pole is seen in 42.5 percent, a configuration apparently unique to children. All fractures heal with immobilization.

Replantation

Jaeger, S.H.; Tsai, T.; and Kleinert, H.E.: Upper extremity replantation in children. Orthop. Clin. North America 12:897-907, 1981.

Sixty replantations in forty-one patients under 16 years of age have an overall survival rate of 85 percent. Guillotine amputations have the best survival and return of function. Avulsion injuries have 74 percent survival with some good results. Growth is an "all-or-none" phenomenon.

O'Brien, B.M.; Franklin, J.D.; Morrison, W.A.; and Macleod, A.M.: Replantation and revascularisation surgery in children. Hand 12:12-24, 1980.

Thirty-five completely and incompletely severed parts including a foot and a leg are reported. Minimal growth retardation is observed when well revascularized. Overall survival is 64.5 percent. Bone shortening should be minimized.

Juvenile Rheumatoid Arthritis

Granberry, W.M., and Mangum, G.L.: The hand in the child with juvenile rheumatoid arthritis. J. Hand Surg. 5:105-113, 1980.

Ulnar deviation and loss of extension of the wrist are frequent. Radial deviation and extension contractures of the metacarpophalangeal joints are characteristic of this disease. Treatment should consist of splinting and therapy; surgery is rarely indicated.

Cerebral Palsy

House, J.H., and Gwathmey, F.W.: Flexor carpi ulnaris and the brachioradialis as a wrist extension transfer in cerebral palsy. Minn. Med. 61:481-484, 1978.

Transfer of the brachioradialis to the radial wrist extensors in addition to tenotomy or lengthening of the flexor carpi ulnaris has produced the best quality of wrist control.

House, J.H.; Gwathmey, F.W.; and Fidler, M.O.: A dynamic approach to the thumb-in-palm deformity in cerebral palsy. J. Bone Joint Surg. 63A:216-225, 1981.

A step-wise approach to the correction of this deformity is described, and the results of surgery are presented. The quality of voluntary muscle control and sensibility are the most important factors predicting the success of surgery. All fifty-six patients have improved function.

Zancolli, E.A., and Zancolli, E.J.: Surgical management of the hemiplegic spastic hand in cerebral palsy. Surg. Clin. North America 61:395-406, 1981.

A thorough discussion of the preoperative evaluation, classification, and surgical treatment of a wide variety of spastic deformities of the hand and wrist is presented.

Tumors

Recurrent Digital Fibrous Tumor

Coskey, R.J.; Nabai, H.; and Rahbari, H.: Recurring digital fibrous tumor of childhood. Cutis 23:359-362, 1979.

A report of two patients and a review of this distinct benign fibrous tumor of childhood are presented. Recurrence is common following excision. Spontaneous regression may occur. Cytoplasmic inclusion bodies are diagnostic.

Lipofibromatous Hamartoma

Patel, M.E.; Silver, J.W.; Lipton, D.E.; and Pearlman, H.S.: Lipofibroma of the median nerve in the palm and digits of the hand. J. Bone Joint Surg. 61A:393-397, 1979.

A discussion of this unusual neural tumor, including etiology, mode of presentation, histology, and treatment is presented. Limited incisional biopsy and carpal tunnel release is the recommended treatment.

21 WRIST AND HAND: TRAUMA

Subjects covered in this section include flexor tendon injuries, posttraumatic carpal instability, and microvascular repair.

Hand

Digital Tip Injuries It has long been appreciated that digital tip injuries in children heal remarkably well when allowed to heal by secondary intention. Recent work indicates that digital tip injuries in adults with no bone exposed also heal quite satisfactorily when treated nonoperatively (Fig. 1). In one series the method used was sterile dressing changes and sulfadiazine occlusive dressings until healing occurred. The results were best with crushing injuries and those involving only soft tissues or the distal one-third of the fingernail. In certain situations, primary repair is preferred, but judgment and experience are required.

Nail Bed Injuries Injuries to the nail bed are extremely common and may lead to unsightly deformities that may be distressing to the patient. The most prevalent injury of this sort is the car door injury. Fracture of the distal phalanx with damage to the nail matrix and a disruption of the overlying nail plate form the typical triad of this type of injury (Fig. 2). Recent anatomical study of the nail bed has documented that much of the deformity following untreated nail bed injuries may be prevented by proper surgical treatment at the time of the incident. Reapproximation of the nail matrix with fine, absorbable sutures is the most important step in the treatment which also includes thorough cleansing and reduction of the fracture and repair or replacement of the nail into the nail fold. This program is effective in lessening nail deformities.

Flexor Tendon Injuries Injuries to the flexor tendons of the fingers and thumb may be divided, according to one author, into five different zones: Zone 1 involves the area distal to the superficialis insertion; zone 2 includes the area distal to the MP joint of the thumb or between the A1 pulley (arising from the volar plate of the MP joint) and the superficialis insertion in the fingers; zone 3 involves the portion of the flexor pollicis longus proximal to the A1 pulley of the thumb and between the transverse carpal ligament and the A1 pulley of the finger; zone 4 is the area of the carpal tunnel; and zone 5 is the area proximal to the transverse carpal ligament.

Many factors, including the nature and location of the injury and the patient's motivation, affect the results following flexor tendon repairs. Historically, the area of zone 2, or "no man's land," has been the most unpredictable in achieving satisfactory functional results.

The blood supply to the flexor tendons in the digital sheaths is through a series of vincula that approach the flexor tendons on their dorsal surface and transmit blood vessels arising from the appropriate digital arteries. Microangiographic visualization of these vessels demonstrates the blood supply to the flexor tendons is more abundant on the dorsal surface of the tendons than on the

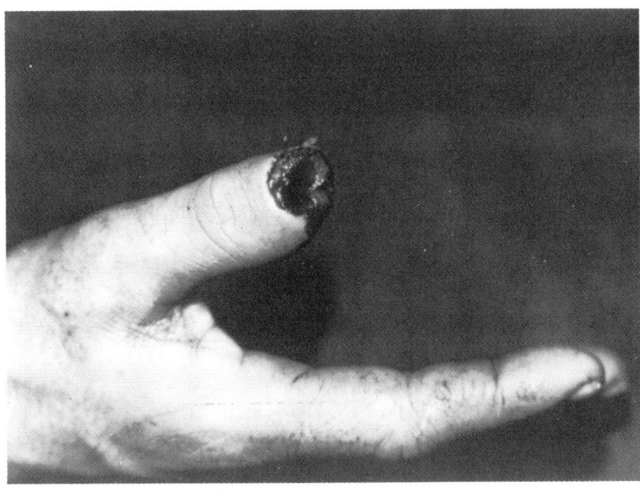

Figure 1-A

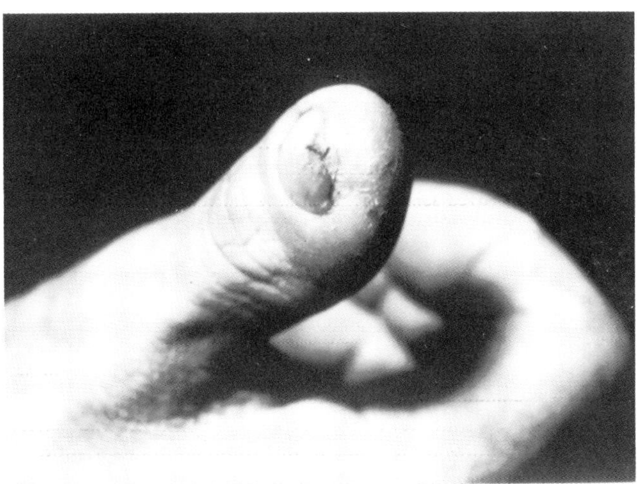

Figure 1-B

Figure 1: (A) Thumb tip cut off in a power saw injury is allowed to heal by secondary intention with frequent dressing changes. (B) Four and one-half years after the open treatment of the injury. The tip of the thumb has recontoured and is not painful.

Figure 2-A

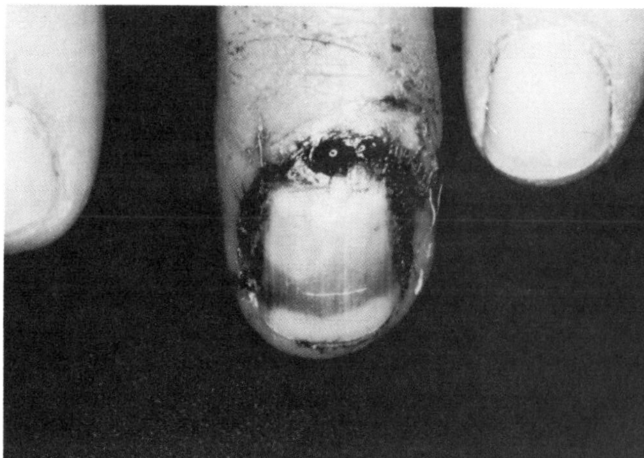

Figure 2-B

Figure 2: (A) A typical car door fingertip injury with a fracture of the distal phalanx, injury to the nail matrix, and avulsion of the nail plate out of the eponychial fold. (B) Ten days following treatment of this injury. Fracture was thoroughly irrigated and reduced, the nail matrix was repaired utilizing 6-0 absorbable suture, and the nail was replaced in the nail fold after it had been thoroughly cleansed. This method of management lessens late nail deformities.

volar surface. In addition, there is some evidence indicating that the volar aspects of flexor tendons in the areas of the fibrous digital pulleys may be relatively avascular. Recent studies suggest that the nutrition of the flexor tendons may be dependent upon both direct vascular permeation and diffusion through the synovial fluid.

On this basis, it is advocated that suture placement be in a more volar position within the tendon during flexor tendon repairs so as to be less injurious to the blood supply. It is also suggested that less damage to the vincula occurs if exposure for flexor tendon repair is through a volar zig-zag incision rather than a mid-axial approach. However, this has not been proved nor has it been proved that this approach gives a better result in tendon surgery than a mid-lateral incision.

Several authors have reported their results after secondary or delayed repair of flexor tendons. Secondary tendon repair generally is considered a suitable method of treatment when primary repair is not possible or, for a justifiable reason, could not be accomplished at the time of injury. Repair can be performed up to 3 weeks after injury, but there is some evidence suggesting the result may be better if the repair is accomplished within 6 to 10 days after injury.

Postoperative management programs following repair of flexor tendon injuries currently are being directed toward early (less than 5 days postoperative) passive range of motion of the repaired digit. Established techniques provided for early (3 weeks postoperative) protected active extension of the involved digit to promote passive gliding of the repaired flexor tendon within the fibrous digital sheath. In one recent study it appears that controlled passive motion may be better.

The management of partial tendon lacerations of the digital flexors is controversial, with repair being the usual practice. However, satisfactory results have been reported when repair was not performed and the digit mobilized by active, nonresisted motion beginning 1 week after injury. To avoid triggering, beveled lacerations that will pass under a fibrous flexor sheath should probably be excised if less than 25 percent of the cross-sectional area of the tendon or repaired if larger.

Nerve Injury The possibility of complete restoration of motor and sensory function following peripheral nerve injury and repair in the adult patient seems limited. The advent of microsurgical techniques gives the surgeon an opportunity to appreciate the grossness of nerve repair performed without use of magnification and appropriate instrumentation. When there is no contraindication to doing primary repair (such as severe contamination, extensive crushing, avulsion injuries, or other more serious concomitant problems), it is considered preferable to repair a sharply lacerated peripheral nerve within the first 24 hours following injury. Both epineurial and group fascicular repair are advocated for the management of acute peripheral nerve injuries. To date there is no convincing study that substantiates the superiority of either of these methods; thus many surgeons advocate epineurial repair because it is easier and requires less time.

Joint Injuries

Fracture-Dislocations of the Carpometacarpal Joints Forces directed longitudinally down the length of the metacarpals are believed to be primarily responsible for fractures and dislocations involving the carpometacarpal joints. Because of the deforming pull of the extensor carpi ulnaris, percutaneous pinning or open reduction is considered the treatment of choice for fracture-dislocations of the base of the fifth metacarpal.

Fracture-dislocations involving multiple carpometacarpal joints are usually the result of severe trauma, and these patients may have other serious injuries. Treatment for multiple carpometacarpal dislocations or fracture-dislocations involves some form of internal fixation, usually with multiple Kirschner wires.

Chronic sprains of the carpometacarpal joints have been identified recently as a separate clinical entity and are responsible for a symptom complex consisting of localized pain and weakness of grip. Physical examination following trauma may reveal tenderness over the bases of the metacarpals. Routine radiographs are usually of little value. Trispiral tomography may reveal joint abnormalities. Local injections of lidocaine may help to clarify the diagnosis. The possibility of such an acute injury should be kept in mind so that appropriate early treatment (cast immobilization for 4 weeks) may prevent the development of a chronic symptomatic sprain.

Complex Dislocation of the Metacarpophalangeal Joint Dimpling of the palmar skin at the metacarpophalangeal joint of the affected digit and radiographic distortion of the joint space with or without interposition of a sesamoid are well-recognized clinical findings of complex dislocation of metacarpophalangeal joints. Although this injury may be approached through a volar or dorsal incision, the neurovascular structures frequently are tented over the subcutaneous metacarpal head and are prone to injury when the volar approach is used to reduce the joint dislocation. The dorsal approach, with exposure to the joint accomplished by retraction of the extensor tendons, recently has been advocated. The volar plate is slit longitudinally to accomplish reduction in this approach. Some surgeons routinely use extension block splinting of the finger postoperatively because they believe the result will be better if controlled active motion is permitted immediately after reduction of the dislocation.

Ligamentous Injury to the Metacarpophalangeal Joint of the Thumb Injuries to the ulnar collateral ligament of the thumb are five times more frequent than injuries to the radial collateral ligament. The collateral ligaments of the thumb are lax in full extension or hyperextension and are taut in maximum flexion of the metacarpophalangeal joint. Testing for collateral ligament injuries is best performed with the metacarpophalangeal joint fully flexed (Fig. 3). Radial or ulnar stressing with the metacarpal fixed in extension and the proximal phalanx in flexion will reveal opening of the joint greater than 35 degrees if there is complete disruption of the radial or ulnar collateral ligament. When a ligament is avulsed with or without bony attachment and when the joint opens more than 35 degrees, surgical reattachment of the ligament still is considered the treatment of choice by many surgeons. The surgical finding that the adductor aponeurosis sometimes prevents the ulnar collateral ligament from reapproximating itself to the site of avulsion prompts this approach. Reconstructive efforts with tendon grafting or dynamic transfers yield mixed results.

Proximal Interphalangeal Joint Fractures and dislocations involving the proximal interphalangeal (PIP) joint are some of the most common injuries seen in the hand and may be among the most difficult to treat. The volar plate has strong, dense attachments at its lateral margins both proximally and distally. These lateral attachments distally are confluent with the attachments of the collateral ligament complex. The attachments of the volar plate proximally are confluent with the proximal one-half of the first cruciate pulley that is attached to bone. The distal one-half of the C1 pulley is confluent with the volar plate and the accessory collateral ligaments (Fig. 4). The major central portion of the plate is attached loosely both proximally and distally.

Experimental studies using variable loading rates suggest that during slow loading there is a gradual attenuation of the proximal attachments of the volar plate, whereas a rapid loading rate produces a distal rupture of the lateral distal attachments of the plate. When dislocation of the PIP joint occurs, the line of separation within

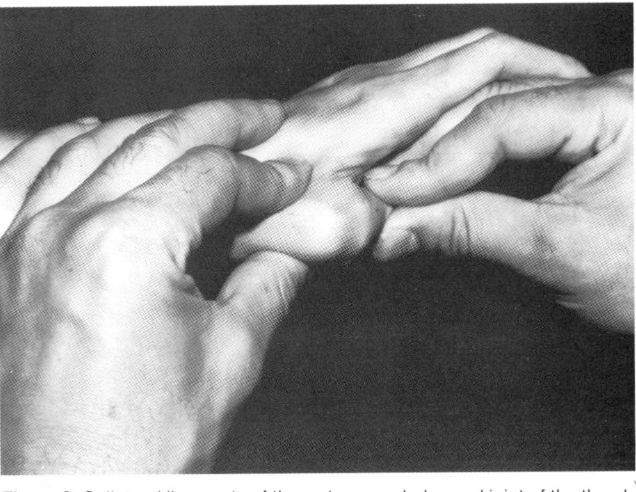

Figure 3: Collateral ligaments of the metacarpophalangeal joint of the thumb are taut in full flexion. Testing for stability of the collateral ligaments of the thumb should be performed as shown. The metacarpal is held in extension, the proximal phalanx is placed in full flexion, and the radial and/or ulnar stresses can be applied, depending upon which ligament is being evaluated. If the ulnar collateral ligament of the thumb is avulsed, the joint can open more than 35 degrees by this maneuver.

the collateral ligament complex is between the proper and the accessory collateral ligament.

Restoration of normal or near normal joint motion and subsequent hand function depends upon recognition of the potential problems associated with fractures and dislocations about the PIP joint. Both late flexion and hyperextension deformities may result from these acute injuries. When stability is in question, a digital block followed by examination is extremely helpful in guiding subsequent treatment. Those injuries that are stable when examined under anesthesia usually do well with a program of early protected motion. When examination under anesthesia reveals an unstable injury, extension block splinting, percutaneous pinning, or open reduction is necessary.

Infections Many street-acquired infections are now resistant to penicillin. As a consequence, cephalosporins are advocated as the initial drug of choice for most infections of the hand prior to specific organism identification and sensitivity testing. *Pasteurella multocida* is a gram-nega-

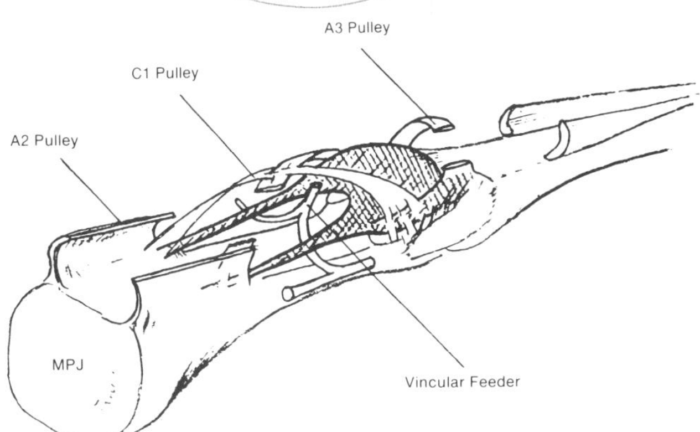

Figure 4: Anatomy of the volar plate of the proximal interphalangeal joint is quite complex. This demonstrates the proximal attachments of the volar plate with its prolonged extensions attaching in confluence with the A2 and C1 pulleys.

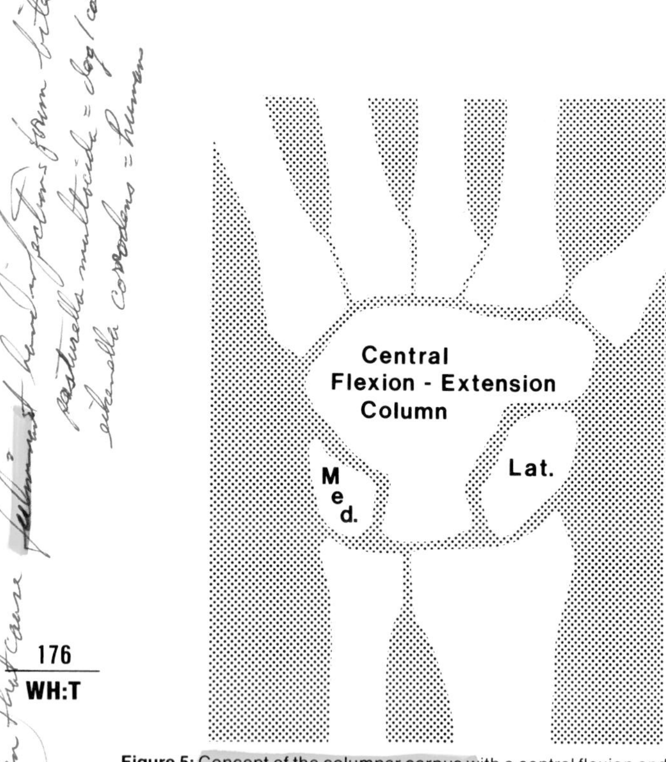

Figure 5: Concept of the columnar carpus with a central flexion and extension column, and medial and lateral rotation columns. This corresponds very closely to the instability patterns that are seen clinically. Disruption between the lateral rotation column and the central flexion-extension column leads to dorsal instability patterns whereas disruption between the medial rotation column and the central flexion-extension column leads to volar instability patterns. (Adapted with permission from Post-traumatic carpal instability, by J. Taleisnik, Clin. Orthop. 149:74, 1980.)

tive rod that is sensitive to penicillin and has been cultured from the oral cavity of up to 70 percent of domestic cats and dogs. It may produce an infection which is fulminating within the first 24 hours with rapid onset of cellulitis, lymphangitis, and purulent drainage. *Eikenella corrodens* is likewise a gram-negative rod that is a primary pathogen in human bite infections of the hand. It is a particularly virulent organism and may cause chronic pyarthrosis and even osteomyelitis. It grows best as a facultative anaerobe and is cultured with increased carbon dioxide tension. It is susceptible to penicillin, and, like *Pasteurella multocida*, appropriate surgical wound management and drainage should be undertaken where indicated. Patients with human bites in which the skin of the hand has been penetrated should be considered for admission to the hospital and receive appropriate antibiotics. One of the family of cephalosporins most closely covers the broad spectrum of organisms likely to be encountered. Thus, selection of a cephalosporin is most appropriate until specific cultural identification and specific sensitivities have been obtained.

Simple hand lacerations probably do not require prophylactic antibiotics; meticulous wound management is satisfactory.

Wrist

Fractures of the Distal Radius One current system of fracture classification divides distal radial fractures into four groups: a type 1 fracture is a nondisplaced extra-articular fracture of the distal radius; a type 2 fracture is not only displaced but also extra-articular; a type 3 fracture is nondisplaced and intra-articular; and a type 4 fracture is displaced and intra-articular.

Although fractures of the distal radius are common, there is no uniform agreement regarding effective methods of treatment. One study reports satisfactory results following functional bracing of displaced distal radius fractures without articular involvement. The results of intra-articular displaced fractures of the distal radius are believed superior in those patients who were functionally braced in supination as compared to those braced in pronation. Recently repopularized, external fixation currently is being modified to allow limited joint motion. One study suggests that functional results correlate best with the adequacy of the initial reduction rather than the position in which immobilization is achieved.

Carpal Fractures

Fractures of the Scaphoid Most often encountered in young male adults, the scaphoid is the most frequently fractured carpal bone. The most common site of fracture is through the scaphoid waist, but horizontal and vertical oblique fractures also may occur. In addition, there are fractures which may involve the tuberosity and are intra-articular, involving the scaphotrapezial joint. Fractures of the proximal and distal poles are the least commonly encountered. An acute fracture of the scaphoid may not be detectable on initial, plain radiographs. Radionuclide imaging is a useful diagnostic technique, and increased local uptake over the scaphoid can be seen as early as 24 hours after trauma.

Plaster immobilization in a short-arm cast including the thumb in a position of palmar abduction is usually sufficient treatment for a nondisplaced scaphoid fracture. Healing time varies considerably depending upon the site of the fracture. Those of the tuberosity and distal pole tend to heal in the shortest time. Fractures of the proximal pole take the longest time to show evidence of radiographic union.

Trapezial Ridge Fractures Fractures of the trapezial ridge are a rare cause of persistent chronic symptoms following a fall on the outstretched hand. The diagnosis is based on clinical examination which shows localized tenderness over the ridge of the trapezium, pain on active wrist flexion against resistance, and radiographic documentation with a carpal tunnel view. Treatment involves

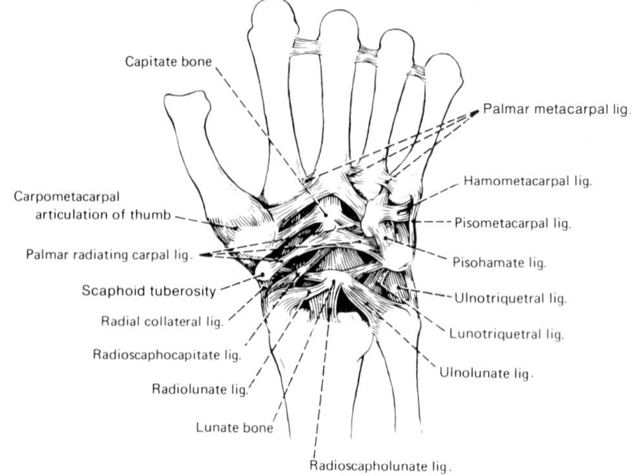

Figure 6: Volar intercarpal ligaments form a complex intertwining network providing stability and normal congruent relationships between the intercarpal bones. Disruption of these ligaments causes various instability patterns.

immobilization until the patient becomes asymptomatic. In some patients, union may not occur, and excision of the avulsed fragment may be necessary.

Scaphocapitate Fractures Fractures involving both the scaphoid and capitate are a well-recognized complex. These appear to result most commonly from severe dorsiflexion injury, but they also may occur with extreme volar flexion. In this circumstance, the proximal pole of the capitate is fractured in conjunction with a fracture through the scaphoid waist. The fragment consisting of the head of the capitate usually rotates at least 180 degrees and loses its proper relationship with the lunate. Attempts at closed reduction of this fracture complex are not successful. The prognosis for function following treatment depends primarily upon the accuracy of the initial reduction as well as the extent of the original trauma.

Posttraumatic Carpal Instability Recent clinical and experimental studies have differentiated recognizable patterns of intercarpal ligamentous disruption from the more commonly recognized patterns of carpal fractures and dislocations and fractures of the distal radioulnar complex. Four patterns of intercarpal instability have been described: dorsal instability is probably the most frequent pattern to occur; volar instability is probably the next most common pattern; ulnar translocation and dorsal carpal subluxation are the least frequent.

An alternate classification is proposed which divides the carpus into three functionally mobile units (Fig. 5). These units are a central intercarpal flexion and extension column, a medial rotation column, and a lateral rotation column. According to this classification, the instability patterns are categorized as central intercarpal, medial, lateral, and proximal radiocarpal.

An intertwining system of ligaments supports the normal congruent relations and complex motions present at the intercarpal, radiocarpal, and radioulnar joints (Fig. 6). Injury to these ligaments leads to radiographically recognizable patterns of intercarpal instability. The normal scapholunate angle averages approximately 45 degrees with a range from 30 to 60 degrees (Fig. 7). With disruption of the ligaments either at the radio-scapholunate area or at the scapho-trapezio-trapezoid area, lateral column instability (dorsal instability) may result (Fig. 8). When there is disruption along the medial rotation column between the lunate and triquetrum or between the triquetrum and the hamate, a medial column (volar instability) pattern may result (Fig. 9). An ulnar translocation instability pattern often is seen as the result of systemic disease, such as rheumatoid arthritis and only rarely is found as a posttraumatic problem. Proximal (dorsal) instability occurring at the radiocarpal level is most often the result of a fracture-dislocation (such as Barton's fracture) or the rare radiocarpal dislocation.

An understanding of the possible forms of intercarpal instability is extremely important for accurate, early diagnosis since most of these injuries are not diagnosed until at least 2 months following the initial injury. At such time the patient may present with pain, limitation of motion, and/or clicking and popping in the wrist. Routine radiographs may not demonstrate any distortion of intercarpal relationships, but several other studies may be useful. Fluoroscopic and cineradiographic studies of radiocarpal and intercarpal motion usually reveal the specific instability pattern. Fist clenching (compression loading) may create a diastasis between the scaphoid and the lunate, as seen in the most common instability pattern (Fig. 10). This dynamic effect also may show instability between the other carpal bones. These motion studies may be stored on videotape and reviewed for further study. In addition, arthrography may be useful in demonstrating

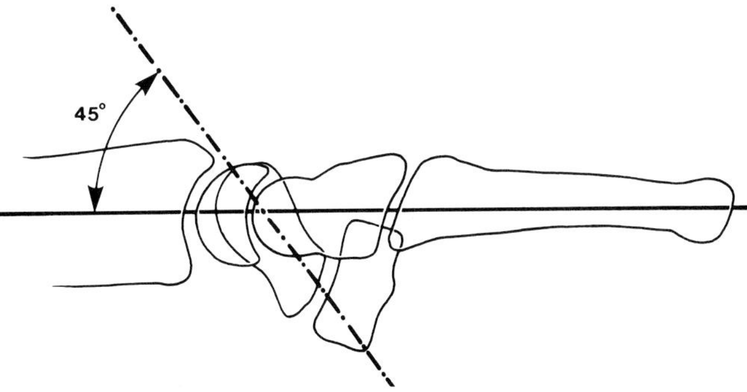

Figure 7: Lateral radiograph of the wrist taken in the neutral position serves as the basis for understanding normal intercarpal relationships. A line drawn through the third metacarpal, the capitate, and the lunate normally should bisect the radius and intersect with a line drawn through the longitudinal axis of the scaphoid at approximately 45 degrees, with the normal range being from 30 to 60 degrees. (Adapted with permission from Traumatic instability of the wrist, by R.L. Linscheid, et al., J. Bone Joint Surg. 54A:1614, 1972.)

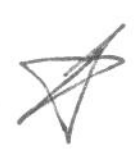

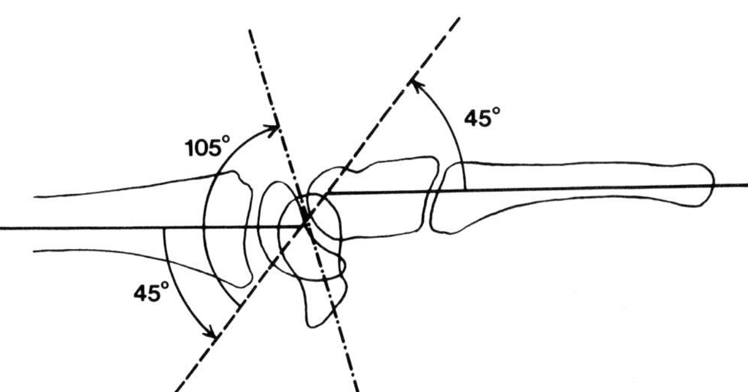

Figure 8: When the dorsiflexion instability pattern occurs, the scaphoid rotates in a volar direction and the lunate rotates in a dorsal direction, so that the scapholunate axis changes markedly and is one of increasing angularity. This angle is 105 degrees. (Adapted with permission from Traumatic instability of the wrist, by R.L. Linscheid, et al., J. Bone Joint Surg. 54A:1615, 1972.)

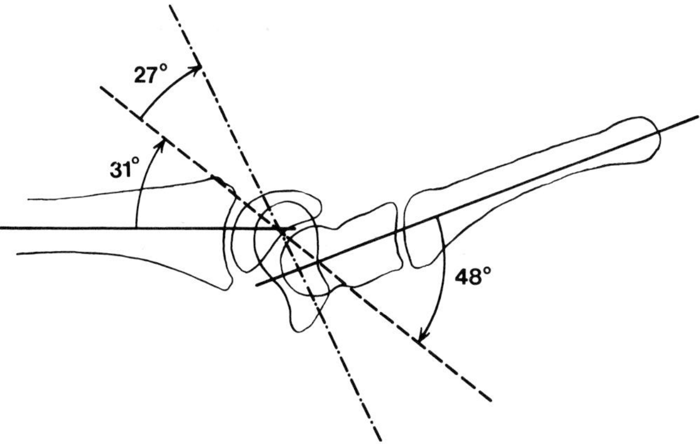

Figure 9: In the volar instability pattern, the distal surface of the lunate rotates in a volar direction and approaches colinearity with the scaphoid axis. This shows decreasing angularity of 27 degrees. (Adapted with permission from Traumatic instability of the wrist, by R.L. Linscheid, et al., J. Bone Joint Surg. 54A:1615, 1972.)

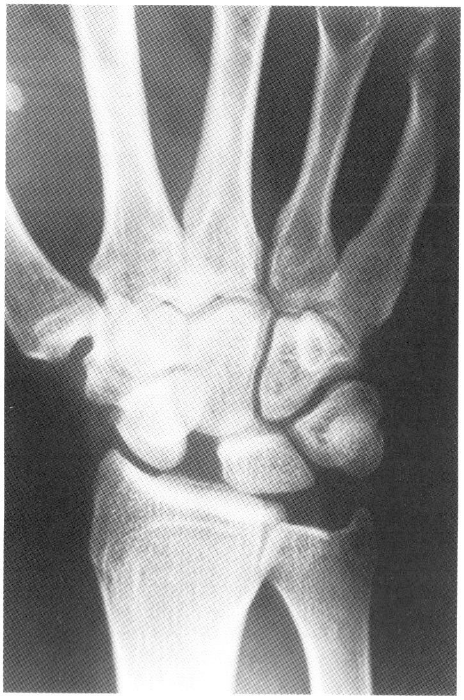

Figure 10: In patients with advanced instability, an anteroposterior radiograph, even without compression, will demonstrate a gap between the scaphoid and the lunate. Normally this distance is not greater than 2 mm. If this diagnosis is suspected but not demonstrable on plain radiographs, fluoroscopic evaluation with compression is useful.

abnormal passage of contrast material in the presence of ligamentous injury (Fig. 11).

When intercarpal instability is identified, acute closed reduction (with or without percutaneous pinning) and cast immobilization for an interval of 6 weeks is the recommended treatment. Earlier recognition and treatment is important because late reconstructive efforts attempting to substitute tendon for ligament have uniformly failed necessitating intercarpal arthrodesis with resultant limitation of wrist motion.

Subluxation of the Extensor Carpi Ulnaris Tendon The extensor carpi ulnaris is restrained in its groove in the distal ulna by a septum that is distinct from the extensor retinaculum. With forced supination, palmar flexion, and ulnar deviation, this ligament may become attenuated so that the tendon may begin to subluxate or dislocate. During pronation of the forearm, the tendon may snap back into its normal position. Subluxation or dislocation of the extensor carpi ulnaris tendon may result from a specific traumatic event or may follow chronic repetitive activities. It also may cause symptoms about the wrist that are initially obscure in their etiology. Reconstruction of the ligament may be effective.

Distal Radioulnar Joint Subluxation Dorsal subluxation is more common than volar and is considered to be the result of a pronation injury. Supination results in reduction, and immobilization in this position for 6 weeks is satisfactory for acute injury. Treatment of chronic subluxation or dislocation is more difficult. The recently described ulnotriquetral augmentation tenodesis with imbrication of the dorsal radioulnar ligament appears to be a reliable method of reconstruction.

Microvascular Surgery

Replantation During the past decade replantation of amputated parts has become a frequent surgical procedure. Long-term follow-up studies show that tissue survival is not synonymous with function, and the results of replantation have narrowed the indications for these procedures. Individual factors may modify the general indications for replantation.

Sharp and clean amputations generally are better suited to replantation than crushing or avulsing injuries. The following are the indications for replantation: (1) any sharp or clean amputation of the thumb may be replanted regardless of the patient's age; (2) except for the thumb, end results do not warrant replantation of a single amputated digit; (3) amputation of multiple digits on the same hand or both hands is an indication for attempted replantation of as many digits as possible; and (4) amputation through the midpalm or of the entire hand is an indication for replantation.

With improved surgical technique, replantation of amputations distal to the proximal interphalangeal joint not only are possible but also yield good functional results in selected patients.

Microvascular Management of Ring Avulsion Injuries Use of microvascular techniques for management of ring avulsion injuries is a logical extension of this surgical technique. One classification of ring avulsion injuries divides them into three types. Type 1 is associated with adequate circulation. Treatment for these injuries is by the usual soft-tissue management. Type 2 includes those

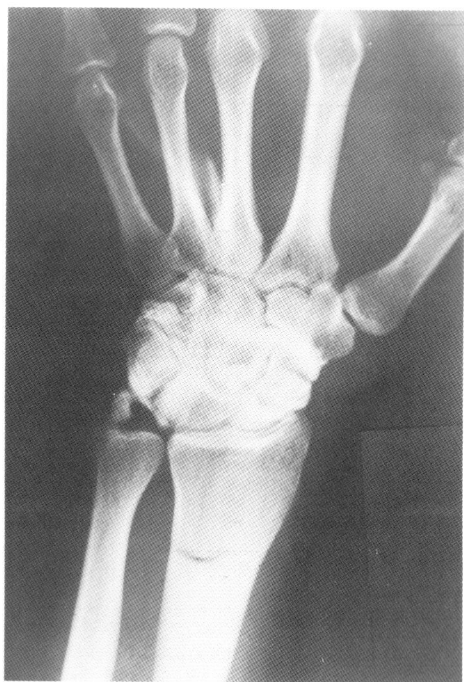

Figure 11: Arthrography may be useful when intercarpal ligamentous disruption is suspected; however, it is not always diagnostic. Normally dye injected into the radiocarpal joint will not flow into the radioulnar joint or into the intercarpal areas. This example shows dye dispersed through the intercarpal ligaments, indicating a ligamentous tear. In this example, the tear is between the triquetrum and the lunate. When the arthrogram is performed, it is useful to monitor the injection under fluoroscopy to watch the pattern of dye flow since radiographs taken after the dye is dispersed may not identify the site of abnormal dye passage.

injuries where the circulation is inadequate, either on the arterial side, the venous side, or both, and where the digit is still in physical continuity with the remainder of the hand. It is possible to have a digit devascularized by a ring injury without disruption of the skin. It is, therefore, important to evaluate thoroughly the circulatory status of a digit injured by a ring. These injuries are managed by microvascular techniques to reestablish satisfactory circulation to the digit. Type 3 injuries are those in which the finger has been either completely amputated or degloved. In this group, although technically possible, replantation usually is not performed because the functional results have been poor.

ANNOTATED BIBLIOGRAPHY

Hand

Digital Tip Injuries

Chow, S.P., and Ho, E.: Open treatment of fingertip injuries in adults. J. Hand Surg. 7:470-476, 1982.

One hundred fingertip injuries greater than 1.0 cm^2 in area were treated by initial cleansing and dressing change until healing was complete. The healing time was 2 to 9 weeks. Except for a 27 percent incidence of nail deformity, there were few complications.

Nail Bed Injuries

Zook, E.G.; Van Beek, A.L.; Russell, R.C.; and Beatty, M.E.: Anatomy and physiology of the perionychium: A review of the literature and anatomic study. J. Hand Surg. 5:528-536, 1980.

This is an anatomical description of the growth and development of the nail. Attention to anatomical factors important in the repair of nail bed injuries is emphasized as the best way to prevent late nail deformity following injury.

Flexor Tendon Injuries

Ejeskär, A.: Flexor tendon repair in no man's land. II. Early versus late secondary tendon repair ad modum Kleinert. Scand. J. Plast. Reconstr. Surg. 14:274-283, 1980.

Delayed repair of flexor tendon injuries in zone II is comparable to primary repair when done within the first 4 weeks after injury. When repair is delayed beyond this point, the results rapidly deteriorate.

Matev, I.; Karagancheva, S.; Trichkova, P.; and Tsekov, P.: Delayed primary suture of flexor tendons cut in the digital theca. Hand 12:158-162, 1980.

The results of delayed primary flexor tendon repair are comparable to primary repair with 70 percent good to excellent results when repair is performed within 6 days of injury.

McClinton, M.A.; Curtis, R.M.; and Wilgis, E.F.S.: One hundred tendon grafts for isolated flexor digitorum profundus injuries. J. Hand Surg. 7:224-229, 1982.

A one-stage repair in which the graft motor was mobilized to gain 30 mm passive motion and the graft almost always placed around the superficialis tendon decussation was utilized. Satisfactory results were obtained in eighty-three of the ninety-six patients and were not affected by patient age. Patient motivation and surgical experience appear to be directly correlated with the results.

Strickland, J.W., and Glogovac, S.V.: Digital function following flexor tendon repair in zone II: A comparison of immobilization and controlled passive motion technique. J. Hand Surg. 5:537-543, 1980.

Twenty-five patients were treated by each technique and the results, based on return of motion at the proximal and distal interphalangeal joints, were excellent or good in 12 percent treated by immobilization and 56 percent in those treated by controlled passive motion. Rupture occurred in 16 percent and 4 percent, respectively. When only those with both profundus and sublimus repair were compared, the excellent and good results were 6 percent and 53 percent respectively.

Wray, R.E., Jr., and Weeks, P.M.: Treatment of partial tendon lacerations. Hand 12:163-166, 1980.

Twenty-six patients with thirty-four partial flexor tendon lacerations varying between 25 and 95 percent of the cross-sectional area were managed by not suturing and active nonresisted motion beginning 1 week after injury. Twenty-four patients obtained satisfactory results, no tendons ruptured, and one trigger finger resolved spontaneously.

Nerve Injury

Braun, R.M.: Epineurial nerve suture. Clin. Orthop. 163:50-56, 1982.

The rationale and techniques of epineurial nerve suture are reviewed.

Gaul, J.S., Jr.: Intrinsic motor recovery: A long-term study of ulnar nerve repair. J. Hand Surg. 7:502-508, 1982.

Forty-one of sixty-five patients were available for study 1 to 6 years after epineurial suture. Young patients with low lesions did best. Older patients with low lesions rarely showed intrinsic recovery at 1 year but often did 2½ to 6 years after repair.

Urbaniak, J.R.: Fascicular nerve suture. Clin. Orthop. 163:57-64, 1982.

The pertinent anatomy, physiology, and surgical technique for peripheral nerve suture are presented with emphasis on fascicular technique.

Joint Injuries

Fracture-Dislocations of the Carpometacarpal Joints

Joseph, R.B.; Linscheid, R.L.; Dobyns, J.H.; and Bryan, R.S.: Chronic sprains of the carpometacarpal joints. J. Hand Surg. 6:172-180, 1981.

The relatively rigid second and third joints are usually involved. Acute sprains respond to casting, and chronic sprains with minimal symptoms respond to steroid injection and splinting and casting. The results in twenty-seven of twenty-eight patients with disabling chronic symptoms treated by arthrodesis were satisfactory.

Complex Dislocations of the Metacarpophalangeal Joint

Bohart, P.G.; Gelberman, R.H.; Vandell, R.F.; and Salamon, P.B.: Complex dislocations of the metacarpophalangeal joint. Operative reduction by Farabeuf's dorsal incision. Clin. Orthop. 164:208-210, 1982.

Dorsal exposure for reduction of complex dislocations is advocated.

Gamekeeper's Thumb

Palmer, A.K., and Louis, D.S.: Assessing ulnar instability of the metacarpophalangeal joint of the thumb. J. Hand Surg. 3:542-546, 1978.

An anatomical and biomechanical study of the stabilization of the MP joint of the thumb. Emphasis is upon testing the MP joint in full flexion to determine the presence of ligamentous injury.

Proximal Interphalangeal Joint

Bowers, W.H.: The proximal interphalangeal joint volar plate. II: A clinical study of hyperextension injury. J. Hand Surg. 6:77-82, 1981.

This suggests that volar plate rupture from its distal attachment is the result of hyperextension injuries at the PIP joint.

Bowers, W.H.; Wolf, J.W.; Nehil, J.L.; and Bittinger, S.: The proximal interphalangeal joint volar plate. I. An anatomical and biomechanical study. J. Hand Surg. 5:79-88, 1980.

The anatomy of this important joint is reviewed with emphasis on the variability of the volar plate attachments to adjacent structures. The biomechanical study suggests that the site of volar plate injury is dependent upon the rate of application of load.

Infections

Arons, M.S.; Fernando, L.; and Polayes, I.M.: *Pasteurella multocida*—The major cause of hand infections following domestic animal bites. J. Hand Surg. 7:47-52, 1982.

The gram-negative coccobacillus, *Pasteurella multocida*, may be a primary pathogen in hand infections caused by cat or dog bites. This organism leads to a fulminating infection within 24 hours of injury. It is sensitive to penicillin.

Grossman, J.A.I.; Adams, J.P.; and Kunec, J.: Prophylactic

antibiotics in simple hand lacerations. J. Am. Med. Assn. 245:1055-1056, 1981.

The incidence of infection (three patients of 265) did not appear to be altered by prophylactic antibiotics, thus making them unnecessary and no substitute for meticulous wound management.

Wrist

Fractures of the Distal Radius

Cooney, W.P., III; Dobyns, J.H.; and Linscheid, R.L.: Complications of Colles' fractures. J. Bone Joint Surg. 62A:613-619, 1980.

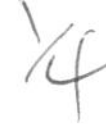

One hundred twenty-eight of 565 patients had at least one serious complication. Complications seemed to be most frequently associated with incomplete restoration of radial length, secondary loss of reduction position, and reduction under local anesthesia.

Engkvist, O., and Lundborg, G.: Rupture of the extensor pollicis longus tendon after fracture of the lower end of the radius: A clinical and microangiographic study. Hand 11:76-86, 1979.

The portion of the tendon passing around Lister's tubercle was demonstrated to be poorly vascularized, suggesting a vascular (nutritional) rather than a mechanical etiology of rupture. Early mobilization of the thumb may facilitate the nutrition of this tendon portion.

Van Der Linden, W., and Ericson, R.: Colles' fracture: How should its displacement be measured and how should it be immobilized? J. Bone Joint Surg. 63A:1285-1288, 1981.

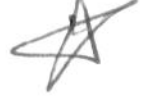

This study suggests that anatomic reduction is more important in determining final results than the method used to obtain reduction.

Carpal Fractures

Ganel, A.; Engel, J.; Oster, Z.; and Farine, I.: Bone scanning in the assessment of fractures of the scaphoid. J. Hand Surg. 4:540-543, 1979.

The bone scan between 24 and 72 hours after injury was a helpful adjunct in determining which patients had fractures when conventional radiography was equivocal. The test appears to be very specific as no fracture occurred in thirty patients with positive clinical symptoms but negative bone scans.

Palmer, A.K.: Trapezial ridge fractures. J. Hand Surg. 6:561-564, 1981.

Fractures of the trapezial ridge are rare and the diagnosis is frequently delayed. Localized tenderness over the trapezium should be followed by a carpal tunnel view.

Rand, J.A.; Linscheid, R.L.; and Dobyns, J.H.: Capitate fractures: A long-term follow-up. Clin. Orthop. 165:209-216, 1982.

Fractures of the capitate should be reduced anatomically, with open reduction if necessary, to ensure the best functional result.

Posttraumatic Carpal Instability

Mayfield, J.K.; Johnson, R.P.; and Kilcoyne, R.K.: Carpal dislocations: Pathomechanics and progressive perilunar instability. J. Hand Surg. 5:226-241, 1980.

This spectrum of injuries was studied by loading thirty-two cadaver wrists to failure. The injury mechanism was extension, ulnar deviation, and intercarpal supination. Scapholunate diastasis was the least severe and lunate dislocation the most severe perilunar instability.

Taleisnik, J.: Posttraumatic carpal instability. Clin. Orthop. 149:73-82, 1980.

In this review of the history, anatomy, pathomechanics, and clinical patterns of carpal instability, the concept of columnar carpus is proposed.

Extensor Carpi Ulnaris Subluxation

Eckhardt, W.A., and Palmer, A.K.: Recurrent dislocation of extensor carpi ulnaris tendon. J. Hand Surg. 6:629-631, 1981.

Four patients are presented as well as anatomic dissection to show separate ECU tendon sheath from the extensor retinaculum. A repair is suggested.

Distal Radioulnar Joint Subluxation

Hui, F.C., and Linscheid, R.L.: Ulnotriquetral augmentation tenodesis: A reconstructive procedure for dorsal subluxation of the distal radioulnar joint. J. Hand Surg. 7:230-236, 1982.

Eight patients were satisfactorily reconstructed utilizing this procedure. In addition to tenodesis, the forearm is fixed in supination by Kirschner wire transfixion at the distal ulna and the ulna and dorsal radiocarpal ligament is imbricated tightly.

Microvascular Surgery

Replantation and Microvascular Surgery

Tamai, S.: Twenty years' experience of limb replantation. Review of 293 upper extremity replants. J. Hand Surg. 7:549-556, 1982.

A review of indications, contraindications, and results during a 16-year period by one of the pioneers of the technique of microvascular surgery.

Urbaniak, J.R.; Evans, J.P.; and Bright, D.S.: Microvascular management of ring avulsion injuries. J. Hand Surg. 6:25-30, 1981.

A classification of ring avulsion injuries is proposed. A follow-up on those injuries treated by microsurgical technique reveals that many more useful digits are salvaged.

22 WRIST AND HAND: RECONSTRUCTION

Topics covered in this section include arthroplasties of the proximal interphalangeal, thumb carpometacarpal, and wrist joints; tendon transfers; carpal tunnel syndrome; thumb reconstructions; Dupuytren's contracture; the triangular fibrocartilage complex; limited wrist arthrodesis; and Kienböck's disease.

Hand

Proximal Interphalangeal Joint Arthroplasty Volar plate advancement hemiarthroplasty has proved effective for acute and chronic fracture-dislocations of the PIP joint. This difficult procedure is indicated when there is disruption of the volar articular surface of the middle phalanx. Technical aspects of the procedure are diagrammed in Figure 1. Postoperatively a functional range of motion and pain relief can be anticipated in most patients.

The most extensively used PIP joint arthroplasty is the silicone rubber implant arthroplasty (Swanson). In a recent report on 100 posttraumatic patients with an average follow-up of 7.4 months, more than 95 percent had relief of pain while obtaining a 43 degree arc of motion. A common complication was extension lag. Less common complications included infection, persistent pain, lateral instability, prosthetic fracture, and bone erosion. Because of the short follow-up and complications, this procedure continues to be relatively contraindicated in young patients and in the index finger PIP joint.

With the exception of a flexible rubber-titanium core implant currently being tested, all cemented PIP joint arthroplasties have proved unsatisfactory and have been withdrawn from use.

Metacarpophalangeal Arthroplasty Presently, the Silastic rubber arthroplasty is the most popular procedure for replacement of the metacarpophalangeal joint. Concurrent soft-tissue surgeries, such as collateral ligament reconstruction, ulnar intrinsic releases, synovectomy, and extensor tendon centralization, remain important adjuncts to this procedure. Currently, clinical trials with a new cemented flexible rubber-titanium core implant and another noncemented carbon prosthesis are being conducted, but long-term follow-up of a large series is not yet available.

Thumb Carpometacarpal Joint Arthroplasty When thumb carpometacarpal arthritis is restricted to the trapeziometacarpal joint, the surgical alternatives are arthrodesis or hemiarthroplasty. Arthrodesis remains an acceptable procedure in young patients who expect to do heavy labor. Some limitation of motion (such as inability to flatten the hand) and occasional nonunions can be anticipated. The silicone concave condylar hemiarthroplasty (Swanson) for arthritis restricted to the trapeziometacarpal joint is a relatively new procedure. This prosthesis requires minimal bone resection. Stabilization does not appear to be as difficult as it is after total trapezial silicone replacement. However, long-term follow-up studies are not available.

Unfortunately, many patients with basal joint arthritis have pantrapezial arthritis which makes the choice of surgical treatment more difficult and controversial. The options are trapezial resection arthroplasty with a silicone spacer, trapezial resection arthroplasty with tendon interposition, or cemented total joint arthroplasty with metal and polyethylene components.

Trapezial resection arthroplasty with a silicone spacer is the most frequently performed procedure. It gives adequate range of motion, improves grip and pinch strength, and relieves pain in most patients. Potential complications include radial nerve injury, infection, subluxation, and dislocation. In early reports the dislocation rate approached 25 percent. The following recent surgical modifications have significantly reduced the dislocation rate: K-wire fixation, suturing the prosthesis to the scaphoid, tendon reinforcement of the capsule, partial resection of the trapezoid, and/or stabilization of the prosthesis by passing a slip of the abductor pollicis longus through a preformed hole in the implant (Fig. 2). Correction of associated metacarpophalangeal joint hyperextension, abductor pollicis longus advancements, and release of associated adductor contractures may also be needed to reduce the likelihood of dislocation.

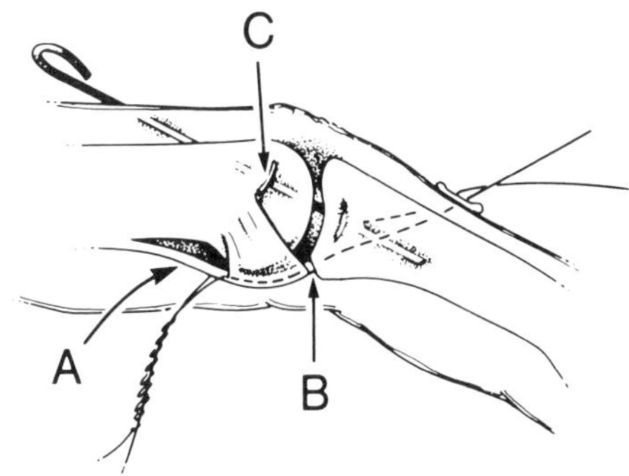

Figure 1: Volar advancement hemiarthroplasty technique. (A) Proximal edges of fibrous volar plate released with preservation of central vascular tissue. (B) Fracture fragments excised and trough made in volar base of middle phalanx. Trough must have a constant depth to prevent postoperative angulation. Volar plate held in place with pull-out wire. (C) Joint temporarily immobilized by a K-wire in no more than 35 degrees flexion. In reconstructions, collateral ligaments are excised.

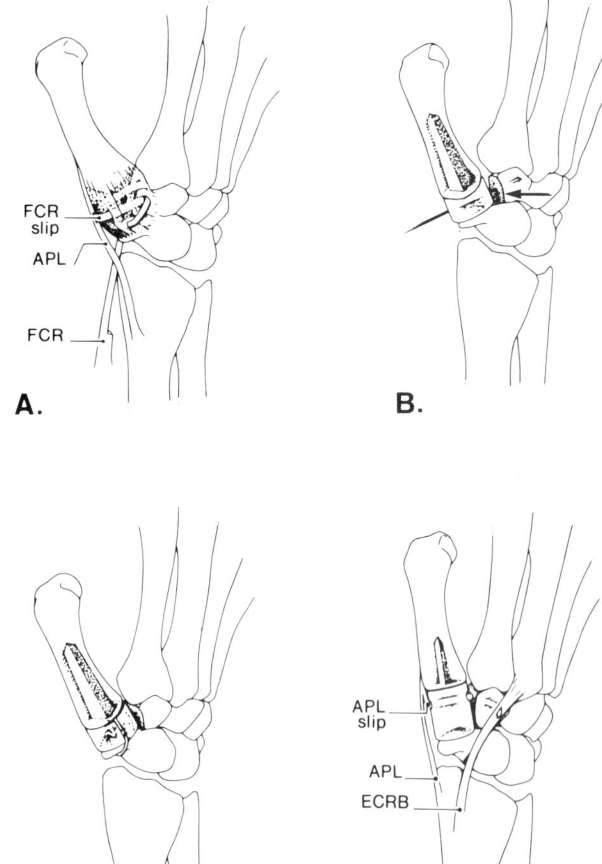

Figure 2: Silicone spacer stabilization. (A) Flexor carpi radialis slip (FCR slip) provides tendinous reinforcement of capsule. Abductor pollicis longus (APL). (B) Temporary K-wire percutaneous fixation and partial resection of trapezoid (arrow). (C) Prosthesis sutured to scaphoid tuberosity. (D) Slip of the abductor pollicis longus (APL slip) is passed through a preformed hole in the prosthesis, into the trapezoid and sutured to the extensor carpi radialis brevis (ECRB).

Trapezial resection arthroplasty with tendon interposition also results in satisfactory preservation of motion, relief of pain, and increased grip and pinch strength. Complications include infection, radial nerve injury, and, occasionally, de Quervain's tenosynovitis. There also may be a slight shortening of the thumb, but this does not represent a significant functional loss. With these arthroplasties it has not been necessary to simultaneously correct thumb MP joint hyperextension or release adduction contractures. A recent report compared trapezial resection arthroplasties with silicone spacers to those with tendon interposition. No statistically significant differences in the grip and pinch strength, range of motion, or pain relief were found. It was concluded that trapeziectomy, with or without silicone spacers, could be expected to give similar and satisfactory results.

Cemented total joint replacements of the thumb carpometacarpal joint have not been uniformly successful. Although long-term follow-up of these procedures is not available, early reports indicate that loosening and bone erosion remain significant problems.

Tendon Transfers Although based on a small number of specimens, a recent study represented the first biomechanical data on forearm and hand muscles that may be of practical use in planning tendon transfers. A list of the mechanical characteristics of all hand and forearm muscles was compiled: muscle mass, average muscle fiber length, and total cross-sectional area of all fibers. The mass is proportional to the work capacity, the average fiber length is proportional to the potential excursion, and the total cross-sectional area is proportional to the maximum tension (tension fraction). Muscles with similar fiber lengths have similar excursion capacities whereas muscles of similar cross-sectional areas have similar force potential.

The persistence of inadequate thumb opposition after nerve repair and in association with peripheral nerve disorders is a common reason for reconstructive tendon transfers. After elimination of contractures, successful opponensplasties require motors that have adequate potential force, potential excursion, and the ability to provide short flexion action in addition to opposition. Without restoration of short flexion action, a collapsing, unstable thumb can develop.

The extensor pollicis longus opponensplasty fulfills these criteria even in patients with progressive disease and high median and combined median and ulnar nerve palsies. In this procedure the normal secondary actions of the extensor pollicis longus, which cause a thumb adduction supination deformity in the paralytic hand, can be combined with thumb MP arthrodesis and extensor pollicis longus transfer to provide a functional opponensplasty (Fig. 3). This transfer provides pronation and abduction of the thumb and satisfactory power. Functioning flexor pollicis longus and extensor pollicis brevis muscles are required. Patients cannot flatten their hands after this procedure, and the refined motion of some other opponensplasties is not obtainable.

An extensor pollicis brevis displacement opponensplasty is another new procedure that may be useful in combined median and ulnar nerve lesions. The extensor pollicis brevis is released from the first dorsal compartment, displaced ulnarly, and relocated in the carpal canal which is also opened through the same incision. Once the extensor brevis has been displaced into the tunnel, the flexor retinaculum is resutured to provide a pulley. Be-

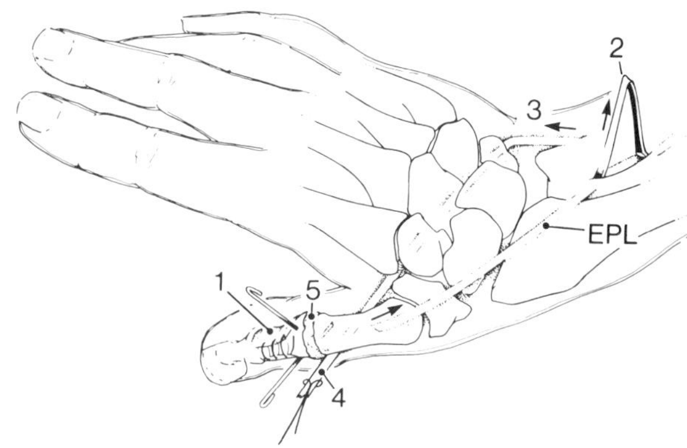

Figure 3: Extensor pollicis longus (EPL) opponensplasty. (1) EPL excised from central portion of extensor hood with remaining intrinsic components sutured. (2) EPL withdrawal into a second incision over dorsal forearm. (3) EPL rerouted subcutaneously around ulnar aspect of wrist and across volar surface of the hand. (4) End of EPL emerging from lateral subcutaneous tunnel. Tendon to be sutured to dorsum of MP joint. (5) MP joint arthrodesis with K-wire fixation.

EIP then Hubert are 1st & 2nd choice

cause neither the origin nor the insertion of the extensor pollicis brevis is divided, early motion is allowed, retraining of the transferred tendon is easy, and satisfactory thumb opposition is obtained quickly.

Previous assessment of opponensplasties has been rather subjective because it is difficult to quantitate the rotation of the thumb as it passes through its 360 degrees arc of motion. A clinically useful technique allowing quantitation of opposition has been described. The abduction axis of the thumb is multiplied by the length of the extension-flexion axis of the thumb and then divided by twice the length of the thumb metacarpal. In the normal hand, this ratio should be approximately one. After an opponensplasty, the ratio will only approach one; therefore, the result can be expressed as a percentage of the anticipated normal.

Carpal Tunnel Syndrome The pathogenesis of carpal tunnel syndrome remains unclear, but localized nerve ischemia probably is a major etiological factor. In a study of normal patients, Wick catheter carpal tunnel pressures averaged 2.5 mm Hg. If external pressure increased this to 30 mm Hg, patients experienced paresthesias. In patients with carpal tunnel syndrome, pressures averaged 32 mm Hg but immediately fell to normal after carpal tunnel release. The localized ischemia hypothesis also correlates with intraoperative conduction studies demonstrating an immediate reduction in prolonged distal latencies after carpal tunnel release.

It is not unusual to find an increased incidence of cervical arthritis and diabetes in patients with carpal tunnel syndrome. The phenomenon of the "double-crush" syndrome has been suggested as an explanation for this association (Fig. 4). In this syndrome a partial proximal compression or a "sick neuron" interferes with axoplasmic flow, thus making the distal nerve more susceptible to compression. It has been shown that this syndrome is present in patients with combined carpal tunnel syndrome and cervical arthritis or diabetes. Patients with carpal tunnel syndrome and the double-crush syndrome have less predictable results following carpal tunnel release than those with carpal tunnel compression alone. Finally, carpal tunnel syndrome is not related to thoracic outlet neurovascular compression, and the combination of these two syndromes does not represent an example of the double-crush phenomenon.

Surgical release of the carpal tunnel remains the most consistently successful treatment of this syndrome. However, some have suggested that carpal tunnel syndrome represents a vitamin B_6 deficiency and that prolonged vitamin B_6 treatment will relieve paresthesias and pain. Other investigators have tried to substantiate this in patients with carpal tunnel syndrome and diabetes, but they have found no evidence of vitamin B_6 deficiencies.

Carpal tunnel syndrome also can be treated by a combination of cortisone injection and splinting. After injection, it has been shown that only 40 percent of mildly symptomatic patients will be symptomfree at the end of 12 months.

Thumb Reconstruction *Pollicization* is indicated in selected patients with traumatic loss of the thumb. An injured digit, a partially amputated digit, or a normal digit can be pollicized in a posttraumatic situation. Pollicization provides stability, length, sensibility, strength, independent motion, and acceptable cosmetic result. Disadvantages include loss of a normal finger, narrowing of the hand, and, in adults, the frequent failure of cerebral reeducation to identify the pollicized digit as a thumb. Additionally, pollicization is technically demanding, and the risk of digit loss always exists. Prior to pollicization, pedicle flaps should be applied if excessive scarring or inadequate skin cover is present in the stump area. If there is any question of previous vascular injury, preoperative angiograms are indicated. In posttraumatic situations, secondary procedures after pollicization, such as tenolysis, may be necessary.

Metacarpal lengthening is an excellent method for regaining thumb function after amputation at the metacarpophalangeal joint level. Prerequisites include good stump skin coverage and a cooperative patient who can participate with the complicated elongation procedure. The thumb metacarpal can be lengthened 2 to 4 cm. Secondary bone grafting of the created gap is usually necessary. The additional length improves grasp and maximizes the use of the existing sensibility. Recent technical refinements have increased the reliability of the procedure.

Osteoplastic reconstruction of the thumb generally is defined as a bone graft covered by a tube pedicle flap. Microsurgical advancements have allowed the develop-

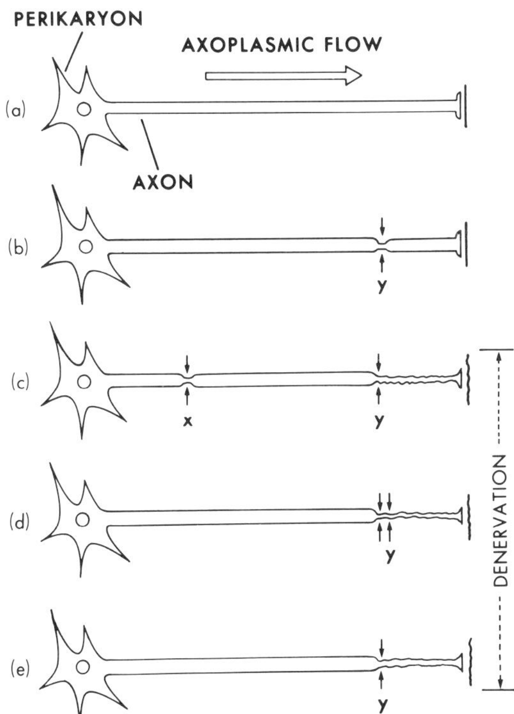

Figure 4: "Double-crush" syndrome. (a) Normal neuron. (b) Partial distal compression (y) without denervation. (c) Partial proximal compression (x) with partial distal compression (y) results in denervation. (d) Severe distal compression (y) with resulting denervation. (e) "Sick" neuron secondary to diabetes with partial distal compression results in denervation. (Redrawn with permission from The double-crush in nerve entrapment syndromes, by A.R.M. Upton, et al., Lancet II:361, 1973.)

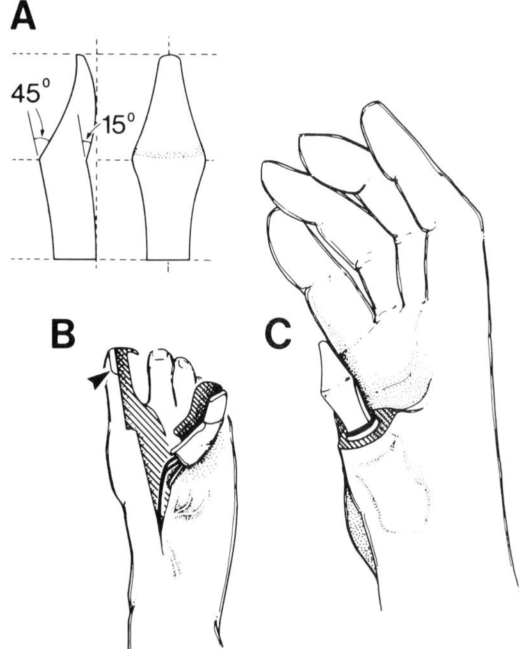

Figure 5: Free neurovascular wrap-around flap from the big toe. (A) An iliac-crest bone graft is shaped to look like a combined distal and proximal phalanx. (B) Toe flap is elevated with dorsal vessels and nerves. Toe distal phalanx shortened. The donor site coverage is from local flaps, skin grafts, and crosstoe flap. (C) Graft arthrodesed to remaining portion of thumb phalanx. Wrap-around flap covers graft.

ment of the newest osteoplastic technique, called a neurovascular "wrap-around" flap from the big toe. This procedure provides a more aesthetically acceptable thumb and decreases the donor site morbidity. The flap uses an iliac graft for internal support. The medial plantar nerves are sutured to the thumb digital nerves, and the deep peroneal nerve is sutured to the radial sensory nerve. The dorsal vein is anastomosed to the cephalic vein, and the dorsalis pedis artery is anastomosed to the radial artery or to the princeps pollicis artery (Fig. 5). This procedure is technically demanding, and there is some resulting limitation of motion because joints are not reconstructed.

Dupuytren's Contracture Recently, the pathogenesis of Dupuytren's contracture has been studied extensively. The Dupuytren's nodules contain large numbers of modulated fibroblasts called myofibroblasts. These cells have ultrastructural properties similar to smooth muscle cells including intercellular contractile myofilaments which are driven by an ATPase energy system. Nodular myofibroblasts are attached to each other by tight junctions. In addition, they are attached to each other and the surrounding collagen by glycosaminoglycan macromolecules. Predicted residual postsurgical contracture and recurrence appear to be related to the numbers of nodular myofibroblasts present (Fig. 6).

Scanning electron microscopy has demonstrated that collagen in Dupuytren's contracture occurs in a helical formation with a shortened wave length. Biochemical analysis has revealed increased amounts of type III collagen and of reducible cross-links indicating immature collagen. Previous histological studies of the grossly uninvolved aponeurotic tissue have shown findings consistent with normal fascia. However, biochemical analysis of the uninvolved aponeurotic collagen has revealed biochemical changes that are qualitatively identical to those in the diseased portions of the aponeurosis. These biochemical abnormalities may account for the relatively high rate of recurrence after surgical excision of the visibly affected area. Despite these findings, present treatment of this disorder remains partial fasciectomy because of the higher morbidity associated with total fasciectomies.

The appropriate treatment of Dupuytren's contracture and coexistent carpal tunnel syndrome recently has been studied. Combined carpal tunnel release and partial fasciectomy for Dupuytren's contracture cause compromised long-term results. Poor results can be avoided by treating the Dupuytren's contracture surgically while treating the carpal tunnel syndrome nonoperatively. If carpal tunnel syndrome symptoms persist, subsequent separate operative intervention is recommended.

Wrist

Anatomy—Triangular Fibrocartilage Complex (TFCC) The triangular fibrocartilage complex consists of the triangular fibrocartilage (articular disc), meniscus homologue (lunocarpal meniscus), ulnar collateral ligament, dorsal radioulnar ligament, volar radioulnar ligament, and sheath of the extensor carpi ulnaris (Fig. 7). The TFCC arises from the ulnar aspect of the lunate fossa of the radius and inserts on the caput ulnae and base of the ulnar styloid. Additional insertions occur on the triquetrum, hamate, and base of the fifth metacarpal. Volarly, the strongest attachment is to the lunotriquetral interosseous ligament and the triquetrum.

The TFCC contains a consistent perforation ulnarly and volarly that extends into the prestyloid recess. A perforation in the central horizontal portion also occurs in 53 percent of specimens. A large proportion of these perforated triangular fibrocartilage complexes are associated with ulnolunate abutment, lunotriquetral ligament tears, and ulna-neutral or ulna-plus variants. Although perforations of this complex do not cause painful instability, the associated ulnolunate abutment syndrome can be painful because of ulnar cartilage erosion and malacia.

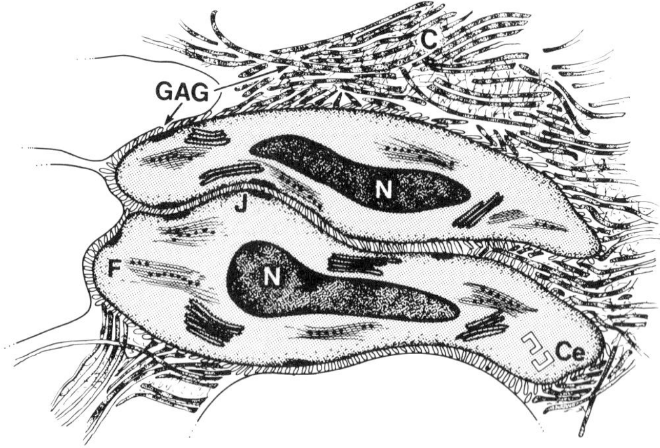

Figure 6: Schematic nodular myofibroblasts of Dupuytren's contracture showing myofibroblasts' ultrastructural relationship to surrounding collagen. Myofilaments with ATPase reaction precipitate (F), collagen (C), junction membrane complex (J), glycosaminoglycans (GAG, arrows), centrioles (CE), and nucleus (N). (Reprinted with permission from The pathogenesis of Dupuytren's contracture: Contractile mechanisms of the myofibroblasts, by M.A. Badalamente, et al., J. Hand Surg. 8:241, 1983.)

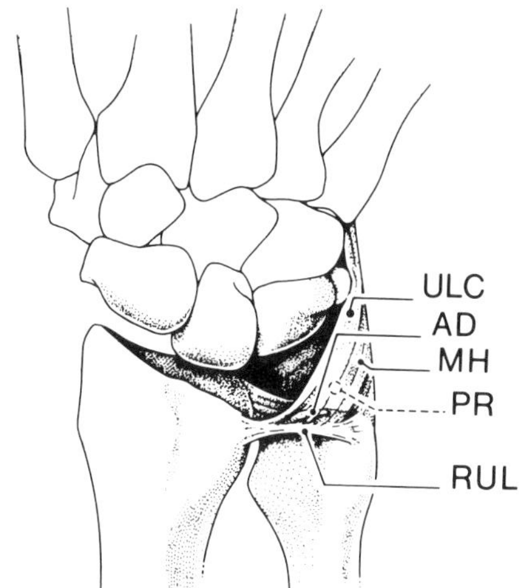

Figure 7: Triangular fibrocartilage complex (TFCC): the ulnar collateral ligament (UCL), the articular disc (AD), the meniscus homologue (MH), the prestyloid recess (PR), and the radioulnar ligaments (RUL). The extensor sheath is not shown.

The TFCC has important biomechanical implications. In normal loading, the radius bears 60 percent of the axial load and the ulna 40 percent. However, when the cushioning effect and force transmitting effect of the TFCC are removed by excision, the radius carries 95 percent of the axial load. The TFCC is also the major stabilizer of the distal radioulnar joint. Its excision results in complete instability of this joint.

Wrist Arthroplasty Patients with severe rheumatoid arthritis are the most frequent candidates for wrist arthroplasty because they generally have bilateral disease and compromise of other upper extremity joints. Arthrodesis does relieve pain, but in these handicapped patients the loss of motion severely interferes with their eating, personal hygiene, and other activities of daily living. In addition to preserving motion, arthroplasty augments grip and pinch strength by preserving the tenodesis effect.

There are two types of wrist arthroplasties available: a flexible silicone interposition prosthesis (Fig. 8) and a cemented metal-on-plastic total wrist prosthesis.

In rheumatoid patients, the silicone rubber arthroplasty (Swanson) usually provides a flexion-extension arc of approximately 60 degrees and relief of pain. Increased strength should not be expected, but correction of deformity, preservation of motion, and decreased pain result in improved hand function. In patients with one wrist arthrodesis and one wrist arthroplasty, the majority preferred the side with the wrist arthroplasty, citing the improved hand function. The long-term results in patients with progressive disease are not known.

Complications after silicone rubber arthroplasties have included skin slough, superficial infection, late attritional extensor tendon ruptures, and a small but significant number of prosthetic fractures even with the new high-performance material. Persistent ulnar deviation and postoperative carpal tunnel syndromes have not been a problem. If needed, revision to wrist arthrodesis is not difficult because minimal bone has been resected. This prosthesis should be considered part of a wrist reconstruction which also includes synovectomy, capsuloligamentous repair, tendon transfer, and tendon repair.

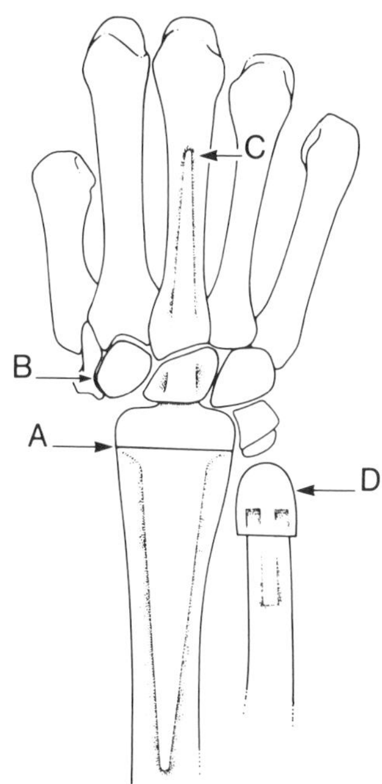

Figure 8: Swanson flexible silicone interposition prosthesis. (A) Distal radius squared off and the proximal carpal row is partially resected. (B) Trapezial-trapezoid joint is preserved. (C) Distal stem passes through the capitate and into the third metacarpal. Distal stem must be shortened if metacarpophalangeal arthroplasties are anticipated. (D) Swanson ulnar head implant is usually inserted during the same procedure.

A trunion-type, 3-part ball-and-socket joint (Meuli) is a cemented total wrist prosthesis. It must be carefully centered to prevent postoperative ulnar deviation. During implantation, the prosthetic stems must be bent to adapt them to individual skeletal variations. Postoperative flexion-extension arcs average 65 degrees. Pain relief is usually excellent. Complications have included deep infection, loosening, dislocation, carpal tunnel syndrome, and persistent ulnar deviation. Postoperative ulnar deviation appears to be related to malalignment of the prosthetic and anatomic centers of rotation. This problem has been partially eliminated by prosthetic redesign. Carpal tunnel syndrome is related to the rather large anteroposterior dimension of this prosthesis.

The other cemented total wrist prosthesis (Volz) has a radial component with a polyethylene articulating surface and a metacarpal component with a highly polished hemispherical metal articulating surface. Both components are cemented into bone with methyl methacrylate. Carpal height is 2 cm. The theoretical flexion-extension arc is 90 degrees. Initially, the distal component had two prongs which were seated in the second and third metacarpals. The present model has a single-prong distal component which is seated in the third metacarpal. With the new single-prong model, alignment of the prosthetic and anatomic centers of rotation is easier. It is hoped that this design change will decrease the incidence of postoperative ulnar deviation. Functional integrity of the extensor carpi radialis brevis is an important prerequisite for success of this arthroplasty. With this total wrist prosthesis, patients obtained pain relief, an average flexion-extension arc of 55 degrees, and improved hand function. Complications have included infection, loosening, dislocation, carpal tunnel syndrome, hematoma, postoperative ulnar deviation, and perforation of the radius.

Limited Wrist Arthrodesis (Scapho-trapezio-trapezoid Arthrodesis) Arthrodesis of the scapho-trapezial-trapezoid joints, which collectively may be called the triscaphoid joint, is indicated for localized degenerative arthritis, trauma to the radial side of the wrist, and chronic rotary subluxation of the scaphoid. Significant technical details include scaphoid reduction prior to arthrodesis, preservation of a small amount of the volar cartilage and bone at the triscaphoid joints, maintenance of the normal carpal bone architecture, and Kirschner wire internal fixation to stabilize the reduction and arthrodesis (Fig. 9). With rotary subluxation of the scaphoid, reduction eliminates the perpendicular scaphoid attitude, closes the scapholunate diastasis, and decreases the potential for late scapholunate arthritis. The volar edge of the trapezium, trapezoid, and scaphoid are preserved to maintain the normal external dimensions of the fusion mass. This may help avoid unnecessary changes in wrist kinematics. The Kirschner wire should not be passed through nonarthrodesed joints because slight motion of these joints minimizes the stress on the joints involved in the arthrodesis. Postoperative plaster immobilization is necessary for 6 to 12 weeks.

Eighty percent of the wrist flexion-extension arc and 60 percent of the radioulnar deviation arc are preserved after triscaphoid limited wrist arthrodesis. Most reported patients have become asymptomatic and have been able to return to routine activities, including heavy labor. Complications have included infection and an occasional nonunion.

Postoperative cineradiographic studies of wrist kinematics after triscaphoid arthrodesis have shown markedly decreased capitoscaphoid motion, loss of reciprocal motion between the proximal and distal carpal rows, but preservation of the lunocapitate motion. Despite this, no degenerative arthritis has been noted in the remaining carpal joints during the 2-year follow-up period. Although the triscaphoid arthrodesis currently is very popular, it must be emphasized that long-term follow-up studies are not yet available.

Kienböck's Disease (Lunatomalacia) The lunate has an excellent extraosseous blood supply with nutrient vessels entering volarly and dorsally. Unfortunately, the interosseous vessels are less abundant, especially in the proximal central pole which lies behind the delicate anastomosis of the dorsal and volar interosseous vessels.

The osteonecrosis of Kienböck's disease is probably secondary to repeated trauma. In one recent study, 67 percent of the patients had identifiable fractures (Fig. 10A). There is also a definite relationship between Kienböck's disease and negative ulnar variance (Fig. 10B). Negative variance is more common among Caucasians and less common in Oriental populations in whom Kienböck's disease is also rare. Despite this clear association, negative ulnar variance is probably a predisposing rather than a causative factor. Further, it is important to note that previous studies on ulnar variance have been based on nonstandardized radiographic techniques. Negative variance of 1 to 2 mm may predispose the lunate to osteonecrosis; however, forearm rotation, wrist deviation, and x-ray beam incident angle can cause as much as 2 mm variation in the measured ulnar variance. To make an accurate assessment of variance, standardized films should be used. The standardized posteroanterior is a zero rotation, ulnar deviation view, and the lateral is done in zero rotation, neutral deviation. In both films the elbow is flexed at 90 degrees, and the x-ray beam is perpendicular to the wrist. Because previous studies have not used standardized views, the reliability of the data is questionable.

In most patients, Kienböck's disease is slowly progressive, and surgical treatment may be necessary. Surgical alternatives include revascularization, bone grafting, ulnar lengthening, shortening of the radius, capitohamate arthrodesis, other limited carpal arthrodeses, proximal row carpectomy, and lunate implant resectional arthroplasty. The two most commonly performed procedures are limited carpal arthrodesis and implant arthroplasty (Fig. 10B). Lunate implant arthroplasty can be complicated by limited wrist motion, decreased grip strength, prosthetic fragmentation, prosthetic dislocation, and rotary subluxation of the scaphoid. Some complications can be avoided by fascial arthroplasty; however, a simultaneous capi-

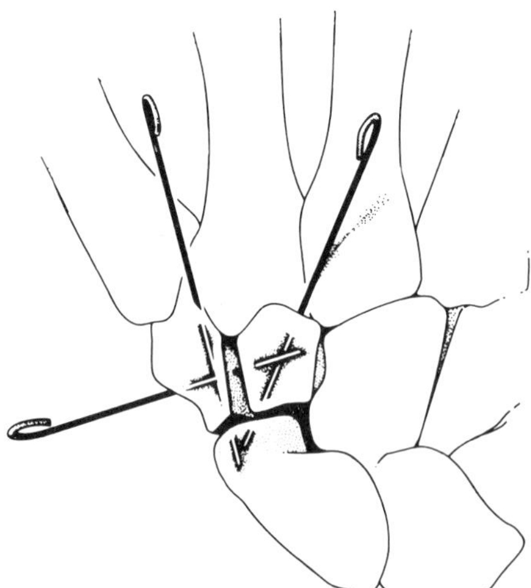

Figure 9: Scapho-trapezio-trapezoid arthrodesis. Joints resected, preserved volar edges, and ready for bone graft. K-wire fixation of arthrodesed joints. If the scaphoid is reduced for rotatory subluxation, K-wire fixation of the scaphoid to the capitate also may be required.

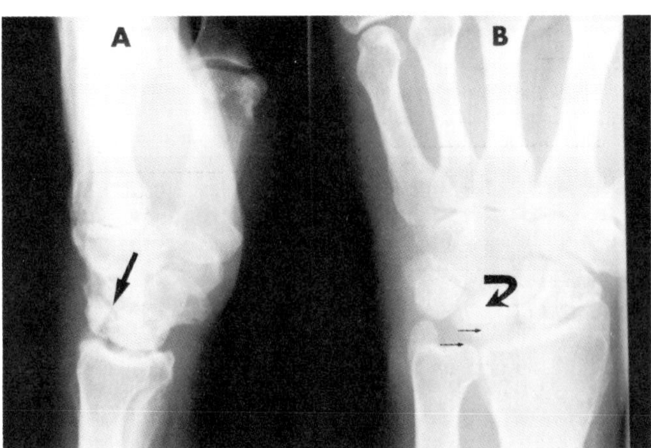

Figure 10: Kienböck's disease. (A) Osteonecrosis of the lunate (lunatomalacia) with fracture of the dorsal pole (arrow). (B) Note the negative ulnar variance (double small arrows), but also note this is not a standardized posteroanterior because the ulnar styloid is not in the maximum lateral position and the wrist is not ulnarly deviated. Swanson implant has been inserted (curved arrow).

tohamate arthrodesis may be needed to prevent late capitate migration. Limited carpal arthrodeses are complicated by limited motion, occasional nonunions, and ultimately an increased incidence of arthritis in the nonarthrodesed carpal joints.

ANNOTATED BIBLIOGRAPHY

Hand

Proximal Interphalangeal Joint Arthroplasty

Eaton, R.G., and Malerich, M.M.: Volar plate arthroplasty of the proximal interphalangeal joint: A review of ten years' experience. J. Hand Surg. 5:260-268, 1980.

During a 10-year period, twenty-four patients had volar plate advancement hemiarthroplasty for acute or chronic fracture-dislocations. Final range of motion averaged 78 degrees. Complications included digital angulation, extensor tendon adherence, and recurrent subluxation.

Strickland, J.W; Dustman, J.A.; Stelzer, L.; Stromberg, W.B.; Steichen, J.B.; and Bell, J.L.: Post-traumatic arthritis of the proximal interphalangeal joint. Orthop. Rev. XI: 8:75-83, 1982.

Ninety-one patients underwent proximal interphalangeal joint arthroplasties for fracture, fracture-dislocation, crush injuries, or simple dislocations. The reason for disability did not correlate with postoperative result or increasing surgical experience.

Thumb Carpometacarpal Joint Arthroplasty

Amadio, P.C.; Millender, L.H.; and Smith, R.J.: Silicone spacer or tendon spacer for trapezium resection arthroplasty: Comparison of results. J. Hand Surg. 7:237-244, 1982.

Twenty-five consecutive trapeziectomies with silicone spacers were compared to 25 trapeziectomies with tendon interposition. All patients were females over the age of 35 years who were housewives or clerical workers. All had osteoarthritis. In those with the silicone spacer, 90 percent reported pain relief, mean thumb abduction was 42.5 percent, and pinch strength averaged 5 kg. With tendon interposition, 95 percent reported pain relief, mean abduction was 46.8 percent, and average pinch strength was 4.6 kg. There was no statistically significant difference between the two groups.

Eaton, R.G.: Replacement of the trapezium for arthritis of the basal articulations: A new technique with stabilization by tenodesis. J. Bone Joint Surg. 61A:76-82, 1979.

Fifty-six patients had trapezial resection arthroplasty with a silicone spacer that incorporated a local tendon strip to stabilize the device. Dislocation rate was 10 percent. All patients obtained painfree, improved motion with pinch strength averaging 6 kg to 8 kg.

Swanson, A.B.; Swanson, G.D.; and Watermeier, J.J.: Trapezium implant arthroplasty: Long-term evaluation of 150 cases. J. Hand Surg. 6:125-141, 1981.

This article contains a long-term evaluation of 150 patients with trapezial resection arthroplasty with silicone spacer. Prosthetic development is reviewed, and techniques of adjunct procedures needed to prevent dislocations are described. There is a brief discussion of silicone condylar hemiarthroplasty implant.

Tendon Transfers

Brand, P.W.; Beach, R.B.; and Thompson, D.E.: Relative tension and potential excursion of muscles in the forearm and hand. J. Hand Surg. 6:209-219, 1981.

The relative mass (work capacity), fiber length (potential excursion), and cross-sectional areas (potential forces) are tabulated for all muscles of the forearm and hand. This original biomechanical data may be of practical use in planning tendon transfers.

Browne, E.Z., Jr.; Teague, M.A.; and Gruenwald, C.: Method for measurement of circumduction of the thumb to evaluate results of opponensplasty. Plast. Reconstr. Surg. 64:204-207, 1979.

Obtaining a numerical expression of thumb circumduction is difficult. An easy clinical technique for quantitating circumduction (opposition) is described.

Matev, I.B.: Restoration of thumb opposition by displacement of extensor pollicis brevis. Hand 13:279-284, 1981.

Twelve patients underwent extensor pollicis brevis opponensplasties and had follow-ups of 1 to 6 years. Restoration of opposition was obtained. All patients could oppose to the long or ring finger.

Riley, W.B., Jr.; Mann, R.J.; and Burkhalter, W.E.: Extensor pollicis longus opponensplasty. J. Hand Surg. 5:217-220, 1980.

Eleven patients underwent EPL opponensplasties. All patients obtained satisfactory function without secondary operations. Surgical details are described and illustrated.

Carpal Tunnel Syndrome

Carroll, R.E., and Hurst, L.C.: The relationship of thoracic outlet syndrome and carpal tunnel syndrome. Clin. Orthop. 164:149-153, 1982.

The relationship of these syndromes was studied retrospectively in 1,000 patients with carpal tunnel syndrome and sixty-three patients with thoracic outlet syndrome. Thoracic outlet is rare and difficult to diagnose. Carpal tunnel syndrome is often still inaccurately diagnosed as thoracic outlet syndrome. The simultaneous occurrence of these syndromes is extremely rare. Initial treatment should be directed at the carpal tunnel.

Ellis, J.; Folkers, K.; Levy, M.; Takemura, K.; Shizukuishi, S.; Ulrich, R.; and Harrison, P.: Therapy with vitamin B_6 with and without surgery for treatment of patients having idiopathic carpal tunnel syndrome. Res. Comm. Chem. Path. Pharm. 33:331-344, 1981.

Twenty-nine patients with idiopathic carpal tunnel showed vitamin B_6 deficiencies. Twelve weeks of vitamin B_6 therapy relieved pain and paresthesias but did not affect muscle atrophy. Life-long replacement is needed if symptomatic relief is to persist.

Eversmann, W.W., and Ritsick, J.A.: Intraoperative changes in motor nerve conduction latency in carpal tunnel syndrome. J. Hand Surg. 3:77-81, 1978.

Nerve conduction latencies were studied prospectively in forty-seven patients. Latencies immediately corrected to normal after carpal tunnel release, suggesting a mechanical or metabolic block such as ischemia. Distal latencies that did not correct from transverse carpal ligament release alone appear to be improved by the addition of internal neurolysis.

Gelberman, R.H.; Aronson, D.; and Weisman, M.H.: Carpal tunnel syndrome: Results of a prospective trial of steroid injection and splinting. J. Bone Joint Surg. 62A:1181-1184, 1980.

Prospective study of fifty patients treated with a single cortisone injection and 3 weeks of splinting. Forty percent of the patients with minimally prolonged distal latencies were free of symptoms at the end of 1 year.

Lundborg, G.; Gelberman, R.H.; Minteer-Convery, M.; Lee, Y.F.; and Hargens, A.R.: Median nerve compression in the carpal tunnel: Functional response to experimentally induced controlled pressure. J. Hand Surg. 7:252-259, 1982.

Sixteen normal volunteers were studied with Wick catheter carpal tunnel pressure monitoring while controlled external compression was applied. Sensory and motor conduction and two-point discrimination were monitored. Nerve fiber viability is jeopardized by pressures greater than 30 mm Hg.

McCann, V.J., and Davis, R.E.: Carpal tunnel syndrome, diabetes, and pyridoxal. Australian New Zealand J. Med. 8:638-640, 1978.

Twenty-five patients with carpal tunnel syndrome and diabetes were studied. No vitamin B_6 deficiency was noted in these patients or in a similar group with diabetic peripheral neuropathy.

Upton, A.R.M., and McComas, A.J.: The double crush in nerve-entrapment syndromes. Lancet 2:359-360, 1973.

An explanation for the association of diabetes or cervical arthritis with carpal tunnel syndrome is presented.

Thumb Reconstruction

Matev, I.B.: Thumb reconstruction through metacarpal bone lengthening. J. Hand Surg. 5:482-487, 1980.

A 12-year experience with thirty-five patients who underwent thumb metacarpal lengthening is described. Four to 8-year follow-up revealed no osteolysis or other trophic changes. Sensibility was good.

Morrison, W.A.; O'Brien, B.M.; and MacLeod, A.M.: Thumb reconstruction with a free neurovascular wrap-around flap from the big toe. J. Hand Surg. 5:575-583, 1980.

The use of a free neurovascularized (wrap-around) flap from the big toe was described in five patients. This procedure does not require the sacrifice of the large toe. It is not indicated if growth is needed or if the trapezial metacarpal joint is absent.

Stern, P.J., and Lister, G.D.: Pollicization after traumatic amputation of the thumb. Clin. Orthop. 155:85-94, 1981.

Nineteen pollicizations were performed. Seven normal finger pollicizations gave very satisfactory results. Eleven previously damaged pollicized digits all showed diminished motion. Seventy-four percent required secondary procedures.

Dupuytren's Contracture

Badalamente, M.A.; Stern, L.; and Hurst, L.C.: The pathogenesis of Dupuytren's contracture: Contractile mechanisms of the myofibroblasts. J. Hand Surg. 8:235-243, 1983.

Fascia excised from twenty patients was investigated by light and electron microscopic histochemical techniques. The energy mechanisms of the myofibroblasts were identified and described in detail. The degree of ATPase activity, as determined by cell counts, appeared to correlate with the residual contracture as predicted by the Legge-McFarland outcome standard formula.

Brickley-Parsons, D.; Glimcher, M.J.; Smith, R.J.; Albin, R.; and Adams, J.P.: Biochemical changes in the collagen of palmar fascia in patients with Dupuytren's disease. J. Bone Joint Surg. 63A:787-797, 1981.

Palmar fascia from 400 patients and 100 controls were studied biochemically. Modifications of the collagen in Dupuytren's disease did not appear to be the cause of the contracture but represented changes similar to rapidly synthesized new collagen that might be seen in the active stages of wound repair.

Nissenbaum, M., and Kleinert, H.E.: Treatment considerations in carpal tunnel syndrome with coexistent Dupuytren's disease. J. Hand Surg. 5:544-547, 1980.

Twenty-nine patients with coexistent Dupuytren's contracture and carpal tunnel syndrome were studied. There was a high proportion of females with dominant hand involvement and a history of trauma. Simultaneous surgical treatment is not recommended.

Wrist

Anatomy—Triangular Fibrocartilage Complex (TFCC)

Palmer, A.K., and Werner, F.W.: The triangular fibrocartilage complex of the wrist: Anatomy and function. J. Hand Surg. 6:153-162, 1981.

The anatomy and biomechanics of the TFCC were studied by dissecting sixty-one specimens. The triangular fibrocartilage was found to be a homogeneous structure composed of several components that are not separately dissectable. Because of its biomechanical functions, excision of the TFCC is not recommended.

Wrist Arthroplasty

Beckenbaugh, R.D.: Total joint arthroplasty: The wrist. Mayo Clin. Proc. 54:513-515, 1979.

Meuli total wrist arthroplasty was performed in 102 patients. The procedure relieved pain and improved mobility in deformed wrists involved with rheumatoid arthritis. The procedure is not appropriate for posttraumatic arthritis.

Davis, R.F.; Weiland, A.J.; and Dowling, S.V.: Swanson implant arthroplasty of the wrist in rheumatoid patients. Clin. Orthop. 166:132-137, 1982.

Twenty-six Swanson radiocarpal implant arthroplasties were performed in twenty-three patients with rheumatoid arthritis with average follow-up of 33 months (5 to 47 months). Pain relief and increased ability to cope with activities of daily living were achieved. Strength and fine motor control were not improved.

Goodman, M.J.; Millender, L.H.; Nalebuff, E.D.; and Philips, C.A.: Arthroplasty of the rheumatoid wrist with silicone rubber: An early evaluation. J. Hand Surg. 5:114-121, 1980.

Thirty-seven arthroplasties were performed for rheumatoid arthritis. Prosthetic fracture rate was 8 percent. Contraindications included marked deformity, instability, bone loss, or multiple tendon ruptures. Ten patients had contralateral arthrodesis.

Lamberta, F.J.; Ferlic, D.C.; and Clayton, M.L.: Volz total wrist arthroplasty in rheumatoid arthritis: A preliminary report. J. Hand Surg. 5:245-252, 1980.

Twenty Volz total wrist arthroplasties were performed for rheumatoid arthritis. Seventy percent retained good or excellent results.

Limited Wrist Arthrodesis (Scapho-trapezio-trapezoid Arthrodesis)

Kleinman, W.B.; Steichen, J.B.; and Strickland, J.W.: Management of chronic rotary subluxation of the scaphoid by scapho-trapezio-trapezoid arthrodesis. J. Hand Surg. 7:125-136, 1982.

Triscaphoid arthrodesis was done in twelve patients for rotary subluxation of the scaphoid. Nine patients were relieved of pain, had preservation of 80 percent of their preoperative motion, and returned to prior activities. Postoperative wrist kinematics were abnormal.

Watson, H.K., and Hempton, R.F.: Limited wrist arthrodeses. I. The triscaphoid joint. J. Hand Surg. 5:320-327, 1980.

Thirteen patients underwent triscaphoid arthrodesis. Eighty percent of the flexion-extension arc and 67 percent of the radioulnar deviation arc of motion were preserved after surgery. Local bone graft donor sites were utilized.

Kienböck's Disease (Lunatomalacia)

Beckenbaugh, R.D.; Shives, T.C.; Dobyns, J.H.; and Linscheid, R.L.: Kienböck's disease: The natural history of Kienböck's disease and consideration of lunate fractures. Clin. Orthop. 149:98-106, 1980.

Forty-six patients with Kienböck's disease were studied with follow-up of 2 to 27 years. Seventy-two percent had a history of wrist injury. Ten patients were not treated. Thirty-six had surgical treatment. Ultimately, relief of pain and functional wrists were present in both the treated and nontreated patients.

Epner, R.A.; Bowers, W.H.; and Guilford, W.B.: Ulnar variance: The effect of wrist positioning and roentgen filming technique. J. Hand Surg. 7:298-305, 1982.

Ulnar variance is the radiographic distance between the articular surfaces of the radiocarpal and ulnocarpal joints. Variance changes with wrist and x-ray incident angle. Supination increases negative variance whereas pronation decreases it. On the standardized lateral film, the ulnar styloid is exactly in the center of the ulna, and the radius is superimposed. On the standardized posteroanterior film, the radial and ulnar styloids are at the extreme lateral and median margins of the radiographic image.

Gelberman, R.H.; Bauman, T.D.; Menon, J.; and Akeson, W.H.: The vascularity of the lunate bone and Kienböck's disease. J. Hand Surg. 5:272-278, 1980.

Vascularity of the lunate was studied in thirty-five fresh cadaver specimens which were injected with latex. Interosseous vascularity presented as either a Y, X, or I pattern. The relative avascularity of the proximal pole supports the theory of compression fractures from repeated trauma as the cause of Kienböck's disease.

23 CERVICAL SPINE: PEDIATRIC

Subjects considered in this section include cervical instability, congenital anomalies of the odontoid, torticollis, and cervical fractures.

Congenital and Developmental

Cervical Instability in Children

Upper Cervical Spine The C1-2 articulation is the most mobile joint of the vertebral column and is, consequently, the least stable. Anatomically its integrity is dependent upon supporting ligaments, particularly in flexion and rotation. Only in extension does the odontoid provide a block to subluxation. Instability may follow inflammation which causes apparent or actual softening of the ligaments or their attachments (e.g., rotatory instability following pharyngitis, instability associated with juvenile rheumatoid arthritis, or infection). The Down's syndrome patient has a unique propensity (25 percent) for laxity of this articulation. Congenital problems such as atlantooccipital fusion (associated with C2-3 fusion), basilar impression, and anomalies of the odontoid can increase the stress on the C1-2 articulation and lead to hypermobility and eventual frank instability. Certain bone dysplasias (achondroplasia, spondyloepiphyseal dysplasia, diastrophic dysplasia, Morquio's syndrome, and Larsen's syndrome) are similarly prone to occipitocervical problems.

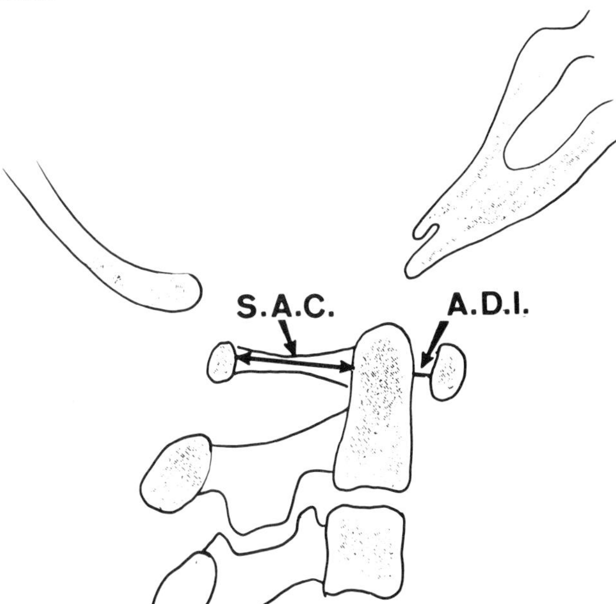

Figure 1: Drawing of the atlantoaxial joint, demonstrating the atlanto-dens interval (ADI) and the space available for the spinal cord (SAC).

The atlanto-dens interval (ADI), the space between the anterior aspect of the dens and the posterior aspect of the ring of C1 (Fig. 1), in children may normally measure as much as 5 mm because portions of the odontoid and C1 ring are unossified. In acute injury a subtle increase in the ADI in the neutral position may indicate complete disruption of the transverse atlantal ligament. In chronic atlantoaxial joint instability, the odontoid frequently is hypermobile and the ADI widened, particularly in flexion (Fig. 2), but most children with this finding are asymptomatic and require no surgical stabilization. Attention should be directed toward the space available for the spinal cord (SAC), the distance from the posterior aspect of C2 to the nearest posterior structure, the foramen magnum or the posterior ring of C1. This is particularly helpful when evaluating patients who develop instability

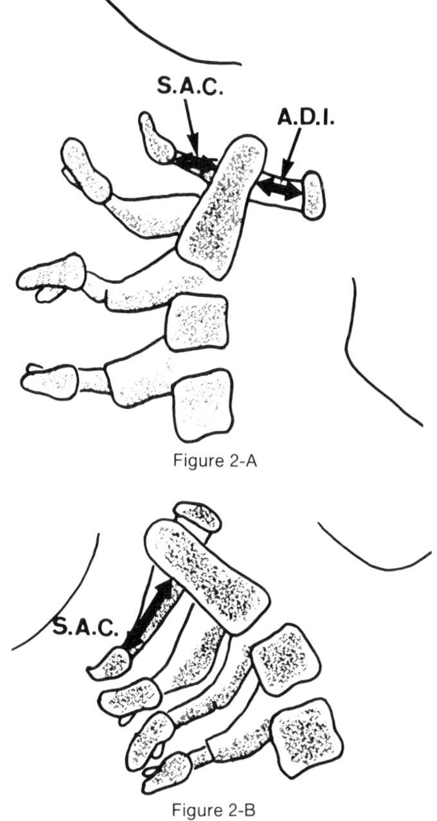

Figure 2: Atlantoaxial joint instability with intact odontoid. (A) Flexion: forward sliding of the atlas with an increase of the ADI and a decrease in the space available for SAC. (B) Extension: ADI and SAC return to normal as the intact odontoid provides a bony block to posterior subluxation.

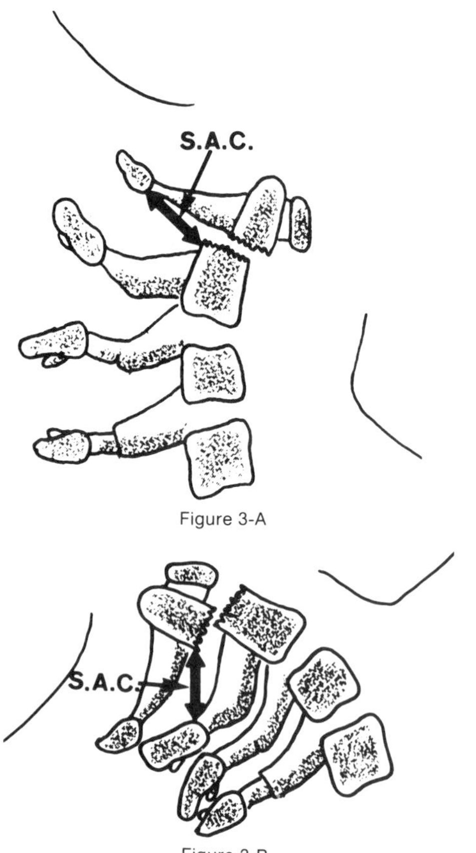

Figure 3: (A,B) Atlantoaxial instability with nonunion of the odontoid, os odontoideum, or absent odontoid. ADI remains unchanged in (A) flexion, and (B) extension. However, SAC is reduced in both positions. Spinal cord impingement can be either posterior from the ring of C1 or anterior from the body of C2.

due to a nonunion of the odontoid, os odontoideum, or absent odontoid. In this situation, the ADI remains constant, and the SAC may narrow considerably in flexion, extension, or both. Spinal cord impingement can be either posterior from the ring of C1 or anterior from the body of C2 (Fig. 3). It generally is agreed that a reduction of the lumen of the spinal canal to 13 mm or less may be associated with neurologic problems. Even those with an absent ring of C1 are in jeopardy because the spinal cord can be stretched over the body of C2 in flexion or indented by a fibrous band which has replaced the arch of C1.

The anterior portion of the C1 ring is unossified at birth, and the ossification center may not be visible until 1 year of age. Similarly, the apex of the odontoid is not ossified at birth and may not appear until the age of 3 years. Thus, in extension, C1 appears to subluxate on the odontoid, so that more than two-thirds of the ring may lie above the superior margin of the ossified portion of the dens.

Obtaining a satisfactory radiograph may be hampered by the patient's limited ability to cooperate, fixed bony deformity, and overlapping shadows from the mandible, occiput, and foramen magnum. A helpful guide is that the atlas moves with the occiput and if the x-ray beam is directed 90 degrees to the lateral of the skull, a satisfactory view of the occipitocervical junction usually results. Visualization may be further enhanced with flexion-extension or tomographic views. Carefully supervised motion studies often are necessary to establish cervical spine instability. Computed tomograms, especially those providing coronal and sagittal reconstructions, are helpful in evaluating the occipitocervical junction. Careful clinical correlation is necessary as the cross-sectional bony anatomy is not only as confusing as the sagittal anatomy but also less familiar.

Once atlantoaxial joint instability occurs in children, it seldom can be controlled nonoperatively and surgical stabilization is often necessary. Reduction of the articulation should be attempted by simple positioning or traction with the patient awake. Operative reduction is associated with increased morbidity and mortality. If the reduction is unstable, surgical stabilization should be performed and maintained until the neurologic status has stabilized. Sublaminar wire fixation and interposing bone graft are favored for stabilizing this articulation. When the ring of C1 is incomplete or malformed, in situ fusion from the occiput to C2 is preferred and alignment maintained postoperatively with a halo cast. Similarly, if reduction is not achieved by preoperative traction, then in situ fusion is preferred rather than manipulative reduction or sublaminar wire fixation, a hazardous procedure in this instance.

ROTATORY SUBLUXATION OF C1-2: Rotatory subluxation presents with spontaneous onset of torticollis, usually following an upper respiratory tract infection, surgery in the upper pharynx (such as a tonsillectomy), or trauma. Inflammation and local edema in the retropharyngeal region leads to laxity of the ligamentous restraints, allowing for greater motion of C1-2. Diagnosis is difficult with standard radiographic techniques, and tomography and computed tomography have proved very helpful (Fig. 4). Early treatment consists of recumbency, aspirin, and a soft collar. Head halter or halo traction may be necessary in long-standing problems or when the torticollis does not resolve with simple measures. If there are recurrent episodes or the condition becomes subacute or chronic (beyond 3 weeks), postreduction immobilization in a Minerva cast or halo is indicated. Rarely, in chronic cases, surgical stabilization may be required.

Lower Cervical Spine The soft tissue of a child's spine

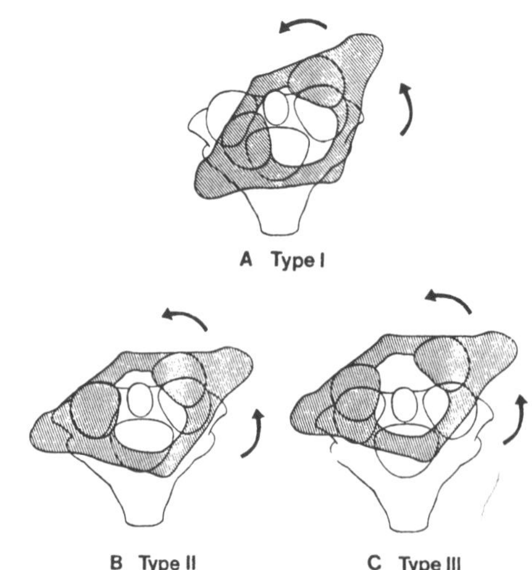

Figure 4: Classification of rotatory displacement. (A) Type I: simple rotatory displacement without anterior shift. (B) Type II: rotatory displacement with anterior shift of 5 mm or less. (C) Type III: rotatory displacement with anterior shift greater than 5 mm. (Adapted with permission from Atlanto-axial rotatory fixation, by J.W. Fielding, et al., J. Bone Joint Surg. 59A:37, 1977.)

is much more flexible than an adult's. The soft tissue shadow of the retropharyngeal space as measured from the anterior-inferior border of C2 is normally less than 5 mm in adults. This distance is not reliable if the child is talking, crying, or has an inflammation of the upper respiratory tract. The cervical spine can be stretched considerably in the young child without permanent injury. However, the spinal cord is not as elastic as the spinal column. Surgical removal of the posterior elements (laminectomy) typically leads to an unstable cervical spine in children under 14 years of age. The majority will develop a significant deformity (kyphosis) and require surgical stabilization.

Prior to 8 years of age, the motion patterns of the cervical spine demonstrate considerable variation in radiographic appearance as compared to the adult. Pseudosubluxation of C2 on C3 (in flexion) secondary to the normal mobility in this area can be so pronounced as to be mistaken for a dislocation. Specific measurements of the normal flexion-extension movement of the bodies of C2 on C3 have proved unreliable. The straight line relationship of the posterior elements in flexion (the posterior cervical line) is found helpful in differentiating physiologic from pathologic anterior displacement of C2 on C3 (Fig. 5).

The orientation of the facet joints of the cervical spine changes with growth. In the young child the angle of the upper cervical facets (C2-4) is nearly horizontal (30-35 degrees) in the sagittal plane, permitting more slide in flexion-extension. As the child approaches adolescence, the facet angles become more vertical (75-80 degrees) and less mobile. The orientation of the lower cervical facets changes from 55 to 70 degrees during the same period.

Thus, the combination of incomplete ossification, relative ligament laxity, and shallow facet joint angles result in a greater radiographic translational motion. In addition, the firm ligamentous fixation of C1 to the skull and the relatively larger weight of the child's skull result in a cervical fulcrum at a higher level (C2-3) as compared to the C5-6 level in the adult.

The configuration of the immature spine continues to pose problems in evaluating the effects of trauma, anomalies, tumor, or infection. Consequently, information continues to be accumulated concerning the normal child's spine. For instance, one recent study on the sagittal diameter of the cervical canal in those under 10 years of age reported that widening is not a reliable indicator of intraluminal pathology since there is considerable, normal width variation throughout the entire canal.

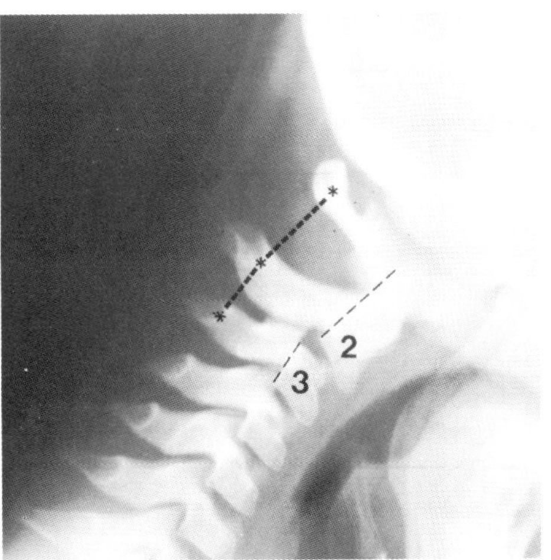

Figure 5: Pseudosubluxation of C2 on C3. Hypermobility is common in children under the age of 8 years. Specific measurements of the movement of the vertebral bodies (thin dotted line) is unreliable whereas the relationship with the posterior elements (thick dotted line) is more consistent. In flexion the posterior arch of C2 normally aligns itself in a straight line fashion with C1 and C3.

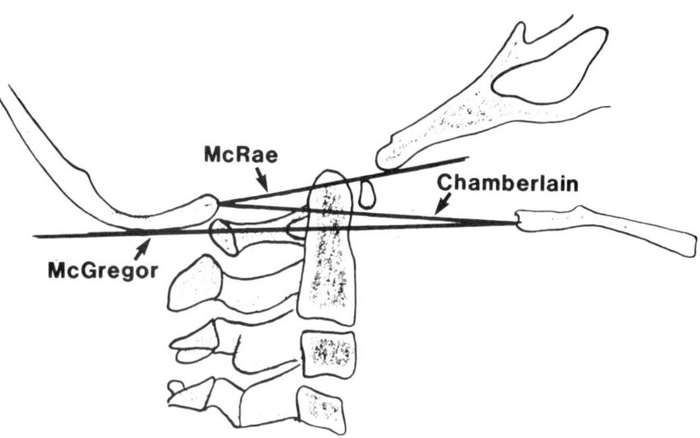

Figure 6: Lateral craniometry. The drawing indicates the three lines used to determine basilar impressions: (1) Chamberlain's line (1939) drawn from the posterior lip of the foramen magnum (opisthion) to the dorsal margin of the hard palate; (2) McGregor's line (1948) is drawn from the upper surface of the posterior edge of the hard palate to the most caudal point of the occipital curve of the skull (the most reliable for screening) and the tip of the odontoid normally does not extend more than 4.5 mm above this line; (3) McRae's line (1953) defines the opening of the foramen magnum, the most clinically relevant.

Basilar Impression (Basilar Invagination) This is a deformity of the osseous structures forming the base of the skull at the margin of the foramen magnum. The floor of the skull appears indented by the upper cervical spine. The tip of the odontoid is positioned more cephalad and may protrude into the foramen magnum, encroach on the brain stem, and interfere with the vertebral arteries or with the flow of cerebrospinal fluid (Fig. 6). The condition is rare. It is difficult to evaluate, but computed tomography and other image-enhancing techniques have made identification easier. Clinically, patients with this deformity closely resemble those with many acquired neurologic diseases: tumor of the posterior fossa, bulbar palsy of polio, syringomyelia, amyotrophic lateral sclerosis, spinal cord tumor, spastic paraplegia, and multiple sclerosis.

There are two types of *basilar impression.* The *primary* basilar impression is a congenital abnormality often associated with other vertebral defects such as atlantooccipital fusion, hypoplasia of the atlas, odontoid abnormalities, and Klippel-Feil syndrome. It also may be seen with various skeletal dysplasias (particularly achondroplasia, spondyloepiphyseal dysplasia, and Morquio's syndrome). *Secondary* basilar impression is a developmental condition secondary to softening of the osseous structures at the base of the skull which develops in later life. This may be recognized in such conditions as severe osteoporosis, osteomalacia, rickets, renal osteodystrophy, Paget's disease, osteogenesis imperfecta, rheumatoid arthritis, neurofibromatosis, or following trauma.

Basilar impression by itself is of little consequence. However, it is important because of its frequent association with various treatable neurologic problems, such as syringomyelia, cerebellar herniation (Arnold-Chiari syn-

MRI

drome), atlantoaxial instability, and spinal cord compression in the region of the foramen magnum. If instability develops, the odontoid may encroach on the medulla oblongata as with altantooccipital fusion. Similarly, if posterior impingement occurs, the presenting symptoms may be increased intracranial pressure and hydrocephalus due to a block of the aqueduct of Sylvius, compression of the cerebellum or herniation of cerebellar tonsils, impingement on the posterior columns and pyramidal tract associated with weakness, hyperreflexia, and spasticity. The vertebral arteries may be compressed as they pass through the stenotic foramen. Additionally, there is a higher incidence of vertebral artery malformations associated with basilar impression and atlantooccipital fusion.

Although it is recognized more frequently now, there is little information as to the indications for surgical intervention or, for that matter, the preferred operative procedure.

Atlantooccipital Fusion (Occipitalization; Assimilation of the Atlas) This most commonly recognized anomaly of the cranio-vertebral junction poses few clinical problems by itself but is typically associated with several hazardous conditions. If accompanied by C2-3 fusion or anomalies of the odontoid, the patient is likely to develop marked instability of the C1-2 articulation (Fig. 7) with the resultant potential for neurologic compromise.

Tomograms often are necessary to demonstrate bony continuity of the atlas with the occiput. Similarly, computed tomography and/or myelography may be necessary to further delineate the degree and site of spinal cord impingement. In the young child, radiographic interpretation may be difficult since a significant portion of the ring of C1 is not ossified at birth and will not be completely ossified until 7 to 10 years of age.

Approximately one-half of the patients have relative basilar impressions due to the diminished vertical height of the ring of the atlas. This brings the tip of the odontoid closer to the opening of the foramen magnum and the medulla oblongata (Fig. 7). Thus, the position of the odontoid is a key factor in the development of neurologic problems. If the odontoid projects into the opening of the foramen magnum, the patient will probably be symptomatic and if below, asymptomatic. The odontoid itself often has an abnormal shape and direction (frequently longer), and its angle with the body of the axis is directed more posteriorly. If instability develops, the ADI will be increased in flexion from the normal of 3 to 4 mm to as much as 12 mm (Fig. 2). Similarly, the SAC will be significantly decreased.

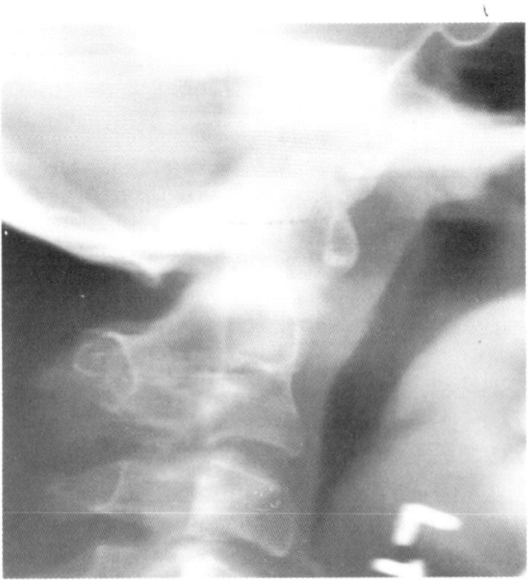

Figure 7: Atlantooccipital fusion and C2-3 fusion. Tomogram demonstrating relative basilar impressions due to diminished vertical height of the ring of the atlas. The tip of the odontoid protrudes into the foramen magnum. The odontoid has become hypermobile due to disruption of the transverse atlantal ligament with an increase in the ADI and reduction of the SAC.

Nonoperative measures (cervical collars, traction, and Minerva casts) are helpful, particularly in patients becoming symptomatic after mild trauma or inflammation of the upper pharynx. If instability is documented, surgical stabilization is usually necessary. If anterior cord symptoms predominate, they usually stem from hypermobility of the odontoid and can be controlled by posterior occiput to C2 fusion. This extensive procedure typically involves fixation to the occiput and requires the combined talents of anesthesia, orthopaedics, and neurosurgery. Success can be predicted if preliminary traction reduces the odontoid and the patient's symptoms improve. Operative reduction should be avoided. If reduction cannot be achieved and the majority of symptoms originate from posterior spinal cord compression, then suboccipital craniectomy, excision of the posterior arch of the atlas, and removal of the thickened dural band, if present, is preferred. If the majority of symptoms originate from anterior spinal cord compression, anterior decompression, a procedure reported in a few centers, may be considered.

Congenital Anomalies of the Odontoid There are several anomalies of the odontoid (aplasia, hypoplasia, and os odontoideum), and they share the same signs, symptoms, and treatment. Os odontoideum is the most common. Its clinical significance lies in its potential to produce serious neurologic sequelae due to atlantoaxial instability.

ETIOLOGY: The cause of os odontoideum is controversial. Some investigators favor traumatic etiology, particularly in children. An injury occurring before 4 years of age may result in a fracture of the odontoid, and as the child grows, the alar ligaments gradually carry the fragment upward, away from its base (Fig. 8). Those studying an older population continue to favor a congenital origin.

PATIENT EVALUATION: Many congenital anomalies of the odontoid are discovered on routine radiographic studies and are asymptomatic. Symptomatic patients generally have instability of the atlantoaxial joint with local pain and torticollis. Neurologic symptoms (such as spasticity, increased deep tendon reflexes, clonus, loss of proprioception, and sphincter disturbances) may originate from either anterior or posterior spinal cord compression. Few patients have symptoms and signs of cerebral ischemia (seizures, mental deterioration, syncope, vertigo, and vestibular disturbances) secondary to vertebral artery compression.

Radiographically, lateral flexion-extension views best demonstrate and document the degree of anteroposterior displacement of the atlas on the axis (Fig. 3). If there are other bony anomalies in the occipitocervical region, flexion-extension tomograms are helpful (Fig. 9). If the instability increases to 10 mm or more of motion, the lumen of the spinal canal will be significantly compromised, reducing the space available for the SAC (see preceding discussion under Upper Cervical Spine).

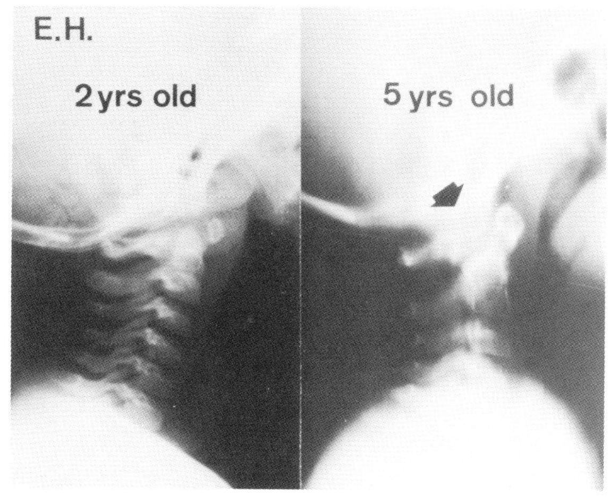

Figure 8: Os odontoideum. (A) Two-year-old male with torticollis after falling from a couch. Lateral radiograph demonstrates normal appearing odontoid and cervical spine. (B) The child was asymptomatic until age 5 years, when he developed increasing neck pain and stiffness. An os odontoideum is now noted with 7 mm of flexion-extension motion. (Reprinted with permission from Os odontoideum, by J.W. Fielding, et al., J. Bone Joint Surg. 62A:378, 1980.)

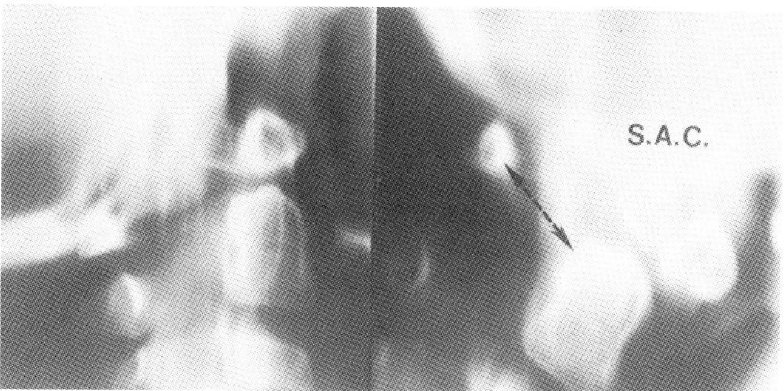

Figure 9: Os odontoideum with C1-2 instability. (A) Extension and (B) flexion tomograms demonstrating instability and a decrease of the lumen of the spinal canal in both positions. Compression of the spinal cord can occur at two points, anterior from the body of C2 or posterior from the ring of C1.

Treatment: Nonoperative treatment is sufficient for the patient presenting with relatively stable os odontoideum, little compromise of the SAC, and only minor mechanical symptomatology. Those with significant diminution of the SAC (13 mm or less) or excessive instability (greater than 10 mm), history of myelopathy, or progressive neurologic deterioration should be considered for surgical stabilization.

The C1-2 articulation should be reduced by simple positioning or traction prior to surgery. The suggested method of stabilization is posterior cervical fusion of C1-2 employing wire fixation and iliac bone graft. When wire fixation is employed, excessive tightening of the wire must be avoided. The articulation is usually unstable in both flexion and extension, and overzealous correction can pull the C1 ring and the odontoid fragment against the anterior aspect of the spinal cord. If the C1 ring is deficient or malformed, the fusion may have to be extended to the occiput and reduction maintained postoperatively in a halo cast.

Patients in whom the C1-2 dislocation cannot be reduced by preoperative traction pose a difficult problem. Manipulative reduction during the surgery is extremely hazardous and should be avoided. Similarly, attempting to pass the wire through the narrow space under the arch of C1 is dangerous and not recommended. Posterior decompression and laminectomy alone has been associated with increased C1-2 instability, and significant morbidity and mortality. Therefore, in those patients who are neurologically intact, a posterior in situ C1-2 fusion is the least hazardous procedure. If there is anterior cord compression, an anterior decompression should be considered after an adequate posterior stabilization.

Klippel-Feil Syndrome This syndrome includes all congenital failure of segmentation of the cervical vertebrae, whether it be two segments, congenital block vertebrae, or the entire cervical spine. Anomalies of the occipitocervical junction (atlantooccipital fusion, basilar impression, and abnormalities of the odontoid) are considered separately as their significance is dependent upon their influence on the atlantoaxial joint. Thus, their prognostic and therapeutic implications differ distinctly.

Congenital fusion is a result of failure of segmentation of the cervical somites during the third to eighth weeks in utero. The etiology is undetermined; however, the defect is not confined to the cervical spine. The patient with Klippel-Feil syndrome, even with minor cervical lesions, may have accompanying anomalies of the genitourinary, nervous, cardiopulmonary, and auditory systems.

Patient evaluation: The classic signs of the syndrome (low posterior hairline, short neck, and limitation of neck motion) are not consistent as less than one-half the patients have all three signs. The most common finding is limitation of neck motion. However, many patients with marked cervical involvement are able to maintain a deceptively good range of motion (Fig. 10). Sprengel's deformity frequently is associated (25-30 percent) and may be unilateral or bilateral.

Except for anomalies involving the atlantoaxial joint, there are no symptoms directly attributed to the lower fused cervical vertebrae. All symptoms commonly associated with this syndrome are due to compensatory hypermobility of the adjacent unfused segments. Due to increased stress on these joints or in response to trauma, hypermobility can lead to frank instability and/or osteoarthritis. Those at greatest risk of developing symptoms have the following anatomic characteristics: (1) massive involvement with more than four fused vertebrae (Fig. 11); (2) fusion of the occiput to the atlas and a C2-3 fusion leading to excessive demands on the atlantoaxial articulation; and (3) an open articulation between two zones of vertebral fusion particularly at the C3-4 and C4-5 levels (Fig. 12) which may lead to degenerative changes.

Radiographic evaluation can be frustrating and time-consuming but is essential. The unossified end plates in the child may give the false impression of a normal disc space. If fusion is suspected, it may be confirmed with lateral flexion-extension views. In the young child, fusion of the lamina posteriorly is more often apparent and a helpful clue to the presence of a block vertebra. Narrowing of the spinal canal, if it occurs, usually develops in adult life and is due to degenerative changes or hypermobility at levels adjacent to the congenital fusion.

The bony defects may extend into the upper thoracic area, particularly in the severely involved patient. A disturbance of the upper thoracic spine on routine chest radiograph may be the first clue to unrecognized cervical

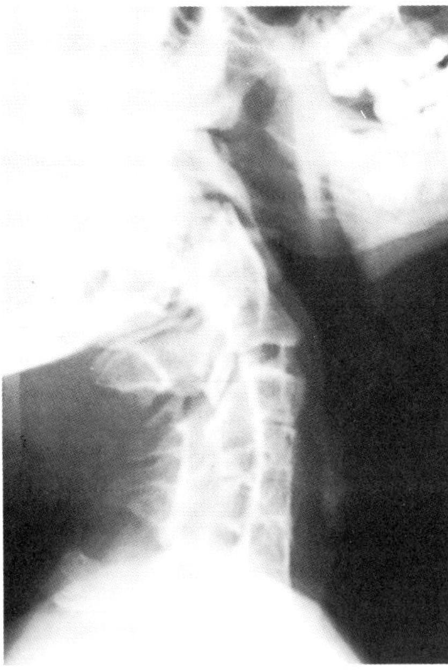

Figure 10-A

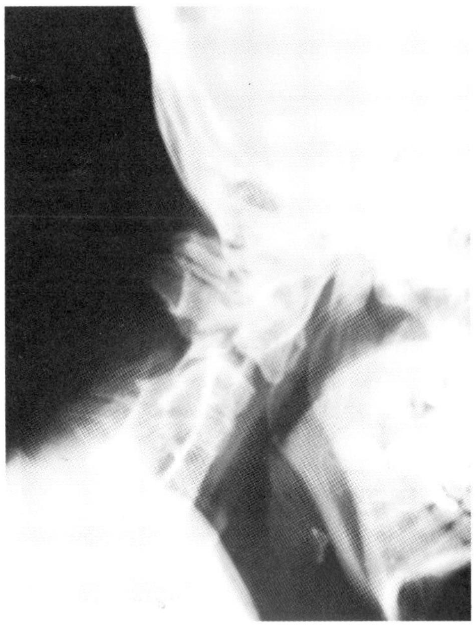

Figure 10-B

Figure 10: (A,B) Klippel-Feil syndrome. Clinically the patient maintains near normal extension and flexion. Radiographically, the majority of neck motion is occurring at the C3-4 disc space. With aging, this hypermobility can lead to frank instability and/or degenerative osteoarthritis.

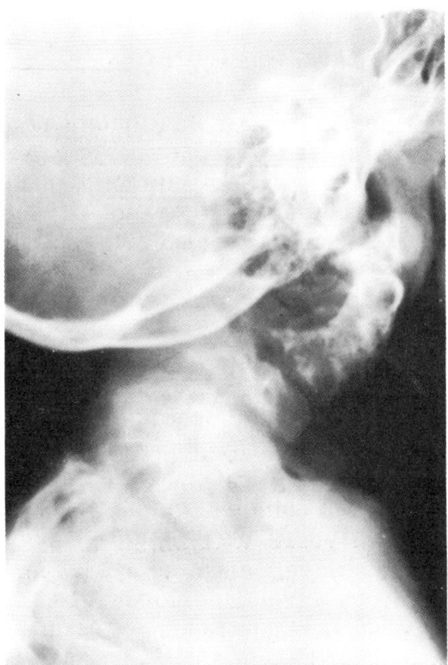

Figure 11: Klippel-Feil syndrome. Twelve year old with an extensive fusion of the cervical spine (C2-6) and an abnormal occipitocervical articulation. This patient is at significant risk of developing symptoms due to increased demands on the abnormal occipitocervical junction.

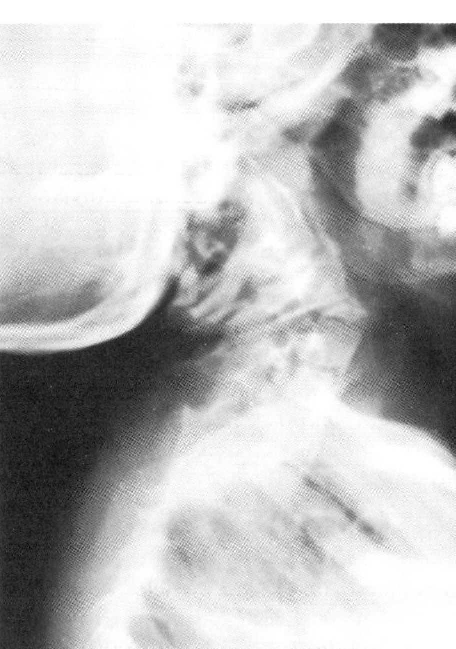

Figure 12: Klippel-Feil syndrome. Seven year old demonstrating an open articulation between two long zones of vertebral fusion. The cervical spine appears to angle or hinge at this movable segment. This may lead to early degenerative changes and osteoarthritis or instability and narrowing of the spinal canal.

synostosis. Radiographic evaluation of high thoracic congenital scoliosis should include lateral views of the cervical spine.

ASSOCIATED CONDITIONS: Scoliosis and/or kyphosis are found in 60 percent of patients with this syndrome. More than one-half require treatment, and these should be followed until skeletal maturity. One-third of the patients have significant urinary tract anomalies. Since this condition is often asymptomatic in the young child, intravenous pyelography or ultrasound should be obtained routinely. There also is a 14 percent incidence of associated congenital heart disease, and 30 percent have varying degrees of hearing loss.

MANAGEMENT: A child with a minimal Klippel-Feil syndrome can be expected to lead a normal active life with no, or only minor, restrictions or symptoms. If cervical spine symptoms occur, they usually develop in adult life due to degenerative spondylosis or instability of the segments adjacent to the areas of synostosis. The majority respond to nonoperative treatment measures, but a small percentage may require surgical stabilization. Cosmetic surgery is of limited benefit in the treatment of the neck deformity. The relatively good prognosis of the cervical lesion overshadows the hidden or unrecognized associated anomalies (scoliosis, renal anomalies, hearing impairment, and neurologic malformations). Early recognition and treatment of these problems may be of substantial benefit, sparing the patient further deformity or serious illness.

Torticollis Torticollis or wryneck, a common childhood deformity, can be caused by various conditions.

CONGENITAL MUSCULAR TORTICOLLIS: This is a painless, congenital condition, usually discovered in the first 6 to 8 weeks of life. It is caused by contracture of the sternocleidomastoid muscle. The head tilts toward the involved (typically, the right) side, and the chin rotates to the contralateral shoulder. It is not accompanied by bony abnormalities or neurologic deficit and is believed to be caused by ischemia of the sternocleidomastoid muscle, particularly the sternal head, due to intrauterine positioning or increased pressure during passage through the birth canal.

Typically a soft, nontender enlargement or "tumor" lies beneath the skin and is attached to the body of the sternocleidomastoid. The tumor usually resolves (6-12 weeks), and the contracture of the sternocleidomastoid muscle becomes apparent. Recent pathologic studies suggest that with time the fibrosis of the sternal head may entrap and compromise the branch of the accessory nerve to the clavicular head of the muscle, further increasing deformity.

Differential diagnosis in the newborn of soft-tissue problems includes abnormal skin webs or folds (pterygium colli) that maintain the torticollis posture and tumors in the region of the sternocleidomastoid (cystic hygroma, branchial cleft cysts, and thyroid teratomas) which, though rare, must be considered.

It also should be remembered that there is a 20 percent incidence of congenital hip dysplasia in these children.

If the contracture does not improve, deformities of the face and skull (plagiocephaly) can result and are usually apparent within the first year (Fig. 13). Flattening of the face on the side of the contracted sternocleidomastoid, due to sleeping position, may be particularly impressive. Thus, if the child sleeps supine, the flattening occurs on the back of the head, and if prone, on the face. The use of a helmet aids in reducing the deformity and hastening face and skull remodeling.

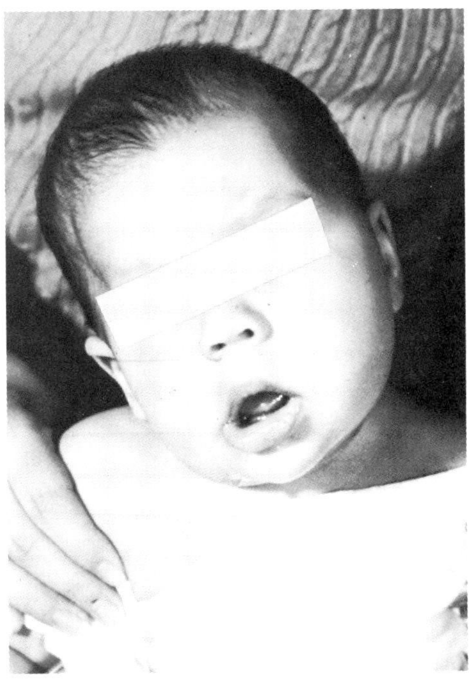

Figure 13: Congenital muscular torticollis. Six month old demonstrates the typical posture with the head tilted toward the involved side and the chin rotated to the contralateral shoulder. Note the flattening of the face and skull (plagiocephaly) on the side of the contracted muscle.

TREATMENT: In the first year of life treatment consists of stretching exercises, range of motion, and positioning. Approximately 85-90 percent of patients respond satisfactorily. If nonoperative measures are unsuccessful by 18 to 24 months of age, surgical intervention is needed to prevent further facial flattening and poor cosmesis (Fig. 14). Surgery usually consists of resection of a portion of the distal sternocleidomastoid muscle. The incision should be positioned transversely in the neck to coincide with the normal skin folds. Placement of the incision near the clavicle should be avoided since scars in this area tend to hypertrophy and spread. The postoperative regimen includes passive stretching exercises and occasionally an orthosis or cast to maintain the corrected position.

MISCELLANEOUS TYPES: If posturing of the head and neck is noted shortly after birth, congenital anomalies of the cervical spine, particularly those involving the occipitocervical junction, should be considered. Clinical findings of torticollis may be present in patients with Klippel-Feil syndrome, basilar impression, and atlantooccipital fusion. Unlike muscular torticollis, the sternocleidomastoid muscle is not contracted in these patients.

Intermittent torticollis can occur in the young child. A seizure-like disorder called *benign paroxysmal torticollis of infancy* is due to many neurologic causes, including drug intoxication. Similarly, Sandifer's syndrome involving gastroesophageal reflux with sudden posturing of the trunk and torticollis is being recognized more often.

In later childhood, bacterial or viral pharyngitis with

involvement of the cervical nodes is a primary cause of torticollis. Spontaneous atlantoaxial rotatory subluxation can occur following acute pharyngitis. Since radiographic confirmation is difficult, computed tomography is helpful in evaluation. Torticollis may accompany a number of inflammatory conditions such as juvenile rheumatoid arthritis, infection of the cervical spine, and acute calcification of a cervical disc.

Traumatic causes should be considered and carefully excluded in the evaluation. If unrecognized, they may have serious neurologic consequences. Torticollis most commonly follows an injury to the C1-2 articulation. Since fractures and dislocations of the odontoid may not be apparent on initial radiographic views, a high degree of suspicion with careful follow-up is required. Children with bone dysplasias, Morquio's syndrome, spondyloepiphyseal dysplasia, and Down's syndrome have a high incidence of C1-2 instability with accompanying torticollis.

Neurologic disorders, particularly space-occupying lesions of the central nervous system (e.g., posterior fossa tumors, tumors of the spinal column, cordoma, and syringomyelia), are often accompanied by torticollis. Uncommon neurologic causes include dystonia musculorum deformans and problems of hearing and vision that can result in head tilt. Though uncommon, hysterical and psychogenic causes exist but should be diagnosed only after carefully excluding other causes.

Vertebral Disc Calcification In this uncommon childhood problem, cervical involvement (typically the C6-7 level) occurs most frequently, with 30 percent of patients having a history of trauma and 15 percent an upper respiratory infection. Usually the onset of symptoms is abrupt with torticollis, neck pain, and limitation of motion the usual presenting complaints. Only 25 percent of the patients are febrile. Rarely, the disc may herniate posteriorly, causing spinal cord compression. If the disc herniates anteriorly, dysphagia may result. Rapid clinical and gradual radiographic resolution is the typical course of the illness. Two-thirds of the children are symptomless within 3 weeks and 95 percent within 6 months. Neurologic improvement can be expected in 90 percent of the patients.

Fractures

Cervical spine fractures in children are uncommon, representing only 2.5 to 3.0 percent of all spine trauma. Familiarity with normal variations in radiographic appearance of the cervical spine in children is essential. Similarly, awareness of the commonly injured sites and clinical signs is helpful in the management of these potentially severe injuries. Fractures of the upper cervical spine most commonly involve the C1-2 articulation and result in C1-2 instability. Fracture of the odontoid and atlantoaxial rotatory displacement are the most prevalent types. Less frequent are the hangman's fracture with C2-3 subluxation and fracture-dislocations of the lower cervical vertebrae.

Cervical spine injuries always should be suspected in children with head injuries, facial lacerations, loss of consciousness, or neck pain and torticollis following injury. Cervical spine radiographs should be taken. However, it is important to realize that the child's cervical spine is more elastic than the spinal cord, and most children under

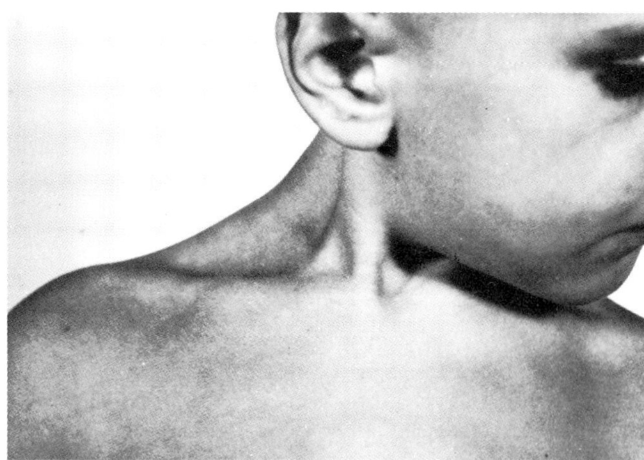

Figure 14: Six year old with untreated congenital muscular torticollis. Both the sternal and clavicular heads of the muscle are involved. Surgical release should be considered after 18 months to 2 years of age when nonsurgical measures are no longer expected to result in improvement.

10 years of age presenting with complete quadriplegia following trauma have no detectable bony injury.

It is now recognized more frequently that cervical spine injuries can occur during delivery. Children who have traumatic deliveries, those who are hypotonic in the newborn period, or those with respiratory problems should be examined for cervical injury.

Child abuse is one cause of injuries to the neck and head (e.g., the whiplash-shaken infant syndrome). Excessive shaking may cause intracranial and intraocular hemorrhages and death (see Section 7, General: Trauma).

Certain conditions, such as Down's syndrome and some bone dysplasias, including spondyloepiphyseal dysplasia, osteogenesis imperfecta, achondroplasia, and diastrophic dysplasia, predispose a child to cervical injury. With Down's syndrome there appears to be a 25 percent incidence of C1-2 instability, believed to be due to laxity of the transverse atlantal ligaments.

Incomplete ossification continues to pose a problem in radiographic interpretation. Variations in ossification are often confused with fracture, and, conversely, nondisplaced fractures may be misinterpreted as variations in ossification. Compression fractures are rare or at least rarely recognized, due to the normal anterior wedge-shaped appearance of the unossified vertebral bodies. By 8 to 10 years of age the cervical spine has attained the adult radiographic appearance except for the fusion of the vertebral end plates. Injuries due to distraction and/or shear forces tend to involve the cartilaginous vertebral end plates or, less commonly, the pars interarticularis. The intervertebral discs in children typically are stronger than bone and consequently are rarely disrupted.

Odontoid fractures in children usually represent epiphyseal slips through the synchondrosis, the lucent cartilaginous line that represents the embryologic base of the odontoid. The synchondrosis is normally present in children at age 3 years and is absent in most, but not all, by 6 years of age. The average age at injury is 4 years; thus, the injury can be easily overlooked. Fracture of the odontoid frequently is associated with head trauma (falls and motor vehicle accidents) in which force is transmitted to the upper cervical spine usually resulting in anterior displacement of the odontoid. The problem can be managed nonoperatively if recognized early, but if not recognized, the child may develop a nonunion.

The hangman's injury (C2-3 subluxation) is reported with increasing frequency and must be differentiated from C2-3 pseudosubluxation. If the fracture is recognized early and reduced, it can be expected to heal satisfactorily. Injuries in the lower cervical spine usually occur in the older child and can be treated as in an adult. A continuing problem is late recognition of significant soft-tissue injuries with resultant late angulation and cervical kyphosis.

Neoplasms

Spontaneous collapse of a vertebral body with only minor or no trauma should lead one to suspect a neoplasm or infection. Involvement of the vertebral body by an eosinophilic granuloma typically results in complete flattening (vertebrae plana). A wedge-shaped collapse is more typical of Ewing's tumor or infection. Involvement of the spine with neurofibromatosis can be devastating with considerable loss of bone substance and resulting instability. This is more common in those who have other areas of spine involvement (scoliosis/kyphosis). The cervical spine should be surveyed radiographically if traction or general anesthesia is considered.

ANNOTATED BIBLIOGRAPHY

Congenital and Developmental

Cervical Instability

Dawson, E.G., and Smith, L.: Atlanto-axial subluxation in children due to vertebral anomalies. J. Bone Joint Surg. 61A:582-587, 1979.

The authors note unusual manifestations and difficulties involved in diagnosing C1-2 instability. Children with instability are at risk of neurologic problems either from a natural increase in subluxation or from minor trauma.

Gangemi, M.; Renier, D.; Daussange, J.; Hirsch, J.F.; and Rigault, P.: Children's cervical spine instability after posterior fossa surgery. Acta Neurol. (Napoli) 37:39-43, 1982.

The essential factor leading to instability is the number of levels involved. Instability is rare when the lamina of C2 is respected, and increases in frequency when more than 20 percent of C2 is resected.

Geehr, R.B.; Rothman, S.L.G.; and Kier, E.L.: The role of computed tomography in the evaluation of upper cervical spine pathology. Comput. Tomogr. 2:79-97, 1978.

The CT scan is useful in diagnosing a variety of pathologic conditions in the upper cervical spine, particularly when they involve subtle neural arch fractures, rotational deformities, and conditions that compromise the neural canal.

Holmes, J.C., and Hall, J.E.: Fusion for instability and potential instability of the cervical spine in children and adolescents. Orthop. Clin. North America 9:923-943, 1978.

Abnormal motion in an immature spine or the potential for such motion should be viewed cautiously, for it may herald severe neurologic compromise. In children, surgical fusion is often the only satisfactory means of obtaining stability.

Nordt, J.C., and Stauffer, E.S.: Sequelae of atlantoaxial stabilization in two patients with Down's syndrome. Spine 6:437-440, 1981.

Two patients developed quadriplegia after manipulative reduction and fusion with sublaminar wiring. Traction should be used preoperatively to reduce the deformity and surgically to maintain alignment. If reduction cannot be obtained, then avoid sublaminar wiring and fuse in situ.

Ogden, J.A.: Postnatal development of the cervical spine. EOA Spinal Research Award. Orthop. Trans. 6:89-90, 1982.

A study of the growth and development of the cervical spine. Normal change in anatomy due to growth predisposes certain patterns of injury at different ages and must be considered in both diagnosis and treatment.

Swischuck, L.E.: Anterior displacement of C2 in children: Physiologic or pathologic? A helpful differentiating line. Radiology 122:759-763, 1977.

The straight line relationship of the posterior elements in flexion (the posterior cervical line) is more constant than specific measurements of the anterior displacement of the vertebral bodies.

Yasuoka, S.; Peterson, H.A.; and McCarty, C.S.: The incidence of spinal deformity and instability after multiple-level laminectomy: Its difference in children and adults. Orthop. Trans. 6:11, 1982.

The majority of children (89 percent) having a cervical laminectomy develop a spinal deformity. Less often deformity follows a thoracic laminectomy (36 percent), and none follow lumbar laminectomy.

Yousefzadeh, D.K.; El-Khoury, G.Y.; and Smith, W.L.: Normal sagittal diameter and variation in the pediatric cervical spine. Radiology 144:319-325, 1982.

A gradual widening of the sagittal diameter of the lower cervical canal and even ballooning in the mid-canal is common in normal children. Thus, sagittal widening of the canal in children is not a reliable sign of an expansile intraspinal lesion.

Os Odontoideum

Fielding, J.W.; Hensinger, R.N.; and Hawkins, R.J.: Os odontoideum. J. Bone Joint Surg. 62A:376-383, 1980.

Nine patients had a normal odontoid prior to the development of os odontoideum, suggesting a traumatic etiology. Twenty-two had anterior instability (average 1.03 cm). Five had posterior instability (average 0.84 cm) and eight had combined instability (average 1.37 cm).

Spierings, E.L., and Braakman, R.: The management of os odontoideum: Analysis of 37 cases. J. Bone Joint Surg. 64B:422-428, 1982.

Patients with local symptoms should not undergo surgical stabilization unless the SAC is less than 13 mm, as then they are at significant risk of developing permanent or progressive cord signs. Patients with progressive signs or myelopathy should be treated surgically.

Torticollis

Canale, S.T.; Griffin, D.W.; and Hubbard, C.N.: Congenital muscular torticollis. A long-term follow-up. J. Bone Joint Surg. 64A:810-816, 1982.

If the condition persists beyond 1 year of age, it does not resolve spontaneously, and nonoperative therapy is rarely successful. Established facial asymmetry and limitation of motion of more than 30 degrees usually precludes a good result.

Ramenofsky, M.L.; Buyse, M.; Goldberg, M.J.; and Leape, L.L.: Gastroesophageal reflux and torticollis. J. Bone Joint Surg. 60A:1140-1141, 1978.

Sandifer's syndrome is a combination of hiatal hernia and abnormal posturing of the head and neck. The abnormal posturing has been attributed as an attempt to decrease the pain of esophagitis resulting from gastroesophageal reflux and hiatal hernia.

Sarant, J.B., and Morrissy, R.T.: Idiopathic torticollis: Sternocleidomastoid myopathy and accessory neuropathy. Muscle and Nerve 4:374, 380, 1981.

The unique blood supply to the sternal head of the muscle predisposes it to ischemia, resulting in focal myopathy and fibrosis. The clavicular head demonstrates progressive denervation due to entrapment of the accessory nerve as it traverses the sternal head, resulting in further deformity.

Vertebral Disc Calcification

Sonnabend, D.H.; Taylor, T.K.F.; and Chapman, G.K.: Intervertebral disc calcification syndromes in children. J. Bone Joint Surg. 64B:25-31, 1982.

Cervical involvement is most common. There is an abrupt onset of symptoms: pain in the neck, torticollis, and reduced range of motion.

Neurologic symptoms are rare. Rapid clinical and gradual radiographic resolution is expected.

Fractures

Fielding, J.W., and Hawkins, R.J.: Atlanto-axial rotatory fixation (Fixed rotatory subluxation of the atlanto-axial joint). J. Bone Joint Surg. 59A:37-44, 1977.

All have torticollis and restricted, often painful, neck motion. Some with long-standing deformity have facial flattening. The deformity may compromise the SAC and even a minor injury to the neck may be catastrophic. If reduction cannot be achieved or recurs, fusion is indicated.

Sherk, H.H.; Nicholson, J.T.; and Chung, S.M.K.: Fractures of the odontoid process in young children. J. Bone Joint Surg. 60A:921-924, 1978.

The children who are recognized early and treated properly can be expected to do well. The fracture can usually be reduced by passive manipulation or the hanging head technique.

Neoplasms

Yong-Hing, K.; Kalamchi, A.; and MacEwen, G.D.: Cervical spine abnormalities in neurofibromatosis. J. Bone Joint Surg. 61A:695-699, 1979.

Thirty percent of patients with neurofibromatosis have cervical spine involvement, particularly those with scoliosis and/or kyphosis (44 percent). The cervical spine should be evaluated prior to general anesthesia or skull traction.

24 CERVICAL SPINE: TRAUMA

Topics considered in this section include patient evaluation and management of cervical spine subluxations, dislocations, and fractures.

Patient Evaluation

Patients sustaining injuries to the cervical spine require careful evaluation. Particular attention should be directed toward the mechanism of injury, the patient's neurologic status, and an adequate radiographic examination.

Mechanism of Injury Cervical fractures and dislocations from direct blows are rare. They usually occur as a result of blows to the head, as in diving. Any patient presenting with evidence of trauma to the head and/or pain in the neck should be considered as having a cervical spinal injury until proven otherwise. Fractures and dislocations of the cervical vertebrae may be missed in patients sustaining multiple trauma unless specifically considered, especially in the unconscious patient.

Sudden acceleration forces applied to the stationary body and head (i.e., struck from behind while sitting in an automobile) may cause rapid extension-flexion forces to the flexible cervical spine, causing painful strains of the musculoligamentous complex without objective evidence of fracture or subluxation.

Neurologic Evaluation The most serious consequence of fractures and dislocations of the cervical spine is injury to the enclosed spinal cord and/or nerve roots. Due to the intimate relationship of the spinal cord and nerve roots within the vertebral canal and neural foramina, documentation of the integrity of the cervical nerve root and spinal cord function is necessary, including the upper and lower extremities, perianal sensation, and rectal-sphincter control. Pathologic reflexes (ankle clonus and Babinski sign) may indicate an occult injury in an otherwise normal examination.

Documentation of neurologic injury is necessary to determine the extent and prognosis of the lesion and for communication among the members of the health care team. Spinal cord lesions are described by the lowest level of injury to the spinal cord and nerve root. For example, a C4 quadriplegic has no function below C4.

CLASSIFICATION OF NEUROLOGIC INJURY: The American Spinal Injury Association has suggested a classification of spinal cord injury based upon anatomical involvement and functional impairment and also a method of documenting recovery or deterioration of function.

ANATOMICAL CLASSIFICATION: With *complete* injury there is no motor or sensory function below the zone of injury. With *incomplete* injury there is partial preservation of motor or sensory function below the zone of injury.

Incomplete spinal cord injuries are further subdivided. In the *anterior cord syndrome,* there is motor paralysis below the zone of injury with hypesthesia, hypalgesia, and preservation of posterior column sensory function only (no sharp/dull, hot/cold discrimination). In the *central cord syndrome* there is dissociation in degree of motor paralysis with lower limbs stronger than upper limbs and sacral sensory sparing, specifically sharp/dull discrimination. With modified hemisection of cord *(Brown-Séquard syndrome),* there is motor paralysis greater on the homolateral side and sensory loss greater on the contralateral side. A *mixed syndrome* is an unclassifiable combination of the above.

FUNCTIONAL CLASSIFICATION: Five levels of function have been defined based on the extent of neurologic injury. These are: (1) *complete paralysis* (see preceding description); (2) *incomplete–sensory only* with preservation of objective sensory function below the zone of injury (trunk, lumbar, or sacral areas) and no voluntary motor function; (3) *incomplete–motor useless* with preservation of "useless" motor function below the zone of injury (lumbar and sacral innervated areas) and trace and/or poor muscle grades; (4) *incomplete–motor functional* with preservation of useful, voluntary motor function below the zone of injury and fair and/or good grade muscles; and (5) *normal* with normal voluntary motor power and sensory function preserved or recovered following injury although residual abnormal reflexes or paresthesias may be present.

Quantitative motor recovery is documented by an extremity trauma motor index score. Using standard physical therapy muscle testing techniques, selected muscles are tested to document functional motor levels and preservation or recovery of voluntary muscles following a spinal injury.

Using the anatomical and functional classifications and the extremity trauma motor index, an accurate assessment of the initial neurologic injury and the degree of recovery (or deterioration) can be documented (Table I).

Radiographic Evaluation Documentation of skeletal injuries is necessary for determining those injuries that are mechanically stable and those that are unstable. Unstable injuries may jeopardize the spinal cord and nerve root function in the acute phase or lead to late instability with pain and/or neurologic deterioration in the chronic phase.

In general, patients with paralysis have a higher degree of instability than patients with a normal neurological examination. Standard radiographs and computed tomography provide the best documentation of the ligamentous-osseous injury.

Spine Fracture Study

Surgeon's Name ____________

Patient ____________ Age ______ Gender ______ Occupation ____________ MR# ____

Injury level ______ Type ____________ Cause ____________

Date of injury ______ Date of adm. ______ Date of surgery ______ Date disch. home ______

Non-surgical treatment ____________

(Days bedrest, type brace or cast, etc.)

Surgical treatment ____________

____

(Instruments used, levels fused, bone graft type, p.o. immobilization)

Date								TRAUMA MOTOR INDEX			Date						
2yr	1yr	6mo	3mo	1mo	1wk	init.	RIGHT	Muscles		LEFT	init.	1wk	1mo	3mo	6mo	1yr	2yr
							+/-	Diaphragm	C-4	+/-							
							0-5	BICEPS	C-5	0-5							
							0-5	WRIST EXT	C-6	0-5							
							0-5	TRICEPS	C-7	0-5							
							0-5	FLEX PROF	C-8	0-5							
							0-5	INTRINSIC	T-1	0-5							
							+/-	Intercost	2-9	+/-							
							+/-	Abdominal	10-12	+/-							
							0-5	ILIOPSOAS	L-2	0-5							
							0-5	QUADRICEP	L-3	0-5							
							0-5	TIB ANTER	L-4	0-5							
							0-5	EX HALLIC	L-5	0-5							
							0-5	GASTROC	S-1	0-5							
							+/-	Blad sph	S-2	+/-							
							+/-	Anal sph	S-3	+/-							
							+/-	B-C reflex		+/-							
							50	TOTAL		50							
								BILATERAL TOTAL		100							
								FRANKEL CLASS (A-E)									
								INCOMPLETE SYNDROME (ant, cent, B.S., mx conus, cauda)									

200

C:T

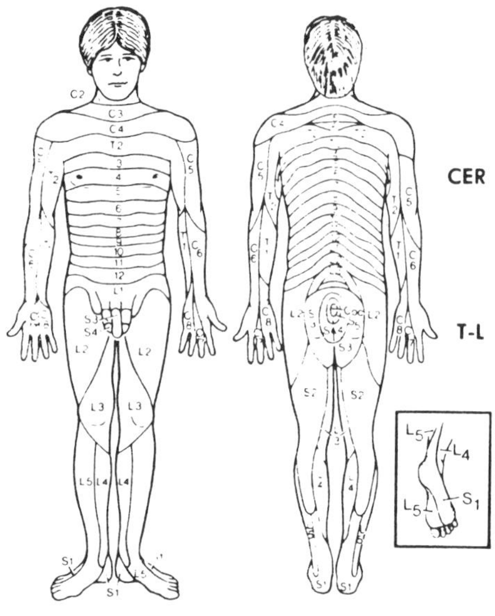

CER	Jefferson	Hangman	Odontoid (I, II, III)	Facet Dx	Body Comp	Burst	Other
T-L	Comp	Slice	Burst (ant body)	Burst (post body)	Chance	Dislocation	Other

ADAPTED FROM AUSTIN

NORMAL ☐

ABSENT

IMPAIRED

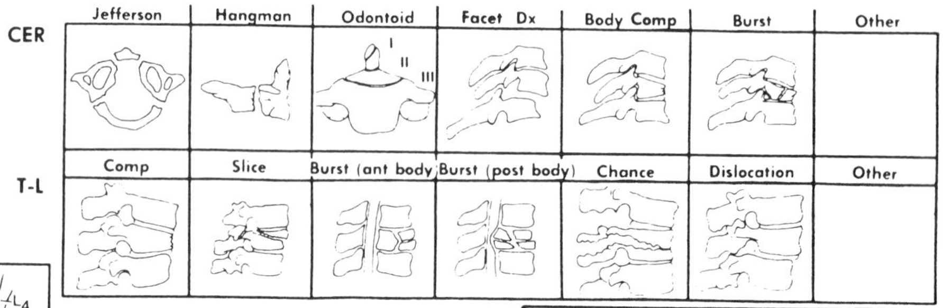

X-Ray Evaluation	Date: init.	1wk	1mo	3mo	6mo	1yr	2yr
KYPHOS ANGLE-degree							
ANTERIOR DISP-mm							
LAT SCOLIOSIS ANGLE-degree							
LAT DISPLACEMENT-mm							
MYELOGRAM % BLOCK							
REG TOMOG % BLOCK							
COMPT TOMOG % BLOCK							

Summary (treatment, results, complications)

3rd mo | 6 mo | 1 yr

Total hosp. days ______

Table I: Flow sheet used to document the initial motor trauma index, Frankel classification, incomplete anatomic syndrome, sensory level, type of fracture, reduction, and residual displacement for patients with spine fractures.

Skeletal deformity on lateral radiographs is quantitated by measuring the displacement of the bony elements in millimeters (i.e., separation of the spinous processes and the anteroposterior displacement of the vertebra) and the degree of angulation of kyphosis. Use of computed tomography may lead to more accurate quantitative descriptions of bony displacement and spinal canal encroachment.

All patients with suspected injuries of the cervical spine should have adequate radiographic evaluation of the entire cervical spine prior to any manipulation or movement of the head. First, a lateral radiograph to include C1 through T1 should be taken. If a fracture or dislocation is seen, application of skeletal traction tongs to further immobilize the spine (beyond the collar and spine board) should be considered prior to further radiographic evaluation. If the lateral radiograph is normal, anteroposterior, open-mouth, and oblique views are taken. A stretch test radiograph may be considered if all static radiographs are normal. This is a lateral view taken with 12 kg traction on a cervical halter to confirm ligamentous integrity. It has been recommended that the weight be increased in increments of 5 kg every 5 minutes up to a total of one-third the body weight, or 30 kg. Any change in neurologic status, interspace separation greater than 1.7 mm, or angulation greater than 7.5 degrees is considered positive. If the preceding radiographs are negative, flexion-extension views may be considered but, because of protective muscle spasm, are rarely of value in the acute postinjury period.

If routine radiographs are not adequate to explain the symptoms or physical findings, *computed tomography* of the occipitocervical junction (C1-2, see Fig. 1) and the cervicothoracic junction (C7-T1) may demonstrate junctional injuries. Computed tomography is much more accurate with less radiation exposure than conventional tomography or "swimmer's views."

Myelography is indicated in the acute phase only if there is a neurologic deficit that cannot be explained by noninvasive radiographic technique or if the patient demonstrates progressive neurologic deterioration. The myelogram may show soft tissue encroachment on the spinal cord, such as a herniated disc, extramedullary tumor, or epidural abscess, which may be responsible for an incomplete paralysis syndrome. If the patient has an unexplained paralysis and there is no detectable bone or ligament injury, a conventional myelogram with Pantopaque introduced by a lumbar puncture provides a more detailed evaluation of the cervical spinal cord. If there is a potentially unstable skeletal lesion, a "minimyelogram" with 2 to 3 cc of Pantopaque introduced from above the lesion by a C1-2 lateral puncture with the patient in traction in the "head-up" inclined position demonstrates the location of a significant cervical canal block.

Metrizamide (water soluble) may be used for lumbar and thoracic myelography. It is not routinely used in the cervical spinal canal because of central nervous system irritation and poor visualization difficulties due to dilutional dispersion.

Patient Management

Strains A strain is defined as a tearing or stretching beyond physiological limits of a muscle-tendon unit. The diagnosis is based on tenderness to palpation and pain on motion of muscles without evidence of associated ligament or bony injury.

The management of patients with injuries to the cervical area without evidence of fracture, ligament rupture, or neurologic loss is based upon control of pain and prevention of both muscle atrophy and joint stiffness with loss of motion. The etiology of the chronic pain which follows muscular strains is elusive. Temporary immobilization by a cervical collar is frequently beneficial in relieving pain. However, this must be accompanied by assisted progressive isometric and isotonic exercises to maintain strength, regain flexibility of the muscles, and maintain motion. Cervical halter traction in the supine or sitting position also may provide symptomatic relief by relaxation of tense muscles. Physical modalities (such as heat, ultrasound, diathermy, or icing techniques) may be used for pain relief and muscle relaxation in preparation for exercises, but these have no healing capabilities of their own. Injection of tender "trigger points" around the area of the insertion of the levator scapulae and rhomboid muscles on the vertebral border of the scapula may provide temporary relief of the local pain in the area, but the results are usually short-lived. Nonsteroidal anti-inflammatory medications as well as muscle relaxants and tranquilizers often are prescribed. These are frequently helpful in managing the patient's overall symptom complex, but the specific mechanism of relief is unclear. Although the occasional strain may precipitate a chronic pain syndrome which lasts several years, these injuries are usually self-limiting and improve with time.

Sprains Sprain is defined as a tearing or a rupture of a ligament(s). There are four classes: I, partial tears with no defect or instability; II, defect in the ligament but no instability; III, complete tear with instability; and IV, dislocation.

Class I sprains are diagnosed by local tenderness isolated to the space between specific spinous processes on the posterior aspect of the neck. This is a clinical diagnosis in view of normal radiographic findings. Class II sprains, which may demonstrate a palpable gap between spinous processes, are identified on radiographs as an increased distance between adjacent spinous processes or widening induced by the stretch test without subluxation or instability.

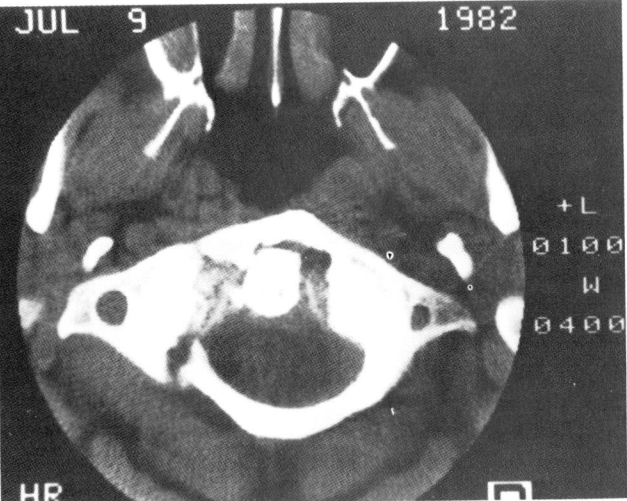

Figure 1: Computed tomogram demonstrating fractures of the ring of C1

Class I and II sprains are stable and should be treated with bracing in the extended position and follow-up at 2 and 3 months to detect potential late instability.

Strains may occur in combination with class I and II sprains. Generalized tenderness over the extensor muscles is indicative of a strain, whereas localized tenderness of spinous processes is indicative of a sprain.

The management of these stable injuries is symptomatic, i.e., analgesics and collar immobilization. The prognosis for recovery from muscular strains is usually slower than for sprains.

Class III sprains are identified by subluxation of the facet joints without dislocation. Class IV sprains demonstrate complete ligamentous rupture, instability, and facet dislocation. Class III and IV sprains allow abnormal motion beyond physiological limits of the affected joints and are unstable. These injuries are discussed under facet subluxations and dislocations in this section.

Disc injuries and associated radiculopathies are discussed in Section 25, Cervical Spine: Reconstruction.

Upper Cervical Spine

Occipital C1 Separation The occiput can be separated from the spine by severe flexion-extension or twisting forces applied to the head. The occipital-C1 junction is primarily maintained by the joint capsules, as there is no posterior longitudinal ligament and only a thin anterior longitudinal ligament. When the capsules are torn and the head is separated from the neck, the injury is usually fatal due to brain stem damage. If the patient does survive, the diagnosis must be suspected prior to the application of skull traction. If any displacement is seen between the occiput and C1, traction should be avoided. Rigid immobilization in a halo-body cast, followed by early occipital C1-2 fusion, is indicated.

C1-2 Subluxation Subluxation of C1 on C2 without fracture of the odontoid may result in a displacement of C1 anterior on C2 due to rupture of the transverse and other supporting ligaments or a rotary subluxation of one C1-2 facet joint which dislocates anteriorly in a rotary fashion and remains fixed in place. They tend to recur after reduction and immobilization and usually require a C1-2 posterior fusion to prevent recurrence. C1-2 dislocations are rare.

Fractures of C1 Computed tomography has provided a clearer image of fracture of C1 than conventional radiographic images or anteroposterior and lateral tomography (Fig. 1). C1 is a rigid bony ring and (depending upon the applied forces) if it breaks at one site there is usually another fracture(s) of the ring. If only one break in the ring is identified, a congenital failure of complete ossification should be suspected. Undisplaced fractures of the ring of C1 may heal rapidly with cervical orthotic immobilization. However, delayed union with persistent symptoms may warrant halo-jacket immobilization, especially when there is any displacement. To allow adequate healing of the atlas cortical bone ring, immobilization, including limitation of rotatory motion, should continue for 12 weeks and until the patient is pain free.

Fractures of the Odontoid Fractures of the odontoid are caused most often by automobile accidents and falls and are usually associated with trauma to the head. As reflected by the divergent results reported in the literature, there is no consensus about the nonoperative treatment of these fractures. Fracture location and displacement as well as patient age are prognostically important. Type I (the upper tip) and type III (across the base extending down into the body of C2) fractures have a high union rate with immobilization, rarely requiring fusion. On the other hand, type II fractures (across the waist) have nonunion rates of 20 to 80 percent. Undisplaced fractures in young adults have the lowest nonunion rate. Those displaced more than 4 mm in patients over 50 years of age have the highest nonunion rate. If the type II fracture is nondisplaced or can be reduced, it should be treated with 8 to 12 weeks in a halo-jacket, followed by an additional 8 to 12 weeks in a cervical orthosis. It may take 6 months to demonstrate bony union of this peg of bone. If the fracture cannot be reduced to within 4 mm of normal, especially in the older patient, early C1-2 posterior fusion should be considered. An advantage of early posterior C1-2 fusion is that it allows mobilization of the patient in a cervical orthosis instead of a halo, some motion of the other joints of the cervical spine, and exercise of the cervical spine muscles. Immobilization in a halo for 12 weeks, on the other hand, frequently results in stiffness of the cervical spine and atrophy of cervical muscles. Many months of rehabilitation may be required to regain strength of the muscles and flexibility of the cervical spine.

Delayed union of type II fractures may eventually heal. However, if at 16 weeks there is motion or dissolution of bone at the fracture site and continued cervical pain, posterior C1-2 fusion is recommended.

Occasionally, an odontoid fracture is accompanied by a posterior C1 ring fracture. This should be ruled out prior to attempting a C1-2 posterior fusion because wiring it to C2 does not reestablish stability and may lead to a nonunion of the fracture of the ring of C1.

Posterior C1-2 fusion is performed by exposure of the central part of the posterior ring of C1 and exposure of the spinous process and lamina of C2. Lateral exposure is to be avoided because of the presence of the vertebral arteries. A double loop of wire is passed under the arch of C1 and tightened around the spinous process of C2. The dorsal arches of C1 and C2 are decorticated with a double-action bone rongeur or air-driven burr. These methods are safer than the use of gouges or osteotomes. Strips of iliac corticocancellous bone are then added to the decorticated posterior elements of C1 and C2. Some investigators recommend passing two double loops of wire beneath the lamina of C2 as well as under the arch of C1, but others believe this adds unnecessary risk to the spinal cord and vertebral arteries. There is no added advantage of attempting arthrodesis to the occiput or the spinous process of C3 when treating isolated fractures of the odontoid.

Fracture of C2 (Traumatic Spondylolisthesis of C2, "Hangman's Fracture") This injury is characterized on the lateral radiograph as a fracture through the pedicles of C2 with forward displacement of the body of C2 on C3. The inferior facet joints of C2 remain normally articulated with the superior facets of C3. A fracture of C2 is most frequently caused by hyperextension forces. The injury is often unstable, and, although it may be reduced with traction, it usually returns to its original displaced position. Nonunion is uncommon. These fractures heal with

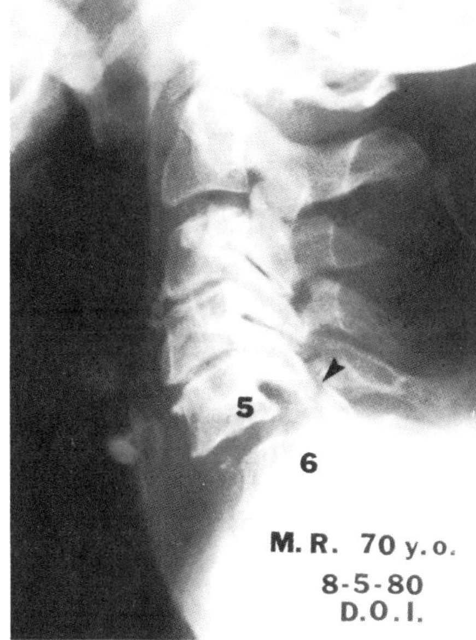

Figure 2-A

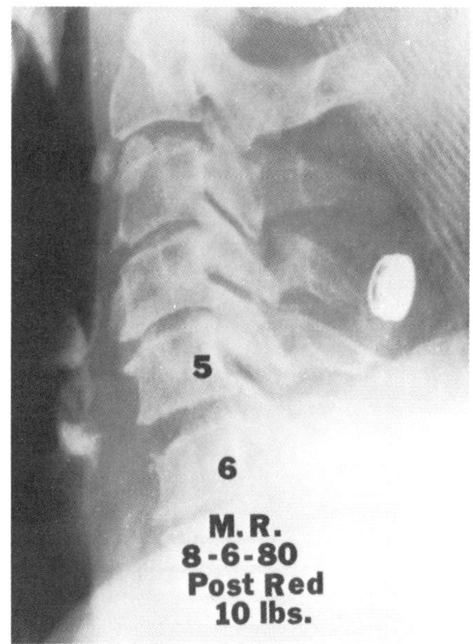

Figure 2-B

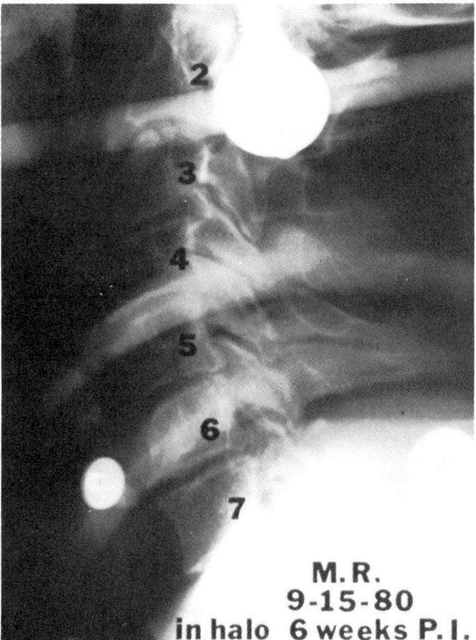

Figure 2-C

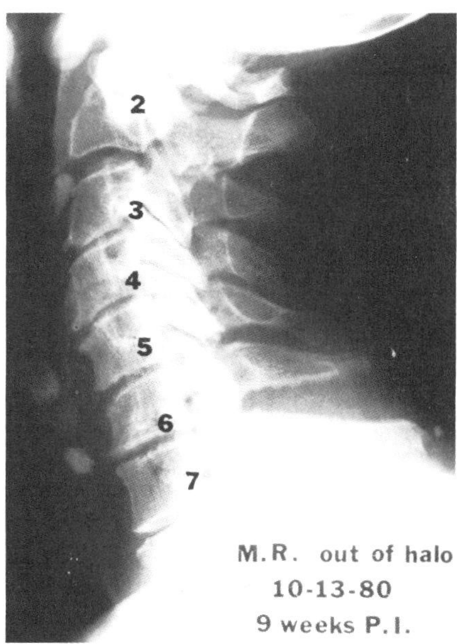

Figure 2-D

Figure 2: (A) Lateral radiograph demonstrating bilateral facet dislocation with fracture of facet. (B) Dislocation reduced with halo traction. (C) Stable healing in halo-body jacket. (D) Healed and stable, 9 weeks postinjury.

Figure 3-A

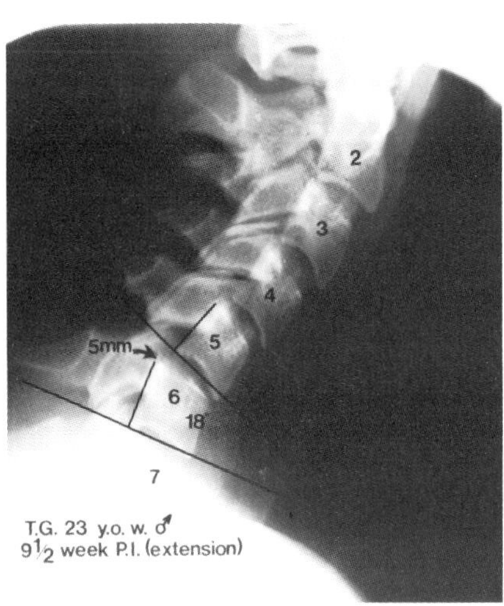

Figure 3-B

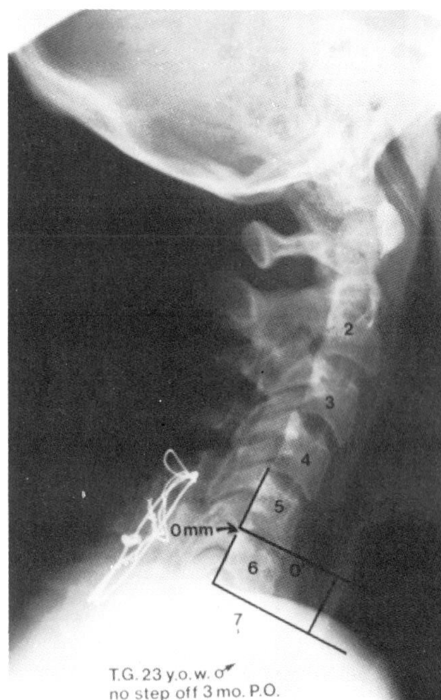

Figure 3-C

Figure 3: (A) Lateral radiograph demonstrating compression fracture of the body of C6 with widening of the interspinous distance. Displacement is 3 mm and angulation is 8 degrees between C5 and C6. There is also a fracture of the arch of C2 (note arrow). (B) Same patient, 9½ weeks postinjury, treated with a Somi brace. Five mm anterior displacement and 18 degrees angulation exceed the criteria for prediction of instability. Kyphosis angulation of greater than 11 degrees more than adjacent disc spaces and/or more than 3.5 mm of anterior vertebral body displacement indicate progressive instability. (C) Lateral radiograph of same patient illustrating posterior interspinous wire fixation and fusion.

union of the pedicles and often with associated spontaneous anterior ankylosis between C2 and C3 with external immobilization in a halo-body jacket for a period of 8 weeks. If delayed union or late instability results, anterior C2-3 fusion is preferred to posterior C1-2 fusion because it stabilizes the C2 body to C3 without the loss of rotation that accompanies a posterior C1-2 fusion. Posterior fusion to C3 is usually not necessary because the posterior elements of C2 are in normal alignment with C3.

Lower Cervical Spine (C3-7 Injuries) In addition to neurologic evaluation and radiographic analysis, management of cervical fractures and dislocations is guided by a knowledge of their natural history.

If there is neurologic loss, the neck should be immobilized by skeletal traction, and any malalignment of the spine reduced by appropriate traction. A halo may be used for initial traction if the type of injury is amenable to definitive halo-jacket immobilization therapy.

Facet Dislocation in the Spinal Cord Injured Patient If spinal alignment cannot be obtained by guided traction to reduce the unilateral or bilateral dislocated facets, early open reduction should be considered. Unless it can be shown that more immediate surgery is advisable, 12 to 24 hours are allowed to obtain closed reduction with traction and muscle relaxation. If this is unsuccessful, open reduction and spinous process wiring is advised, thus allowing early removal of traction tongs and mobilization of the patient in an orthosis within several days of injury. It must be realized, however, that even careful open reduction under anesthesia carries a small, but definite, risk of increasing the neurologic deficit in patients with partial cord injury.

If closed reduction is accomplished by traction, the patient may be treated with bed rest in continual traction or mobilized in a halo-body jacket and rehabilitation begun. An elective posterior "in situ" fusion of the dislocation reduced in traction may be considered to allow early mobilization in a cervical orthosis without the necessity of a halo-body jacket, virtually assuring a straight, stable spine. Unfortunately, ligamentous healing in a halo-body jacket without fusion is poor and frequently results in persistent instability and late redisplacement. Closed reduction, if possible, is desirable as there is less risk of added neurologic damage while the patient is awake when compared with attempted reduction of dislocated locked facets under anesthesia. When closed reduction is unsuccessful, open reduction and fusion is necessary. Incomplete lesions generally show progressive recovery of neurologic function. Complete lesions usually show recovery only of nerve root function at the zone of injury. Posterior fusion is preferred to anterior fusion for these injuries since the instability is due to the disrupted posterior ligaments, and the dislocation may be reduced under direct vision. Anterior fusions for posterior instability have a high incidence of postoperative graft displacement.

Facet Dislocations Without Neurologic Loss Facet dislocations without neurologic loss are treated in a similar manner with more time and effort spent obtaining closed reduction with traction. The application of a halo to obtain better control of flexion-extension and rotation may help achieve reduction in patients with difficult injuries. Closed reduction with traction in the conscious patient is infrequently associated with spinal cord or nerve root function deterioration.

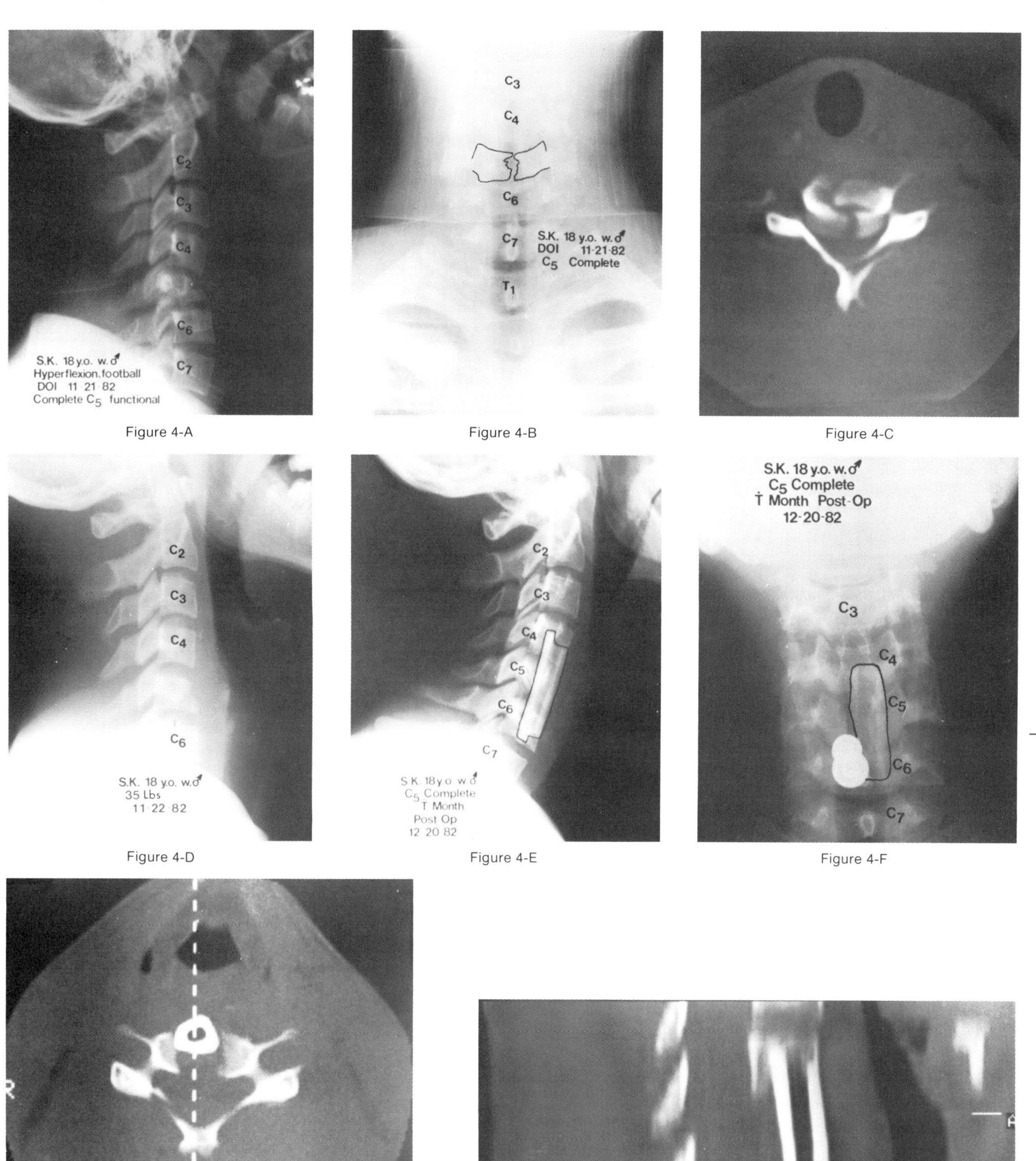

Figure 4-G

Figure 4-H

Figure 4: (A) Lateral radiograph of an 18-year-old patient demonstrating comminuted ("burst") body fracture of C5. (B) Anteroposterior radiograph demonstrating an increase in the interpedicular width and a sagittal fracture of the body of C5. (C) Computed tomogram demonstrating comminuted vertebral body fracture and left laminar fracture. (D) Lateral radiograph demonstrating improvement of alignment of fracture fragments and integrity of the posterior ligaments with 35 pounds of longitudinal traction in Gardner-Wells tongs. (E) Lateral radiograph demonstrating full-thickness fibular strut graft reconstruction for the burst fracture of the body of C5. (F) Anteroposterior radiograph following anterior fibular strut stabilization. (G) Computed tomogram following fibular strut stabilization. (H) Sagittal reconstruction demonstrating self-locking position of the posterior cortex of the fibula into the body of C4 superiorly and C6 inferiorly and the support position of the anterior cortex of the fibula supporting the anterior cortex of the body of C4 and resting on the anterior cortex of the body of C6.

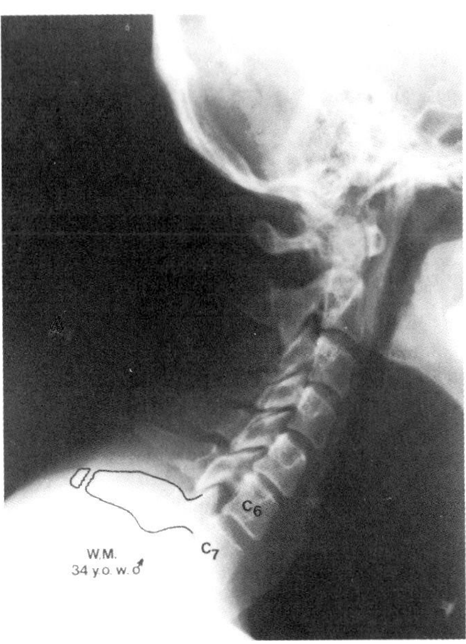

Figure 5: Radiograph demonstrating avulsion fracture of the spinous process of C7 (clay shoveler's fracture). These fractures have no significant influence on stability or neurologic damage.

Facet dislocations with facet or lateral mass fractures frequently heal spontaneously in traction or halo-jacket immobilization (Fig. 2).

Ligamentous injuries with facet subluxations or dislocations without evidence of posterior element fracture heal poorly with a high percentage of late instability. Early elective posterior internal fixation with interspinous process wiring and bone grafting should be strongly considered to allow early mobilization in an orthosis. If nonoperative management is elected, radiographic follow-up at 6 and 12 weeks is necessary to evaluate stable healing. If the subluxation recurs or there is pain or persistent motion, elective posterior fusion should be considered.

Facet Subluxation Without Dislocation Because of protective muscle spasm, these apparently "benign" injuries may not be obvious on the original radiographs. With a widening between the spinous processes, any anterior subluxated position of the vertebral body or angulation at the disc space must be carefully evaluated for potential persistent instability. Lesions considered unstable are those with angulation of more than 11 degrees and/or more than 3.5 mm anterior displacement of the vertebral body (Fig. 3). Any patient with subluxation, angulation, displacement, or spinous process widening should be protected in an orthosis or halo-body jacket and followed. If symptoms persist or displacement increases during the healing period of approximately 16 weeks, a posterior fusion should be performed. If progressive displacement occurs, it can be demonstrated at 16 weeks by flexion-extension radiographs.

Comminuted Vertebral Body Fractures Axial load forces on the cervical spine resulting in comminuted vertebral body fractures with or without posterior facet dislocation usually cause severe spinal cord damage with resultant permanent paralysis (Fig. 4A). The anterior portion of the vertebral body is split off and displaced anteriorly. The posterior portion of the vertebral body is split off posteriorly into the spinal canal, impacting the cord. The middle mass of the vertebral body is split sagittally (Fig. 4B), producing a widening of the interpedicular distance on the anteroposterior radiograph. There is usually an accompanying fracture through the posterior arch, either through one or both of the pedicles or laminae (Fig. 4C). By tensing the ligamentous attachments, straight longitudinal traction will often pull these fragments into improved alignment, thereby decreasing pressure on the spinal cord (Fig. 4D). Healing may be accomplished in traction but requires 12 to 16 weeks in the recumbent position. These injuries, if minimally displaced, may be treated with halo-jacket immobilization. However, if there is significant displacement requiring reduction in traction, the halo-jacket cannot be depended upon to maintain the reduction.

Surgical removal of the comminuted vertebral body fragments and replacement strut graft stabilization by the anterior approach (Figs. 4E, F) provides adequate stability for early mobilization in a cervical orthosis. Prior to anterior reconstructive surgery, stability must be evaluated on the maximum traction lateral radiograph with a stretch test (traction increments of 5 kg up to a maximum of 30 kg or one-third the body weight, Fig. 4D). If the posterior interspinous ligament complex remains intact and the facet joints are not dislocated, anterior strut grafting is sufficient to reestablish stability. If the posterior ligamentous complex is disrupted in addition to the comminuted anterior body fracture, anterior strut grafting should be followed by halo-body jacket immobilization for 6 to 12 weeks or a second stage posterior interspinous process wiring and bone grafting should be performed.

Several sources of bone grafts are suitable for the anterior strut graft. A corticocancellous iliac-crest graft is probably the most common choice. A tibial or fibular cortical graft can be used as a strut. The iliac-crest graft demonstrates earliest radiographic evidence of union and host replacement. Stability is not as rigid, however, as with fibular graft (Figs. 4E-H). Replacement by host bone requires a longer period of time with a tibial or fibular graft. It is important to use a one-piece strut graft rather than several bone grafts placed in individual disc spaces. Multiple grafts at several disc levels are associated with a higher level of failure of fusion than strut grafts. The strut graft is placed under compression which aids healing.

The avoidance of prolonged bed rest or halo-jacket immobilization in the quadriplegic patient prevents muscle atrophy of the functioning muscles, other metabolic complications, and psychological depression which accompanies long-term bed immobilization. Rehabilitation time and hospital stay are decreased with early surgical stabilization. Some retrospective studies indicate that anterior decompression may result in improved neurologic recovery in some patients with incomplete quadriplegia, but this has not yet been shown statistically in an adequately matched series of surgical versus nonsurgical management.

Isolated fractures of the spinous processes of the lower cervical vertebrae are stable avulsion fractures (Fig. 5). They do not displace or cause neural damage. They are treated symptomatically and do not cause long-term problems, even though they may heal by a fibrous union.

ANNOTATED BIBLIOGRAPHY

Patient Evaluation

Allen, B.L., Jr.; Ferguson, R.L.; Lehmann, T.R.; and O'Brien, R.P.: A mechanistic classification of closed, indirect fractures and dislocations of the lower cervical spine. Spine 7:1-27, 1982.

This comprehensive classification identified six common patterns of injury from a retrospective analysis of 165 fractures and dislocations. The radiographs of each group are further subdivided into stages according to anatomic damage. The authors state that in using their classification, it is possible to formulate a rational treatment plan, although treatment is not discussed.

Carol, M.; Ducker, T.B.; and Byrnes, D.P.: Minimyelogram in cervical spinal cord trauma. Neurosurgery 7:219-224, 1980.

Fifty-eight patients are presented who had Pantopaque "minimyelograms" after spinal realignment was achieved by closed methods. Fourteen had myelographic defects, five of which were believed to be indicative of operative intervention; two patients operated upon demonstrated improvement greater than that predicted. The authors state their protocol for the Pantopaque minimyelogram in the immediate management of spinal cord injured patients.

Lucas, J.T., and Ducker, T.B.: Motor classification of spinal cord injuries with mobility, morbidity and recovery indices. Am. Surg. 45:151-158, 1979.

The authors suggest a neuro-trauma motor index for the initial evaluation and recovery of spinal cord injured patients using standard muscle test scores of selected muscles; 436 patients were evaluated in regard to their initial and recovery indices. This system allows a quantitative documentation of the degree of paralysis and recovery rates following injury to the spinal cord.

Post, M.J.D.; Green, B.A.; Quencer, R.M.; Stokes, N.A.; Callahan, R.A.; and Eismont, F.J.: The value of computed tomography in spinal trauma. Spine 7:417-431, 1982.

Sixty patients with spinal trauma were reviewed with regard to information obtained by computed tomography, plain films, tomograms and/or myelograms. Forty patients had metrizamide CT scans. CT scans were particularly helpful in diagnosing neural arch fractures and spinal canal compromise. The addition of metrizamide helps to differentiate extrinsic cord pressure and cord edema. The authors recommend CT for routine use along with plain films in the evaluation of spine trauma. There is less manipulation of the patient, less radiation exposure, and fewer complications than encountered with conventional myelography.

Patient Management

Upper Cervical Spine

Böhler, J.: Anterior stabilization for acute fractures and non-unions of the dens. J. Bone Joint Surg. 64A:18-27, 1982.

Union was achieved in twenty-seven odontoid fractures treated with two compression screws through the body of C2 into the odontoid from the anterior approach. This procedure does not significantly limit head rotation as is frequently seen after posterior C1-2 arthrodesis.

Brooks, A.L., and Jenkins, E.B.: Atlanto-axial arthrodesis by the wedge compression method. J. Bone Joint Surg. 60A:279-284, 1978.

The authors advocate sublaminar passage of wires under C1 and C2 with compression of bone graft between the arch of C1 and the spinous process of C2 followed by a Minerva cast or four-poster brace. In fifteen patients, twelve of the thirteen nonrheumatoid patients achieved a fusion without apparent complication; both rheumatoid patients had complications with one nonunion and one intraoperative axis fracture necessitating fusion to the occiput. Although this modification of the conventional Gallie-type fusion provides more stability, there may be an added risk to the intradural contents by passage of the wire beneath the laminae of C2. The authors caution against its use in patients with severe osteopenia.

Griswold, D.M.; Albright, J.A.; Schiffman, E.; Johnson, R.; and Southwick, W.O.: Atlanto-axial fusion for instability. J. Bone Joint Surg. 60A:285-292, 1978.

Fifty-nine patients with atlantoaxial instability secondary to trauma were reviewed, using the criteria of the atlantodens interval exceeding 4 mm. Nineteen were treated nonoperatively, and eleven were treated with a posterior Gallie wiring and onlay bone graft. Thirty were treated with the fusion described by Brooks and Jenkins. Although comparison was difficult due to many variables, the incidence of solid fusion was higher after the Brooks fusion, despite less postoperative immobilization.

Schweigel, J.F.: Halo-thoracic brace management of odontoid fractures. Spine 4:192-194, 1979.

Thirteen adult patients with odontoid fractures were treated for at least 60 days in the halo-thoracic brace. Healing occurred in all patients, as evidenced by tomographic trabecular bridging of the fracture site. Although five of the thirteen fractures were undisplaced, all healed regardless of fracture type, degree or direction of displacement, or patient age.

Southwick, W.O.: Current concepts review. Management of fractures of the dens (odontoid process). J. Bone Joint Surg. 62A:482-486, 1980.

The author presents the current concepts of management of fractures of the odontoid process with a discussion of the current literature describing the nonoperative and operative methods of treatment. Treatment of children nonoperatively with a halo device or a Minerva jacket is recommended. It is suggested that the halo was not adequate treatment for type II adults odontoid fractures, and posterior C1-2 wiring that incorporates iliac crest graft is recommended.

Lower Cervical Spine

Bohlman, H.H.: Acute fractures and dislocations of the cervical spine. An analysis of 300 hospitalized patients and review of the literature. J. Bone Joint Surg. 61A:1119-1142, 1979.

This study of 300 patients hospitalized for acute cervical injuries revealed that no patient with complete quadriplegia that had persisted for 48 hours had recovery of spinal cord function. Those who underwent a laminectomy had a higher mortality rate and loss of function than those with closed treatment. The use of steroids did not improve neurologic recovery. The author recommended treating subluxation and dislocation with closed or open reduction followed by posterior wiring and bone graft arthrodesis. Compression and burst fractures of the vertebral bodies should be treated with anterior decompression and strut graft fusion to provide the best chance for recovery of neurological function in the incomplete spinal cord lesions and restoration of stability of the spine.

Johnson, R.M.; Owen, J.R.; Hart, D.L.; and Callahan, R.A.: Cervical orthoses: A guide to their selection and use. Clin. Orthop. 154:34-45, 1981.

This study documents the effectiveness of seven cervical orthoses in restricting cervical motion in flexion-extension, lateral bending, and rotation in normal subjects. The orthoses tested ranged from the soft collar to the halo cast. The total restriction of motion at each cervical segment by the various orthoses was documented. The authors provide a guide for the selection of the appropriate orthosis to control cervical motion in specific clinical situations.

Textbooks and Monographs

Bedbrook, G.M.: The Care and Management of Spinal Cord Injuries. New York, Springer-Verlag, 1981.

The author describes practical, day-to-day medical management of individuals with spinal paralysis, placing emphasis on the team approach and the nonoperative reduction of spinal injuries.

Bohlman, H.H.; Ducker, T.B.; and Lucas, J.T.: Spine and spinal cord injuries. *In* The Spine, edited by R.H. Rothman and F.A. Simeone, Ed. 2, 2:661-756. Philadelphia, W.B. Saunders, 1982.

The general principles, clinical assessment, and treatment of spine and spinal cord injuries are discussed in the light of clinical experience and potential complications. An extensive current reference list is included.

Cloward, R.B.: Acute cervical spine injuries. *In* Clinical Symposia, Vol. 32, no. 1, pp. 1-32. Summit, New Jersey, CIBA Pharmaceutical, 1980.

The philosophy and technique of early operative anterior decompression and stabilization are presented and illustrated.

Donovan, W.H., and Bedbrook, G.M.: Comprehensive management of spinal cord injury. *In* Clinical Symposia, Vol. 34, no. 2, pp. 1-36. West Caldwell, New Jersey, CIBA Pharmaceutical, 1982.

This is an illustrated monograph underscoring the need for a comprehensive multidisciplinary approach to the management of the spinal cord injured patient. It documents the long-term results of nonoperative treatment and acknowledges that a controlled study of surgical versus nonoperative treatment remains to be done.

MacNab, I.: Acceleration extension injuries of the cervical spine. *In* The Spine, edited by R.H. Rothman and F.A. Simeone, Ed. 2, 2:647-660. Philadelphia, W.B. Saunders, 1982.

The frequent exasperating clinical entity of the "whiplash symptom complex" is presented. Particular emphasis is placed on preventing iatrogenic neurosis and managing litigation neurosis.

Stauffer, E.S.: Rehabilitation of the spinal cord injured patient. *In* The Spine, edited by R.H. Rothman and F.A. Simeone, Ed. 2, 2:1118-1131. Philadelphia, W.B. Saunders, 1982.

This chapter points out the current concepts of comprehensive rehabilitation of the spinal cord injured patient, emphasizing prevention of medical, physical, and psychological complications and the rehabilitation goals attainable for the various levels of spinal paralysis.

Tator, C.H.: Early management of acute spinal cord injury. *In* Seminars in Neurological Surgery. New York, Raven Press, 1982.

This symposium on the management of acute spinal cord injuries provides a guide to the current methods of diagnosis and treatment based on clinical and laboratory research.

25 CERVICAL SPINE: RECONSTRUCTION

Topics considered in this section include evaluation and treatment of the patient with neck pain due to cervical disc disease, segmental instability, tumors, arthritis, and thoracic outlet syndrome.

Introduction

Chronic pain problems involving the adult cervical spine are usually due to encroachment on neural elements, mechanical or structural instability, or nerve inflammation and irritation. Most of these problems result from congenital abnormalities, aging, or trauma. Treatment is directed toward relief of neural encroachment, provision of stability, or reduction of inflammation. An understanding of the functional anatomy, the biomechanical function, and the disease processes pertaining to the cervical spine aids in effective treatment.

Patients with cervical spine disability often are involved with insurance claims, litigation, and emotional overreaction. However, many have a structural cause for their symptoms.

Structure and Function

Anatomy The cervical spine differs from the remainder of the axial skeleton in that it has a greater range of motion, is surrounded by less musculoskeletal mass and thus is less protected, and protects the most vital portion of the spinal cord.

The neuroanatomy of the cervical spine is complex, and the clinical implications are incompletely understood. For example, the descending tract of the fifth cranial nerve (trigeminal nerve) is joined by fibers of the seventh, ninth, and tenth cranial nerves. Fibers from all three divisions of the fifth cranial nerve have been found in the upper cervical spine, e.g., the fibers of the ophthalmic division at least as low as C4. These findings *may* account for some of the seemingly bizarre symptoms (such as facial pain or blurring of vision) frequently accompanying neck injuries.

Pain syndromes associated with the cervical ventral rami from C3 through C8 are well recognized and described in standard texts. Recently there has been interest in the cervical dorsal rami and their possible involvement in cervical pain by a referred pain mechanism. However, it is still not clear that disorders of the cervical dorsal rami result in clinical pain syndromes. Long-term documentation of the results of trigger point injection and radiofrequency coagulation are not as yet available.

Biomechanics The normal motion pattern of each segment on flexion and extension is a rocking, pivotal motion with the nucleus of the intervertebral disc serving as the fulcrum. It has been shown that any rotation of the vertebral body that occurs with flexion or extension or with angulation of 11 degrees more than the adjacent segments represents instability (i.e., a 20 degree measurement compared with an 8 degree measurement at an adjacent segment, see Fig. 1A).

The normal limit of anteroposterior translation at each level in the adult may be up to 3.5 mm, although at most levels it is zero (Fig. 1B).

If a cervical spine segment exhibits segmental motion patterns which exceed these normal limits, a structural disruption of the supporting soft tissues should be considered, including a disruption within the substance of the intervertebral disc. Abnormal segmental motion may be masked if total motion is restricted by pain and muscle spasm. Examination at a later stage or under the influence of some analgesic may provide a more accurate assessment for instability.

Normally, the intervertebral disc provides a constraint as well as a "cushion" between the vertebral bodies. Investigations have demonstrated disruptions of the intervertebral disc-vertebral body bond in experimental animals (primates) subjected to forces that exceed or distort the normal intervertebral motion and in autopsy studies of the cervical spine in individuals sustaining fatal head injuries.

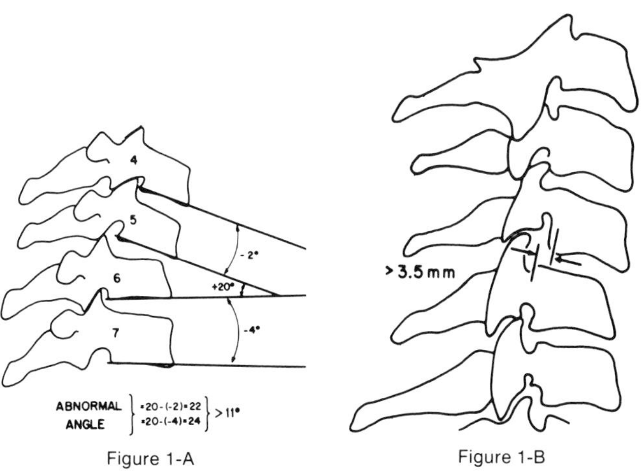

Figure 1: (A) Diagram of lateral radiograph showing rotation (or angulation) of C5 on C6 measuring 11 degrees more than either adjacent intervertebral joint is interpreted as demonstrating instability. (B) Diagram of lateral radiograph showing horizontal displacement of a vertebral body measuring more than 3.5 mm is interpreted as representing instability. (Reprinted with permission from Biomechanical analysis of clinical stabilization in the cervical spine, by A.A. White, et al., Clin. Orthop. 109:93, 94, 1975.)

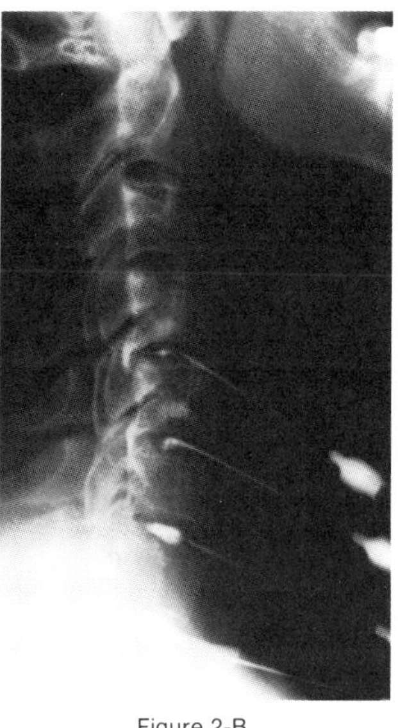

Figure 2-A Figure 2-B

Figure 2: (A) Cervical discogram. Anteroposterior view performed with 60 percent Renografin, 0.2 cc at each level in a male age 36 years. Note normal findings at C6-7 and C7-T1; abnormal findings of significance at C4-5 and C5-6. (B) Cervical discogram. Lateral view of patient in Figure 2A. Note normal appearance at C6-7 and C7-T1; posterior (posterolateral) concentration of contrast fluid at C4-5 and C5-6.

Evaluation

Certain areas of the body are always sensitive to firm palpation (e.g., the tip of the spinous process of C2, the superomedial angle of the scapula, the coracoid process, the insertion of the deltoid, and the extensor mass over the lateral aspect of the elbow). However, specific muscle discomfort may have localizing value. Biceps or pectoralis major discomfort may occur with a C5-6 lesion. The latter may also mimic a costal chondritis. Pain in the elbow or shoulder may be the presenting complaint of the patient with cervical injury. There may be tenderness over the tip of the ipsilateral transverse process, and pressure there may result in referred pain to the arm.

Lateral bending of the cervical spine may be more free in the supine and relaxed position and quite limited in the erect position. In a patient with emotional overreaction, the motion may be equally restricted in the supine position.

With nerve root compression, a combination of rotation and extension may aggravate pain on the involved side, whereas motion to the opposite side may relieve the pain. The recently described shoulder abduction relief (SAR) sign may also be helpful in the diagnosis of radicular pain due to cervical extradural compression. The presence of this sign is of prognostic value in that it correlates well with the results of surgical decompression. Approximately 70 percent of a series of twenty-two patients demonstrated this sign. The suggested explanation is that abduction of the arm at the shoulder (as by placing the hand on the head) shortens the distance between the transverse process of C5 and the coracoid process by approximately 3 cm, thus relieving stretch on cervical nerve roots. This test may prove valuable to differentiate a radiculopathy from thoracic outlet syndrome, which may be aggravated by this maneuver.

Radiologic Examination The radiographic evaluation should be tailored to the patient's physical examination. If radicular symptoms and signs are present, oblique views should be included. Lateral flexion and extension views should be obtained if instability is suspected. Also, a technique has been described in which lateral radiographs are taken in five positions: one in full extension, one in full flexion, and three in intermediate positions. These views may demonstrate abnormalities of cervical spine motion in patients who show no structural abnormalities on routine radiographic examination.

Myelography is most helpful when there are clear radicular symptoms or findings. However, because of the short distance that the subarachnoid space extends along the nerve root, it may fail to demonstrate posterolateral cervical disc protrusions. Also, extradural defects may be identified that have no clinical significance.

At present, computed tomography provides an accurate study of spinal canal geometry. With improved resolution, study of the canal contents is possible, thus compensating for some of the shortcomings of myelography.

Although still controversial, some believe that awake discography with attention to the injection pain response is helpful in the diagnosis of symptomatic cervical disc disease, especially with instability or multiple level changes on plain radiographs and without clear radicular findings. Volumes as small as 0.1 to 0.2 cc of 60 percent Renografin have been shown to give a satisfactory clinical response and radiographic study (Fig. 2). The injection of the abnormal disc itself with local anesthetic (preferably 2 percent lidocaine) gives valuable additional information and confirmation of the pain source during discography.

Confirmation of nerve root involvement by local anesthetic infiltration has proved helpful in those cervical syndromes with associated upper extremity pain. The correlation with discography is high. However, cervical nerve root blocks combined with myelography (or computed tomography) are even more helpful to avoid misinterpretation of false positive myelographic findings.

Congenital and Developmental

Os Odontoideum There is evidence to suggest that os odontoideum may be an acquired lesion due either to an ununited and perhaps unrecognized fracture of the odontoid process or to a traumatic disruption of the blood supply and absorption at the level of the facets. It may also be a congenital lesion, possibly associated with other anomalies of the cervical spine. Its significance is that it may be a site of structural weakness and even instability, especially when there is ankylosis or fusion of a portion of the lower cervical spine. The stress and motion resulting from normal activity and varying degrees of trauma may result in transmission of force and movement to the weak or unstable segment, thereby jeopardizing the spinal cord. Such a patient has been reported, with a fatal outcome, in a 71-year-old male. Neurologic deficit, even if transient, and/or instability greater than 5 mm in the presence of neck complaints are indications for C1-2 fusion.

See Section 23, Cervical Spine: Pediatric for further discussion of os odontoideum.

Congenital Cervical Block Vertebrae Congenital fusion of cervical vertebrae is most common at the C2-3 level. Isolated block vertebrae below C2 have very little clinical resemblance to the Klippel-Feil syndrome, which is a

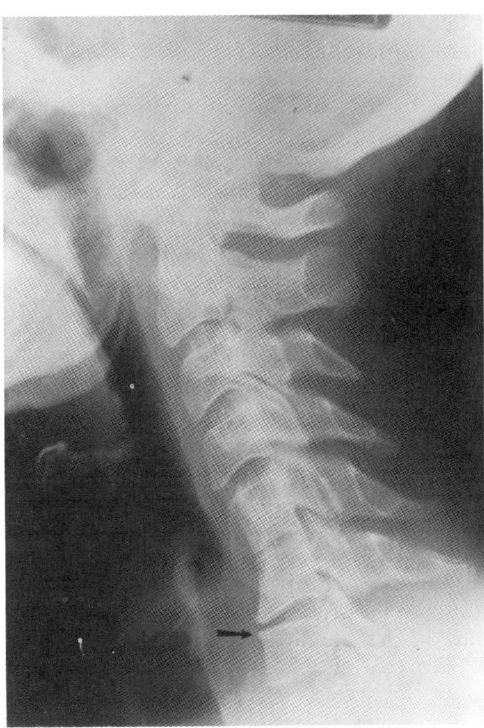

Figure 3: Lateral radiograph of cervical spine showing congenital block vertebra C5 and C6 segments. Note degenerative changes at intervertebral joint below with flexion attitude. This was the site of an acute cervical disc protrusion with radiculitis.

more extensive congenital failure of segmentation.

Congenital block vertebrae are rare and most commonly constitute an incidental, asymptomatic radiologic finding. It is not known how often isolated block vertebrae below the axis are associated with neurologic problems. The congenital "fusion" is apparently a defect in development and as such can be expected to demonstrate a "wasp waist" appearance. The posterior elements are usually also fused, and some underdevelopment or stenosis of the spinal canal or lateral foramina may occur. Serious neurologic symptoms can occur with or without injury.

A review of ten previous patients and three new patients with congenital block vertebrae with significant neurologic symptoms and findings was recently presented. Associated conditions of congenital spinal stenosis and degenerative arthritis or subluxation of the adjacent segments were believed to be major contributing causes of neurologic involvement (Fig. 3). These conditions were not associated with the acquired cervical block vertebrae that followed cervical fusion. The discovery of a congenital block vertebrae, especially below the axis, is best followed by assessment of the cervical spine for other anomalies, evidence of segmental instability, progressive degenerative changes at adjacent joints, and evidence of spinal or foraminal stenosis.

Mixed Etiology

Acute Cervical Disc Protrusion Cervical disc protrusion has been described as only one element of the general process of disc degeneration. Little has been added to the literature in the past 3 years to add to our understanding and management of this condition.

A characteristic of the acute cervical disc protrusion syndrome is an acute sudden stinging pain radiating into the upper extremity, often associated with a turning, stretching, or reaching activity. Usually the stage is set by some preliminary disc degeneration or prior injury.

The principles of treatment are limited activity (most often bed rest) and immobilization to allow resolution of the acute inflammatory response to disc herniation. Physical therapy to relieve muscle spasm, mild analgesics, and muscle relaxants are helpful. Traction may aggravate the symptoms if the amount of traction and the direction of pull are not ideal.

There continue to be differences of opinion (or at least preferences) regarding the merits of the operative procedures. The anterior approach has proved to be a relatively safe and effective method of removing abnormal disc material or extruded disc fragments. As the purpose and function of the disc are to serve as a bond between the vertebral bodies and as a fulcrum of movement between the bodies, it is difficult to justify removal of significant amounts of disc tissue without substituting some form of stability. However, some neurosurgical reports indicate equally good results with anterior discectomy with or without fusion. A randomized prospective study of military patients showed a 92 percent success rate whether or not fusion was added to discectomy. However, there was only a 6-month follow-up. Stabilization in the presence of advanced degenerative changes seems advisable.

Instability and/or Painful Intervertebral Segments This category represents the great majority of patients with "chronic cervical syndrome." Generally these patients have a history of a significant soft-tissue injury. Most such injuries heal within a matter of weeks. After soft-tissue healing, a conditioning period is necessary to restore function. This often requires several months, and symptoms may persist during this time. Supportive symptomatic treatment and reassurance are important. If symptoms persist beyond 12 months, or if they are unusually severe, more extensive investigation is indicated. Myelography is seldom helpful unless there is evidence of a definite radiculopathy. Some believe that cervical discography with addition of local anesthetic into the suspected disc and/or the corresponding nerve root or cervical dorsal ramus may provide valuable diagnostic information.

Intradiscal corticosteroids have proved to be of limited value when injected following discography. They may be worthwhile in individuals who are not good surgical candidates or as a means for further evaluation. Twenty to 25 percent of patients with either pure discogenic pain or radicular pain can be expected to achieve satisfactory long-term relief following intradiscal steroid injection. Those who had some relief with injections were all significantly improved with later anterior fusion. Two-thirds of those who did not get relief with injections obtained satisfactory relief with anterior fusion.

Studies have indicated that most people can tolerate chronic pain for approximately 3 months but thereafter may develop some emotional overreaction and chronic pain behavior. Depression is common. Although they may require surgical treatment, patients who exhibit emotional overreaction may have less than a gratifying outcome from surgery, and their emotional problems may require treatment as well.

Instability following extensive posterior cervical laminectomy occurs late and is usually accompanied by

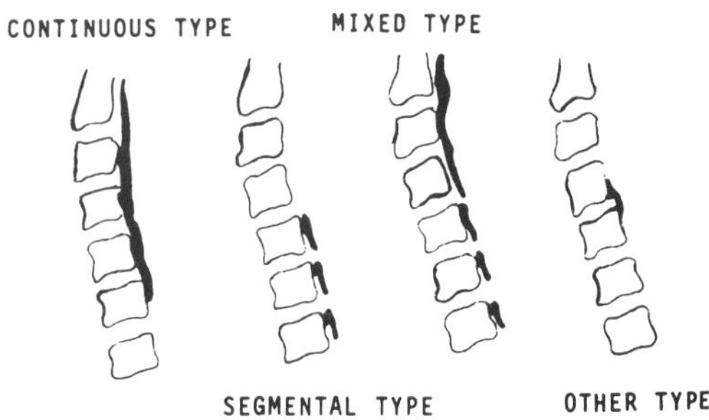

Figure 4: Types of ossification of the cervical posterior longitudinal ligament. (Adapted with permission from Operative results and postoperative progression of ossification among patients with ossification of cervical posterior longitudinal ligament, by K. Hirabayashi, et al., Spine: 6:355, 1981.)

symptoms. Posterior facet fusion with strut grafts and facetal wiring is technically demanding but may provide a strong and durable fusion. Anterior fusion in the presence of posterior instability carries the risk of added instability. A posterior cervical spinal fusion is indicated when an extensive posterior decompressive laminectomy is performed.

Cervical Spondylotic Myelopathy Patients often present with a wide variety of symptoms, many atypical. Common symptoms, in addition to neck pain and upper extremity pain, are gait disturbances, unsteadiness, clumsiness, weakness, impotence, and sphincter disturbances. Common signs are nerve root signs (often multiple), long tact signs, Lhermitte's sign (sudden transient, electric-like shocks spreading down the body with cervical flexion), Horner's syndrome, and cord hemisection syndrome. Occasionally, various demyelinating diseases may be misdiagnosed.

Although there are normal variations in the dimensions of the cervical spinal canal, there are relatively simple measurement techniques available that should alert the clinician to the likelihood of cervical myelopathy. The diameter of the cervical spinal cord is approximately 10 mm. A cervical spinal canal measuring 15 mm or less allows little or no leeway for any other space-occupying tissue or distortion of the neural canal. The distance between the posterior margin of the vertebral body and the cortical bone line at the base of the spinous process on the routine lateral radiograph is a reliable measure of the anteroposterior diameter of the spinal canal. Computed tomography is an accurate diagnostic test when cervical spinal stenosis is suspected.

If symptoms and stenosis are severe, adequate posterior decompression offers the best opportunity for recovery. If the stenosis is marginal and the posterior ridges or spondylosis are prominent, anterior decompression and fusion may be most effective. However, regression of the intraforaminal osteophytes is often disappointing. Anterior stabilization alone gives good results if the duration of symptoms is less than 6 months, if major posterior column damage in the cord is not present by examination, and if a single level is involved. Laminectomy has recently been reported to give better results when multiple levels are involved, but long-term follow-up (7 to 20 years) indicates a tendency for late worsening. Anterior fusion, on the other hand, shows a tendency for slow and late improvement. Some evidence exists to support a combined two-stage procedure in some circumstances.

Ischemia of the spinal cord by external compressive forces has been considered to play a role in cervical myelopathy and account for some of the less than satisfactory results. Experimental studies show that compression or ischemia alone had less adverse effect on neurologic function and blood flow patterns than did a combination of the two factors. Spinal cord ischemia seems to play a role in the pathogenesis of cervical spondylotic myelopathy, and more aggressive decompression and stabilization should be considered.

The "finger escape" sign may be noted in patients with cervical myelopathy. When the hand is extended and pronated, the little finger assumes an abducted position or cannot maintain an adducted position. More severe myelopathy may produce involvement of more fingers. This sign is present in 25 to 50 percent of the patients and occurs irrespective of the cause or localization of the myelopathy. It is considered to be a pyramidal tract sign. Early disappearance of this sign after surgery predicts a satisfactory recovery.

Ossification of the posterior longitudinal ligament of the cervical spine (OPLL) is common in Japan and is recognized as a cause of cervical myelopathy. Thickening of the ossified ligament may exceed 60 percent of the sagittal diameter of the spinal canal. It is less commonly recognized in the United States (Fig. 4).

Myelopathy has been demonstrated in Caucasians by computed tomography in twelve of twenty-five patients with this ligament ossification. OPLL is generally not visible on lateral radiographs but is demonstrated by lateral tomograms and is quite evident on CT scanning. In some patients, the ossification measures as much as 4.5 mm. Laminectomy provides satisfactory decompression in a lordotic spine, but anterior fusion with or without laminectomy is suggested with a kyphotic spine.

Neoplasms

Bone tumors of the spine are rare (only 7 percent of all bone tumors). Of 282 extradural spinal tumors studied, approximately 13 percent occurred in the cervical region. Primary malignant tumors are even rarer, the most frequent being myeloma, followed by metastatic tumors from the breast, lung, thyroid, prostate, and bowel. Under 20 years of age, benign tumors are most common. Pain and neurologic loss are indications for decompression and/or stabilization.

Polytomography, computed tomography, and angiograms have value in demonstrating paravertebral expansion. Surgical biopsy is indicated to establish a diagnosis so that a treatment plan can be established. Decompression by resection of the tumor usually relieves symptoms but is palliative at best, considering the aggressive nature of most primary malignant tumors.

Infection

Osteomyelitis of the cervical spine is uncommon but may be associated with severe cervical problems. It may infrequently occur following discography. Anterior surgery is recommended to: (1) establish a bacteriologic diagnosis; (2) drain abscesses; and (3) decompress the spinal cord and simultaneously add bone graft for stability. Laminectomy is not indicated in vertebral osteomyelitis. The general principles of treating infections, preventing deformity, providing stability, and protecting neural elements are the same as for infections elsewhere in the spine.

Arthritis

The inflammatory and destructive processes associated with *rheumatoid arthritis* have serious implications for the cervical spine, especially the atlantoaxial joint.

Odontoid impaction through the foramen magnum occurs much less frequently than instability of the atlas on the axis but is likely to result in more severe symptoms. Generally, these patients improve and even show reduction and good alignment in halo traction. Although transoral odontoidectomy has been performed in some centers, combined anterior and posterior cervico-occipital fusion has recently been recommended in this instance. Halo cast or halo-pelvic immobilization during healing is recommended.

Atlantoaxial instability, due to rheumatoid destruction of the ligamentous constraints, is a frequent clinical problem. There has been much disagreement about the indications for surgical stabilization. On one hand, C1-2 instability can lead to sudden death following a fall or jolt in the rheumatoid. On the other hand, C1-2 fusion in the rheumatoid carries a high risk of surgical complications, including reported mortality rates ranging from 10 to 15 percent. The degree of anterior displacement of C1 on C2 noted on flexion-extension radiographs does not correspond with symptoms or prognosis. Currently C1-2 fusion is recommended in those patients with demonstrable instability and any resulting neurologic deficit. Those without neurologic problems must be watched carefully to detect developing cord compression and should wear a protective orthosis (e.g., Philadelphia collar) when involved in activities in which they might be at risk for a jolt or jar to the neck.

In *ankylosing spondylitis* with a "chin-on-chest" deformity, corrective osteotomy is possible. The deformity must be in the cervicothoracic junction to be amenable to this technique. With the patient in a preoperative halo cast, laminectomy is performed under local anesthesia in the upright position, completely exposing the C8 nerve roots. Then under general anesthesia, the cervical spine is extended to approximate the resected margins of the laminae of C7 and T1, thus correcting the deformity. The technique is demanding, hazardous, and, fortunately, is not commonly indicated.

Current Concepts of Surgical Treatment

The anterior approach to the cervical spine offers a relatively safe access to the vertebral bodies, disc, and anterior spinal cord. The Smith-Robinson technique is a commonly used procedure for performing anterior interbody fusion. Avoiding the necessity for decortication of the vertebral end plates adds stability but may delay union and make it difficult to assess union. Reversal of the iliac graft with the cortical portion placed posteriorly seems to provide maximum distraction of the vertebral bodies and good stability (Fig. 5).

A keystone graft probably provides the most stable fusion configuration but its performance is technically demanding. The Cloward procedure is generally favored by neurosurgeons and has the advantage of employing rather precise instrumentation. Maximum distraction and contact of the vertebral cortices is necessary to prevent collapse. Banked bone and even bovine processed bone are used by some, but they do not seem as effective as autogenous bone. Exposure of the ilium on the abdominal side affords a more perpendicular approach to the cortical surface of the ilium and results in less postoperative pain than occurs when the lateral muscles are stripped from the ilium. Careful hemostasis is recommended when the medial approach to the ilium is used.

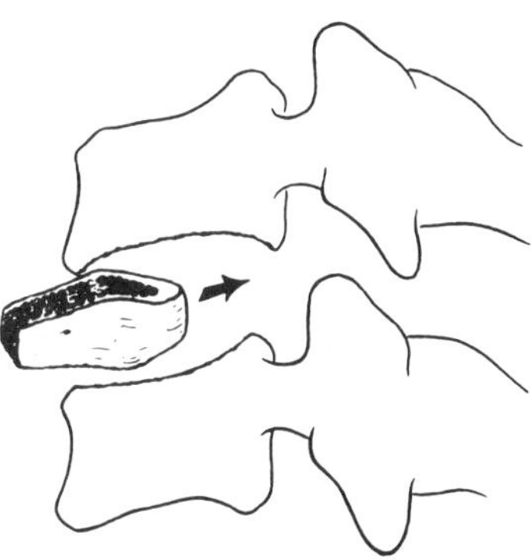

Figure 5: Reversal of Smith-Robinson iliac bone graft placing the strong iliac cortex in the posterior part of the intervertebral space. (Reprinted with permission from Anterior intervertebral fusion of the cervical spine, by M.H. Bloom, et al., J. Bone Joint Surg. 63A:842, 1981.)

For strut grafts to span multiple segments or defects of entire vertebral bodies, the fibula is well suited and often preferable to iliac-crest struts. A useful technique is the insertion of a longitudinal Steinmann pin through an iliac strut, protruding a few millimeters on either end to facilitate keying into the superior and inferior vertebrae. Lateral posterior strut grafts with segmental facetal wiring is technically demanding but may provide a secure fusion without interfering with decompressive laminectomy (Fig. 6).

High posterior cervical spine fusions are often required for rheumatoid arthritis and other serious problems, but they carry a higher incidence of failure and associated complications than fusions carried out in the mid- and lower cervical regions.

Difficult cervical spinal fusion in patients with rheumatoid arthritis, extensive destructive neoplasms, or gross instability has been successfully accomplished with the supplemental use of methyl methacrylate either anteriorly to replace a significant defect or posteriorly combined with wiring to reinforce the fusion construct. This is an especially helpful technique if postoperative irradiation is planned. However, an excessively large composite (methacrylate-metal-bone graft) mass may interfere with primary wound healing. Long-term results confirm the efficacy of these techniques.

Thoracic Outlet Syndrome

Thoracic outlet syndrome is an enigmatic and controversial condition that may cause chronic neck, shoulder, and arm pain. Thus, it requires differentiation from cervical spine disease.

Anatomy Seven types of fibromuscular bands have been identified in the thoracic outlet. Types I and II are ligamentous bands associated with a cervical rib or broad C7 transverse process, representing the anlage of the rudimentary rib. Type III is a short bowstring band across

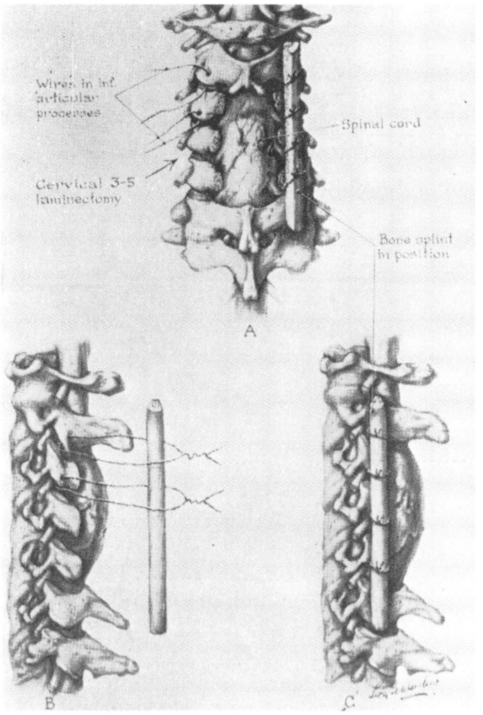

Figure 6: Lateral facet fusion with segmental wiring through facets and lateral masses securing cortical strut grafts. (Reprinted with permission from Indications and technics for early stabilization of the neck in some fracture dislocations of the cervical spine, by R.A. Robinson, et al., Southern Med. J. 53:574, 1960.)

the posterior curve of the rib. Type IV is a fascial sling joining the anterior and middle scalene muscles under the neurovascular bundle. Types V and VI are either a muscular scalenus minimus or a fibrous band to the fascia separating the subclavian artery and the nerve plexus. Type VII is a fibrous or fascial band extending from the posterior fascia of the anterior scalene muscle to the posterior aspect of the sternum. Two additional types have been added to this list as further variations.

More recently the syndrome has been divided into upper and lower types (Table I). The upper type involves C5, C6, and C7 roots; the lower type is predominantly C8 and T1.

Many of the recurrent syndromes following first rib resection are due to the upper type. Five additional anomalies of the scalene musculature have been recognized to account for the upper type: (1) fusion of anterior scalene muscle fibers in the perineurium of the major nerves; (2) pencil-sized muscle bundles connecting the anterior to the middle scalene muscle, interdigitating between the nerves of the plexus; (3) abnormal origin of the anterior scalene muscle arising behind and under the roots of C5 and C6 but over or anterior to the roots of C7, C8, and T1; (4) a single mass of scalene muscle not separated into anterior and middle divisions with the individual nerves separately perforating the muscle; and (5) taut, strong fibrous bands crossing the cervical nerves vertically behind the anterior scalene muscle. Types 1, 2, 3, and 4 may be minor variations of the same basic muscle anomaly. Some of the variations suggest they result from healing of torn muscle fibers following acute trauma.

Patient Evaluation The most frequently described symptoms of thoracic outlet syndrome are paresthesias in the arm and ulnar three digits. However, pain in the arm, shoulder and scapular region, and even into the side of the neck and head occur (Table I).

Vascular signs of obstruction have been stressed. However, experience has shown that they are not significant or necessary for the diagnosis. Obliteration of the radial pulse and the presence of a subclavian bruit may be manifested even in normal individuals. To require these signs to establish the diagnosis is not logical and to require them to support the decision for surgical treatment is misleading.

The anomalies described explain the predominance of neurologic symptoms without vascular involvement.

EMG abnormalities are rare but may occur, especially with the upper type.

Nerve conduction studies including the F-wave response are inconsistent and unreliable. The F-wave response is not a spinal reflex response, as initially believed, but is a result of recurrent motor neuron discharges. A prolonged value may be obtained only when the symptoms are otherwise aggravated. Evoked somatosensory responses show promise of eventually being developed as a reliable objective study. This is because it is a sensory measurement and thoracic outlet syndrome is predominantly a sensory syndrome.

A careful clinical history and physical examination are the best methods of establishing a diagnosis. Infiltration of the anterior or middle scalene muscle with local anesthetic has been described as the best confirmatory test.

Treatment Nonoperative measures include postural and muscle strengthening exercises. These may control or alleviate mild to moderate neurologic symptoms. When the symptoms are more severe or advanced so that they interfere with employment, sleep, or daily life, surgical treatment should be considered. The surgical procedure should remove, not merely divide, the abnormal structures to provide adequate decompression. The introduction of the transaxillary approach for first rib resection contributed greatly to the successful results since it afforded release of many of the abnormal structures whether or not they were clearly recognized. Many series report 80 to 90 percent satisfactory results with this procedure.

Several large series have reported as much as a 15 percent recurrence rate. If there still appears to be evidence of costoclavicular compression, repeating the transaxillary decompression may be indicated. However, most recurrences are best treated by anterior scalenectomy which requires a careful dissection of the major nerve trunks and branches of the brachial plexus with excision of the entire anterior scalene muscle to its tendinous origins on the transverse processes. Recurrences are most common with the upper type of thoracic outlet syndrome.

In a series of ninety-three scalenectomies performed over a 6-year period for upper plexus type thoracic outlet syndrome (either primary or recurrent), every patient obtained relief of symptoms, although 21 percent of the recurrent group still had significant residuals. Combined resection of the first rib and scalenectomy, where indicated, afforded the best results.

One report advocates middle scalenectomy as well as anterior scalenectomy rather than first rib resection. However, the reported results with this procedure are no better

Table I

Symptoms and Signs of Upper and Lower Thoracic Outlet Syndromes (TOS)

Upper Type TOS	Lower Type TOS
I. Pain	I. Pain
A. Lateral neck and head	A. Suprascapular
B. Rhomboid and suprascapular regions	B. Posterior neck and shoulder
C. Outer shoulder and arm	C. Inner arm through elbow and forearm
II. Aggravation by:	II. Aggravation by:
A. Turning head to opposite side	A. Elevating the arm
B. Tilting head	B. Reaching
C. Lifting and straining	C. Lifting
III. Weakness	III. Weakness
A. Arm	A. Arm
B. Wrist	B. Hand grip
	IV. Paresthesias
	A. Inner or entire arm
	B. Long, ring, and little fingers
	C. Spread to entire hand and arm
	D. Sensation of heaviness, tiredness and coldness

(Reprinted with permission from The place for scalenectomy and first-rib resection in thoracic outlet syndrome, by D.B. Roos, Surgery 92:1078, 1982.)

than rib resection alone so the search for the optimal procedure continues.

ANNOTATED BIBLIOGRAPHY

Structure and Function

Anatomy

Bogduk, N.: The clinical anatomy of the cervical dorsal rami. Spine 7:319-330, 1982.

A detailed description of the anatomy of the cervical dorsal rami is provided. Their clinical significance is discussed in relation to headache, occipital neuralgia, and neck pain and in relation to target points suitable for diagnostic blocks or facet denervation.

Brain, L., and Wilkinson, M.: Cervical Spondylosis. Philadelphia, W.B. Saunders, 1967.

A monograph that considers the specific anatomy of the cervical spine, membranes, spinal cord, nerve roots, and brachial plexus. Extensive review of the symptoms, pathology, and treatment is included.

Biomechanics

Brunton, F.J.; Wilkinson, J.A.; Wise, K.S.H.; and Simonis, R.B.: Cine radiography in cervical spondylosis as a means of determining the level for anterior fusion. J. Bone Joint Surg. 64B:399-404, 1982.

Cineradiography demonstrated two types of abnormal movement described as the single-rock and the double-rock movement. The demonstration of irregular motion is a significant finding.

White, A.A.; Johnson, R.M.; Panjabi, M.M.; and Southwick, W.O.: Biomechanical analysis of clinical stabilization in the cervical spine. Clin. Orthop. 109:85-96, 1975.

Laboratory stress studies were conducted on cadaver specimens related to systematic section of supporting structural anatomical elements. The criteria for determining clinical instability of the adult cervical spine are described.

Congenital and Developmental

Congenital Cervical Block Vertebrae

Lee, C.K., and Weiss, A.B.: Isolated congenital cervical block vertebrae below the axis with neurological symptoms. Spine 6:118-124, 1981.

Three patients were reported and an additional ten reviewed. The significance of coexisting spinal stenosis and segmental instability is emphasized and is related to the symptoms presented and to the decisions for treatment.

Mixed Etiology

Acute Cervical Disc Protrusion

Davidson, R.I.; Dunn, E.J.; and Metzmaker, J.N.: The shoulder abduction test in the diagnosis of radicular pain in cervical extradural compressive monoradiculopathies. Spine 6:441-446, 1981.

Of twenty-two patients requiring myelography for unremitting radicular pain, fifteen experienced relief with shoulder abduction. This shoulder abduction relief sign has not been commonly elicited in the past. It not only is a valuable clue to the origin of pain but also to the excellent prognosis if surgical treatment is elected.

Spetzler, R.F.; Roski, R.A.; and Kaufman, B.: Microsurgical approach to the anterior cervical spine. Orthop. Trans. 5:117-118, 1981.

This seems an appropriate technique when the cause of the radiculopathy or myelopathy is clearly and discreetly localized since it does not utilize a fusion. It has the advantage of a lower morbidity as do other microsurgical techniques.

Instability and/or Painful Intervertebral Segments

Kikuchi, S.; MacNab, I.; and Moreau, P.: Localisation of the level of symptomatic cervical disc degeneration. J. Bone Joint Surg. 63B:272-277, 1981.

Every patient in whom discography reproduced the symptoms noted that infiltration of the nerve root abolished the pain in the arm. The correlation was not as good when associated with myelography. Nerve root infiltration is a valuable adjunct to determining the level for surgical fusion.

LaRocca, H.: Acceleration injuries of the neck. Clin. Neurosurg., Proceedings of the Congress of Neurological Surgeons 25:209-217, 1978.

Review of clinical, experimental, and therapeutic facts. Hyperextension may produce muscular or soft-tissue tears, apophyseal joint injury, or intervertebral disc avulsion. Twelve percent of such patients have long-term symptoms.

Martins, A.N.: Anterior cervical discectomy with and without interbody bone graft. Orthop. Trans. 1:144, 1977.

A prospective study of 51 patients randomly selected to one of two treatment groups. There was no difference in the success rate between the two groups. Ninety-two percent had very satisfactory results.

Cervical Spondylotic Myelopathy

Bohlman, H.H.: Cervical spondylosis with moderate to severe myelopathy. Treatment of 17 cases by anterior cervical discectomy and fusion without removal of osteophytes. Orthop. Trans. 1:148, 1977.

Significant recovery can be obtained in patients with cervical myelopathy if the patient's symptoms have been present for less than 6 months and if major posterior column damage is not present by examination.

Gui, P.L.; Merlini, L.; Savini, R.; and Davidovits, P.: Cervical myelopathy due to ossification of the posterior longitudinal ligament in Caucasians. Orthop. Trans. 6:180, 1982.

Ossification was generally not clearly visible on lateral radiographs, more visible on lateral tomograms, and quite evident on CT. In the lordotic spine, a modified but rather extensive hemilaminectomy was done. For a kyphotic cervical spine, anterior fusion with or without hemilaminectomy was preferred.

Robinson, R.A.; Afeiche, N.; Dunn, E.J.; and Northrup, B.E.: Cervical spondylotic myelopathy. Orthop. Trans. 1:146, 1977.

Review of 120 patients in whom surgery was done for signs of progressive deterioration. Results were generally disappointing. Treatment, however, consisted of distraction of the disc spaces anteriorly and fusion to cause regression of the osteophytes.

Veidlinger, O.F.; Colwill, J.C.; Smyth, H.S.; and Turner, D.: Cervical myelopathy and its relationship to cervical stenosis. Spine 6:550-552, 1981.

All thirty-five patients with myelopathy encountered over 10 years had a canal diameter below average. A relatively simple measurement of the cervical canal can alert the clinician to the presence of cervical myelopathy.

Neoplasms

Weidner, A., and Immenkamp, M.: The operative management of extradural tumors of the cervical spine. Orthop. Trans. 5:116, 1981.

Tumors of the cervical spine are rare, representing 1 percent of all tumors. CT scanning is helpful in determining paravertebral extension. Surgical biopsy is indicated in primary tumors. Decompression by resection of the tumor may be palliative, depending upon the character of the tumor.

Infection

Eismont, F.J., and Bohlman, H.H.: Pyogenic vertebral osteomyelitis of the cervical spine. Orthop. Trans. 5:124, 1981.

The basic principles of anterior surgery to identify an organism, drain abscesses, decompress the spinal cord, and provide stability are stressed. The condition is rare but serious and potentially catastrophic.

Ono, K.; Okade, F.; Fuji, T.; and Ojina, S.: Finger escape sign—An objective sign signifying pyramidal tract involvement of the cervical spinal cord. Orthop. Trans. 6:181, 1982.

Abduction of the little finger in the pronated hand was found in 52 percent of patients with cervical myelopathy. A disappearance of the sign postoperatively indicated a good prognosis.

Arthritis

Simmons, E.H.: Flexion deformities of the neck and ankylosing spondylitis. J. Bone Joint Surg. 51B:193, 1969.

Cervicothoracic junction extension osteotomy performed under local anesthesia is described.

Verbiest, H.: Transoral surgery in the upper cervical spine. Orthop. Trans. 5:117, 1981.

Halo traction resulted in reduction of the odontoid from intracranial protrusion, and the transoral approach was used to remove the odontoid.

Whitesides, T.E., Jr.: Odontoid protrusion through the foramen magnum in severe rheumatoid arthritis. Orthop. Trans. 1:143, 1977.

Reduction in halo traction relieved symptoms and neural deficits in all of the reported patients, but a combined anterior and posterior cervico-occipital fusion was believed necessary. Stability and relief of neural deficits can be obtained, but the inexorable progression of the disease continues.

Current Concepts of Surgical Treatment

Bloom, M.H., and Raney, F.L., Jr.: Anterior intervertebral fusion of the cervical spine. J. Bone Joint Surg. 63A:842, 1981.

Reversal of the Smith-Robinson graft placed the cortical portion posteriorly to provide maximum distraction and stabilization.

Bryan, W.J.; Inglis, A.E.; Sculco, T.P.; and Ranawat, C.S.: Methylmethacrylate stabilization for enhancement of posterior cervical arthrodesis in rheumatoid arthritis. J. Bone Joint Surg. 64A:1045-1050, 1982.

Immediate internal splinting by metal and methacrylate aids healing of autogenous bone grafts in difficult instances.

Callahan, R.A.; Johnson, R.M.; Margolis, R.N.; Albright, J.A.; Keggi, K.; and Southwick, W.O.: Cervical facet fusion for control of instability following laminectomy. Orthop. Trans. 1:144, 1977.

Cortical strut grafts placed posterolaterally with segmental intrafacetal wiring provide a secure fusion without interfering with decompressive laminectomy.

Harrington, K.D.: The use of methylmethacrylate for vertebral-body replacement and anterior stabilization of pathological fracture-dislocations of the spine due to metastatic malignant disease. J. Bone Joint Surg. 63A:36-46, 1981.

Anterior decompression allows excision of the tumor and direct neural decompression. However, postoperative irradiation often interferes with bone healing and the use of methyl methacrylate as a space filler facilitates patient care and relieves symptoms.

Thoracic Outlet Syndrome

Glover, J.L.; Worth, R.M.; Bendick, P.J.; Hall, P.V.; and Markand, O.M.: Evoked responses in the diagnosis of thoracic outlet syndrome. Surgery 89:86-93, 1980.

Nineteen previously untreated symptomatic patients were evaluated and followed, some with and some without operation. Because this is primarily a sensory neurogenic syndrome, this diagnostic test may prove useful.

Roos, D.B.: The place for scalenectomy and first-rib resection in thoracic outlet syndrome. Surgery 92:1077-1085, 1982.

From evaluation of 3,630 patients for possible thoracic outlet syndrome, two distinct patterns of neurologic symptoms seem apparent: that affecting the upper roots of the brachial plexus (C5, C6, and C7) and that affecting the lower roots (C8 and T1). Additional congenital anomalies are described. Anterior scalenectomy, specifically designed to relieve the upper plexus type, is described. Ninety-three scalenectomies are reported.

Weber, R.J., and Piero, D.L.: F-wave evaluation of thoracic outlet syndrome: A multiple regression derived F-wave latency predicting technique. Arch. Phys. Med. Rehab. 59:464-469, 1978.

For thirty-eight control and sixteen patients with clinical evidence of thoracic outlet syndrome (TOS), the ulnar nerve forearm velocity, as determined by F-wave response, was measured. Using multiple regression analysis, a formula (using ulnar nerve velocity and arm length) was developed that consistently identified control patients and correctly identified some patients with clinical TOS. The TOS patients not identified may represent primary vascular TOS, or the clinical diagnosis may have been incorrect.

26 THORACOLUMBAR SPINE: PEDIATRIC

Pediatric spinal problems in the thoracic and lumbar areas center around the various causes for and treatment of scoliosis and kyphosis, spondylolisthesis, disc problems, infection, and tumor.

Adolescent Idiopathic Scoliosis The etiology of this, the most common form of scoliosis, remains unknown, but some clues to its causation are beginning to emerge.

The original description of abnormal balance systems in these children has been investigated further in several laboratories. A consistent pattern has emerged indicating that these children have abnormal balance in the labyrinthine rather than the ocular system. It does not appear to be secondary since patients with other scoliosis etiologies (e.g., congenital) do not have the abnormality. Nonscoliotic siblings of scoliosis patients also show abnormal sway tests. Caloric stimulation tests demonstrate that the increased sway occurs with stimulation of the labyrinth on the convex side of the scoliosis.

NATURAL HISTORY: Much knowledge has been gained by the increased use of school screening for scoliosis and several studies on the natural history of these patients. School screening by visual or Moire screen evaluation can detect scoliosis early and with minimal cost.

About 1.2 percent of those screened are found to have structural scoliosis. Most idiopathic scolioses do not progress. Progression is related to the size of the curve (bigger curves progress more than smaller curves), the area of the spine involved (thoracic and double primary curves progress more than single lumbar or thoracolumbar curves), and the physiologic age of the child (those with Risser signs of 0, in which the iliac epiphyses are not visible, or 1 progress much more than do children with Risser signs of 2, 3, or 4 as determined by the ossification of the iliac epiphyses from lateral to medial). For example, a girl with a Risser sign of 0 or 1 with a curve of 20 degrees to 29 degrees has a 68 percent probability of progression, whereas a boy with a Risser sign of 3 or 4 with a curve of less than 20 degrees has only a 2 percent probability.

Knowledge of these risk rates can lead to more rational patient management. Low-risk patients need be seen less frequently and far fewer radiographs need be taken. Some patients previously placed in orthoses to prevent progression are no longer braced.

RADIATION EXPOSURE: Increased awareness of the problem of spine deformity has resulted in an increased concern for the potential risk of repeated radiographic exposure.

The most radiosensitive tissues appear to be the breast, thyroid, and bone marrow in that order, with the breast being even more sensitive during childhood and adolescence. An early report of skin exposure (including the breasts) of over 1,000 millirems per exposure stimulated a considerable effort to reduce exposure to the radiosensitive organs. The simplest step to reduce breast (and thyroid) exposure has been to change from the anteroposterior to posteroanterior projection, a step that reduces radiation to the breast by twenty times or more. Concern that radiographic quality would be sacrificed has not been realized, and the alteration in curve size has been found to be a few degrees at most. However, the posteroanterior projection does increase the bone marrow exposure. Thus, some physicians have continued to use an anteroposterior projection with the addition of lead breast and thyroid shields, which also effectively reduces radiation exposure.

In addition, whole body exposure has been reduced overall by many other technical changes. As a result, breast exposure (as measured by surface dosimeters) should be quite small, on the order of 10 millirads or less, and entrance beam skin exposure should be less than 75 millirads. Based on these levels of radiation per exposure, the accumulative exposure during follow-up is believed to result in a very small (less than 0.1 percent) relative increase in the risk of breast cancer. It should be noted that an actual increase in the incidence of neoplasia in patients followed for scoliosis is unproved. Because of the low projected increase in incidence due to scoliosis radiographs, it may be difficult (if not impossible) to determine a statistically significant change in incidence, even if one existed.

TREATMENT: For smaller curves, treatment has become chiefly *observation*, with active treatment being applied only to curves of 20 to 29 degrees that are showing actual progression. Curves of 30 to 40 degrees are treated when first seen (if Risser 3 or less).

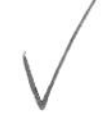

Exercise treatment is of no value. The few improving patients were those of spontaneous improvement, occurring in 5 to 10 percent of the reported series.

The *nonoperative treatment* of choice for these small, but progressive, curves is bracing. Several studies of the long-term results of Milwaukee brace treatment are now available. Although the original belief that this orthosis could provide permanent improvement in most patients has not proved valid, most patients, who were still actively growing at the beginning of treatment and with curves between 20 and 40 degrees, have had successful stabilization of the curve and have avoided surgery. Those patients who wore the orthosis longer and were weaned out more

slowly did better than those with shorter duration and earlier removal.

Underarm orthoses, either custom-made or prefabricated, have been popular in the past decade. These orthoses are highly effective and are the treatment of choice for lumbar and thoracolumbar curves and curves between 20 and 40 degrees (Fig. 1). The treatment of thoracic curves with such an orthosis is controversial.

An alternative method still under investigation is the treatment of these progressive curves of less than 40 degrees with electrical stimulators. Skin adherent electrodes are placed on the convex side of the curve, and the device is used only while sleeping. Early results indicate stabilization of progressive curves in about 75 percent of patients.

Surgical treatment is the procedure of choice for adolescent idiopathic scoliosis of 50 degrees or greater. The standard method is posterior spine fusion with Harrington instrumentation. Anterior procedures, such as the Dwyer or Zielke methods, are not of any particular value for adolescent idiopathic curves.

Analysis of curve patterns shows that lumbar curves need fusion only when they are the primary curve or part of a true double-primary pattern. Lumbar curves that are structural, yet definitely secondary to a primary thoracic curve, need not be fused. Preservation of lumbar mobility is highly advantageous for the patient. Low back pain can be avoided since fusion to L4 is associated with a significant increase of low back pain in later years (Fig. 2).

Scheuermann's Disease Although of unknown etiology,
218 histologic and histochemical studies of this condition
TL:P indicate a marked alteration in the cartilage growth plate
of the vertebral bodies. Bone growth is stunted in these areas, and disc material penetrates into the vertebral bodies. There have been no inflammatory findings or evidence of necrotic bone.

Recent studies of "normal" individuals reveal a wider range of thoracic kyphosis than the 20 to 40 degrees previously accepted. Location of the kyphosis is as important as its magnitude. Treatment is probably best limited to those children with painful deformity, documentation of progressive apical vertebrae wedging, and at least 2 years of growth remaining.

Milwaukee brace treatment continues to be the method of choice for the typical thoracic deformity. Underarm orthoses are effective only for thoracolumbar curves. The duration of treatment remains controversial, but those with an average of 18 months lose more correction than those with longer periods of treatment (Fig. 3). Electrical stimulation is under experimental investigation, and no results are available.

Surgical treatment rarely is required in children or young adolescents due to the extremely high percentage of good results with dedicated orthosis treatment. Infrequently an older adolescent with a severely painful kyphosis may benefit from surgery, with best results achieved by staged anterior discectomy and fusion and posterior instrumentation and fusion.

Scheuermann's disease in the lumbar or thoracolumbar spine is associated with low back pain in 78 percent of patients, but spontaneous resolution most often occurs.

Congenital Spine Deformity There has been considerable research on this deformity, especially in the induction of anomalies of the spine in mouse embryos with a period of anoxia to the pregnant mother. Typical anomalies occur with great regularity, are noted in the mesenchymal stage, and persist throughout the chondrification and ossification stages. Further research centers on the specific tissues involved and specific mechanisms of induction of anomalies.

Congenital scoliosis progresses in about 75 percent of patients. The rate of progression and severity of the eventual deformity can vary widely. The particular lesions involved and the importance of the area of the spine involved are becoming better delineated. The prognosis is poorest for those patients with unilateral unsegmented bar with a contralateral hemivertebra, especially if located in the thoracic or thoracolumbar spine. Prognosis is next

Figure 1: (A) Pretreatment radiograph of a 10-year-old girl with a progressive 27 degree idiopathic scoliosis. (B) Same patient 5 years later after 4 years of treatment with a custom-molded underarm orthosis.

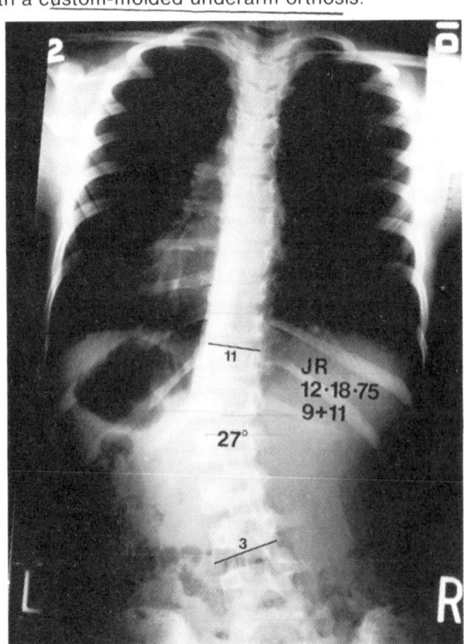

Figure 1-A

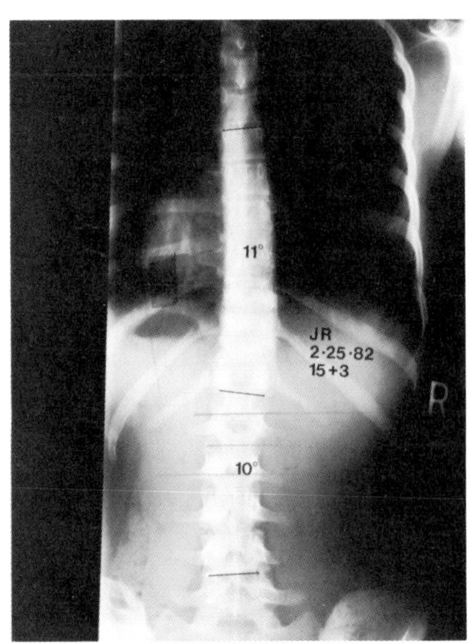

Figure 1-B

Figure 2-A

Figure 2-B

Figure 2: (A) Pretreatment radiograph of a 15-year-old girl with a 75 degree right thoracic primary curve (idiopathic) and a 57 degree left lumbar secondary curve. The supine side-bending films show the upper curve to correct to 50 degrees and the lower to 37 degrees. (B) The same patient 12 years after fusion of only the thoracic curve.

poorest for the unilateral unsegmented bar, followed by double hemivertebrae on the same side, single hemivertebrae, wedged vertebrae, and the least progressive is the block vertebrae (Fig. 4).

TREATMENT: The standard of treatment for congenital scoliosis remains posterior spine fusion, preferably done at an early age and without rods. Fears of universal bending and progressive lordosis following fusion are unfounded. Use of Harrington distraction instrumentation tends to increase the incidence of paraplegia, even in smaller curves. Preoperative myelography (water-soluble) and intraoperative neurologic evaluation substantially reduce the risks of using Harrington rods.

Hemivertebrae excision is a valid technique for an occasional patient, particularly with a severely decompensated spine due to a lumbosacral hemivertebra. Newer techniques used for congenital scoliosis emphasize early convex anterior and posterior hemiarthrodesis and hemiepiphysiodesis (Fig. 5).

Congenital kyphosis is best treated surgically by combined anterior and posterior fusion. However, only a posterior fusion is necessary before the age of 5 years as spontaneous improvement of the kyphosis usually occurs.

Neuromuscular Spine Deformity

Spinal Muscular Atrophy In this relatively common disorder, the most frequently encountered orthopaedic problem is progressive spine deformity. Far more children survive than previously known. Many deaths previously believed due to the disease process were actually due to scoliosis and probably were preventable.

The frequency of scoliosis and the age at onset are directly related to the severity of muscle weakness. Many believe bracing should begin at the first sign of structural scoliosis (curve present on the supine radiograph). Curves

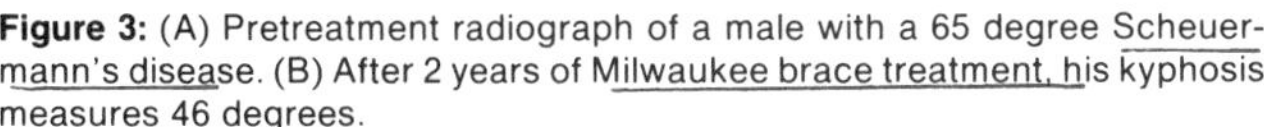
Figure 3: (A) Pretreatment radiograph of a male with a 65 degree Scheuermann's disease. (B) After 2 years of Milwaukee brace treatment, his kyphosis measures 46 degrees.

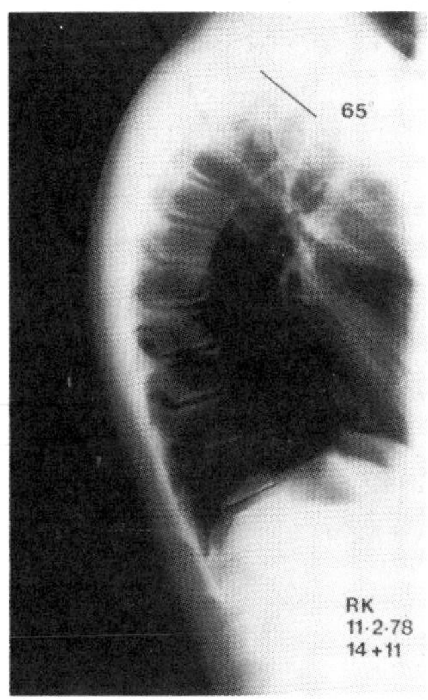

Figure 3-A

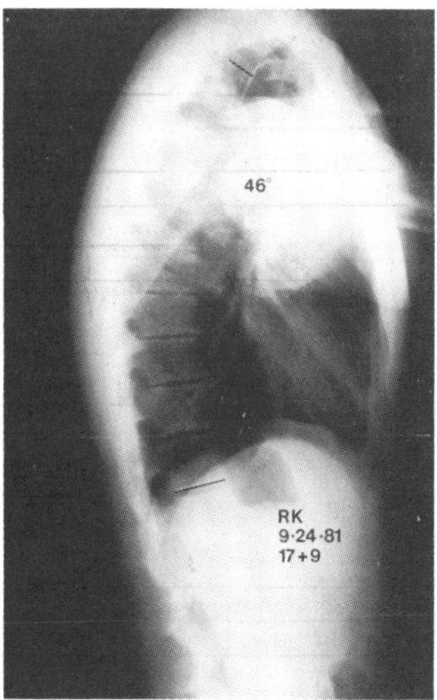

Figure 3-B

Figure 4-A

Figure 4-B

Figure 4: (A) Girl first seen for her congenital scoliosis at age 1 year. A unilateral unsegmented bar can be seen on the right side from T10-L3. The scoliosis measures 48 degrees. No treatment was given. (B) (Reprinted with permission from Congenital Deformities of the Spine, by R.B. Winter, New York, Thieme-Stratton, p. 60, 1983.) When seen at age 11 years, her curve had increased to 133 degrees. She had severe pelvic obliquity and respiratory insufficiency.

progressing beyond 60 degrees should be treated surgically. Posterior fusion combined with Harrington rods has been the time-honored approach, but recent experience suggests the Luque technique is preferable. Curves progressive at young ages despite bracing can be salvaged by instrumentation without arthrodesis. The final fusion is done when adequate torso length is achieved, usually at the onset of the adolescent growth spurt.

Cerebral Palsy Scoliosis is rare in ambulatory, minimally involved patients but very common in severely involved, spastic quadriplegics. Treatment techniques for these problems have improved tremendously.

Functional sitting can be achieved in many patients with body jackets or molded wheelchair inserts. Surgical stabilization is the treatment of choice for progressive structural curves. Thoracic and thoracolumbar curves without pelvic obliquity, most often seen in the ambulatory individual, can be treated adequately by posterior instrumentation and fusion. Severe curves with marked pelvic obliquity require combined anterior and posterior instrumentation and fusion for adequate results. Treatment is directed toward functional goals, such as sitting balance and pain relief, rather than cosmesis.

Myelomeningocele These spine deformities remain the most difficult to treat. Progressive deformity is common, bracing is difficult, and surgery is subject to many complications.

Progressive paralytic scoliosis may be due to disturbed

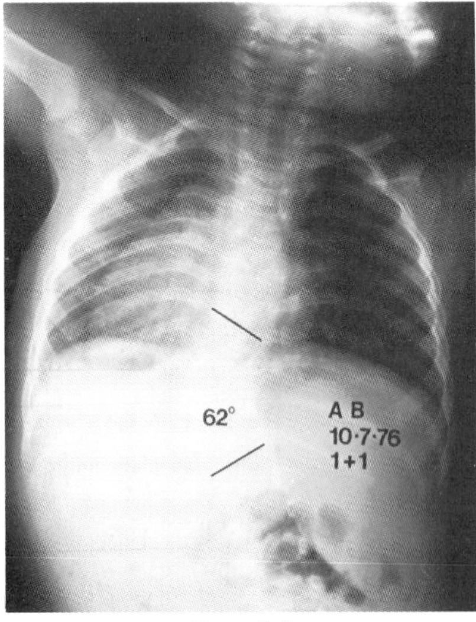

Figure 5-A

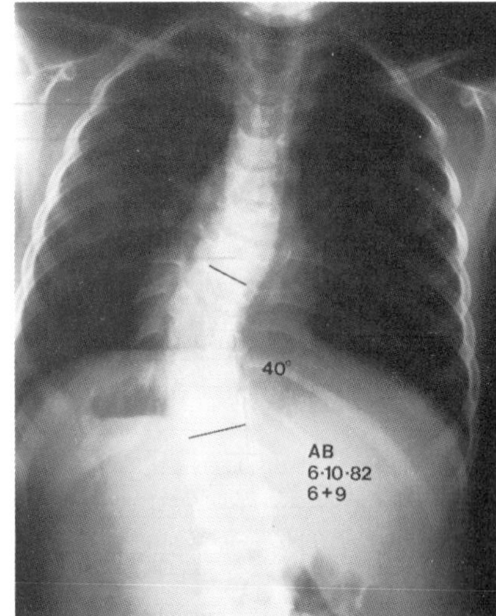

Figure 5-B

Figure 5: (A) (Reprinted with permission from Convex anterior and posterior hemiarthrodesis and hemiepiphysiodesis in young children with progressive congenital scoliosis, by R.B. Winter, J. Pediat. Orthop. 1:365, 1981.) One-year-old girl has a congenital scoliosis due to hemivertebrae on the left side. Her curve has increased from 50 degrees at age 6 months to 62 degrees at age 1 year when she underwent anterior and posterior hemiepiphysiodesis and hemiarthrodesis. Maximal correction in a postoperative cast was to 54 degrees. (B) A follow-up at age 6 years shows gradual improvement of the curve to 40 degrees.

ventricular shunt mechanics and a progressive hydromyelia or syringomyelia. It may be possible to relieve this problem by revision of the ventricular shunt, thus halting or reversing the progressive scoliosis, particularly if detected before the curve reaches 50 degrees.

For established paralytic scoliosis, best results are obtained by anterior fusion and instrumentation combined with posterior fusion and secure internal fixation plus bank bone grafting (Fig. 6). Pseudarthrosis at the lumbosacral level may be improved with use of Luque instrumentation to the pelvis using the "Galveston" technique.

For early myelomeningocele kyphosis, total fusion of the lumbar spine at an early age can prevent progression but leaves the patient with an extremely short torso. Partial resection of the apical vertebra and of the proximal lordotic curve without fusion of the whole lumbar spine has given encouraging early results.

Segmental Spinal Instrumentation (Luque Technique) This technique, first introduced in 1974, has brought about a profound change in spine deformity surgery. It presents a significant advantage in that no external immobilization is necessary. There are those who believe it is the best method available for surgical treatment of virtually all spinal deformities. Conversely, there are those who believe its efficacy is not yet confirmed.

Since the procedure is new, the recent literature has very limited follow-up. A large amount of instrumentation is involved, and it may require much time before pseudarthroses become evident and the rods break.

The amount of correction obtained in the average curvature depends upon the flexibility of the curve, not upon the type of instrumentation used. No attempt should be made to correct beyond the amount demonstrated on bending or distraction films (Fig. 7 D-F). Dual L-shaped rods should be used, and each should be secured to each lamina and then to each other (Fig. 7 A-C). Thorough facet excision and bone grafting are critical for ultimate arthrodesis.

Fixation to the pelvis is most secure using the "Galveston" technique wherein the rods pass downward and outward between the iliac cortices to just above the hip joints.

Severe curves, particularly those with poor flexibility, are best managed by preliminary multiple-disc excision and anterior bone chip fusion followed 1 to 2 weeks later by posterior instrumentation and fusion.

The technique has been adapted to both lordosis and kyphosis in addition to scoliosis. Until it became available, there was no satisfactory procedure for the treatment of thoracic lordosis.

Some surgeons have experienced an increased incidence of neurologic deficit with the use of segmental wiring, presumably due to entry of the spinal canal.

Biomechanical testing of the Luque system against more conventional methods with Harrington rods indicates that a single Harrington rod is the least stable. A single Harrington rod with multiple sublaminar wires is equal to a Harrington distraction rod connected by transverse approximators to the multiple hook Harrington compression system. Both of the above systems are similar in stability to dual L-rods with wiring except that the 3/16 inch dual L-rods tend to fail by bending.

Miscellaneous Spine Problems

Neurofibromatosis There are two types of spine deformity, the dystrophic and the nondystrophic. Dystrophic neurofibromatosis demonstrates rib penciling, vertebral body scalloping, dural ectasia, and adjacent soft-tissue masses. Dystrophic curves do not respond to any form of bracing and require surgical stabilization. For pure scoliosis, posterior fusion (preferably with internal fixation) is satisfactory. For kyphoscoliosis problems, both anterior and posterior fusion are required. Even then, pseudar-

Figure 6-A

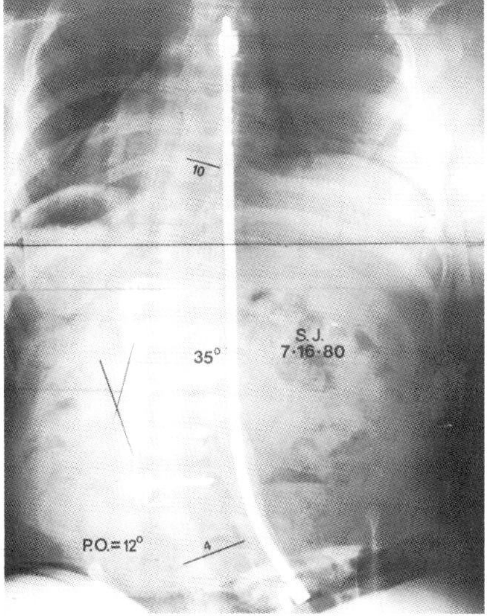

Figure 6-B

Figure 6: (A) Nine-year-old girl (skeletal age 12) has a 119 degree paralytic myelomeningocele scoliosis with severe (57 degrees) pelvic obliquity. She is treated by anterior discectomy and fusion with Zielke instrumentation followed 2 weeks later by posterior fusion from T6 to the sacrum with Harrington instrumentation and bone graft. (B) Two and one-half years later, the fusion is solid, the scoliosis is 35 degrees, and the pelvic obliquity 12 degrees. (Reprinted with permission from Surgical treatment of scoliosis associated with myelomeningocele, by W.R. Osebold, J. Bone Joint Surg. 64A:851, 1982.)

Figure 7-A

Figure 7-B

Figure 7-C

Figure 7: (A) Excision of the ligamentum flavum. (B) Passing the wire loop. (C) Drawing of the upper three vertebrae with the rods wired in position. Note how the L of the left rod passes over the right rod and both are stabilized to the lamina. This is important for rotational stabilization. (Reprinted with permission from Congenital Dislocation of the Spine, by R.B. Winter, New York, Thieme-Stratton, pp. 126-127, 1983.) (D) A 13-year-old girl with severe spinal muscle atrophy and a 114 degree scoliosis. She is unable to sit. (E) A traction film showed her to be correctable to 73 degrees. The Luque rods should be bent to conform to this amount of curve. (F) Arthrodesis from T2 to the sacrum is performed with Luque rods and segmental stabilization. A 2-year follow-up shows no loss of correction, and she has unlimited sitting ability.

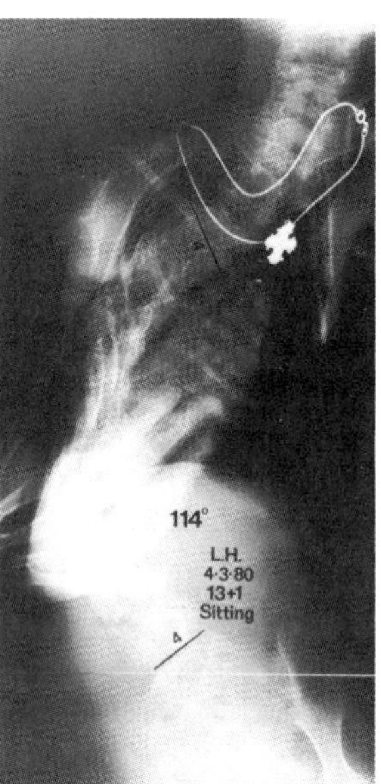

Figure 7-D

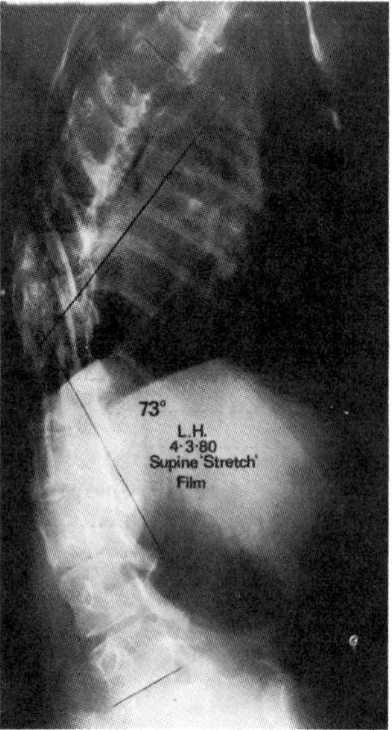

Figure 7-E

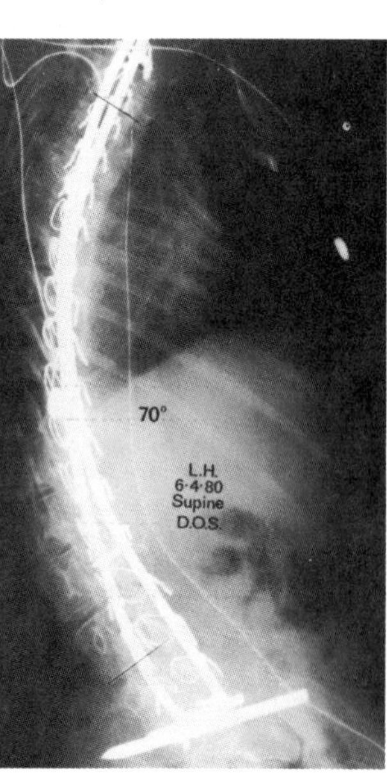

Figure 7-F

throsis may occur, and repair be required. Neurologic deficits may occur due to intraspinal neoplasms, kyphosis, or both. Preoperative myelography is recommended.

Dwarfism Spinal deformity and instability of the upper cervical spine are quite common in patients with dwarfism. Kyphosis is more prevalent than scoliosis. The incidence and pattern of deformity and instability vary according to the type of dwarfing disorder.

Irradiation This can cause deformity in the survivors of childhood malignancies, especially Wilms' tumor and neuroblastoma. Although scoliosis long has been recognized, kyphosis has been emphasized recently. Marked increases in the deformity can occur at the adolescent growth spurt, long after the period of radiation. Careful monitoring of such patients until the end of growth is necessary. Significant kyphotic deformities require both anterior and posterior fusion.

Laminectomy Laminectomy may be a significant cause of spinal deformity in children and may occur independently of other factors also causing spinal deformity. Progressive kyphoses require anterior and posterior fusion. Instrumentation may be impossible due to the extent of the laminectomy. Children having extensive laminectomies, especially when facet excision is included, require long-term follow-up because they may develop deformities due to instability.

Disc Herniation Disc excision in children is infrequently performed, and postoperative deformity usually does not occur. Children differ from adults in the form of presentation, and objective neurologic deficits are rare. Initial results are good but may deteriorate slightly. Long-term results are good in approximately 75 percent of patients. Subsequent operations, either repeat laminectomy or lumbosacral fusion, may be necessary.

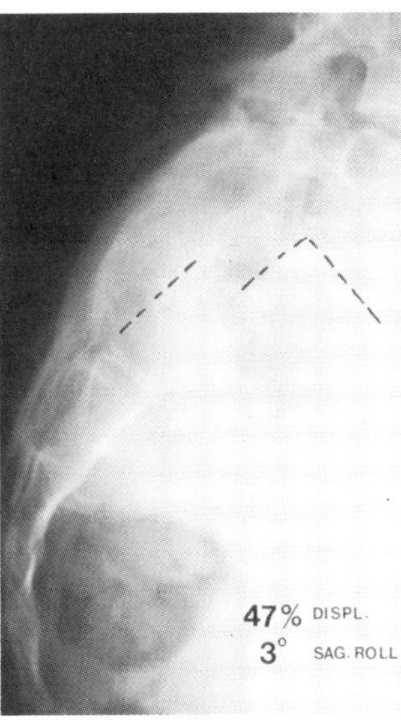

Figure 8-A Figure 8-B

Figure 8: (A) A 12-year-old girl with severe hamstring spasm shows a spondylolisthesis with a displacement of 67 percent and a "roll" (slip angle) of 23 degrees. Treatment consists of an alar-transverse process fusion (L4-S1) and postoperative immobilization in a double pantaloon cast with the hips in extension. (B) Two years after surgery the fusion is solid, the displacement is 47 percent, and the roll (slip angle) is 3 degrees. All complaints are gone and the hamstring tightness no longer exists.

Spondylolisthesis Management of spondylolysis and spondylolisthesis in children and adolescents is unsettled. The defect usually appears by 5 to 7 years of age and is influenced strongly by genetic factors. Repetitive hyperextension microtraumas are increasingly encountered. Individuals who have never ambulated do not develop spondylolysis. Children with spondylolysis may be asymptomatic and not develop spondylolisthesis. The polyphosphate radioisotope bone scan is useful in detecting impending pars interarticular defects before apparent on conventional radiographs. Patients with spondylolisthesis may range from being totally asymptomatic to totally incapacitated.

TREATMENT: Nonoperative management is appropriate for most patients.

Operative management is reserved for patients with persistent back and/or radicular pain especially for patients with progressive slip of greater than 50 percent (Fig. 8). The major considerations are arthrodesis, decompression, and reduction. Most patients can be managed successfully with an in situ posterolateral arthrodesis. Posterior element excision is unneccessary unless there are objective neurologic deficits. Posterior element excision alone is not recommended in children as further slip has been documented. The indications for reduction are unclear, but generally it should be reserved for symptomatic patients with larger degrees of slip angle (lumbosacral kyphosis). The forces involved are longitudinal traction and lumbosacral hyperextension. Although there are several techniques available, no single one has emerged as being clearly superior.

The major cause of failure of spondylolisthesis surgery has been the lack of high-quality alar-transverse process fusion and the adequate postoperative immobilization of the patient. Children differ from adults in that they are more prone to increase the amount of slip. Adolescents being fused from L5 to S1 because of pain (not progression of the slip) do not require casting. Patients with slips of more than 50 percent or those having surgery because of progression need immobilization in a cast with one or both legs included.

Disc Space Infection Disc space infection is relatively uncommon but still must be considered in any child presenting with back pain, particularly if febrile. Radioisotope bone scans are very useful since they are positive before conventional radiographs show any abnormality. The causative organism is usually staphylococcus. Many believe that antibiotics should be administered, that culture by needle aspiration is usually unnecessary, and that spinal immobilization is desirable.

Tuberculosis of the Spine Unlike disc space infection in children, tuberculosis affects the vertebral bodies and does not destroy the disc until very late in the disease. Currently there seems to be an increase in this condition, probably due to the influx into North America of large numbers of children from Southeast Asia and Mexico, both areas of high endemic tuberculosis.

If detected early (before collapse of more than one vertebral body), drug treatment alone is adequate. More advanced disease, presenting with an abscess and a kyphosis, usually requires anterior abscess removal, anterior spine fusion, posterior spine fusion, and antituberculous therapy.

Tumors of the Spine Tumors of the vertebral bony elements are rare but must be considered in any child with back pain. Radioisotope bone scans are useful for the diagnosis of a lesion but do not specify the type of tumor. Painful scoliosis may be caused by osteoid osteoma, osteoblastoma, or aneurysmal bone cyst (Fig. 9). Excision of the specific lesion results in elimination of pain and curve straightening. Arthrodesis is necessary only in very long-standing deformities. Irradiation should not be used for benign lesions. Spinal cord tumors also should be considered in children with back pain.

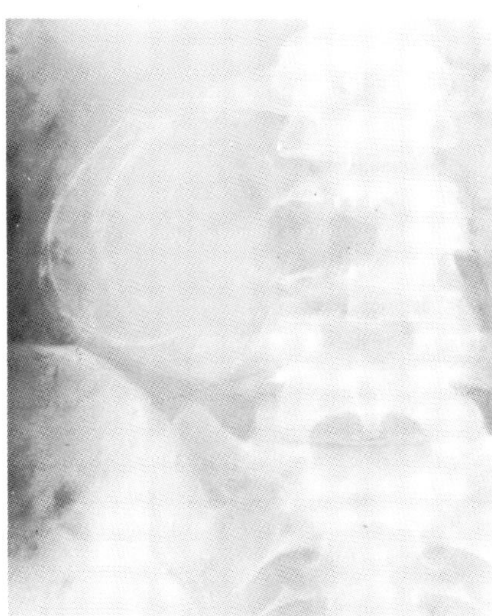

Figure 9: An aneurysmal bone cyst. The presenting complaint was low back pain in an adolescent.

ANNOTATED BIBLIOGRAPHY

Adolescent Idiopathic Scoliosis

Brown, J.C.; Axelgaard, J.; and Howson, D.C.: Multicenter trial of a noninvasive stimulation method for idiopathic scoliosis. Orthop. Trans. 7:10, 1983.

A preliminary analysis of 548 patients treated in fifty-four investigational clinics shows that 78 percent of progressive curves are stabilized by this technique. Only 22 percent progress and require other treatment.

Bunnell, W.P.: A study of the natural history of idiopathic scoliosis. Orthop. Trans. 7:6, 1983.

This study of the natural history in 326 patients reveals no correlation of progression with family history, thoracic kyphosis or lordosis, lumbar lordosis, decompensation, or pregnancy. Positive correlations are noted with female sex, immature Risser sign, and degree of curvature.

Carr, W.A.; Moe, J.H.; Winter, R.B.; and Lonstein, J.E.: Treatment of idiopathic scoliosis in the Milwaukee brace. J. Bone Joint Surg. 62A:599-612, 1980.

Results are analyzed 5 years or more after brace removal. Of 133 original patients, 29 had surgery, 30 were lost to follow-up, and 74 had follow-up without surgery. Eighty percent of these seventy-four showed some curve progression. Curves over 40 degrees did less well than curves under 40 degrees. Curves showing a good initial response to the brace did better.

Edmonson, A.S., and Smith, G.R.: Long-term follow-up study of Milwaukee brace treatment in patients with idiopathic scoliosis. Orthop. Trans. 7:10-11, 1983.

A follow-up 10 years after brace removal shows good results with very little loss (average 1 degree) as compared to 2 years after brace removal. No harmful effect on the curve from childbearing is noted.

Gray, J.E.; Hoffman, A.D.; and Peterson, H.A.: Reduction of radiation exposure during radiography for scoliosis. J. Bone Joint Surg. 65A:5-12, 1983.

By adopting six changes in technique the exposure to breast and thyroid was reduced to 6 millirems or less per exposure. The most important single factor was changing from anteroposterior to posteroanterior exposure. Other changes further reduced exposure and at the same time retained or improved radiograph quality.

Herman, R.; Stuyck, J.; Yamamoto, H.; MacEwen, D.; Maulucci, R.; and Herr, B.: Vestibular functioning in idiopathic scoliosis. Orthop. Trans. 3:218-219, 1979.

Testing of adolescent idiopathic scoliosis patients for sway control indicates a definite abnormality as compared to both normal children and children with congenital scoliosis. Blindfold testing locates the abnormality in the vestibular system, not the ocular.

King, H.; Moe, J.; Bradford, D.; and Winter, R.: Selection of fusion levels in thoracic idiopathic scoliosis. Orthop. Trans. 5:25, 1981.

Four hundred forty-five patients are analyzed as to the proper selection of fusion levels. The only time a lumbar curve should be fused is if it is part of a true double-primary pattern. Secondary lumbar curves need not be fused even if they have some structural characteristics.

Lidström, J.; Sahlstrand, T.; and Örtengren, R.: Defective postural control: A possible clue to the etiology of adolescent idiopathic scoliosis. Orthop. Trans. 5:20, 1981.

Stabilometry testing of adolescent idiopathic scoliosis patients indicates increased sway if vision is excluded. There is also noted increased sway in the nonscoliotic siblings.

Lonstein, J.E.; Bjorklund, S.; Wanninger, M.H.; and Nelson, R.P.: Voluntary school screening for scoliosis in Minnesota. J. Bone Joint Surg. 64A:481-488, 1982.

School screening for scoliosis continues for 8 years with 250,000 children examined each year. Of these children 3.4 percent are referred for evaluation and, 1.2 percent are found to have scoliosis. The cost is 6.6¢ per student examined. A marked decrease in patients needing surgery is noted.

Lonstein, J.E., and Carlson, J.M.: Prognostication in idiopathic scoliosis. Orthop. Trans. 5:22, 1981.

The risk of progression is studied in 727 patients; 558 are nonprogressive and 169 progress. Double thoracic curves and single thoracic curves progress most and single lumbar curves least. A curve of 20 degrees to 29 degrees in a Risser 0-1 patient has a 68 percent chance of progression, while a curve less than 20 degrees in a Risser 2-4 patient has only 1.6 percent chance of progression.

McCollough, N.C., III; Schultz, M.; Javech, N.; and Latta, L.: Miami TLSO in the management of scoliosis: Preliminary results in 100 cases. J. Pediat. Orthop. 1:141-152, 1981.

This study of a custom-molded polypropylene underarm brace in 100 patients shows in-brace improvement of 36 percent in thoracic curves, 56 percent in thoracolumbar curves, and 63 percent in lumbar curves. Results out of the brace show one-third better by 5 degrees or more, and two-thirds unchanged. None progress 5 degrees or more from the initial curve.

Sahlstrand, T.; Petruson, B.; and Örtengren, R.: Vestibulospinal reflex activity in patients with adolescent idiopathic scoliosis: Postural effects during caloric labyrinthine stimulation as recorded by stabilometry. Acta Orthop. Scand. 50:275-281, 1979.

Postural sway with caloric labyrinthine stimulation is evaluated by stabilometry in forty-nine patients (thirty-two controls). Scoliotic patients tend to have increased sway with stimulation of the labyrinth on the convex side of the scoliosis.

Stone, B.; Beeckman, C.; Hall, V.; Guess, V.; and Brooks, H.L.: The effect of an exercise program on change in curve in adolescents with minimal idiopathic scoliosis. Phys. Ther. 59:759-763, 1979.

This controlled study of the effectiveness of an exercise program shows that the treated patients do no better than the nontreated patients.

Torell, G.; Nordwall, A.; and Nachemson, A.: The changing pattern of scoliosis treatment due to effective screening. J. Bone Joint Surg. 63A:337-341, 1981.

A 10-year program was evaluated as to its effectiveness. A threefold increase in the number of patients treated is noted with a significant decrease in the curve severity at diagnosis. Most patients needing treatment do not require surgery due to the early diagnosis.

Scheuermann's Disease

Bradford, D.S.; Ahmed, K.B.; Moe, J.H.; Winter, R.B.; and Lonstein, J.E.: The surgical management of patients with Scheuermann's disease: A review of twenty-four cases managed by combined anterior and posterior spine fusion. J. Bone Joint Surg. 62A:705-712, 1980.

Combined anterior and posterior fusion gives better correction and especially much better maintenance of correction. Loss of correction is usually due to too short a fusion. Heavy compression rods with many hooks are best.

Ippolito, E., and Ponseti, I.V.: Juvenile kyphosis: Histological and histochemical studies. J. Bone Joint Surg. 63A:175-182, 1981.

A 16-year-old male with Scheuermann's disease was killed in a car accident, allowing pathologic spine evaluation. Abnormal cartilage was found. Vertebral bone growth was stunted under the areas of abnormal vertebral and growth plates. Necrotic bone was not seen. Disc material had herniated into the vertebral bodies (Schmorl's nodes).

Kehl, D.K.; Lovell, W.W.; Silva, J.; and MacEwen, G.D.: Scheuermann's disease of the lumbar spine. Orthop. Trans. 6:343, 1982.

Ninety-eight patients with findings in the lumbar or thoracolumbar spine are evaluated and findings in the lumbar or thoracolumbar spine are evaluated and followed for 4 years. Seventy-eight percent have low back pain on presentation (none with radiation) but all resolved.

Montgomery, S.P., and Erwin, W.E.: Scheuermann's kyphosis—long-term results of Milwaukee brace treatment. Spine 6:5-8, 1981.

A follow-up study of thirty-nine patients indicates an end of brace value of 41 degrees as compared to 62 degrees pretreatment. However, later follow-up at 15 months out of brace shows relapse to 56 degrees, indicating that lasting results require brace treatment for longer than 18 months.

Stagnara, P.; de Mauroy, J.C.; Dran, G.; Gonon, G.P.; Costanzo, G.; Dimnet, J.; and Pasquet, A.: Reciprocal angulation of vertebral bodies in the sagittal plane: Approach to references for the evaluation of kyphosis and lordosis. Spine 7:335-342, 1982.

This study of sagittal plane alignment analyzes the thoracic kyphosis and lumbar lordosis in 100 patients. Radiographs are taken with a highly standardized positioning. Averages are calculated but the very wide extremes make "normalcy" difficult to define.

Congenital Spine Deformity

McMaster, M.J., and Ohtsuka, K.: The natural history of congenital scoliosis: A study of 251 patients. J. Bone Joint Surg. 64A:1128-1147, 1982.

The worst lesion is a unilateral unsegmented bar with a contralateral hemivertebra, next a unilateral segmented bar, next double hemivertebrae on the same side, next a free hemivertebra, and then a wedge vertebra. Thoracic lesions are worse than lumbar for progression.

Montgomery, S., and Hall, J.: Congenital kyphosis: Surgical treatment at Boston Children's Hospital. Orthop. Trans. 5:25, 1981.

Thirty-four patients with congenital kyphosis are treated surgically, eight having preoperative neurologic deficit. Ten have combined anterior and posterior fusion. Eight require reoperation for neurologic deficit, failed fusion, or dislodged anterior graft.

Rivard, C.; Narbaitz, R.; and Uhthoff, H.: Congenital vertebral malformations: Time of induction in human and mouse embryos. Orthop. Rev. 8:135, 1979.

Hypoxia on the ninth and tenth days of gestation in the pregnant mouse results in a high percent of embryos with congenital spinal anomalies. These anomalies are present in the mesenchymal stage and persist through the cartilaginous and ossification stages.

Winter, R.B.: Convex anterior and posterior hemiarthrodesis and epiphysiodesis in young children with progressive congenital scoliosis. J. Pediat. Orthop. 1:361-366, 1981.

Ten young children are treated by this technique. All achieve solid fusion, none progress, and two improve with time. There are no complications.

Winter, R.B., and Moe, J.H.: The results of spinal arthrodesis for congenital spine deformity in patients younger than five years old. J. Bone Joint Surg. 64A:419-432, 1982.

Forty-nine patients fused under 5 years of age are reviewed for success of arthrodesis and for complications of fusion at a young age. Early posterior fusion is ideal for kyphosis since progressive improvement results. Most patients fused for scoliosis have good results with little tendency for late progression and no tendency for late lordosis.

Neuromuscular Spine Deformity

Evans, G.A.; Drennan, J.C.; and Russman, B.S.: Functional classification and orthopaedic management of spinal muscular atrophy. J. Bone Joint Surg. 63B:516-522, 1981.

Fifty-four patients are divided into four groups based on the severity of neurologic deficit. Forty-nine of the fifty-four survive. Progressive spinal deformity is noted in all except one-half of those with late onset disease. The more severe the weakness, the earlier is the onset of scoliosis. Spine fusion is the treatment of choice for curves of 60 degrees or more.

Hall, P.; Lindseth, R.; Campbell, R.; Kalsbeck, J.; and DeSousa, A.: Scoliosis and hydrocephalus in myelocele patients: The effects of ventricular shunting. J. Neurosurg. 50:174-178, 1979.

Eleven patients with progressive paralytic scoliosis are treated by ventricular shunting. Four progress, but seven improve. Progressive scoliosis may be due to shunt malfunction.

Lindseth, R.E., and Stelzer, L., Jr.: Vertebral excision for kyphosis in children with myelomeningocele. J. Bone Joint Surg. 61A:699-704, 1979.

Partial resection of the apical vertebra and the proximal lordotic curve done in twelve patients gives persistent correction and allows continued growth of the remaining lumbar vertebrae.

Lonstein, J.E.: Deformities of the spine in children with cerebral palsy. Orthop. Rev. 10:33-44, 1981.

The incidence of scoliosis ranges from 6 percent in ambulatory, minimally involved patients to 64 percent in severely involved patients. Bracing and specialized seating devices can improve function and delay curve progression. Surgical stabilization is effective and should be done to regain or preserve function, especially sitting balance.

Osebold, W.R.; Mayfield, J.K.; Winter, R.B.; and Moe, J.H.: Surgical treatment of paralytic scoliosis associated with myelomeningocele. J. Bone Joint Surg. 64A:841-856, 1982.

The best results are achieved by anterior instrumentation and fusion combined with long posterior instrumentation and fusion to the sacrum. Pseudarthrosis at the lumbosacral area remains a problem. Postoperative management is upright in bivalved plastic body jackets.

Segmental Spinal Instrumentation (Luque Technique)

Allen, B.L., and Ferguson, R.L.: The Galveston technique for L-rod instrumentation of the scoliotic spine. Spine 7:276-284, 1982.

The technique for fixation to the sacrum and pelvis is described.

Luque, E.R.: Segmental spinal instrumentation for correction of scoliosis. Clin. Orthop. 163:192-198, 1982.

Sixty-five consecutive patients with an average follow-up of 18 months are reviewed. The average curve preoperatively is 69 degrees with an average correction at surgery of 74 percent. There is only a 2 percent (1.5 degree) loss at follow-up. Complications include two infections and two pseudarthroses.

Wenger, D.; Wanters, M.; Herring, J.; and Carollo, J.: Comparative mechanics of segmental spinal instrumentation versus traditional Harrington instrumentation in scoliosis treatment: Laboratory analysis. Orthop. Trans. 5:16, 1982.

In vitro analysis of dissected calf spines subjected to various forms of spinal instrumentation and then subjected to various acute stresses shows the single Harrington distraction rod to be the least stable. A Harrington distraction rod with a multiple hook compression assembly and transverse approximators is much more stable and equal to a similar rod with sublaminar wiring. Luque L-rods and wiring tend to bend but not acutely fail.

Miscellaneous Spine Problems

Bethem, D.; Winter, R.B.; Lutter, L.; Moe, J.H.; Bradford, D.S.; Lonstein, J.E.; and Langer, L.O.: Spinal disorders of dwarfism: Review of the literature and report of eighty cases. J. Bone Joint Surg. 63A:1412-1425, 1981.

Abnormal kyphosis is seen in fifty-seven and scoliosis of more than 30 degrees in twenty-one patients. Ten patients have C1-2 instability. Thirteen patients have neurologic damage, paraparesis in ten, and quadriparesis in three.

DeOrio, J.K., and Bianco, A.J.: Lumbar disc excision in children and adolescents. J. Bone Joint Surg. 64A:991-996, 1982.

Fifty-six patients 16 years of age or younger are reviewed with an average follow-up of 19 years. Ninety-four percent got good relief after the original surgery, but twelve needed a further operation. Seventy-four percent had a good result on late follow-up.

Dubousset, J.: Spine deformities induced by irradiation of Wilms' tumors. Rev. Chir. Orthop. 66:441-451, 1980.

Of fifty-nine consecutive patients treated between 1950 and 1963, 65 percent of the survivors develop a kyphosis and 40 percent develop a scoliosis.

Winter, R.B.; Moe, J.H.; Bradford, D.S.; Lonstein, J.E.; Pedras, C.V.; and Weber, A.H.: Spine deformity in neurofibromatosis: A review of 102 patients. J. Bone Joint Surg. 61A:677-694, 1979.

Eighty patients have dystrophic bone changes which are prognostically important. Brace treatment of dystrophic curves is universally unsuccessful. Posterior fusion is best for scoliosis problems and anterior and posterior fusion best for kyphotic problems. Sixteen patients have neurologic deficit due to the deformity.

Yasuoka, S.; Peterson, H.A.; and MacCarty, C.S.: The incidence of spinal deformity and instability after multiple level laminectomy: Its difference in children and adults. Orthop. Trans. 5:11, 1981.

Fifty-eight patients from birth to age 24 years are reviewed. In the group of twenty-six between birth and the age of 15 years, twelve (46 percent) develop a spinal deformity necessitating fusion in eight. In the group of thirty-two patients aged 15 to 24 years, only two develop a deformity and neither requires a fusion.

Spondylolisthesis

Boxall, D.; Bradford, D.S.; Winter, R.B.; and Moe, J.H.: Management of severe spondylolisthesis in children and adolescents. J. Bone Joint Surg. 61A:479-495, 1979.

Forty-three patients with a 50 percent or greater slip are reviewed. Slip angle is found of as great importance as the percentage of slip. There is no correlation of hamstring tightness with neurologic deficit. Fusion alone gives excellent functional results. Progression after solid fusion may occur.

Bradford, D.: Treatment of severe spondylolisthesis: A combined approach for reduction and stabilization. Spine 4:423-428, 1979. Orthop. Trans. 5:410-411, 1981.

Patients with severe spondylolisthesis are treated by posterior decompression and alar-transverse fusion, halo-femoral traction with hyperextension, and anterior fusion. Significant reductions are achieved and maintained. Complications are frequent.

McPhee, I.B., and O'Brien, J.P.: Reduction of severe spondylolisthesis: A preliminary report. Spine 4:430-434, 1979.

Eight patients with spondylolisthesis of Grade III or IV are treated by laminectomy, root decompression, alar-transverse process fusion, halo-femoral traction with hyperextension, and anterior fusion. Very significant reductions are achieved and maintained.

Sevastikoglou, J.A.; Spangfort, E.; and Aaro, S.: Operative treatment of spondylolisthesis in children and adolescents with tight hamstrings syndrome. Clin. Orthop. 147:192-199, 1980.

Ten patients are reviewed. All present with sciatic-like complaints and five exhibit objective neurologic findings. Nine are treated by anterior fusion. One also has a laminectomy. One has a posterior fusion only. All have excellent results with totally normal functional activity at follow-up.

Velikas, E.P., and Blackburne, J.S.: Surgical treatment of spondylolisthesis in children and adolescents. J. Bone Joint Surg. 63B:67-70, 1981.

Thirty-six children and adolescents with slips of more than 10 percent are reviewed. No progression of slip after fusion is seen. Posterolateral fusion relieves symptoms in 75 percent, achieves sound fusion in 83 percent, and prevents more slip in 100 percent of patients.

27 THORACOLUMBAR SPINE: TRAUMA

Adult and pediatric spinal injuries in both the acute and chronic stages are considered in this section.

Adult Thoracolumbar Spinal Injuries

Acute Phase Holdsworth's classification, based upon subdividing the spine into two columns, has been useful in appreciating the complexity of spinal injuries. Originally, it was believed that rupture of the posterior column was sufficient to create instability of the spine. However, recent experimental evidence indicates that instability or the ability to subluxate or dislocate a spinal motion segment occurs only after additional rupture of the posterior longitudinal ligament and the anulus fibrosus. Thus, it has been suggested that the two-column theory be replaced with a three-column theory in which the third or middle column is represented by structures which must be torn in addition to the posterior ligamentous complex to create instability (Fig. 1). The middle column structures are the posterior longitudinal ligament, posterior anulus fibrosus, and posterior half of the vertebral body. The posterior column includes the pedicles, facet joints, laminae, spinous process, interspinous ligaments, and supraspinal ligaments. The anterior column is formed by the anterior longitudinal ligament, anterior anulus fibrosus, and anterior half of the vertebral body.

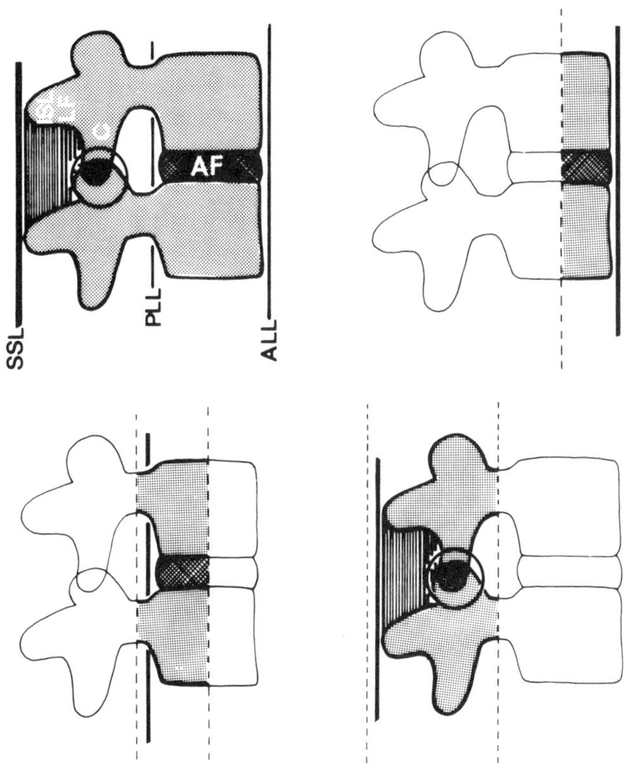

Figure 1: Anterior, middle, and posterior columns. (Figures 1-13 are reprinted with permission from The three column spine and its significance in the classification of acute thoracolumbar spine injuries, by F. Denis, Spine (In press).)

Classification of Spinal Column Injury

COMPRESSION FRACTURES: These are the result of compression failure of the anterior column. The middle column remains intact and acts as a hinge. When the amount of anterior collapse of the vertebral body reaches approximately 50 percent of its height, the posterior ligamentous column begins to fail under tension. The two main subtypes of compression fractures are the anterior compression (Fig. 2) and the lateral compression (Fig. 3).

The vertebral body is wedged anteriorly and the posterior part of the body remains intact and well aligned with the bodies above and below. The interspinous distance is increased in geometrical proportion to the anterior wedging at that level. The posterior wall of the vertebral body appears normal (as can be demonstrated by CT scan) indicating that the vertebral ring around the neural elements is intact (Fig. 4).

BURST FRACTURES: These are the result of axial compression forces on the vertebral body with resultant failure

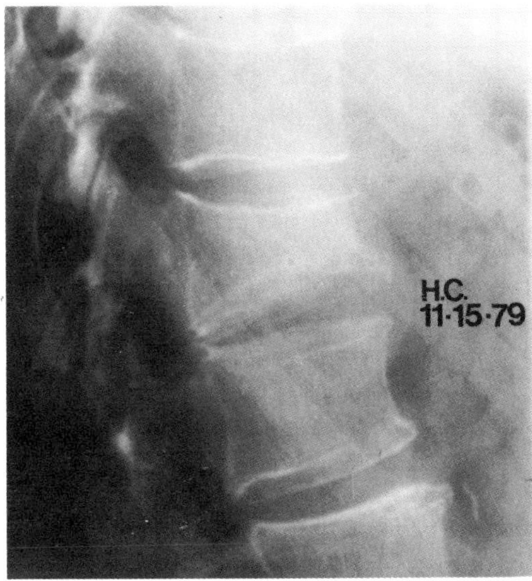

Figure 2: Anterior compression fracture with disruption of the inferior end plate. Note the normal height of the posterior part of the vertebral body.

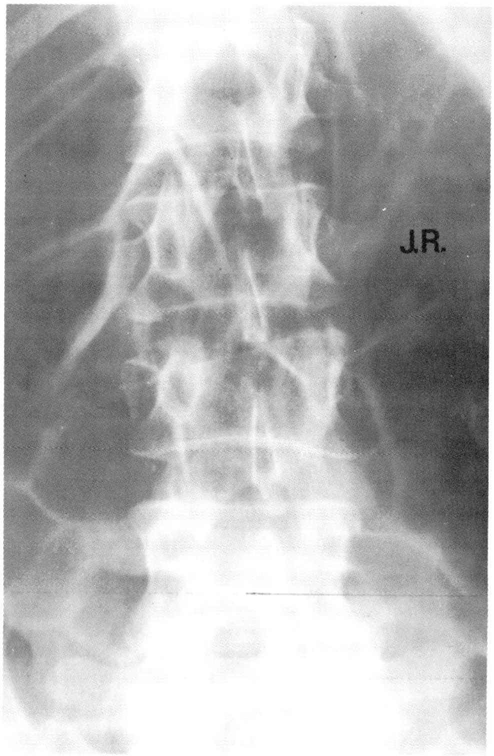

Figure 3: Lateral compression fracture.

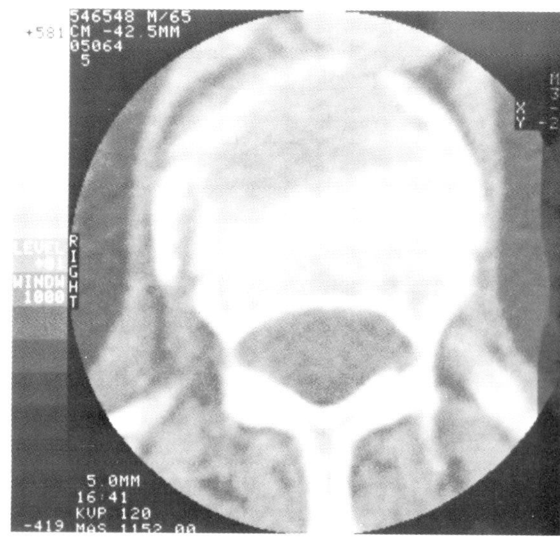

Figure 4: Computed tomogram of compression fracture. Note anterior end plate fracture and totally intact posterior wall of the vertebral body.

of both the anterior and middle columns (Figs. 5, 6, and 7). The crushing of the vertebral body is accompanied by forces that tend to open the posterior arch, frequently causing an increase of the interpediculate distance, a greenstick fracture of the anterior cortex of the lamina, and splaying of the posterior facet joints with rupture of the capsule. Radiographic examination of the fracture may demonstrate all these signs. Computed tomography in burst fractures demonstrates the break of the posterior wall of the vertebral body with retropulsion of bone into the canal and usually a fracture of the posterior arch at the level of the lamina.

SEAT-BELT TYPE INJURIES: These injuries are represented by failure of both the posterior and middle columns under tension forces generated by flexion (Fig. 8). The intact anterior column acts as a fulcrum. The anteroposterior radiograph usually shows a symmetrical rupture of the posterior arch with a split extending through the spinous process, laminae, transverse processes, and pedicles. In a Chance fracture, this horizontal fracture continues into the vertebral body. In other pa-

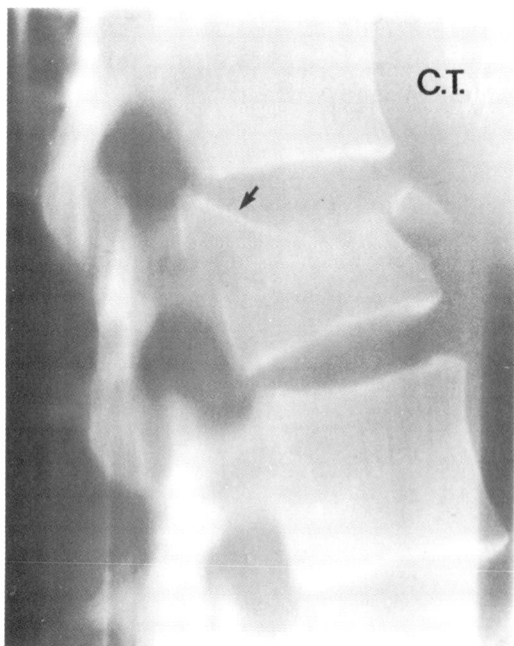

Figure 5: Lateral tomogram of a burst fracture (type B). Note severe disruption of superior end plate, loss of height of posterior vertebral body, and fracture of posterior wall of body. The arrow indicates the large fragment retropulsed into the canal.

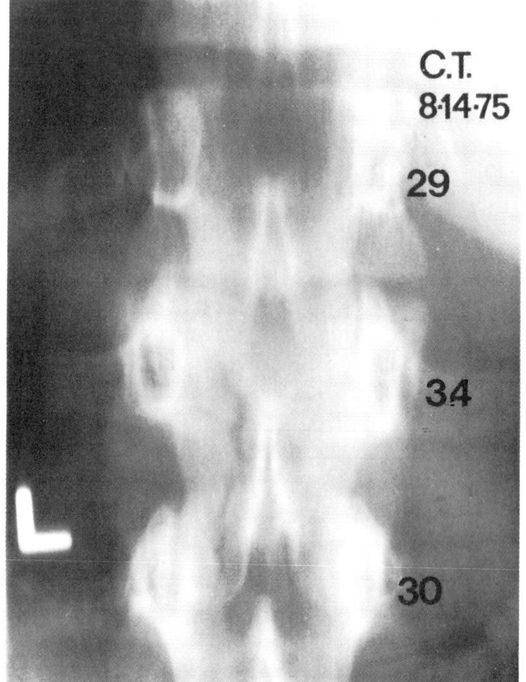

Figure 6: Anteroposterior tomogram of a burst fracture. Note the increased interpedicular distance (34 mm) and the vertical laminar fracture.

tients, it may pass through the disc. Computed tomography does not provide much information about these spinal injuries since the plane of exploration lies parallel to the plane of disruption, and, thus, the scan may miss them. But, anteroposterior and lateral tomograms provide a view perpendicular to the fracture and allow identification of the different components.

FRACTURE-DISLOCATIONS: The main characteristic of fracture-dislocations is that all three columns have failed under compression, tension, rotation, or shear. There are three recognized mechanisms of fracture-dislocations: flexion-rotation, shear, and flexion-distraction.

In *flexion-rotation injuries* the posterior and middle columns are ruptured totally due to tension and rotational forces (Fig. 9). The anterior column has failed under a combination of compression and rotation, occasionally leading to a rupture of the anterior column through bone (slice fracture) or disc. The lateral radiograph shows subluxation or dislocation. There is frequently an increase of the interspinous distance seen both on anteroposterior and lateral views. Careful scrutiny discloses a displaced fracture of the superior articular process on one side, the proof of rotational failure of the posterior column. Multiple transverse process and rib fractures may accompany this injury. Computed tomography may demonstrate reduction in the size of the neural canal caused by the offset of the superior segment on the inferior (Fig. 12). It also may show a fragment of bone avulsed from one of the bodies, sitting in the spinal canal. This fragment usually is smaller than those seen with burst fractures.

In *shear type fracture-dislocations,* (Figs. 10 and 11) all three columns are disrupted, including the anterior longitudinal ligament. The radiographic findings usually are represented by a frank dislocation without wedging of the vertebral bodies anteriorly and multiple fractures of the posterior arches posteriorly.

The *flexion-distraction injury* resembles the seat-belt type injury where both the posterior and middle columns rupture under tension (Fig. 13). However, in this injury the anterior anulus fibrosus also is disrupted with subluxation of the segment above on the vertebra below. It usually is accompanied by stripping of the anterior longitudinal ligament without rupture. Radiographic characteristics are similar to those of the seat-belt type injury but also include subluxation and dislocation.

Classification of Neurologic Injury

SPINAL SHOCK: This injury is represented by a total loss of motor, sensory, and reflex function of all the lumbar and sacral segments following a cervical or thoracic cord lesion. It is usually transient, sometimes persisting up to 24 hours. The end of spinal shock is demonstrated by the return of the bulbocavernosus reflex or the anal reflex. This occurs because an upper motor neurone lesion accompanied by an intact lower motor neurone allows return of the distal cord reflexes. Diagnosis of severity of the cord injury cannot be made until the bulbocavernosus reflex returns, at which time it becomes possible to separate complete from incomplete paraplegia.

INCOMPLETE PARAPLEGIA: This may present in different ways depending upon the level of spinal injury. With upper motor neurone lesions, diagnosis can be made after return of the bulbocavernosus reflex. Incomplete paraple-

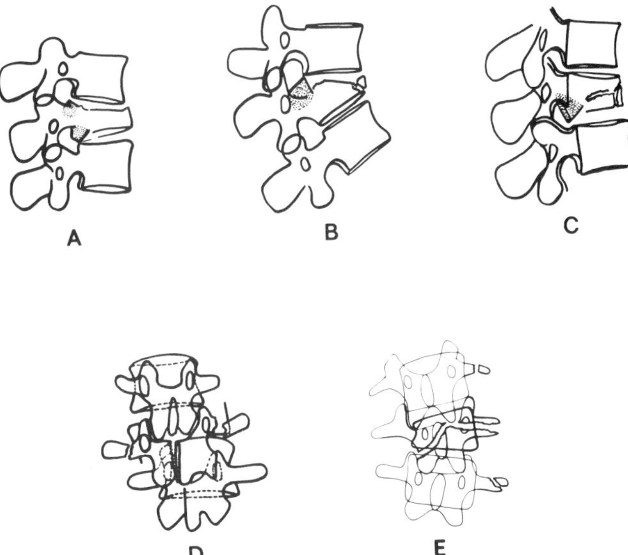

Figure 7: Classification of burst fractures. (Top left) Type A—Fracture of both end plates (axial load). (Top middle) Type B—Fracture of superior end plate (axial load and flexion). (Top right) Type C—Fracture of inferior end plate (axial load and flexion). (Bottom left) Type D—Burst rotation (axial load and rotation). (Bottom right) Type E—Burst lateral flexion (axial load and lateral flexion). Types A, B, and C are diagnosed mainly on lateral radiographs. Anteroposterior radiographs reveal the basic pathognomonic features seen on type B. Types D and E are diagnosed on anteroposterior radiographs. The lateral film of a type D looks like a type A, whereas the lateral film of a type E may look like type A, B, or C.

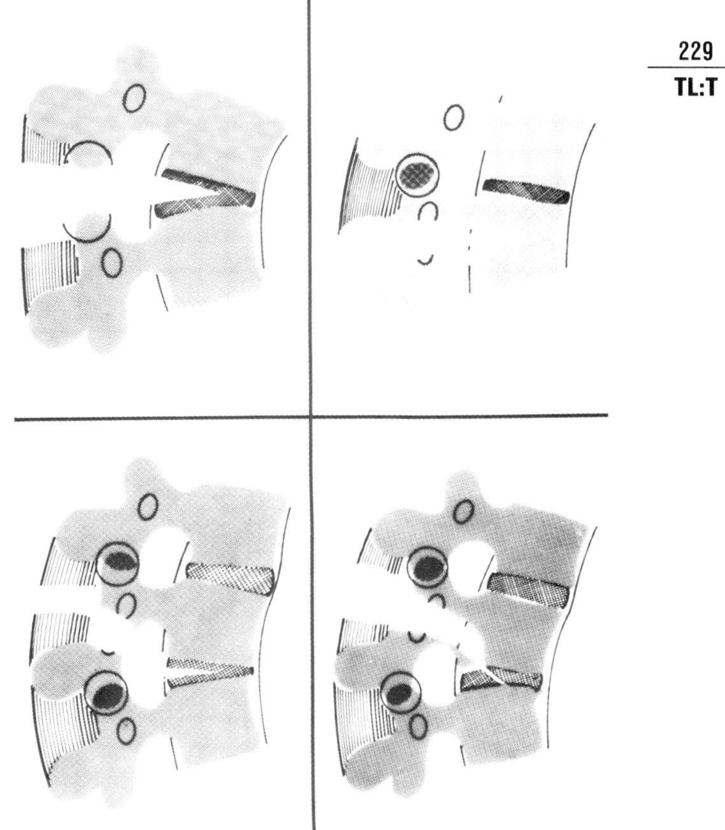

Figure 8: Classification of seat-belt type injuries. (Top left) One-level, seat-belt type injury through ligaments. (Top right) One-level, seat-belt type injury through bone (Chance fracture). (Bottom left) Two-level, seat-belt type injury through ligaments at the level of the middle column. (Bottom right) Two-level, seat-belt type injury through bone at the level of the middle column.

gia is indicated by any evidence of sacral sparing on initial examination. Preservation of perianal skin sensation, a patchy sensitivity to sharp and dull pin pricks, isolated toe flexion, or rectal sphincter control indicate a partial lesion and a better functional prognosis.

The area of the conus medullaris differs from the spinal cord not only in that it contains the tip of the cord but also because the cauda equina acts similarly to peripheral nerves in terms of its physiology. The lower part of the conus contains the S2-3-4 myelomeres, responsible for the bulbocavernosus and the anal reflex, which in patients with severe injury at that level would not be expected to return.

The cauda equina is composed of lower motor neurones. The complete absence of motor, sensory, and reflex function distal to a cauda equina lesion cannot be called a complete paraplegia since its prognosis is dissimilar to that of spinal cord repair and more resembles that of peripheral nerve regeneration.

Complete paraplegia: At the end of spinal shock when the bulbocavernosus reflex or the anal reflex returns, complete absence of motor and sensory function distal to the lesion indicates that the cord has been anatomically or physiologically transected and that no functional return is expected. The term *complete paraplegia* should not be used in association with fractures of T12 or the lumbar vertebrae as these injuries are associated with lesions of the conus and cauda equina or pure lesions of the cauda equina.

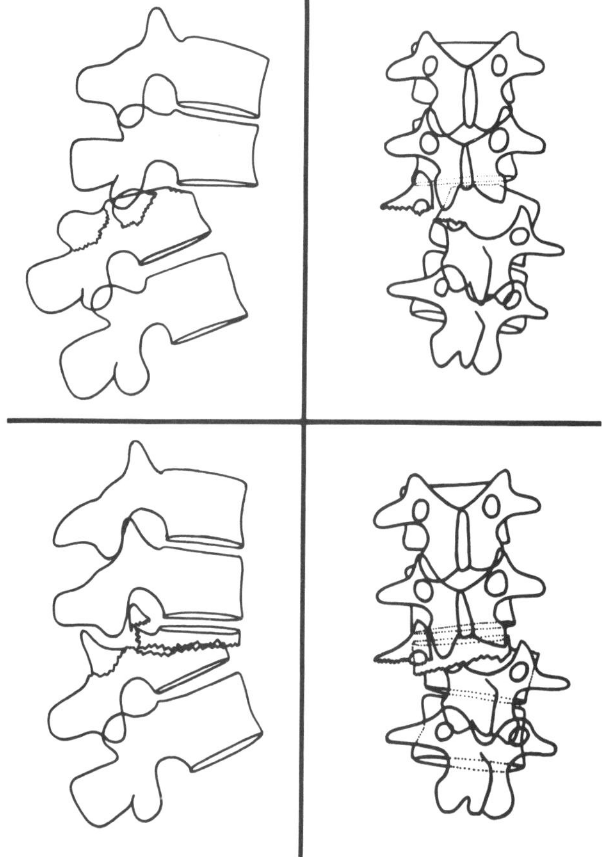

Figure 9: Classification of flexion-rotation injuries. (Top left) Lateral diagram of a fracture-dislocation of the flexion-rotation type through the disc. Note the superior articular process fracture on one side only. (Top right) Anteroposterior diagram of a fracture-dislocation of the flexion-rotation type through the disc. Note the fracture of the left superior articular process. (Bottom left) Lateral diagram of a fracture-dislocation of the flexion-rotation type through bone (slice fracture). (Bottom right) Anteroposterior diagram of a fracture-dislocation of the flexion-rotation type through bone (slice fracture). Note the rotation between both spinal segments.

Ascending paraplegia: The common type of neurologic deterioration occurring during the first 4 days after injury is a rise in the level of the lesion usually by one segment, occasionally by two. This deterioration is very significant at the cervical level where the loss of one further segment represents a drastic change in the function of the upper extremity. At the thoracic level, deterioration involving the first thoracic segment would be most significant because of the relationship to the interossei muscles of the hand. In the lower thoracic levels, a deterioration of one level has only a sensory significance with no further loss of motor function in the involved patient. This phenomenon usually reverses itself and the final neurological lesion becomes the same as that noted immediately after injury.

A rarer form of deterioration has been described as a spinal cord lesion appropriate to the bony injury which rises by several segments in the first few weeks after the original injury. This has been associated both with complete and incomplete lesions, most frequently at the conus level associated with T11, T12, or L1 fractures, with ascending neurologic loss up to the midthoracic or upper thoracic cord. This form of deterioration is usually irreversible although it may regress by one or two levels. The incidence is low, estimated at 1 percent in acute spinal cord injuries in general. However, it is more common with lesions in front of the conus, where its incidence increases to about 2 percent in the T11 or T12 and L1 fractures.

Patient Evaluation A careful history provides information about the mechanism of injury as well as some clues about the presence of a spinal cord injury. For instance, a patient with a burst fracture of T12 may present with a normal neurological examination but with a history of an inability to move the legs for 5 minutes following the injury. This is equivalent to a loss of consciousness accompanying a head injury. The patient should be observed more carefully, and the injury consid-

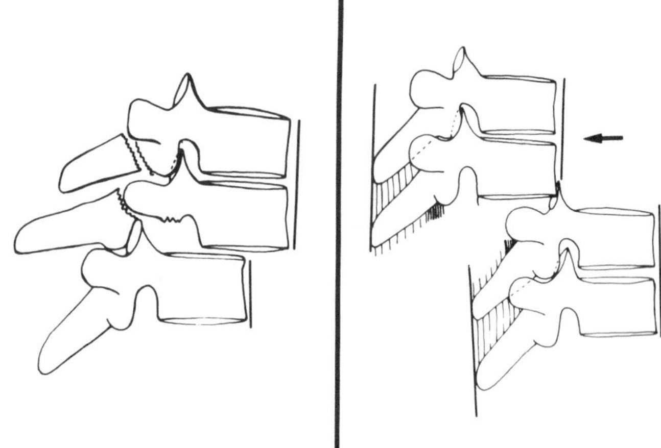

Figure 10: Shear injuries. (Left) Lateral diagram of a posteroanterior shear injury. A large part of the posterior arch may be left behind (floating lamina). (Right) Lateral diagram of an anteroposterior shear injury. The posterior arches and anterior vertebral bodies may be entirely intact, but the three ligamentous columns are disrupted.

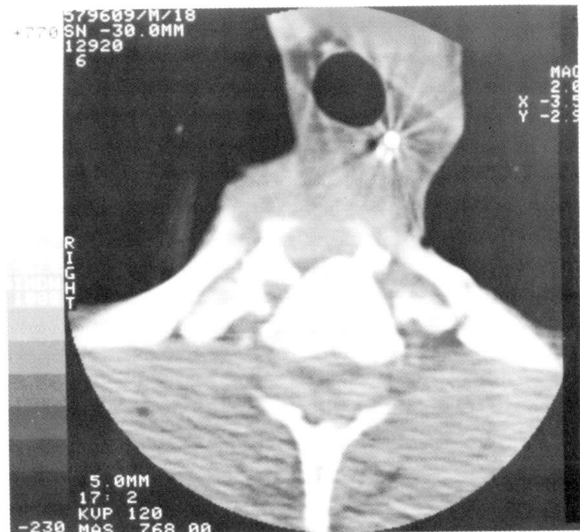

Figure 11: Computed tomogram of a fracture-dislocation of the anteroposterior shear type. Note the anterior aspect of the superior vertebral body locked on the superior facets of the inferior vertebral body.

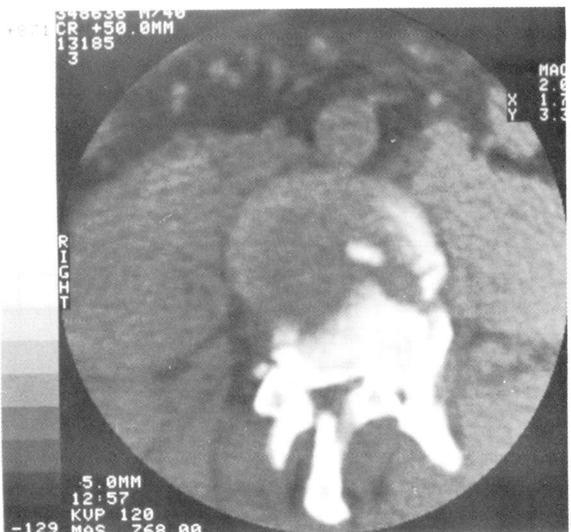

Figure 12: Computed tomogram of a flexion-rotation fracture-dislocation showing reduction of canal size due to dislocation offset.

ered more unstable than the patient presenting with a T12 burst fracture, who was able to walk after the injury. Another important feature to be clarified by history is progressive neurologic deficit. Such a patient might remember being able to move the feet immediately following an accident, only later to lose that ability.

INDICATIONS FOR FURTHER RADIOLOGICAL EVALUATION: Computed tomography is useful in the diagnosis of most spinal fractures. With burst fractures particularly, the CT scan adds a new dimension to the bony obstruction of the canal and allows a more comprehensive approach to treatment. However, computed tomography has limitations. In spinal injuries presenting a line of fracture in the horizontal plane (e.g., seat-belt type injuries), the cut obtained by CT scan may miss the fracture. The tomogram taken in a plane perpendicular to the plane of fracture allows more complete visualization of the injury. Postoperative computed tomography is not invalidated by the presence of metallic rods in the spine. The scattering effect induced by metal decreases soft-tissue definition significantly, but bony definition remains sufficient to indicate reduction or sequestration of a bony fragment displaced into the neural canal.

Treatment: General Of the 18,000 to 38,000 spinal injuries occurring annually in the United States, approximately 4,700 result in paraplegia. Eighty percent of spinal cord injury victims are males younger than 40 years of age. In the United States, there has been a significant trend toward incomplete injuries. This dramatic change may be attributed in part to the sophistication of the emergency medical services systems. The cost of treatment and lifetime follow-up of spinal cord injuries is great. The economic impact in terms of lost wages and loss of production for these patients is even greater. It is important for them to undergo appropriate treatment to attain their fullest potential. Basic and clinical research must continue in this area to reduce the devastating impact of spinal cord injury both to patients and society.

The relative roles of nonoperative versus operative treatment of acute spinal injuries remain unclear. British spinal cord injury centers have tended to favor nonoperative treatment, whereas surgical intervention tends to be emphasized in North America. Early clinical comparisons between nonoperative and operative treatment of spinal cord injuries have yielded several important observations.

Isolated laminectomies have produced poor results. In patients with fracture-dislocations, laminectomy increases spinal instability with the risk of further neurologic damage. In patients with burst fractures, laminectomy does not permit adequate removal of bony fragments responsible for anterior compression of the spinal cord. Laminectomies increase the incidence of posttraumatic kyphosis and chronic instability of the spine.

In a burst fracture with neurologic deficit, blind realignment of the spine with rods or plates may decompress the neural elements. However, in many patients it may not. To ensure neural decompression during instrumentation, a cross-table lateral radiograph, perioperative mye-

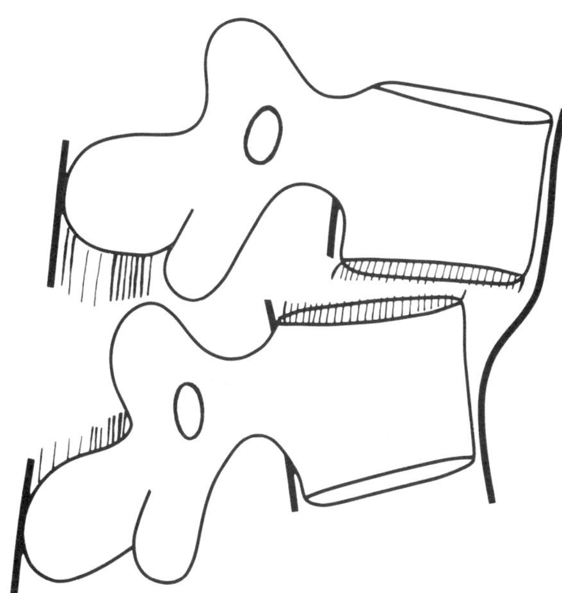

Figure 13: Lateral diagram of a fracture-dislocation of the flexion-distraction type. The posterior, middle, and anterior ligamentous columns are disrupted, and the anterior longitudinal ligament is stripped off the vertebral body below.

logram, or even careful exploration of the neural canal may be necessary.

The significance and extent of neural compression and its deleterious effects upon neural recovery are controversial. The radiographic definition of significant neural compression is unsettled. Some believe that a complete block on myelographic examination is necessary to be significant. Others believe that a root may be compressed in a lateral recess without the presence of a complete block. Differences of opinion between the proponents of anterolateral decompression and of posterior or posterolateral decompressions in the treatment of burst fractures emphasize this uncertainty.

It is anticipated that much uncertainty associated with the treatment of acute spinal injuries will be dispelled in the near future when treatment protocol data from the regional spinal injury centers in the United States become available.

The value of emergency versus delayed surgical intervention has not been fully answered. Experimental canine data demonstrate that functional recovery after acute extradural compression of the spinal cord depends upon the magnitude of the compressive force as well as its duration. With large compressive forces, full recovery of function occurred when compression was released within 1 minute. When such compression was applied for longer periods, functional recovery usually did not occur. The cause of these irreversible changes was destruction of the spinal cord at the compression site. When minimal spinal cord compressive force was used to produce complete motor and sensory loss in hind limbs, recovery occurred with periods of compression up to 2 hours.

Compression of the cauda equina by large balloons for as long as 5 hours was compatible with full functional recovery after release. Failure of recovery within this period and probably after longer periods of compression was due to hemorrhage within the conus medullaris which diffused upwards to destroy the adjacent segment or two of the spinal cord innervating the hind limbs. Although functional recovery in dogs may begin as early as 1 to 5 days after spinal cord or cauda equina compression, it may be delayed as long as 30 days after spinal cord compression and 59 days after cauda equina compression. Pain sensation persisted after motor function of the hind limbs was lost after compression of the spinal cord and the cauda equina. During recovery, pain sensation returned before motor power and position sense. The duration of spinal cord compression compatible with recovery was much longer (up to 1 week or more) in animals that showed complete loss of motor function but preserved pain sensation.

Some may argue that human spinal cords differ significantly from canine. In the absence of clear evidence to the contrary, it seems logical for the clinician to accept some similarity between the experimental model and the clinical situation. One possible implication from the experimental data is that in burst fractures of T12 or L1, emergency decompression within 5 hours of the accident may yield improved results when compared to later decompressions. As yet there is no human data to support this.

There are no convincing answers to the following perplexing questions: whether a distraction rod, compression rod, or a Luque rod should be used; whether there should be a fusion and if it is to be done, whether it should go the entire length of the distraction instrumentation, be inserted two levels above and two levels below, or three above and three below; whether a round-ended rod should be used in the lumbar spine or a square-ended rod contoured into lordosis; and whether steroids should be used in the patient with acute spinal cord injuries. Answers may be forthcoming from the prospective studies now being performed in the regional spinal injury centers.

At this time there is no evidence that any mechanical (except possibly early reduction) or chemical treatment has a spinal cord sparing effect. Despite this, steroids frequently are given following injury although some investigators do not use steroids because of the risk of causing gastroduodenal ulcers. When used, the dosage is usually 15 mg per kg of body weight of methylprednisolone succinate intravenously, given initially as a loading dose and followed by the same quantity administered in four equally divided doses for 10 days. Cimetidine is given prophylactically.

Treatment: Specific

COMPRESSION FRACTURES: In an osteoporotic elderly patient with a simple compression fracture without neurologic injury, treatment consists of observation and symptomatic therapy. Hospitalization is not required as long as the trauma is minimal. Admission occasionally may be necessary to investigate a suspected pathological fracture or for ileus. Any attempt to reduce a compression fracture in an elderly patient almost always fails as the comminution of osteoporotic bone is "irreversible." The use of a hyperextension orthosis or a corset for symptomatic treatment occasionally is helpful.

In severe compression fractures (50 percent or more loss of vertebral height), the posterior ligamentous structures are ruptured at least partially. There is an increased rate of posttraumatic pain and kyphosis in these patients. Adequate reduction can be obtained and maintained in active, healthy patients when the spine is immobilized for a sufficient period of time (3 to 6 months). A recent trend has been to immobilize those patients in a body cast without reduction until healing occurs. Patients who develop late complications, such as pain, kyphosis, and neurologic change, may be treated surgically. When kyphosis is an acute problem, Harrington instrumentation with contoured distraction rods and spinal fusion has been recommended. The fusion should extend the entire length of the instrumentation in the thoracic spine (minimal motion, low rate of pseudarthrosis). In the lumbar spine, it is recommended that only the levels involved in the injury be fused to preserve lumbar motion. It must be remembered that the incidence of pseudarthrosis is higher in the lumbar spine. Subsequent degenerative changes of the mobile lumbar spine tend to increase with longer lumbar fusions.

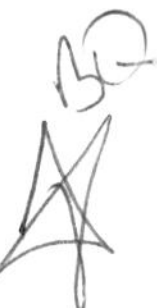

BURST FRACTURES WITHOUT NEUROLOGIC DEFICIT: Computed tomography often shows a significant obstruction of the neural canal without neural deficit. This most frequently occurs in the region of the cauda equina where the canal is wide. Late neurologic changes necessitating surgical intervention have been reported in about 20 percent of patients. Provided that the patient has been informed of the potential neurologic risk, nonoperative treatment with application of a body cast followed by

Figure 14-A

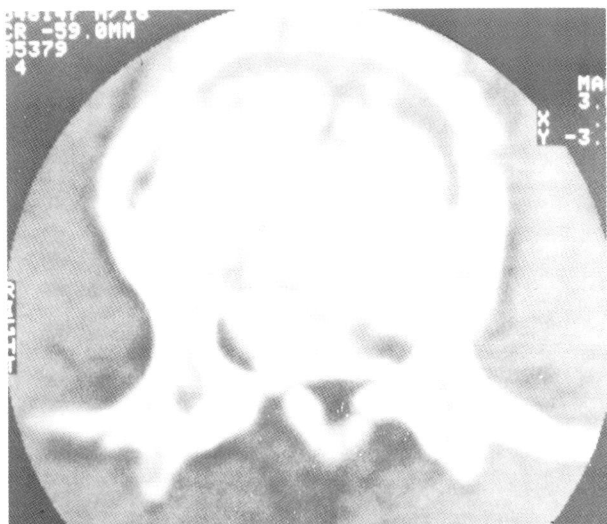

Figure 14-B

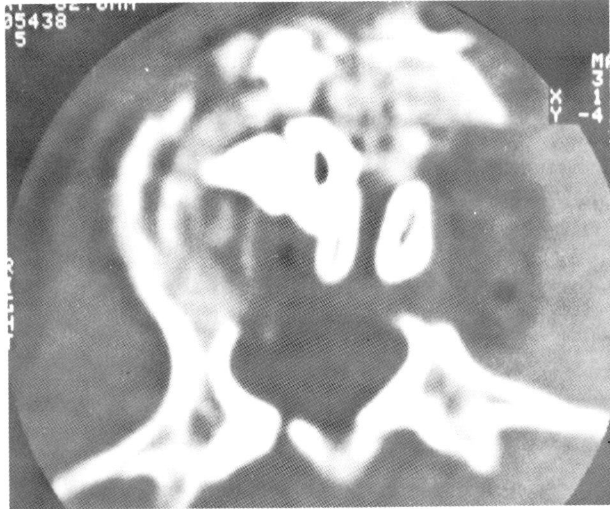

Figure 14-C

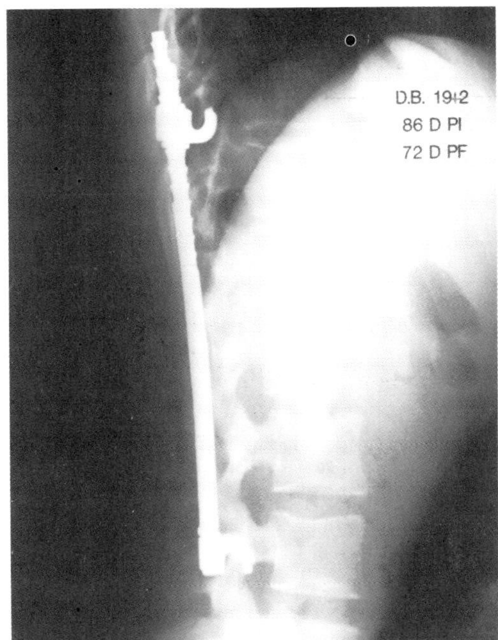

Figure 14-D

Figure 14: (A) Lateral radiograph of a type B burst fracture in a patient with "pseudocomplete" paraplegia at the L1 level. (B) CT scan showing, in the same patient, an 80 percent obstruction of the canal by retropulsion of bone from the vertebral body. (C) CT scan after anterior decompression and anterior fusion. (D) About 3 months after anterior decompression and anterior fusion followed by posterior stabilization 2 weeks later. The patient is able to walk without crutches with a minimal limp with bilateral AFO's.

early or delayed ambulation (3 to 6 weeks) is appropriate. The cast should be worn for about 3 to 6 months depending upon comminution of the fracture as well as its radiographic appearance at 3 months. An alternative to nonoperative treatment is prophylactic open reduction and internal fixation with square-ended rods contoured into lordosis and a localized fusion carried out at the levels of involvement. Rods are removed between 12 and 18 months after insertion. Compression rods should not be used with acute burst fractures since they may precipitate neurologic damage by collapse of the middle column. Luque rods have been demonstrated to be ineffective in those fractures since they cannot control axial collapse.

Burst fractures with neurologic deficit: When damage to the conus medullaris accompanies this injury, it is difficult to carry out adequate decompression from posterolaterally as retraction on the conus damages it further. Some recommend anterior decompression of burst fractures of L1 and above accompanied by neurologic deficit. Posterior instrumentation with square-ended rods and localized spinal fusion is carried out 2 weeks later (Fig. 14). Others recommend instrumentation with a distraction rod allowing some reduction of the retropulsed fragment from the tension on the posterior longitudinal ligament. An intraoperative myelogram, cross-table lateral radiograph, or a small hemilaminectomy may be needed to confirm the adequacy of the decompression. When decompression is judged insufficient, some investigators proceed with posterolateral decompression. Others recommend carrying out an anterolateral decompression either during the same operation or 2 weeks later. Fractures below L1 can be treated from posterior with distraction rods since posterolateral decompression is easier at that level. The instrumentation used for stabilization includes dual square-ended distraction rods contoured into lordosis. Postoperative immobilization is maintained in a Risser body cast or a bivalved thoraco-lumbo-sacral orthosis (TLSO). Burst fractures of L4 and L5 are difficult to immobilize (as evidenced by frequent rod dislocations) unless the cast is extended to include one thigh.

SEAT-BELT TYPE INJURIES: A Chance fracture (without subluxation or dislocation) is best treated with a hyperextension body cast. However, one-level posterior and middle ligamentous column disruption is best managed with open reduction and internal fixation with a one-level compression instrumentation and fusion. Postoperative immobilization in a body cast for 3 months is recommended.

In two-level injuries, an attempt at closed reduction in a body cast is appropriate. If an adequate reduction cannot be achieved, open reduction and internal fixation with short compression instrumentation and spinal fusion are indicated.

FRACTURE-DISLOCATIONS: In a patient with complete paraplegia, spinal instrumentation and spinal fusion may be delayed for several days. Surgery does not assist neurologic recovery but does stabilize the spine, permitting the patient to proceed more rapidly with rehabilitation. In a patient with incomplete paraplegia, as well as with "pseudocomplete" paraplegia (below T11), open reduction, spinal instrumentation, and careful inspection of the spinal canal are recommended. Neural compression in these patients may be related to the offset of the already smaller canal in the thoracic spine than in the lumbar spine and avulsed bone fragments from the posterior vertebral bodies at the time of dislocation. These fragments of bone cannot be reduced or even contained by the posterior longitudinal ligament since this ligament is torn (unlike that observed in burst fractures).

Osteotomizing the superior facets of the lower vertebrae to allow reduction is not indicated in fracture-dislocations unless necessary to obtain reduction since this tends to decrease stability of the spine after reduction. The instrumentation consists of bilateral square-ended distraction rods contoured into lordosis, combined with a metallic posterior tension band (stainless steel wire or a small compression system inserted on the midline at the level of disruption). In shear type fracture-dislocations, the anterior longitudinal ligament is torn completely and bilateral distraction instrumentation alone leads to overdistraction, making use of a midline compression rod at the level of disruption of the posterior column necessary.

Chronic Stage

With Progressive Neurologic Deficit

POST FRACTURE-DISLOCATION INSTABILITY: Fracture-dislocations not surgically stabilized are unstable and may progress to further neurologic deficit with more displacement. Deformities encountered in these patients include kyphosis, scoliosis, or a combination of both. Recommended treatment is decompression followed by spinal stabilization. A combination of anterior and posterior surgery may be required in some patients. In other patients, if seen early enough, both decompression and stabilization may be obtained through a posterior approach.

POST BURST COLLAPSE: Twenty percent neurologic complications have been recorded in patients with burst fractures who were neurologically intact initially, but in whom the fracture collapsed following nonoperative treatment. Surgical goals for these patients are to decompress the neural elements anteriorly and perform anterior fusion with either immediate anterior instrumentation or a posterior stabilization with square-ended distraction rods and fusion 2 weeks later. In some chronic stable situations, posterior compression after conservative anterior decompression may be considered, although this probably is not as mechanically secure as square-shouldered distraction rods contoured into lordosis.

POSTTRAUMATIC KYPHOSIS: This may progress to neurologic deficit as the cord becomes tented over the apex of a severe kyphosis. A 50 percent failure rate with anterior spinal fusion alone indicates the need for combined anterior and posterior fusions with posterior instrumentation. Late posttraumatic kyphosis may be treated successfully by a combined anterior decompression, anterior fusion, and posterior instrumentation and fusion using either distraction or compression rods. However, decompression in the critical vascular zone between T5 and T9 carries some risk since 20 percent of patients may develop an increased neurologic deficit in the immediate postoperative period.

POSTTRAUMATIC LATERAL RECESS STENOSIS: A severe obstruction associated with a burst fracture in the mid-lumbar spine may occur without neurologic deficit acutely. During the chronic stage, degenerative changes at the posterior facets may lead to further narrowing of the lateral recess with stenosis of the most lateral root in the spinal canal. These patients may require posterior or anterior decompression with spinal fusion.

POSTTRAUMATIC SYRINGOMYELIA: These patients with complete or incomplete paraplegia develop a slow proximal migration of their sensory level several months or years after trauma and often complain of intractable pain. Radiological diagnosis is best made by metrizamide myelography with standard films followed by immediate postmetrizamide computed tomography (CT). This must be repeated about 3 or 4 hours later to demonstrate the metrizamide in the posttraumatic syrinx. If significant motor function is at risk, the syrinx should be decompressed.

Without Progressive Neurologic Deficit

NONDECOMPRESSED SPINAL CANAL WITH POOR NEUROLOGIC RETURN: The efficacy of late decompression in terms of neurologic return has now been demonstrated in patients with severe canal obstruction and incomplete paraplegia who have been operated upon during the first year or two after injury. The procedure consists of anterior decompression and anterior fusion. Anterior or posterior instrumentation is usually required.

POSTTRAUMATIC KYPHOSIS: This condition may occur with pain without neurologic deficit and is treated by correction and fusion without anterior decompression. Depending upon the degree of kyphosis, a combination of anterior and posterior surgery or posterior approach alone may be required.

PAIN WITH CHRONIC INSTABILITY: Chronic instability following certain fracture-dislocations may be suggested in a patient complaining of pain accompanied by a feeling of weakness or subluxation of the spine. In the absence of kyphosis, these patients may be treated by a one-level posterolateral fusion or a posterior instrumentation with spinal fusion in the more severe deformities.

Pediatric Thoracolumbar Spinal Injuries

Acute Stage

Peculiarities of the Pediatric Spine The relative rarity of spinal fractures in children may be partially due to reduced accident risk but is mainly the result of both increased elasticity of the vertebral column and the lesser mass of the child's body. A special feature of the growing vertebral column is the presence of epiphyseal plates and ring apophyses which may be the site of traumatic separation. During clinical and radiographic examination, a pediatric patient's spine may appear intact when a dislocation actually had occurred at the time of injury. Many spinal cord injuries occur in children without evidence of associated fracture or dislocation. The mechanism of neural damage in these patients remains difficult to determine. It appears that children younger than 8 years of age sustain more serious neurologic damage and suffer a larger number of upper cervical cord lesions than children over that age. It should also be noted that 52 percent of children presenting with spinal cord injury without radiographic abnormalities show delayed onset of paralysis up to 4 days after injury. Most of these children recall experiencing transient paresthesias, numbness, or subjective paralysis. This raises the probability of an unrecognized instability occurring which led to acute, but temporary, malalignment of the spine with subsequent neural damage.

Classification of Bone and Neurologic Injury

BONE INJURY WITHOUT NEURAL INJURY: The same fractures seen in adults may occur in children without neural injury. Carefully supervised flexion-extension films may demonstrate a spinal instability not apparent on plain films.

NEURAL INJURY: Categories of spinal injury are similar for adults and children. Children, however, may show neural injury without radiographic changes.

Indications for Further Radiological Evaluation Burst fractures and fracture-dislocations may occur in pediatric patients. Lateral tomograms, myelography, and computed tomography have been shown to be quite effective in both the differential diagnosis and the delineation of the extent of the spinal injury.

Treatment Except for the need to be aware of the potential for instability in the child, treatment of acute spinal injuries is the same as for adults. If an incomplete neurologic deficit is present, neural decompression and spinal stabilizaton should be performed. The only difference may be the need for smaller instrumentation because of the smaller size of the pediatric spine.

Any child who sustains a spinal injury and gives a history of transient paresthesias, numbness, or subjective paralysis also should be immobilized in a plaster cast even if the neurologic and radiologic examinations are negative.

Chronic Stage Clinical implications of chronic spinal instability in adolescents are the same as in adults. In contrast, spinal cord injuries in prepubertal patients result in spinal deformity in all. Sixty percent of these patients ultimately require spinal fusion with Harrington or Luque instrumentation. Scoliosis will develop in 90 percent of these patients with approximately one-half of them developing significant pelvic obliquity with ineffective sitting balance. Fifty percent of these patients will develop kyphosis extending progressively from the upper thoracic spine to the lower lumbar spine or the sacrum. Excessive lumbar lordosis will occur in approximately 20 percent of these patients, who will also develop severe hip flexion contracture.

TREATMENT: An infantile or juvenile patient with spinal cord injury should be braced prophylactically with a thoraco-lumbo-sacral orthosis (TLSO) to attempt to prevent development and progression of spinal deformity. If successful, this treatment should be continued until spinal growth ceases. Surgical treatment is indicated in the patient in whom spinal deformity continues to progress despite bracing. Harrington rod or Luque rod instrumentation with spinal fusion are recommended for those patients whose pelvic obliquity is supple enough to allow correction of sitting balance through a posterior approach. If a more severe or inflexible pelvic obliquity is present, a combination of anterior and posterior surgery is necessary. Fusion in all patients should extend to the sacrum as failure to do so inevitably leads to recurrence of pelvic obliquity at the unfused levels. Unlike juvenile patients, only about one-third of adolescent patients require spinal fusion and stabilization because of the inherent spinal stability that accompanies growth.

ANNOTATED BIBLIOGRAPHY

Adult Thoracolumbar Spinal Injuries

Acute Phase

Bazilevskaia, Z.V.: State of vertebral canal in vertebral and spinal cord injuries. Zh Vopr Neirokhir 4:54-59, 1978.

This analysis of 128 patients who died after cervical or thoracolumbar spinal cord injury shows damage to the walls of the spinal canal in all patients. In 85 percent the injury involved only the ligaments and disc surrounding the canal.

Daniels, A.U., and Dunn, H.K.: Anterior spine stabilization: An implant system. Orthop. Trans. 5:18-19, 1981.

This is a report on type III anterior instrumentation which appears to render stability similar to that of dual Harrington rods utilized posteriorly. This negates the need for a secondary procedure to stabilize the spine posteriorly following anterior decompression of burst fractures.

DeLaTorre, J.C.: Spinal cord injury: Review of basic and applied research. Spine 6:315-335, 1981.

This review of recent spinal cord injury research includes experimental and clinical monitoring tools and therapeutic possibilities. A discussion of the rationale of corticosteroid administration is included.

Denis, F.: Updated classification of thoracolumbar fractures. Orthop. Trans. 6:8, 1982.

This retrospective study of 412 thoracolumbar spinal injuries introduces the new concept of a three-column system which allows the identification of failure of each column. The new classification correlates well with neurological findings and treatment plans.

Denis, F., and Armstrong, G.W.D.: Burst fractures in the lumbar spine. Orthop. Trans. 5:417, 1981.

This is a review of fifty-nine patients with burst fractures. Thirty were treated operatively and twenty-nine nonoperatively. Twenty percent of nonoperative patients developed a neurologic deficit due initially to collapse of the fracture and laterto posttraumatic lateral recess stenosis.

Flesch, J.R.; Leider, L.L.; Erickson, D.L.; Chou, S.N.; and Bradford, D.S.: Harrington instrumentation and spine fusion for unstable fractures and fracture-dislocations of the thoracic and lumbar spine. J. Bone Joint Surg. 59A:143-153, 1977.

Of forty patients with unstable fractures and fracture-dislocations treated with Harrington instrumentation and fusion, thirty-five had a neural deficit. Twenty-three patients had posterior or posterolateral decompression prior to instrumentation, and thirteen were decompressed at the time of stabilization. All but one patient obtained solid fusion. Advantages were effective stabilization, early mobilization, and prevention of late deformity.

Frankel, H.L.; Hancock, D.O.; Hyslop, G.; Melzack, O.J.; Michaelis, L.S.; Ungar, G.H.; Vernon, J.D.S.; and Walsh, J.J.: The value of postural reduction in the initial management of closed injuries of the spine with paraplegia and tetraplegia. Paraplegia 7:179-192, 1969.

This series of 612 patients with spinal injuries evaluates nonoperative therapy in terms of its neurofunctional results. It is a good baseline comparison of operative methods to the nonoperative Guttman's method.

Gelfan, S., and Tarlov, I.M.: Physiology of spinal cord nerve root and peripheral nerve compression. Am. J. Physiol. 185:217-229, 1956.

The reversible conduction block produced by maintained mechanical deformation of spinal cord, nerve root, or peripheral nerve is due to mechanical deformation of the neuronal tissue and not to lack of oxygen as suggested by distinctly different patterns of recovery.

Ito, H., and Bassett, C.A.L.: Effects of pulsing electromagnetic fields (PEMF) on motor function after transaction of the rat sciatic nerve. Orthop. Trans. 5:202-203, 1981.

The findings in this study suggest that PEMF's accelerated neural regeneration and return of motor power after transection of the rat sciatic nerve. The authors suggest controlled studies of PEMF effects in humans.

Jacobs, R.R., and Ghista, D.N.: A biomechanical basis for treatment of injuries of the dorsolumbar spine. *In* Osteoarthromechanics, pp. 435-471, edited by D.N. Ghista. New York, Hemisphere, McGraw-Hill, 1981.

When the anterior bone is sufficiently intact to resist compressive loads, a compression instrumentation is suitable. Otherwise, distraction rods contoured to resist bending are necessary. Spinal fusion is required because ligamentous healing is not sufficiently strong.

Miller, F.; Reger, S.I.; Wang, G.J.; and Boychuck, L.: Biomechanical analysis of segmental spinal fixation in a fracture model. Orthop. Trans. 6:23, 1982.

There does not appear to be any increase in strength by fixing more levels than the ends of the rods, nor is there any increase in strength by fixing more than two levels above and below the fracture site.

Nagel, D.A.; Koogle, T.A.; Piziali, R.L.; and Perkash, I.: Stability of the upper lumbar spine following progressive disruptions and the application of individual internal and external fixation devices. J. Bone Joint Surg. 63A:62-70, 1981.

Flexion of L1 on L2 of 20 degrees or a lateral bend of 10 degrees indicate that all posterior ligaments, including the posterior longitudinal ligament and part of the anulus fibrosus, must be disrupted.

Nash, C.L., Jr.; Lorig, R.A.; Schatzinger, L.A.; and Brown, R.H.: Spinal cord monitoring during operative treatment of the spine. Clin. Orthop. 126:100-105, 1977.

This report on use of somatosensory-evoked potentials in thirty-four patients undergoing spine surgery indicates that a positive correlation seems to exist between evoked potentials and clinical conditions.

Posner, I.; White, A.A.; Edwards, W.T.; and Hayes, W.C.: A biomechanical analysis of the clinical stability of the lumbar and lumbosacral spine. Orthop. Trans. 5:287, 1981.

In the flexion instability sequences, all functional spinal units failed when all the posterior components plus one anterior component had been destroyed.

Purcell, G.A.; Markolf, K.L.; and Dawson, E.G.: Twelfth thoracic-first lumbar vertebral mechanical stability of fractures after Harrington-rod instrumentation. J. Bone Joint Surg. 63A:71-78, 1981.

When using distraction rods for stabilizing fractures, hook placement three laminae above and two laminae below is recommended. This allows instrumentation to maintain increased stability in a flexion mode.

Reger, S.I.; Anderson, C.P.; Wang, G.J.; and Stamp, W.G.: Long-term quantitive correlation of spinal evoked potentials with cord injury. Orthop. Trans. 5:299-300, 1981.

Spinal evoked potentials were recorded clinically and experimentally. Results show that the amplitude of postinjury potentials correlated directly with functional recovery whereas latency correlated inversely. Early return of one indicated an expected significant long-term recovery.

Tarlov, I.M.; Klinger, J.; and Vitale, S.: Spinal cord compression studies: 1. Experimental techniques to produce acute and gradual compression. 2. Time limits for recovery after acute compression in dogs. Arch. Neurol. and Psychiat. 71:271-290, 1954.

This study of acute extradural compression of spinal cord and cauda equina demonstrates the significance of the magnitude of compression and its duration. Compression of cauda equina for 5 hours was compatible with full recovery.

Chronic Stage

Bohlman, H.H., and Eismont, F.J.: Surgical techniques of anterior decompression and fusion for spinal cord injuries. Clin. Orthop. 154:57-67, 1981.

One hundred patients treated by late spinal cord decompression demonstrated beneficial effects on neurologic recovery.

Osborne, D.R.S.; Vavoulis, G.; Nashold, B.S., Jr.; Dubois, P.J.; Drayer, B.P.; and Heinz, E.R.: Late sequelae of spinal cord trauma: myelographic and surgical correlation. J. Neurosurg. 57:18-23, 1982.

This article describes six patterns of myelograms in posttraumatic paraplegia. The main problems were unrecognized bony obstructions of the canal and posttraumatic syringes in four patients. Combinations of metrizamide myelogram and computed tomography allowed diagnosis.

Whitesides, T.E., Jr.: Traumatic kyphosis of the thoracolumbar spine. Clin. Orthop. 128:78-92, 1977.

Persistent and progressive kyphosis can impede rehabilitation by causing progressive neural loss, inhibiting potential neural recovery, and causing a painful deformity which precludes a supine sitting or standing posture.

Pediatric Thoracolumbar Spinal Injuries

Acute Stage

Benner, B.; Moiel, R.; Dickson, J.; and Harrington, P.: Instrumentation of the spine for fracture dislocations in children. Child's Brain 3:249-255, 1977.

Thirteen children with severe thoracolumbar injuries and neurological deficits were treated by Harrington instrumentation and spinal fusion with posterior decompressions when necessary. Indications for spinal instrumentation for the pediatric group are similar to those for adults.

Pang, D., and Wilberger, J.E.: Spinal cord injury without radiographic abnormalities in children. J. Neurosurg. 57:114-129, 1982.

Among children with this syndrome, 52 percent have delayed onset of paralysis up to 4 days after injury. Most recall transient paresthesia, numbness, or subjective paralysis. There is a review of the possible mechanisms of neural damage.

Chronic Stage

Mayfield, J.K.; Erkkila, J.C.; and Winter, R.B.: Spine deformity subsequent to acquired childhood spinal cord injury. J. Bone Joint Surg. 63A:1401-1411, 1981.

In this study all juvenile patients with spinal cord injuries developed spine deformities. Eighty-six percent had progression of deformity. Paralytic scoliosis was associated with pelvic obliquity in all patients. Collapsing kyphosis and hyperlordosis were noted in 57 percent and 18 percent of patients, respectively.

28 THORACOLUMBAR SPINE: RECONSTRUCTION

Subjects covered in this section include idiopathic scoliosis and neuromuscular (mainly postpoliomyelitis) and congenital curves. Adult kyphosis, most frequently postmenopausal, and Scheuermann's disease are also discussed.

Scoliosis

PREVALENCE: The number of adults in the United States with significant scoliosis of over 30 degrees is estimated to be 450,000 to 500,000. Only a small percentage of these present with clinical complaints. In a study evaluating intravenous pyelograms in 5,000 patients, most of whom were in the sixth to eighth decades, 3.9 percent were found to have lumbar curves over 10 degrees, with 59 percent having back pain. The pain was unrelated to age and occupation but was more common in curves over 45 degrees and curves exhibiting facet sclerosis radiographically.

NATURAL HISTORY: Scoliosis in adults over 20 years of age usually begins in childhood or adolescence. Progression of these curves may or may not occur with aging. Pregnancy has no direct effect on curve progression in the untreated adult, and curves increasing during pregnancy would have progressed anyway. Some curves seem to stabilize by the age of 20 years and others during the twenties or even the thirties. A long-term follow-up shows that curves most likely to progress in adulthood are thoracic curves of 50 to 80 degrees at skeletal maturity and the lumbar component of double thoracic and lumbar curves of 50 to 74 degrees. Currently no factors are known that will help predict which of these curves will progress and which will not.

Lumbar scoliosis can appear in adulthood in a previously normal spine because of multiple disc degeneration and collapse of the intervertebral space. If this process is unusually severe at one space, lateral or rotatory subluxation can occur (Fig. 1). The relationship between osteoporosis and the de novo development of scoliosis in adults is still controversial.

Adults who were treated with a Milwaukee brace during adolescence tend to lose correction after its discontinuance so that 10 years later the curve approximately matches the

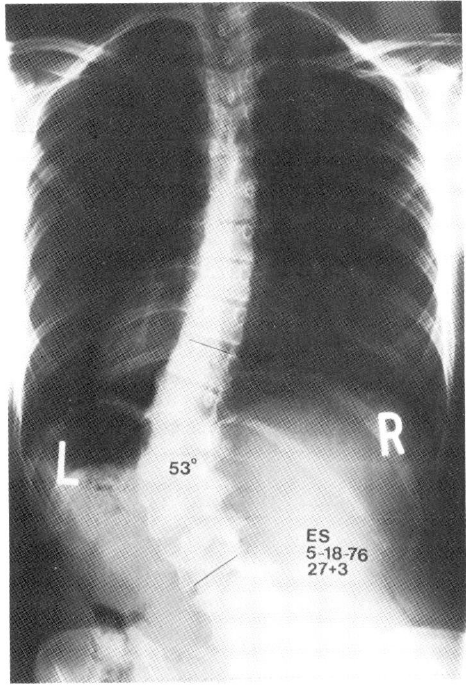

Figure 1-A

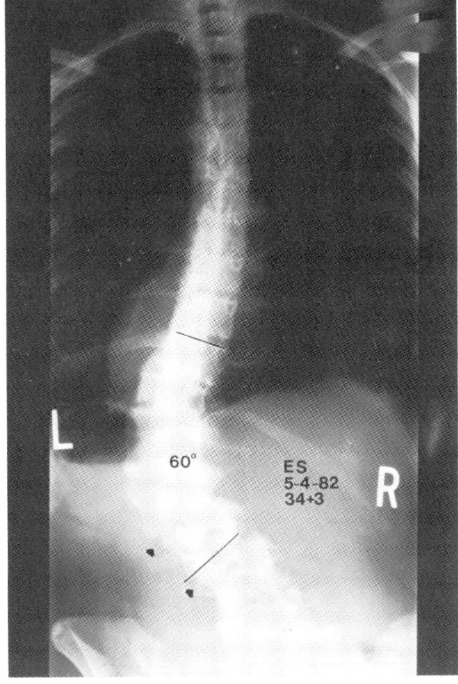

Figure 1-B

Figure 1: (A) With a lumbosacral fusion at age 19 years for spondylolysthesis, the patient presented at age 27 years, 3 months with mild low backache and a 53 degree left thoracolumbar curve. (B) Over the next 7 years pain gradually increased until it altered her lifestyle. The curve also increased to 60 degrees. Rotatory subluxation indicated by the arrows.

original curve. In brace-treated patients, pregnancy (especially before 23 years of age) may be associated with an increased likelihood of curve progression.

Long-term follow-up of scoliosis patients fused *without* instrumentation indicates less low back pain than the general population (or unfused scoliosis) but increased degenerative disease in the lumbosacral area as demonstrated radiographically by narrow L5-Sl discs and facet sclerosis. These radiographic changes do not correlate with low back pain or the lower limit of the fusion. Patients fused *with* instrumentation to the lumbar spine demonstrate an increasing incidence of low back pain the closer the fusion gets to the sacrum, i.e., the fewer discs remaining for motion, the higher is the incidence of low back pain.

PRESENTATION AND EVALUATION: Adults with scoliosis present with pain, deformity (with or without curve progression), cardiopulmonary problems, functional loss in neuromuscular curves, and, rarely, with neurological problems. Pain, the most common symptom, is associated more frequently with lumbar curves and may be localized to the curve (either on the concave or convex side) or below the curve (lumbosacral). Neurological problems usually are due to nerve root entrapments in the concavity of the fractional lumbosacral curve or in the concavity of the main curve. In lumbar curves, an apparent kyphosis caused by vertebral rotation (the "kyphosing scoliosis" described by Stagnara) is a common presenting problem. Adults who had previous surgery may present with problems related to pseudarthroses, a too-short previous fusion, progression of the deformity, decompensation, or loss of lumbar lordosis.

In adults the relationship of scoliosis to pain is difficult to determine because of the high incidence of back pain in the general population. Radiographic changes of facet sclerosis and disc degeneration in lumbar curves do not correlate with the occurrence of low back pain. Discography has proved useful in identifying the source of the pain particularly in the following instances: (1) above or below the curve, (2) lumbosacral, (3) discs below a previous fusion, or (4) discs above a lumbosacral fusion. Metrizamide myelography aids in the differentiation of disc herniation and root compression by pedicle shifts or facet sclerosis in patients with marked degenerative changes.

TREATMENT: General treatment principles of low back pain apply to the adult with scoliosis and pain. In the symptomatic older patient with primary degenerative disease or degeneration superimposed on a preexisting scoliosis, a custom-fabricated thoraco-lumbo-sacral orthosis (TLSO) helps to relieve the lumbar pain. The TLSO is fabricated without any attempt at correction and is worn for support when upright. Commonly prescribed extension exercises for myoligamentous or discogenic low back pain may aggravate the pain if it is due to degenerative facet arthritis.

Surgical treatment of adult scoliosis differs for the previously untreated adult and the adult having a failed spinal fusion.

In the *previously untreated* adult, accurate assessment of the presenting problems as well as the curve pattern and flexibility is necessary. Pain relief and curve stabilization are the prime surgical objectives. Curve correction is secondary. The posterior approach with instrumentation is adequate for most single curves or double, balanced curves (double thoracic or double thoracic and lumbar). The techniques of halo-femoral traction or preliminary releasing operations do not obtain additional correction over that shown on an initial supine, side-bending, flexibility radiograph or over an initial traction radiograph. Additional internal fixation with compression rods and transverse fixation devices or with segmental (Luque) wiring is proving useful. The compression instrumentation helps to reduce kyphosis.

Anterior fusion and instrumentation without a subsequent posterior fusion is employed in selected patients with single thoracolumbar and lumbar curves because a shorter fusion is required as compared to a posterior fusion. Dwyer instrumentation has been used most frequently; a disadvantage is its tendency to produce kyphosis. Zielke instrumentation with a rod instead of the Dwyer cable is useful as it controls this tendency better. However, the role of anterior fusion and instrumentation alone is still controversial since no long-term, comparative studies are available.

The combined two-stage anterior and posterior approach is helpful for adult patients with neuromuscular and idiopathic scoliosis with significant lumbar or thoracolumbar curves, either single curves or part of a double curve pattern with more progression and pain in the lumbar than the thoracic curve. Both curves need treatment, but to achieve a balanced spine and a low pseudarthrosis rate, it is best to treat the lumbar or thoracolumbar curve anteriorly and both curves posteriorly (Fig. 2).

Anteriorly, the fusion can be achieved by a discectomy alone or a discectomy combined with instrumentation using the Dwyer or Zielke devices. Ten to 14 days later posterior fusion and instrumentation encompassing both curves is performed.

Surgical correction and stabilization may be indicated in selected elderly patients, e.g., those with a progressive or painful curve where a TLSO or another nonoperative means is not successful in relieving pain.

Treatment of nerve root compression syndromes in the fractional lumbosacral curve depends upon the age of the patient and the status of the lumbar curve. In the elderly, simple nerve root decompression is an adequate treatment. With a symptomatic lumbar curve and flexible lumbosacral curve, straightening and fusion of the lumbar curve alone (often with anterior fusion and instrumentation) can decompress the root by straightening the curve. If the fractional curve is rigid, fusion of the lumbar curve to the sacrum with root decompression is necessary.

In adults who have had *previous spinal fusions,* treatment selection is dependent upon the underlying problem: pseudarthroses are repaired with compression instrumentation, too-short fusions are extended, and the "flat back" syndrome of lumbar lordosis loss is corrected with posterior closing-wedge lumbar osteotomies with compression instrumentation (Fig. 3). In more complex problems, staged treatment may be necessary with multiple osteotomies performed to correct the deformity. The osteotomy, combined with traction (either halo-femoral or, more commonly, halo-wheelchair), obtains this correction. A second-stage posterior approach stabilizes the obtained correction with the addition of multiple instrumentation. For patients with true kyphosis, an anterior fusion is also necessary. With more secure internal fixation, TLSOs have replaced casts for postoperative immobilization.

Halo-femoral or halo-wheelchair traction generally plays a small role in the treatment of adult scoliosis. Preoperative traction is only beneficial for patients presenting in cor pulmonale. Curve correction in traction with improvement in cardiopulmonary status improves the health of the patient and is indicative that surgical

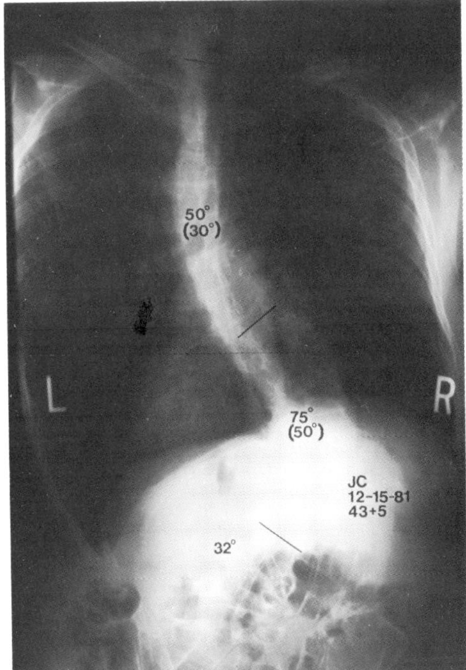

Figure 2-A

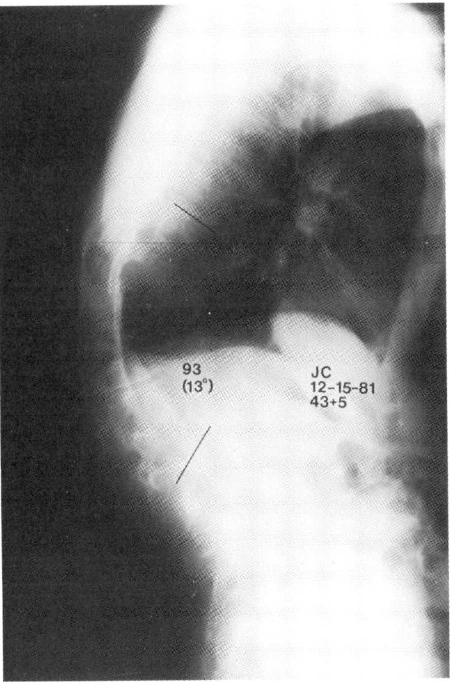

Figure 2-B

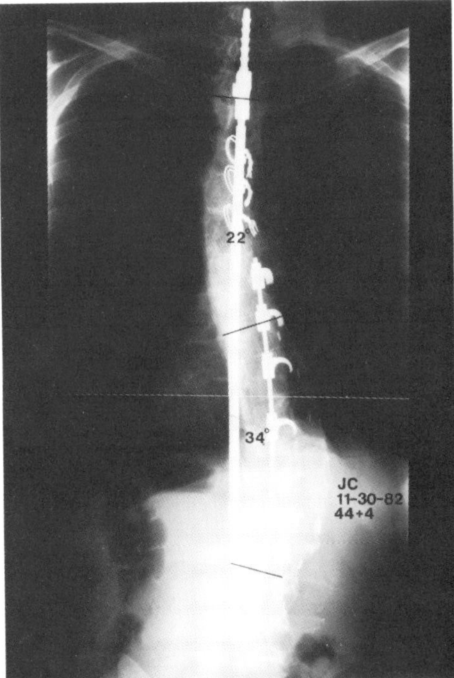

Figure 2-C

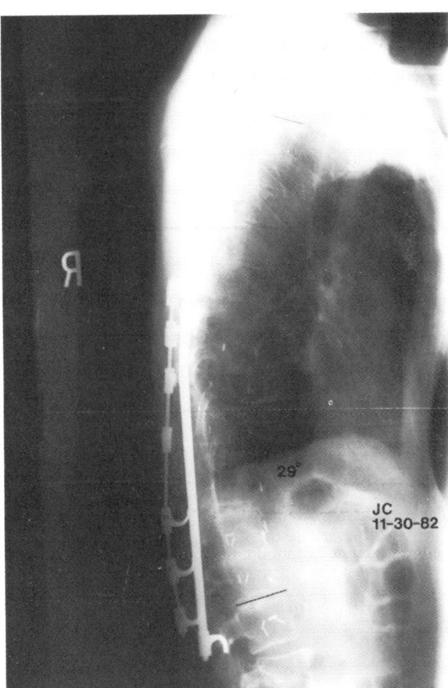

Figure 2-D

Figure 2: Forty-three-year-old male presented with a history of poliomyelitis at age 13. He wore an orthosis for 3 years subsequent to onset for scoliosis. He had a history of progressive back tiredness and a height loss of 3 inches in 3 years. (A) Standing posteroanterior radiograph shows a T2-T10 left thoracic curve of 50 degrees and a T10-L3 right thoracolumbar curve of 75 degrees, the curves bending to 40 and 50 degrees respectively on supine side-bending. (B) Lateral standing radiograph shows a rotatory thoracolumbar kyphosis of 93 degrees. He underwent a two-stage correction and fusion consisting of anterior interbody fusion from T10-L4 and posterior fusion and instrumentation from T4-L4. The upper hook displaced 10 days later and was replaced being secured with three sublaminar wires after increasing the bend in the rod for the residual kyphosis. He was immobilized in a one-piece polypropylene orthosis, and 7 months later the fusion was solid with only 5 degrees loss in the correction of the scoliosis and absence of back pain. (C) Posteroanterior standing radiograph shows the balanced curves of 22 and 34 degrees and solid fusion. (D) Lateral view showing correction of the kyphosis to 29 degrees.

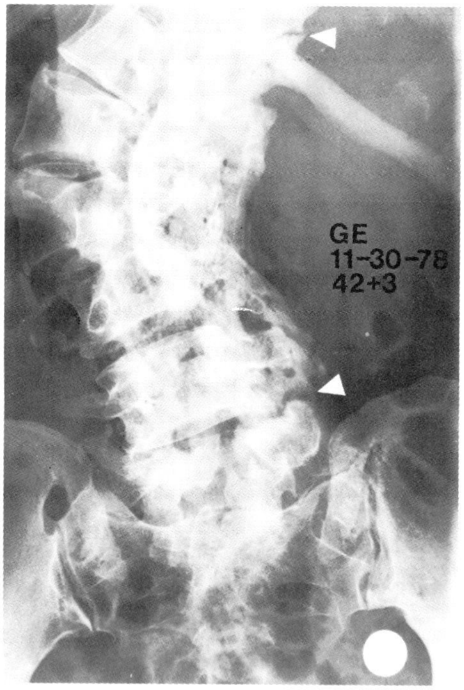

Figure 3-A

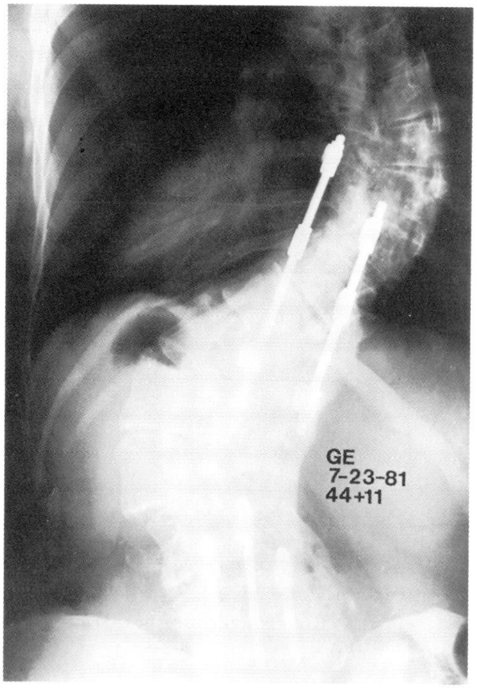

Figure 3-B

Figure 3: Originally fused for idiopathic scoliosis, the patient presented at the age of 36 years with a pseudarthrosis and progressive back pain. She underwent a two-stage reconstruction with Harrington instrumentation and three additional procedures for reinsertion of the lower hook. Severe pain persisted and the instrumentation was removed. (A) At the age of 42 years, 3 months there was residual back pain and two pseudarthroses were visible on the supine radiograph at T10-T11 and L4-L5. (B) One year later she underwent pseudarthrosis repair with bone grafting and internal fixation using 1/4" Harrington compressing instrumentation. She was immobilized for 6 months in a cast, being supine for the first 3 months in an underarm cast with a single-thigh extension. Two years later she is pain-free with a solid fusion.

stabilization will be helpful. In multiple-stage corrective surgery with osteotomies, traction obtains the correction. The second-stage surgical procedure stabilizes the correction.

When a solid fusion is achieved, pain relief occurs in 68 to 70 percent of patients. Discography aids in classifying pain patterns and selecting the lower limit of the fusion. With lumbosacral pain, discography of the lower lumbar discs may differentiate pain arising from the curve from that arising from degeneration of the lower lumbar or lumbosacral intervertebral disc. This aids in deciding whether the curve alone needs fusion or whether the fusion should extend to the sacrum. Combined anterior and posterior fusion reduced the pseudarthrosis rate in one series from 11 percent to 0.5 percent.

The *complication* rate of 53 to 71 percent is high. The major complications are pseudarthroses, pulmonary problems, urinary tract infections, thrombophlebitis, and instrumentation problems. The complication rate rises with increasing age. Paraplegia and mortality rates are significantly higher than those found with spinal fusion in children or adolescents.

Kyphosis

Kyphosis is less common than scoliosis in younger adults. True kyphosis can occur in the presence of scoliosis or at the junction of two scoliotic curves. Apparent, or rotational, kyphosis is much more common especially in lumbar or thoracolumbar curves.

Symptomatic kyphosis in adults may be associated with Scheuermann's disease, osteoporosis, ankylosing spondylitis, or, more uncommonly, congenital vertebral anomaly or tuberculosis. The rare patient with kyphosis and neurological loss (usually congenital, posttuberculosis, neurofibromatosis, or posttraumatic) will require anterior spinal cord decompression and anterior fusion. In some patients, posterior fusion is necessary to stabilize the deformity.

Scheuermann's Disease Scheuermann's disease seldom presents in adulthood with progressive deformity or pain. The pain may be in the area of kyphosis or in the compensatory lumbar lordosis. With progressive deformity or incapacitating pain, surgical correction using the two-stage approach of an anterior release and fusion combined with posterior fusion using compression Harrington instrumentation gives the best results.

Osteoporosis After age 40, bone mass in the skeleton tends to decrease in both black and white males and females, but most rapidly in white females. About one-half of white females aged 45 years or older exhibit radiographic evidence of osteoporosis in their lumbar spines, with the prevalence rising to almost 90 percent above the age of 75 years. This loss is probably related to hormonal changes occurring at menopause (see Section 3, General: Bone Metabolism).

Bone loss itself does not cause symptoms, but associated fractures with vertebral collapse may cause considerable back pain. Additionally, vertebral collapse can cause increased thoracic kyphosis. The presentation is thus back pain, kyphosis, or a combination of the two.

There is clinical evidence that estrogen replacement therapy protects the postmenopausal female against osteoporosis. Currently, the roles of fluorides, calcium, vitamin D, and vigorous physical activity in the protection against osteoporosis are being studied. In a patient presenting with pain or kyphosis, the treatment is symptomatic. Analgesics are used for pain and a supporting orthosis occasionally is indicated with severe progressive kyphosis. The role of estrogen replacement therapy at this stage of the disease is unclear.

Ankylosing Spondylitis Severe flexion (kyphotic) deformity may occur in patients with ankylosing spondylitis. Prevention with bracing or early posterior fusion in active spondylitis would be ideal, but no reports of this treatment are available.

Thus, the patient presents with marked functional disability due to inability to be in a more upright position. The deformity can be in the hips or spine, but the cervical or lumbar areas are most commonly involved. The kyphosis may include the whole spine. Careful identification of the primary site of the deformity (such as hip joints, lumbar spine, thoracic spine, or cervical spine) is necessary. The area of the main deformity should be corrected. In some patients with kyphosis and severe hip flexion deformity, bilateral hip replacements improve function to a degree that spinal surgery is not required.

Surgery in these patients is hazardous. Since intubation is difficult when the cervical spine is rigid, cervical and lumbar osteotomies are performed under local anesthesia in some centers. With the rigid kyphosis, prone positioning may be impossible so the patient may be placed on the side. Postoperative pulmonary complications are common due to the rigid chest.

A posterior closing-wedge midlumbar osteotomy is used for correction of lumbar kyphosis. The disc fractures anteriorly when the osteotomy is closed, and the correction is held with interspinous wiring or Harrington compression instrumentation. The removed bone is used as bone graft, and an extension cast is used postoperatively. In some patients with kyphosis of the whole spine, function may be improved with a single lumbar osteotomy without requiring thoracic or cervical osteotomies.

Very infrequently patients with localized or major thoracic kyphosis may require correction of the kyphosis with a two-stage approach consisting of anterior spinal osteotomies and fusion and posterior osteotomies and fusion with compression instrumentation.

Miscellaneous

Infections Spine infections in adults may be classified as pyogenic, hematogenous, or due to direct invasion (such as following surgery) or tuberculous. The site of the infection from hematogenous seeding is the end plate of the vertebral body. The process either remains localized or spreads to the disc secondarily.

Pyogenic Infections The hematogenous type of pyogenic, or nontuberculous, infection occurs usually as a complication of dialysis, genitourinary tract instrumentation, in drug abusers, or following infection at another site with bacteremia and septicemia. The presentation may be localized back pain alone or general signs of infection such as anorexia, fever, malaise, and weight loss.

A bone scan is invaluable in early diagnosis before radiographic changes are apparent. After 2 to 4 weeks, radiographs may show a soft-tissue paraspinal inflammatory mass, a narrow disc space, and end plate irregularity and sclerosis. The sedimentation rate is virtually always elevated, but the leukocyte count may or may not be elevated at this stage of the disease process. Bacteriologic diagnosis is important due to the many unusual or resistant organisms found (e.g., gram-negative bacteria and fungi). If blood cultures and needle biopsies are negative, open biopsy via a costotransversectomy or anterior approach may be necessary.

Appropriate intravenous antibiotics with bed rest is the initial treatment. Once the pain has diminished, the patient may be ambulated in an orthosis or cast and continued on parenteral antibiotics, usually for 3 to 6 weeks.

Disc space infection following disc excision is a rare complication. If it occurs, there is a recurrence of severe back pain with signs of an acute infection. Diagnosis and treatment are the same as for pyogenic vertebral osteomyelitis.

Tuberculous Infections Spinal tuberculosis presents in adults either with an active infection or a kyphotic deformity following treated tuberculosis. This problem is common in the developing countries and is seen today in certain parts of the United States.

Tuberculous infection presents either with back pain or paraplegia. As tuberculosis is a chronic infection, radiographic changes are marked and may include a paravertebral mass with multiple vertebral involvement, vertebral collapse, kyphosis, and evidence of new bone formation (repair).

Treatment is aimed at eradicating the infection and preventing late deformity. Long-term studies of the British Medical Research Council in Korea, Hong Kong, Rhodesia (later Zimbabwe), and South Africa show that very similar infection eradication was obtained with long- or short-course antituberculous therapy, inpatient or outpatient therapy, bed rest or ambulatory therapy, and surgical debridement with or without anterior fusion. However, late kyphosis with subsequent danger of spinal cord compression occurred in all groups except those treated with debridement and anterior fusion.

Treatment of spinal tuberculosis is thus tailored to available facilities. If possible, an anterior approach with debridement and bone grafting is performed with postoperative immobilization in a cast, combined with appropriate antituberculous therapy.

Acute infection with cord compression is best treated with anterior decompression and fusion. In the patient with late kyphosis and spinal cord compression, an anterior decompression is performed with removal of the anterior compressing bone. A fusion also is done when no spontaneous anterior fusion is present.

Tumors Primary bone tumors of the spine are rare in adults. The most common is myeloma. Often vertebral involvement is the first manifestation, presenting as deep, unremitting pain. Radiographically the lesion is lytic with vertebral collapse and demineralization of the vertebrae. The proliferating plasma cells manufacture an abnormal protein, making the serum protein electrophoresis determination diagnostic. Treatment involves radiation therapy and chemotherapy.

Metastatic disease to the spine is more common in

adults with primary sites of breast, lung, kidney, and prostate. The presentation is with pain and/or neurological loss, commonly paraparesis or paraplegia. The pain can be caused either by tumor invasion and proliferation or by marked bone loss with spinal instability. In the early stages the radiographs appear normal, and a bone scan is diagnostically valuable. Computed tomography, useful at this point to show the extent of bone destruction, is most helpful in delineating the exact extent of the tumor spread when there is neurological loss. When neurological signs

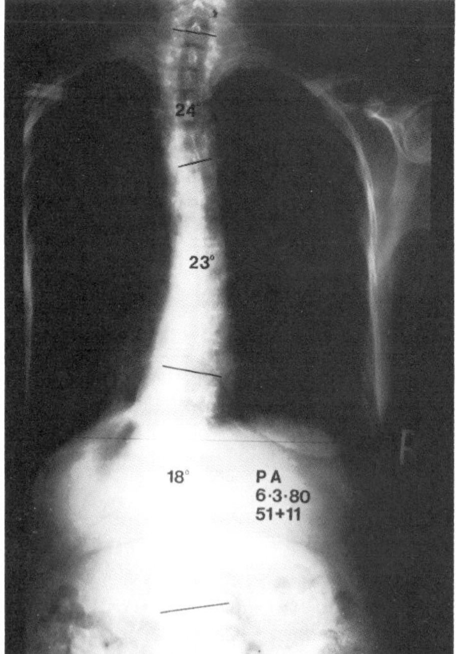

Figure 4-A

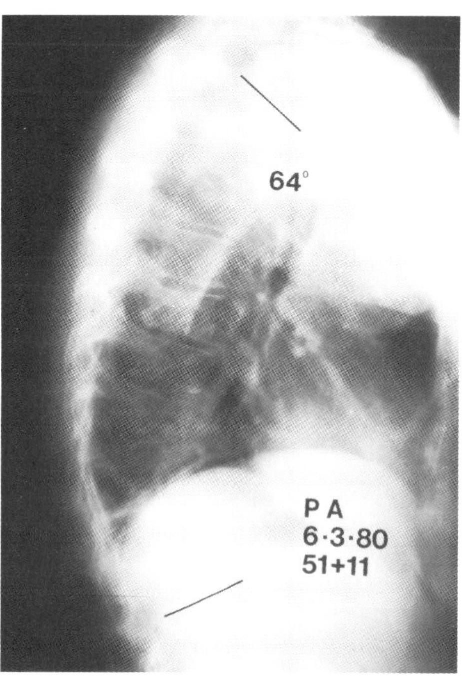

Figure 4-B

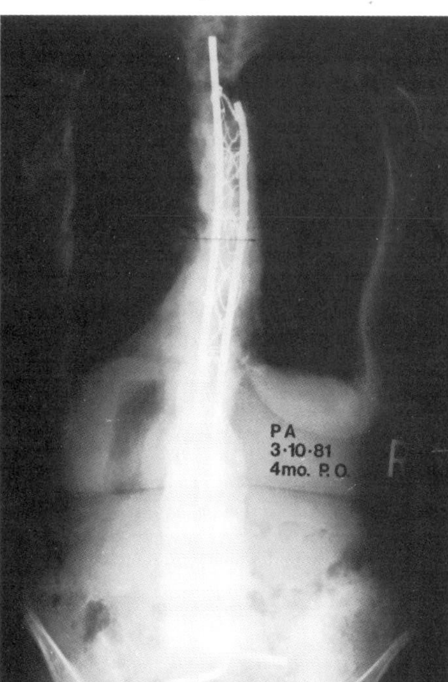

Figure 4-C

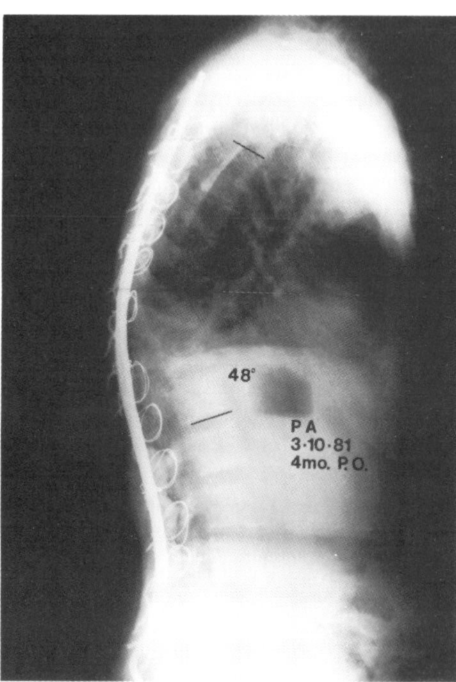

Figure 4-D

Figure 4: Presenting at the age of 51 years, 11 months, 3 years after undergoing a mastectomy for breast carcinoma, the patient had multiple metastases to the spine, pelvis, and femurs and had received maximum megavoltage radiotherapy doses at all sites. She had pain in her back and a history of height loss. (A, B) Standing radiographs showed minimal scoliosis and thoracic kyphosis of 64 degrees with multiple vertebral involvement and vertebral collapse. Placed in an underarm orthosis which initially relieved her symptoms, over the next 6 months the disease progressed with increases in the vertebral involvement, kyphosis, and pain. Pain was only present when she was upright and was not controlled by narcotics. Posterior stabilization was performed from the upper thoracic spine to the sacrum using Luque rod, multiple sublaminar and inter-rod wiring, and methyl methacrylate. The extent of the procedure was determined by the marked vertebral involvement present. The pain was improved, and she was able to decrease the narcotic dosage and resume many activities. (C,D) Standing radiographs 4 months postoperatively show the instrumentation in place, with the methyl methacrylate well seen on the posteroanterior view.

are present in a patient with multiple vertebral body involvement, a myelogram may localize the exact site of spinal cord compression.

In early vertebral body involvement with pain, radiation therapy often is effective in controlling the vertebral spread. However, with more extensive involvement resulting in kyphosis and vertebral instability, radiation therapy seldom relieves pain. A custom-fabricated polypropylene orthosis often affords some degree of pain relief. With more marked instability or kyphosis, surgical treatment may be indicated to achieve pain relief and a better quality of life. With extensive vertebral involvement or mechanical instability, posterior stabilization with dual instrumentation (Luque or Harrington), sublaminar wires, and methyl methacrylate augmentation provide instant rigid stability (Fig. 4). In localized involvement with marked vertebral destruction and localized instability, vertebral body replacement with methyl methacrylate may provide anterior stabilization and pain relief.

The presence of neurological loss usually is caused by tumor extension from the vertebral body. Anterior spinal cord decompression and vertebral body replacement with methyl methacrylate may provide cord decompression and anterior stability. A laminectomy is indicated in the rare instance of a patient with an epidural metastasis causing cord compression.

Thoracic Disc Herniation Rare and perhaps difficult to diagnose, these herniations occur equally in males and females and are most common in the lower thoracic spine, usually below T9. A history of trauma (sometimes mild) is found in one-third of the patients. The presentation varies depending upon whether the protrusion is acute or chronic and whether the herniation is central or posterolateral. The complaints are vague and may include back pain, dermatomal pain, sensory disturbances, or motor complaints ranging from vague weakness with a feeling of the legs giving way to frank paraparesis. Sphincter disturbances with bowel or bladder symptoms are infrequent.

Physical findings often are absent unless gross motor weakness is present, and because of this, the diagnosis often is delayed. Radiographs may be normal or the disc space may be narrowed. In chronic protrusions, disc calcification and/or vertebral end plate sclerosis are often present. Electromyography and cystometrography may aid in this difficult diagnostic problem. The latter test frequently is abnormal even when no bladder difficulty is mentioned by the patient. A myelogram demonstrates the disc herniation, but careful positioning is needed so that the lower thoracic area is visualized adequately.

The treatment for these herniations is surgical. Affording better exposure, a transthoracic approach yields the best results, but a wide costotransversectomy posterolateral approach is an alternative. Numerous reports indicate that laminectomy is an inadequate approach for disc excision in the thoracic area because of the small canal and anterior nature of the pathology.

ANNOTATED BIBLIOGRAPHY

Scoliosis

Prevalence and Natural History

Blount, W.P., and Mellencamp, D.D.: The effect of pregnancy on idiopathic scoliosis. J. Bone Joint Surg. 62A:1083-1087, 1980.

Stable curves do not progress with pregnancy in patients in the second decade whereas unstable scoliosis progresses in patients even into the third decade.

Kostuik, J.P., and Bentivoglio, J.: The incidence of low-back pain in adult scoliosis. Spine 6:268-273, 1981.

A review of IVPs in 5,000 patients (the majority in the sixth to eighth decades) shows a 3.9 percent incidence of lumbar curves over 10 degrees. Fifty-nine percent had back pain, a figure similar to the general population. Pain was more common in patients with facet sclerosis (not osteophytes) and was more severe in patients with curves over 45 degrees.

Moskowitz, A.; Moe, J.H.; Winter, R.B.; and Binner, H.: Long-term follow-up of scoliosis fusion. J. Bone Joint Surg. 62A:364-376, 1980.

Sixty-one patients reviewed after an average follow-up of 26 years following posterior spinal fusion show stable fusions with low back pain not a significant problem. The incidence of low back pain below the fusion is unrelated to the lowest limit of the fusion and the presence of osteophytes. Patients with marked facet sclerosis have more low back pain than those with mild or no sclerosis.

Nachemson, A.: Adult scoliosis and back pain. Spine 4:513-517, 1979.

Surgery for scoliosis in the adult is unusual. Some curves arise de novo in the adult due to disc degeneration and osteoporosis. The incidence of back pain in adults with scoliosis is no different from that in adults with straight spines.

Nachemson, A.; Cochran, T.P.; Irstram, L.; and Fallstrom, K.: Pregnancy after scoliosis treatment. Orthop. Trans. 6:5, 1982 (Abstract).

Of eighty-five Milwaukee brace and ninety-five surgically treated patients, eight of the braced and three of the operated patients' (nonfused secondary) curves progressed. All who progressed had at least one full-term pregnancy before 23 years of age whereas none with first full-term pregnancy after 23 years of age did.

Robin, G.C.; Span, Y.; Steinberg, R.; Makin, M.; and Menczel, J.: Scoliosis in the elderly: A follow-up study. Spine 7:355-359, 1982.

Scoliosis of a minor degree is very common in the elderly, many curves arising de novo. Curves do progress in the elderly. There is no relationship between scoliosis and osteoporosis, back pain, or degenerative changes in the spine.

Weinstein, S.L.; Zavala, D.C.; and Ponseti, I.V.: Idiopathic scoliosis: Long-term follow-up and prognosis in untreated patients. J. Bone Joint Surg. 63A:702-711, 1981.

One hundred and ninety-four patients reviewed with a follow-up of 39.3 years show an incidence of backache slightly less than that in the general population. In some patients, progression occurs during adulthood, especially in thoracic curves that measure between 50 and 80 degrees at the end of growth.

Presentation and Evaluation

Kostuik, J.P.: Decision making in adult scoliosis. Spine 4:521-525, 1979.

This is a review of 350 adult patients, the majority between ages 25 and 40. In the over-30 age group, lumbar and thoracolumbar curves are most common. Discography is discussed and improvement in pain relief is found with the use of discography in decision making.

Kostuik, J.P.: Recent advances in the treatment of painful adult scoliosis. Clin. Orthop. 147:238-252, 1980.

Discography is useful in the assessment of the adult presenting with painful lumbar or thoracolumbar scoliosis. Evaluation of pain within a curve, pain below a curve (especially lumbosacral), pain below a previous fusion, and pain unrelated to the curve is possible with discography. The use of anterior fusion with Dwyer instrumentation in lumbar or thoracolumbar curves reduces the incidence of pseudarthrosis and loss of lumbar lordosis.

Treatment—Untreated Adult

Simmons, E.H., and Jackson, R.P.: The management of nerve root entrapment syndromes associated with the collapsing scoliosis of idiopathic lumbar and thoracolumbar curves. Spine 4:533-541, 1979.

Root entrapment syndromes occur in the compensatory lumbosacral curve. Treatment is by nerve root decompression by laminectomy or by straightening the lumbosacral as well as the more proximal curve by curve correction and fusion. Dwyer anterior instrumentation is an effective method in selected cases.

Swank, S.; Lonstein, J.E.; Moe, J.H.; Winter, R.B.; and Bradford, D.S.: Surgical treatment of adult scoliosis. A review of 220 cases. J. Bone Joint Surg. 63A:268-287, 1981.

Scoliosis surgical treatment in 222 adults with an average 3.6 years follow-up shows pain relief in 68 percent and a solid fusion in all but six patients. Preoperative traction does not result in increased correction. The complication rate is high (53 percent), increasing with age.

Swank, S.; Winter, R.B.; and Moe, J.H.: Scoliosis and cor pulmonale. Spine 7:343-354, 1982.

Severe scoliosis causes cor pulmonale. Nine patients had surgical correction after curve correction in halo-femoral traction, during which the cor pulmonale improved. Best results are found in the postpoliomyelitis patients. Poor results are found with congenital and infantile idiopathic scoliosis.

Treatment—Previous Surgery

Cummine, J.L.; Lonstein, J.E.; Moe, J.H.; Winter, R.B.; and Bradford, D.S.: Reconstructive surgery in the adult for failed scoliosis fusion. J. Bone Joint Surg. 61A:1151-1161, 1979.

Fifty-nine patients requiring surgery for a failed previous fusion show reduction in pain in 67 percent of patients but with a high complication rate of 71 percent. After posterior osteotomies, traction helps obtain correction. The subsequent second-stage operation stabilizes this condition.

Kyphosis

Lonstein, J.E.; Winter, R.B.; Moe, J.H.; Bradford, D.S.; Chou, S.N.; and Pinto, W.C.: Neurologic deficits secondary to spinal deformity. Spine 5:331-355, 1980.

Neurological complications are rare and occur with severe kyphosis. Decompression by laminectomy is ineffectual. Anterior spinal cord decompression is the most effective way to remove the bone compressing the neural tissue.

Osteoporosis

Nordin, B.E.; Horsman, A.; Crilly, R.G.; Marshall, D.H.; and Simpson, M.: Treatment of spinal osteoporosis in postmenopausal women. British Med. J. 280:451-454, 1980.

Ninety-five women with postmenopausal osteoporosis are studied with seven different treatment plans to investigate the prevention of further osteoporosis. Initial data suggest that the addition of calcium and vitamin D to estrogen therapy may be beneficial.

Ankylosing Spondylitis

Simmons, E.H.: Kyphotic deformity of the spine in ankylosing spondylitis. Clin. Orthop. 128:65-77, 1977.

This report assesses the deformity and treatment principles of kyphotic deformities. The technique of osteotomy is well described.

Miscellaneous

Infections

Reports of the Medical Research Council Working Party on Tuberculosis of the Spine. J. Bone Joint Surg. 58B:399, 411, 1976. J. Bone Joint Surg. 60B:163-177, 1978. J. Bone Joint Surg. 64B:393-398, 1982.

Reports of an ongoing study of different regimens in the treatment of spinal tuberculosis presents results 5 to 10 years after completing active treatment of acute disease.

Tumors

Harrington, K.D.: The use of methylmethacrylate for vertebral-body replacement and anterior stabilization of pathological fracture-dislocations of the spine due to metastatic malignant disease. J. Bone Joint Surg. 63A:36-46, 1981.

In this report of treatment in fourteen patients, all but two have pain and neurological deficits. Good pain relief in twelve patients and improvement in the neurological deficit in ten patients point to the good results possible with this technique. There was one postoperative death due to a myocardial infarct.

Thoracic Disc Herniation

Albrand, O.W., and Corkill, G.: Thoracic disc herniation: Treatment and prognosis. Spine 4:41-46, 1979.

The seven patients studied point out the varied presentation and difficulty in making a diagnosis of thoracic disc herniations. Treatment by the transthoracic approach in six patients yields good results.

29 LUMBOSACRAL SPINE: RECONSTRUCTION

This section deals with the diagnosis and treatment of low back pain in the adult. It opens with a brief review of the epidemiology of low back pain and is organized on the basis of possible causative factors.

Epidemiology

Low back pain affects 80 percent of all people at some time during their lives. It is the most frequent cause of time lost from work and is first among all diseases or conditions as a cause of disability in people under 45 years of age. In the United States the annual cost of treatment and compensation for low back pain exceeds $14 billion, and, in addition, the loss of productivity is estimated at 4 hours per year, per worker.

The annual incidence of work-disrupting low back pain for workers is approximately 2 percent, peaking in the late fourth and early fifth decades of life. Males and females of working age appear to have an equal incidence of low back pain, but females have far fewer compensable back injuries. This may be related to job description. In the older age group, the incidence of back pain resulting in medical consultation may be even higher, approaching 5 percent in the sixth decade of life. In this age group, females are more commonly affected than males.

Workers most at risk are those performing repetitive, lifting tasks, especially with a torsional component. The majority are able to return to work within 2 to 3 weeks, but the recurrence rate is high. Factors predisposing to recurrence include traumatic origin of the first attack, sciatica, alcoholism, and specific job situations.

Physical fitness and conditioning, as well as good job design, have been identified as important preventative factors. Preemployment strength testing appears to be an effective method of screening whereas preemployment radiographs have not.

Congenital Anomalies

The *sacrohorizontal angle (Ferguson's angle)* describes the relationship between the superior border of S1 and the horizontal plane, as measured on a standing lateral radiograph (Fig. 1). An increased sacrohorizontal angle is statistically associated with an increased incidence of low back pain only if it exceeds 70 degrees.

Population studies have shown that congenital or gradually developing *leg length discrepancy* of up to 4 cm is not associated with an increased incidence of low back pain. However, for the patient who has over 2.5 cm of congenital shortening and low back pain, a small lift of comfortable height under the short leg is advised. An attempt to completely level the pelvis is not desirable. Acquired, acute shortening, such as that following a fracture, of as little as 1.3 cm may increase the incidence of back trouble and should be corrected at least partially by a shoe lift.

Facet tropism is present when the facet joints of the same vertebral level are oriented in different planes. At the extreme, one facet is in a coronal and the other in a sagittal plane. Population studies do not show an increased incidence of low back pain related to tropism. However, facet asymmetry may alter the normal kinematics of the affected vertebral segment. Some investigators have shown increased motion (especially rotation) on the side of the more coronally oriented facet. Because of the cam action that is created, the disc at that level may degenerate sooner, and, if there is a disc rupture at that level, it nearly always will be on the side of the coronally oriented facet. Some believe that with injury the level of the facet tropism is predisposed to nucleus pulposus herniation.

Transitional vertebra between the lumbar and the sacral areas do not increase the incidence of low back pain according to population studies. With chronic injury, it is the motion segment above that may be damaged. *Congenital end plate defects* permit prolapse of nuclear material into the spongiosa of the vertebral body (see end plate injuries). The defects are not statistically associated with low back pain.

Degenerative

Intervertebral Disc Degeneration of the intervertebral disc is a physiological process which is universal. The first

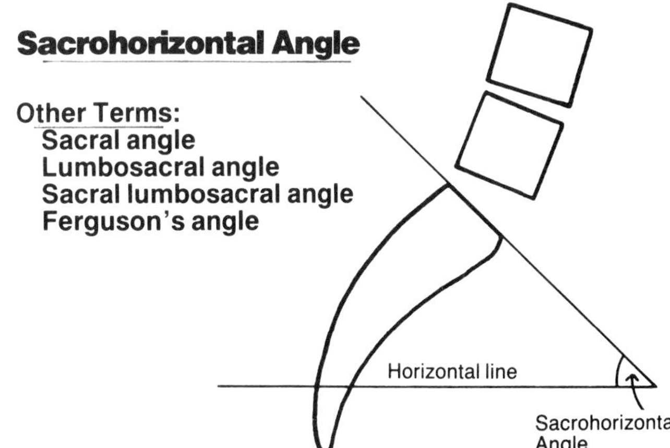

Figure 1: The sacrohorizontal angle is the angle between the superior border of S1 and the horizontal plane. It is a fairly important angle. To call this the lumbosacral angle is incorrect because the lumbar area is not involved. (Adapted with permission from Terminology and measurement of spondylolisthesis, by L. Wiltse, et. al., J. Bone Joint Surg. 65A:771, 1983.)

signs can be detected as early as the beginning of the second decade of life. Radiographic signs of disc degeneration are not statistically related to low back pain. Some people with severe degenerative changes noted on radiographs have no back pain, and others with minimal changes have severe pain. The reasons for this paradox are unclear, but it may be due to certain "modifying" factors, such as muscular control of the vertebral segment, activity level, pain modulation, and psychological factors. The difference between disc disease and physiological disc degeneration is not distinct. The rate of disc degeneration varies, and there appears to be a hereditary component.

Severe, and especially early, disc degeneration of several levels is related to an increased incidence of low back pain. As degeneration progresses and annular tears occur, disc herniation or extrusion may result.

Biochemical Aspects Collagen is the main structural component of the annulus and the nucleus pulposus. In the annulus, there is principally type I collagen, and in the normal nucleus pulposus, there is predominantly type II. Collagen possesses great tensile strength and is largely responsible for resisting the stresses to which the disc is exposed. The annulus has alternating lamellae of collagen, set at angles much like latticework. As the disc narrows, these collagen fibers become lax and resist loads poorly, especially in torsion.

As aging progresses, the boundary between the nucleus and the annulus becomes less well defined, the cellular content of the nucleus sparser, and the fibrous components more prominent. Gradually desiccation and even cavitation of the nucleus are noted. There occurs a progressive lowering of hydration of the nucleus from 88 percent water content in the first decade to 60 percent in the eighth. The high water content and hydrostatic properties of the nucleus are directly attributable to the concentration of proteoglycans consisting of a protein core and side chains of chondroitin-4-sulphate, chondroitin-6-sulphate, and keratan sulphate. With aging there is a decrease in chondroitin sulphate and an increase in keratan sulphate.

Biomechanical Aspects Studies in healthy subjects have shown that lumbar intradiscal pressures vary with body position during the performance of various tasks. In certain positions, intradiscal pressure seems to have a positive correlation with symptoms. Compared with the upright standing, a reclining position reduced intradiscal pressure by 50 to 80 percent, unsupported sitting increased the pressure by 40 percent, forward leaning and weight lifting increased the pressure by more than 100 percent, and a position of forward flexion and rotation increased the load by 400 percent. Large increases in pressure were also observed in subjects performing various commonly prescribed abdominal strengthening exercises.

The same hydrodynamic properties of the normal disc have been found in the moderately degenerated disc but not in the severely degenerated disc.

With disc degeneration and consequent disc space narrowing, the stabilizing intersegmental ligaments become lax. This may result in *instability,* defined as abnormal deformation brought about by physiological load. There appears to be a positive correlation between identifiable instability and back pain. On lateral flexion and extension radiographs, anteroposterior translation greater than 2.5 mm, tilt of more than 12 degrees, or more than 25 percent change in disc height is associated with an increased likelihood of back pain (Fig. 2). Torsion has been shown to be resisted about equally by the intervertebral disc and the facet joints. With disc narrowing, more torsion is transmitted to the facet joints. Torsion displacements have been shown to be significantly higher in patients with back pain. It is possible that dynamic muscle

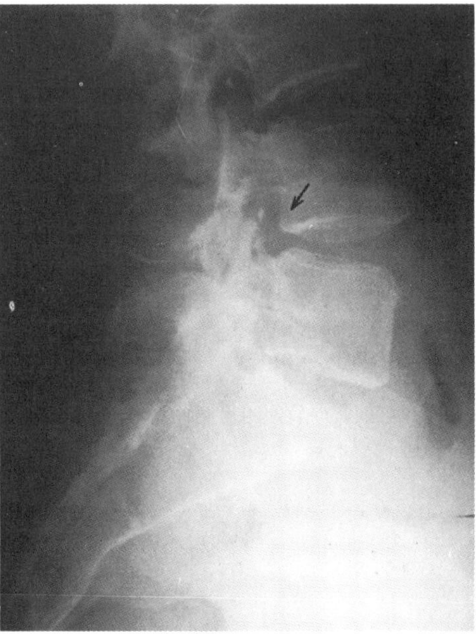

Figure 2-A

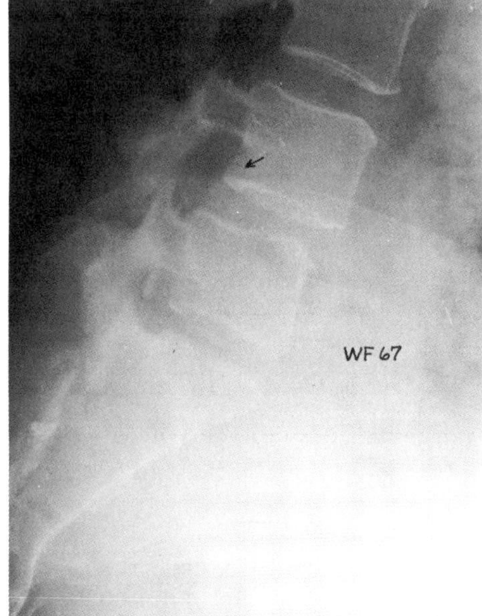

Figure 2-B

Figure 2: (A,B) Knutsson test for instability. This type of instability may cause symptoms. 2.5 mm of anteroposterior slip or 10 to 15 degrees tilt are considered abnormal and may produce pain. To take the extension exposure, the patient stands with the buttocks against a firm support and bends backward while a lateral radiograph is taken. To take a flexion exposure, the patient sits on a stool with the feet on a lower stool and then flexes as far as possible. (Reprinted with permission from The instability associated with disc degeneration in the lumbar spine, by F. Knutsson, Acta Radiol. 25:593-609, 1944.)

Posterior Longitudinal Ligament
Nuclear Material
DEGENERATED DISK

Figure 3-A

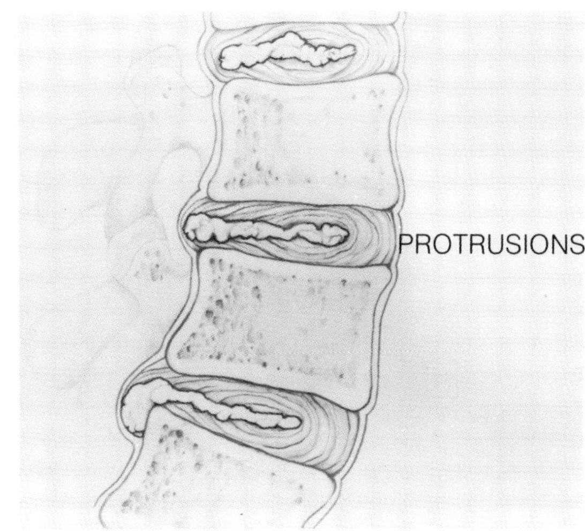

Figure 3-B

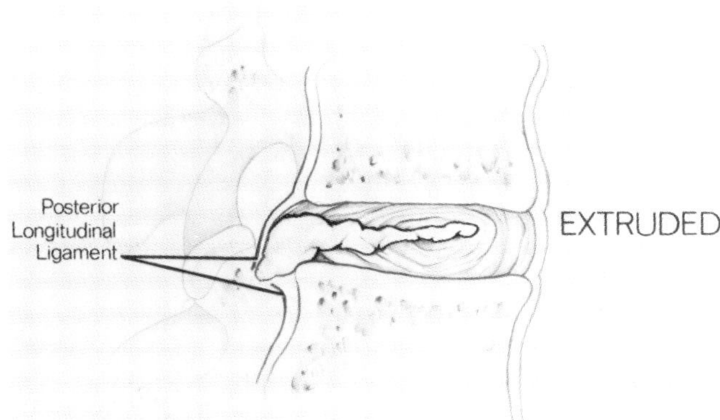

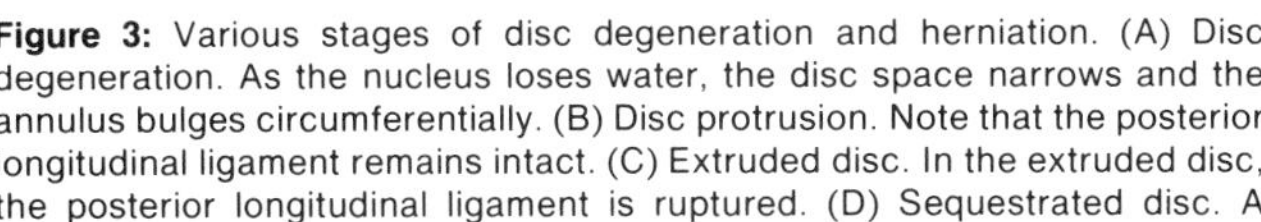

Figure 3-C

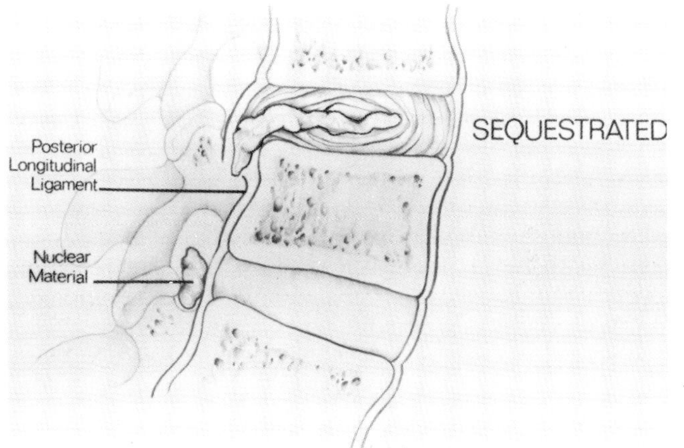

Figure 3-D

Figure 3: Various stages of disc degeneration and herniation. (A) Disc degeneration. As the nucleus loses water, the disc space narrows and the annulus bulges circumferentially. (B) Disc protrusion. Note that the posterior longitudinal ligament remains intact. (C) Extruded disc. In the extruded disc, the posterior longitudinal ligament is ruptured. (D) Sequestrated disc. A fragment has left the point of extrusion and has lodged somewhere a short distance away. Some believe that to be sequestrated the pathway between the sequestrated fragment and the opening in the posterior longitudinal ligament and annulus must have sealed off.

control of segmental vertebral motion may substitute for ligamentous laxity and result in normal stability of the segment despite disc degeneration and narrowing. This may at least partially explain the lack of correlation between radiographic findings and the presence of low back pain.

Herniated Disc The degenerative process may result in disc space narrowing (Fig. 3A), annulus bulging with an intact posterior longitudinal ligament (Fig. 3B), disc extrusion with rupture of the posterior longitudinal ligament (Fig. 3C), or disc sequestration in which the disc fragment is located at a distance from the point of extrusion (Fig. 3D).

PATIENT EVALUATION: There are several techniques (some developed recently) that have made it possible to provide a more exact diagnosis than previously possible. Several *physical examination* tests to separate the hysteric or outright malingerer have been described. The flip test is performed with the patient sitting erect and legs dangling at 90 degrees knee flexion. In the presence of sciatic irritation, passive knee extension results in lumbar lordosis reversal and backward flexion of the trunk. The test is negative when the spine remains erect with normal lumbar lordosis when the knee is extended. The Burns test is illustrated (Fig. 4). The flexed thigh test is performed by pushing the flexed knee and thigh toward the abdomen. The reverse sciatic tension test is performed by plantar flexing rather than dorsiflexing the foot. If these maneuvers result in a complaint of pain, the patient may be malingering or hyperreacting. The Hoover test is performed by having the patient attempt to raise the painful leg with the knee straight. Normally the patient pushes down with the contralateral heel. If not, the test is positive, and the patient's symptoms or cooperation may be questioned.

Laboratory studies that may be helpful in evaluation include psychological tests, biochemical tests, plain radiographs, electromyography, myelography, computed tomography, discography, and nuclear magnetic resonance.

A pain drawing completed by a patient provides insight into the perception of pain and is a quick, easy way of surveying the areas of pain. Magnified or exaggerated pain perception may be indicated by nonanatomic distribution of pain, "whole body" pain patterns, or amplifying words or symbols drawn outside the body silhouette.

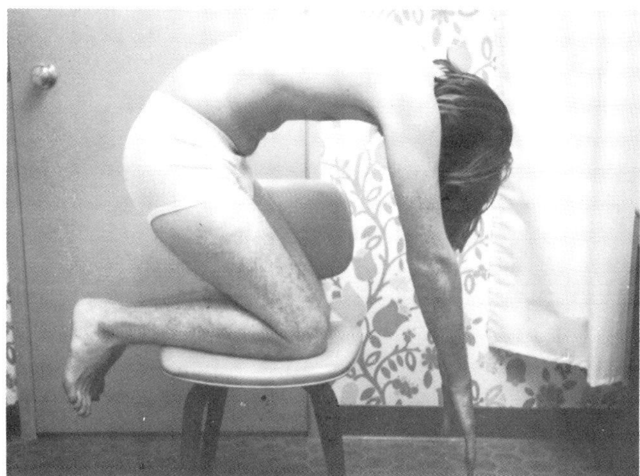

Figure 4: Burns test. The patient with chronic back pain (unless hip disease is also present) should be able to touch the floor. If the patient cannot, then the back pain is probably feigned or exaggerated.

An "arthritis" panel consisting of a sedimentation rate, nonfasting blood uric acid, latex fixation, and, in young males, an HLA-B27 determination may be helpful.

Lumbosacral spine radiographs on the first visit for back pain are often desirable, but the necessity for these is controversial. Current literature supports the practice of not obtaining the radiographs on the first visit for an *acute* episode of back pain. By waiting 8 weeks, the vast majority of patients will have recovered and do not need radiographs.

Acute disc syndrome is a clinical diagnosis made on the basis of history and physical examination. Various adjunctive tests are available to help confirm and localize the diagnosis. Although electromyography may supply ancillary diagnostic data, it is not diagnostic and a negative electromyographic study does not exclude a herniated nucleus pulposus.

Computed tomography is the best test for detecting spinal stenosis, especially of the lateral canal. CT techniques have developed to the point that a herniated disc can be well demonstrated. It is now considered reasonable to operate or inject with chymopapain without a myelogram if the CT is diagnostic and there is no evidence of other problems, such as spinal cord tumor or arachnoiditis.

Nuclear magnetic resonance (NMR) reveals the distribution of atoms in the body without the use of radiographs. NMR signals evoked by radiofrequency are detected by a coil and forwarded to a computer for analysis. The image is especially helpful in evaluating soft tissues, such as the brain and spinal cord. Although still not widely available, rapid strides are being made in its development and distribution for diagnosis of spinal diseases.

Discography requires good fluoroscopy equipment (Fig. 5). Ideally, two-plane instantaneous imaging, with a memory for each plane, should be available. Correlation of an abnormally appearing discogram with the patient's pain syndrome is still subject to error. However, this technique is useful in some diagnostic situations.

TREATMENT—NONOPERATIVE: For the patient believed to have a herniated nucleus pulposus, nonoperative treatment should be pursued as long as possible, unless there are absolute indications for surgery. Cauda equina dysfunction or progressive neurologic deficits do indicate surgery.

The cornerstones of nonoperative treatment are bed rest, nonaddicting analgesics, and physical therapy consisting of isometric trunk muscle exercises, training in biomechanics, and low back care. In addition, epidural steroids may be helpful. Traction, bracing, short wave diathermy, heat and cold, anti-inflammatory medication, sedatives, and muscle relaxants are advocated by some, but their effectiveness in shortening the period of disability has not been proved.

Patient education in low back care is especially important. This may be facilitated by a back school in which the patient is given detailed instructions in back care and maintenance. The formats of existing back schools vary, but all consist of several sessions of personalized education and instruction. Recently, McKenzie extension exercise techniques have been advocated but must be used with care by a technician well-trained in their application.

The herniated disc is not ordinarily considered for surgical treatment, unless there is a significant true sciatic component. An exception may be a large midline disc rupture presenting without sciatica. However, usually there are striking accompanying signs, such as severe list or a very flat lumbar spine. The levels most prone to this presentation are L3 and L4. Also, it is now recognized that pain referred from deranged facet joints may closely mimic sciatica.

Absolute indications for surgery are progressive paralysis of the legs or cauda equina syndrome. Relative indications are severe pain intractable to adequate nonsurgical treatment, moderate motor weakness in the legs, and recurring incapacitating episodes of sciatica. As long as the absolute indications for laminectomy are not present, the patient may be treated nonoperatively for an indefinite period. Foot drop and reflex and sensory changes are not affected in the long-term regardless of whether surgery is done or not.

TREATMENT—SURGICAL: The options are: (1) classic laminectomy, (2) microdiscectomy, (3) chemonucleolysis with chymopapain (or intradiscal collagenase which is still experimental), or (4) removal with a modified arthroscope.

Laminectomy continues to be the standard operation for disc removal. A small circle of bone is removed from the two contiguous laminae (Fig. 6). The spinal nerve is moved in the appropriate direction, usually medially, and a cruciate or rectangular opening is made in the annulus.

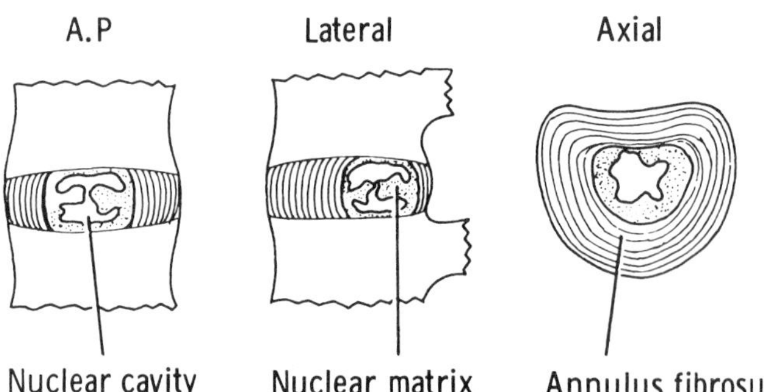

Figure 5: There is a dumbbell-shaped cavity in the normal nucleus pulposus. If the needle tip is in the cavity, it will be a normal discogram. If the tip is in the matrix (stippled area), a spherical mass of contrast may be seen. If the tip is placed in the annulus, an abnormal discogram is produced but the disc may be normal. (Reprinted with permission from An investigation of artefacts in lumbar discography, by R. Quinnell, et al., British J. Radiol. 53:835, 1980.)

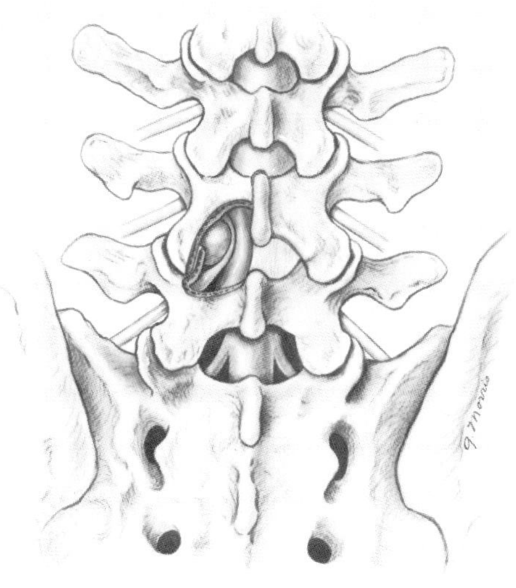

Figure 6: Classical discectomy. Note that the medial swing of the superior articular process of L5 has been nipped off. (Reprinted with permission from Surgery for intervertebral disk disease of the lumbar spine, by L.L. Wiltse, Clin. Orthop. 129:27, 1977.)

As much nuclear material as possible is removed, but the end plates should not be severely curetted. It is generally possible to remove no more than one-half of the actual nuclear material. If there is lateral recess narrowing, care should be taken to decompress the nerve roots by removing the medial portion of the superior articular process of the vertebra below.

The kneeling position is helpful to decrease bleeding from the epidural veins (Fig. 7). No serious complications have been reported with the use of the kneeling frame.

If sciatica is unilateral, only the painful side should be explored, unless the myelogram or the CT scan is strikingly positive on the painless side. If the pain is bilateral and there is evidence of nuclear bulging on the other side, both sides are exposed. If the patient presents with a bulging disc at two levels, the second level should be explored and discectomy and decompression carried out only if clinically indicated.

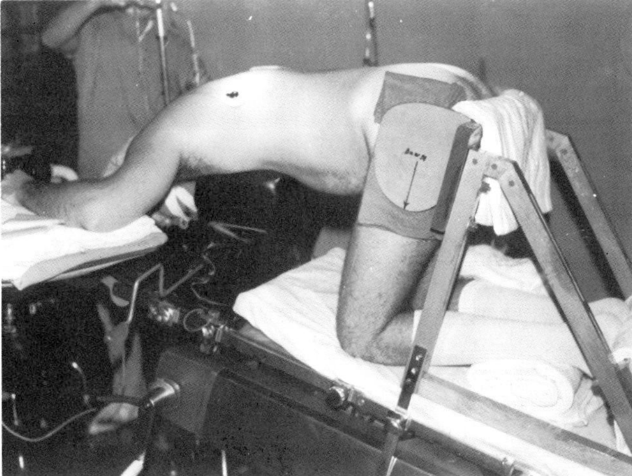

Figure 7: This frame was designed by Hastings and others. The patient is in a kneeling position (never knee-chest). This position is extremely helpful when working around the spinal nerves since it nearly eliminates the pressure in the veins of Batson. The chest support can be raised or lowered by turning the removable crank. (Reprinted with permission from Surgery for intervertebral disk disease of the lumbar spine, by L.L. Wiltse, Clin. Orthop. 129:26, 1977.)

Laminectomy may be performed through a midline or paraspinal muscle-splitting approach.

Free fat grafts and pedicle fat grafts applied over the dura in a laminectomy defect are being widely used, but studies of their ultimate effectiveness are not yet available.

Microdiscectomy seems to be a useful procedure, especially for the young patient. There appears to be less postoperative pain and the incision is certainly smaller than with classic laminectomy. With the release of chymopapain, the indications for microdiscectomy could be reduced.

Chemonucleolysis with chymopapain offers the patient with a herniated disc that is not sequestrated an alternative to laminectomy and discectomy. The indications are the same. Chymopapain appears to depolymerize the aggregated proteoglycans of the nucleus, resulting in loss of water and subsequently decreasing the turgidity and intrinsic pressure of the nucleus. However, the exact mechanism of action remains unknown. In animals, studies have shown that the disc returns chemically and mechanically to its preinjection status in 6 months to 1 year.

Chemonucleolysis should not be attempted without good fluoroscopic equipment and special training. An anesthesiologist should be present throughout the entire procedure, even if it is being performed under local anesthesia. Anaphylaxis and anaphylactoid reactions are by far the most serious complications and occur in about 1 percent of patients. Females with elevated sedimentation rates appear to be especially at risk. Patients with a history of sensitivity to either papaya and papaya extracts should be excluded. Methods for controlling anaphylaxis are available and should be followed scrupulously. They include pretreatment with H^1 and H^2 histamine receptor antagonists (cimetidine and diphenhydramine), secure intravenous infusion routes, 100 percent oxygenation preinjection, and immediately available epinephrine.

The indications for the number of disc spaces to be injected is the same as for laminectomy.

The patient may be allowed up immediately after injection. Postinjection back care is about the same as for surgical discectomy, but the morbidity is often less. However, postinjection muscle spasm is the rule.

Collagenase, as an agent of chemonucleolysis, is being studied under Food and Drug Administration control. Very early reports indicate that the results are quite satisfactory. The indications at this time seem to be the same as those for chymopapain.

Arthroscopic removal of disc fragments is being performed in a few centers. Although the results appear to be favorable, they are not equal to those reported with chemonucleolysis or laminectomy. It is known that stenosis of the neural canal or foramina is present as a contributory factor in about two-thirds of all patients with acute disc syndrome. Arthroscopy does not allow adequate visualization or decompression in these patients. Therefore, this technique may be of questionable value.

Spinal fusion is rarely, if ever, indicated for degenerative disc disease. However, it may be done for postlaminectomy instability and spondylolisthesis, especially if there is concern about further vertebral displacement. It is not necessary after uncomplicated discectomy. In large pub-

Figure 8-A

Figure 8: Technique of bending films to determine fusion. (A) The patient is horizontal on the table and then flexes and extends without rolling. (B) Lines are drawn on the sacrum and vertebral bodies at strategic points. If these lines superimpose perfectly, the fusion is believed to be solid.

lished series comparing discectomies with discectomy and fusion, results are very little, if any, better following disectomy and fusion. Fusion may be complicated by pseudarthrosis. This complication may be painful, but it has been noted that some patients with radiographic evidence of pseudarthrosis have no complaints of back pain.

Techniques for improving the success of lumbar fusion are being studied. Various types of allograft material have been advocated but have yet to be proved equal to autografts. Different forms of internal fixation have been utilized to stabilize lumbar segments. Thus far, evidence is inconclusive that any of these devices are effective in improving fusion rates. Electrical stimulation is in clinical trial, but as yet there is no proof that it improves fusion rates over autogenous bone grafting alone. At this time no substitute has been found for meticulous preparation of the fusion bed and ample autogenous corticocancellous bone graft.

Bending films of good quality to determine the solidity of fusion may be taken at 1 year postfusion (Fig. 8). It should be possible to draw lines across critical points on the vertebral bodies that superimpose perfectly. This cannot be done with standing exposure without special equipment. Recumbent exposure is satisfactory for bending views if the technician takes special care not to let the patient roll when bending. Right and left lateral (anteroposterior) bending exposures are not nearly as helpful as flexion and extension views.

COMPLICATIONS: Those peculiar to discectomy include spinal nerve injury, injury to the great vessels, and postoperative epidural bleeding of sufficient degree to cause cauda equina syndrome. If this occurs, prompt reexploration to obtain hemostasis with closure over suction drainage is recommended.

Since the advent of metrizamide, the incidence of new patients with arachnoiditis has dropped precipitously. To date, no patient with clinical arachnoiditis secondary to metrizamide has been reported. Metrizamide causes some microscopic arachnoidal scarring in monkeys after high concentrations are injected (but not with the usual clinical

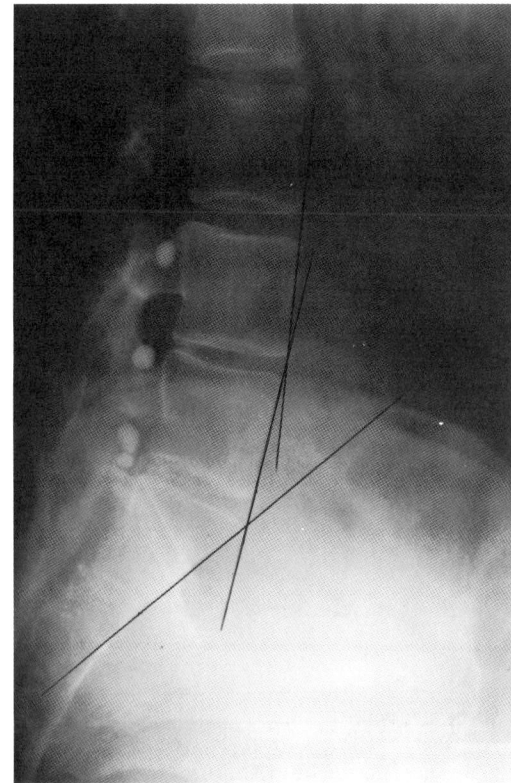

Figure 8-B

concentrations). There remains a considerable residuum of patients with arachnoiditis from the use of Pantopaque. These patients should be evaluated carefully to differentiate between arachnoiditis, spinal stenosis, or herniated nucleus pulposus.

If the condition appears to be only arachnoiditis, surgical treatment is very unsatisfactory. Opening the dura and microscopically dissecting the nerve roots may help temporarily, but long-range relief has not been the rule. Recent study indicates that deep brain stimulation may be of help, but long-term results are not available. Epidural implants have not been very satisfactory.

Other Disc-Related Diseases

IDIOPATHIC VERTEBRAL SCLEROSIS: This condition has been called by many names, e.g., discogenic vertebral sclerosis, aseptic discitis, pseudoinfectious discitis, nonpyogenic discitis, benign vertebral sclerosis, aseptic postlaminectomy discitis, nonneoplastic sclerosis, internal disc disruption, and isolated disc resorption. It is believed that in its classic form, it represents a distinct clinical entity of unknown etiology. It may simply represent increased bone formation adjacent to an unstable vertebral segment. It occurs most commonly at L4. It appears more frequently in the female and is characterized by back rather than leg pain. Usually, only one level is involved and the other disc spaces appear quite normal.

Treatment is nonoperative until the severity of pain necessitates surgery. Preoperative discograms may be done above and below the involved level, and then at the level of vertebral sclerosis. If the involved level reproduces the pain and the disc above and below do not, there is reason to believe that the sclerotic level is the site of the pain. A culture is done at the time of the discogram, and if

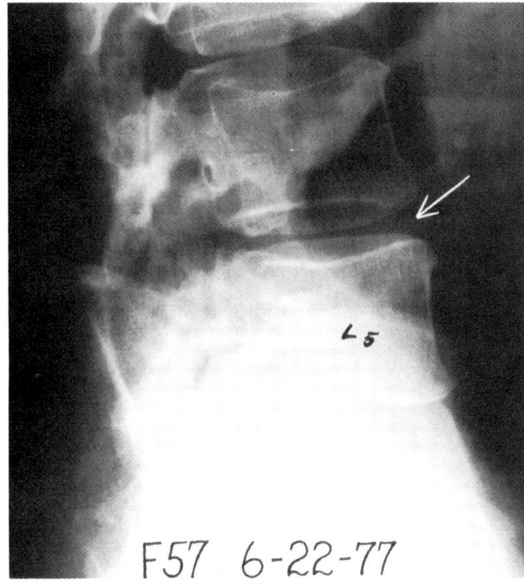

Figure 9-A

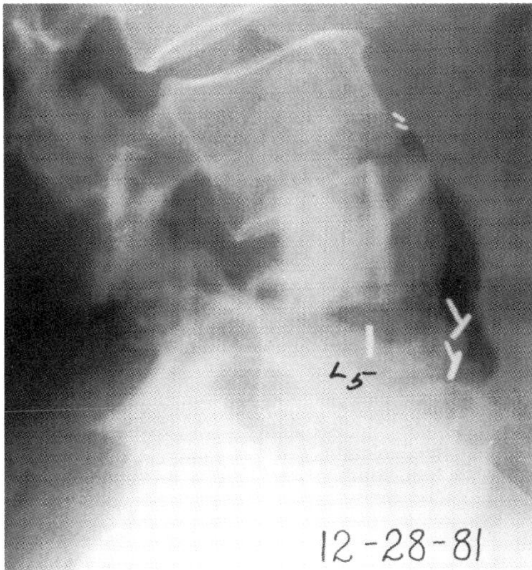

Figure 9-C

Figure 9: Idiopathic vertebral sclerosis. (A) Female, 57-year-old patient who had severe back pain for 3 years. This lateral radiograph was taken 2 years before, 1 year after the onset of pain. Note that the L4 disc space looks fairly normal. (B) Twenty months later there is marked change at L4, characteristic of what has been described as discogenic vertebral sclerosis. (C) About 23 months after interbody fusion with fibular grafts. The patient was immediately and completely relieved of her pain by fusion.

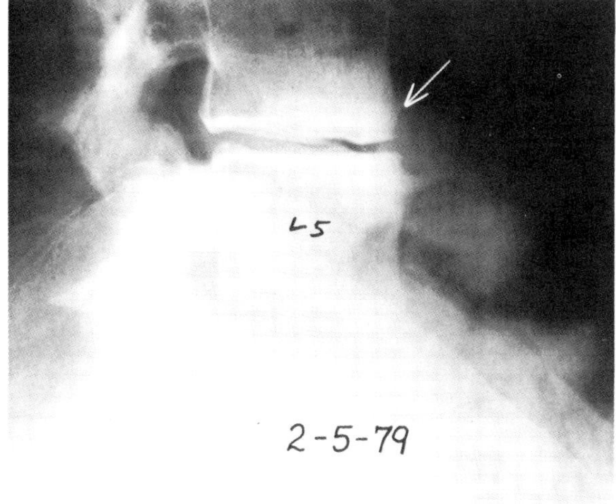

Figure 9-B

it is negative, the diagnosis is idiopathic vertebral sclerosis (Fig. 9). Material removed from the disc space at surgery may show inflammatory reaction. Treatment is fusion of the involved interspace which may be performed either through a posterior or anterior approach. Where there is a large bulge of nuclear material posteriorly, the Cloward operation (posterior lumbar interbody fusion, PLIF) has been advocated and theoretically should be effective. However, a high complication and low fusion rate have been reported with this technique.

Premature widespread disc degeneration (congenitally inadequate discs): Some patients in the third or fourth decades of life are encountered with low back pain believed to be due to multiple disc space narrowing without osteoarthritis (Fig. 10). Typically these patients complain of back pain for many years. It is not clear whether this represents a distinct clinical entity of unknown etiology or is a severe form of degenerative disc disease. Many of these patients have been treated by L4-S1 fusions early in life in an effort to stop their unremitting back pain. After fusion, pain may be relieved for a few months but may recur due to degenerative changes and instability at segmental levels above the fusion.

Facet Arthrosis Moderate degenerative changes in the facet joints that are noted on radiographs are not believed to be associated with an increased incidence of back pain, except in patients with ankylosing spondylitis. Severe osteoarthrosis throughout the lumbar spine correlates somewhat with increase in back pain, but whether it is due to facet arthrosis is not clear. In ankylosing spondylitis, facet arthrosis may be the cause of at least part of the pain.

Facet arthrosis may be effectively treated with nonsteroidal anti-inflammatory drugs. Other semi-invasive procedures which may be helpful include: (1) facet or posterior ramus injection with a local anesthetic, such as bupivacaine, and a steroid, such as dexamethasone, under fluoroscopy; (2) chemical rhizolysis of the posterior ramus with 10 percent phenol in glycerine; and (3) posterior ramus rhizolysis with diathermy. It must be remembered, however, that many of these techniques have not been subjected to clinical trials.

Spinal Stenosis There are multiple causes for spinal stenosis (Table I). The most common form is the "combined" in which there is some congenital narrowing of the central or lateral canals but where degenerative disc disease and osteophytic buildup have contributed to further narrowing. Central canal stenosis is less commonly the cause of pain than is lateral canal stenosis.

Symptoms: Spinal stenosis causes back and leg pain, especially leg pain on walking. The leg pain can be either of the sciatic or the claudicatory type. The sciatic type is more common. Pain of the claudicatory type characteristically begins after walking a short distance. When pain becomes severe, the patient is forced to stop and bend forward or sit. One of the differentiating points between

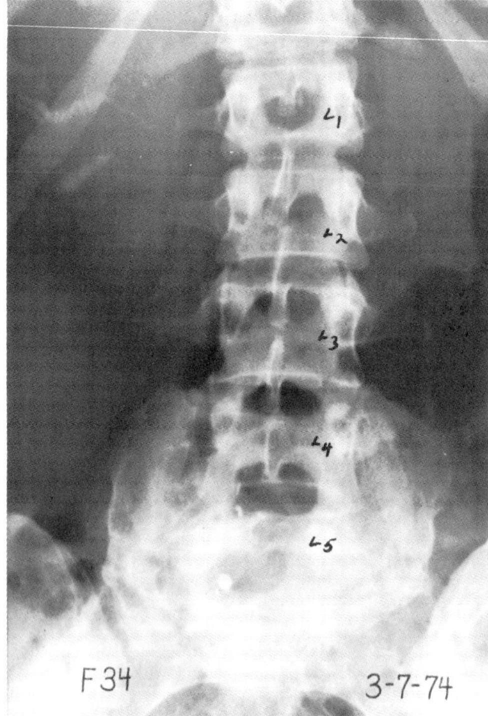

Figure 10-A

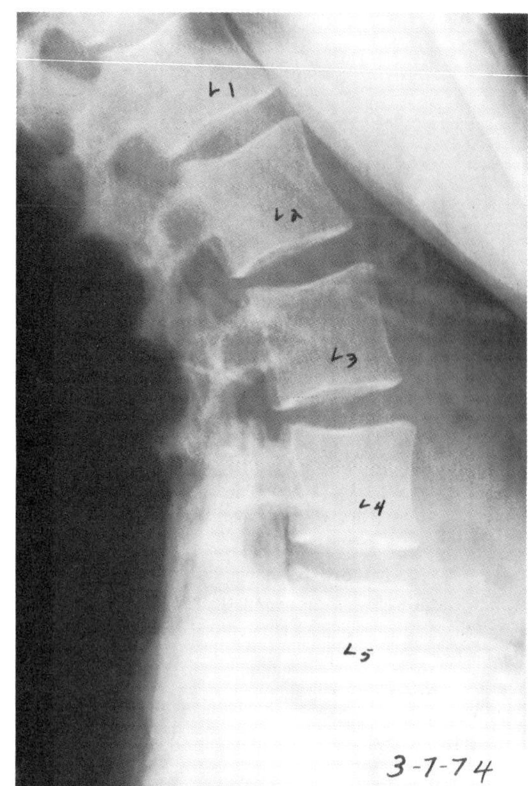

Figure 10-B

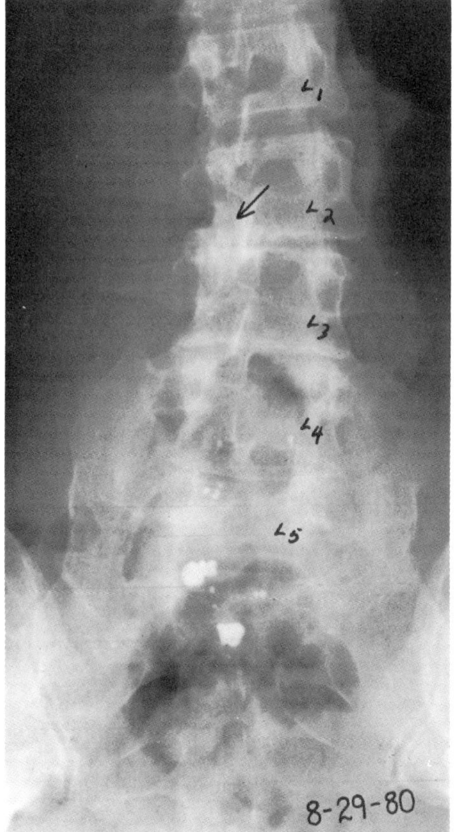

Figure 10-C

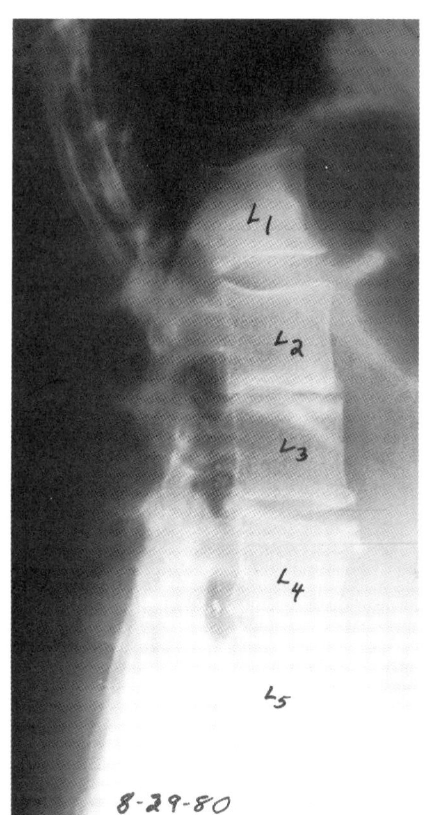

Figure 10-D

Figure 10: Congenitally inadequate discs. (A) When first seen, this patient had had a two-level L4-S1 fusion. For 4 years previously she had had unremitting back pain with right-sided sciatica. She was negative neurologically. (B) Note the disc spaces are of about normal width. (C) In 4½ years her discs have degenerated at several levels, far more than average. Her back pain had stopped for a few months after the fusion and then typically recurred with equal severity. (D) Note the marked several-level disc degeneration but mild osteoarthritis. This degree of disc degeneration is far more than average for only 6 years.

Table I
Spinal Stenosis Classification

- I. Congenital–Developmental Stenosis
  - A. Idiopathic
  - B. Achondroplastic
- II. Acquired Stenosis
  - A. Degenerative
    - 1. Central portion of spinal canal
    - 2. Peripheral portion of canal, lateral recesses, and spinal nerve canals
    - 3. Degenerative spondylolisthesis
    - 4. Disseminated idiopathic skeletal hyperostosis (DISH)
  - B. Combined: Any possible combinations of congenital–developmental stenosis, degenerative stenosis, and herniations of the nucleus pulposus.
  - C. Isthmic or dysplastic spondylolisthesis
  - D. Iatrogenic
    - 1. Postlaminectomy
    - 2. Postfusion (anterior and posterior)
    - 3. Postchemonucleolysis
  - E. Posttraumatic, late changes
  - F. Miscellaneous
    - 1. Paget's disease
    - 2. Fluorosis

neurogenic and vascular claudication is that the patient with vascular claudication can rest a certain length of time in a standing position and then go on. The distance walked is almost exactly the same each time, as is the rest period. However, with neurogenic claudication, the patient more often has to sit to get the back into a flexed position. Lying down might even be required, and considerable time may have to pass before walking can be resumed. The exact cause of neurogenic pain has not been discovered.

The sciatic type of leg pain with spinal stenosis closely resembles sciatica associated with a ruptured disc, whereas the claudicatory type may present with back ache, with leg pain noted only when the patient walks. Either type may exhibit few objective findings, such as reflex change, motor weakness, or inability to stoop. However, hyperextension is virtually always markedly limited and painful. Often normal reflexes disappear after the patient exercises to the point of severe pain, and numbness and weakness also may appear.

TREATMENT: Surgical treatment usually is associated with a satisfactory outcome, but some patients may continue to have back pain even though the leg pain has been relieved. The major problem in surgical treatment is to decompress adequately and still maintain spinal stability. The indications for concurrent spinal fusion are not clear.

Lateral spinal nerve compression can occur as far out as the lateral border of the pedicle and even beyond. Compression beyond the lateral border of the foramen has recently been described and termed the *far-out syndrome* (Fig. 11). This syndrome refers to compression of the spinal nerve between the transverse process and ala of the sacrum. To adequately decompress these patients, the caudal one-half of the pedicle along with the caudal one-half of the transverse process must be removed. With this surgical destabilization of the posterior elements, some type of fusion is usually necessary or olisthesis may occur.

As the population ages, it seems likely there will be more patients needing surgery for spinal stenosis. Since stenotic phenomena are well recognized, it should not be necessary to accept this type of disability as a natural consequence of age.

Some form of lumbar spinal stenosis is frequently present along with a ruptured disc as the cause of low back pain and sciatica. Because several levels usually show changes on myelogram and CT studies, diagnosis of the symptomatic level remains difficult. Myelography has been the traditional test for diagnosing spinal stenosis, but CT has proved to be more useful because it shows the dimensions in the lateral canals, even to the tips of the transverse processes. To show the transverse processes, it is necessary to increase the field of exposure.

Combined use of the metrizamide myelogram and CT provides a very good demonstration of the points of compression. At the present time, no study exists correlat-

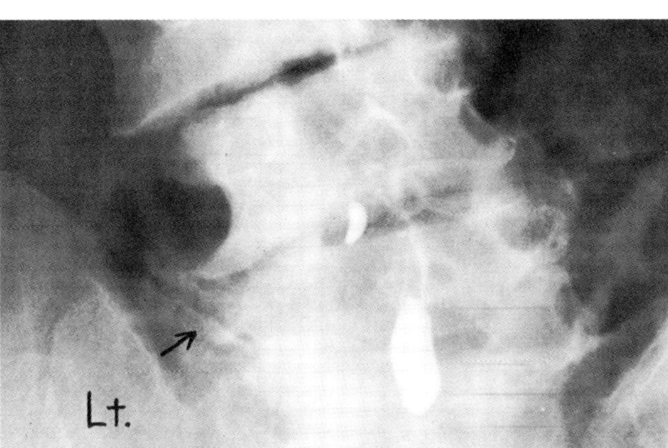

Figure 11-A

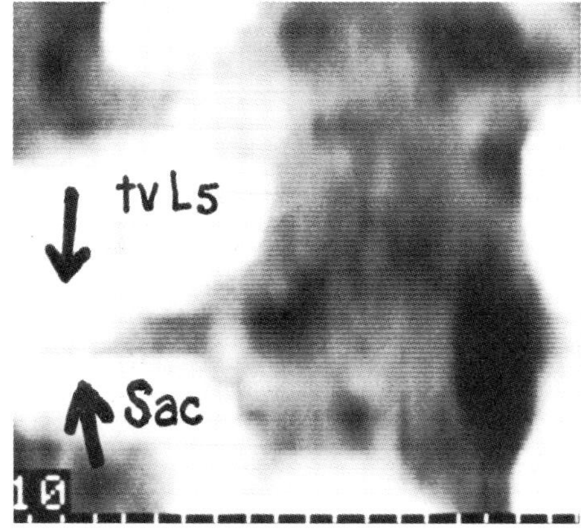

Figure 11-B

Figure 11: The far-out syndrome. (A) Radiograph showing the left transverse process impinging upon the ala. Symptoms, neurologic finding, and EMG findings indicated L5 spinal nerve involvement. Total decompression with removal of the left L5 transverse process relieved the symptoms. A right-sided fusion was also done from L2 to S1 using Harrington rods. (B) Coronal reconstruction of a lumbosacral CT scan of the patient. Note that transverse process of L5 (TV L5) lies against sacral ala (SAC). (Reprinted with permission from Alar transverse process impingement syndrome, by L. Wiltse, et al., Spine (in press).

ing the degree of spinal compression with symptoms. There are published studies dealing with neural canal measurements, but they are merely guidelines.

To make the best use of CT, sagittal and coronal as well as horizontal reconstructions should be made. The radiologist should report in very concise terms each point of constriction. A grading system is helpful in determining the severity of compression.

Trauma

Acute Low Back Injury It is difficult to know what actually happens when a patient "sprains" or "strains" the back, since no dissections of the area have been made for pathological examination. The patient often describes the incident as the back "going out." The possibilities include: (1) intervertebral disc disease; (2) facet joint injury (compression fracture of an articular process, transverse facet fracture, or synovial pinch); (3) end plate injury; (4) intraspinous or supraspinous ligamentous injury ("sprung back" of Newman); (5) muscle tear; and (6) compression fracture of a vertebral body.

The patient most commonly describes the injury that set off the acute low back pain as a combined stooping and twisting injury. Slipping and falling injuries are the next most common.

In a large study of patients with first time acute back injuries secondary to minor trauma, 90 percent were relieved of pain in 6 weeks and 95 percent in 3 months. It made no difference what treatment was used: drugs, manipulation, hot packs, massage, steady or intermittent traction, bed rest, or simple observation.

Once a patient has had a severe attack of back pain, there seems to be a predisposition to further episodes. The best predictor of further back pain is a history of previous back trouble (with surgery in particular).

Injection of trigger points with 1 percent lidocaine and a corticosteroid is a simple and valuable adjunct in the treatment of acute low back pain and one that has been overlooked to some extent in recent years. If a tender point can be located, marked temporary relief is often the rule, and even prolonged relief is not uncommon. If no tender spot can be found, injection is not likely to be of value. Whether the addition of a corticosteroid to the injection actually helps is unclear.

Facet Fractures (Fractures of the Articular Processes) There is often question about the origin of the ossicles at the low tips of the facets that are seen on radiographs. They could be traumatic in origin, representing nonunited fractures but are more likely a failure of fusion of the secondary centers of ossification which form the articular processes. Since the advent of computed tomography, apparent fractures at the base of the articular processes have been noted frequently in postdiscectomy patients. These are not true facet fractures, nor are they in the middle of the pars as in spondylolysis.

End Plate Injuries Injuries of the vertebral end plate usually occur in older people with osteoporotic bone. There is considerable disagreement as to whether end plate injuries and Schmorl's nodules are synonymous. It appears that in the young patient, nuclear material can creep through the end plate and into the vertebral body through a congenital defect at the point where a vessel enters. Other investigators believe these nodules are congenital cartilaginous rests. There seems little doubt that a severe injury can cause a break in the end plate and force nuclear material into the body. Thus, it appears that there are two explanations for Schmorl's nodules: congenital end plate defects and end plate fractures.

Table II

Classification of Spondylolisthesis

I. Dysplastic (congenital): Congenital abnormalities of the upper sacrum or the arch of L5 permit the olisthesis to occur.

II. Isthmic: The lesion is in the pars interarticularis. Three types can be recognized:
   A. Lytic—fatigue fracture of the pars.
   B. Elongated but intact pars.
   C. Acute fracture of the pars (not to be confused with "traumatic," see IV).

III. Degenerative: Due to long-standing intersegmental instability.

IV. Posttraumatic: Due to fractures in areas of the bony hook other than the pars. (Fracture-dislocation is not considered in this type of spondylolisthesis, but the differentiation may not always be clear.)

V. Pathologic: There is generalized or localized bone disease.

Spondylolisthesis Spondylolisthesis is discussed under trauma because, except for the relatively rare dysplastic and pathological types, it is largely due to either chronic or acute trauma. Even the degenerative type results from a combination of degenerative disc disease and chronic trauma to the articular processes. The currently accepted classification is shown in Table II (see Section 26: Thoracolumbar Spine: Pediatric).

Dysplastic This type is very much less common than the isthmic type and when symptoms do occur, they usually occur during childhood or early adolescence. Because there is no defect in the pars interarticularis and the posterior elements follow along with the main body of the vertebra, slip cannot progress to more than about 30 percent of the S1 body width before the patient begins to have pain due to compression of the cauda equina.

Bilateral posterolateral fusion, either by the midline or paraspinal approach, from L5-S1 is recommended for symptomatic patients. If the top of L5 is more than 60 degrees with the horizontal in the standing position (L5-horizontal angle), L4 should be included in the fusion.

Isthmic Spondylolisthesis The basic lesion is in the pars interarticularis. Secondary changes, such as alteration in the shape of the body of L5 or change in the sacrohorizontal angle, may occur, but these are not fundamental to its etiology.

Subtype A, Lytic. This type is caused by a fatigue fracture in the pars interarticularis. It is seen in young children, usually by age 7 years of age. The incidence is about 3.3 percent. Between this age and adulthood, another 0.8 percent manifest themselves, most commonly between 10 and 13 years of age when adolescents begin to engage in strenuous athletics that might produce stress fractures of the pars. Boys develop the defect about twice as frequently as girls.

Subtype B, Elongation of the pars without separation. This is fundamentally the same as subtype A and is secondary to microfractures that heal in a somewhat elongated position as the vertebra slides forward.

Subtype C, Acute pars fractures. These are rare and are secondary to severe trauma. Olisthesis may be present, but mild hyperextension should reduce it. Most patients with this acute fracture heal if immobilized in a "knee-to-nipples" cast with the back in some hyperextension.

TREATMENT: The nonoperative treatment of adults with isthmic spondylolisthesis is basically the same as that for back pain from other causes.

Most studies of adult populations indicate that the presence of spondylolisthesis with less than 10 percent slip is not associated with increased incidence of low back pain, whereas high-grade spondylolisthesis is. Adolescent athletes, however, differ from adults in that spondylolisthesis is more apt to be symptomatic. These children develop stress fractures that unquestionably cause pain. A bone scan shows these developing stress fractures even before they become obvious on radiographs. Treatment consists of prohibition of athletics and a low back corset or brace if activity limitation does not eliminate the pain. Healing can be expected to occur in about 8 months if there is only a stress reaction seen on the bone scan or if the stress fracture is not established. Knees-to-nipple casts for 3 months have been suggested but may be unwarranted for what is usually a relatively mild disease.

The principal reason for *surgical treatment* in the adult is relief of pain, not prevention of progression of slip (as slip rarely increases in the adult). If further slip does occur, the percent progression is small and not an indication for surgery. A one-level posterolateral fusion is usually sufficient. Whether to extend the fusion to L4 depends upon the status of the L4 disc. This is evaluated by computed tomography, myelography, and discography. Some believe the pain reproduction test done at the time of discography is particularly helpful.

The rate of arthrodesis in the adult is about 94 percent if limited to one level but drops to 84 percent for two-level arthrodeses.

Removal of the loose element without fusion (Gill's operation) is not recommended in a child and should be reserved for the older person (over 60 years of age) with a markedly narrowed and osteoarthritic L5 space and sciatica as a prominent pain component. Fortunately, sciatica in patients with spondylolisthesis is usually unilateral or severe on one side but mild on the other. Only the painful side requires decompression. On the painful side, the L5 nerve root should be traced laterally, totally freeing the root. If the slip is more than 30 percent, removing part of the pedicle and the caudal half of the transverse process is generally required. It is not wise to fuse over this area of wide decompression; rather, a unilateral fusion on the other less painful side is preferred. An anterior interbody fusion could be added 1 week to 10 days later if there is concern about instability or inadequacy of fusion.

Retrograde ejaculation after anterior interbody fusion has been reported. The exact incidence is not known but is believed to be about 2 percent. This complication may cause the patient to be sterile. Fortunately, it is usually temporary, lasting 6 to 12 months. There is no practical way of proving its presence or its recovery, thus making its treatment a difficult problem for both patient and doctor. The following precautions are suggested in the sexually active male: (1) carefully inform him of the risks with a witness present; (2) have a patient sign a very specific consent; (3) record if the patient says he wants no more children and if he has had a vasectomy; (4) at surgery dissect carefully, avoid cautery, and try to push the presacral sympathetic nerves laterally off the lumbosacral prominence.

Degenerative Spondylolisthesis This lesion is caused by long-standing intersegmental instability. It most commonly involves a slip of L4 on L5. There is remodeling of the articular processes at the level of involvement which may become more horizontal as slip progresses. Multiple small compression fractures of both the inferior articular processes of L4, and to a much less extent the superior articular processes of L5, may occur. Because of the slip and resulting incongruity, severe degenerative arthritis develops in the facets. Some investigators believe that degenerative arthritis of the facets may be the primary cause of the degenerative spondylolisthesis. One side virtually always slips more than the other, thus rotation at the level of olisthesis is characteristic. This type occurs after the age of 40 years and is four times as frequent in females as in males. It occurs four times more frequently when the L5 vertebra is sacralized or is well distal to the intercrestal line. When the lesion occurs at L4, the L5 vertebra is more stable and in less lordosis than average, thus concentrating more stress at L4, a fact important in its causation. Olisthesis has not been noted to exceed 33 percent unless there has been surgical intervention.

TREATMENT: Nonsurgical treatment of degenerative spondylolisthesis is preferable and generally successful. The long-term use of isometric exercises, combined with activity alterations and occasional use of a corset for bothersome activities is recommended. If sciatic pain is severe, canal and root decompression removing all or part of the lamina of L4 and L5, but saving the pars and articular processes may be carried out (Fig. 12). A one-level bilateral posterolateral arthrodesis with autogenous iliac-crest bone graft is recommended if the patient can tolerate the procedure. It is important to save the pars and an adequate amount of articulating facet or pars fracture may occur, resulting in severe olisthesis.

Other techniques are being used in various parts of the world, including: (1) Luque rods and wires posteriorly from L3-4 and fusion with no decompression; (2) as above with decompression at L4 and passage of wire around lateral masses at L4; (3) anterior interbody fusion at L4; (4) posterior lumbar interbody fusion; (5) Farfan facet fusion at L4 only; and (6) various combinations of the above.

Posttraumatic Spondylolisthesis Spondylolisthesis can occur infrequently following single impact (acute) fractures. These fractures generally involve the articular processes or rarely the pedicles. Treatment is usually surgical and is the same as recommended for isthmic spondylolisthesis.

Pathological Spondylolisthesis Spondylolisthesis may occur due to various diseases of bone, such as Paget's disease. This is rare and seldom requires surgical treatment, but when it does, the same treatment principles are utilized.

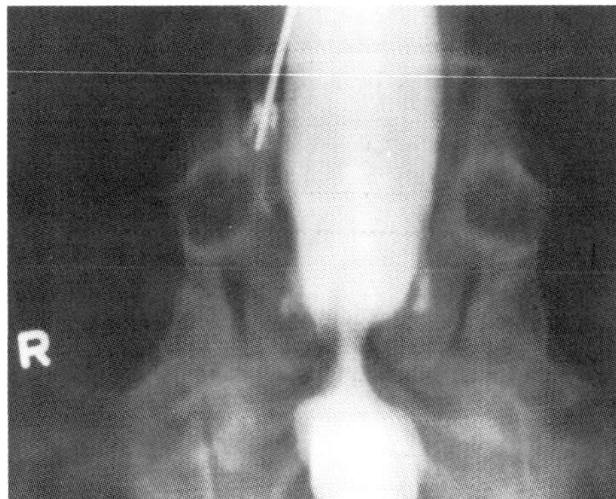

Figure 12-A

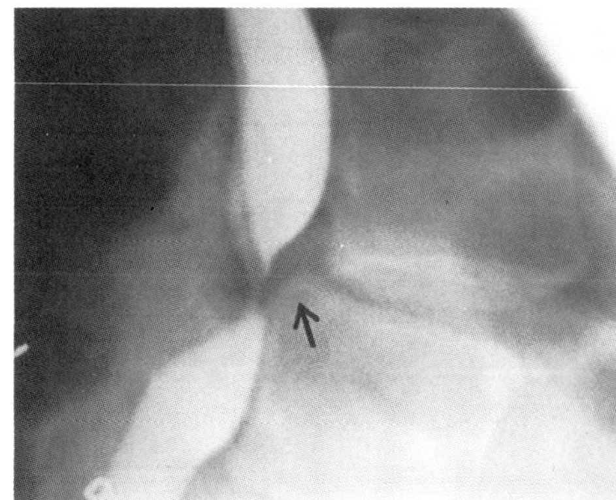

Figure 12-B

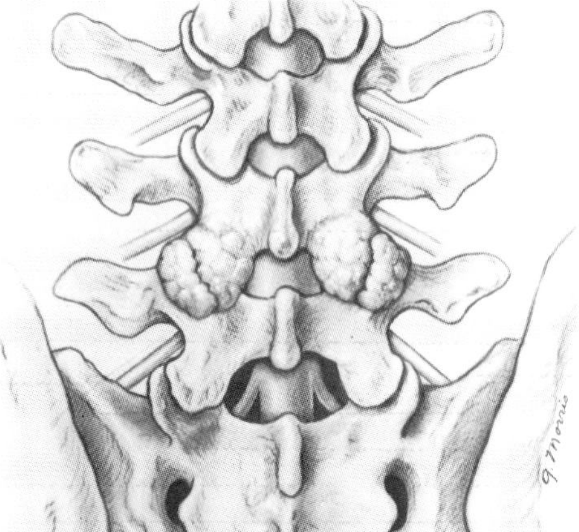

Figure 12-C

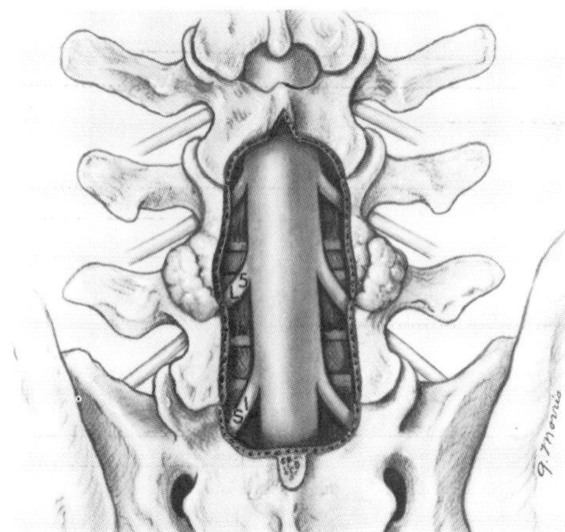

Figure 12-D

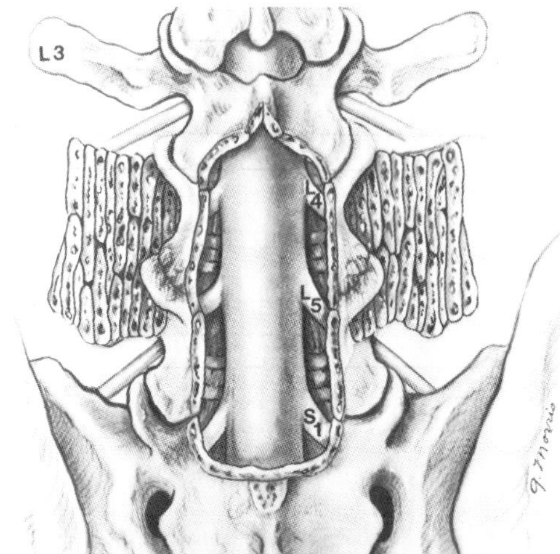

Figure 12-E

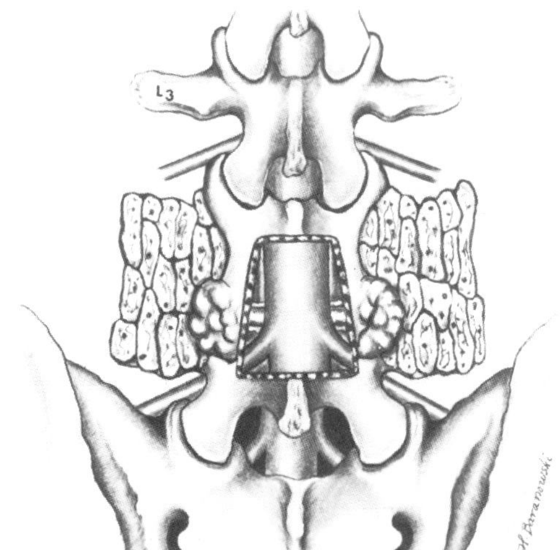

Figure 12-F

Figure 12: Degenerative spondylolisthesis. (A) Anteroposterior myelogram standing. (B) Lateral myelogram standing. (C) Drawing of degenerative spondylolisthesis. (Adapted with permission from AAOS Symposium of Lumbar Spine, p. 164. St. Louis, C.V. Mosby, 1981.) (D) Drawing of a commonly used decompression technique. The pars and at least two-thirds of the articulating surfaces of the facets between L4 and L5 are saved. (Reprinted with permission from Surgery for intervertebral disk disease of the lumbar spine, by L.L. Wiltse, Clin. Orthop. 129:28, 1977.) (E) A type of fusion. The L5 vertebra is usually strong and the sacrohorizontal angle is reduced. The sacrum need not be included in the fusion. (F) All of the laminae of L4 and L5 need not be removed in every patient. There is, however, probably no advantage in saving these slivers of laminae.

ANNOTATED BIBLIOGRAPHY

General

AAOS Symposium on Idiopathic Low Back Pain. Edited by A.A. White, III and S.L. Gordon. St. Louis, C.V. Mosby, 1980.

Proceedings of a 1980 symposium committed to the discovery of the cause of "man's most important nonlife-threatening disease." The twenty-six papers are divided into five sections: (1) epidemiology, (2) anatomy and ultrastructure, (3) biomechanics, (4) biochemistry, and (5) neuromechanisms. Each section is followed by a summary statement that includes proposals for future investigation.

Epidemiology

Frymoyer, J.; Pope, M.; Costanza, M.; Rosen, J.; Goggin, J.; and Wilde, D.: Epidemiologic studies of low-back pain. Spine 5:419-423, 1980.

Of 3,920 patients entering a family practice unit over a 3-year period, an episode of low back pain occurred in 11 percent of males and 9.5 percent of females. Increased incidence was associated with truck driving and heavy lifting, cigarette smoking (especially with chronic cough), anxiety, and depression.

Kelsey, J., and White, A.A., III: Epidemiology and impact of low-back pain. Spine 5:133-142, 1980.

The impact on society of six disorders of the lumbar spine are reviewed. These are disc prolapse, disc degeneration, apophyseal osteoarthrosis, vertebral fractures and dislocations, osteoporosis, and spondylolisthesis. The authors conclude that there is a great need for allocation of more resources for prevention, diagnosis, and treatment of these disorders.

Congenital Anomalies

Cyron, B., and Hutton, W.: Articular tropism and stability of the lumbar spine. Spine 5:168-172, 1980.

In the loaded spine, the joints with articular tropism were found to rotate toward the side of the more coronal facet. This could cause early disc degeneration at that level because of the instability and cam action.

Gross, R.H.: Leg length discrepancy: How much is too much? Orthopedics 1:307-310, 1978.

Patients with less than 2.0 cm discrepancy did not consider their short leg to be a problem. There was no critical "cutoff" point. A survey of pediatric orthopaedists reflected a wide variety of opinion regarding indications for equalization of leg length. There seems little indication for equalization of discrepancies of less than 2 cm. "Clinical judgment" must be weighed on an individual basis.

Nachemson, A.: The lumbar spine: An orthopaedic challenge. Spine 1:59-71, 1976.

This is a review of knowledge of the lumbar spine up to 1976. The author believes that most of the anomalies, either congenital or acquired, seen on plain radiographs have no relationship to the incidence of low back pain.

Wigh, R., and Anthony, H., Jr.: Transitional lumbosacral discs: Probability of herniation. Spine 6:168-171, 1981.

In forty-two patients in whom a transitional lumbosacral vertebra existed, none showed myelographic evidence of herniation. Before transitional discs are operated on, proof of herniation should be incontrovertible.

Degenerative

Intervertebral Disc

Biochemical and Biomechanical

Posner, I.; White, A.A., III; Edwards, W.; and Hayes, W.: A biomechanical analysis of the clinical stability of the lumbar and lumbosacral spine. Spine 7:374-389, 1982.

The authors studied lumbar and lumbosacral spinal units under conditions which simulate maximum physiological flexion and extension with preloads which are analagous to lying and standing. The sagittal plane translations and rotations of transected functional spinal units were measured and compared with the measurements of the intact spinal unit.

Schultz, A.; Andersson, G., Örtengren, R.; Haderspeck, K.; and Nachemson, A.: Loads on the lumbar spine. Validation of a biomechanical analysis by measurements of intradiscal pressures and myoelectric signals. J. Bone Joint Surg. 64A:713-720, 1982.

The authors studied the validity of predictions of compressive loads on the lumbar spine and contraction forces in lumbar trunk muscles based on a biomechanical mode. The predictions were validated by quantitative measurements of myoelectric activities. The model predicted that the tasks imposed mean compressive loads on the spine of as much as 2,400 newtons and required contraction forces of the posterior muscles on the back of as much as 1,800 newtons. Intradiscal pressures of as much as 1,600 kilopascals were also measured.

Herniated Disc

Bernick, S., and Cailliet, R.: Vertebral end-plate changes with aging of human vertebrae. Spine 7:97-102, 1982.

There is a gradual reduction in the width of the growth cartilage up to adulthood. From 60 to 73 years of age, the end plates consist of only articular cartilage that undergoes calcification followed by resorption and replacement by bone. This impedes passage of nutrients from the blood to disc. Collagen fibers arise from the older vertebral end plates to course into the midregion of the disc.

Hilton, R.; Ball, J.; and Benn, R.: Annular tears in the dorsolumbar spine. Ann. Rheumat. Dis. 39:533-538, 1980.

The distribution and severity of anterior and posterior annular tears are assessed by charting the tears in sagittal slabs of 117 fresh specimens. The number of specimens with tears in multiple discs increases with age. Posterior tears at L4 and L5 do not predict tears at other levels. The severity of anterior tears corresponds with increased mobility in the L4-5 disc at least from 50 to 70 years.

Patient Evaluation:

Fairbank, J.; O'Brien, J.; and Davis, P.: Intraabdominal pressure rise during weight lifting as an objective measure of low-back pain. Spine 5:179-184, 1980.

Twenty-three male patients with low back pain swallowed a transducer, then lifted weights. The patients who experienced extra pain during lifting had higher rises of pressure than normal controls and also higher than those who did not experience extra pain. The authors suggest this as a method of objectively measuring pain.

Liang, M., and Komaroff, A.: Roentgenograms in primary care patients with acute low back pain: A cost effectiveness analysis. Arch. Internat. Med. 142:1108-1112, 1982.

The authors compared the benefits, risks, and costs of obtaining a radiograph of the lumbar spine routinely at the initial visit with performing a radiograph only if the patient's pain does not improve during an 8-week follow-up period. The risks and costs of obtaining lumbar radiographs at the initial visit in patients with acute low back pain do not justify the relatively small associated benefit.

Ooi, Y.; Satoh, Y.; Inoue, K.; Mikanagi, K.; and Morisaki, N.: Myeloscopy with special reference to blood flow changes in the cauda equina during Lasègue's test. Internat. Orthop. 4:307-311, 1981.

Two hundred eight patients were myeloscoped without complications. It is possible to watch blood flow changes during Lasègue's test. Direct observation of the nucleus pulposus can also be achieved.

Pykett, I.; Newhouse, J.; Buonanno, F.; Brady, T.; Goldman, M.; Kistler, J.; and Pohost, G.: Principles of nuclear magnetic resonance imaging. Radiology 143:157-168, 1982.

Nuclear magnetic resonance reveals the distribution of atoms in the body without the use of radiographs. NMR signals evoked by radio frequency pulses are detected by a coil and forwarded to a computer. It may be particularly good to detect tissue in which the blood supply has been mechanically obstructed.

Quinnell, R., and Stockdale, H.: An investigation of artefacts in lumbar discography. British J. Radiol. 53:831-839, 1980.

Depending upon where the tip of the discography needle is, even in a normal disc, the discogram may look normal, grossly abnormal, or totally artefactual.

Treatment:

Bromley, J.W., and Gomez, J.G.: Lumbar intervertebral discolysis with collagenase. Spine 8:322-324, 1983.

Fifty-two patients treated under experimental protocol were followed for 2 years. Seventy-eight percent were markedly improved. There were no adverse effects.

Farfan, H., and Kirkaldy-Willis, W.: The present status of spinal fusion in the treatment of lumbar intervertebral joint disorders. Clin. Orthop. 158:198-214, 1981.

The shortcomings of the available information on spine fusion are reviewed and a protocol designed to identify the specific pathological problem is presented.

Goald, H.: Microlumbar discectomy: Follow-up of 477 patients. J. Microsurg. 2:95-100, 1980.

Microlumbar discectomy in 477 patients over a 4.3-year period is presented. A good result was obtained in more than 90 percent. Postoperative pain was minimal and did not require narcotics. Early ambulation was possible, and there was no need for transfusion.

McKenzie, R.: The lumbar spine: Mechanical diagnosis and

therapy. New Zealand, Spinal Publications, 1981.

This book describes the author's method of using hyperextension to relieve the pain in certain types of back pain with sciatica. Special training is necessary to use this technique effectively.

Nachemson, A.: Low back pain. Its etiology and treatment. Clin. Med. 1:18-24, 1971.

The various treatments for the acute attack, such as bed rest, manipulation, traction, and physical therapy, yield about the same results. The back school diminished the number of doctor visits.

Troisier, O.; Dewerpe, P.; and Pelleray, B.: Evaluation of five years of nucleolysis treatment in 150 cases of radiculalgia and ten cases of lumbago of disc origin. Rev. Rhum. Mal. Osteoartic. 49:377-383, 1982.

Problems were assessed on the basis of four parameters: root pain, neurological deficit, residual lumbar pain, and spinal mobility. Good or excellent results were about 75 percent.

White, A.H.; Derby, R.; and Wynne, G.: Epidural injections for the diagnosis and treatment of low-back pain. Spine 5:78-86, 1980.

Three hundred and four consecutive patients were given epidural anesthetic and steroid injections. A prospective study demonstrated that 87 percent had short-term success and 34 percent had relief of pain for as long as 6 months. No patient was cured by these injections. Unless fluoroscopy was used, needle placement, even in experienced hands, was incorrect 25 percent of the time.

Wiesel, S.; Cuckler, J.; DeLuca, F.; Jones, F.; Zeide, M.; and Rothman, R.: Acute low-back pain. Spine 5:324-330, 1980.

The roles of bed rest, anti-inflammatory, and analgesics in the treatment of acute low back pain were analyzed. Bed rest was the best single treatment but was better when combined with analgesics in getting patients to full activities. Anti-inflammatory drugs added nothing.

COMPLICATIONS:

Haughton, V.; Eldevik, P.; Khang-Cheng, H.; Larson, S.; and Unger, G.: Arachnoiditis from experimental myelography with aqueous contrast media. Spine 3:65-69, 1978.

Metrizamide myelography in monkeys caused microscopic arachnoiditis when twice the concentration ordinarily used clinically in humans was used but did not with the usual concentration.

Other disc-related diseases

Fairbank, J.; Park, W.; McCall, I.; and O'Brien, J.: Apophyseal injection of local anesthetic as a diagnostic aid in primary low-back pain syndromes. Spine 6:598-605, 1981.

The authors proposed that patients who responded well to facet injections probably had some anatomic source in the facet joint for their pain. Those nonresponders may well have had pain arising from the nerve root. The pain patterns in the two groups were different. The nonresponders had pain patterns resembling dermatomal patterns and the responders sclerotomal.

Sauser, D.; Goldman, A.; and Kaye, J.: Discogenic vertebral sclerosis. J. Canadian Assn. Radiol. 29:44-50, 1978.

Narrowing of a disc space, sclerosis of the adjacent vertebral bodies, and irregularity of the vertebral end plates constitute a roentgen complex. In some individuals the reactive sclerosis is sufficiently intense to resemble infection.

Spinal Stenosis

Kirkaldy-Willis, W.; Wedge, J.; Yong-Hing, K.; Tchang, S.; de Korompay, V.; and Shannon, R.: Spinal nerve lateral entrapment. Clin. Orthop. 169:171-178, 1982.

Computed tomography makes it possible to diagnose lateral entrapment with accuracy. Surgery is bilateral minimal laminectomy with removal of medial portions of the superior articular processes.

Tsuyama, N.: The ossification of the posterior longitudinal ligament of the spine: OPLL. J. Japanese Orthop. Assoc. 55:425-440, 1981.

There are about 4,000 patients with OPLL in Japan. The incidence in Japanese, for unknown reasons, is many times higher than in Caucasians. The CT scan is the best diagnostic tool. OPLL seldom gives low back symptoms, but often gives cervical symptoms.

Julkunen, H.; Knekt, P.; and Aromaa, A.: Spondylosis deformans and diffuse idiopathic skeletal hyperostosis (DISH) in Finland: Incidence and pathogenic factors. Scand. J. Rheumat. 10:193-203, 1981.

Incidence of DISH was 0.7 patients per one hundred person years in males and 0.4 in females. DISH was equally common in all types of population. Diabetes mellitus and glucose intolerance were associated with DISH.

Wiltse, L.; Guyer, R.; Spencer, C.; Glenn, W.; and Porter, I.: Alar transverse process impingement of L5 spinal nerve (the far-out syndrome). Spine (in press).

The L5 spinal nerve can be trapped between the ala and the L5 transverse process in two special situations: (1) degenerative lumbar scoliosis, and (2) spondylolisthesis with more than 20 percent slip. Levels other than L5 can also occasionally show far lateral nerve entrapment. Transitional vertebrae do not produce this syndrome.

Trauma

Acute Low Back Injury

Ahlgren, S., and Hansen, T.: The use of lumbosacral corsets prescribed for low back pain. Prosthet. Orthot. Internat. 2:101-104, 1978.

Two hundred and one patients (109 women and 92 men) fitted with their first lumbosacral corsets because of low back pain were interviewed after 3.5 to 4.5 years. Only three-quarters of them wore the corsets even regularly immediately after prescription. Of those who still had symptoms (about one-half of the original group) 105 were still wearing a corset. Women doing heavy work tended to use their corsets more frequently. The frequency with which the corsets were used was not influenced by the clinical diagnosis or the type of corset prescribed.

Omar, M.M., and Levinson, E.M.: An unusual fracture of the vertebral articular process in a skier. J. Trauma 19:212-213, 1979.

An unusual vertical fracture through the superior articular process of L5 is described in a professional skier. Follow-up radiographs after 14 months demonstrated a nonunion of the fracture.

Spondylolisthesis

Farfan, H.: The pathological anatomy of degenerative spondylolisthesis. A cadaver study. Spine 5:412-418, 1980.

The morbid anatomy of nineteen spines demonstrating degenerative spondylolisthesis were studied to define the precise changes which produced this lesion and radiographic appearance. The studies indicated that the olisthesis is basically a persistent rotary deformity and not a simple forward displacement. There is no general constriction of the neural canal at the site of the olisthesis.

Semon, R., and Spengler, D.: Significance of lumbar spondylolysis in college football players. Spine 6:172-174, 1981.

Two groups of athletes were compared as to time lost from games and practices. One group had low back pain and lumbar spondylolysis. The randomly selected control group had low back pain but no spondylolysis. There was no significant difference in practice or playing time lost between these two groups. Lumbar spondylolysis is of minimal clinical significance at least over a short period.

30 PELVIS, HIP, AND FEMUR: PEDIATRIC

Subjects covered in this section include femoral anteversion, congenital dislocation of the hip, Legg-Calvé-Perthes disease, slipped capital femoral epiphysis, hip problems encountered with myelodysplasia and cerebral palsy, and trauma to the hip and femur.

Congenital and Developmental

Increased Femoral Anteversion There is no conclusive documentation of any long-term adverse effects (such as degenerative arthritis) from persistent increased idiopathic femoral anteversion. Unless the limitation of external rotation is severe (zero or less degrees) or at least moderate (less than 15 degrees), functional hip performance in adolescents and adults is usually uncompromised. Only if functional hip performance is compromised is treatment necessary.

Orthotic treatment has not been effective. However, for cosmetic reasons it is advisable to avoid the reverse tailor sitting position.

Operative treatment by femoral derotational osteotomy is advocated only for the child who has functional disability combined with a significantly increased femoral anteversion. Since the majority of the excess anteversion naturally tends to decrease and the gait to improve during the first 8 years of life, surgical correction before this age rarely is indicated.

Anteversion measurement by radiographic technique is probably unnecessary as postoperative normalization of gait is well correlated with clinical assessment of internal and external hip rotation. There appears to be no difference in the result whether the osteotomy is performed in the subtrochanteric or the supracondylar portion of the femur.

In patients in whom anteversion is a component of a more complex deformity (such as spastic dislocation of the hip), computed tomography has been utilized to determine anteversion because it provides assessment of the femoral head-acetabulum relationship as well as the acetabular inclination. However, computed tomography does not allow determination of the true neck shaft angle in the coronal plane and requires more radiation exposure than biplanar radiographs.

Congenital Dislocation of the Hip (CDH) Examination of each newborn's hips in the nursery effectively detects the majority with dislocated hips. However, newborn examination is not effective in detecting every patient with dislocated hips, and follow-up examination during well-baby checks should be encouraged. Beyond the newborn period the Ortolani test becomes progressively less reliable because of the development of adductor muscle contracture, and limited hip abduction in flexion becomes the most frequent physical finding. Bilateral dislocation may be particularly difficult to diagnose since the diagnostic signs dependent upon asymmetry are not reliable.

It is also important to recognize the epidemiological factors associated with congenital dislocation of the hip, such as firstborn white females carried or delivered in the breech position, other associated deformities (e.g., muscular torticollis or substantial postural or structural foot deformities), and certain ethnic groups (e.g., the Navajo Indians). For these particular infants, repeat examination and radiographs at 6 months are appropriate.

Radiographic evaluation in the newborn is not diagnostic (of CDH) but does identify teratologic dislocations and provides an impression of acetabular development.

TREATMENT: In the newborn, abduction splinting is recommended for both the dislocatable (positive Barlow's or Palmén test) and the dislocated hip. A stable concentrically reduced hip can be expected in about 95 percent of patients treated by abduction splinting. Splinting done without excessive abduction carries very little risk of osteonecrosis. Weekly visits are advisable initially for adjustment of the splint and confirmation of maintenance of reduction. The dislocated hip generally stabilizes and presents a normal radiographic appearance by 6 to 8 weeks.

When clinical examination indicates that the child's thighs are properly positioned, radiographic examination is useful to confirm proper relationship between the proximal femur and acetabulum.

Satisfactory results following abduction splinting have been reported with the vonRosen splint, the Craig splint, the Pavlik harness, and others.

The Pavlik harness has recently been popularized and very low complication and failure rates have been reported. However, osteonecrosis and failure of concentric reduction may occur. The important principles when using the Pavlik harness (or any other splint) are to determine the stable zone (i.e., the degrees of abduction in 90 to 100 degrees flexion between maximum unforced abduction following reduction and redislocation when moving toward adduction) and to splint the hip within that zone (Fig. 1).

The patient with a dislocatable or dislocated hip should continue to be examined clinically and radiographically after treatment to confirm normal growth and development. Abnormal growth patterns may be due to osteonecrosis, inadequate reduction, or instability. These conditions require an individualized treatment program.

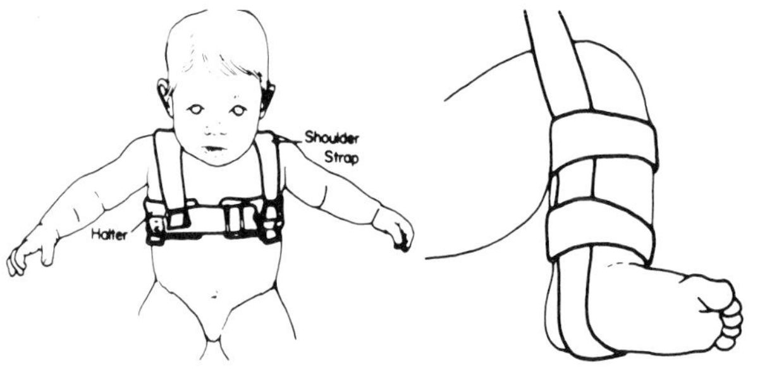

Figure 1-A

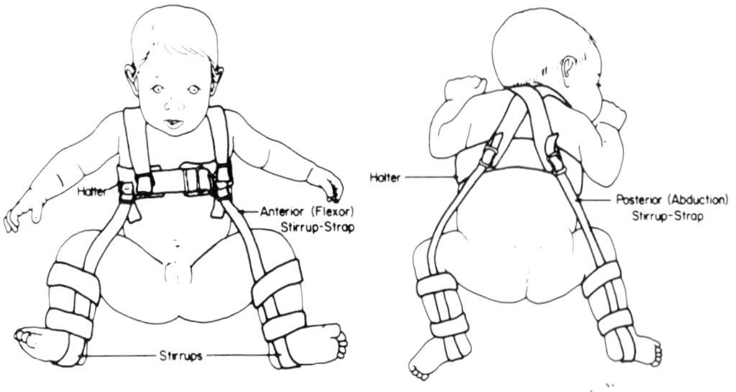

Figure 1-B

Figure 1: (A) The halter is applied across the nipple line to prevent abdominal compression. The straps supporting the foot are just below the popliteal fossa to prevent bowstringing. (B) The anterior (flexion) strap is located over the anterior axillary line. They are adjusted so that hip flexion is between 100 and 110 degrees. The shoulder straps cross in the back to prevent them from slipping off the child's shoulders. The posterior (abduction) buckle is over the scapula. The posterior stirrup straps are adjusted so that the hips have free abduction and there is approximately 5 to 8 cm between the knees when both hips are adducted. (Reprinted with permission from Pitfalls in the use of the Pavlik harness for treatment of congenital dysplasia, subluxation, and dislocation of the hip, by S. Mubarak, et al., J. Bone Joint Surg. 63A:244, 1981.)

The dislocated hip detected after the perinatal period sometimes can be reduced gradually in a Pavlik harness. Closed reduction becomes necessary for those that do not. Prereduction skin traction is usually recommended in the child younger than approximately 18 months. Traction in hip flexion of 45 degrees generally is considered adequate to neutralize the effect of the neonatal hip flexion contracture.

Following traction, an atraumatic reduction should be performed under general anesthesia. If the hip joint is stable following reduction, it should be immobilized in a position of adequate abduction to maintain reduction but less than the maximum position of abduction. Occasionally an adductor tenotomy may be necessary to extend the safe zone. Forced abduction is unphysiologic and is associated with a higher incidence of osteonecrosis. A bilateral hip spica cast is applied with the hips flexed 90 to 110 degrees and abducted within the safe zone.

When the adequacy of reduction is in doubt, an arthrogram with examination under anesthesia should be performed prior to application of the cast. This allows determination of the most stable position, aids in visualizing any soft-tissue obstruction within the acetabulum, and defines any capsular constriction or laxity. Slight lateral displacement of the femoral head due to acetabular fossa soft tissue may be acceptable if the reduction is stable. As not all such hips eventually achieve a concentric reduction, close follow-up is necessary.

When closed reduction is not possible or cannot be maintained, open reduction is indicated. Arthrotomy through the anterolateral approach generally is used to expose and correct the soft-tissue abnormalities responsible for failure of closed reduction. This procedure includes excision of the ligamentum teres, removal of the fibrofatty tissue from the acetabular fossa, division of the transverse acetabular ligament, reduction of the femoral head into the acetabulum, and capsulorrhaphy. Excision of the labrum is discouraged; if infolded, it should be turned out or radially incised but preserved.

The anterolateral approach also facilitates femoral shortening which may be necessary to accomplish reduction in the older child. Femoral shortening of 2 or 3 cm decompresses the hip and lessens the risk of osteonecrosis by lengthening all the musculature about the joint. The resulting limb length inequality generally resolves with growth during the 1- to 2-year period after reduction.

The medial approach should be restricted to children under approximately 24 months of age who have not responded to abduction splintage or in whom a stable closed reduction cannot be accomplished. This approach has not been satisfactory in patients with teratologic dislocations (e.g., arthrogryposis and high stiff dislocations) and following previous surgery.

Indications for osteotomy continue to undergo change and must be individualized. Recent studies have shown that acetabular development improves for several years following concentric reduction. Therefore, pelvic or proximal femoral osteotomy at the time of open reduction is used less frequently. Proximal femoral osteotomy probably should be done only if there is documented significant anteversion and coxa valga. A preoperative full range of motion is necessary.

Persistent acetabular dysplasia in the age group between 2 and 5 years can be corrected either by the pericapsular osteotomy (Pemberton) or innominate osteotomy (Salter). Pericapsular osteotomy is particularly helpful with larger degrees of acetabular inclination and with a relatively flattened acetabulum as compared to the femoral head. Older children whose triradiate cartilage and symphysis pubis are less flexible require more extensive procedures to accomplish acetabular redirection. Two useful procedures are the double innominate (Sutherland) and the triple innominate (Steele) osteotomies. Direct rotation of the acetabulum (Eppright or Wagner) is demanding and difficult to achieve but is theoretically attractive for the treatment of acetabular dysplasia in the adolescent. The Chiari osteotomy or shelf procedure may be reasonable alternatives as a salvage procedure when acetabular reconstruction is not possible. However, in one recent series the long-term results of the shelf procedure were unsatisfactory.

Osteonecrosis of the femoral head remains a major complication in the treatment of congenital dislocation of the hip. The effect of osteonecrosis on the growth of the upper femur has been studied recently. Growth disturbance depends upon the site of necrosis and may produce either a varus or valgus deformity with or without shortening of the femoral neck and overgrowth of the greater

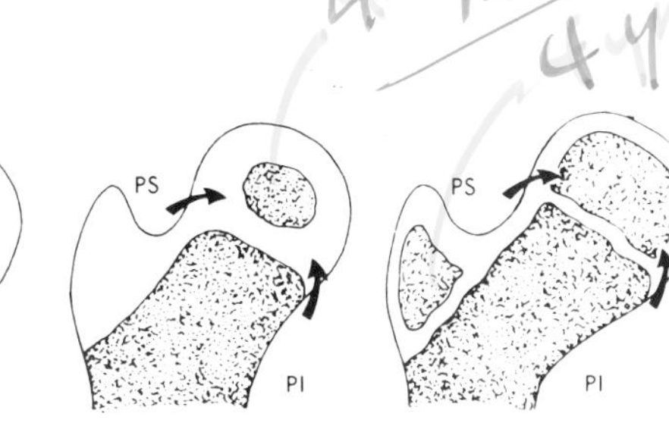

Figure 2-A

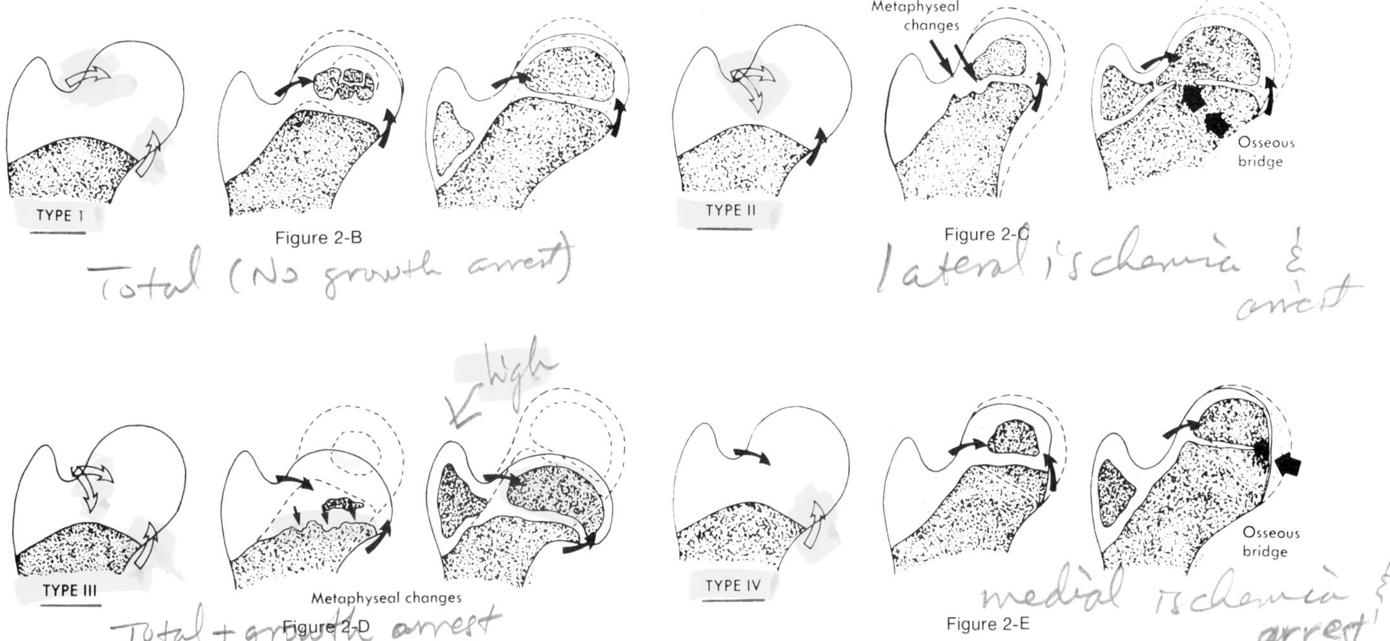

Figure 2-B

Figure 2-C

Figure 2-D

Figure 2-E

Figure 2: (A) Schematic of normal proximal femur at 2 months, 1 year, and 9 years of age. *PS,* posterosuperior vessels; *PI,* posteroinferior vessels. (B) Schematic of type I ischemic necrosis at 2 months, 1 year, and 9 years of age. The broken lines represent anticipated contours if growth had continued normally. The open arrows represent the sites of temporary vascular occlusion. (C) Schematic of type II ischemic necrosis at 2 months, 1 year, and 9 years of age. The broken lines represent anticipated contours if growth had continued normally. The open arrows represent the probable primary site of vascular occlusion. Note localized irregularity in the lateral metaphysis and physis and subsequent premature epiphysiodesis in the same region, both of which occur at the site of presumptive vascular ischemia to the epiphyseal vessels supplying this region of the physis. (D) Schematic of type III ischemic necrosis at 2 months, 1 year, and 9 years of age. The broken lines represent anticipated contours if growth had continued normally. The open arrows represent the sites of temporary vascular occlusion causing impaired longitudinal growth throughout the capital femoral physis, as well as the intraepiphyseal physis. The trochanteric region continues relatively normal longitudinal growth. (E) Schematic of type IV ischemic necrosis at 2 months, 1 year, and 9 years of age. The broken lines represent anticipated contours if growth had continued normally. The open arrow represents the sites of temporary vascular occlusion, which corresponds to the region of impaired longitudinal and latitudinal growth and premature epiphysiodesis. (Adapted with permission from Patterns of ischemic necrosis of the proximal femur in nonoperatively treated congenital hip disease by Bucholz, et. al., *In* The Hip—Proceedings of the Sixth Open Scientific Meeting of the Hip Society, pp. 48, 50, 53, 55, St. Louis, C.V. Mosby, 1978.)

trochanter (Fig. 2). Treatment planning depends upon an assessment of these factors. Sequential radiographic evaluation is valuable for selecting the proper time for osteotomy or epiphysiodesis, should surgery become necessary.

Irritable Hip Syndrome The cause of irritable hip syndrome is unknown. The major diagnostic concern is to exclude septic arthritis. Other differential diagnostic considerations include arthritis, trauma, appendicitis, hemorrhage into the iliopsoas (as seen in hemophilia and Schönlein-Henoch purpura), and closed disc space infection.

A strong correlation with later Perthes' disease has not been established. However, as some (possibly 1 to 3 percent) of these patients subsequently appear to develop Perthes' disease, follow-up for 1 year is recommended.

Legg-Calvé-Perthes Disease Epidemiologic studies have identified a patient profile associated with an increased incidence of Perthes' disease. Factors frequently encountered include retarded bone growth, low socioeconomic background, breech delivery, and children of older parents. In patients with bilateral hip involvement the differential diagnoses should include dysplasia epiphysealis multiplex, dysplasia epiphysealis capitus femoris (Meyer's dysplasia), sickle cell disease, and hypothyroidism.

Most theories of etiology assume an interruption of blood supply to the femoral head. Some of the proposed

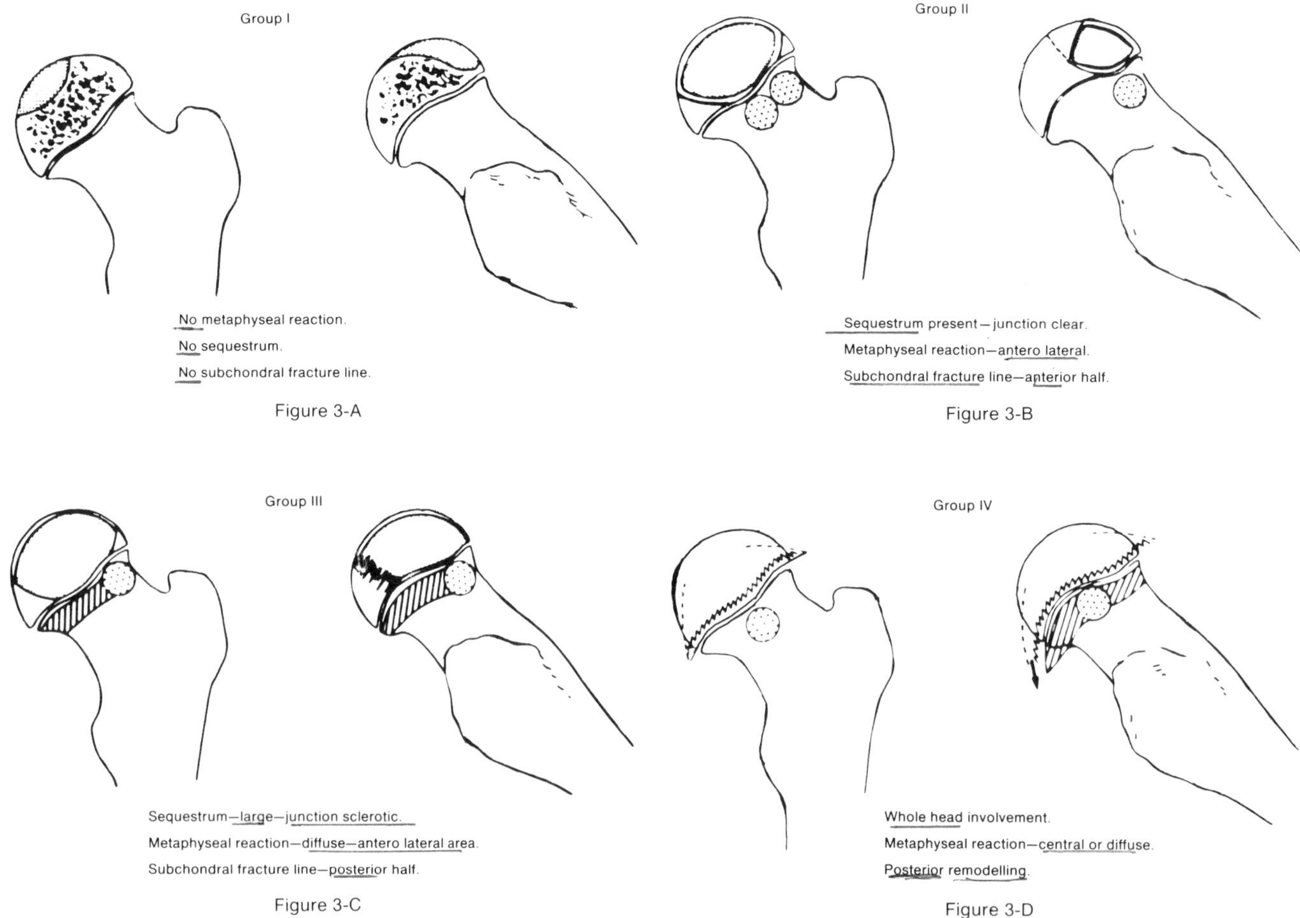

Figure 3: Catterall classification of the extent of necrotic involvement of the femoral head with Legg-Calvé-Perthes syndrome. (A) Drawing of Group I. (B) Drawing of Group II. (C) Drawing of Group III. (D) Drawing of Group IV. (Reprinted with permission from Legg-Calvé-Perthes syndrome, by Catterall, Clin. Orthop. 158:42, 43, 1981.)

mechanisms include intraosseous venous hypertension, increased blood viscosity, cytotoxic agents, synovitis, double infarction, and constitutional defect of growing bone predisposing the patient to a force-oriented hip lesion.

In the initial stage of the disease, a bone scan may show a "cold" area, presumably due to avascularity, within the epiphysis of hips with suspected Perthes' disease. However, this area of decreased radioisotope uptake may not correlate with the later radiographic appearance of the area of necrosis. Magnification and quantitative radioisotope techniques are being developed that may prove to be more valuable diagnostic tools.

Classification: Currently, Catterall's classification is the standard description of the extent of necrotic involvement of the femoral head (Fig. 3). It correlates well with long-term prognosis. However, this classification has been criticized as not being sufficiently prospective as the extent of involvement often is not established for up to 6 to 8 months after diagnosis.

Four radiographic stages in the evolution of the disease process have been described (Waldenström). Stage 1 is the initial stage characterized by failure of the ossific nucleus to grow and by widening of the joint space. Stage 2 is the fragmentation stage characterized by areas of radiolucency and fragmentation. Collapse occurs during this phase. Stage 3 is the reossification stage characterized by areas of new bone formation. Stage 4 is the healed phase.

Natural history: Studies of the untreated disease process indicate that results are good in approximately one-third, fair in one-third, and poor in one-third of the patients. Those with partial head involvement (Catterall I and II) have a much better prognosis than those with nearly total or total head involvement (Catterall III and IV). In Catterall's series of untreated patients, 90 percent of the poor results occurred in patients in groups III and IV whereas 92 percent of the good results occurred in patients in groups I and II. Fifty percent of the patients in group III and 71 percent of group IV had poor results.

There are certain clinical and radiographic at-risk signs that are predictive of a poor result. The clinical signs are: (1) age greater than 6 years, (2) obesity, (3) progressive loss of hip motion, and (4) adduction contracture. The radiological signs are: (1) a defective area of ossification in the lateral epiphysis, (2) calcification in the epiphysis lateral to the area of coverage, (3) diffuse metaphyseal reaction, (4) lateral subluxation of the hip (defined as a portion of the bony epiphysis lying lateral to the margin of the bony acetabulum), and (5) a horizontal growth plate which occurs when the femoral head lies in a position of adduction and external rotation. At-risk signs may occur in any of the four Catterall groups but are much more common in groups III and IV. If two or more of the

Figure 4: Standing anteroposterior radiograph of the pelvis of a patient with Legg-Calvé-Perthes disease being treated with a bilateral hip abduction orthosis (Scottish Rite) demonstrates that the hips are adequately abducted and that coverage of the femoral head is present.

radiographic at-risk signs are consistently present during stage 1, 2, and 3 of the disease, the child can be predicted to have a poor result if not actively treated.

TREATMENT: Treatment in the early stages of the disease while the head is still reasonably round affords the best opportunity for a satisfactory result. During stage 2 it is generally believed that the overall shape of the femoral head may be preserved by containment. Once reossification has occurred, further treatment will probably not alter the shape of the head.

Maintenance of hip range of motion is a high treatment priority. Abduction of the lower extremities so that the lateral portion of the femoral head is completely beneath the coverage of the acetabulum has been described as the principle of "containment." However, the femoral head, which represents about 75 percent of the sphere, cannot be totally "contained" by the acetabulum which is only 50 percent of the sphere. The usual criteria for determining adequate containment are: (1) centering of the femoral head within the acetabulum and (2) covering the entire epiphysis with the acetabulum so that the lateral epiphyseal plate margin lies at or inside the acetabular margin.

Best reported results are in children treated by prolonged bed rest (2 years) combined with splinting in abduction. Although effective, this form of treatment is no longer used because of its restrictions and expense. Therefore, for patients requiring treatment, ambulation with weight-bearing either in an abduction orthosis (Fig. 4) or following osteotomy of the femur or pelvis is recommended. Devices not providing hip abduction and therefore not containing the femoral head are probably ineffective in altering the disease process and actually may have a negative effect because they tend to adduct and subluxate the hip.

Abduction treatment in an ambulatory orthosis, which keeps the hip abducted so that the physeal plate is at the margin of the acetabulum, should be continued until reossification is demonstrated by serial radiographs. Splinting can be safely discontinued only with evidence of reossification of the femoral head (generally 12 to 18 months after onset of the disease process) and satisfactory range of hip motion.

Varus osteotomy of the femur can accomplish the goal of containment of the femoral head and free the patient from orthotic wear. Two operations are necessary, the femur is shortened (usually temporarily), and the resting length of the hip abductors are decreased, resulting in a temporary limp.

Similar results have been reported whether containment is obtained by a carefully supervised orthotic program or by femoral osteotomy.

Innominate osteotomy (Salter) has also been performed but in fewer patients. This procedure may be considered in those patients who have an excellent range of motion and whose femoral head is still spherical. However, range of motion limitation, pain, and joint space narrowing may be more frequent than following femoral osteotomy.

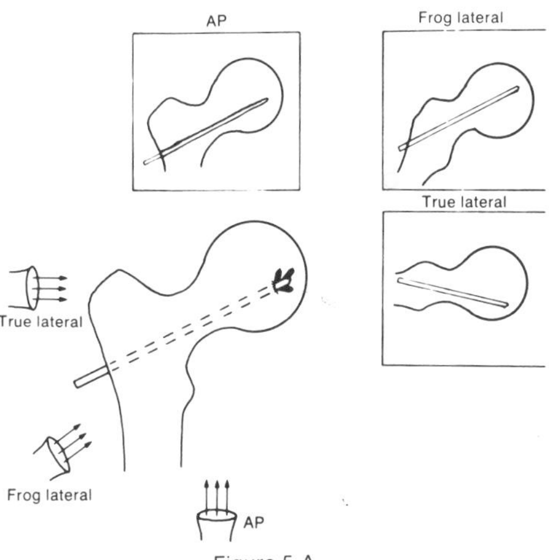

Figure 5-A

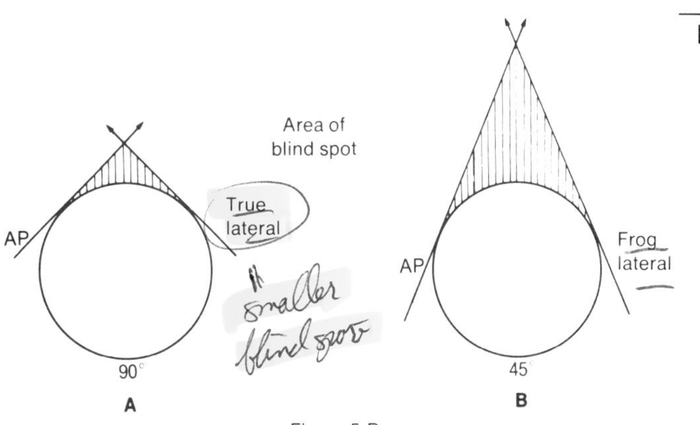

Figure 5-B

Figure 5: (A) The arc of the circle seen on any radiograph projection is the surface of the femoral head where the x-ray beam passes tangential to the surface; that is, the plane passing through the center of the head perpendicular to the x-ray beam. Pin tips not located in these planes and projecting beyond the femoral head can go undetected. (B) Method of estimating the maximum area of blind spot and the magnitude of pin protrusion. Note that although the position for the frog lateral radiograph rotates the femur 90 degrees and creates a plane passing through the femoral head perpendicular to the anteroposterior radiograph plane, A, the tangent of this radiograph to the femoral surface intersects the anteroposterior radiograph at approximately a 45 degree angle, creating a large blind spot, B. (Reprinted with permission from Joint destruction: A sequela of unrecognized pin penetration in patients with slipped capital femoral epiphyses by Walters, et. al., *In* The Hip—Proceedings of the Eighth Open Scientific Meeting of the Hip Society, pp. 148, 151. St. Louis, C.V. Mosby, 1980.)

Slipped Capital Femoral Epiphysis Many biochemical alterations have now been demonstrated in the physeal plate of patients with slipped capital femoral epiphysis. These include increased width of the zone of hypertrophy as well as abnormalities in collagen and proteoglycan concentration and distribution. However, the etiology of these changes remains unknown, and it is not clear whether these changes are primary or secondary.

Slipped capital femoral epiphysis patients usually present with pain in the groin, medial thigh, or knee.

TREATMENT: The primary goal of treatment is prevention of further displacement of the capital femoral epiphysis. This can be accomplished by internal fixation with pins or screws or by epiphysiodesis.

Excellent results have been reported with both techniques. Because of the disadvantages of a more difficult operation and the postoperative spica cast accompanying epiphysiodesis, pin fixation continues to be the most popular technique. As the femoral head is posteriorly displaced, such pinning may necessitate pin insertion through the anterior portion of the neck rather than through the greater trochanteric area. If the pins penetrate into the intra-articular space, there is a higher risk of chondrolysis with subsequent narrowing of the joint space. Therefore, the pins should be placed into the central portion of the epiphysis. The pins should cross the growth plate only far enough to gain fixation and avoid penetration of the articular cartilage. Image intensification allows the surgeon to move the head through a full range of motion under radiographic control to determine that the pins are well placed (Fig. 5). In patients with bilateral slipped capital femoral epiphysis whose hips cannot be positioned satisfactorily to allow radiographic visualization of the femoral heads, open epiphysiodesis should be considered.

Two or three finely threaded Knowles pins, threaded Steinmann pins, or screws approximately 5/64 inch in diameter provide sufficient rigidity for immobilization. The pins should be removed once closure of the growth plate has been radiographically documented. Therefore, pins used should permit removal, preferably having reverse cutting threads. The Craig pin extractor or Knowles pin sleeve can facilitate removal in difficult situations.

In acute slips of the epiphysis it is unclear whether to attempt reduction. Although it is reasonable to use traction or manipulation to return the epiphysis to anatomic position prior to pinning, they have been associated with an increased risk of osteonecrosis, particularly if the slip is overreduced. It usually is preferable to accept the reduction obtained by placing the patient on a fracture table without any specific manipulation other than the traction necessary to straighten the knee after the foot has been secured into place. Osteonecrosis may be the result of damage to the blood supply at the time of the acute slip and not be related to the method of treatment.

Since chronic slips have some capacity for remodeling, fixation in situ generally is recommended. However, primary biplanar osteotomy in the intertrochanteric area may be considered for chronic slips presenting with very severe deformity. Even in these situations pinning in situ is usually performed. Reconstructive osteotomy is possible for patients with severe deformity or with insufficient remodeling after healing. If osteotomy is required, it usually is performed in the intertrochanteric area since osteotomy at a more proximal level (particularly in the subcapital area) is associated with a high incidence of osteonecrosis of the femoral head.

Chondrolysis is manifested clinically by stiffness and a decreased joint space. It most commonly occurs postoperatively but may occur without operation. Therefore, the preoperative patient with a decrease in the range of motion of the hip out of proportion to the degree of slip should be noted. Plain radiographs should demonstrate a normal joint space of approximately 4 to 5 mm. If the joint space is 3 mm or less, chondrolysis may be present. Before proceeding with treatment, it is desirable to counsel the family about the potential long-range problems associated with chondrolysis.

Since chondrolysis is associated with intra-articular pin penetration in as many as 90 percent of patients, it should be suspected whenever persistent postoperative pain is present.

Osteonecrosis presents the most difficult problem in management. If the necrosis is partial (involving less than 50 percent of the femoral head), a valgus osteotomy can occasionally produce a satisfactory hip. However, arthrodesis is usually necessary in these young, active individuals for whom prosthetic arthroplasty is inappropriate.

Idiopathic Chondrolysis Although uncommon, chondrolysis not associated with slipped capital femoral epiphysis is a distinct entity. It occurs primarily in adolescent girls and is characterized by the insidious onset of hip pain and limitation of motion with joint space loss of a variable extent. The cause is believed to be a localized autoimmune response to cartilage. Treatment is directed toward maintaining as much functional range of motion as possible using rest, traction, physical therapy, and non-narcotic analgesics. Reconstruction occasionally may be necessary, and vitallium-mold arthroplasty is a consideration.

Neuromuscular

Myelodysplasia Although paralytic hip deformity and dysplasia in the myelomeningocele patient are common, a completely satisfactory treatment plan has not yet emerged. A concentrically reduced and stable hip with a functional range of motion would seem to be ideal, but to date consistent achievement of this goal has not been possible. In fact, this ideal does not appear to be necessary for optimum function in certain patient groups. These observations have stimulated studies to define the variables affecting patient function (particularly ambulation), define treatment groups, and improve treatment methods.

The most important variable affecting ambulatory function is the level of paralysis. Other important variables include age, obesity, and other musculoskeletal deformities (spine, pelvic obliquity, and lower extremity alignment). There are probably other important factors, such as motivation, that need to be considered when planning treatment for the individual patient.

Most studies have shown that patients who do not have good (4+) quadriceps function have limited long-term ambulatory potential and that the status of hip reduction/subluxation/dislocation does not affect ambulation. However, those patients with a functional range of motion, particularly hip extension, appear to do better than those who do not. Although there is no consensus, many investigators believe that patients with good (4+) quadriceps function have better ambulatory potential if their hips are concentrically reduced and stable, in addition, of course, to having a functional range of motion, particularly full extension.

Patients without good (4+) quadriceps function can be subdivided into a thoracic group with no functional lower extremity motion and an upper lumbar group with variable degrees of hip flexion and adduction strength with or without antigravity (but not more than 3+) quadriceps function. Subluxation and dislocation are uncommon in the thoracic group and common (50 percent or more) in the upper lumbar group. Hip abduction and external rotation deformities are common in the thoracic group, whereas flexion deformity is common in the upper lumbar group. Although the deformity in the two groups differs, the goal is the same: maintenance of a functional range of motion through positioning, therapy, and surgical release without attempting to reduce the subluxated or dislocated hip or hips.

Patients with good (4+) quadriceps function can be subdivided into a lower lumbar level paralysis group with hamstring and occasionally anterior tibial function and a sacral level paralysis group with at least fair (3+) triceps surae function. Hip deformity is very uncommon in the sacral level paralysis group, but when present the treatment principles are the same as those for idiopathic congenital dislocation of the hip. Hip deformity in the lower lumbar level paralysis group is very common (75 percent or more), and it is this group for which treatment of paralytic hip dysplasia is most important.

The principles of hip deformity management in the lower lumbar paralysis group are to maintain or obtain stable concentric reduction, to realign bone deformity that either interferes with stable concentric reduction or that cannot be expected to improve with time, and to balance muscle forces. In addition, suprapelvic obliquity needs to be controlled or corrected.

If a closed reduction or operation is done at an early age, only tendon transfer to obtain better muscle balance may be necessary. Release of the adductor deformity or transfer of the adductors to the ischium has been combined with external abdominal oblique transfer to the greater trochanter to provide abduction force. The iliopsoas can be lengthened to correct deformity and provide better balance in the sagittal plane. An alternative approach to achieve muscle balance is to transfer the iliopsoas through the ilium to the greater trochanter (Sharrard). Since results of this procedure are somewhat unpredictable, many surgeons favor simple tenotomy or advancement to the anterior hip capsule.

In the child over 3 years of age, there is frequently sufficient femoral deformity that upper femoral varus rotational osteotomy as well as tendon transfer should be performed. If these procedures are done early and the hip is concentrically reduced, acetabular remodeling can be expected. In children older than 4 to 5 years of age, acetabular remodeling probably will not occur. In these children, acetabular deformity also may require treatment, usually by pericapsular osteotomy (Pemberton) or innominate osteotomy (Chiari), although the latter may be associated with an increased incidence of posterior subluxation. The former procedure is more appropriate for the younger child, and the latter for the older child. Innominate osteotomy (Salter) is generally inappropriate because the acetabulum is deformed rather than maldirected.

Cerebral Palsy The child with spastic cerebral palsy may develop progressive deformity of the hip with dislocation. The more severe the spastic involvement, the higher the risk for dislocation. Adduction and flexion contractures of the hip may impair walking ability in less spastic patients. Internal rotation deformity due to femoral anteversion or muscle imbalance also may be a significant problem.

Subluxation of the hip may occur in the first few years of life whereas dislocation generally presents at about 4 to 8 years of age and is frequently painful. Other problems may result from or be associated with spastic paralytic hip dislocation, including increased spasticity, impaired sitting balance, pelvic obliquity, and scoliosis. Although ischial skin breakdown may occur, the intact sensation appears to be partially protective, and sitting pressure necrosis occurs infrequently (a distinct difference from the experience with the myelodysplasia patient).

TREATMENT: Principles of treatment are to maintain and obtain concentric reduction, proper joint alignment, and muscle balance.

Correction of an adduction deformity that restricts abduction to less than 40 degrees should be considered. Adductor myotenotomy has been the standard procedure in these patients. Recent studies comparing release with adductor transfer to the ischial tuberosity have reported better results with transfer, particularly in the ambulatory patient. This operation, however, is associated with a somewhat high complication rate and is technically more demanding.

Internal rotation deformity may be treated by posterior transfer of the origin of the internal rotators or rotational osteotomy, either supracondylar, subtrochanteric, or, if a component of varus is to be added, intertrochanteric.

For the child with early evidence of subluxation of the hip, soft-tissue release of the deforming muscular forces should be performed. This includes releasing the necessary adductors to obtain 80 to 85 degrees of passive abduction. To avoid overcorrection, selective release may be necessary and the need for anterior obturator neurectomy requires individual assessment. Neurectomy is performed less frequently now as it may result in overcorrection. Following soft-tissue release, the hips should be concentrically reduced. If, after soft-tissue release, the hips cannot be concentrically reduced but are reduced with abduction and internal rotation, an intertrochanteric varus derotation osteotomy utilizing secure internal fixation is advisable.

When severe subluxation or dislocation is present, the principles of concentric reduction, bony deformity correction, and muscle balance may be satisfied by: (1) open reduction (using an anterolateral approach), (2) an intertrochanteric varus derotation shortening osteotomy of the proximal femur (using a standard lateral approach), (3) pelvic osteotomy, and (4) occasionally myotenotomy. The pericapsular osteotomy (Pemberton) is appropriate up to the time of closure of the triradiate cartilage. In the older patient, innominate osteotomy (Chiari) is an alternative but is associated with problematic posterior subluxation.

Innominate osteotomy (Salter) is generally not recommended as it results in loss of posterior coverage and perhaps in posterior dislocation of the hip.

The completely dislocated hip may present late, near skeletal maturity, or after unsuccessful attempts at maintaining reduction of the hip. These patients have painful, deformed hips which interfere with nursing care. Subtrochanteric resection of the upper femur and suture of a muscle cuff over the resected femur has been reported to be more successful than the original Girdlestone procedure (not a satisfactory procedure for this purpose). Prolonged postoperative skeletal traction may be helpful in allowing the protective soft-tissue cuff to heal adequately and separate the pelvis from the resected end of the femur.

Occasionally, arthrodesis of the hip may be utilized for patients with severe degenerative changes. The position of the hip must be adapted to the patient's function. More extension is appropriate (in the range of 30 to 35 degrees of flexion) in the patient who is ambulatory. If the patient is wheelchair-bound, flexion to 45 or 50 degrees is more desirable. In those who have had a spine fusion as well, flexion must be to 65 to 70 degrees to allow sitting and perineal care.

Infection

Pyogenic arthritis during childhood commonly involves the hip joint. Nearly one-half of the patients are 1 year of age or less, and it is in this group that the poorest results have been reported. This finding seems to be related to the frequency with which diagnosis and treatment is delayed and to the presence of vessels across the epiphyseal plate until 9 to 18 months of age. Although pyogenic arthritis of the hip may be primary, it is probably usually secondary to osteomyelitis of the femoral neck that has decompressed into the hip joint.

Diagnosis involves maintaining a high index of suspicion in the irritable child with limited hip motion. Treatment includes early aspiration followed by surgical drainage (usually posteriorly with either a gravity drain or closed suction) if positive, immobilization (traction or bivalved cast), and appropriate parenteral antibiotics (Table I). In infancy a second antibiotic is necessary because 10 to 30 percent of *H. influenzae* are resistant to ampicillin. Local instillation of antibiotics is no longer considered necessary (see Section 6, General: Infection for the principles of duration of parenteral antibiotic management).

Permanent damage to the epiphysis and epiphyseal plate may occur. It has recently been recognized that the triradiate cartilage may be damaged as well.

Osteomyelitis of the ilium and septic arthritis of the sacroiliac joint are uncommon. Diagnosis is often delayed. Early diagnosis may be made with a high index of suspicion, technetium bone scan, and aspiration of the involved area utilizing fluoroscopic guidance. *Staphylococcus aureus* is the most common organism, and appropriate intravenous antibiotic treatment is usually effective.

Trauma

Pelvic Fractures For a discussion of pelvic fractures, see Section 31, Pelvis and Acetabulum: Trauma.

Traumatic Dislocation Traumatic dislocation of the hip in children requires less force than in adults. Manipulative reduction and Buck's traction for approximately 2 weeks, followed by avoidance of hip flexion and adduction, is usually satisfactory treatment. Open reduction is indicated either when a stable closed reduction cannot be achieved and maintained or in the presence of bone fragments in the hip joint (as visualized by plain radiography and/or computed tomography). Sciatic nerve injury occurs somewhat less frequently than in the adult.

Posterior dislocation in association with ipsilateral femoral fracture may not be apparent. Most are amenable to closed reduction with conventional methods of management of the femoral fracture.

Traumatic anterior dislocation is less common than posterior and has a higher complication rate. Closed treatment is usually possible.

Hip Fractures Fractures of the hip in children are rare, usually result from severe trauma, and frequently present with associated injuries. Unlike most other fractures in children, complications are common. Because of the

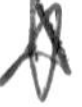

Table I
Etiology and Initial Treatment of Septic Arthritis From Birth Through Childhood**

Clinical conditions	Etiology	Initial Therapy
Septic arthritis, neonatal	*S. aureus*, coliform bacilli	Methicillin 100-150 mg/kg/day I.V. in 2 or 3 doses *and* gentamicin 5-7.5 mg/kg/day I.M. in 2 or 3 doses
Septic arthritis, infancy	*H. influenzae*	Ampicillin 150 mg/kg/day I.V. in 4 doses *plus* chloramphenicol* 100 mg/kg/day in 4 doses
Septic arthritis, childhood	*S. aureus*, Group A Streptococcus, gonococcus	Nafcillin 150 mg/kg/day I.V. in 4 doses
Septic arthritis	Unknown etiology	Nafcillin and chloramphenicol* until cultures available

*Chloramphenicol may be substituted by 2nd generation cephalosporins (e.g., cefamandole, cefuroxime) or 3rd generation cephalosporins (e.g., moxalactam).
**Courtesy Cheng T. Cho, M.D., Kansas City, Kansas.

tenuous blood supply to the femoral head, there is a high incidence of osteonecrosis. Malunion (usually coxa vara), nonunion, and growth disturbance are among the other complications.

Treatment principles for adult hip fractures do not apply to pediatric patients because of the significant anatomic and physiological differences. Children have denser bone which, although it holds a fixation device well, is more difficult to penetrate. The epiphyseal plate allows for remodeling but is prone to early closure after fracture. Finally, the small diameter of the femoral neck limits the number and size of fixation devices that may be introduced.

Recommendations for treatment depend upon the type of femoral neck fracture. For the transepiphyseal fracture, closed reduction and internal fixation are recommended. If the femoral head fragment is dislocated, open reduction and internal fixation with smooth pins should be performed. In this instance the incidence of osteonecrosis approaches 100 percent. For the displaced or nondisplaced transcervical fracture, closed reduction and internal fixation generally are recommended to prevent the complications of coxa vara and nonunion. Supplemental spica cast immobilization for 4 to 6 weeks is recommended. Osteonecrosis occurs in 15 to 50 percent of these patients. The nondisplaced base of neck fracture may be treated in a spica cast whereas the displaced should be treated as is the transcervical fracture. The intertrochanteric fracture usually can be treated with traction and spica cast immobilization.

Osteonecrosis is the major complication occurring in 30 to 50 percent of patients. The incidence of osteonecrosis rises in children over 8 years of age and with severe displacement. Unfortunately, there is no satisfactory method of preventing this complication.

Premature epiphyseal plate closure may occur in 15 to 60 percent of patients (see Section 34, Knee and Leg: Pediatric for treatment principles). Coxa vara occurs in 20 to 30 percent of patients and frequently can be prevented by accurate reduction and internal fixation. Remodeling tends to occur in a high percentage of patients even though the neck shaft angle may be temporarily reduced. One to 2 years should elapse before considering valgus osteotomy.

Nonunion is unusual but may occur due to loss of reduction in a spica cast or with poor initial reduction and fixation. Treatment usually involves subtrochanteric osteotomy with or without bone graft to the nonunion. Nonunion is frequently accompanied by osteonecrosis and/or premature plate closure.

Other complications that may possibly occur include coxa valga and shortening of the extremity.

Femoral Shaft Fractures Femoral shaft fractures in children generally can be treated closed. Immediate spica cast application has been advocated recently for the uncomplicated femoral shaft fracture in a child younger than approximately 7 to 10 years. To assess the patient for possible accompanying injuries, a period of traction may be appropriate prior to cast application.

Reduction prior to spica application is facilitated by general anesthesia, and radiographic control with an image intensifier is beneficial. A 1½ spica cast is utilized with the limbs abducted to 30 degrees and externally rotated 20 to 30 degrees with flexion of a variable amount depending upon the level of the fracture. The thigh portion is applied first, utilizing the principles of total contact (over a stockinette or a fracture brace liner) and three-point molding. Alignment should be checked on a regular basis throughout the cast period of approximately 8 weeks.

In the child older than approximately 10 years, distal femoral traction with a skeletal pin inserted proximal to the epiphysis is necessary. Spica cast application generally should be delayed for 2 to 3 weeks until early callus formation and stability develop. Angulation in plaster as well as shortening are more common in this group.

Internal fixation may be considered in the older child approaching skeletal maturity or the child with multiple injuries, particularly head injury. In involved children older than 10 years, intramedullary fixation carries only a small risk of disturbance of growth of the greater trochanter. For the patient with decerebrate rigidity or with frequent seizures, the internal fixation stabilizes the femur and aids treatment of the other problems.

Late problems of limb length inequality due to overgrowth are well recognized. In children younger than 6 to 7 years, 1 cm of overriding in reduction of the fractures is ideal. Rotation alignment of the fracture fragments should also be carefully evaluated to prevent an external rotation deformity.

ANNOTATED BIBLIOGRAPHY

Congenital and Developmental

Increased Femoral Anteversion

Ogata, K., and Goldsand, E.M.: A simple biplanar method of measuring femoral anteversion and neck-shaft angle. J. Bone Joint Surg. 61A:846-851, 1979.

A technique allowing calculation of both the true coronal and horizontal plane alignment of the femoral neck and proximal femoral shaft is described. Anteroposterior and lateral radiographs are obtained utilizing positioning techniques not requiring special equipment.

Staheli, L.T.; Clawson, D.K.; and Hubbard, D.D.: Medial femoral torsion: Experience with operative treatment. Clin. Orthop. 146:222-225, 1980.

Seventy-eight patients were reviewed who had femoral derotational osteotomy for increased anteversion. Complications were frequent (15 percent). There is a lack of evidence for any long-term adverse effects if moderate medial femoral torsion is uncorrected.

Congenital Dislocation of the Hip

Kalamchi, A., and MacEwen, G.D.: Avascular necrosis following treatment of congenital dislocation of the hip. J. Bone Joint Surg. 62A:876-888, 1980.

One hundred and nineteen patients with osteonecrosis were reviewed in an attempt to identify factors of prognostic significance. Changes confined to the ossific nucleus were of little long-term significance. In contrast, changes in the physis were pivotal in predicting residual deformity. Greater trochanteric overgrowth, limb length inequality, and varus/valgus inclination of the neck shaft angle may result. Preliminary traction not only reduces the incidence but also the severity of osteonecrosis. The child under 6 months of age is at higher risk for osteonecrosis than the older child.

Kalamchi, A., and McFarlane, R., III: The Pavlik harness: Results in patients over 3 months of age. J. Pediat. Orthop. 2:3-8, 1982.

One hundred and twelve patients with 114 dysplastic subluxated hips and twenty-five dislocated hips were reviewed. All those whose hips reduced upon initial application of the harness developed satisfactory hips with 3 months full-time and 1½ months part-time wear. Five of twenty-five dislocated hips did not reduce in the harness. Those that did reduce were treated for an average of 8 months.

Lindstrom, J.R.; Ponseti, I.V.; and Wenger, D.R.: Acetabular development after reduction in congenital dislocation of the hip. J. Bone Joint Surg. 61A:112-118, 1979.

In 148 patients with 185 dysplastic hips, the acetabular index improved for 2 to 8 years after reduction. Therefore, reconstructive acetabular procedures can be delayed until the normal acetabular developmental process has ceased.

MacKenzie, I.G., and Wilson, J.G.: Problems encountered in the early diagnosis and management of congenital dislocation of the hip. J. Bone Joint Surg. 63B:38-42, 1981.

Of 53,033 infants screened for congenital dislocated hip, 0.11 percent of live births were not diagnosed at neonatal examination.

Mubarak, S.; Garfin, S.; Vance, R.; McKinnon, B.; and Sutherland, D.: Pitfalls in the use of the Pavlik harness for treatment of congenital dysplasia, subluxation, and dislocation of the hip. J. Bone Joint Surg. 63A:1239-1248, 1981.

Eighteen infants were reviewed who had problems with the Pavlik harness including: failure to obtain reduction (12); poor quality harness (9); and poor compliance (6). Proper construction of the Pavlik harness consists of straps which cross in the back, the anterior (flexion) buckle at the anterior axillary line, the posterior (abduction) buckle over the scapula, and Velcro for the leg strap located just below the popliteal fossa.

Renshaw, T.S.: Inadequate reduction of congenital dislocation of the hip. J. Bone Joint Surg. 63A:1114-1121, 1981.

After being held in an appropriate position for 2½ months, eleven patients had persistent hip lateralization. Arthrography was used to confirm the lack of concentric reduction. Open reduction is necessary when there is lack of concentric reduction.

Westin, G.W.; Dallas, T.G.; and Watanabe, B.M.: Skeletal traction versus femoral shortening in treatment of older children with congenital hip dislocation. Isr. J. Med. Sci. 16:318-322, 1980.

Treatment methods in the older child were compared. Osteonecrosis was found in 57 percent of the skeletal traction group (thirty hips in twenty-two patients), whereas none were found in the open reduction, femoral shortening group (seventeen hips in twelve patients).

Weinstein, S.L., and Ponseti, I.V.: Congenital dislocation of the hip: Open reduction through a medial approach. J. Bone Joint Surg. 61A:119-124, 1979.

In twenty treated hips of sixteen patients (1 day to 32 months of age), two developed osteonecrosis and two subluxated (one requiring operation). The acetabular index improved rapidly during the first year after reduction and at a slower rate after that.

White, R.E., Jr., and Sherman, F.C.: The hip-shelf procedure. A long-term evaluation. J. Bone Joint Surg. 62A:928-932, 1980.

Poor long-term results (pain in fifteen of twenty-two patients) were found in patients treated with this procedure.

Irritable Hip Syndrome

Sharwood, P.F.: The irritable hip syndrome in children. A long-term follow-up. Acta Orthop. Scand. 52:633-636, 1981.

One hundred and one children were seen between 1962 and 1972 with irritable hip syndrome. Radiologic changes were found in four patients at follow-up. Two of these four were considered to be incidental findings. One patient with Perthes' disease and one with coxa magna were found.

Legg-Calvé-Perthes Disease

Calver, R.; Venugopal, V.; Dorgan, J.; Bentley, G.; and Gimlette, T.: Radionuclide scanning in the early diagnosis of Perthes' disease. J. Bone Joint Surg. 63B:379-382, 1981.

Fifty children with irritable hips and normal plain radiographs had bone scans, five of whom were found to have ischemia. All five later developed Perthes' disease.

Catterall, A.: Legg-Calvé-Perthes syndrome. Clin. Orthop. 158:41-52, 1981.

This review emphasizes radiographic evaluation of the hip and the current indications for treatment.

Green, N.E., and Griffin, P.P.: Intra-osseous venous pressure in Legg-Perthes disease. J. Bone Joint Surg. 64A:666-671, 1982.

Twenty-three patients with Perthes' disease and twenty-three controls were studied. An abnormal venous drainage pattern was demonstrated in the Perthes' disease patients. The authors believed that this may aid in early diagnosis.

Harrison, M.H.M., and Burwell, R.G.: Perthes' disease: A concept of pathogenesis. Clin. Orthop. 156:115-127, 1981.

The authors hypothesize that Legg-Perthes' disease is a force oriented hip lesion predisposed to by a constitutional defect of growing bone. Observation supporting this hypothesis includes skeletal immaturity, disproportionate growth patterns, elevated levels of somatomedin, and frequency of abnormalities in the contralateral hip.

Kehl, D.K., and Coleman, S.S.: An evaluation of Perthes' disease: Comparison of nonsurgical and surgical treatment. Orthop. Trans. 5:407, 1981.

Of nintey-six hips with Catterall class III and IV involvement studied after skeletal maturity, better radiographic and functional results were found in contained than noncontained hips. Radiographic results were comparable for nonoperatively and operatively (Salter innominate osteotomy) contained hips, but functional results were better following nonoperative containment.

Kleinman, R.G., and Bleck, E.E.: Increased blood viscosity in patients with Legg-Perthes' disease: A preliminary report. J. Pediat. Orthop. 1:131-136, 1981.

Twenty-two patients with Legg-Perthes' disease were found to have significantly increased blood viscosity when compared to twenty-one control subjects. Diminished blood flow of the capital femoral epiphysis is proposed as a mechanism of pathogenesis of this disease.

Sutherland, A.D.; Savage, J.P.; Paterson, D.C.; and Foster, B.K.: The nuclide bone-scan in the diagnosis and management of Perthes' disease. J. Bone Joint Surg. 62B:300-306, 1980.

Scans were found to have a greater sensitivity and specificity than plain radiographs in the diagnosis of Perthes' disease.

Thompson, G.H., and Westin, G.W.: Legg-Calvé-Perthes disease: Results of discontinuing treatment in the early reossification phase. Clin. Orthop. 139:70-80, 1979.

Eighty-one consecutively treated patients with Perthes' disease had their treatment discontinued when there was evidence of subchondral reossification. This was compared to another group treated until complete reossification was present. Discontinuance with early reossification did not compromise the result.

Van Dam, B.E.; Crider, R.J.; Noyes, J.D.; and Larsen, L.J.: Determination of the Catterall classification in Legg-Calvé-Perthes disease. J. Bone Joint Surg. 63A:906-914, 1981.

Of fifty hips, twenty (40 percent) changed Catterall classification before entering the fragmentation stage. After entering the fragmentation stage, only three (6 percent) changed classification.

Wynne-Davies, R.: Some etiologic factors in Perthes' disease. Clin. Orthop. 150:12-15, 1980.

The role of the environment in the etiology of Perthes' disease was studied. Socioeconomically deprived children, those born breech, and born to older parents are at increased risk. Delayed growth and skeletal maturation are often present at the time of diagnosis. There is no evidence for genetic factors in most patients.

Slipped Capital Femoral Epiphysis

Bishop, J.O.; Oley, T.J.; Stephenson, C.T.; and Tullos, H.S.: Slipped capital femoral epiphysis. A study of 50 cases in black children. Clin. Orthop. 135:93-96, 1978.

Fifty black children with seventy involved hips developed chondrolysis in 6 percent, all related to pin penetration. Osteonecrosis occurred in 7 percent, all after valgus reduction of an acute slip.

Boyer, D.W.; Mickelson, M.R.; and Ponseti, I.V.: Slipped capital femoral epiphysis: Long-term follow-up study of 121 patients. J. Bone Joint Surg. 63A:85-95, 1981.

This is perhaps the largest long-term follow-up (21-47 years) of patients with this problem. Satisfactory results were obtained with in situ fixation, even with severe slips. The risk of osteonecrosis was greatest for hips reduced by manipulation more than 3 weeks after slippage (eleven of twenty-six).

Ippolito, E.; Mickelson, M.R.; and Ponseti, I.V.: A histochemical study of slipped capital femoral epiphysis. J. Bone Joint Surg. 63A:1109-1113, 1981.

The slipped epiphysis has a normal resting zone but abnormal proliferative (loose and fibrilated, increased proteoglycans) and hypotrophic (disarrayed and thickened, increased structural glycoprotein) zones, through which the slippage occurs. Enchondral ossification was disturbed and the metaphysis contained many large uncalcified cartilage columns.

Melby, A.; Hoyt, W.A.; and Weiner, D.S.: Treatment of chronic slipped capital femoral epiphysis by bone graft epiphysiodesis. Orthop. Trans. 2:209, 1978.

In a series of 106 hips there was no cartilage necrosis or osteonecrosis. Graft resporption, with or without slip progression occurred in 4 percent.

O'Brien, E.T., and Fahey, J.T.: Remodeling of the femoral neck after in situ pinning for slipped capital femoral epiphysis. J. Bone Joint Surg. 59A:62-68, 1977.

Sixty-two patients followed over a 36-year period had in situ pinning as their only treatment. Two failed to remodel. These two patients had closure of the triradiate cartilage at the time of their slip.

Walters, R., and Simon, S.R.: Joint destruction: A sequelae of unrecognized pin penetrations in patients with slipped capital femoral epiphysis. *In* The Hip—Proceedings of the Eighth Open Scientific Meeting of the Hip Society, pp. 145-164. St. Louis, C.V. Mosby, 1980.

One hundred and two patients with grade I and II slips whose plain intra- and postoperative radiographs were considered to show no pin penetration were studied. Upon review, 10 percent were found to have evidence of penetration, usually noted only on a single view. When the "true distance" was calculated, using methods described in this article, only forty of 102 were found to have all pins located safely within the femoral head. Forty penetrated 5 mm less and had a 35 percent incidence of chondrolysis at follow-up. Twenty-two had greater than 5 mm of pin penetration and a 77 percent incidence of chondrolysis at follow-up.

Idiopathic Chondrolysis

Duncan, J.W.; Nasca, R.; and Schrantz, J.: Idiopathic chondrolysis of the hip. J. Bone Joint Surg. 61A:1024-1028, 1979.

The article is a report of eight patients (9 hips) and a review of the literature.

Neuromuscular

Myelodysplasia

Drummond, D.S.; Moreau, M.; and Cruess, R.L.: The results and complications of surgery for the paralytic hip and spine in myelomeningocele. J. Bone Joint Surg. 62B:49-53, 1980.

Forty patients were reviewed who had had at least one major procedure to correct a deformed spine or hip. Sixty-nine operations were done on twenty-seven patients to stabilize the hips. Stability was achieved in 69 percent (sixteen of twenty-three). Walking ability improved in 26 percent (six of twenty-three). Poor motor function in those with lesions at L3 or above were associated with a poor prognosis. In contrast thirty-eight operations were carried out on eighteen patients to stabilize the spine. Stability was achieved in all.

Menelaus, M.B.: The Orthopaedic Management of Spina Bifida Cystica. Ed. 2, pp. 125-152. New York, Churchill Livingstone, 1980.

A comprehensive program of hip deformity management is presented. The importance of maintaining motion, especially extension, is emphasized.

Sherk, H.H., and Ames, M.D.: Functional results of iliopsoas transfer in myelomeningocele hip dislocations. Clin. Orthop. 137:181-186, 1978.

Paralytic hip dislocations in thirty-seven patients were reviewed. At follow-up less than one-half were community ambulators and had maintained reductions. Ambulatory potential is more related to the level of the spinal lesion, alignment of the lower extremities and trunk, and the presence of scoliosis and/or pelvic obliquity than to the status of hip reduction.

Yngve, D.A., and Lindseth, R.E.: Effectiveness of muscle transfers in myelomeningocele hips measured by radiographic indices. J. Pediat. Orthop. 2:121-125, 1982.

In a study of thirty-five lower lumbar level paralysis patients, best results were obtained following combined abductor and adductor procedures.

Cerebral Palsy

Castle, M.E., and Schneider, C.: Proximal femoral resection-interposition arthroplasty. J. Bone Joint Surg. 60A:1051-1054, 1978.

Fourteen dislocated hips in twelve severely mentally retarded and physically handicapped patients were treated with this procedure. The results were satisfactory in all, as opposed to three patients treated by femoral head and neck resection, where results were universally unsatisfactory.

Root, L., and Spero, C.R.: Hip adductor transfer compared with adductor tenotomy in cerebral palsy. J. Bone Joint Surg. 63A:767-772, 1981.

In a 10-year study on two groups of patients, fifty patients with ninety-eight adductor transfers were compared with fifty-two patients with 102 adductor tenotomies and/or obturator neurectomies. Overall improvement was considered greater and better maintained in the transfer group. In addition, the transfer was believed to provide greater hip stability and decreased hip flexion contracture.

Infection

Beaupré, A., and Carroll, N.: The three syndromes of iliac osteomyelitis in children. J. Bone Joint Surg. 61A:1087-1092, 1979.

Of 867 children with hematogenous osteomyelitis, twenty (2.3 percent) had involvement of the ilium. The three syndromes were: (1) gluteal buttock pain, (2) abdominal signs and symptoms similar to acute appendicitis; (3) lumbar disc back, hip, and thigh pain. Direct palpation can clinically localize the affected area. Technetium bone scans are useful for early diagnosis and localization. With early diagnosis, intravenous antibiotic treatment alone was found to be effective.

Jackson, M.A., and Nelson, J.D.: Etiology and medical management of acute suppurative bone and joint infections in pediatric patients. J. Pediat. Orthop. 2:313-323, 1982.

This review is based on experience with 471 patients over a 26-year period. The hip joint had the highest incidence of significant sequelae (40 percent). Medical aspects are discussed.

Schaad, U.B.; McCracken, G.H., Jr.; and Nelson, J.D.: Pyogenic arthritis of the sacroiliac joint in pediatric patients. Pediatrics 66:375-379, 1980.

Seventy-seven pediatric patients with septic sacroiliac joints were found to have an average 3.9-week delay in diagnosis. A subacute onset was seen in two-thirds. *Staphylococcus aureus* was the most common organism.

Wientroub, S.; Lloyd-Roberts, G.C.; and Fraser, M.: The prognostic significance of the triradiate cartilage in suppurative arthritis of the hip in infancy and early childhood. J. Bone Joint Surg. 63B:190-193, 1981.

In thirty-one children who had suppurative arthritis of the hip, the extent of damage to the femoral head correlated with the presence of narrowing and premature closure of the triradiate cartilage.

Trauma

Traumatic Dislocation

Barquet, A.: Traumatic anterior dislocation of the hip in childhood. Injury 13:435-440, 1982.

One hundred and eleven patients from the literature and four new patients were reviewed. This injury is more severe and has a higher complication rate than posterior dislocation.

Hip Fractures

Canale, S.T.: Traumatic dislocations and fracture-dislocation of the hips in children. *In* The Hip—Proceedings of the Ninth Open Scientific Meeting of the Hip Society, pp. 219-245. St. Louis, C.V. Mosby, 1981.

Dislocation and fracture-dislocation of the hip in the child are reviewed and compared to adults with regard to their complication rate. Management principles are similar to the adult's. Poor results in children are related to delay in reduction, severe trauma, and incongruous reduction. The major causes of poor results are osteonecrosis and myositis ossificans.

Femoral Shaft Fractures

Allen, B.L., Jr.; Schoch, E.P., III; and Emery, F.E.: Immediate spica cast system for femoral shaft fractures in infants and children. Southern. Med. J. 71:18-22, 1978.

Fifty-three children age 3 weeks to 14 years were treated for fifty-five fractures. Rereduction was necessary in two. Healing in satisfactory position was routinely obtained and at a large saving in cost.

Reynolds, D.A.: Growth changes in fractured long-bones: A study of 126 children. J. Bone Joint Surg. 63B:83-88, 1981.

The growth acceleration in the affected tibia and femur following fracture lasted from 40 to 60 months with most occurring during the first 18 to 24 months.

Staheli, L.T., and Sheridan, G.W.: Early spica cast management of femoral shaft fractures in young children. Clin. Orthop. 126:162-166, 1977.

Twenty patients aged 4 months to 8 years were reviewed with a minimal follow-up of 17 months. Limb length discrepancy did not exceed 7 mm. Angulation exceeded 10 degrees in two patients. Anteversion varied 10 to 20 degrees in five patients from the unaffected side.

LAWRENCE A. VIERRA, M.C.
557-66-7688

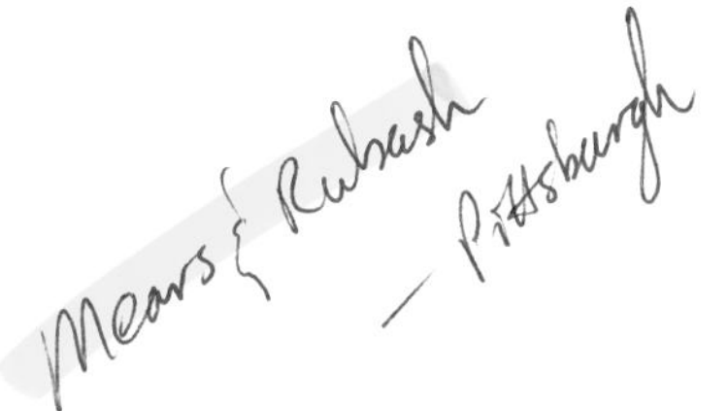

31 PELVIS AND ACETABULUM: TRAUMA

This section deals with the pathophysiology, evaluation, and treatment of pelvic injuries, acetabular fractures, and acetabular and pelvic ring disruptions in both adults and children.

Pelvic Injuries

The *pelvic ring* provides osseous protection for certain intra-abdominal viscera, an effective support for the transmission of weight-bearing forces between the spine and the lower extremities, and anchorage for muscular attachments to the trunk and lower extremities. The pelvic ring consists of two identical hemipelves, composed of the ilium, ischium, and pubis. The anterior aspects of the hemipelves are bridged by a fibrocartilaginous pubic symphysis whereas the posterior hemipelves are spanned by the bony sacrum. Each sacroiliac joint is a diarthrodial joint surrounded by small anterior and dense posterior ligamentous attachments. The posterior sacroiliac ligaments originate broadly from the posterosuperior iliac spine to the posteroinferior iliac spine and fan out obliquely to attach to the lateral sacral crest. The anterior and especially the posterior sacroiliac ligaments provide crucial stabilization for the posterior weight-bearing portion of the pelvic ring. Supplementary sacrospinous and sacrotuberous ligaments extend from the spinous processes and ischial tuberosities posteriorly to the ventral surface of the sacrum. They provide a sling to support the posterior aspect of the pelvic floor.

The close proximity of the intrapelvic viscera, major vessels, and nerves accounts for the complexity of the soft-tissue injuries which frequently complicate pelvic fractures.

The remainder of the pelvic ring is the hemispherical socket or *acetabulum* which articulates with the femoral head. The acetabulum is characterized by two osseous columns: an anterior one which extends from the pubic rami to the articular surface; and a posterior one which courses from the posterior ilium and "dome," or superior weight-bearing portion of the acetabulum, to the ischium. A fibrous capsule originates around the periphery of the acetabular rim and inserts around the base of the femoral neck.

Pathophysiology The nature of a *pelvic fracture* is determined largely by the magnitude and direction of the provocative force. Following a relatively mild injury (e.g., a simple fall, especially in an osteoporotic or elderly individual), a stable, impacted ramus fracture may ensue. Indirect injuries such as avulsion fractures at the sites of principal muscular attachments are documented frequently in athletes. Most serious disruptions of the pelvis, however, are caused by motor vehicle accidents, industrial injuries, or falls from heights. These injuries are characterized by two or more fractures of the pelvic ring and may be classified as stable or unstable. Acetabular fractures form a special group which may occur in isolation or as part of a pelvic ring disruption.

A classification system for pelvic fractures has been devised which is based upon the direction of the provocative force and the degree of instability of the traumatized pelvic ring. Both clinically and radiographically a pelvic fracture may be categorized as an anteroposterior compression injury, a lateral compression injury, or a vertical shear fracture. Most anteroposterior compression injuries result from a blow to the posterior ilium which creates a diastasis of the symphysis pubis. The anterior sacroiliac ligaments of one or occasionally both sacroiliac joints are disrupted although usually the important posterior sacroiliac ligamentous complex is spared. When the posterior ligamentous complex is preserved, this injury is defined as a stable disruption. In a small percentage of these anteroposterior injuries (i.e., in probably less than 10 percent of patients) the posterior ligamentous complex is violated, producing an unstable hemipelvis.

A lateral compression injury arising from a direct lateral blow to the ilium may cause a stable, impacted fracture of the sacrum or rarely the adjacent ilium. However, with an anterolateral or posterolateral force the traumatized hemipelvis usually rotates with disruption of the posterior bony elements or of the crucial posterior ligamentous complex across the ipsilateral sacroiliac joint. Usually the contralateral rami are fractured, although not infrequently the ipsilateral rami or all four rami are disrupted. These disruptions are identified as unstable lateral compression injuries. Both a stable and an unstable lateral compression injury can be complicated by an acetabular fracture.

All vertical shear injuries are unstable and show evidence of posterior ligamentous instability. Most of these injuries are caused by a fall from a height, which disrupts the symphysis pubis and one or both sacroiliac joints. Both the unstable lateral and vertical shear injuries usually present with other types of ligamentous disruptions in the pelvic floor or the base of the spine (e.g., avulsion of the sacrotuberous or sacrospinous ligaments or the lumbosacral ligaments from the transverse processes of L4 or L5). Recognition of the degree of pelvic instability determines the type of treatment for each category of pelvic fracture.

Acetabular injuries can arise from the application of direct or indirect forces. A direct lateral blow to the greater trochanter can provoke a lateral compression pelvic ring fracture and/or a transverse acetabular fracture with displacement of the medial wall. Alternatively, a force can be transmitted indirectly through the lower extremity (i.e., the foot or knee joint). The vector of the force transmitted from the femoral head to the acetabulum and, therefore, the region of the acetabular disruption are determined by the position of the femur and the hip joint at the moment of impact. The magnitude of the impact as well as the direction of the provocative force through the proximal femur and acetabulum determine the specific pattern of acetabular fracture and the degree of comminution. A blow to the flexed knee with the knee and hip flexed at 90 degrees creates a fracture pattern similar to that initiated by a blow to the plantar surface of the foot when the knee is extended and the hip is flexed to 90 degrees.

Patient Management

Associated Injuries and Acute Resuscitation

ASSOCIATED INJURIES: With the large amount of force required to provoke a disruption of the *pelvic ring*, it is not surprising that a patient who sustains such an insult frequently presents with other serious or life-threatening injuries. The remainder of the musculoskeletal system (85 percent) and the respiratory system (65 percent) most often have associated injuries. These are followed in frequency by injury to the central nervous system (40 percent), gastrointestinal system (30 percent), and genitourinary system (12 percent). Management of the patient with a pelvic fracture requires careful planning to treat both the musculoskeletal injury and other major systemic disruptions. Uncontrolled hemorrhage and pulmonary disorders are the most serious complications that arise as immediate and delayed complications. In a series of patients with closed pelvic ring fractures, the mortality ranged between 10 and 20 percent. In an open pelvic fracture (where the fracture site communicates with the vagina, rectum, bladder, urethra, or a cutaneous laceration), the anticipated mortality may approach 40 or 50 percent with hemorrhage as the major initial cause of death. In addition, the potential for bacterial contamination of the fracture site from the intestinal tract, genitourinary tract, and skin is considerable. Sepsis is a major late complication.

From the discussion of the injuries that accompany pelvic ring fractures it is not surprising that numerous associated injuries of the abdomen, thorax, spine, and central nervous system and a large retroperitoneal hematoma frequently complicate disruption of the *acetabulum.* However, although injury to a major intrapelvic vessel frequently complicates a pelvic ring fracture, this catastrophe is uncommonly associated with an acetabular fracture. The only common vascular insult to accompany acetabular fractures is injury to the superior gluteal artery in the presence of a posterior column fracture. In addition to macroscopic and microscopic injury to the femoral head and the capsule of the hip joint, associated fractures of the ipsilateral lower extremity are common. A posterior or central dislocation of the femoral head requires a closed or open reduction on an emergency basis. In this instance, the femoral head is relocated under the undisplaced iliac portion of the fractured acetabulum. A closed reduction is provisionally stabilized with skeletal traction until the adequacy of the reduction can be ascertained. Injury to the sciatic nerve has been recorded in association with up to 12 percent of acetabular fractures. Posterior fracture dislocations of the femoral head are particularly likely to result in injuries to the nerve which can also be injured by bony fragment impalement or by adjacent hematoma. A careful evaluation of the neurologic function of the ipsilateral extremity is necessary. In the presence of sciatic nerve dysfunction, an operative approach to the acetabulum includes examination of the proximal portion of sciatic nerve and possible removal of impaling bony fragments and neurolysis.

ACUTE RESUSCITATION: As a part of the initial evaluation of the patient who sustains a pelvic or acetabular fracture, consideration of the potential for massive hemorrhage is very important as this is responsible for fatalities. Blood loss following a pelvic fracture may range from 2 to 20, or even 80 units. Average blood loss of 20 to 30 units has been documented in patients who die in the immediate posttraumatic period.

Initial treatment protocol includes volume resuscitation by the use of suitable intravenous fluids (Fig. 1). At the accident the paramedic team is advised to apply a MAST (military antishock trousers) suit to an unstable, bleeding patient. The MAST suit increases cardiac output by the supplementation of venous return to the heart. Immobilization of the pelvic fracture may prevent further damage to the retroperitoneal tissues by sharp bony fragments. Such external compression of the pelvic ring impacts bone fragments against one another and retards bleeding from cancellous bone. It may also partly reduce the pelvic fracture and, thereby, decrease the intrapelvic volume so that effective tamponade of the retroperitoneal hematoma is achieved with the smallest size of blood clot.

Once the patient arrives in the emergency department,

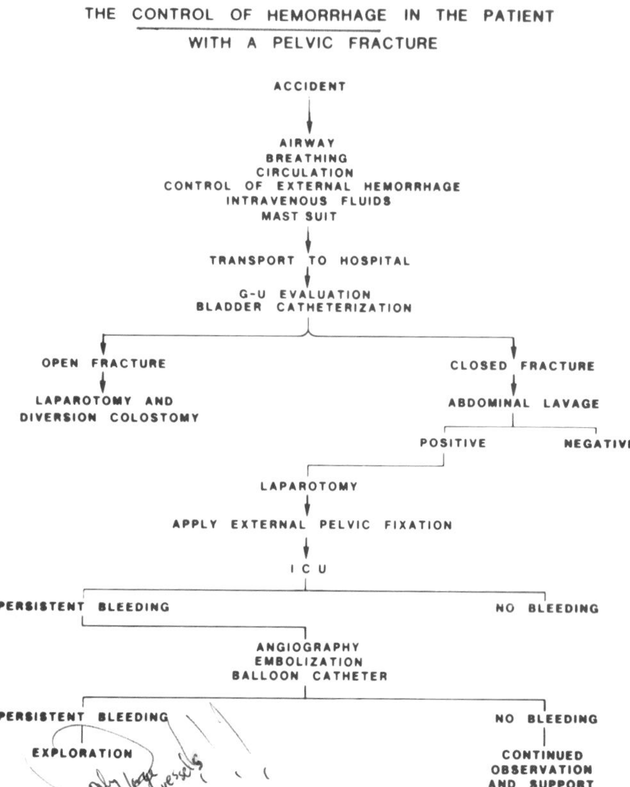

Figure 1: The control of hemorrhage in the patient with a pelvic fracture.

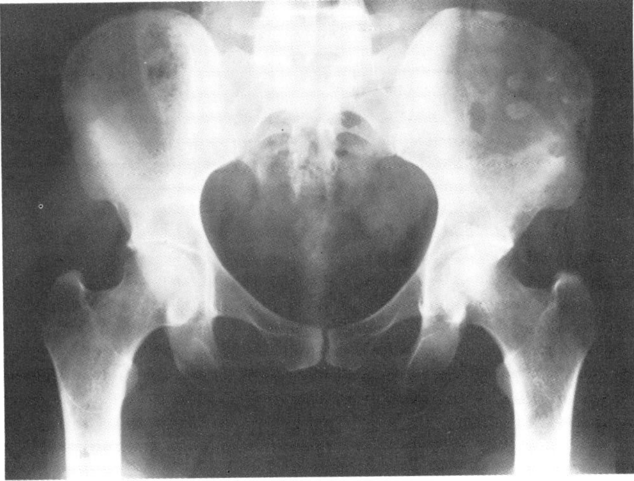

Figure 2-A

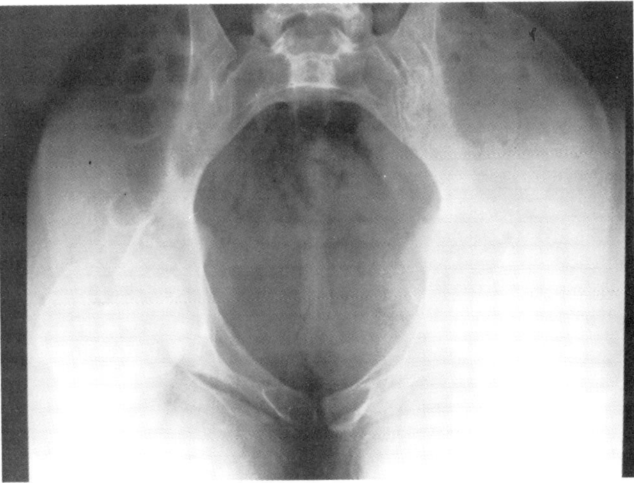

Figure 2-B

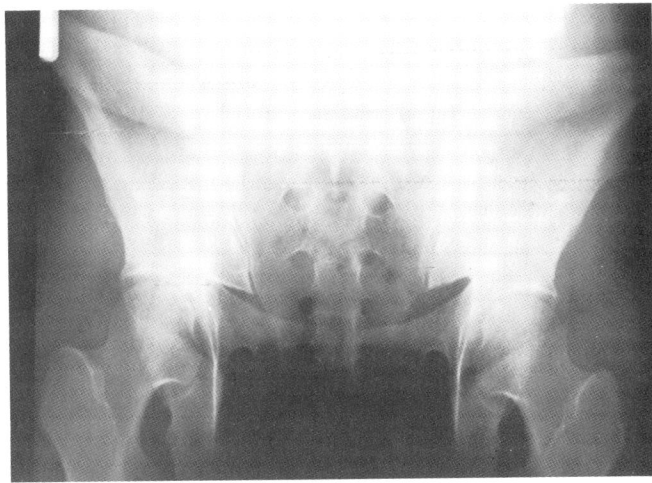

Figure 2-C

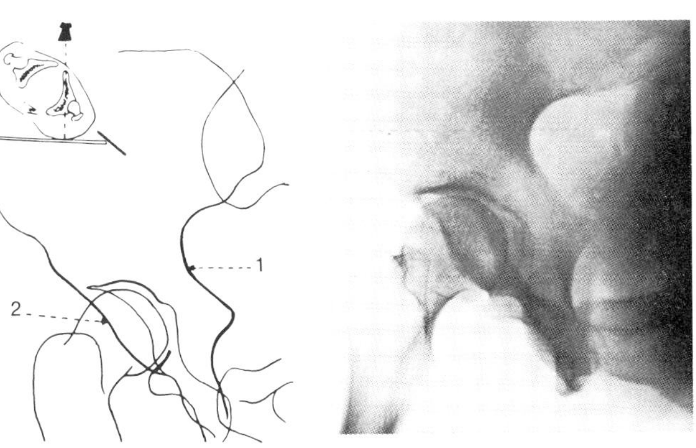

Figure 2-D

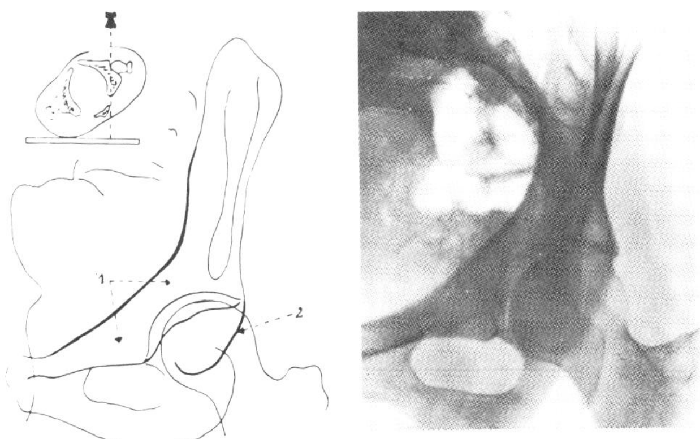

Figure 2-E

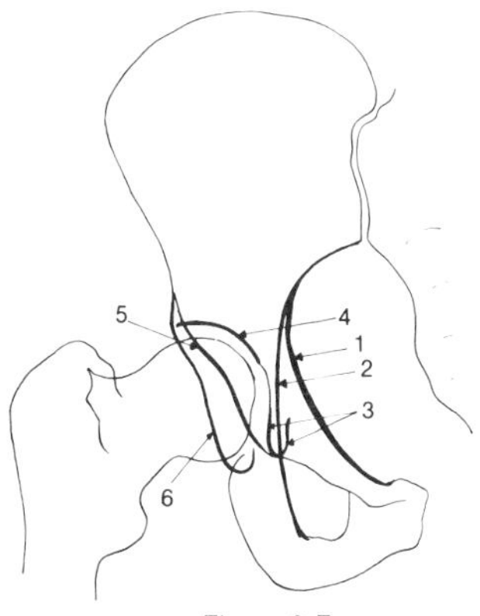

Figure 2-F

Figure 2: Standard radiographic views of the pelvis. (A) Anteroposterior view. (B) Inlet view. (C) Outlet view. (D) Iliac oblique view. (1) Posterior border of the pelvic bone. (2) Anterior edge of acetabulum. (E) Obturator oblique view. (1) Anterior column and superior pubic ramus. (2) Posterior edge of acetabulum. (F) Radiographic features of anteroposterior acetabular view. (1) Brim of true pelvis. (2) Ilioischial line. (3) Teardrop. (4) Roof. (5) Anterior border of acetabulum. (6) Posterior border of acetabulum.

Figure 3-A

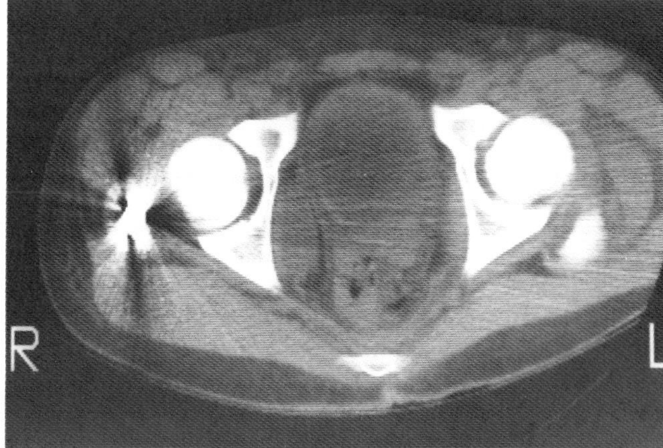

Figure 3-B

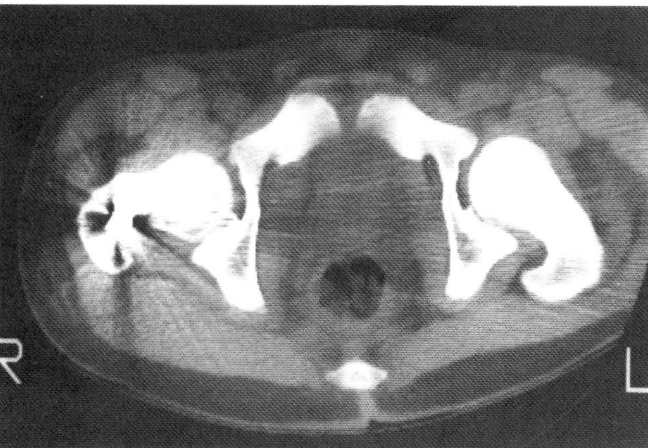

Figure 3-C

Figure 3: Computed tomographic views of the pelvis. (A) Sacroiliac joints and sacrum. (B) Medial acetabular wall and femoral head. (C) Femoral head and superior ramus. (Other helpful sections: superior portion of sacroiliac joints and iliac wings, acetabular dome and symphysis.)

extreme caution should be exercised during the deflation of the MAST suit. At this time the patient requires blood replacement as well as infusion of lactated Ringer's solution. In a volume-depleted patient, type specific or O-negative blood can be employed within 15 minutes after the blood specimen has been collected. In contrast, more time is needed to obtain a suitable cross-match. Persistent hypotension despite the application of an inflated MAST suit indicates either inadequate volume resuscitation, continued hemorrhage, or both.

Catheterization of the urinary bladder to document urinary output allows an important measurement of adequate volume replacement but requires special care. Concomitant injury to the bladder or urethra occurs in about 20 percent of the patients. Features of the physical examination indicating a possible bladder or urethral injury include bloody drainage from the meatus and an abnormally positioned or highly mobile prostate. Microscopic hematuria indicates a genitourinary injury. A Foley catheter can be placed directly into the bladder of a female patient, but in a male a urethrogram should first be performed. If there is passage of contrast medium into the bladder without extravasation, the catheter is advanced into the bladder. A cystogram is performed to exclude a rupture of the bladder. Finally, an intravenous pyelogram is done to assess the kidneys and ureters. If a urethral injury is identified, the patient should have a suprapubic cystostomy. However, this procedure may be complicated by the presence of a large pelvic hematoma.

Frequently, the initial abdominal examination performed upon a patient who presents with a pelvic fracture can be misleading. If the findings are consistent with profuse intra-abdominal hemorrhage or a visceral disruption, an exploratory laparotomy is indicated. Clinical findings (e.g., unexplained hypotension or anemia, or a physical examination of the abdomen which shows questionable findings) indicate the need for peritoneal lavage. This procedure is generally associated with a false positive test of less than 2 to 3 percent. In the presence of an open pelvic fracture, where a completely divided colostomy is mandatory to lessen the likelihood for overwhelming bacterial contamination of the fracture site, peritoneal lavage is unnecessary and is replaced by a formal laparotomy at the time of the colostomy.

In the presence of continued profuse hemorrhage associated with a pelvic fracture, further therapeutic measures are used according to a standard protocol (Fig. 1). The application of external fixation to the pelvis is a rapid and minimally invasive method to reduce and stabilize the fracture. Reduction of the pelvic fracture provides tamponade of intrapelvic osseous bleeding and a substantial reduction in the volume of the true pelvis and, thereby, the size of the retroperitoneal space in which a hematoma may collect. Selective angiography may permit localization of the specific bleeding sites and control of hemorrhage by the injection of one of a variety of embolic anticoagulants or by the insertion of a balloon catheter. This method obviates the need for laparotomy under general anesthesia and, thereby, minimizes the risk of an intra-abdominal infection. Also, the technique preserves the tamponade effect provided by a retroperitoneal hematoma. Admittedly, selective angiography with embolization possesses a small potential risk for misdirected emboli. At present the use of selective angiography with embolization or balloon catheter occlusion is recommended for the patient who continues to bleed profusely despite the previous application of external pelvic fixation. Direct surgical exploration for ligation of a bleeding intrapelvic vessel rarely is undertaken unless angiography shows the presence of an injury to the iliac artery. Surgical ligation of the hypogastric artery as a method to control profuse intrapelvic

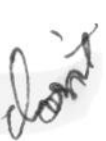

hemorrhage now is recognized as minimally effective and carries a high risk of ischemic necrosis of essential intrapelvic structures.

Radiologic Assessment Prior to initiation of definitive treatment, the pelvic fracture is classified according to its clinical and radiographic features. Sites of ecchymosis or contusion may indicate the direction of the provocative force. In addition, palpation of the hemipelvis with attention to symmetry, stability, and alignment of the iliac crests, antero- and posterosuperior iliac spines, and the superior pubic rami affords an initial impression of the degree of displacement of the pelvic ring.

Special radiographic views have been devised that demonstrate various portions of the pelvic ring (Fig. 2). A standard anteroposterior radiographic view provides the basis for identification of fractures of the pelvic ring as well as acetabular and proximal femoral disruptions. Also, it permits recognition of many avulsion fractures of the lower lumbar transverse processes. The anteroposterior view is supplemented by two oblique views, the pelvic inlet and outlet projections taken 60 degrees obliquely to the anteroposterior plane of the pelvis. The pelvic inlet or obstetric projection may demonstrate the site of disruption of the pelvic ring and sacroiliac joints. In addition, it permits an assessment of the degree of posterior pelvic displacement and the presence of associated avulsion fractures involving the sacrospinous and sacrotuberous ligaments. Also, it documents the degree of medial wall displacement in an acetabular fracture. With a lateral compression injury, it permits recognition of the posterior fracture site. The pelvic outlet view provides optimal visualization of the pubic rami and the degree of superior migration or rotation of the hemipelvis that accompanies a vertical shear injury. It provides the best visualization of ligamentous avulsion fractures from the lower lumbar transverse processes.

Computed tomography is most helpful in determining the stability of a posterior disruption at or adjacent to the sacroiliac joints (Fig. 3). Frequently, computed tomography provides the only available method to recognize an unstable posterior disruption, especially a sacral fracture, which requires operative stabilization. With a concomitant acetabular fracture, serial CT cuts through the acetabulum and proximal femur may facilitate the classification of the injury, recognition of free intra-articular osteochondral fragments, subluxation of the hip, and determination of the optimal surgical approach.

The elaborate *radiological classification* of acetabular fractures devised by Judet and Letournel is briefly summarized here. The two acetabular columns (the anterior, or iliopubic, and posterior, or ilioischial) are assessed in an anteroposterior pelvic view combined with two 45 degree oblique views. The fractures are characterized by region and by the degree of comminution (Table I). A "wall" fracture refers to a portion of the acetabular rim, and a "column" fracture indicates a complete disruption of the anterior or posterior supportive elements of the acetabulum. Another category, a transverse fracture, refers to a disruption of the ilium from the remaining portions of the anterior and posterior columns. A comminuted form of transverse fracture, the so-called T-fracture, indicates a separation of the ischium from the pubis that is in continuity with the obturator foramen. Other such "associated" fractures indicate comminution of two or more regions of the acetabulum.

Table I
Classification of Acetabular Disruptions

Fracture Type	Percentage of Fractures	Radiographic Views
Simple		
Posterior wall	25	anteroposterior obturator oblique
Posterior column	5	anteroposterior iliac oblique
Anterior wall	<5	anteroposterior obturator oblique
Anterior column	<5	anteroposterior obturator oblique
Transverse	10	anteroposterior obturator oblique iliac oblique
*Associated**		
T-shaped	5	anteroposterior obturator oblique iliac oblique
Both column	20	anteroposterior obturator oblique iliac oblique
Others[1]	25	anteroposterior obturator oblique iliac oblique

*CT scan provides additional information for the classification of acetabular fracture pattern and identifies concomitant disruptions of the pelvic ring.
[1]Posterior column + posterior wall; transverse + posterior wall; anterior column or wall + posterior hemitransverse.
Adapted from R. Judet and E. Letournel

Pelvic Stabilization Techniques Pelvic ring fractures have been treated by a wide variety of methods including bed rest, a pelvic sling, a hip spica cast, skeletal traction, and, more recently, by external and internal fixation systems. While the pelvic sling, skeletal traction, and hip spica cast have been used to immobilize many types of pelvic fractures, their application necessitated prolonged recumbency with a greater likelihood of late pulmonary, thromboembolic, urologic, and soft-tissue complications. These methods were assistive in the reduction of an open-book type of anteroposterior compression injury but were unlikely to be helpful in the management of most other pelvic fractures. The use of a hip spica cast, however, remains the most efficacious method for treating a child with an unstable pelvic ring fracture given the smaller size of the patient, shorter immobilization period, and lower incidence of thromboembolic problems.

External fixation: For approximately 20 years, attempts have been made to employ external fixation for immobilization of a pelvic ring fracture. Many external fixation systems have been utilized with a wide variety of frame configurations. Biomechanical and clinical studies indicate that external fixation is the optimal method of

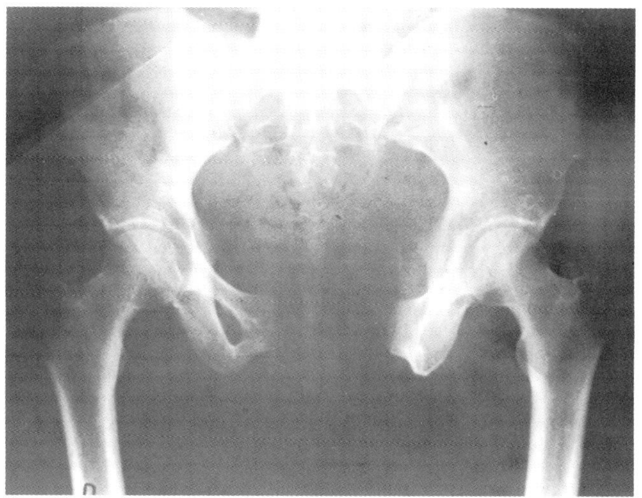

Figure 4-A

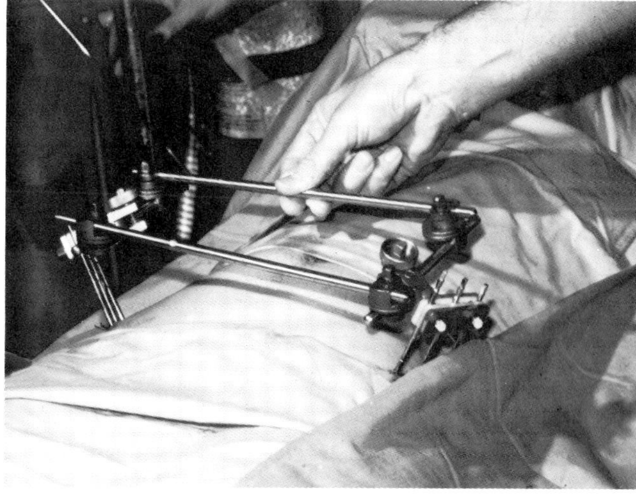

Figure 4-B

Figure 4: (A) Anteroposterior radiograph of the pelvic presents a stable anteroposterior compression injury with a wide diastasis. (B) The simplest form of stabilization. The use of a simple anterior external frame, such as a quadrilateral design, is shown.

treatment for many, if not most, pelvic ring fractures. A striking reduction in posttraumatic bleeding has been documented when an external device is applied during the initial management of the patient. Extensive biomechanical studies of external pelvic fixation methods, as well as comparisons between external and internal pelvic fixation, are now available. The early frame designs were simple anterior polygons anchored to each of the hemipelves by single pin clusters. These frames provided relief of fracture pain and adequate immobilization of stable disruptions, such as a stable anteroposterior compression injury with preservation of the posterior sacroiliac ligamentous complex. This frequently encountered type of pelvic disruption is particularly suited for application of any one of the available simple external frames. Several designs employ two 5-mm or three 4-mm pins inserted into both anterosuperior spines and iliac crests. The frame is erected as a quadrilateral or trapezoidal configuration, or the Wagner device is employed (Fig. 4). Although unique mechanical attributes of the various frames have been claimed, more recent mechanical data indicate that most provide comparable levels of stability. After the pins have been inserted and the wounds have been closed, the patient is turned from a supine to a lateral position which greatly facilitates the closed reduction.

Many investigators have reported the use of one or more of these simple frames for immobilization of unstable pelvic fractures with posterior instability. Several centers have now documented unacceptable loss of fixation and reduction in virtually all these patients, unless the patient is maintained at bed rest for several weeks. Such immobilization tends to defeat a principal objective of pelvic stabilization. As an alternative treatment of an unstable pelvic disruption, a simple frame can be supplemented by the use of appropriate internal fixation for the posterior injury.

For the immobilization of an unstable pelvic ring fracture, clinical and biomechanical studies have suggested the superiority of various three-dimensional frame configurations attached to two clusters of pins on each hemipelvis (Fig. 5). A simple, yet mechanically stable, triangular frame currently is utilized in many centers (Fig. 6). The triangular frame employs standard Hoffmann components and is simple to apply even in the acute situation. It provides approximately three times the stability that is achieved by the use of other frames. Admittedly, the triangular frame affords only one-fourth of the stability of the intact pelvic ring and is not as stable as internal fixation. This design is nevertheless adequate to permit immediate postoperative bed-to-chair activity, even for the patient who sustains an unstable pelvic disruption. No loss of reduction during the period of external fixation with the triangular frame has been reported to date. Satisfactory closed reduction with good approximation of the posterior disruption site is essential; otherwise, the likelihood for a painful nonunion is high. If an acceptable closed reduction cannot be achieved, open reduction with internal fixation of the posterior disruption is performed with temporary removal of the external frame.

Certain pelvic fractures, especially a lateral compression injury, are difficult to classify from the standpoint of stability, particularly in the absence of computed tomography. In such a patient a triangular frame should be applied acutely, or alternatively a simple frame can be used acutely and supplemental internal fixation of the posterior disruption can be undertaken when the patient's general condition has stabilized.

Internal fixation: Since the details of pelvic internal fixation have been reported elsewhere, only the general principles of the most common methods are discussed here.

For *symphysis diastasis* the rami are approached through a Pfannenstiel incision (Fig. 7A). The spermatic cords, or round ligaments, are carefully identified and protected. A tenaculum-type forcep is applied with the jaws inserted into the obturator foramina. While the opposing rami are approximated, the bladder and urethra are retracted gently to ensure that they are not trapped between the rami. For a stable anteroposterior compression injury, one 3.5-mm, 4-hole dynamic compression or reconstructive plate, anchored with cortical screws, suffices. With posterior instability, two 6- to 8-hole plates are applied to the anterior and superior surfaces of the rami.

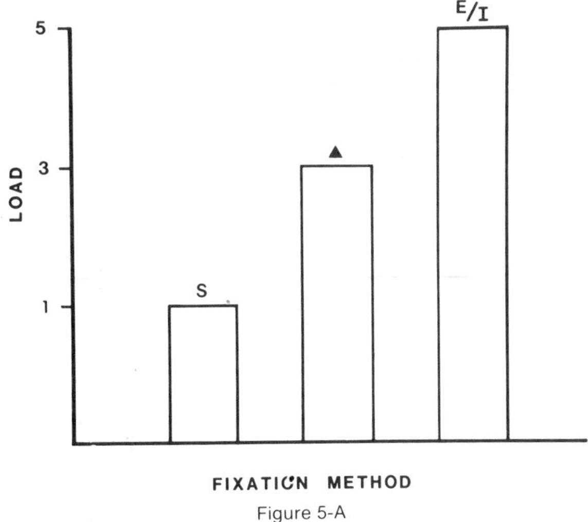

Figure 5-A

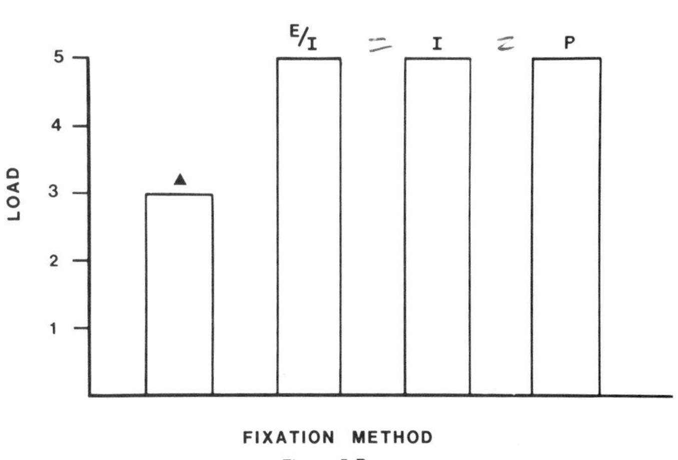

Figure 5-B

Figure 5: (A) Comparison of the degree of stability achieved by the use of a simple anterior trapezoidal or Slatis frame(s) with a biplanar anterior triangular frame (▲) with a combination of an anterior trapezoidal frame with posterior internal fixation of the sacroiliac joint (E/I). "Load" refers to the magnitude of the deforming force applied to a model fracture in a fresh cadaveric pelvis stabilized by an appropriate method and mounted in an Instron tensometer unit. (B) Comparison of the degree of stability achieved by the application of a biplanar triangular frame (▲) with a combination of anterior external and posterior internal fixation (E/I) with anterior and posterior internal fixation (I) with the degree of stability documented in an intact pelvis (P).

For *multiple rami fractures*, open reduction is limited by the complexity and potential anatomical hazards of the approach. If indicated a uni- or bilateral ilioinguinal exposure can be employed (Fig. 7B). The spermatic cords (or round ligaments), femoral nerve, artery, and vein are carefully identified. Appropriate exposure of the superior ramus is achieved by dissection medial to the anteroinferior spine, between the femoral artery and vein and at the symphysis. A curved plate or a suitably contoured 3.5-mm reconstruction plate is applied to the ramus with 4.5-mm or 3.5-mm cortical screws respectively. For a ramus fracture and a diastasis, the plate is extended across the midline for the insertion of two or three screws into the contralateral superior ramus. In the presence of bilateral ramus fractures and a diastasis, one long curved plate is extended across the symphysis along both iliopectineal lines.

The typical displaced *iliac fracture* extending from the anteroinferior spine to the sacroiliac notch may be exposed using a curvilinear incision along the iliac crest (Fig. 7C). After elevation of the superficial soft tissues from the ilium, an accurate anatomical reduction may be achieved. With a moderate to markedly comminuted fracture, multiple 3.5-mm dynamic compression or reconstruction plates are carefully contoured and applied to the various fracture lines on the superficial surface of the ilium. Supplementary plates applied to fracture lines violating the iliac crest may be necessary to provide stable fixation.

A *unilateral sacroiliac dislocation* may be exposed by a longitudinal incision from the posterosuperior to the posteroinferior spines (Fig. 7D). Soft tissues are elevated from the posterior portion of the lateral ilium, including the origin of gluteus maximus. Tenaculum bone-holding forceps are applied from the ilium to the sacrum to correct superior migration of the ilium or widening of the joint. Two or three 6.5-mm short-threaded cancellous lag screws

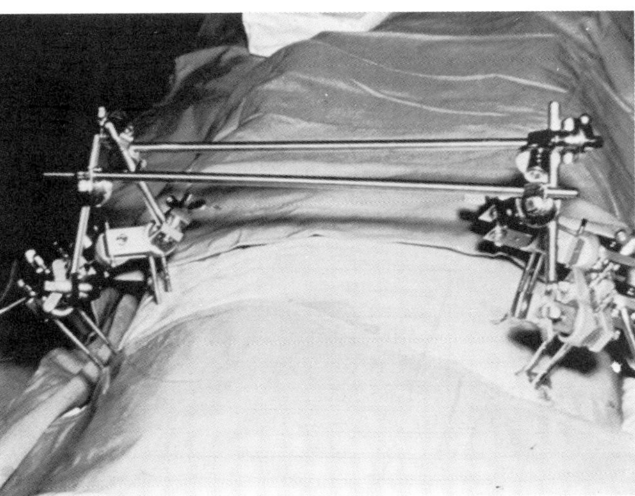

Figure 6-A

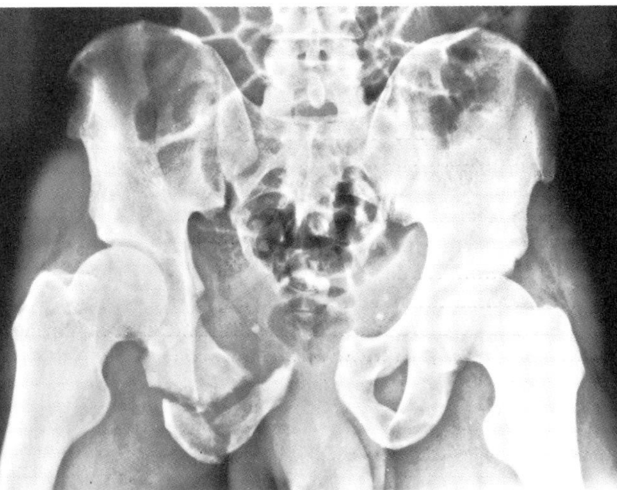

Figure 6-B

Figure 6: (A) A biplanar triangular frame which is suitable for immobilization of an unstable pelvic ring disruption. (B) An anteroposterior radiograph of an unstable lateral compression injury which would be adequately immobilized by the application of a triangular frame.

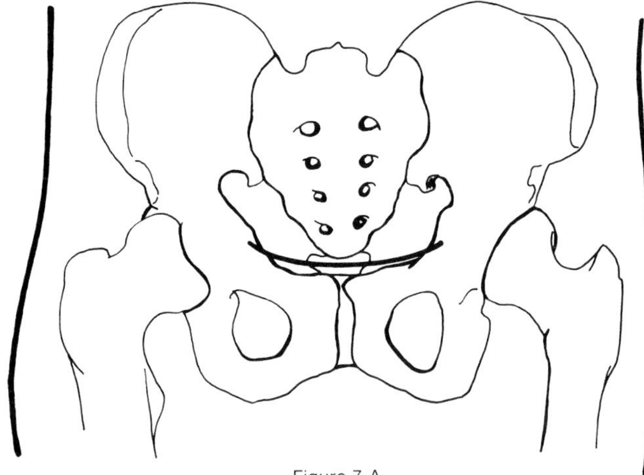

Figure 7-A

are applied through a 4.5-mm dynamic compression plate on the posterior ilium. The screws are directed into the ala of the sacrum for firm anchorage. The plate serves as a washer to increase rotational stability.

An *unstable sacral fracture* or *bilateral sacroiliac disruption* may be exposed by a transverse curvilinear incision across the midportion of the sacroiliac joints (Fig. 7E). After lateral reflection of the origins of both of the gluteus maximus muscles from the posterosuperior spines, a subperiosteal plane is developed on the sacrum below the paraspinous muscles. The bases of the sacral spinous processes are osteotomized. A subperiosteal exposure of the posterior ilia is undertaken. A double Cobra plate of appropriate size is inserted below the paraspinous muscles adjacent to the sacrum. It is first anchored with two 4.5-mm cortical screws to the posterior surface of the sacrum. Then three 6.5-mm cancellous lag screws are

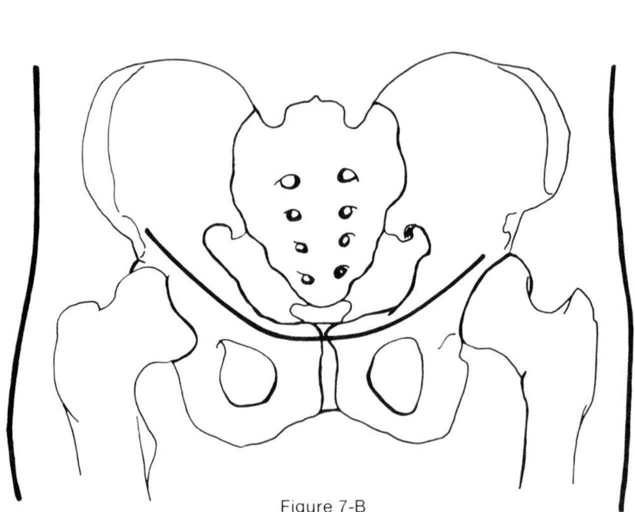

Figure 7-B

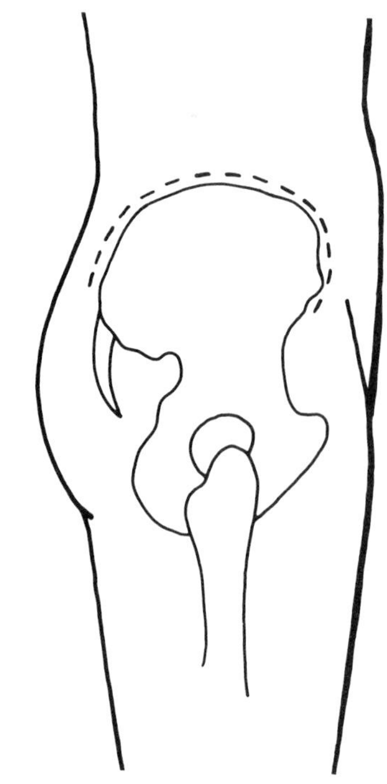

Figure 7-C

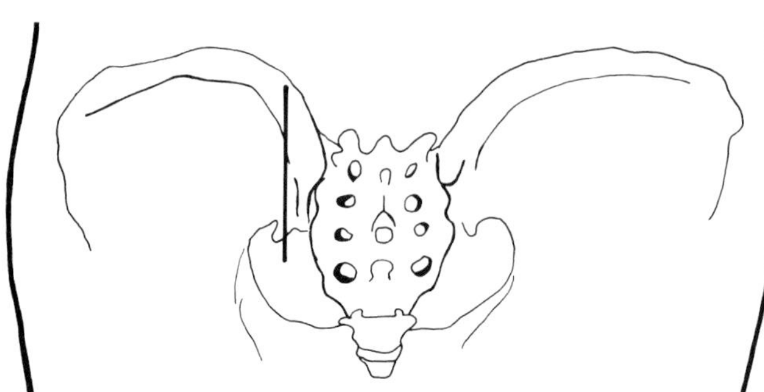

Figure 7-D

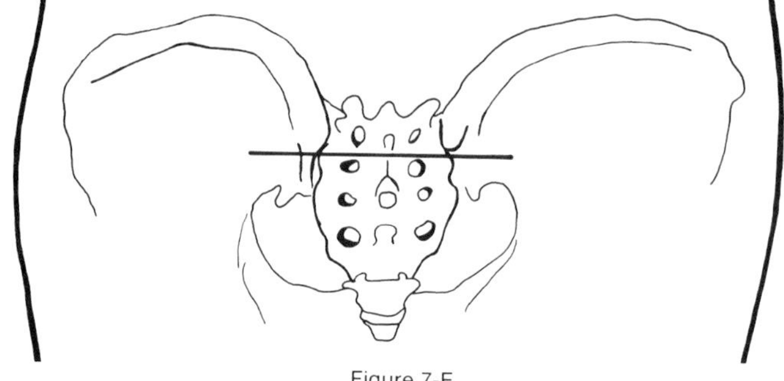

Figure 7-E

Figure 7: Principal surgical approaches to the pelvis for internal fixation. (A) Pfannenstiel approach to the symphysis. (B) Bilateral ilioinguinal approach to both superior rami and the symphysis. (C) Curvilinear iliac crest approach to the ilium. (D) Longitudinal approach to the sacroiliac joint and adjacent posterior ilium. (E) Transverse approach for immobilization of the sacrum or both sacroiliac joints with the application of a double Cobra plate. (Curvilinear extension of this incision permits exploration of one or both sciatic nerves.)

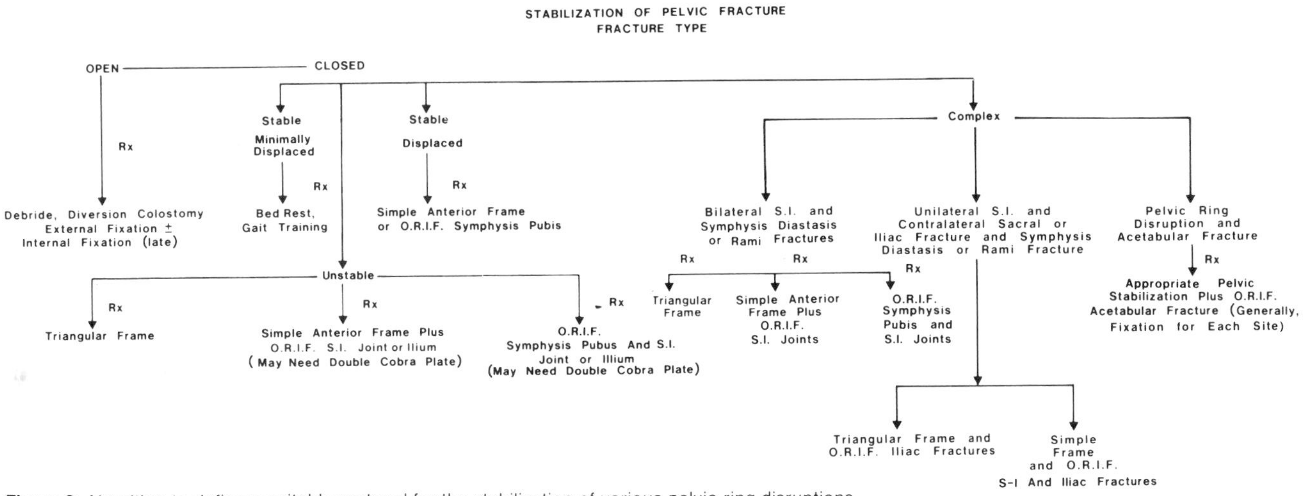

STABILIZATION OF PELVIC FRACTURE
FRACTURE TYPE

OPEN — CLOSED

- OPEN → Rx → Debride, Diversion Colostomy External Fixation ± Internal Fixation (late)
- CLOSED:
  - Stable Minimally Displaced → Rx → Bed Rest, Gait Training
  - Stable Displaced → Rx → Simple Anterior Frame or O.R.I.F. Symphysis Pubis
  - Unstable:
    - Rx → Triangular Frame
    - Rx → Simple Anterior Frame Plus O.R.I.F. S.I. Joint or Ilium (May Need Double Cobra Plate)
    - Rx → O.R.I.F. Symphysis Pubus And S.I. Joint or Illium (May Need Double Cobra Plate)
  - Complex:
    - Bilateral S.I. and Symphysis Diastasis or Rami Fractures → Rx → Triangular Frame; Rx → Simple Anterior Frame Plus O.R.I.F. S.I. Joints; O.R.I.F. Symphysis Pubis and S.I. Joints
    - Unilateral S.I. and Contralateral Sacral or Iliac Fracture and Symphysis Diastasis or Rami Fracture → Rx → Triangular Frame and O.R.I.F. Iliac Fractures; Simple Frame and O.R.I.F. S-I And Iliac Fractures
    - Pelvic Ring Disruption and Acetabular Fracture → Rx → Appropriate Pelvic Stabilization Plus O.R.I.F. Acetabular Fracture (Generally, Fixation for Each Site)

Figure 8: Algorithm to define a suitable protocol for the stabilization of various pelvic ring disruptions.

applied across both sacroiliac joints into the ala of the sacrum. Supplementary iliac fixation may be achieved by the use of 4.5-mm cortical screws.

Classification and Treatment As a result of recent clinical observations, an algorithm has been developed to assist in the selection of the stabilization technique for almost any type of pelvic ring disruption (Fig. 8). Four distinct categories of pelvic fractures are recognized.

The first category comprises *stable minimally displaced injuries* usually resulting from low velocity, lateral compression forces. A temporary period of bed rest followed by a partial weight-bearing gait for a few weeks is usually sufficient treatment. A large subgroup includes most anteroposterior and lateral compression injuries, such as a simple displaced pelvic fracture with preservation of the posterior sacroiliac ligaments and the sacrum. The most suitable treatment for this subgroup is a simple anterior external frame. When an emergency laparotomy is undertaken, possibly for the repair of a ruptured bladder, an alternative method of pelvic immobilization would be the application of plate fixation to the symphysis after closed reduction of the fracture. While plate fixation can be applied to anterior ramus fractures, the surgical approach is difficult. Generally, external fixation is indicated for an anterior injury with multiple displaced rami fractures.

A second category of *displaced pelvic disruption* presents with an unstable posterior injury, either of a sacroiliac joint or a posterior ilium, frequently adjacent to the sacroiliac joint. This includes virtually all vertical shear injuries with a unilateral posterior disruption, many lateral compression injuries, and a few anteroposterior compression injuries. The simplest therapeutic solution is a closed reduction with the application of a triangular external frame. For a vertical shear fracture accompanied by superior migration of a hemipelvis, a satisfactory closed reduction may be achieved by longitudinal traction applied on a fracture table. In the unlikely event that a closed reduction is unsatisfactory, open reduction and internal fixation of the posterior disruptions are indicated. Two other appropriate methods of treatment are the application of a simple external frame combined with open reduction and internal fixation of the sacroiliac joint or the ilium, or internal fixation of both the symphysis and the posterior disruption. A somewhat similar problem is an unstable sacral fracture which can be treated by application of a triangular frame. Alternatively, a double Cobra plate provides highly effective posterior stabilization. The accompanying anterior fractures can be immobilized with a simple external frame or with internal fixation.

Complex ring disruption is the third major category of pelvic fractures. There are four main subgroups: (1) bilateral unstable posterior disruptions and an anterior disruption; (2) a unilateral unstable posterior fracture accompanied by an iliac fracture and an anterior disruption; (3) a unilateral posterior fracture, an anterior disruption, and an acetabular fracture with or without an iliac fracture and; (4) various patterns of comminuted fractures with uni- or bilateral unstable posterior disruptions, bilateral acetabular and/or iliac fractures, and bilateral ramus fractures with or without diastasis of the symphysis.

Most pelvic fractures with bilateral unstable sacroiliac dislocations and a diastasis of the symphysis are due to vertical shear injuries. The simplest technique of immobilization is a closed reduction with the application of a triangular frame followed by open reduction and internal fixation of one sacroiliac joint or of both sacroiliac joints if an adequate closed reduction cannot be attained. A simple external frame is sufficient if bilateral open reduction and internal fixation of the sacroiliac joints are accomplished using lag screw techniques or the double Cobra plate. Plate fixation of the symphysis is satisfactory as an alternative to the external frame.

For an unstable sacroiliac joint with multiple rami fractures or a diastasis and an iliac fracture (lateral compression injury), suitable immobilization may be achieved in one of two ways. A simple external frame can be accompanied by open reduction and internal fixation of the sacroiliac disruption and the iliac fracture. Or, a triangular frame can be employed along with internal fixation of the iliac fracture. Generally, multiple rami fractures hamper the use of anterior internal fixation.

An unstable sacroiliac disruption with multiple rami fractures or a diastasis and an acetabular fracture, with or without propagation into the ilium, is another consequence of lateral compression injury. Open reduction and internal fixation of the acetabulum are generally undertaken through a suitable extensile exposure (see following discussion of the details of acetabular fixation). In the presence of an ipsilateral sacroiliac fracture, such an exposure permits lag screw fixation of that fracture, while the rami are immobilized with a simple external frame. With a contralateral sacroiliac disruption, both that injury and the rami fractures are immobilized by the application of a triangular frame.

Following violent traumatic insults, several patterns of injuries are seen which include uni- or bilateral acetabular fractures, bilateral sacroiliac disruptions or other equivalent posterior injuries, and bilateral ramus fractures with or without a diastasis of the symphysis. In most of these patients virtually all the principal ligamentous supports for the pelvic ring are severely compromised. As a rule, each site of pelvic disruption should be stabilized by the use of an appropriate method of internal or external fixation.

Open injury is the fourth major category of pelvic fracture. These injuries are best managed by an immediate, thorough debridement, external fixation, and a complete diversion colostomy. Even in the presence of an intact colon and anal sphincter, colostomy is mandatory to minimize the risk of fecal contamination of the open wounds. In certain patients with marked pelvic instability, delayed supplementary internal fixation, especially of unstable posterior disruptions, is necessary.

Although the use of external fixation as part of the emergency treatment for hemorrhage and pain control is well established, the optimal timing of supplementary pelvic internal fixation for closed fractures remains unclear. Whenever the general condition of the patient (including the hemodynamic status) is questionable, open reduction with its potential for considerable blood loss is deferred for 24 to 48 hours after injury. Further delay is likely to result in pulmonary, thromboembolic, and urological complications. When the general condition of the patient is satisfactory, early surgical intervention may provide for the most rapid recovery with the least likelihood for the complications associated with enforced recumbency. In one recent reported series which documented more than 200 consecutive patients who underwent early surgical intervention without the use of routine anticoagulation, just one relatively minor case of pulmonary embolus was documented.

Postoperative Care Following pelvic external fixation, the patient initially is best monitored in an intensive care unit. Pin tracks are cleansed daily with hydrogen peroxide-soaked swabs. Radiographs are taken to document the accuracy of the reduction. When necessary, and before the formation of abundant granulation tissue and callus, one carefully planned alteration of the closed reduction may be performed within a few days after the operation under heavy sedation or a short-acting general anesthetic. The external frame is loosened and the uprights are manipulated until a satisfactory realignment is confirmed under radiographic control. When the status of other injuries permits, the patient is encouraged to sit up the day after the operation. Within another 2 to 3 days, the patient is encouraged to initiate bed-to-chair transfers. If the original fracture is stable, a touchdown gait is permitted; but if the fracture is unstable, a touchdown gait is deferred for 6 to 8 weeks. The same procedure is utilized when open reduction and internal fixation of the pelvic ring are performed. A posterior fracture generally is healed 6 weeks after stabilization, but a sacroiliac disruption requires an 8- to 10-week period. At that time, the patient is readmitted for removal of the pelvic frame under general anesthesia. During this procedure, the stability of the pelvis can be assessed by manipulation of the pins. Upon removal of the pins, the pin sites are irrigated with Betadine solution and dry dressings are applied. Subsequently, the patient begins partial weight-bearing and progresses to full weight-bearing as tolerated. When a patient undergoes internal fixation or a combination of internal and external fixation of a pelvic fracture, the postoperative mobilization program depends upon the degree of pelvic stability that is achieved surgically. If both anterior and posterior internal fixation are used or if posterior internal fixation is supplemented by anterior external fixation, the patient is permitted to undertake immediate bed-to-chair transfers and a touchdown gait. If the pelvic fixation is of questionable stability, a touchdown gait is deferred for 6 to 8 weeks.

Pelvic Nonunion and Malunion Nonunion of the pelvis may present with posterior or, less frequently, anterior pelvic pain and instability. A malunion may cause complaints due to an apparent leg length discrepancy, pelvic obliquity, tender osseous prominences, or cosmetic problems. Most of these problems arise as complications of inadequate initial pelvic stabilization of unstable injuries, especially when bed rest, a pelvic sling, skeletal traction, or hip spica immobilization were employed. A symptomatic nonunion requires rigid stabilization and supplementary bone grafting of both the posterior and the anterior disruptions, even though the symptoms may be limited to one area. Treatment of a symptomatic malunion or nonunion with malalignment requires a formidable reconstructive procedure with pelvic osteotomy, realignment, and internal fixation. With experience, pelvic reconstruction can achieve highly satisfactory results although referral to an appropriate orthopaedic center is advised.

Acetabular Fractures

Acetabular fractures should be managed similarly to other intra-articular fractures. Anatomical restoration of the articular surfaces and early initiation of active motion exercises are principles of management not only for most intra-articular fractures but also acetabular fractures. Undisplaced or minimally displaced fractures are best managed by early active exercises and protected weight-bearing. In the presence of multiple fragments when the capsular attachments between the acetabular fragments and the proximal femur remain intact, skeletal traction can provide an accurate closed reduction and permit early active motion exercises in traction. If a loose interposed osteochondral fracture fragment is present, early surgical excision is required to avoid abrasive damage to the cartilage of the acetabulum and femoral head. With an imperfect closed acetabular reduction, certain types of deformity are less acceptable than others. Long-term studies have shown that the less acceptable deformities possess a greater potential to progress to traumatic arthritis. A "step-off" in the superior weight-bearing portion of the acetabulum of greater than 1 to 2 mm possesses a particularly poor prognosis. Comminuted acetabular fractures may demonstrate several osseous fragments

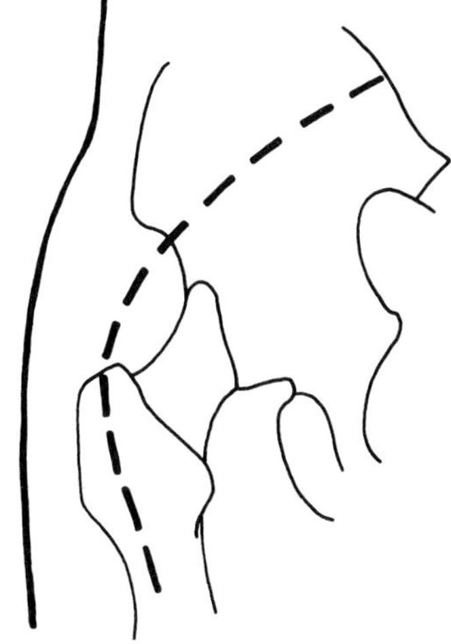

Figure 9-A

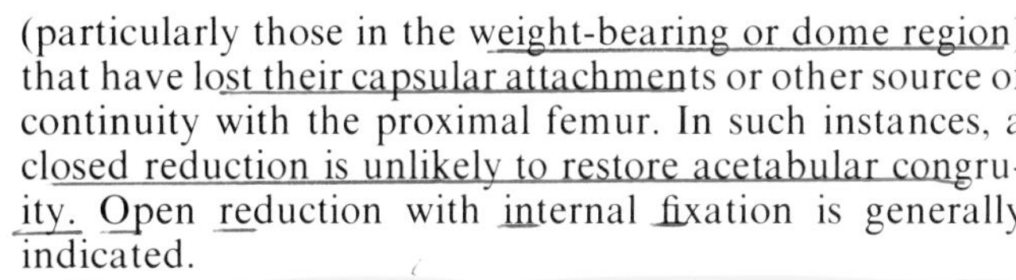

(particularly those in the weight-bearing or dome region) that have lost their capsular attachments or other source of continuity with the proximal femur. In such instances, a closed reduction is unlikely to restore acetabular congruity. Open reduction with internal fixation is generally indicated.

There are at least two contraindications to open reduction. Marked osteoporosis may render available techniques of internal fixation ineffective, and substantial acetabular comminution may preclude effective internal fixation. An open grade III acetabular and pelvic fracture is a contraindication to early open reduction and internal fixation of the acetabulum although a secondary reconstruction may be indicated. Preexisting arthritis of the hip joint may dictate the use of closed methods, followed by a total hip joint replacement after union of the acetabulum. However, if the acetabular fragments are markedly displaced so that subsequent union would provide poor support for an acetabular component, open reduction is indicated.

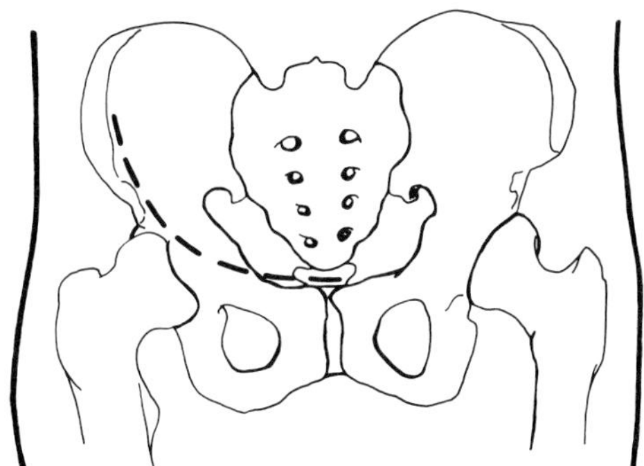

Figure 9-B

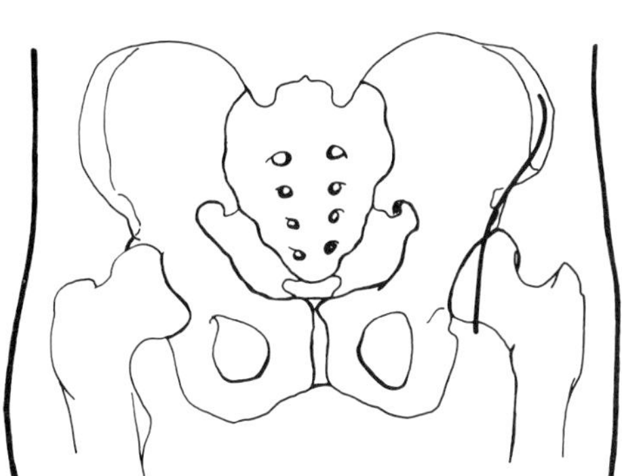

Figure 9-C

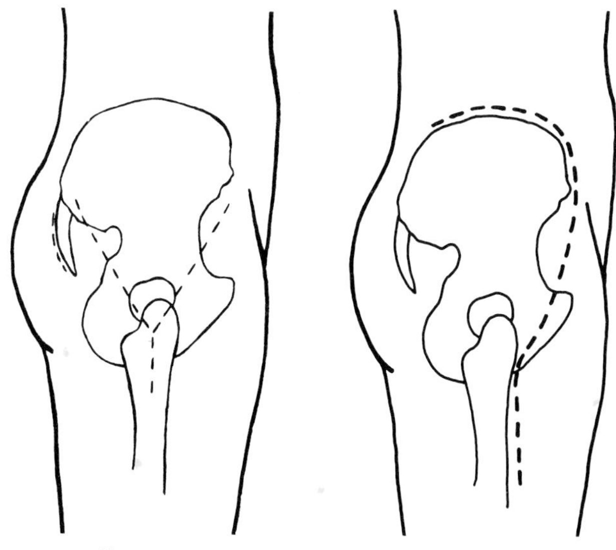

Figure 9-D

Figure 9-E

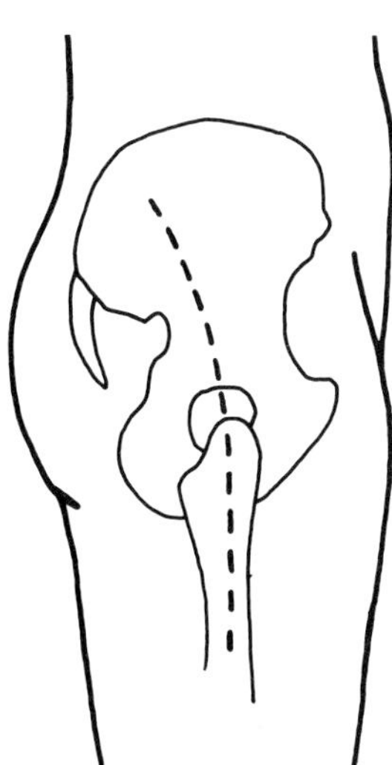

Figure 9-F

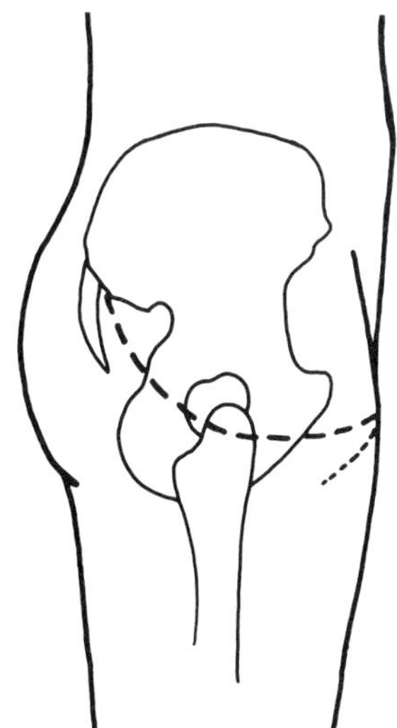

Figure 9-G

Figure 9: Principal surgical approaches to the acetabulum. (A) Kocher-Langenbeck (posterolateral). (B) Ilioinguinal (anterior). (C) Smith-Petersen (anterior). (D) Triradiate (Y, extensile visualization of the anterior and posterior columns, lateral ilium and hip joint). (E) Iliofemoral (extensile visualization comparable to triradiate approach). (F) Lateral longitudinal transtrochanteric (visualization of lateral ilium, posterior column and hip joint). (G) Senegas (extensile visualization of lateral ilium, posterior column and hip joint).

Table II
Surgical Treatment of Acetabular Disruptions

Fracture Type	Operative Approach	Reduction Techniques	Stabilization
Simple			
Posterior wall	Kocher-Langenbeck	tenaculum forceps K-wire	lag screw(s) buttress plate
Posterior column	Kocher-Langenbeck	tenaculum forceps Farabeuf-Lambotte forceps K-wire	lag screw(s) neutralization plate
Anterior wall	Smith-Petersen	tenaculum forceps Farabeuf-Lambotte forceps K-wire	lag screw(s)
Anterior column	Smith-Petersen ilioinguinal	tenaculum forceps Farabeuf-Lambotte forceps K-wire	lag screw(s) ± neutralization plate
Transverse fracture	Kocher-Langenbeck ± ilioinguinal lateral transtrochanteric triradiate iliofemoral	tenaculum forceps Farabeuf-Lambotte forceps K-wire	lag screw(s) ± neutralization plate
Associated			
T-shaped	Kocher-Langenbeck ± lateral transtrochanteric triradiate iliofemoral	tenaculum forceps Farabeuf-Lambotte forceps K-wire	lag screw(s) neutralization plate(s)
Both column	Kocher-Langenbeck ± lateral transtrochanteric triradiate iliofemoral	tenaculum forceps Farabeuf-Lambotte forceps K-wire	lag screw(s) neutralization plate(s)
Other*			

*See Table I, page 275.

In summary, for most displaced acetabular fractures where a brief period of 24 to 48 hours of skeletal traction fails to provide an accurate reduction, open reduction and internal fixation should be seriously considered. More complex variants of acetabular fractures generally need internal fixation.

Initial Management On presentation, the patient should receive a thorough clinical examination to elicit evidence of other potential systemic injuries. A complete radiological examination of the pelvis, including anteroposterior pelvic inlet and outlet and Judet or oblique acetabular views, is obtained (Fig. 2). Computed tomography (Fig. 3) of the pelvis is strongly recommended. If not available, conventional tomography may permit visualization of loose osteochondral fragments in the hip joint or malaligned acetabular fragments. Drawings of the fracture lines on the radiographs may facilitate identification of the type of injury according to the classification of Judet and Letournel. Subsequently, a suitable treatment protocol should be devised. If a dislocated hip joint is present, a closed or open reduction should be undertaken immediately. In the presence of a displaced acetabular fracture, skeletal traction may be tried through either a distal femoral or proximal tibial pin. With a complex fracture in which it is unlikely that an acceptable closed reduction can be obtained, early open reduction and internal fixation is considered provided that the general condition of the patient is stable. Table II gives an outline of the preferred types of acetabular reconstruction, progressing from the simpler, more frequently encountered acetabular fractures to the more complex and less commonly encountered. The principal surgical approaches to the acetabulum are shown schematically in Figure 9.

Surgical Reconstruction A *posterior wall fracture* can be visualized through a Kocher-Langenbeck or equivalent posterior or posterolateral approach with retraction of the short external rotators. After irrigation of the hip joint and removal of any loose osteochondral fragments, the fracture is reduced and provisionally stabilized by a tenaculum forceps or Kirschner wires. Immobilization of a small fragment (less than 3 cm) can be achieved by the use of lag screws whereas larger fragments are buttressed with a 3.5-mm reconstruction or dynamic compression plate.

A *posterior column fracture* can be visualized through a posterior or posterolateral approach to the entire posterior column from the ischial tuberosity to the greater sciatic notch and the lateral ilium. A blunt-tipped retractor is inserted into the greater sciatic notch. The hip and knee are maintained in extension and flexion respectively to protect the sciatic nerve. Tenaculum forceps are applied to

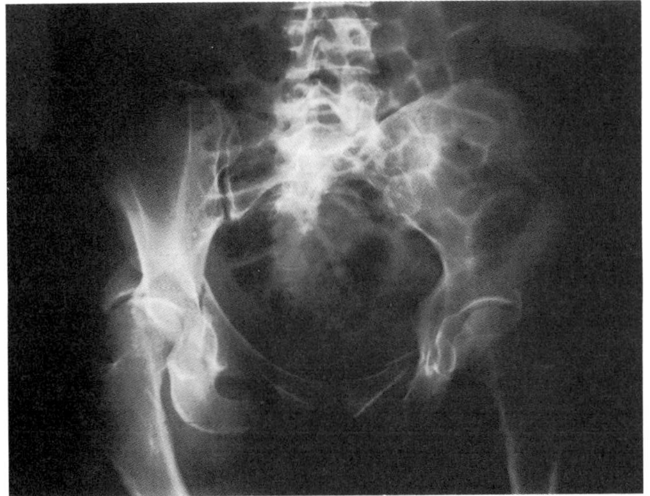

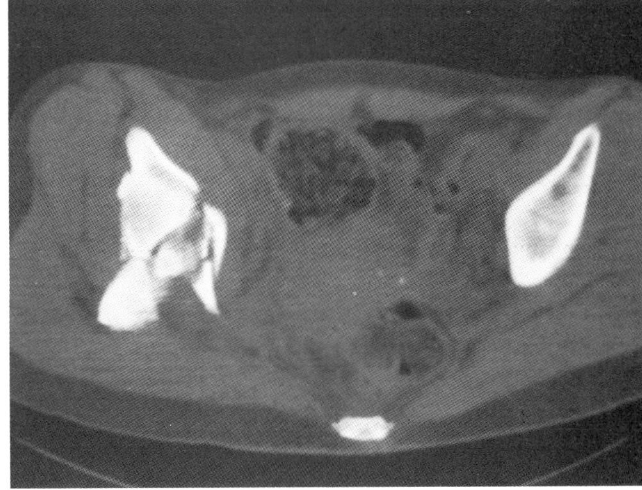

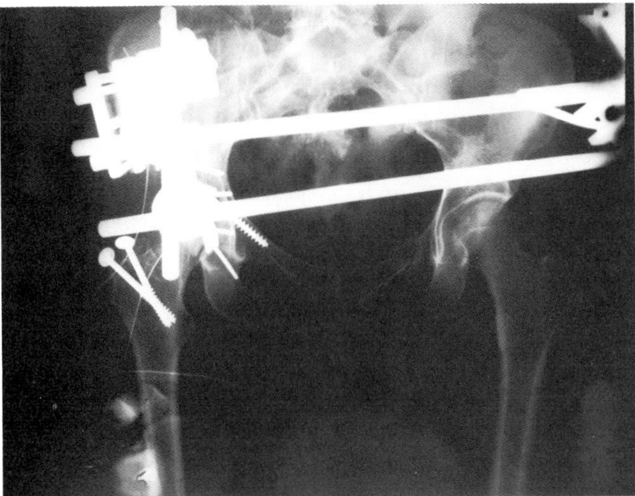

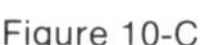

Figure 10-C

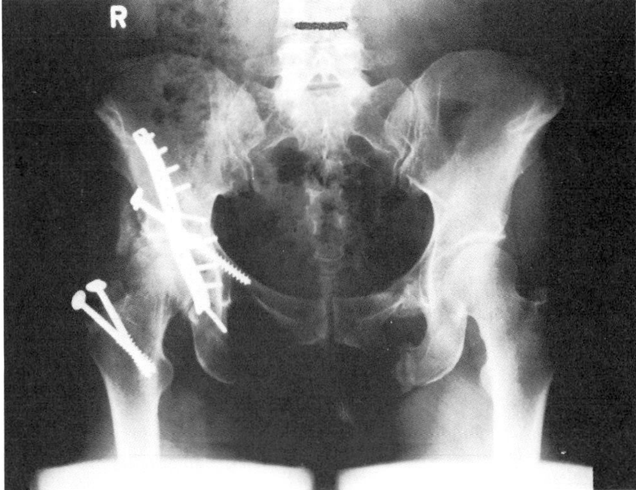

Figure 10-D

Figure 10: Radiographic views and CT scan show a complex right acetabular disruption with posterior subluxation of the femoral head. (A) Anteroposterior view visualizes posterior wall fragment with T-type fracture. (B) CT scan illustrates comminuted dome region with displacement of posterior wall fragment. (C) Immediate postoperative anteroposterior radiograph reveals the acetabular reconstruction with greater trochanteric lag screws and external fixation of the pelvis. A triradiate incision was used to approach the acetabular fracture. (D) Anteroposterior radiograph taken 6 months after surgery and following the removal of the external frame. A precise anatomical reduction is evident, along with a small amount of lateral ectopic bone.

achieve the reduction. A 3.5-mm reconstruction or dynamic compression plate is applied from the ischial tuberosity to the lateral ilium. The plate is positioned adjacent to the sciatic notch so that the screws are least likely to violate the hip joint. If a large supplementary posterior wall fragment is present, a second buttressing plate is used to immobilize that fragment.

An *anterior wall fracture* is uncommon. It can be approached through a Smith-Petersen or ilioinguinal incision. Generally the small fragments are stabilized temporarily with a tenaculum forcep or Kirschner wires, prior to lag screw immobilization.

An *anterior column fracture* can be visualized through an ilioinguinal, Smith-Petersen or the anterior half of a triradiate or Y-incision (Watson-Jones). A simple fracture can be immobilized with a 6.5-mm cancellous lag screw and a washer. More comminuted fractures are best visualized through an ilioinguinal approach. A buttress plate is applied along the iliopectineal line. Whenever possible, supplementary lag screws should be used.

For a *transverse fracture* the previously preferred exposure was a posterolateral incision for the application of a plate along the posterior column, with or without a supplementary posterior lag screw. Although this is the least complicated method, it encourages a "yawning" apart of the most anterior portion of the fracture line of 2 to 4 mm. Recently, a lateral longitudinal transtrochanteric approach has been recommended. A buttress plate is applied to the posterior column. A long 6.5-mm cancellous screw is inserted across the anterior portion of the fracture. With this method an exact anatomical reduction is possible. In the presence of a comminuted transverse fracture a triradiate approach provides the optimal visualization.

T- and both column fractures are complex injuries and are visualized best by a triradiate incision, an iliofemoral approach of Letournel, or occasionally a lateral longitudinal transtrochanteric approach. Generally the preferred sequence of reduction is the anterior column fragment to the ilium, followed by the posterior column fragment. Interfragmentary lag screws may be supplemented by a posterior column buttress plate.

In more *complex fracture patterns*, such as transverse fractures, T-fractures and combined anterior and posterior column fractures, one of several extensile exposures may be employed. Examples of these transtrochanteric approaches include a modified Ollier approach, an extended iliofemoral exposure, and the triradiate or Y-approach. In these approaches both the anterior and posterior columns can be visualized, reduced, and stabilized. In the extended iliofemoral and triradiate approaches, the abductor muscles of the hip are elevated from the iliac crest and lateral ilium until most of the lateral ilium, including any comminuted fragments, can be visualized. The more extensile approaches require a prolonged operative time with increased blood loss; but anatomic reduction can be achieved, and this translates into good clinical results in the long-term.

Acetabular and Pelvic Ring Disruptions

These rare and highly complex fractures are best treated in special trauma centers (Fig. 10). In general, the lateral ilium is reconstructed first through an appropriate extensile exposure, followed by repair of the acetabular fracture. An ipsilateral sacroiliac fracture can be stabilized by lag screws inserted through the same exposure, superior to the greater sciatic notch. A contralateral sacroiliac fracture is immobilized most simply by the use of external fixation. Bilateral acetabular fractures are managed by sequential open reductions and internal fixation performed through suitable incisions.

Following stable internal fixation, active mobilization of the hip is encouraged within 1 or 2 days after surgery. Supplementary physiotherapy with bed-to-chair transfers, crutch walking, and a touchdown gait is begun in 1 to 2 weeks. Progression to full weight-bearing is not allowed until about 12 weeks when there is radiological evidence of fracture healing.

The results of surgical reconstruction for acetabular nonunions and/or malunions by osteotomy with open reduction and internal fixation have been reported. Preliminary results seem highly encouraging, both as an attempt to reconstruct a functional hip joint and to provide optimal bone stock for later reconstructive procedures, such as total hip arthroplasty.

Pelvic and Acetabular Fractures in Children

From the limited number of documented studies of pediatric patients, the provocative forces and the radiologic methods of assessment of these injuries appear to be similar to adult injuries. Anteroposterior and vertical shear injuries produce disruptions that are similar to those seen in adults. In the child, however, a lateral compression force frequently injures the vulnerable triradiate cartilage.

Most of the unstable displaced pelvic ring fractures without acetabular involvement are best managed by the use of a closed reduction under general anesthesia and the application of a well-molded, double-hip spica cast. Generally, the fractures heal uneventfully. While radiologic evidence of a partial growth arrest of the ilium or rami and fusion of the sacroiliac joint has been reported, late symptomatic problems in such children appear to be uncommon.

A more difficult problem is premature fusion or partial growth arrest of the triradiate cartilage following an acetabular disruption. Recent published reviews show that age of the patient at the time of injury and degree of damage sustained by the triradiate cartilage are the prognostic factors that determine the severity of subsequent growth arrest. Acetabular deformity with incongruity of the hip joint may not become symptomatic for years or even decades. Nevertheless, given the potential for such problems, a child who sustains an acetabular fracture should be followed until skeletal maturity. With the recently recognized potential for acetabular maldevelopment in a child who sustains such an injury, the treatment should be directed toward the restoration of a congruent acetabulum with accurate realignment of the triradiate growth plate. Initially, closed reduction with skeletal traction may be undertaken. If an accurate reduction is obtained, hip spica immobilization can be employed. If closed methods fail to restore acetabular congruity, an open reduction with Kirschner wire fixation is recommended. Supplementary cast immobilization is required for 6 weeks.

ANNOTATED BIBLIOGRAPHY

Pelvic Injuries

Lansinger, O.; Romanus, B.; and Goldie, I.F.: Fracture mechanism in central acetabular fractures: An experimental study. Arch. Orthop. Trauma Surg. 94:209-212, 1979.

The relationships between the vectors of disruptive forces and resultant acetabular fracture patterns are described.

Patient Management

Associated Injuries and Acute Resuscitation

GENERAL

McMurtry, R.; Walton, D.; Dickinson, D.; Kellam, J.; and Tile, M.: Pelvic disruption in the polytraumatized patient: A management protocol. Clin. Orthop. 151:22-30, 1980.

A detailed protocol is given for the management of polytrauma patients with pelvic fractures, based upon the author's experience with seventy-nine such patients. A correlation between the "injury severity score" and the anticipated amount of resuscitative effort is emphasized.

VASCULAR

Flint, L.M., Jr.; Brown, A.; Richardson, J.D.; and Polk, H.C.: Definitive control of bleeding from severe pelvic fractures. Ann. Surg. 189:709-716, 1979.

A group of forty patients with severe pelvic fractures is discussed with reference to the optimal protocol to control profuse hemorrhage. The roles of the MAST suit, selective arteriography with embolotherapy, and surgical intervention are discussed.

Riska, E.B.; von Bonsdorff, H.; Hakkinen, S.; and Jaroma, H.: Operative control of massive hemorrhage in comminuted pelvic fractures. Internat. Orthop. 3:141-144, 1979.

In forty-two patients who presented with massive hemorrhage complicating comminuted pelvic fractures, operative exploration was undertaken through various surgical exposures. The principal sources of bleeding were the superior and inferior gluteal, pudendal, and obturator arteries. In certain patients, temporary compression of the abdominal aorta was helpful prior to ligation of the injured vessels.

Rothenberger, D.A.; Fischer, R.P.; and Perry, J.F.: Major vascular injuries secondary to pelvic fractures: An unsolved clinical problem. Am. J. Surg. 136:660-662, 1978.

Operative exploration of the pelvis to control profuse hemorrhage following pelvic ring disruption is discussed. In the presence of iliac and femoral arterial or venous injuries, early operative exploration is strongly recommended.

Sclafani, S.J., and Becker, J.A.: Traumatic presacral hemorrhage: Angiographic diagnosis and therapy. Am. J. Roentgenol. 138:123-126, 1982.

Identification of bleeding from the iliolumbar and lateral sacral branches of the hypogastric artery by the use of arteriography is described. Bleeding was controlled by small particulate embolotherapy.

Stock, J.R.; Harris, W.H.; and Athanasoulis, C.A.: The role of diagnostic and therapeutic angiography in trauma to the pelvis. Clin. Orthop. 151:31-40, 1980.

The general principles for diagnostic and therapeutic arteriography of intrapelvic vessels to identify vascular injuries for embolotherapy are outlined.

Intra-abdominal

Murr, P.C.; Moore, E.E.; Lipscomb, R.; and Johnston, R.M.: Abdominal trauma associated with pelvic fracture. J. Trauma 20:919-928, 1980.

The intra-abdominal injuries in 16 percent of seventy consecutive patients who survived pelvic fractures are discussed. The injuries are characterized, and an initial diagnostic protocol is suggested.

Zannis, V.J., and Wood, M.: Laparotomy for pelvic fracture. Am. J. Surg. 140:841-846, 1980.

Following a review of 224 patients who were managed for pelvic fractures, the criteria for laparotomy were established. In this series, the relatively low reliability (57 percent) for peritoneal lavage as an index is in marked contrast to the reliability (90 percent) of clinical findings upon abdominal examination.

Urologic

Colapinto, V.: Trauma to the pelvis: Urethral injury. Clin. Orthop. 151:46-55, 1980.

An account of the diagnostic and therapeutic protocol for urethral injuries accompanying pelvic fractures is given. The crucial role of retrograde urethrography in the male is emphasized.

Weems, W.L.: Management of genitourinary injuries in patients with pelvic fractures. Ann. Surg. 189:717-723, 1979.

After a study of 282 male patients with urethral injuries complicating pelvic fractures, a therapeutic protocol was devised which defines nonoperative and operative methods of treatment and the role of early versus late urethral repair.

Neurologic

Thakkar, D.H., and Porter, R.W.: Heterotopic ossification enveloping the sciatic nerve following posterior fracture-dislocation of the hip: A case report. Injury 13:207-209, 1981.

In addition to the previously described mechanisms of sciatic nerve injury that complicate acetabular and pelvic fractures, the delayed onset of nerve compression, secondary to heterotopic bone formation, is described.

Skeletal

Browne, R.S., and Mullan, G.B.: Intertrochanteric fracture of the femur with ipsilateral central fracture of the acetabulum. Injury 11:251-253, 1980.

Examples of ipsilateral femoral fractures complicating acetabular fractures are described, including methods of treatment.

Radiologic assessment

Hansen, S.T., Jr.: CT for pelvic fractures. Am. J. Roentgenol. 138:592-593, 1982.

An account of the optimal cross-sectional views of the pelvic rings and relevant findings is provided. Unstable disruptions of the sacrum may be visualized that are not readily apparent on plain radiographs.

Letournel, E.: Acetabulum fractures: Classification and management. Clin. Orthop. 151:81-106, 1980.

The accepted classification of acetabular fractures based upon 22 years of experience with analysis of over 700 patients is provided.

Mack, L.A.; Harley, J.D.; and Winquist, R.A.: CT of acetabular fractures: Analysis of fracture patterns. Am. J. Roentgenol. 138:407-415, 1982.

A study of thirty-one patients who sustained acetabular fracture-dislocations is presented which defines the CT findings and correlates them with conventional radiographs for various fracture patterns.

Pennal, G.F.; Tile, M.; Waddell, J.P.; and Garside, H.: Pelvic disruption: Assessment and classification. Clin. Orthop. 151:12-21, 1980.

A correlation between mechanisms of injuries, radiographic findings, and therapeutic protocols for pelvic ring fractures based upon more than 20 years of experience are presented.

Pelvic stabilization techniques

Brown, T.D.; Stone, J.P.; Schuster, J.H.; and Mears, D.C.: External fixation of unstable pelvic ring fractures: Comparative rigidity of some current frame configurations. Med. and Biolog. Eng. and Comput. 20:727-733, 1982.

(See following annotation.)

Rubash, H.E.; Brown, T.D.; Nelson, D.D.; and Mears, D.C.: Comparative mechanical performance of some new devices for fixation of unstable pelvic ring fractures. Med. and Biolog. Eng. and Comput. 20:1182-1189, 1983.

These two articles present biomechanical characterizations of a variety of external and internal fixation techniques applied to several types of pelvic ring fractures prepared on instrumental cadaveric pelves.

Mears, D.C.; Rubash, H.E.; and Nelson, D.D.: External fixation of the pelvis using the Pittsburgh triangular frame. Contemp. Orthop. 5:21-38, 1982.

The indications for use and the technique for assembly of the triangular frame, applicable to unstable pelvic ring fractures, are reviewed.

Slätis, P., and Karaharju, E.O.: External fixation of unstable pelvic fractures: Experiences in 22 patients treated with a trapezoid compression frame. Clin. Orthop. 151:73-80, 1980.

The biomechanical basis and clinical experience with the Slätis frame is presented. The role of external pelvic fixation to control hemorrhage and pain and to permit mobilization of the patient is confirmed.

Classification and Treatment

Letournel, E.: Surgical fixation of displaced pelvic fractures and dislocations of the symphysis pubis. Rev. Chir. Orthop. 67:771-782, 1981.

Ninety-three patients with pelvic ring fractures managed by surgical fixation are reviewed with emphasis on the selection of the optimal approach.

Rubash, H.E.; Steed, D.; and Mears, D.C.: Fractures of the pelvic ring. Surg. Rounds 5:16-30, 1982.

The general principles of management as well as the role of external and internal fixation of the pelvis are presented.

Tile, M., and Pennal, G.F.: Pelvic disruptions: Principles of management. Clin. Orthop. 151:56-64, 1980.

A complete protocol for the management of pelvic ring disruption including nonoperative and operative techniques of stabilization is provided.

Pelvic Nonunion and Malunion

Pennal, G.F., and Massiah, K.A.: Nonunion and delayed unions of the pelvis. Clin. Orthop. 151:124-129, 1980.

Forty-two examples of pelvic nonunion are described, indicating how frequently this problem can occur and how disabling it is to a patient. Methods of treatment are discussed.

Acetabular Fractures

Jungbluth, K.H.; Sauer, H.D.; and Schöttle, H.: Results of the surgical reconstruction of acetabular fracture-dislocations. Hefte Unfall. 140:154-160, 1979.

The results of collected statistics by a German study group investigating fixation of acetabular fractures are given.

Letournel, E., and Judet, R.: Fractures of the Acetabulum. New York, Springer-Verlag, 1981.

Surgical treatment of acetabular fractures in regard to radiographic description, surgical approach, and stabilization is presented.

Mears, D.C., and Rubash, H.E.: The use of an extensile exposure of the pelvis. Contemp. Orthop. 6:21, 1983.

An extensile transtrochanteric exposure for visualization of the posterior and anterior columns, lateral ilium, and hip joint is presented along with a review of clinical results.

Tile, M.: Fractures of the acetabulum. Orthop. Clin. North America 11:481-506, 1980.

The selection of suitable surgical exposures for various types of acetabular fractures is illustrated along with pre- and postoperative care.

Pelvic and Acetabular Fractures in Children

Bryan, W.J., and Tullos, H.S.: Pediatric pelvic fractures: Review of 52 patients. J. Trauma 19:799-805, 1979.

A systematic review of juvenile pelvic fractures documented in an urban medical center over a 5-year period is presented.

Bucholz, R.W.; Ezaki, M.; and Ogden, J.A.: Injury to the acetabular triradiate physeal cartilage. J. Bone Joint Surg. 64A:600-609, 1982.

The pathogenesis of triradiate disruption is clarified. The role of open reduction and internal fixation of displaced triradiate fractures is emphasized so that late problems with malunion and growth arrest are minimized.

Reichard, S.A.; Helikson, M.A.; Shorter, N.; White, R.I., Jr.; Shemeta, D.W.; and Haller, J.A., Jr.: Pelvic fractures in children: Review of 120 patients with a new look at general management. J. Pediat. Surg. 15:727-734, 1980.

This account of the management of pelvic disruption in a child is based upon an unusually large clinical experience. It documents the care of the accompanying visceral injuries and hemorrhage as well as pelvic stabilization.

32 HIP AND FEMUR: TRAUMA

Among the topics considered in this section are hip dislocations and fractures and treatment techniques for femoral shaft fractures.

Hip

Hip Dislocations

Anterior Dislocations Anterior traumatic dislocation accounts for only 10 to 20 percent of all traumatic dislocations of the hip. Femoral head damage is common (in up to 87 percent of patients), including transchondral and indentation fractures which often require polytomography for visualization. Indentation fractures deeper than 4 mm have a poor prognosis. Osteonecrosis occurs in 15 percent of these dislocations, and a majority of anterior dislocations eventually progress to degenerative arthritis.

Posterior Dislocations Most of these dislocations can be reduced by closed methods with adequate anesthesia. In some patients with posterior dislocation without apparent fracture, the femoral head may be buttonholed through the capsule, or the piriformis muscle may be interposed, necessitating open reduction.

Once reduced, the hip must be evaluated carefully to ascertain that the reduction is concentric. Computed tomography is probably more useful for this purpose than arthrography or conventional tomography. Inversion of the labrum or osteocartilaginous loose bodies is the cause of nonconcentric reduction and necessitates surgical correction.

The long-term outlook for simple posterior dislocations is directly correlated with the severity of injury. In the more severe, the incidence of posttraumatic arthritis increases from 33 percent at 10 years to 100 percent at 30-year follow-up. Osteonecrosis may occur in 10 percent.

Posterior dislocations or fracture-dislocations are occasionally unrecognized (e.g., hip dislocations with ipsilateral femoral shaft fracture). By 3 weeks postinjury, the acetabulum fills with fibrous tissue, making closed reduction impossible. Even with open reduction, the success rate is less than 25 percent. Osteonecrosis occurs in more than 50 percent. In the younger patient, an attempt to reduce the hip (and repair an acetabular fracture, if present) is probably justified, even as late as 3 months postinjury. In older patients with untreated dislocations, primary reconstructive surgery (arthrodesis or arthroplasty) seems to offer the best prognosis.

Posterior Dislocations With Femoral Head Fractures This injury usually results from high-speed vehicular accidents and accounts for approximately 7 percent of all hip dislocations. Pipkin's classification is most useful in categorizing the femoral head fracture (Fig. 1). The injury probably occurs with the hip flexed less than 60 degrees, and the femoral head is driven into the thicker posterior superior rim of the acetabulum.

Careful evaluation of the initial radiographs is mandatory to exclude an associated femoral neck fracture (Pipkin 3) and to avoid displacing such a fracture during a closed reduction. CT scans provide valuable information, particularly in regard to the presence or absence of free chondral or osteochondral fragments. Closed reduction can be attempted in Pipkin 1, 2, and 4 injuries, and if concentric, the extremity can be held in traction for 6

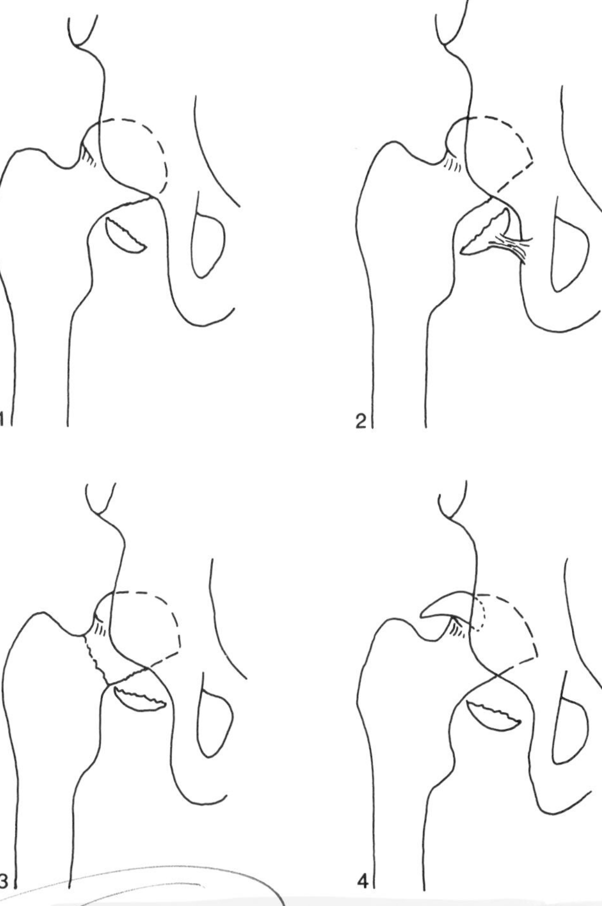

Figure 1: Pipkin's classification of grade IV hip fracture dislocations. (Type 1) Dislocation with a fracture of the femoral head caudad to the fovea. (Type 2) Dislocation with larger femoral head fragment cephalad to the fovea and attached to the ligamentum teres. (Type 3) Type 1 or 2 with a femoral neck fracture. (Type 4) Type 1 or 2 with a fracture of the posterior acetabulum. (Redrawn with permission from Treatment of grade IV fracture-dislocation of the hip, by G. Pipkin, J. Bone Joint Surg. 39A:1027-1042, 1957.)

weeks with the likelihood of good results. Open reduction may be done anterolaterally with trochanteric osteotomy to avoid further injury to the posterior retinacular vessels. However, it is believed by some that the surgical approach should be posterolateral to preserve the undisturbed anterior vessels. By exposing the hip anteriorly, the femoral head may be completely devascularized. Also, open reduction is preferable to closed reduction because of the likelihood of the presence of free intra-articular fragments and the resulting high incidence of coxarthrosis. Small head fragments should be excised, but with large fragments the ligamentum teres should be sectioned and the fragment reattached with two screws, one through the fovea and one inferiorly. The type 3 injury probably should have initial open reduction with pinning of the femoral neck fracture and screw fixation of the head fragment. If a femoral neck fracture is unrecognized and displaced by attempted closed manipulation, a primary endoprosthetic replacement is generally recommended. Others believe that open reduction and internal fixation should be attempted, particularly in the younger age group.

Hip Fractures

General Considerations

EPIDEMIOLOGY: The social and economic costs of hip fractures are staggering. Approximately 200,000 hip fractures occur annually in the United States, resulting in health care costs of $1 billion or more. Hip fractures account for 30 percent of all patients hospitalized for the treatment of fractures and more than one-half of hospital bed days for all patients with fractures. Females experience 70 to 80 percent of these fractures, and there is a doubling of the fracture rate for each decade of life above age 50 years. Hip fracture incidence is lower among blacks. The rate of subcapital and intertrochanteric fractures is approximately equal. Mortality rates of 20 percent within 6 months of hip fracture are reported. Those patients who survive longer than 6 months retain the life expectancy of their age group. Among males over the age of 75 years, mortality increases.

The literature presents conflicting evidence on the incidence of hip fractures. One study finds no indication of a rise in incidence over the past 35 years whereas another study from Sweden predicts that if present trends continue, incidence will double in the next 20 years. It is known that as life expectancy grows, the number of hip fractures occurring annually will increase, imposing even greater burdens on the health care system. Rehabilitation of these patients to their prefracture social status is difficult, with perhaps only one-half returning to their former degree of independence. This adds another dimension to the economic cost of hip fractures.

ETIOLOGY: Cardiac disease and senility frequently are associated with hip fractures. Although only one patient in five has overt clinical signs of these problems on admission, over one-half have abnormal EKG findings, and nearly one-third may have occult episodic arrhythmias on continual EKG monitoring. These arrhythmias are serious enough to cause dizziness, syncope, and falls resulting in hip fractures. These associated problems convey a decreased prognosis for survival.

Osteoporosis is accepted widely as an important factor in the etiology of hip fractures, and several recent studies demonstrate that estrogen administration in postmenopausal patients lowers the incidence of hip and wrist fractures. However, a recent investigation from Australia compares femoral heads from fracture patients with femoral heads removed at autopsy. The findings are that: (1) the Singh index is not reliable as an indicator of the bone content of the femoral head; (2) the bone content of the femoral heads in the two groups does not differ; (3) osteomalacia is not a factor; and (4) the distribution of trabecular microfractures does not implicate progressive fatigue as a cause of femoral neck fracture. The study concludes that the single most important factor in the etiology of femoral neck fracture is injury due to falling.

INFECTION: Incidence of wound infection in hip fractures is higher than in any other type of orthopaedic surgery. Several reports show the value of prophylactic antibiotics. A recent double-blind prospective study shows infection rates of 4.7 percent in the placebo group versus 0.7 percent in the group given antibiotics. In addition, treated patients have fewer positive urine cultures and a lower mean peak in postoperative temperature. Use of an appropriate broad spectrum antibiotic beginning during or just prior to surgery and continuing for 1 to 2 days postoperatively is recommended in these high-risk patients.

THROMBOEMBOLIC DISEASE: This may occur more frequently in hip fracture patients than in those undergoing total hip arthroplasty. Low-dose heparin does not appear to be effective in preventing thrombosis and embolism in the hip fracture patient. Some studies report that aspirin has a prophylactic value especially in males, whereas others find it ineffective. Warfarin is probably the best prophylactic agent, but its administration must be monitored closely to prevent bleeding complications. Dextran probably is effective but increases the risk of congestive heart failure in the elderly patient. Prophylaxis for thromboembolic disease is recommended, but a totally safe, effective treatment is not currently available.

SPECIAL PROBLEMS: The senile, institutionalized patient presents a particular challenge. If ambulatory before fracture, surgery should be aimed at restorating function in the patient rather than normal anatomy. This approach suggests percutaneous pinning of Garden I and II (undisplaced) fractures and hemiarthroplasty for Garden III and IV as the treatments of choice. Intertrochanteric fractures in these patients are perhaps best treated with condylocephalic techniques. Since the bedridden, severely osteoporotic patient is likely to lose fixation of the fracture regardless of the surgical device used, nonsurgical treatment with traction for a few days seems preferable to internal fixation. Senile patients should be returned to their prehospital environments as rapidly as possible.

Hip fractures in patients with rheumatoid arthritis may be complicated by the usually associated osteoporosis and rheumatoid involvement of the hip joint. Displaced subcapital fractures may be treated with hemiarthroplasty or with total hip arthroplasty if the acetabulum is involved.

Hip fractures in neurologically impaired patients have a poor prognosis. In one series of patients with Parkinson's disease, the mortality rate was 80 percent (twelve of fifteen) in patients treated with endoprosthesis as compared with the 47 percent rate among all other patients with hip fracture. When dislocation of the prosthesis occurred (in 37 percent), all patients died within 6 months. Efforts should be made to internally fix these fractures, but if endoprosthesis is necessary, the prosthesis should be inserted through an anterolateral approach to help avoid dislocation.

PATHOLOGIC FRACTURES: These present special problems. If there is a reasonable life expectancy, surgical therapy is indicated for pathological and impending fractures. Criteria for stabilizing impending fractures include a lytic lesion more than 2.5 cm in size, destruction of 50 percent or more of the cortex of a long bone, and persistent pain with ambulation after irradiation. Surgical stabilization of an impending fracture is technically easier, and the patient is spared the pain and disability of a fracture.

Patients treated prophylactically tend to have less operative mortality, fewer complications, less stabilization failure, and more successful rehabilitation than those who suffer pathologic fracture before surgery.

Preoperative irradiation therapy should be administered whenever possible. Most commonly 300 rads per day for 10 days are delivered to the metastatic deposit with minimal late normal tissue effects. If rapid therapeutic effects are desired, a total dose of 2,000 rads can be delivered over 4 to 5 days; the normal tissue effects, however, are greater.

Polymethyl methacrylate (PMMA) used as an adjunct to internal fixation in pathologic fractures provides pain relief and facilitates rehabilitation. PMMA in long bones helps to prevent telescoping and nail protrusion. Generally, it is difficult to achieve good filling of the medullary canal with PMMA unless the pathologic area is approached directly, the tumor removed, and PMMA packed in or injected. Bone grafts do not heal well when subjected to irradiation and are not useful in pathologic fractures unless at least 9 months have elapsed since completion of local irradiation.

Tumor involvement of the femoral head and neck can be treated by hemiarthroplasty, often employing a long-stem prosthesis. PMMA can be injected retrograde from below through a portal in the femur once the prosthesis is in place. This is perhaps better than filling the medullary canal with PMMA and trying to insert a long-stem prosthesis, which risks incomplete insertion if the PMMA cures too rapidly. In one report of 160 long-stem prostheses, the median survival time was 5.6 months, and the deep infection rate was 1.2 percent.

If the acetabulum is involved by tumor, total hip arthroplasty can be done using a standard or long-stem prosthesis. The tumor must be cleaned out of the ilium, and the acetabular cup can be stabilized by some combination of metallic mesh, Steinmann pins or screws, PMMA, and a protrusio shell. Technical improvisations under these difficult circumstances are often necessary. These modified arthroplasties may last only a limited time but provide immediate stability and pain relief.

A tumor in the subtrochanteric region is best treated by a Zickel nail (intramedullary rod with triflanged nail) with or without cement (Fig. 2).

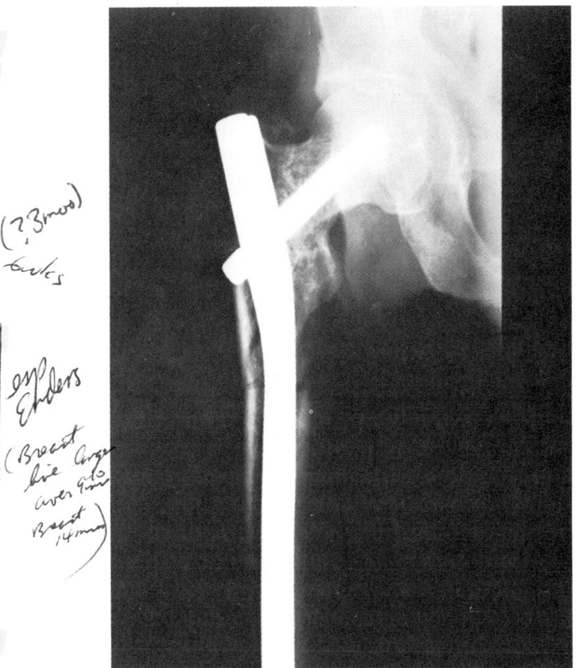

Figure 2: Zickel nail used to stabilize a pathologic fracture (lung primary) in the trochanteric-subtrochanteric region.

Intracapsular Fractures There is no consensus regarding the optimal treatment of this difficult fracture. There are strong advocates of internal fixation and equally strong proponents of prosthetic replacement. There are even a few supporters of primary total hip replacement in fit patients with subcapital fractures. Success rates of various treatment modalities vary widely in the literature, and critical interpretation is necessary. Garden I and II fractures may achieve a 90 percent success rate with multiple pinning, nail, or screw fixation. Controversy arises in the treatment of displaced femoral neck fractures.

REDUCTION AND INTERNAL FIXATION: Accurate reduction of the fracture in anatomic position or slight valgus may be the key to success. Accurate placement of a fixation device that allows fracture impaction by sliding or telescoping is the second major determinant of success or failure. The type of fixation device is less important than the quality of reduction and correct usage of the implant. Multiple pins inserted parallel to each other either by percutaneous or open operation can achieve 75 percent success rates. The rate of successful fracture fixation by sliding nails ranges from 50 to 84 percent. The Pugh sliding nail achieved the highest rate, although some asymptomatic patients with osteonecrosis are included in this series.

The compression screw is not a universally successful device for the displaced femoral neck fracture. Malrotation of the head fragment can be prevented by stabilizing the femoral head with two Kirschner wires prior to the insertion of the screw. Threads of the screw should be entirely in the femoral head fragment and not across the fracture line (thereby preventing impaction).

Other adjuncts to treatment include open reduction and bone grafting. In patients under 40 years of age with imperfectly reduced fractures, open reduction is suggested. A posterior approach aids in reduction and replacement of posterior comminution of the femoral neck. A muscle pedicle bone graft of the quadratus femoris may be used to buttress the posterior neck and may provide more blood supply to the femoral head fragment. Like open reduction, the muscle pedicle graft may be used in younger patients. When using the C-arm and videodisc recorder to assess fracture reduction, technically satisfactory images should be obtained. Quality of reduction is generally best judged with permanent radiographs.

The incidence of osteonecrosis and segmental collapse of the femoral head varies, but it seems dependent upon accuracy of reduction and stability of fixation. Most femoral heads in displaced fractures are devascularized at least partially by the injury, but revascularization occurs occasionally. Although serial technetium bone scans may predict osteonecrosis, their prognostic value is unclear.

PROSTHETIC REPLACEMENT: There is controversy concerning use of the conventional (Moore or Thompson) or the bipolar (Bateman, Giliberty, etc.) prosthesis and whether they should be cemented. There is little evidence documenting the superiority of either of these methods. A report on the bipolar (Christiansen) prosthesis shows a decrease in walking ability and radiographic deterioration at 5-year follow-up. Another report concludes there is no advantage of the Bateman universal proximal femoral endoprosthesis over the Moore prosthesis at 2.5-year follow-up.

In a comparison of the Moore and Thompson prostheses, it was apparent that technical problems were related to improper neck length and head size, varus position of the stem, and poor seating of the prosthesis on the femoral neck. The results of 63 percent of 600 prostheses were considered excellent or good. The incidence of infection and dislocation seems higher when a posterior approach is used, whereas femoral fracture and prosthetic malalignment occur more often with the anterolateral approach. The question of the efficacy of routine cementing of these prostheses is unresolved. If a good "press fit" is not achieved, PMMA can be used but may pose an additional hazard to the frail, elderly patient.

Disassembly of the commonly used bipolar prostheses occasionally has occurred in vivo. When dislocated, it is much more difficult to reduce closed than is a conventional prosthesis. Bipolar prostheses generally are cemented into the femur based on the assumption that conversion to a total hip could be done more easily should acetabular wear occur. Whether this will be necessary or practical is unknown. Another means of fixation is porous coating of the prosthetic stem to encourage bone ingrowth. This remains experimental but may solve the problems associated with PMMA use.

Primary total hip arthroplasty for subcapital fracture occasionally has been recommended assuming that the quality of the result is superior to an endoprosthesis and that only one operation is necessary. In one series, the dislocation rate was 15 percent. In another group of eighty-five patients at 1-year follow-up, thirteen patients were more active than before fracture whereas thirty-three were less active. A frail, elderly patient with an intracapsular fracture is probably not a candidate for a total hip unless there is accompanying disease of the acetabulum.

INTERNAL FIXATION OR ENDOPROSTHESIS: Several studies have attempted to evaluate this question. The advantages of internal fixation are shorter hospitalization time, less expense, and lessened morbidity. Endoprosthetic replacement seems a more definitive procedure with fewer reoperations and better results at 1 year. However, these studies are flawed in that none used a compression screw or sliding nail in the internal fixation group. Neither method seems to have any clear superiority. Even though their advantages and disadvantages vary, the documented percentage of good to excellent results for both is similar. A well-conceived, prospective, randomized study done by experienced surgeons comparing the compression screw or sliding nail to the Moore prosthesis is needed. Lacking this, a well-reduced and accurately fixed fracture may be slightly preferable, especially in the patient under 70 years of age.

Intertrochanteric Fractures The major need in unstable intertrochanteric fractures is a bone implant composite capable of providing firm fixation of the fragments and withstanding the bending moment occurring at the neck shaft junction of the femur. Many investigators have studied the biomechanics of this problem. The variable factors include bone quality, comminution, reduction, implant choice, and implant placement. The surgeon can control the type of reduction as well as implant selection and insertion. The available implants are of three major types: rigid nail plates, telescoping or collapsing nails and screws, and the newer condylocephalic nails.

RIGID NAILS: The Jewett nail remains the most commonly used of this type of implant. One series of over 1,000 fractures, anatomically reduced, showed a complication rate of nail penetration or cutting out in 9 percent. Poorly reduced fractures had more nail-related problems. The infection rate was 3.5 percent and virtually all (98.7 percent) healed. However, another report showed a 38 percent rate of femoral head penetration by Jewett nails. Many believe the rigid one-piece nail does not satisfactorily stabilize the unstable intertrochanteric fractures.

TELESCOPING IMPLANTS: These devices allow for fracture impaction and thus appear to be superior to one-piece nails in unstable comminuted fractures. Impaction at or following surgery aids the formation of a more stable load transmission system. Biomechanically, there does not appear to be any significant advantage of the compression screw over the sliding nail. The average collapse (impaction) in stable fracture was 14.9 mm and 19.6 mm in unstable fractures in one study. If the fracture is mechanically impacted at surgery, less postoperative collapse occurs. Surgical impaction seems advantageous in that better bone contact is obtained, thereby decreasing the chances of fracture displacement.

These devices are available with 135 and 150 degree nail plate angles. In the very unstable fractures, a valgus reduction can be achieved and the 150 degree implant used. Most believe this is superior to and should replace the displacement osteotomy. The end of the nail or screw should be positioned in the center of the femoral head about 1 cm from the joint.

CONDYLOCEPHALIC NAILS: Increasingly popular in the past few years, both the multiple nail (Ender) and single nail (Harris) methods of fixation are available. Their foremost advantage is that they bear less mechanical stress at the neck shaft junction (Fig. 3). Other benefits are decreased operative time, infection rate, and blood loss as

Figure 3: The bending movement (d) is greater on a nail plate than on a condylocephalic device.

compared to standard hip nailing. However, these advantages are offset by a high incidence of problems about the knee (e.g., pain, backing out of the nails) in up to 40 percent of patients (Fig. 4), reoperation in 20 percent or more, external rotation deformity, and an occasional supracondylar fracture of the femur at the point of nail insertion. Some believe that condylocephalic nails should be used only for stable fractures.

The surgical technique may be as demanding as conventional nailing, a fact supported by the high incidence of technical problems in the early cases in virtually all series. The Harris condylocephalic nail is diamond-shaped and only one is used. One report suggests that the complication rate is lower than with the Ender method. There are several comparative analyses of conventional nailing and the Ender method. The consensus is that a compression screw or sliding nail is equal or superior to the Ender technique, particularly in unstable fractures.

Condylocephalic nailing requires image intensification and a videodisc recorder with a suitable fracture table. Although the collimation of these units is excellent, there is some backscatter from the patient's thigh when the C-arm is in the lateral position. The x-ray tube should be positioned on the side of the thigh opposite to the surgeon.

Other treatment adjuncts: Acrylic cement has been recommended for use in unstable intertrochanteric fractures, particularly in patients over 70 years of age and those with severe osteoporosis. Its routine use, however, is probably unnecessary if a sliding implant is used.

Endoprosthetic replacement occasionally is advocated for intertrochanteric fractures but does not seem to offer any particular benefit and adds potential for complications.

Subtrochanteric Fractures Mechanical stresses, especially tensile stresses on the lateral femoral cortex, are highest in the subtrochanteric region of the femur. This results in a high rate of implant failure, particularly for nails with a long side plate. Intramedullary devices have become the treatment of choice. Immediate cancellous bone grafting is recommended for comminuted fractures without medial contact.

The Zickel nail provides immediate stability, is technically demanding to insert, and requires an extensive operative exposure (Fig. 5). Addition of cerclage wires or bands may be helpful to control comminuted fragments.

A stepped, fluted intramedullary rod (Sampson) has been introduced, and initial results seem promising. This rod does not give as secure a purchase in the proximal fragment as do the Zickel nail and Ender nails.

The Ender technique is used widely for subtrochanteric fractures. Often, nails are inserted from both medial and lateral portals in the supracondylar area. In comminuted fractures, Ender nailing does not give good immediate stability, and the patient should be kept in skeletal traction for 3 weeks after nailing. This method is less invasive and therefore less injurious to the soft-tissue attachments of the fracture fragments (Fig. 6).

Closed treatment of these fractures usually requires skeletal traction for several months. A modification of functional bracing introduced recently may make nonoperative care a viable option without necessitating prolonged bed rest. After several weeks of 90-90 degrees traction, the leg is lowered to horizontal over 7 to 10 days when a single-leg hip spica cast is applied with the hip abducted 20 degrees. Knee hinges are added to the cast,

Figure 4: A frequent complication of Ender fixation with the nails backing out and leading to: (A) varus deformity at the fracture site; and (B) knee pain from the prominent nails.

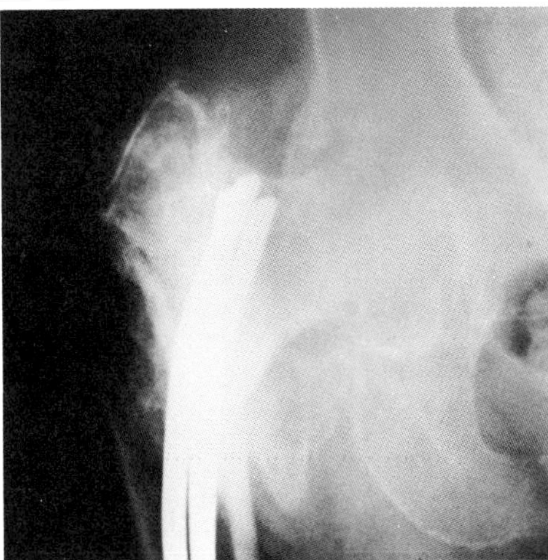

Figure 4-A

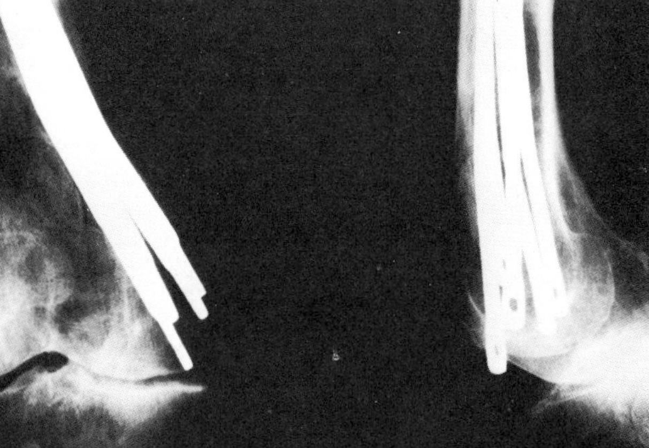

Figure 4-B

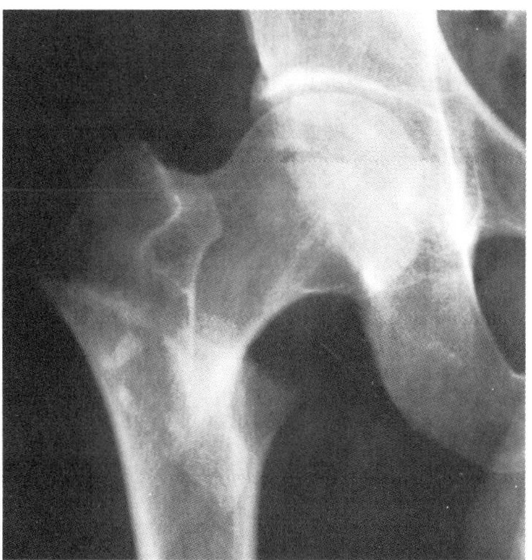
Figure 5-A

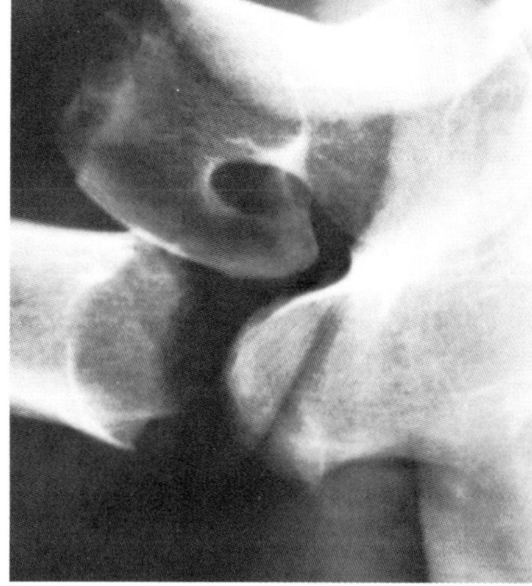
Figure 5-B

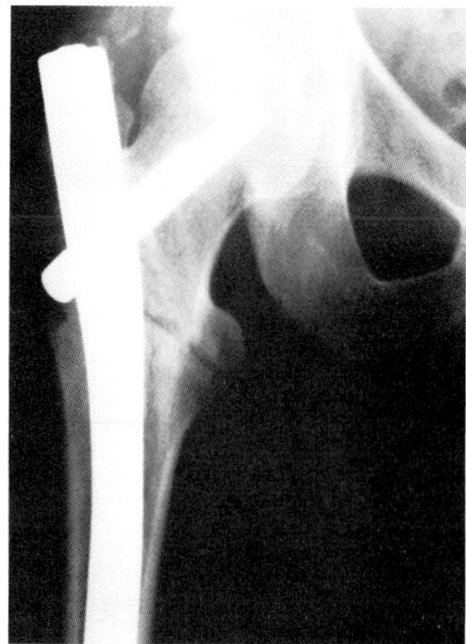
Figure 5-C

Figure 5: (A,B) Initial anteroposterior and lateral views of an unstable fracture. (C) At 4 weeks, callus is visible, and the fracture healed anatomically after Zickel nailing.

and 5- to 7-cm shoe lifts are inserted in the contralateral shoe. Varus angulation may be corrected by wedging. Close follow-up with weekly radiographs is required. Hip and knee function are good, and there is no need to remove an implant later.

The nail plate in the care of subtrochanteric fractures rapidly is being replaced by implants that maintain alignment while allowing for impaction of the fracture fragments. The Zickel, Ender, and Sampson devices are most appropriate. Traction and modified functional bracing seem to offer an alternative to surgery, but the risk of angulation deformity is high.

Femoral Shaft Fractures

General Considerations Fractures of the femoral shaft are amenable to various treatment options including traction, functional bracing, plating, and closed or open intramedullary nailing. Traction avoids the risk of infection at the expense of longer hospitalization as well as greater rates of nonunion and angulation. Functional bracing avoids infection but is more likely to result in limb shortening due to angulation, particularly when used in treatment of fractures above the middle third of the femur. Short-term loss of knee motion may also be a problem. Closed nailing shortens the hospital stay, prevents angulation, allows good joint motion, and has a very low infection rate. A less than anatomic reduction with closed nailing does not seem to be a disadvantage. Open nailing has similar advantages but involves a higher infection rate. Plating is useful in proximal, distal, and comminuted femoral fractures but carries the highest rate of infection and often necessitates later surgery for removal of the implants.

The femoral shaft is surrounded by a generous soft-tissue envelope and is less subject to infection and nonunion than the tibia. Immediate or early internal fixation of open femoral fractures gives a high percentage of satisfactory

Figure 6: (A) Spiral subtrochanteric fracture in a 38-year-old man struck by a car. (B) After Ender nailing and 3 weeks of postoperative skeletal traction, anatomical healing occurred.

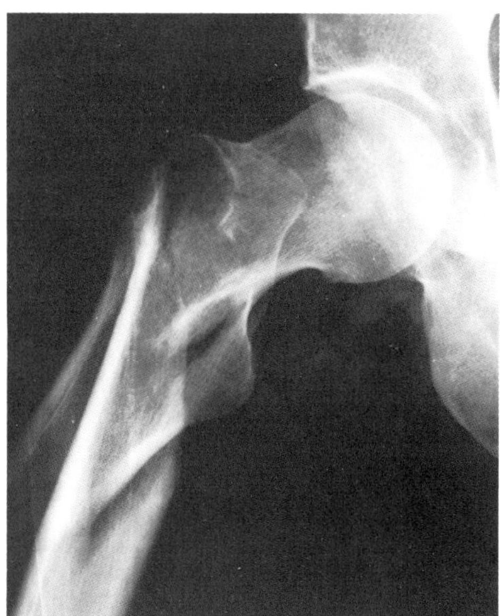
Figure 6-A

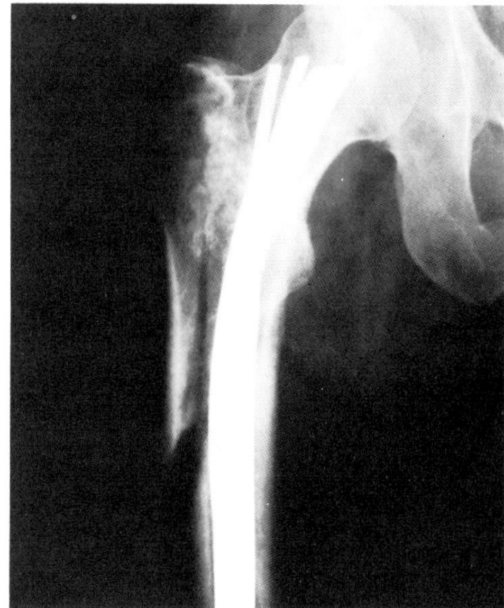
Figure 6-B

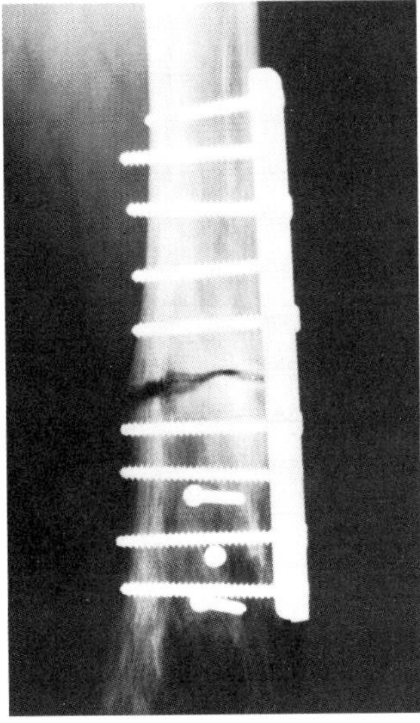

Figure 7-A

Figure 7-B

Figure 7-C

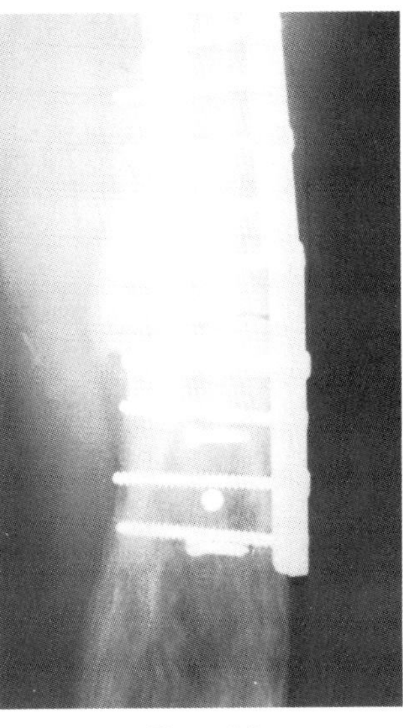

Figure 7-D

Figure 7: Extensive Paget's disease with a transverse femoral shaft fracture in a 58-year-old male. (A) At 1 week, the plate has straightened the lateral bow of the femur, causing the fracture to gap open medially. (B) At 4 months, some callus is visible medially. (C) At 7 months, a fatigue fracture has occurred through the plate, allowing better apposition of the fracture. (D) At 11 months, union is proceeding with trabeculae across the fracture.

results with minimal infection, particularly with a closed nailing technique.

Following open fractures, it is recommended the wound be debrided after the injury and closed secondarily at a later date if there is significant contamination. There currently is a tendency toward early internal fixation in open fractures particularly following polytrauma.

Concomitant Knee Ligament Damage Trauma severe enough to cause a midshaft femoral fracture results in some ipsilateral knee ligament damage in approximately 45 percent of the patients. The anterior cruciate and medial collateral are the most frequently injured ligaments, and recognition of the injury is often delayed due to difficulty in examining the knee joint below a femoral fracture. If ligament damage is suspected, arthroscopy or stress radiographs under anesthesia can be carried out. It is recommended to carefully test knee ligaments after internal fixation of a femoral fracture so that the diagnosis of ligament damage can be made when primary repair is still feasible.

Ipsilateral Femoral Shaft and Neck Fractures Ipsilateral fractures of the femoral shaft and neck are uncommon. Occasionally, a femoral neck fracture is missed because initial radiographs do not include the hip. Often these patients have had multisystem trauma. It is suggested that an abduction force causes the shaft fracture, and impingement of the neck against the lateral acetabulum causes the hip fracture. The shaft fracture frequently is comminuted whereas the neck fracture may be undisplaced. Fixation of both fractures is desirable. The shaft fracture usually can be fixed with an IM nail or plates, and traction will reduce the hip fracture for screws, multiple pins, or a sliding nail or compression screw. Although the Ender technique has been suggested for these fractures, it is technically difficult and not suitable for secure fixation of femoral neck fractures.

Paget's Disease Femoral fractures through pagetoid bone may have a nonunion rate of 40 percent, with subtrochanteric and upper shaft fractures most commonly progressing to nonunion. Callus in these fractures may be involved with Paget's disease and is not a reliable sign of union. Assessment of union should be based upon immobility at the fracture site, absence of pain with weight-bearing, and development of trabeculae across the fracture site by radiograph. Implants may be difficult to apply due to the bowing of pagetoid bone (Fig. 7). Intramedullary devices are probably superior to plates in this disease. An osteotomy occasionally may be performed above or below a fracture to straighten a bowed femur and allow use of an IM nail.

Head Injuries The difficulty of managing a femoral fracture by traction in a head-injured patient with spastic hemiplegia is well recognized. The end result of internal fixation in this group is far superior to that achieved by either traction or traction and a cast. Intramedullary nailing allows faster mobilization, lessens the difficulty of nursing care, results in less shortening and angulation, and provides greater knee motion as compared with traction. However, the incidence of wound infection in the head-injured patient is higher than in other groups.

Fractures Below Femoral Head Prostheses Stress concentration at the tip of a prosthesis may cause a fracture. If the prosthesis is not cemented, it may be possible to insert Ender pins across the fracture and up the medullary canal beside the prosthetic stem (Fig. 8). The same technique can be used for a fracture below a nail plate. A cemented prosthesis presents a more difficult situation. If traction is not possible, cerclage and internal fixation may be carried out, or the prosthesis may have to be removed and replaced with a long-stem prosthesis. The fracture site probably should be bone grafted at the same time.

Treatment Techniques

Traction and Functional Bracing Occasional femoral fractures are not suitable for internal fixation, and non-operative care is necessary. Traction with a Thomas splint

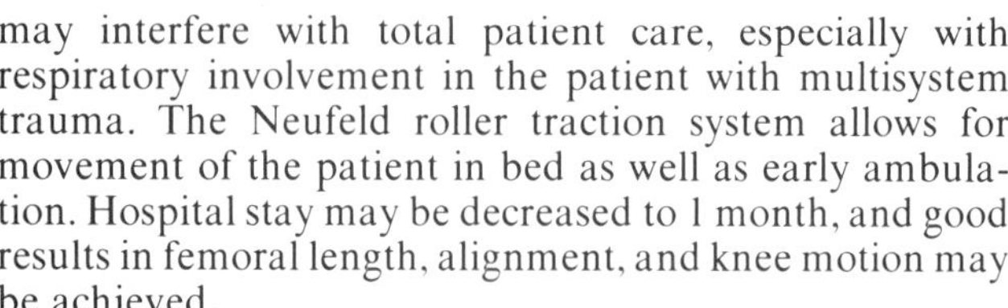

Figure 8

Figure 8: Spiral fracture below a prosthetic stem stabilized with Ender nails inserted through the trochanter and cerclage wires. Uneventful healing occurred.

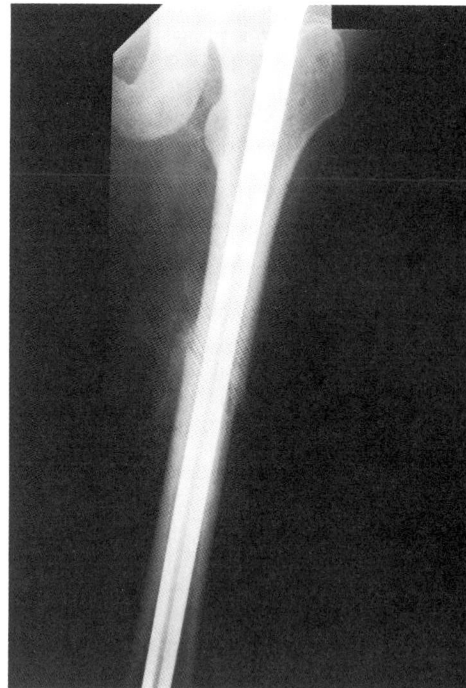

Figure 9

Figure 9: An ideal transverse femoral fracture treated with closed intramedullary reaming and nailing. Good callus at 2 months.

may interfere with total patient care, especially with respiratory involvement in the patient with multisystem trauma. The Neufeld roller traction system allows for movement of the patient in bed as well as early ambulation. Hospital stay may be decreased to 1 month, and good results in femoral length, alignment, and knee motion may be achieved.

The technique of using pins-in-plaster for femoral shaft fractures may not produce good results due to pin tract infection, shortening, angulation, and frequent rehospitalization and reapplication of the cast.

Functional bracing seems to be useful, particularly in fractures of the distal third of the femur. Controversy exists about its feasibility as a treatment for proximal third shaft fractures, but according to some reports if applied in abduction with a pelvic belt and hip hinge, the varus angulation can be reduced in magnitude or prevented.

Biomechanical studies show that 20 to 50 percent of applied weight can be removed from a femoral fracture by use of a snugly fitted functional brace. Good muscle tone aids in this weight transfer. As fracture callus matures, the femur assumes a gradually increasing percentage of the applied load, reaching 90 to 100 percent at the time of union. Failure of stress transfer indicates delayed union or nonunion, with danger of refracture if the functional brace is removed.

Success has been reported in functional brace treatment of ipsilateral fractures of the femur and tibia when open injury or comminution does not safely allow internal fixation. But, bilateral femoral shaft fractures are very difficult to treat in traction and functional braces, and they should be internally fixed if at all possible.

Plating of Femoral Shaft Fractures Plate osteosynthesis for comminuted diaphyseal fractures continues to be advocated by some. When used, rigid fixation and interfragmentary compression should be achieved. Double plating is discouraged now in favor of one dorsolateral plate. Cancellous bone grafting is desirable in patients with cortical deficiency (especially in the medial cortex), devascularized fragments, and without rigid fixation.

Sepsis rates run from 3 to 6 percent in the open treatment of closed fractures. Implant failure and refracture occur in 3 to 7 percent. These mechanical complications are minimized by achieving rigid stabilization, bone grafting cortical defects, and not removing the plate until 18 to 36 months have elapsed. Good to excellent results are achieved in 90 percent of the patients treated with plating for femoral fractures.

Intramedullary Nailing The technique of closed intramedullary reaming and nailing is increasingly popular. Advantages include shorter hospital stay, high rate of primary union (over 99 percent in some studies), lowered sepsis rate compared with open nailing, and faster joint mobilization (Fig. 9).

The image intensifier, videodisc recorder, and special fracture table are necessary. A Steinmann pin inserted through the femoral condyles allows application of traction to distract the femur slightly, while permitting flexion of the hip and knee to prevent sciatic or peroneal nerve damage. Care must be taken with the perineal post to avoid the complication of pudendal nerve palsy. The perineal post should be well padded and can be placed between the genitalia and the intact limb. Curved nails simulating the natural bow of the femur provide better rotational control. However, to pass the curved nail, the proximal fragments must be overreamed slightly to decrease the risk of the nail binding or causing further comminution. In fractures with a segmental defect, it is possible to insert ground up bone graft material through a chest tube into the area of the defect, thereby avoiding opening of the fracture to place the graft.

As the closed technique has been perfected, indications for its use have expanded from the transverse and short oblique midshaft fractures to the more comminuted and those at either end of the diaphysis. In comminuted fractures the nail may serve as an internal splint and require additional treatment such as traction, functional brace, or spica cast.

The Ender technique has been adapted for femoral shaft fractures, using nails inserted both medially and laterally. Reaming is not done, and thus the surgery is faster with less blood loss. Rigid fixation is not obtained by this method, and technical difficulties may be encountered in passing the nails across the fracture site. Although this technique occasionally may be useful, it does not seem likely to supplant closed intramedullary nailing.

ANNOTATED BIBLIOGRAPHY

Hip

Hip Dislocations

Epstein, H.C.: Traumatic Dislocations of the Hip. Baltimore, Williams & Wilkins, 1980.

This book presents a long-term follow-up of a very large experience with various groups of fractures and fracture-dislocations of the hip.

Upadhyay, S.S., and Moulton, A.: The long-term results of traumatic posterior dislocation of the hip. J. Bone Joint Surg. 63B:548-551, 1981.

Eighty-one patients are reviewed with average follow-up of 12.5 years. There was a direct correlation between the severity of the initial injury and the long-term results. The incidence of osteoarthritis was 33 percent at 10 years and 100 percent at 30 years.

Hip Fractures

General Considerations

Harrington, K.D.: New trends in the management of lower extremity metastases. Clin. Orthop. 169:53-61, 1982.

Prophylactic fixation is indicated in lytic lesions 2.5 mm or larger, lesions destroying 50 percent or more of the femoral cortex, and those causing pain with weight-bearing after adequate irradiation. Choice of fixation device, use of methyl methacrylate, and radiation doses are discussed.

Lane, J.M.; Sculco, T.P.; and Zolan, S.: Treatment of pathological fractures of the hip by endoprosthetic replacement. J. Bone Joint Surg. 62A:954-959, 1980.

One hundred and sixty-seven patients with long-stemmed prostheses or total hips are discussed. Pain relief was dramatic and median survival was 5.6 months. Cementing the prosthesis allowed stabilization of the entire femur.

Melton, L.J., III; Ilstrup, D.M.; Riggs, B.L.; and Beckenbaugh, R.D.: Fifty-year trend in hip fracture incidence. Clin. Orthop. 162:144-149, 1982.

Over the last several decades there has been no significant increase in the incidence rates of hip fractures in Rochester, Minnesota. There is no evidence to support the contention that hip fracture incidence has increased in recent years.

Wicks, M.; Garrett, R.; Vernon-Roberts, B.; and Fazzalari, N.: Absence of metabolic bone disease in the proximal femur in patients with fractures of the femoral neck. J. Bone Joint Surg. 64B:319-322, 1982.

The Singh index is an unreliable indicator of the bone content of the femoral head. Decreasing bone density correlates with increasing age, and the primary cause of subcapital fracture is a fall, not osteoporosis.

Intracapsular Fractures

Drinker, H., and Murray, W.R.: The universal proximal femoral endoprosthesis. J. Bone Joint Surg. 61A:1167-1174, 1979.

This study compares 107 Batemans and 160 cemented Thompsons. Five of the nine dislocated Bateman prostheses were irreducible by closed means, and overall the dislocation rate was 14.8 percent for Bateman and 7.5 percent for Thompson with most occurring in patients with previously existing neuromuscular disease.

Fielding, J.W.: The telescoping Pugh nail in the surgical management of the displaced intracapsular fracture of the femoral neck. Clin. Orthop. 152:123-130, 1980.

The Pugh nail appears to be superior to prosthetic replacement based on 84 percent good to excellent results in 256 patients. Seventeen percent had osteonecrosis, but twenty-four were asymptomatic and were considered satisfactory.

Kwok, D.C., and Cruess, R.L.: A retrospective study of Moore and Thompson hemiarthroplasty. Clin. Orthop. 169:179-185, 1982.

In 599 hemiarthroplasties, the 3-month mortality rate was 5 percent, and the dislocation rate 5.3 percent. Technical problems (improper neck length, inaccurate head size, varus or poor seating of prosthesis) account for many failures.

Lucie, R.S.; Fuller, S.; Burdick, D.C.; and Johnston, R.M.: Early prediction of avascular necrosis of the femoral head following femoral neck fractures. Clin. Orthop. 161:207-214, 1981.

The article reports 92.5 percent success in predicting femoral head viability with 99 MTC phosphate scintigraphy. Based on these findings, a rational treatment program can be outlined.

Soreide, O.; Molster, A.; and Raugstad, T.S.: Replacement with the Christiansen endoprosthesis in acute femoral neck fractures, a five-year follow-up study. Acta Orthop. Scand. 51:137-144, 1980.

Patients with a trunion-bearing endoprosthesis were studied at 15 and 67 months postoperatively. The patients noted little change, but objective results showed a decrease in function, more acetabular protrusion, as well as increased prosthetic settling and loosening.

Intertrochanteric Fractures

Chapman, M.W.; Bowman, W.E.; Csongradi, J.J.; Day, L.J.; Trafton, P.G.; and Bovill, E.G., Jr.: The use of Ender's pins in extracapsular fractures of the hip. J. Bone Joint Surg. 63A:14-28, 1981.

A randomized prospective study of Ender nailing and the compression screw. More technical errors, reoperation, and knee problems occurred in the Ender group. Ender nailing is not a simple operative technique.

Harris, L.J.: Closed retrograde intramedullary nailing of peritrochanteric fractures of the femur with a new nail. J. Bone Joint Surg. 62A:1185-1193, 1980.

One hundred and seventy-six cases of inter- and subtrochanteric fractures with at least 8 months follow-up are reviewed. Loss of reduction occurred in only 2.3 percent, and there were no nonunions, implant failures, or infections. Valgus reduction and manual impaction are stressed.

Jensen, J.S.; Sonne-Holm, S.; and Tondevold, E.: Unstable intertrochanteric fractures. A comparative analysis of four methods of internal fixation. Acta Orthop. Scand. 51:949-962, 1980.

McLaughlin, Jewett, sliding screw-plate, and Ender methods are compared in over 1,000 unstable fractures. Technical failures were 48 to 53 percent in Jewett and McLaughlin, and the reoperation rate was 41 percent with Ender technique. The sliding screw is the only suitable implant for unstable intertrochanteric fractures.

Kaufer, H.: Mechanics of the treatment of hip injuries. Clin. Orthop. 146:53-61, 1980.

Variables of bone quality, fragment geometry, reduction, implant choice, and placement of the implant are discussed. Stable reduction, whether anatomic or not, must be achieved.

Wilson, H.J., Jr.; Rubin, B.D.; Helbig, F.E.; Fielding, J.W.; and

Unis, G.L.: Treatment of intertrochanteric fractures with the Jewett nail: Experience with 1,015 cases. Clin. Orthop. 148:186-191, 1980.

Fractures were reduced anatomically or in slight varus. Unsatisfactory nailing occurred in 6.8 percent with complications in virtually all. Wound infection rate was 3.5 percent. Union occurred in 98.7 percent.

Subtrochanteric Fractures

DeLee, J.C.; Clanton, T.O.; and Rockwood, C.A., Jr.: Closed treatment of subtrochanteric fractures of the femur in a modified cast brace. J. Bone Joint Surg. 63A:773-779, 1981.

Reducing the fracture in 90-90 degree skeletal traction for 3 to 4 weeks is suggested. Apply plaster one-leg spica with hip abducted 20 degrees and add knee hinges and lift on sound leg. Fracture reduction plus frequent follow-up to avoid varus angulation are emphasized.

Pankovich, A.M., and Tarabishy, I.E.: Ender nailing of intertrochanteric and subtrochanteric fractures of the femur. J. Bone Joint Surg. 62A:635-645, 1980.

The Ender technique involves simpler and shorter surgery, less blood loss, minimal risk of infection, quicker functional return, and less chance of delayed union or nonunion. Nails are inserted both medially and laterally in virtually all subtrochanteric fractures.

Zickel, R.E.: Subtrochanteric femoral fractures. Orthop. Clin. North America 11:555-568, 1980.

A review of the biomechanical stresses acting on subtrochanteric fractures emphasizing the desirable features of intramedullary fixation.

Femoral Shaft Fractures

General Considerations

Casey, M.J., and Chapman, M.W.: Ipsilateral concomitant fractures of the hip and femoral shaft. J. Bone Joint Surg. 61A:503-509, 1979.

In fifty-two cases in the literature, the hip fracture was initially missed in 31 percent. These are usually associated with complex, multisystem trauma. Intracapsular fracture should be fixed with multiple pins, the shaft fracture with IM rod, plate, or Ender's pins.

Geist, R.W., and Laros, G.S.: Femoral shaft fractures: Editorial comment and comparative results. Clin. Orthop. 138:5-9, 1979.

The results of over 2,300 femoral shaft fractures are reviewed and compared. Suggested minimum standards for reporting results are proposed to enable more accurate comparison between plating, IM rods, traction, and functional bracing.

Treatment Techniques

Hansen, S.T., and Winquist, R.A.: Closed intramedullary nailing of the femur, Küntscher technique with reaming. Clin. Orthop. 138:56-61, 1979.

Of 300 fractures there was only one nonunion and nineteen malunions (most relatively minor). Infection occurred in only 0.7 percent. Technical modifications of the Küntscher method are discussed.

Magerl, F.; Wyss, A.; Brunner, C.; and Binder, W.: Plate osteosynthesis of femoral shaft fractures in adults. Clin. Orthop. 138:62-73, 1979.

Primary cancellous bone grafting is important in fractures with nonrigid fixation, devascularized fragments, or cortical defects. Some of the complications in this series would have been averted by primary bone grafting.

Mooney, V.: Nonoperative care using functional bracing for the fractured femur. *In* Controversies in Orthopaedic Surgery, edited by R.E. Leach, F.T. Hoaglund and E.J. Riseborough, pp. 123-136. Philadelphia, W.B. Saunders, 1982.

The technique and results of Neufeld roller traction are discussed. Patient cooperation is essential for proper use of the system and achievement of optimal results. The system is easily learned and requires minimal equipment.

Rüedi, T.P., and Lüscher, J.N.: Results after internal fixation of comminuted fractures of the femoral shaft with DC plates. Clin. Orthop. 138:74-76, 1979.

Infection occurred in 5.8 percent of closed fractures. The rate of implant failure was 7 percent. Ninety-two percent of these comminuted fractures achieved good results. Bone grafting as a primary part of femoral plating is advised.

33 PELVIS, HIP, AND FEMUR: RECONSTRUCTION

This section includes discussions of biomechanics of the hip, osteotomy, total hip replacement, surface replacement, and cementless prosthetic replacement.

Biomechanics The in vivo hip joint forces on a strain-gauged "English" prosthesis have been recorded, and the compression forces measured were approximately 50 percent lower than those calculated theoretically. The peak hip joint forces coincide exactly with the ground reaction forces during gait. During bed rest and passive motion, the hip force was between 0.5 and 1.0 times the body weight. With assisted walking, the maximum hip force increased to 1.5 times body weight. In walking without external aids, the joint force approached 2.2 times the body weight.

It is possible to reduce hip contact force to 17 to 26 percent of body weight by the use of a cane in the contralateral hand. However, patients rarely place more than 20 percent of their body weight on a cane, and hip contact forces rarely are reduced below 60 percent of body weight.

Prosthetic Reconstruction The clinical experience with hip replacement surgery over the last two decades as well as the more recent theoretical (mathematical, analytical, and computerized finite element studies) and experimental (strain gauge analysis, in vitro, and in vivo testing) information have improved the understanding of the behavior of the prosthetic-bone-cement composite.

Successful prosthetic reconstruction of the hip joint must eliminate pain and restore function. Pain generally is relieved when all components are cemented properly and remain well fixed. If muscle power is normal and adequate joint motion exists, function should be restored. Achievement of these goals is closely related to the geometry of the reconstructed joint.

Geometric alterations should minimize: (1) the muscular effort required to perform normal activities; (2) the joint contact force at the hip; and (3) the bending moment at the prosthetic neck-stem junction. Surgical procedures that satisfy these criteria will maximize the patient's functional level and minimize the incidence of prosthetic loosening, breakage, and wear.

A mathematical model of the hip allows evaluation of the effects of such surgically achievable mechanical alterations as acetabular placement, femoral shaft-prosthetic neck angle, neck length of femoral prosthesis, and transfer of the greater trochanter. The loads on the hip are lowered significantly by placing the center of the acetabulum as far medially, inferiorly, and anteriorly as is anatomically feasible. Increasing the femoral shaft-prosthetic neck angle increases the joint reaction force but decreases the bending moment about the prosthetic stem-neck junction. A neck length of the femoral prosthesis of 35 mm results in moments that are lower than those for a neck length of 45 mm. Lateral transfer of the greater trochanter increases the hip abduction moment and reduces hip joint forces.

The stem of a total hip femoral component transmits and distributes the force developed at the joint center, through the cement, and to the proximal femur. The effects of stem cross-sectional shape on the stresses in the surrounding cement have been examined using a three-dimensional numerical stress analysis. Results indicate that the predicted levels of stress in the cement are often close to failure levels. The magnitude and mode of loading in the cement are affected significantly by stem cross-sectional shape. High compressive stresses in the cement result from prostheses with narrow medial surfaces and small area moments of inertia. High cement tensile stresses are caused by stems with small area moments of inertia. Desirable stress distributions result from prostheses with broad medial surfaces and even broader lateral surfaces (Fig. 1).

Other aspects of the design of the femoral component

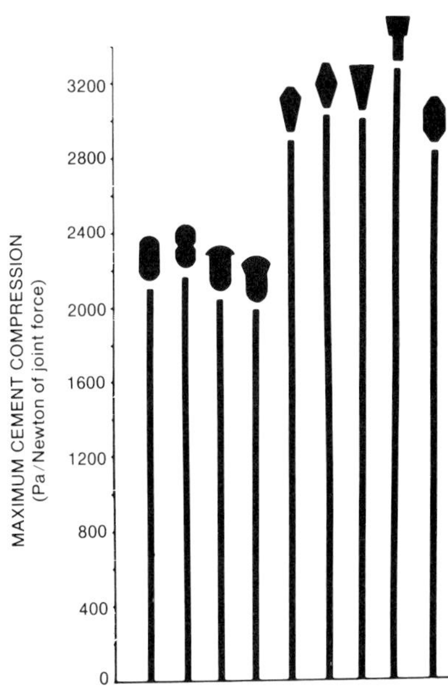

Figure 1: Maximum cement compression (principal stress) resulting from varus stem cross-sectional shapes. Predicted stresses are within the most proximal portion of the structure and result from a one-newton joint load. (Reprinted with permission from: The effect of femoral stem cross-sectional geometry on cement stresses in total hip reconstruction, by R.D. Crowninshield, et al., Clin. Orthop. 146:72, 1980.)

have been analyzed using three-dimensional finite element stress analysis. Increasing the length of the stem increases the stress present in the stem, whereas decreasing stem length increases the stress in the cement. Increasing the cross-sectional size of the stem decreases the stress in both the stem and the cement. Decreasing the modulus of elasticity of the stem material (making it more flexible) decreases the stress in the stem but increases the stress in the cement. Increasing the modulus of elasticity of the stem material (making it stiffer) increases the stress in the stem while decreasing the stress in the cement. Contact of the collar of a femoral component with the calcar femorale increases the longitudinal component of bone stress in the region of the calcar.

The achievement of femoral stem collar-calcar femorale contact has been shown to prevent subsidence in cadaver femora. The larger the surface area of the collar, the greater the support provided to the proximal portion of the stem offset from the loading axis, which deflects elastically as load is being applied to the head of the prosthesis. However, the amount of support provided by the calcar, and hence the proportion of load shared by it, depend upon the degree of fit between the flange and the cortical rim. Since the elastic deflections between the flange and bone are so small (less than 0.1 mm), the resected neck must be crafted flat and parallel to the undersurface of the collar to provide uniform stress transfer to the calcar femorale. Such a precise fit is difficult to obtain consistently in the operating room.

Significant research has been conducted to optimize cement fixation. Pulsating lavage, brushing, pressure injection of the cement with plugging the femoral canal result in a stronger bone-cement interface. Also, the cement is contained in the proximal part of the femur, where the stem will be located, making cement removal easier if revision becomes necessary. Cement syringes have been developed to permit retrograde delivery from the plug proximally. In addition, femoral compactors have been introduced which occlude the proximal femoral opening and further pressurize the cement with a plunger. Similar techniques have been developed for the acetabulum. However, there is as yet no documented evidence that these techniques lower the incidence of prosthetic loosening.

An in vitro study assessing femoral stem thickness, orientation, and insertion pressure on the strength of the stem-cement-bone composite concluded that the main factor determining the failure load was the presence of a distal plug: when no plug was present, failure occurred at the bone-cement interface; when a plug was present, it occurred at the prosthesis-cement interface.

Femoral prostheses with stems of more optimal design and with higher (stiffer) or lower (more flexible) modulus of elasticity have been implanted during the last few years. Stiffer stems should protect the proximal cement, transferring the stress distally. However, this may result in stress shielding of the proximal femur. The more flexible stems will transfer the stress to the proximal cement. Theoretically, the stiffer stem could cause disuse bone resorption of the proximal femur, whereas the more flexible stem may fatigue the proximal cement (the weakest material in the metal-cement-bone composite), causing increased loosening. Clinical experience with these different prostheses (including collar and collarless) has yet to demonstrate radiographic evidence supporting the theoretical predictions. Complicating matters further, the biological response of bone is still poorly understood, surgical and cementing techniques differ among surgeons, and the methodology, interpretation, and reporting of radiographic findings are varied. It would be helpful if unified criteria for radiographic analysis and reporting of clinical data could be established.

Osteotomy The pain-relieving effect of intertrochanteric osteotomy (usually varus or valgus) in osteoarthritis of the hip has been demonstrated by many clinical studies.

Most authors report approximately 75 percent good results at 1-year follow-up. Some report this result to be maintained at 5 years, but others note a deterioration such that only 40 to 50 percent of patients enjoy a good result after 5 years. In most studies, the 10-year results are good for only about 25 percent of the original patients.

It has not been possible to predict consistently the effect of osteotomy from the preoperative clinical or radiographic picture. The operative procedure (varus, valgus, amount of displacement) does not seem to influence the result. Although the effects of osteotomy may not be as long-lasting as previously believed, most investigators believe it has a place in the treatment of osteoarthritis in younger patients, particularly if congruity of the joint can be improved.

Most reports of osteotomy describe the change in angulation with respect to the coronal plane. Since the anterior portion of the femoral head is often relatively free from degenerative changes, flexing the proximal fragment (extension osteotomy), bringing the anterior portion of the femoral head under the roof of the acetabulum, has been suggested. Extension osteotomy is indicated when varus-valgus or derotation does not recenter the femoral head, while flexion does recenter it. A 65 percent incidence of good results at 10-year follow-up has been reported for this procedure. It is less radical than total hip replacement and easily converted, should the necessity arise. Studies have indicated that prior osteotomy does not jeopardize the outcome of subsequent total hip replacement.

Sugioka has reported good results with a transtrochanteric curved varus osteotomy ("rotational" osteotomy) in patients with osteonecrosis of the hip. He believes that this technique is advantageous because shortening is minimal, the vascular supply to the head is not jeopardized by the approach, nonunion is rare, and fixation is "easily" achievable with two or three large screws. Other surgeons have not been able to reproduce the satisfactory results reported.

Salter has extended the indication of his operation of three-dimensional correction of the acetabulum to the young adult with persistent subluxation. The biomechanical and biological function of the abnormal hip is improved by correcting or reducing the subluxation.

Prerequisites include subluxation, reasonable congruity, at least one-half of the normal cartilage thickness, and 60 percent of the normal range of motion (particularly flexion and abduction). In a patient population comprising eighty-one hips operated upon during the last 20 years, 68 percent obtained complete pain relief, and 28 percent had significant decrease of pain; 63 percent improved their gait.

Total Hip Replacement

Long-term Follow-up Ten-year follow-up studies have shown a radiographic loosening from 10 to 29 percent for the acetabular component and from 30 to 41 percent for the femoral component. Symptomatic loosening requiring revision surgery ranges from 1.3 to 12 percent for the acetabular side and from 3 to 20 percent for the femoral side. Variations in design, materials, and surgical techniques probably account for most of these differences.

A West German, Austrian, and Swiss multicenter study assessed the results of total hip replacement in a 10 percent random sample. After 10 years, satisfactory clinical results were noted in 91 percent of the patients. Techniques utilizing trochanteric osteotomy produced 4.9 percent unsatisfactory results, whereas those without osteotomy produced 11.8 percent. Causes for reoperation included loosening in 63.2 percent, technical error in 23.2 percent, and wound complications and heterotopic ossification in the remainder.

The cost effectiveness (benefit to cost ratio) of total hip replacement has been estimated to be about 2.7 to 1.0 (6 to 1 under the age of 59 years, and 2.1 to 1 from 60 to 69 years of age). No monetary benefits are estimated over the age of 70 years, but the improvement in the quality of life cannot be measured in monetary terms.

The long-term survival of total hip replacement units has been analyzed using standard actuarial methods. The probability of survival after 11 years was found to be 53 percent for metal-to-metal prostheses, and the average probability of removal was 5.5 percent per year. The results were better for metal-to-plastic prostheses (88 percent survival and 1.5 percent per year removal).

These studies present the long-term results of earlier surgical techniques that are considered inadequate by present standards. It is reasonable to expect better long-term results with proper selection of patients, improved surgical and cementing techniques, materials, and designs as utilized presently. A recent 3-year follow-up study evaluating the femoral loosening after total hip replacement in patients performed with plugging of the femoral canal and delivery of cement with a gun demonstrated a 1.1 percent incidence of prosthetic migration.

One study reported the results of acetabular pressurization carried out in 162 of 422 hips. No cups were revised for loosening in the pressurized group, whereas five were revised in the nonpressurized group. There was one asymptomatic cup migration in the former and five in the latter group.

An in vivo animal (sheep) study, performed to assess the temporal sequence of radiographic, histologic, mechanical, bacteriologic, and chemical changes at the femoral bone-cement interface, concluded that degenerative changes at the bone-cement interface may be inevitable with time and that these may prove to be significant factors in producing prosthetic loosening.

LOOSENING: According to one report, the rate of loosening of the femoral component appears to decrease with time, while acetabular loosening increases (Fig. 2). Young age, heavier weight, male sex, increased level of activity, stems placed in varus, curved stems with a narrow medial edge and occupying less than one-half of the femoral canal, suboptimal cement technique, and poor bone stock are factors associated with increased femoral loosening.

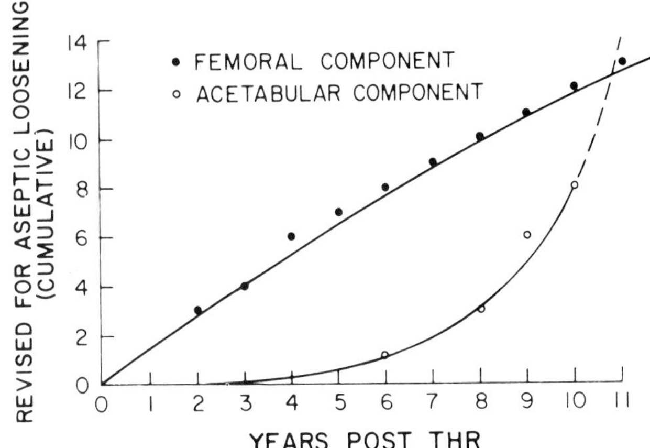

Figure 2: Cumulative revisions required for loosening of the femoral components (dots) and the acetabular components (circles) versus time. (Reprinted with permission from A ten-year follow-up of 100 consecutive Müller curved-stem total hip-replacement arthroplasties, by C.J. Sutherland, et al., J. Bone Joint Surg. 64A:981, 1982.)

Previously failed endoprostheses also have a higher incidence of femoral loosening. The main modes of loosening include pistoning (stem within cement or cement and stem within bone) and bending cantilever. Using a Charnley femoral stem with dorsal flanges (Cobra) significantly reduced subsidence and distal transverse cement fractures according to one report.

The incidence of loosening of the acetabular component increases with longer follow-up and was more of a problem than femoral loosening in Charnley's 15-year follow-up. He predicted that it would be the biggest problem following total hip replacement in the future. Loosening of the acetabular component was associated with protrusio acetabuli, inadequate bony coverage, perforation, and failed cups. Metal sensitivity does not appear to be a significant factor in the incidence of component loosening.

Complications

MATERIAL FAILURE: Acetabular wear, originally a matter of concern, has not proved to be a problem according to follow-ups no longer than 15 years. Clinical studies using a metallic marker in the polyethylene reveal wear rates averaging 0.07 mm per year. Most changes previously attributed to plastic wear appear to be related to plastic deformation, or creep. Rate of wear is inversely related to the molecular weight of the plastic (see Section 12: Polyethylene in Total Joint Replacement). Accelerated wear does not occur with the passage of time.

Fracture of polyethylene acetabular cups rarely occurs through the deep grooves in the old Muller cups, where originally there was a thickness of only 5 mm of polyethylene.

Finite element analyses by various investigators have demonstrated that metal backing of the acetabular component reduces peak stresses in bone, cement, and plastic. An axisymmetric finite element model with nonaxisymmetric loading of an acetabular arthroplasty and surrounding pelvic bone revealed that thinner plastic cups increase maximum stresses in the cement-bone composite. Trabecular bone stresses increase after removal of the subchondral bone. Stiffer metal-backed acetabular cups reduce maximum cement and bone stresses and offset the

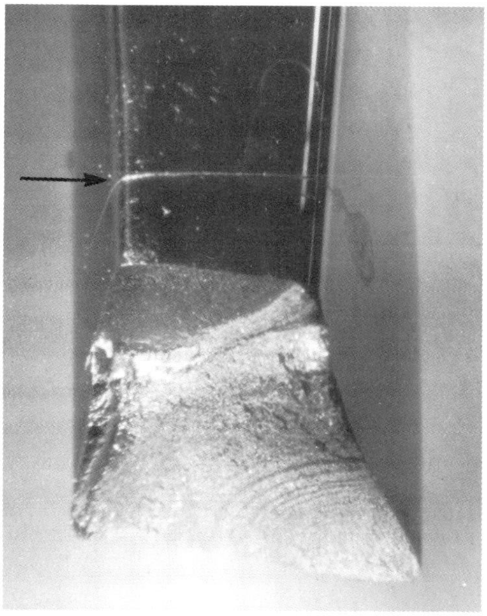

Figure 3: Fractured T-28 stem with the "clamshell" or "beach" markings evident on the fracture surface and a large secondary crack proximal to the fracture surface (arrow). (Courtesy of Timothy Wright, Ph.D.)

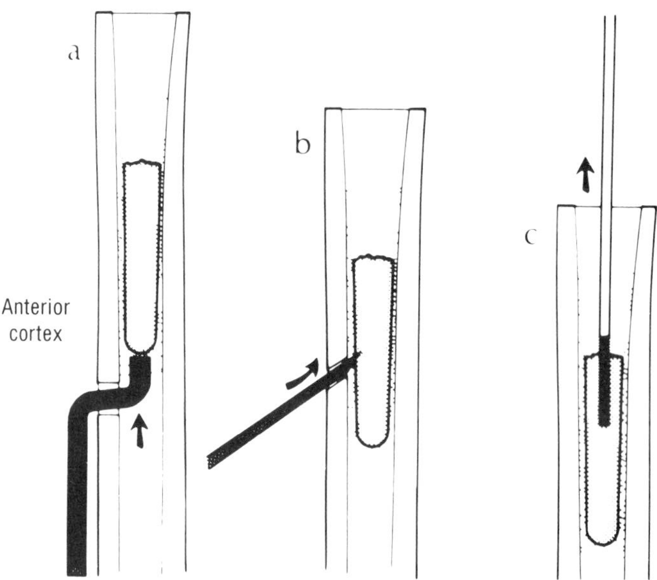

Figure 4: Three different methods for removal of the retained broken stem. (Reprinted with permission from Mechanical failures in total hip replacement requiring reoperation, by P.M. Pellicci, et al., J. Bone Joint Surg. 61A:35, 1979.)

effects of cup thickness and subchondral bone removal. However, there is still insufficient clinical data to support any advantages of metal-backed acetabular cups over the traditional ones.

STEM FRACTURE: It has been reported to be associated with thin stems, a sharp medial edge, metallic defects, or placement in varus position (Fig. 3). Male patients heavier than 76 kg appear to be at greatest risk for stem fracture.

Two-thirds of stems that break do so in the cantilever fatigue mode with proximal loosening. One-sixth fail through a similar mechanism without evidence of proximal loosening (adequate proximal cement) but with inadequate surrounding cortical bone and overstressing of the stem. About one-sixth fail due to defects in the lateral side of the stem, created by wires or the drill bit during reattachment of the greater trochanter. A risk index for prediction of stem fracture has been suggested.

Better bone preparation and cementing techniques, improved stem design, and the use of high strength alloys should reduce the incidence of stem fracture. However, one fracture recently was reported in a high-strength alloy stem of modern, adequate design with good position, surrounding bone, and cement technique. The variation in grain size of this high-strength, forged vitallium alloy was probably responsible for the failure which occurred 20 months after insertion. Early breakage of the stem (within the first 3 years) may be related to metallurgic defects, intermediate breakage (4 to 7 years) fixation failure, and late breakage (8 years or later) may be due to stress failure.

New techniques for removing the retained distal stem fragment have been devised, which obviate the creation of a femoral window. They require drilling into the end of the broken stem with a high-speed air turbine and several special cutting tools and inserting an extractor into the drill hole. They can be used even with high-strength alloys (Fig. 4).

INFECTION: Deep periprosthetic infection is one of the most serious complications of total hip replacement. The use of radionuclide bone scanning to aid in the diagnosis in a patient with a painful endoprosthesis has been advocated. Combined technetium and gallium scanning has been reported to be an accurate and reliable method of demonstrating infection in such patients. Technetium 99 diphosphonate is believed to be absorbed into the hydroxyapatite crystal of bone, and its uptake is proportional to the degree of vascularity and rate of bone remodeling. Its uptake is usually increased in the presence of mechanical loosening or infection, while gallium 67 uptake is increased only in the presence of infection, due to its affinity for polymorphonuclear leukocytes. It also has been helpful in evaluating the presence of osteomyelitis. "Three phase" bone scanning has been recommended for the evaluation of a patient suspected to have a septic joint replacement. A negative bone scan should help to rule out the possibility of infection.

Needle aspiration of the prosthetic joint is a helpful diagnostic procedure. Recovery of the infecting organism must be vigorously sought, either by repeated aspirations or open (or arthroscopic) biopsies.

Treatment is dependent upon factors of wound biology, duration and type of infection, and host factors. When the infection is acute (days), the components still well fixed, and the infecting organism sensitive to antibiotic therapy, it is reasonable to attempt to salvage the prosthesis by open drainage and closure over inflow and outflow tubes, especially if the patient is elderly or otherwise incapable of tolerating extensive surgery. Tubes should be removed after 48 hours to prevent superinfection. The prognosis must be guarded. Complete removal of prosthetic components and acrylic cement remains the accepted treatment for established deep periprosthetic infections.

Infection has been considered an absolute contraindication for reimplantation, but an increasing number of studies report successful results of either one-stage debridement, removal of all foreign material and reconstruction of the joint with another total hip prosthesis, or

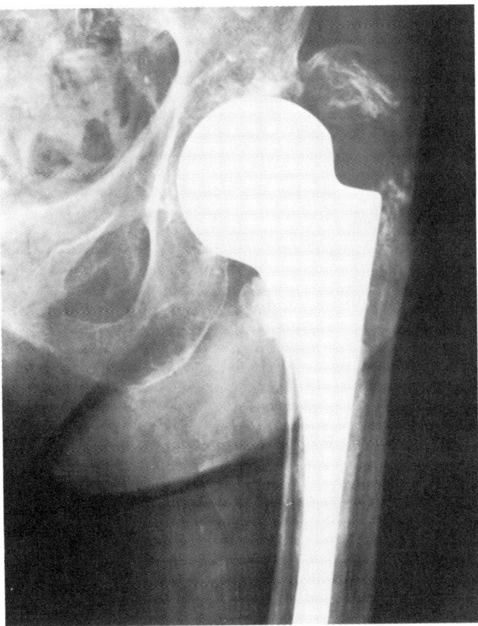

Figure 5-A

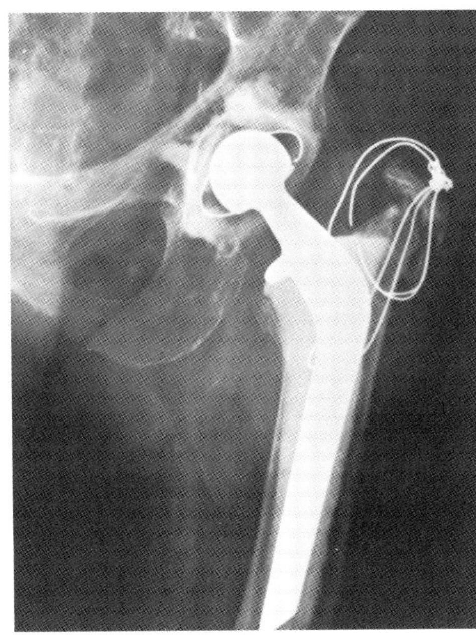

Figure 5-B

Figure 5: (A) Septic loosening of a femoral head prosthesis with absent joint space, subsidence, and proximal migration of the greater trochanter. The infecting organism was enterococcus. (B) Postoperative radiograph obtained 1 year after one-stage reimplantation. At surgery a thorough incision and debridement were performed after removal of prosthesis and cement. The total hip replacement was implanted with gentamicin-impregnated Palacos cement. In addition, the patient received 6 weeks of intravenous penicillin and gentamicin obtaining 1:64 serum bactericidal levels. The result after 2 years of follow-up continues to be excellent.

delay of the reconstruction to a second operative session. Staging of the reconstruction is determined by the pathogenicity of the infecting organism, intraoperative results of Gram stain, frozen section, and the surgeon's observation of the wound. If in doubt, treatment of the infection must take precedence over reconstruction. Adequate antibiotic coverage should begin as soon as the diagnosis is certain and the organism identified. Intravenous antibiotics, obtaining at least 1:8 peak bactericidal serum activity, should be continued postoperatively for 6 weeks. Using these methods, a 90 percent success rate without recurrence of infection has been obtained.

Direct exchange surgery using gentamicin-impregnated acrylic has been performed in Europe over the past several years. The largest series report about 80 percent success rates (Fig. 5). A modified two-stage reimplantation for deep infections due to gram-negative bacteria and/or extensive bone destruction has been recommended. At the primary operation, the prosthetic components are removed, and the cavity is filled with gentamicin-impregnated PMMA beads. Reimplantation is performed 3 to 4 weeks later with gentamicin-impregnated cement (see Section 13: Polymethyl Methacrylate).

It is important to consider reimplantation of a total hip replacement as the results of resection arthroplasty (Girdlestone) are generally unsatisfactory. According to one report the majority of patients have pain with weight-bearing, weakness, instability, and shortening, and they must use crutches or a walker. Some have pain at rest. Few are satisfied with the result.

Late deep wound infection secondary to hematogenous spread of bacteria from a distant focus is an infrequent but serious complication of total joint replacement. Characteristically, the initial operation is uneventful and a long, asymptomatic interval ensues, followed by a definite febrile illness and acute joint pain. The source of the infection often is not recognized.

Prevention of Infection: The surgeon must warn each patient of the risk of late hematogenous seeding from infection elsewhere in the body (see Section 6, General: Infection). It is also important to give special attention to patients who are at high risk, such as those with rheumatoid arthritis or other systemic diseases. According to one report urethral instrumentation for urinary retention after total hip replacement increased the deep sepsis rate to 6.2 percent. A knowledge of the bacterial flora of the various areas of the body is essential in choosing the appropriate prophylactic antibiotic.

A multicenter study of sepsis after 8,000 total hip or knee replacements concluded that when operations were done in ultra-clean air systems, the infection rate was one-half of that which occurred in conventional operating rooms. Furthermore, when whole body exhaust ventilated suits were worn in a theater ventilated by an ultra-clean system, the incidence of sepsis was about one-quarter of that found in conventional operating rooms. A significant reduction of infections was also observed in those patients who received prophylactic antibiotics.

Horizontal laminar airflow may produce either beneficial or adverse effects, depending upon whether the surgical procedure is performed in accordance with the theory of operation of the airflow system. One study reported a significant reduction of infection in total hip replacement, but with total knee replacement, the infection rate was increased, perhaps because members of the surgical team must stand between the source of the horizontal laminar airflow and the open wound. As the surgeons did not use whole body exhaust ventilated suits, they were probably shedding their own bacteria onto the open wound during total knee replacement (Fig. 6).

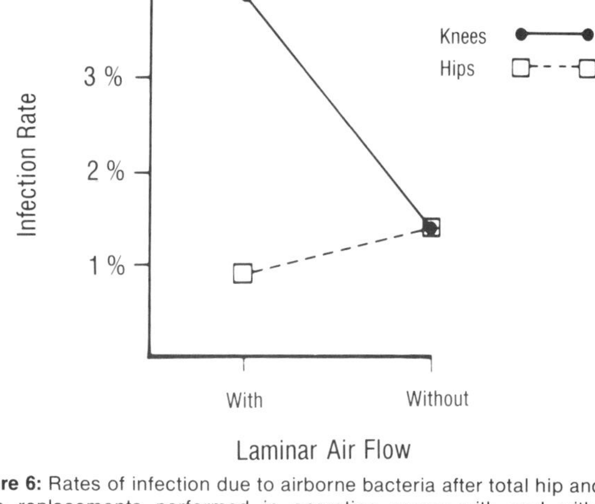

Figure 6: Rates of infection due to airborne bacteria after total hip and total knee replacements performed in operating rooms with and without a horizontal unidirectional flow of filtered air. (Reprinted with permission from Infection rates after 3,175 total hip and total knee replacements performed with and without a horizontal undirectional filtered air-flow system, by E.A. Salvati, et al., J. Bone Joint Surg. 64A:530, 1982.)

Ultraviolet irradiation during total hip replacement significantly reduces airborne bacterial contamination of the operative field. One study reported that with ultraviolet light the rate of infection from possible airborne sources was 0.15 percent after 1,322 total hip replacements.

Perioperative prophylactic antibiotics is the widest used modality to prevent infection, and multiple studies have demonstrated its efficacy, particularly in clean elective surgery.

THROMBOEMBOLISM: During hip surgery there is a strong, systemic activation of the clotting cascade, associated with local vessel injury and local stasis in the femoral vein, an association not found in most general surgical procedures.

Advanced age and previous venous thromboembolism are predictors for an increased incidence of pulmonary embolus and thrombophlebitis. There appears to be no correlation with obesity, varicose veins, diabetes, cigarette smoking, or length of surgery. Plasma concentrations of free fatty acids and the quotient of fibrinogen to serum antithrombin III were higher in patients who developed postoperative deep venous thrombosis (D.V.T.). These may serve as additional parameters in the prediction of postoperative D.V.T.

The peak onset of thrombosis is on the fourth postoperative day. Prophylaxis with subcutaneous heparin might delay the appearance of thrombosis but does not reduce the incidence.

The incidence of pulmonary embolism following total hip replacement is 6 to 8 percent when evaluated by lung ventilation perfusion scans and pulmonary arteriography according to one study. In most instances the patient remained asymptomatic and showed no clinical evidence to support the diagnosis.

Low-dose heparin therapy has not been proved effective in prophylaxis against venous thromboembolism. The data available support the use of aspirin (1.2 gm/day) in males as effective prophylaxis. The efficacy in females is questionable. A recent prospective study demonstrated a 6 percent incidence of pulmonary embolus in those patients treated with low doses of warfarin compared to 19 percent in those receiving aspirin, and there was no difference between females and males regarding the prophylactic efficacy of aspirin.

Treatment with Coumadin, starting the night before or the night of surgery to bring the prothrombin to one and one-half times control, is effective in both males and females. However, the incidence of wound hematoma and other bleeding complications is higher.

Graded pressure stockings and cyclic sequential compression of the lower limbs are believed to be effective in decreasing the incidence of D.V.T.

Pulmonary bone embolism was found at autopsy in both lungs of an 84-year-old patient who underwent two-stage bilateral total hip replacements, 3 months and 10 months prior to death. It was believed that acetabular grindings entered the damaged venous system and were filtered by the lungs.

NEUROVASCULAR: The incidence of sciatic and femoral nerve palsies following total hip replacement is less than 1 percent. The causes are multifactorial and include nerve stretch when the limb is lengthened, hematoma, and damage by cement, instrument, or retractor. Recovery is partial in most patients with some residual motor and sensory symptoms. About one-half such patients are believed to have made a "good" recovery.

If the cause of the nerve palsy seems to be related to hemorrhage, especially in anticoagulated patients, there is some evidence to suggest that surgical decompression can improve the prognosis.

Vascular accidents occurring in the course of hip surgery may be very serious and pose an immediate and sudden threat to life and limb. Arterial injury occurs in only about 0.2 percent of all total hip replacements. Causative factors include damage to the external iliac or common femoral artery with the tip of an anteriorly placed Hohman retractor, intimal tear with appositional thrombosis, intrapelvic intrusion of acrylic cement through medial acetabular defects, and direct injury with knife or osteotome.

The surgeon should be familiar with the exposure of the main vessels proximal to the hip to control severe hemorrhage. A McBurney incision with retroperitoneal exposure and clamping of the external iliac artery will diminish bleeding considerably. Thereafter, careful dissection and placement of snares about the common and deep femoral arteries and, if necessary, the medial and lateral circumflex arteries may allow vascular repair. Transcatheter embolization also has been used for control of bleeding following total hip replacement.

MISCELLANEOUS COMPLICATIONS: Dislocation occurs in 1 to 4 percent of total hip replacements depending upon the reported study. Patients with neuromuscular disease, altered mental status, or after revision surgery are more prone to this complication. Malpositioning of components, proximal migration of the greater trochanter, and shortening of the limb (due to high placement of the cup or low section of the neck) are the major technical problems that may result in dislocation. According to some the posterior approach is associated with a higher incidence of dislocation than the transtrochanteric approach. This dislocation tendency possibly may be decreased by reattachment of the external rotators and posterior capsule. A study reviewing a large number of patients with disloca-

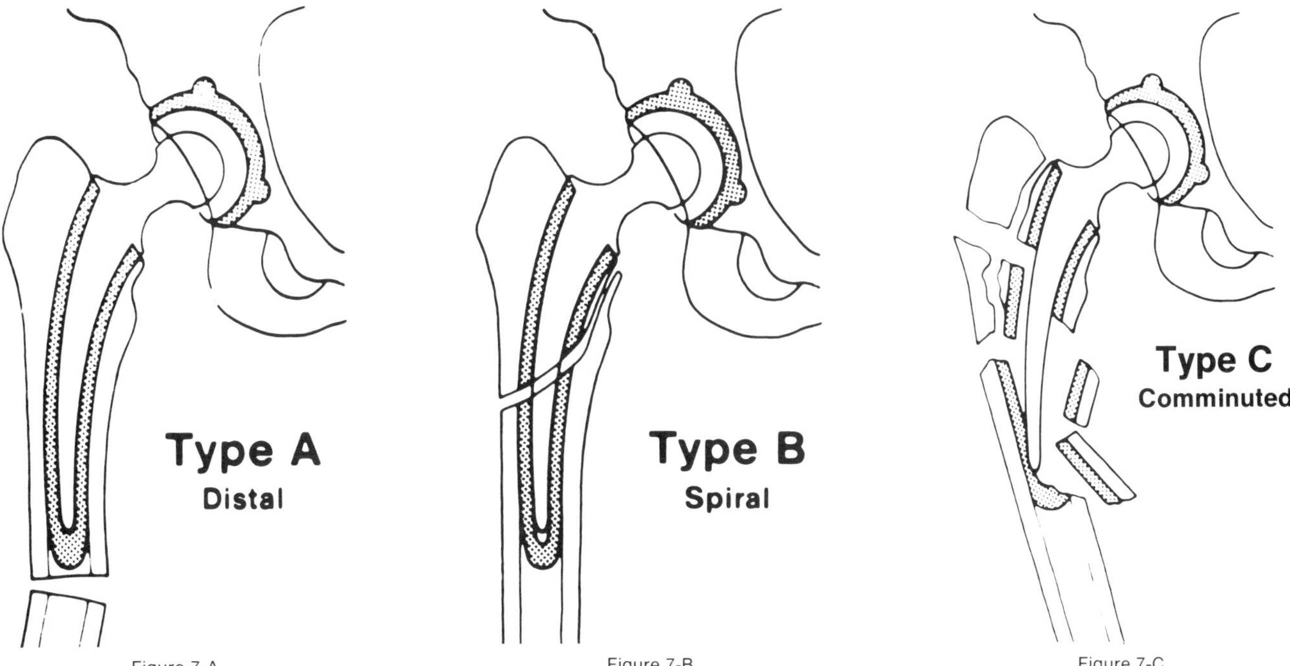

Figure 7: (A-C) Type A, Distal: Type A fracture, at stem tip. Type B, Spiral: Type B fracture, spiral around stem. Type C, Comminuted: Type C fracture, comminuted around stem. (Reprinted with permission from Proximal femoral fractures following total hip arthroplasty, by Bethea, et al., Clin. Orthop. 170:96, 97, 1982.)

tions reported that reoperation for instability was required in one-third of the patients and that one-third of those reoperated on continued to dislocate. Arthroscopy has been employed successfully to identify and remove entrapped acrylic cement within the acetabular cup following reduction of a dislocation.

Nonunion of the greater trochanter is not an uncommon problem. When it occurs, few patients are troubled sufficiently to require reoperation. When symptoms are significant and surgery is deemed necessary, firm fixation of the trochanter to an adequate bony bed is essential to achieve union. The soft tissue at the site of nonunion must be excised. Adequate mobilization of the fragment and bone grafting are necessary. Wiring over wire mesh, if the fragment is osteoporotic, can be performed so that containment and firm fixation are achieved. Multifilament cable has been found to be versatile, easy to work with, and possessing mechanical properties superior to monofilament wire. A cable grip system has been developed that reduces the incidence of trochanteric detachment to 1.5 percent after primary surgery. Adduction stresses must be prevented postoperatively, if necessary, by the use of an orthosis. Surgical attempts to correct nonunion of the osteotomized greater trochanter are frequently unsuccessful.

The reported incidence of heterotopic bone formation following total hip arthroplasty has varied from 5 to 61 percent, the range variance being related to differing methods of patient selection, classification, and radiographic examination. Significant symptoms occur in only 1 to 5 percent, with the major disability being loss of motion. High risk patients include males with hypertrophic osteoarthritis, those with ankylosing spondylitis or Paget's disease, and patients who have developed heterotopic ossification following previous hip surgery.

In these at-risk patients, prophylaxis with diphosphonates (administered orally for 1 month pre- and 3 months postoperatively) or low-dose irradiation (2,000 rads over 10 days immediately postoperatively) have been successful in minimizing this problem. The use of a free fat transplant also has been reported to prevent recurrence following surgical excision.

Fracture of the ipsilateral femur in patients with total hip replacement may present formidable management problems. Certain guidelines have been suggested for the treatment of these patients. Fractures entirely distal to the stem may be managed in standard fashion. Fractures at the tip of the prosthesis (Fig. 7-A) usually require revision with a long stem femoral component. Fractures proximal to the tip of the stem (Fig. 7-B) that do not jeopardize the fixation of the component may be treated in traction if adequate apposition and alignment can be maintained and if the patient can tolerate protracted bed rest. If not, open reduction, fixation with cerclage wires or a plate and screws (directed obliquely to avoid the stem) may be required. For comminuted fractures proximal to the tip of the stem (Fig. 7-C), the surgeon may choose between early or delayed surgical reconstruction, provided adequate alignment can be obtained in traction. The main advantage of delayed replacement (if possible) is working with healed bone, thus avoiding multiple fragments. Although it might be appealing to obtain open reduction and internal fixation at the same operative session, it may be difficult to contain the cement for adequate fixation and avoid interfragmentary cement leakage. This leakage will not only jeopardize fixation but also delay or even prevent bone healing.

Perforation of the femoral shaft by the prosthetic stem is an infrequent complication of total hip replacement. The problem occurs most often in females, in osteoporotic bone, or in patients who have had previous surgery or previous fractures. If the perforation is proximal (peri-

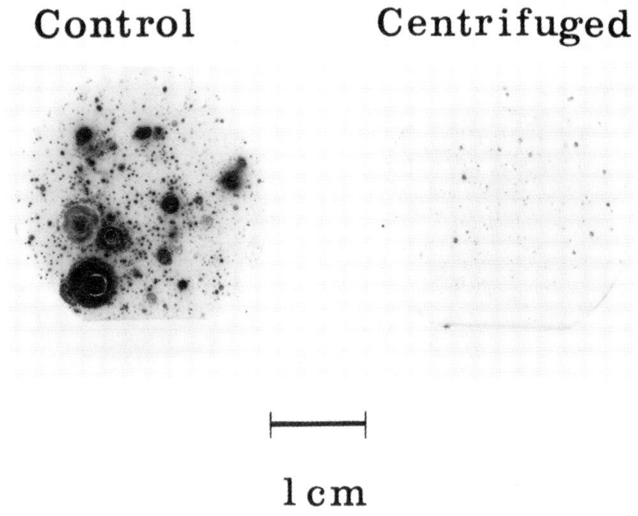

Control Centrifuged

1cm

Figure 8: Close up photograph of polished PMMA discs obtained with India ink from a control and a centrifuged specimen. The striking difference in porosity is obvious. (Courtesy of Dennis Burke, M.D. and Evelyn Gates, B.S.)

trochanteric or subtrochanteric), revision is probably necessary. If penetration is distal (less than 2 cm of stem protruding), fixation may not be seriously compromised, and the patient may not need additional surgery.

Pain following total hip replacement occasionally may be due to a stress fracture of a thin medial acetabular wall or the ipsilateral pubic ramus. A technetium 99 bone scan can aid in the diagnosis.

Techniques Bilateral total hip replacement in a single stage generally has been found to carry no increased risk over bilateral hip replacement performed in two stages. There may, however, be a higher incidence of pulmonary embolus in the single-stage group. A cost reduction of 30 percent may be realized with bilateral total hip replacement done as a one-stage procedure. Considerable experience with total hip replacement is desirable before performing such surgery.

Some studies have advocated autotransfusion as a means of reducing the risks of using bank blood. Decreased blood loss, prolonged postoperative analgesia, and less thromboembolic complications have been reported with epidural anesthesia. However, urinary retention is more frequent. Hypotensive anesthesia does decrease blood loss and with careful monitoring does not seem to be associated with increased risk.

Improvements in the preparation of cement have been suggested, including centrifugation to reduce air voids and porosity (thus increasing its mechanical properties) and the addition of methylene blue to enhance its visibility and facilitate removal during revision surgery (Fig. 8). Graphite fiber reinforcement of plain cement produced a 32 percent increase in fracture toughness; however, decreased intrusion characteristics were observed (Fig. 9). Low viscosity cement has been advocated to increase its intrusion characteristics; however, decreased fracture toughness has been observed when compared to standard cement (see Section 13: Polymethyl Methacrylate).

Special Problems Protrusio acetabuli due to previous surgery, rheumatoid arthritis, or fracture creates a difficult reconstructive problem. The goals to obtain a successful reconstruction include placing the acetabulum in the anatomic position, reinforcing the deficient medial wall with autogenous or allograft bone well fixed to the existing pelvis and, if necessary, providing peripheral support to the acetabular component with a protrusio shell or reinforcement ring.

Total hip replacement for congenital dislocation of the hip gives good results in most patients, but complications such as dislocation and sciatic palsy occur more frequently than in other groups. The acetabular component should be positioned in the true acetabulum; this often requires the use of a very small (34 to 36 mm) cup, so a 22 mm femoral head should be used. Superolateral bone grafting is often necessary to obtain bony coverage of the acetabulum. In patients with severely deficient acetabular bone stock, frozen femoral head allografts may be used for augmentation. These must be securely anchored to the existing pelvis to provide support to the prosthetic component.

Adductor, iliopsoas, and abductor releases may be required to mobilize high iliac dislocations. The femur may require osteotomy at the level of the true acetabulum (often in the subtrochanteric region) to permit a snug reduction which will provide stability and prevent excessive traction on the neurovascular structures. Small, straight femoral components are often necessary to fit the often narrow femoral shaft. Careful preoperative planning is essential to achieve success. Preoperative radiographs obtained with a standard 6-foot tube distance (to reduce magnification) and a radiopaque ruler placed at the level of the proximal femur are essential if custom-made prostheses are to be used.

Total hip replacement for failed femoral hemiarthroplasty is associated with a higher incidence of femoral loosening: 8 percent after 3 years according to one study. Canal preparation and cement technique must be meticulous in these patients. Preoperative hip aspiration to rule out low-grade sepsis is recommended.

Conversion of ankylosed or arthrodesed hips to total hip replacement may be indicated for disabling low back or ipsilateral knee pain. These symptoms often can be

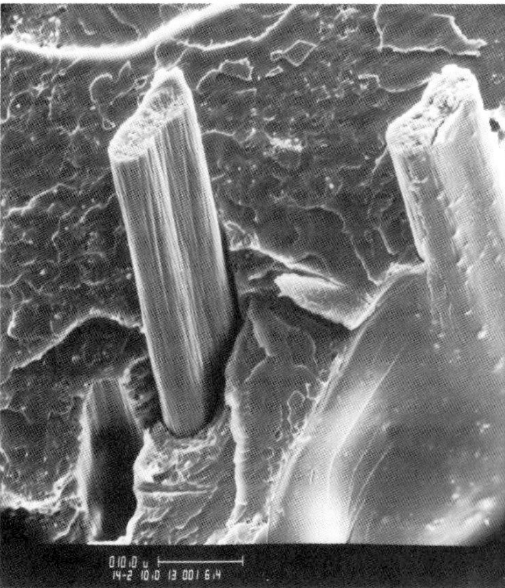

Figure 9: Scanning electron photomicrograph of carbon reinforced bone cement. Carbon fibers can be seen protruding from the fracture surface of this laboratory specimen. A hole from which a fiber has been pulled is also visible. Poor adherence exists between the fibers and the bone cement; this is one of the drawbacks of this material. (Courtesy of Timothy Wright, Ph.D.)

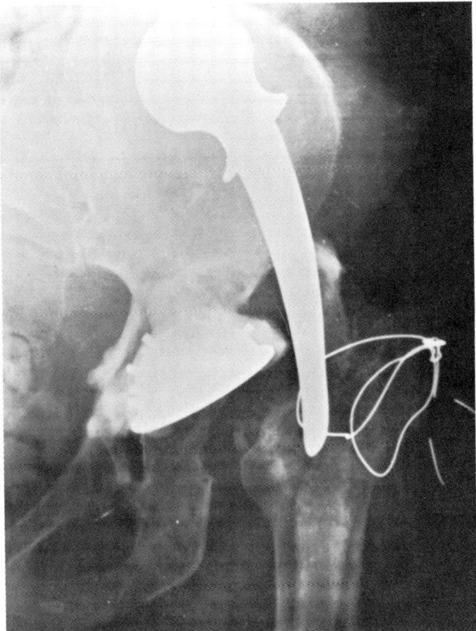

Figure 10-A

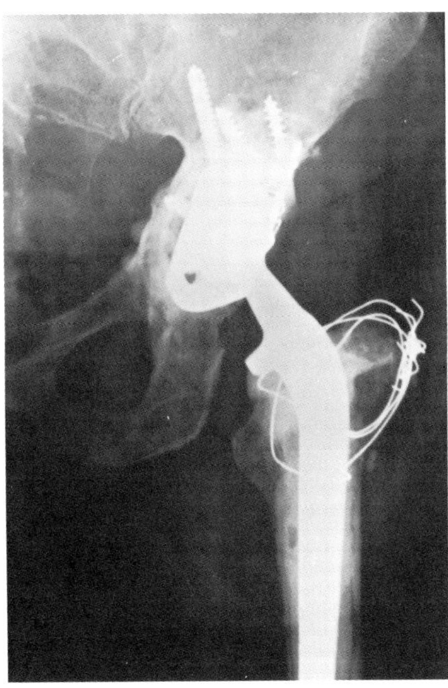

Figure 10-B

Figure 10: (A) Grossly loose femoral and acetabular components. (B) Due to the severe acetabular bone deficit, a large autogenous iliac bone graft was placed bridging the bony defect. In addition, an acetabular reinforcement ring was screwed to the ilium.

relieved by this approach. However, the incidence of dislocation, abductor weakness, and trochanteric nonunion is increased in these patients, many of whom will have a persistent abductor limp and require the use of a cane.

Total hip replacement in juvenile rheumatoid arthritis gives predictably good results which appear to persist over time, although long-term follow-up reports have not yet been published. Advance planning and appreciation of developmental abnormalities are important. In contrast, total hip replacement in other patients younger than 30 years old (without juvenile rheumatoid arthritis) carries a 57 percent failure rate due to actual or potential loosening at 5 years according to one study. Factors that adversely affected the results were an initial diagnosis of osteonecrosis, previous cup arthroplasty, heavy activity, unilateral arthroplasty, and weight of more than 82 kg (180 lbs.). Acetabular loosening occurred more than twice as frequently as femoral loosening. Total hip replacement for Gaucher's disease has shown a higher risk of hemorrhage, infection, and loosening.

Revision Total Hip Replacement Revision total hip arthroplasty has become a topic of major importance not only because of its technical difficulty and decreased predictability as compared to primary total hip replacement but also because of the increasing numbers of patients who require revision.

Several technical points are useful. In patients with severe scarring or shortening, preliminary exposure of the sciatic nerve for protection during the remainder of the procedure is a useful precaution.

Trochanteric osteotomy is recommended by some for revision total hip replacement. It has been suggested that it improves exposure, minimizes the incidence of femoral fracture, and allows better adjustment of the abductor mechanism. Enough pseudocapsule and soft tissue must be resected to completely mobilize the proximal femur from the pelvis.

When the acetabular component loosens, it generally occurs at the bone-cement interface. The cup and a large portion of cement will often lift off with moderate traction, leaving plugs and patches of cement in fixation holes or with mushroom expansions deep to the acetabulum. All loose cement must be removed, or at least enough to provide a clean, dry, cancellous bony bed for the new cement. Care should be taken not to injure large intrapelvic vessels by overly vigorous attempts to remove intruded cement. Large defects should be bone grafted using iliac or banked femoral head grafts. The bone graft may, if necessary for stability, be fixed to the ilium with pins, screws, or bolts prior to implantation of the acetabular component. If the acetabular is very large, an acetabular mesh or preferably a reinforcement ring may be used (Fig. 10). If a nonunion of the anterior and/or posterior column is present, internal fixation, bone graft, and restoration of skeletal continuity should take precedence over the joint replacement.

When a loose femoral stem is removed, a variable amount of cement will come with it. The easily accessible proximal cement usually is removed with few problems. However, removing the distal cement is often difficult and tedious. All loose cement must be removed. Even if the cement is well fixed to bone, enough must be removed to provide sufficient space for the new component to be inserted in proper orientation. This procedure requires experience and is time-consuming. Shortcuts may result in femoral shaft perforation or fracture. If it is necessary to rechannel a previous bone or cement plug to insert a long stem component for bypassing a shaft defect, this can be accomplished using the high-speed air turbine power drill. Extensive exposure of the femur and/or two-plane fluoroscopic or radiographic control may be helpful to avoid perforation in difficult procedures.

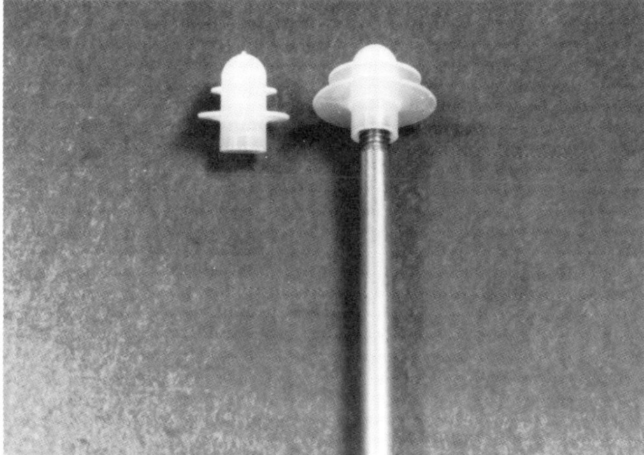

Figure 11: Plastic plugs of different sizes with inserter.

When sufficient cement and bone have been removed to meet the preceding criteria, the canal may be cleaned by pulsating lavage and brush. A new bone or cement plug may be inserted if necessary. A press fit polyethylene plug with a special inserter is also an available alternative (Fig. 11). If osteotomized, the trochanter can be reattached with three or four wires. Wire mesh can be used to cover osteoporotic trochanters.

Defects in the femur, whether created intentionally or inadvertently, should be occluded during insertion of cement and prosthesis. If a window has been made, the bone plate should be replaced. Large defects may be covered by mesh to aid in cement containment and should be visualized to assure that the new component is not passed through the defect. A small defect (e.g., a screw hole) should be bypassed by a length of stem equivalent to the femoral shaft diameter. It has been suggested that a large defect (e.g., a cortical window) should be bypassed by at least two to three shaft diameters to prevent the defect acting as a stress riser.

Revisional arthroplasty may, at times, require special or custom prostheses. A large variety of cup and stem sizes and neck lengths must be available. In patients in whom the proximal femur is deficient (calcar resorption following previous total hip replacement, settling of an endoprosthesis, destruction by tumor or fracture), a calcar replacement prosthesis is recommended. This prosthesis gains bony support distally and can restore leg length (Fig. 12).

A total femoral prosthesis has been utilized as an alternative to amputation or disarticulation, incorporating a total knee in some patients. For patients in whom there is severe acetabular destruction, a saddle prosthesis articulating with the remnant of the ilium has been developed. Long-term follow-up studies of these prostheses are not yet available.

Each patient's problem must be individualized. For instance, the prosthetic needs should be decided early enough prior to operation that customized prosthetic components and assistive devices may be manufactured, if necessary. It is important to avoid compromising the operative outcome through lack of necessary equipment or inadequate preoperative planning (Fig. 13).

The quality of a well-fixed, uncomplicated revision arthroplasty seems to be comparable with that of primary total hip arthroplasty. The former, however, is more difficult to achieve, as evidenced by only a 60 percent incidence of good or excellent results in a major series. The immediate postoperative radiolucent lines that appear in most patients suggest less than optimal fixation. This is not surprising in light of the sclerotic cortical bone that remains when component and cement are removed at the time of revision. The incidence of complications is higher with infection and trochanteric problems being two to three times more frequent than after primary replacement. A high (14 percent) incidence of mechanical failure for total hip arthroplasties that have been revised once (in the absence of infection) has been reported. In addition, of those hips still causing no symptoms, 26 percent have progressive radiolucent zones between cement and bone on serial radiographs. Another study of revision surgery

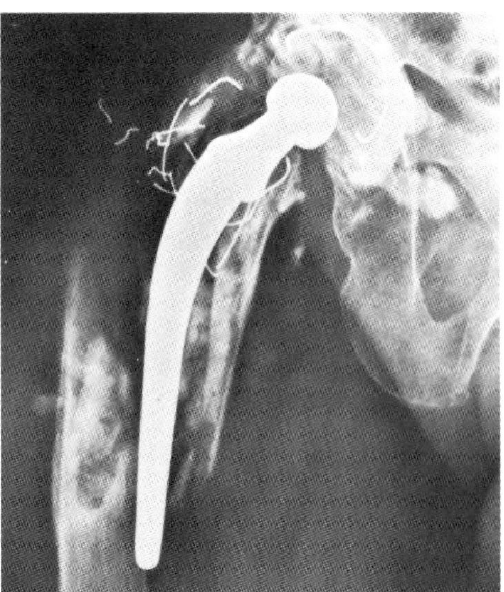

Figure 12-A

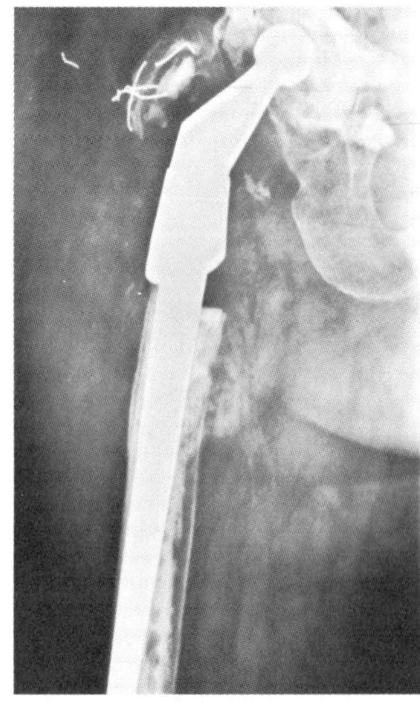

Figure 12-B

Figure 12: (A) Fracture around a grossly loose femoral component. (B) Due to the comminution and poor bone stock of the proximal fragment, a calcar replacement prosthesis was implanted. The abductor mechanism and greater trochanter were sutured to the vastus lateralis.

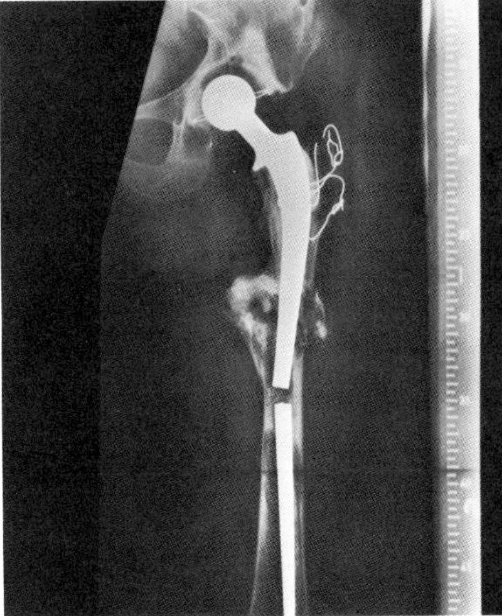

Figure 13-A

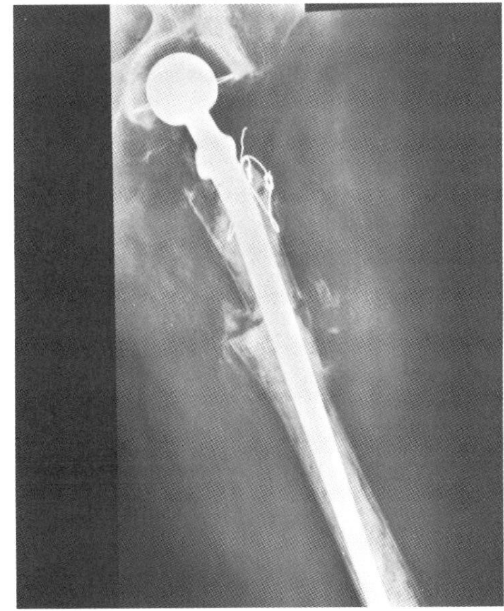

Figure 13-B

Figure 13: (A) Fracture of a long stem prosthesis. This radiograph was obtained with a radiopaque ruler placed at the level of the femoral shaft. A lateral view is obtained with similar technique. They permit exact calculation of the radiographic magnification and precise sizing for a custom design long stem prosthesis. (B) Postoperative radiograph demonstrating adequate alignment and fixation of custom-made, long stem prosthesis.

revealed similar figures and predicted a 25 percent failure rate after 7 years.

Surface Replacement The enthusiasm with which surface replacement arthroplasty was embraced several years ago has decreased due to a number of reports citing high failure rates after relatively short follow-up. Two-year follow-up studies from two major centers reported failure rates of 16 and 34 percent. The main causes are femoral loosening with or without osteonecrosis of the underlying femoral head, femoral neck fracture, and acetabular loosening.

The technical aspects of the surgery are demanding, particularly with reference to preservation of the blood supply to the femoral head, avoidance of notching of the femoral neck when reaming the head, and meticulous cement technique on both the acetabular and femoral sides. Failure rates tend to be higher with osteonecrosis, dysplasia, and inflammatory arthritis. Revision of failed femoral components of surface replacements is easier than conventional total hip replacement revision. However, the acetabular side is more difficult because of the greater sacrifice of bone needed to fit the large surface cup.

Following infection, "stump arthroplasty," in which the reamed femoral head and neck form a fibrous articulation with the acetabulum, is an alternative to Girdlestone arthroplasty or reimplantation.

Cementless Prosthetic Arthroplasty Interest in porous surface implants is increasing, in the hope of obviating the known mechanical problems reported with cemented prostheses. Porous surfaced components have been fab-

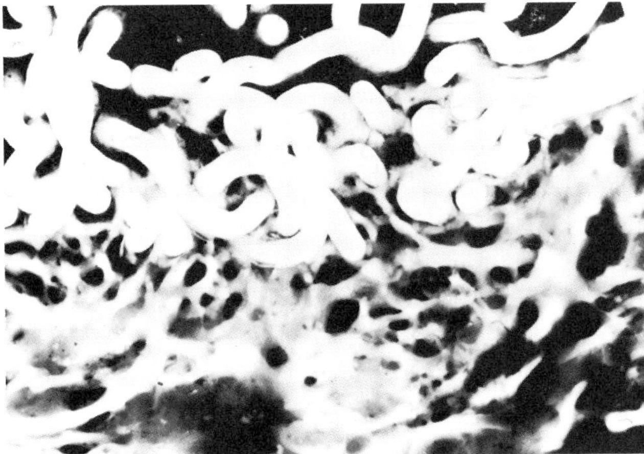

Figure 14: High power view of a microradiograph of the interface between titanium mesh and bone in the acetabulum. The upper portion of the microradiograph indicates how the mesh is interlocked with the polyethylene. Bone permeates the remaining porous mesh up to the polyethylene. Notice the three-dimensional character of the bond achieved between the porous layer and supporting bone stock. (Courtesy of Dr. Anthony K. Hedley)

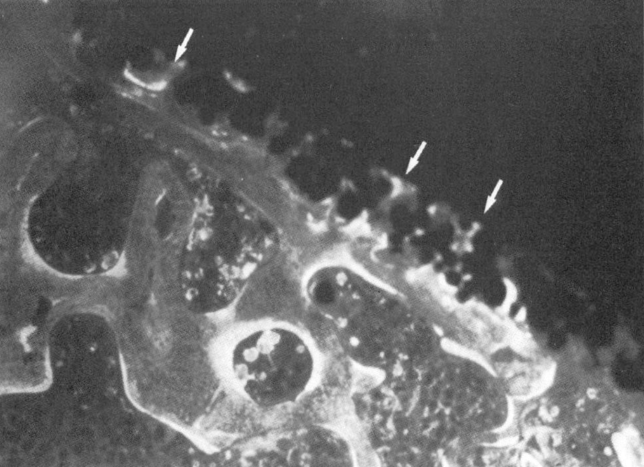

Figure 15: High magnification of the interface between bone and porous surface. The bone has been labeled with fluorochromes and indicates active new calcification within the porous layer. This label was administered 2 weeks postoperatively indicating the rapid ingrowth of calcified tissue within the porous layer marked by arrow. (Courtesy of Dr. Anthony K. Hedley)

ricated from metal, ceramics, polymers, and composite materials. Animal research has been reported (Figs. 14 and 15). However, studies reporting results in human subjects have been limited and of short follow-up.

Three phases of biologic response have been described with porous implants: the early phase requires secure fixation for bone ingrowth to occur; the intermediate phase of bone remodeling as the bone adjusts to the new stress; and, finally, a stable phase.

The increased surface area of porous materials can have deleterious effects on corrosion. Co-Cr-Mo alloy and Ti6Al4V appear suitable, but 316L stainless steel has shown increased corrosion. Porous ceramics are intrinsically brittle and should be limited to components primarily loaded in compression.

Porous polymers have been utilized because of their lower elastic moduli compared with metals. This feature could provide better long-term stability. However, due to material weakness they are prone to creep under sustained load.

Carbon fiber proplast composites do not appear to provide a strong metal composite bond, and coating degloving has been reported.

Good initial fixation seems essential to achieve bone growth. Thus, a variety of component sizes will be required to maximize precise fit and greater contact area. Secure fixation by bone ingrowth alters the stress of the surrounding bone and its remodeling process. It has been shown in animal studies that if good distal bone ingrowth is obtained around a stem, the proximal bone may resorb. This distal fixation could fatigue the stem by a cantilever mode, and, if stem fracture occurred, implant removal would pose a significant challenge.

Most human experience with cementless fixation has been gained in Europe. The early results of "isoelastic" total joint replacements appear promising, and the prosthesis is being utilized increasingly. A follow-up study of 250 cementless acetabular fixations (average 19 months, range 6 months to 4 years) disclosed no loosening.

The clinical use of ceramic prostheses has been complicated by component fractures and, in rare instances, by excessive wear. Improvement in the physical properties of these materials may reduce this problem.

Madreporic arthroplasty has been suggested as an alternative to cemented prostheses. Clinical and radiographic analysis of 300 madreporic arthroplasties demonstrated reliable biological anchoring by endosteal osteogenesis. The frequency of discomfort on weight-bearing is probably greater than with cemented prostheses.

Soft-tissue ingrowth was observed with a porous, low modulus stem coating. Acceptable clinical results were observed in only 50 percent of patients. The major cause of failure (40 percent) was inadequate initial press fit.

One study reported microporous coated metal prostheses with a pore width of approximately 50 μm. Thirty-four patients were followed for 3 years. Four required reoperation (12 percent) and ten (29 percent) demonstrated radiolucent lines, suggesting that ingrowth had not occurred.

Significant clinical and basic research is being conducted in this field, and it is reasonable to expect that important information will become available in the next few years.

ANNOTATED BIBLIOGRAPHY

Biomechanics

Carter, D.R.; Vasu, R.; and Harris, W.H.: Stress distributions in the acetabular region. J. Biomech. 15:165-170, 1982.

A two-dimensional finite element study suggests that increasing cup stiffness, either by additional cement or metal backing, causes a more efficient transfer of the stresses to the ilium. The improvement was more dramatic with metal backing. Its use might help delay or prevent cup loosening and migration.

Crowninshield, R.D.; Brand, R.A.; Johnston, R.C.; and Milroy, J.C.: The effect of femoral stem cross-sectional geometry on cement stresses in total hip reconstruction. Clin. Orthop. 146:71-77, 1980.

Predicted levels of cement stress are often close to failure levels. Prostheses with narrow medial surfaces create higher compressive stresses in the cement.

Osteotomy

Collert, S., and Gillström, P.: Osteotomy in osteoarthritis of the hip: A prospective study. Acta Orthop. Scand. 50:555-561, 1979.

Ninety-one hips were assessed after osteotomy. At 1 year 73.5 percent had no pain, while at 5 years 45 percent did not. Nineteen hips required total hip replacement. Osteotomy has a place in the treatment of osteoarthritis although its effects may not be as long-lasting as previously believed.

Weisl, H.: Intertrochanteric osteotomy for osteoarthritis: A long-term follow-up. J. Bone Joint Surg. 62B:37-42, 1980.

The results of 757 intertrochanteric osteotomies for osteoarthritis were reviewed. Joint space in two-thirds was increased. A similar proportion had pain relief for at least 5 years, declining after some 10 years; only one-quarter had a lasting "good result."

Total Hip Replacement

Total Hip Joint Replacement in the United States. J. Am. Med. Assn. 248(15):1817-1821, October 15, 1982. (NIH Consensus Conference Program, March 1-3, 1982)

Indications, design, materials, performance, fixation, biocompatibility, surgical considerations, results, complications, revision surgery, and future directions are discussed.

Long-Term Follow-up

Salvati, E.A.; Wilson, P.D., Jr.; Jolley, M.N.; Vakili, F.; Aglietti, P.; and Brown, G.C.: A ten-year follow-up study of our first 100 consecutive Charnley total hip replacements. J. Bone Joint Surg. 63A:753-767, 1981.

Good or excellent results were noted in 88 percent, fair results in 6 percent, and poor results in 6 percent. Four percent required reoperation.

Stauffer, R.N.: Ten-year follow-up study of total hip replacement. J. Bone Joint Surg. 64A:983-990, 1982.

Loosening was 11.3 percent for the cup and 29.9 percent for the stem. Revision rate was 7.4 percent. Calcar resorption was not related to loosening.

Sutherland, C.J.; Wilde, A.H.; Borden, L.S.; and Marks, K.E.: A ten-year follow-up of 100 consecutive Müller curved-stem total hip-replacement arthroplasties. J. Bone Joint Surg. 64A:970-982, 1982.

Aseptic loosening was 29 percent for the cup and 40 percent for the stem. Thirty percent were revised.

Complications

Buchholz, H.W.; Elson, R.A.; Engelbrecht, E.; Lodenkämper, H.; Röttger, J.; and Siegel, A.: Management of deep infection of total hip replacement. J. Bone Joint Surg. 63B:342-353, 1981.

Excision of soft tissue, removal of implant and cement, and replacement in one stage is recommended using Palacos R acrylic cement loaded with an appropriate antibiotic and, more recently, systemic antibiotics. An overall 77 percent success rate from a first attempt in 583 patients and a 90 percent success rate after subsequent exchange procedures are reported. Failures include: Pseudomonas group, Streptococcus group D,

Proteus group, and *Escherichia coli*, delay in operation, and inadequate antibiotic dosage in the cement.

Chao, E.Y.S., and Coventry, M.B.: Fracture of the femoral component after total hip replacement: An analysis of 58 cases. J. Bone Joint Surg. 63A:1078-1094, 1981.

Clinical, radiographic, biomechanical, and metallurgical data from fifty-eight fractured stems were analyzed, as well as twenty-seven controls with matching clinical and radiographic data. A risk index in predicting the possibility of fracture or loosening was developed.

Coventry, M.B., and Scanlon, P.W.: The use of radiation to discourage ectopic bone. J. Bone Joint Surg. 63A:201-208, 1981.

Low-dose radiation postoperatively may decrease the incidence of heterotopic ossification complicating total hip replacement. Two thousand rads were given over ten sessions beginning in the early postoperative period.

Harris, W.H.: Revision surgery for failed, nonseptic total hip arthroplasty: The femoral side. Clin. Orthop. 170:8-20, 1982.

The discussion of revision surgical techniques emphasizes wide exposure, including trochanteric osteotomy, femoral component contraction instrumentation, broken femoral stem extraction instrumentation, proximal femoral medullary canal preparation, and reconstruction considerations including optimum replacement component stem length.

Harris, W.H.; Athanasoulis, C.A.; Waltman, A.C.; and Salzman, E.W.: High and low-dose aspirin prophylaxis against venous thromboembolic disease in total hip replacement. J. Bone Joint Surg. 64A:63-66, 1982.

Low-dose aspirin in males is an effective antithrombosis prophylactic regimen. There is no benefit to be gained by high-dose aspirin therapy in males. In females, neither low- nor high-dose aspirin therapy significantly lowers the incidence of venous thromboembolic disease.

Johansson, J.E.; McBroom, R.; Barrington, T.W.; and Hunter, G.A.: Fracture of the ipsilateral femur in patients with total hip replacement. J. Bone Joint Surg. 63A:1435-1442, 1981.

Recommendations for treatment of fractures of the femoral shaft are made based upon a series of thirty-five patients. Fractures proximal to the tip of the prosthesis should be treated nonoperatively if the bone-cement-prosthesis interface is intact. Fractures occurring at or near the tip should be stabilized surgically. Those occurring completely distal to the stem can be managed in the same manner as those occurring in femora without prostheses.

Josefsson, G.; Lindberg, L.; and Wiklander, B.: Systemic antibiotics and gentamicin-containing bone cement in the prophylaxis of postoperative infections in total hip arthroplasty. Clin. Orthop. 159:194-200, 1981.

A multicenter Swedish study demonstrated a reduction in postoperative sepsis (1.6 percent versus 0.4 percent) when systemic antibiotic prophylaxis was compared to the combination of systemic antibiotics and gentamicin-impregnated cement.

Lubahn, J.D.; Evarts, C.M.; and Feltner, J.B.: Conversion of ankylosed hips to total hip arthroplasty. Clin. Orthop. 153:146-152, 1980.

The primary indication for conversion was disabling pain in low back, ipsilateral knee, and contralateral hip. Relief in the lower back was seen in twelve of thirteen patients, in the knee in four out of four, and in the contralateral hip in seven of ten. Complications included heterotopic ossification, infection, perforation of the femur, and trochanteric nonunion with dislocation.

Ranawat, C.S.; Dorr, L.D.; and Inglis, A.E.: Total hip arthroplasty in protrusio acetabuli of rheumatoid arthritis. J. Bone Joint Surg. 62A:1059-1065, 1980.

Thirty-five total hips with an average follow-up of 4.3 years (3 to 7 years) were rated good in 66 percent, fair in 26 percent, and poor in 8 percent. Although 100 percent demonstrated acetabular-cement-bone interface demarcation, only 10 percent showed progression. Eight percent showed femoral loosening or subsidence, 8 percent calcar resorption, and 6 percent a receding cortex with cystic changes. Twenty-three percent had nonunion of the greater trochanter after trochanteric osteotomy.

Salvati, E.A.; Chekofsky, K.M.; Brause, B.D.; and Wilson, P.D., Jr.: Reimplantation in infection: A 12-year experience. Clin. Orthop. 170:62-75, 1982.

A 90 percent success rate in terms of eradication of infection and reimplantation of a total hip has been achieved with stringent patient selection, surgical techniques, and antibiotic regimens (obtaining at least 1:8 peak bactericidal serum activity).

Woo, R.Y.G., and Morrey, B.F.: Dislocations after total hip arthroplasty. J. Bone Joint Surg. 64A:1295-1306, 1982.

Dislocations occurred in 3.2 percent of 10,500 total hip replacements. Previous surgery was the most significant factor predisposing to dislocation (4.8 percent). Dislocation rate was 2.3 percent after anterolateral and 5.8 percent after posterior approach. One-third required surgical revision, and, of these, one-third failed to achieve stability.

Revision Total Hip Replacement

Pellicci, P.M.; Wilson, P.D., Jr.; Sledge, C.B.; Salvati, E.A.; Ranawat, C.S.; and Poss, R.: Revision total hip arthroplasty. Clin. Orthop. 170:34-41, 1982.

Only 60 percent good or excellent results were found in 110 revisions from two major centers. There were 14 percent mechanical failures, 13 percent trochanteric problems, and 3.6 percent infections.

Turner, R.H., and Scheller, A.D., Jr., Editors. Revision Total Hip Arthroplasty. New York, Grune & Stratton, 1982.

This volume is a comprehensive presentation of revision total hip arthroplasty.

Surface Replacement

Amstutz, H.C.; Graf-Radford, A.; Mai, L.L.; and Thomas, B.J.: Surface replacement of the hip with the Tharies system: Two to five-year results. J. Bone Joint Surg. 63A:1069-1077, 1981.

Two- to 5-year clinical results of 200 Tharies were comparable to those of conventional total hip replacement. There were ten patients with aseptic and one patient with septic loosening. Fifty-five percent of patients for whom serial radiographs were available had some progression of radiolucency.

Jolley, M.N.; Salvati, E.A.; and Brown, G.C.: Early results and complications of surface replacement of the hip. J. Bone Joint Surg. 64A:366-377, 1982.

Fifty-five hips with an average follow-up of 36 months were reported. Seven arthroplasties (13 percent) were failures. This is an alarming number in view of the relatively short follow-up. Since publication, the failure rate has increased to 21 percent. This figure only includes failures requiring revision. It excludes impending failure by radiographic criteria.

Cementless Prosthetic Arthroplasty

Bryan, W.J.; McCaskill, B.L.; and Tullos, H.S.: Hip endoprosthesis stabilization with a porous low modulus stem coating: Factors influencing stabilization. Clin. Orthop. 157:125-132, 1981.

A polytetrafluoroethylene/vitreous carbon porous material mechanically fused to the endoprosthesis stem has been shown to promote soft tissue ingrowth. In twenty-nine patients, acceptable clinical results occurred in 50 percent. The major cause of failure (40 percent) was an initially inadequate press fit.

Griss, P., and Heimke, G.: Five years' experience with ceramic-metal-composite hip endoprostheses: I. Clinical evaluation. II. Mechanical evaluations and improvements. Arch. Orthop. Trauma Surg. 98(3):157-171, 1981.

One hundred and thirty ceramic endoprostheses with an average of 5-year follow-up showed satisfactory results in 84 percent, loosening in 2 percent, and breakage in 6 percent. Few showed significant wear. Improvements to reduce these complications are discussed.

Hedley, A.K.: Present state, problems, and future complications of porous coated implants. *In* The Hip Society, Proceedings of the Eighth Open Scientific Meeting of The Hip Society. St. Louis, C.V. Mosby, 1980.

Factors that affect bone ingrowth into porous materials, the effects on the bone, the strength of the bond, inherent problems, and what lies ahead are discussed.

Miscellaneous

Draenert, K.: Histomorphology of the bone to cement interface: Remodeling of the cortex and revascularization of the medullary canal in animal experiments. *In* The Hip Society, Proceedings of the Ninth Open Scientific Meeting of The Hip Society. St. Louis, C.V. Mosby, 1981.

The medullary canal of rabbit femora was filled with cement. Bone remodeling was studied by polychromatic sequential labeling. Casting the vessels allowed to study the revascularization. New bone formation was demonstrated in the gap between bone and cement.

34 KNEE AND LEG: PEDIATRIC

Topics considered in this section include congenital, developmental, inflammatory, traumatic, and neoplastic disorders, such as angular deformities, patellar instability, fractures, soft-tissue injury, and leg length discrepancy.

Congenital and Developmental

Congenital Deficiency Congenital femoral deficiency varies from hypoplasia of the entire bone to a complete absence of the proximal end. Lengthening may be considered for congenital short (hypoplastic) femur with less than 17 cm of discrepancy. In patients with unilateral proximal focal femoral deficiency with severe shortening, arthrodesis of the knee and Syme's amputation of the foot, followed by fitting with an above-knee prosthesis, is generally recommended. This eliminates the contractural deformities of the limb and gives a stable stump. Function in bilateral proximal focal femoral deficient children depends upon inequality of limb length, foot position, and associated anomalies with secondary importance given to pelvifemoral instability or the actual length of the short limb.

Congenital deficiency of the fibula may be divided into two groups: those with hypoplasia and those with complete absence. In the patient with hypoplasia, shortening may be treated by limb length equalization, whereas amputation of the foot and prosthetic fitting are best for optimal function in patients with complete absence (Fig. 1). Associated anomalies, such as ball-and-socket ankle, tarsal coalition, and foot anomalies, are frequent in both groups.

Absent tibia is a severe deformity causing instability of both the knee and ankle. Transfer of the fibula to substitute as a neoarticulation at the knee and ankle is possible in patients when a quadriceps tendon is present (Fig. 2). But, results for this procedure tend to fail in the teenage years due to degeneration of the neoarticulation. Knee disarticulation is the most reliable solution for this problem.

Congenital Angular Deformity Posteromedial bow of the tibia tends to be self-correcting but may represent a cause for progressive limb length discrepancy, generally in the 2.5- to 5.0-cm range.

Anterolateral bow of the tibia usually suggests the presence of congenital pseudarthrosis of the tibia. Fractures occurring at an early age associated with spindling, high mobility, and fracture gap carry a poor prognosis. Three concepts have proved helpful in the treatment of patients with congenital pseudarthrosis. The first is immobilization which should be rigid and is best obtained by transtarsal intramedullary smooth rod fixation of the tibia (and fibula when possible) supplemented with a spica cast for 3 months. The second is removal of abnormal tissue and autogenous bone grafting. A microvascularized free bone transfer may be of additional benefit. The third concept is pulsed electromagnetic fields, which has been reported to produce healing in approximately 50 percent of patients. Long-term success in these patients depends not merely upon healing of the defect but satisfactory growth and function of the extremity including sufficient strength and flexibility of adjacent joints. If bony union cannot be established after a reasonable number of attempts (usually 3), amputation is generally recommended. The Syme amputation is preferable to one through the area of pseudarthrosis. The pseudarthrosis may be managed by a smooth intramedullary pin or simply contained in the prosthetic socket.

Cumulative experience during the last 20 years has shown that amputation and prosthetic replacement of

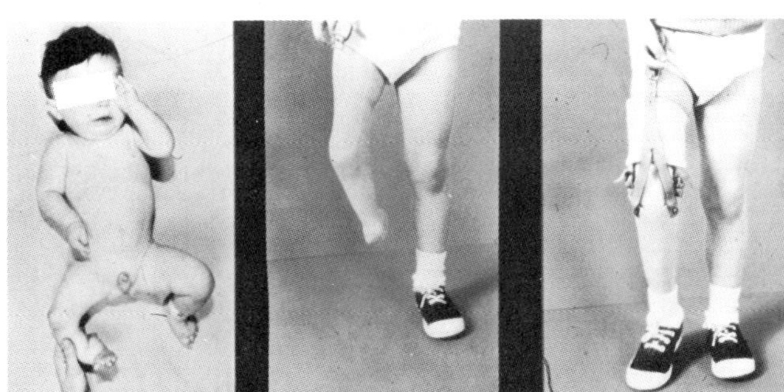

Figure 1: Congenital absent fibula with severe foot deformity and shortening treated by Boyd amputation and below-knee prosthesis.

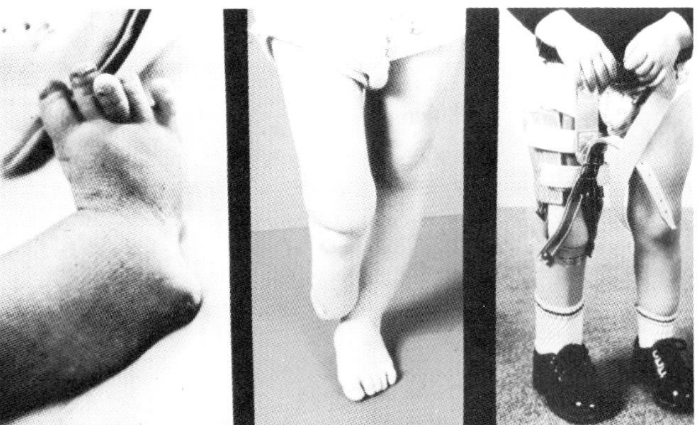

Figure 2: Congenital absent tibia treated by Syme's amputation and Putti-Brown type transfer of proximal fibula. Lateral prosthetic support is necessary for knee stability.

major limb length deficiencies can avoid repetitive operative procedures. Disarticulation is preferable to transdiaphyseal amputation in the child when these are the treatment options.

Patellar Instability Acute dislocation of the patella in children nearly always is associated with structural abnormalities including genu valgum, lateral patellar tilt, patella alta, and hypoplasia of the lateral femoral condyle. Additional abnormalities of the soft tissue are frequent, including lateral capsular contracture and medial capsular laxity, associated with vastus medialis weakness. Only one patient in six with acute dislocation develops recurrent dislocation, approximately one-third have minor symptoms after acute dislocation, and the remainder are asymptomatic. In patients with recurrent dislocation, proximal soft-tissue realignment, including lateral capsular release and medial tightening with or without semitendinous augmentation, usually gives a satisfactory result. Distal and medial transplantation of the tibial tubercle is unattractive because of late degeneration of the joint as well as potential acute complications, such as compartment syndrome and nerve palsies. In the growing child, operative manipulation of the tibial tubercle can cause growth arrest and genu recurvatum.

Painful subluxation of the patella and patellar pressure syndrome due to lateral contracture may be relieved by a vigorous, well-structured exercise program in over 90 percent of patients. Lateral retinacular release is successful in 80 percent of patients who do not respond to exercise.

Exercise programs for the painful patella include straight leg raising in full extension (rather than in flexion) since this loads the patella in a decreased contact position, thus minimizing further patellar irritation. Hamstring stretching exercises to relieve overload due to dynamic flexion contracture are also important.

Tourniquet time should be limited in knee operations to that necessary for hemostasis as EMG changes have been documented in thigh and calf muscles proportional to the duration of tourniquet ischemia. EMG changes can occur in as short a time as 15 minutes and in as high as 85 percent of patients after 60 minutes with the amount of pressure a major factor. Time for the EMG to revert to normal may be up to 60 days. This partially accounts for the quadriceps inhibition frequently seen after arthrotomy.

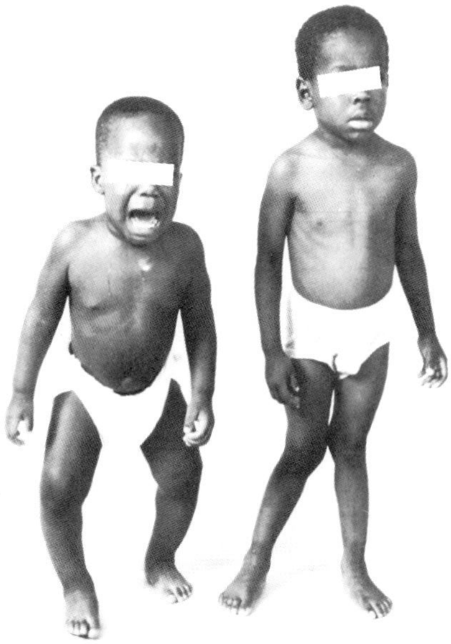

Figure 3: Two brothers demonstrating the normal angular growth of the lower limb. On the left, under 2 years of age with genu varus and on the right at 3 years of age with genu valgus. They illustrate the change from varus to valgus at approximately 2 years.

Sinding-Larsen-Johansson's disease is a condition associated with ossification at the attachment of the ligamentum patellae to the inferior pole of the patella. It tends to be a self-limited syndrome, similar to Osgood-Schlatter's disease.

In the adolescent chondromalacia of the patella with cartilaginous degeneration is nearly always associated with biomechanical abnormality. There is either malalignment of the extensor mechanism, angular deformity, or ligamentous instability. Arthroscopy may aid in the diagnosis of chondromalacia and correlation of the pathologic lesion with symptoms. However, physical examination alone may demonstrate subpatellar tenderness, crepitus, and apprehension on movement of the patella.

Treatment of chondromalacia depends upon successful normalization of biomechanical factors, including realignment of the extensor mechanism and improvement of joint instability.

Quadriceps myofibrosis usually is caused by repeated intramuscular injection of the thigh during early childhood. It causes a painless, progressive loss of flexion. Treatment consists of excising the fibrous band before severe secondary changes occur. Improvement usually ensues.

Developmental Angular Deformity Lateral angular deformities of the knee may be physiologic or pathologic. Physiologic genu varum occurs under 2 years of age with valgus deformity most pronounced at 3 years of age and continuing until about 8 years of age (Fig. 3). Physiologic varus as high as 33 degrees and valgus as high as 20 degrees have been noted to undergo spontaneous correction in growing children. Pathologic genu valgum may be associated with various bone dysplasias such as Morquio's disease.

Pathologic genu varum is most commonly due to Blount's disease, a disturbance of the medial tibial growth plate. The metaphyseal-diaphyseal angle describes the tilt from perpendicular occurring in the tibial metaphysis in this disease (Fig. 4). Bowing deformity in the tibial metaphysis that will pose a later problem is indicated by a metaphyseal-diaphyseal angle greater than 11 degrees. Prior to 9 years of age, tibia vara may improve with osteotomy, but as age progresses and the medial epiphyseal plate closes, osteotomy alone leads to recurrent deformation.

Osteotomy is appropriate for pathologic lateral angular deformities of genu varum or valgum. Distal femoral epiphyseal stapling also has been used to treat angular deformities, although the results may not be as predictable.

Genu recurvatum may be caused by an injury to the anterior tibial growth plate (such as with tibial pin traction) prolonged cast immobilization in extension, and as a side effect of neuromuscular conditions such as cerebral palsy. Treatment of genu recurvatum or flexion contracture depends upon the cause. Release of soft tissues in the early stage of flexion contractures can lead to bone

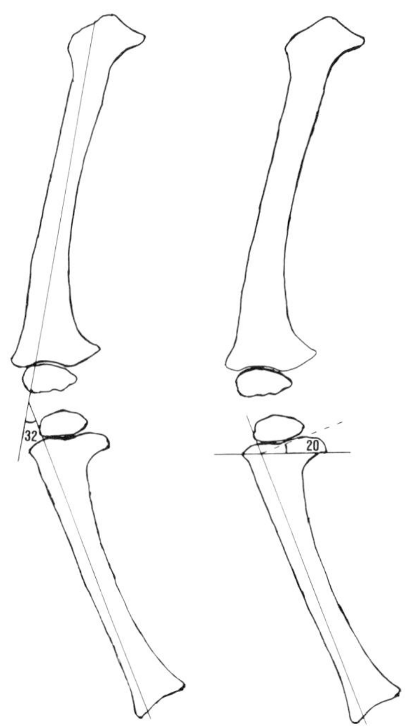

Figure 4-A Figure 4-B

Figure 4: (A) Tibiofemoral angle. Angle between a line along the longitudinal axis of the tibia and of the femur is 32 degrees. (B) Metaphyseal-diaphyseal angle. Dashed line is constructed perpendicular to the longitudinal axis of the tibia. A second line is drawn connecting the two peaks of the metaphysis. Angle between is the metaphyseal-diaphyseal angle, 20 degrees in this patient. (Reprinted with permission from Physiological bowing and tibia vara, by A.M. Levine, et al., J. Bone Joint Surg. 64A:1159, 1982.)

remodeling whereas late deformities may require either femoral or tibial osteotomy depending upon the location of the deformity to produce normal alignment. In ambulatory patients, the hamstring muscles are better lengthened than detached.

Osteochondritis Dissecans There is no consensus about the cause of osteochondritis dissecans, which occurs most frequently in the knee joint. Hereditary factors, short stature, and epiphyseal abnormalities frequently are associated with juvenile osteochondritis dissecans of the knee. Prognosis is poor in those patients in whom frank separation of the fragment occurs with free body formation. Therefore, therapeutic measures should be directed at preventing such a separation.

Two types of lesions are recognized. One occurs in the skeletally immature individual, and healing almost always follows restriction of activity and splinting. The other occurs in the skeletally mature patient in whom there is a high incidence of fragment separation.

Arthroscopy has provided a useful means for delineating the stage of disease either as a fragment in situ, a partially detached fragment (Fig. 5), or a free body (Fig. 6).

There are several treatment options. Drilling the fragment in the young patient in whom healing has been delayed is one possibility. This procedure is ineffectual in the older child where stabilization is necessary.

For the partially detached fragment, encouraging long-term results have been reported with bone grafts either inserted through the articular cartilage or superiorly along a guide pin placed through the lesion. Arthroscopic management of the lesion has included stabilization with pins inserted endoscopically.

Replacement of free fragments should be accomplished when possible. If not possible, trephination and spongilization followed by joint range of motion are recommended.

With completely detached free bodies, removal of fragments can be done by arthroscopy. Fibrocartilaginous healing occurs in the debrided bed (Fig. 7).

Inflammation and Infection

Examination by comparative thigh circumference measurement may be of diagnostic and therapeutic value. If measured 1 cm above the patella, the quantity of synovial effusion can be estimated. If measured 8 to 10 cm above the patella, the status of quadriceps deterioration or recovery can be monitored.

The arthroscope is particularly helpful in patients with pain and persistent swelling to determine the cause of synovitis; in instances of pain associated with impingement to determine the presence of a free body, a loosened osteochondritic lesion, or meniscal injury; and in patients with instability associated with pain to assess injury to the cruciate ligaments. In general, arthroscopic procedures have proved useful in obtaining a more accurate diagnosis prior to a proposed arthrotomy and have changed the treatment in 30 to 40 percent of patients in published studies.

Inflammatory lesions may occur about the knee in youngsters, particularly as a result of overuse in athletic activities. The iliotibial friction syndrome occurs over the lateral femoral condyle where the iliotibial band rubs during running activity and is an overuse syndrome of runners associated with pronated feet. It is improved by rest and a shoe orthosis to reduce subtalar valgus. Breaststroker's knee occurs in swimmers on the medial side and is characterized by tenderness about the patella, medial femoral epicondyle, and medial capsular ligament. It is caused by poor mechanics in making the whip kick.

Septic arthritis of the knee is best treated by incision, drainage, and appropriate antibiotics. Intravenous antibiotics should be continued until clinical and laboratory parameters improve and then changed to oral antibiotics (see Section 6, General: Infection and Section 30, Pelvis, Hip, and Femur: Pediatric).

In tuberculous infection, partial synovectomy and excision of pannus over the cartilage is worthwhile in lesions

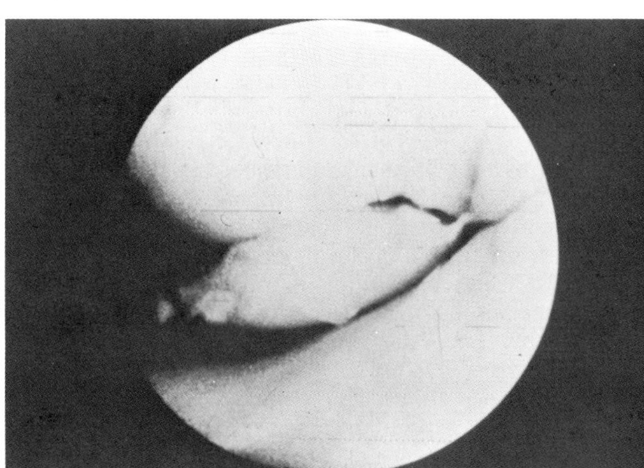

Figure 5: Arthroscopic view of osteochondritis dissecans of the medial femoral condyle. Fragment is partially detached.

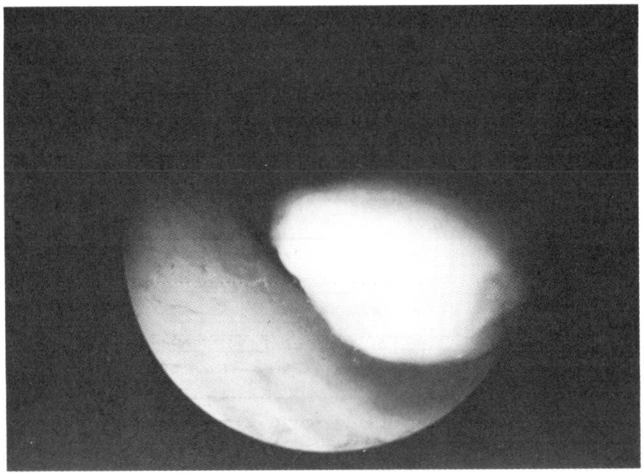

Figure 6: Arthroscopic view of a free body which is a detached fragment of osteochondritis dissecans lying in the lateral gutter where the synovium reflects off the femoral condyle.

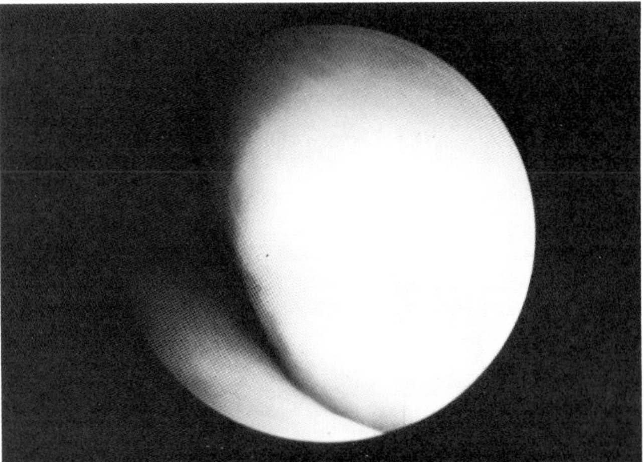

Figure 7: Arthroscopic view of medial femoral condyle 1 year after debridement of osteochondritic crater demonstrating the extent of fibrocartilaginous healing.

without advanced bony and articular damage. More extensive debridement is necessary in patients with more advanced disease.

In patients with puncture wounds, Pseudomonas as well as anaerobes such as Clostridium must be considered. There has been a report of herpetic infection of the joint occurring from skin lesions adjacent to a previously injured knee joint.

In youngsters with hemophilia, synovectomy of the knee may help prevent severe recurrent bleeding.

In patients with juvenile rheumatoid arthritis, treatment is generally nonoperative, utilizing medication and splinting. Synovectomy is helpful in joints with proliferative synovitis which is unresponsive to medical management. Release of soft-tissue contractures is more beneficial in atrophic (dry) joints.

Trauma

Fractures A peculiar type of fracture occurring in the distal femur of the adolescent involves the physis. Salter-Harris type I and II injuries generally have a good prognosis although an average shortening of 1 cm can be expected in most patients and asymmetrical growth arrest may occur. Type II injuries require accurate reduction for a good result. Injuries caused from crushing open wounds or high velocity injuries have a poor prognosis due to multiple fractures and associated injuries, particularly to the adjacent blood vessels, nerve, and muscular compartments. Fracture of the knee physes may be difficult to identify and confused with collateral ligament injuries. Multiple views, stress views, and occasionally tomograms are appropriate when such injuries are suspected.

Chondral and osteochondral fractures may be unrecognized on routine radiographs. These may mimic a torn meniscus, and in such instances arthroscopy is valuable for diagnosis. Injuries resulting in bone being avulsed by either cruciate ligament usually can be better defined by arthroscopy. There has been some success in reducing these fractures by use of the arthroscope, but open reduction is usually necessary, particularly in patients in whom the meniscus is damaged. Open reduction more often is necessitated with injuries produced by posterior cruciate ligament avulsions. Mildly displaced anterior cruciate injuries avulsing the tibial spine frequently can be treated successfully by closed methods.

Injury to the popliteal artery always should be suspected in fracture through the proximal tibial epiphysis. Satisfactory results can be expected with these fractures unless they are associated with open injuries or neurovascular compromise (e.g., lawn mower injuries or high velocity crush injuries). The tibial tubercle may be avulsed by indirect force on the ligamentum patellae, and this is usually seen in adolescents near the end of skeletal growth. Tibial tubercle fractures may involve the articular surface of the upper tibia. Accurate reduction and secure fixation are indicated for displaced fractures or those extending into the joint.

Physeal injury in paraplegic children has a higher incidence of complications, such as growth arrest, malunion, and joint stiffness. It is possible to mistake the overreactive healing callus for a malignant tumor or osteomyelitis. This may lead to unnecessary diagnostic biopsy when the lesion should properly be treated by immobilization and restriction of weight-bearing.

Stress fracture around the knee may not be evident on routine radiographs. A bone scan may be the only positive diagnostic test in some of these patients.

Metaphyseal fractures of the shaft of the tibia can result in valgus deformity. Progression of the deformity occurs for 1 or 2 years after the fracture and subsequently tends to resolve. The growth pattern should be observed before resorting to osteotomy which may restimulate the original valgus deformity process. Diaphyseal fractures of the tibia can stimulate overgrowth of the limb in girls under 10 years of age and boys under 12 years of age. After these ages, undergrowth usually occurs.

Insertion of tibial traction pins may injure the proximal tibial epiphysis resulting in genu recurvatum. For this reason, distal femoral pin traction is preferable in the skeletally immature patient in whom skeletal fixation is deemed necessary.

Soft Tissue

Meniscus The menisci are important for knee stability, load transmission, shock absorption, and lubrication. Meniscectomy in children has been associated with subsequent degenerative arthritis and instability leading to a

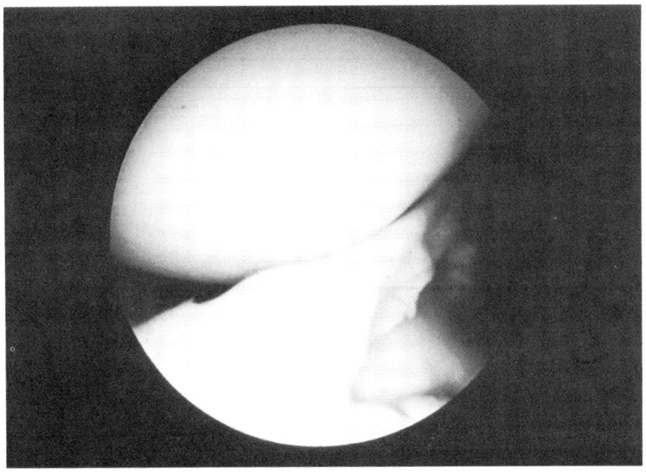

Figure 8: Arthroscopic view of a bucket handle tear of the medial meniscus in a 15-year-old girl. The bucket handle is displaced under the medial condyle. The intercondylar notch is at the right edge of the photograph.

high incidence of narrowing and osteophyte formation on follow-up examination, especially after excision of the lateral meniscus. Fortunately, meniscal tears are very uncommon under 14 years of age and represent only 2 percent of tears in one large series.

The time-related effect from excision of a normal meniscus causes much greater damage to the joint than does a small tear. Therefore, thoughtful evaluation of the knee is necessary prior to meniscectomy. A most valuable technique for this evaluation has proved to be arthroscopy, recommended by many investigators prior to any planned arthrotomy for suspected meniscal lesions, particularly in a child.

Discoid lateral menisci may cause snapping, are not always associated with disability, and are compatible with good joint function if retained. If a significant tear with resulting disability occurs, complete meniscectomy gives better results than partial meniscectomy. This is the exception to the rule that partial meniscectomy has produced less instability and degenerative arthritis and is the procedure of choice for bucket handle tears that are frequently seen in young people (Fig. 8). Repair of the meniscus, particularly following acute trauma, also has proved to be a reliable procedure.

Menisci should be preserved, if possible. Preservation techniques include accurate diagnosis, retention of as much stable, well-contoured tissue as is possible, and repair of peripheral lesions.

Knee Ligamentous Injuries Some suggest that knee joint tightness or laxity correlates with the type of knee ligament injuries. Prospective examination of many teenaged athletes has failed to support this correlation.

Ligament injuries of the knee can occur in children as a major disruption of either the collateral or cruciate ligaments. The cruciate ligaments often are injured along with avulsion of adjacent bone, particularly the tibial spine. When there is cruciate avulsion, collateral ligament injury should be suspected. Failure to recognize and repair these ligament avulsion injuries, whether of the anterior or posterior cruciate, leads to late instability. Surgical repair usually leads to a good or fair result. Accurate diagnosis and open surgical repair form the appropriate course of action for most patients.

Tumors

Tumors of the knee and leg in children are divided into three major groups: benign tumors, a group in whom cellular differentiation is difficult, and malignant tumors (see Section 5, General: Musculoskeletal Neoplasms).

Osteochondroma is the most common benign bone tumor about the knee. Its presence does not produce symptoms unless it causes pressure on adjacent structures resulting in inflammation of the encapsulating bursa. However, if it is frequently traumatized, it should be excised. Excision should be delayed until the lesion is distant from the adjacent physes. Premature excision may result in angular deformity from damage to the growth plate. Lesions that are distant from the physis can be safely excised through the stalk of normal marrow elements. Care should be taken to excise all cartilage tissue.

Fibrous dysplasia of the tibia and fibula recently has become better delineated and should be considered in patients in whom bowing of the tibia is present along with a fibrous lesion. It must be differentiated from ossifying fibroma and adamantinoma of bone. Operative treatment should be delayed as long as possible and restricted to extensive lesions because the tumor tends to persist.

Fibrous cortical defect (of the posterior medial aspect) of the distal femoral metaphysis at the level of insertion of the adductor magnus may create a disturbing radiographic appearance and simulate a malignant bone tumor. Thorough radiographic study makes biopsy seldom necessary. Occasionally, biopsy material from these benign defects have been misinterpreted as osteosarcoma because of the immaturity of reactive bone and fibrous tissue.

Among the difficult-to-classify tumors is *neurofibromatosis* which may behave in a disturbing manner due to its local displacement of bone and nerves. It produces pseudarthrosis of the long bones and damage to nerve supply of the extremity or localized gigantism. The child with extensive involvement by neurofibromatosis is at risk for malignant degeneration to neurofibrosarcoma.

Hemangioma of the lower extremity may produce severe deformity and may be an obscure cause of recurrent hemarthroses of the knee when isolated. Selected embolization of the more serious varieties (e.g., angiodysplasia) should be considered when radical operative treatment such as amputation is being evaluated.

Ollier's disease consists of multiple bones deformed by abnormal proliferating masses of cartilage (enchondromatosis). The disease may lead to severe limb length discrepancy and angular deformities. Frequent osteotomies may be required during the growth period to produce normal alignment at skeletal maturity. Limb lengthening should be considered when the discrepancy is 5 cm or more. Malignant transformation into chondrosarcoma is common but rarely occurs before 20 years of age.

Leukemia, a malignancy of childhood, may present as pain in and about the knee or as a lucency in the metaphysis of the long bone on radiograph. When leukemia is suspected, peripheral blood count and/or bone marrow examination should be part of the laboratory evaluation prior to biopsy.

Limb Length Discrepancy (Anisomelia)

Limb length discrepancy of 2 cm or less produces little or no functional problem with gait, joint pain, back pain, or production of scoliosis. All these symptoms and signs become of increasing concern with further increase in discrepancy.

Causes of leg length discrepancy include trauma, infection, tumor, and congenital anomaly. An accurate treatment plan must be based on prediction of subsequent growth. Vascular inhibition of growth may follow catheterization for cardiac diagnosis. Stimulation of growth may occur in the juvenile rheumatoid arthritic patient under 5 years of age and inhibition of growth over 9 years of age.

Accurate documentation of the pattern of growth is important for making treatment decisions. Such documentation requires sequential assessment of leg length by orthoradiographs and wrist/hand films for bone age to compare the patient's growth with the normal growth charts. The growth pattern in individual patients often varies over time between increase, plateauing, and decrease in discrepancy. Therefore, long-term projection from a single observation can be misleading. The most accurate prediction is based on longitudinal assessment.

Epiphysiodesis continues to be the standard procedure for discrepancies up to 5 cm and for even larger ones according to some investigators. Recent clinical studies show the final result should be within approximately 1 cm of that predicted when accurate data is collected prior to choosing the time for epiphysiodesis.

In instances where the data base is inaccurate and the patient is approaching the end of the expected growth period, adjustment is best made after skeletal growth is completed. The simplest alternative is single-stage shortening with internal fixation.

Limb lengthening is gaining favor recently with the generalized availability and acceptance of the Wagner apparatus and lengthening technique (Fig. 9). Lengthenings of 15 percent of the bone length, or approximately 6 cm for the femur and 5 cm for the tibia, have been obtained in many centers. The high incidence rate of complications includes neurovascular compromise, infection, loss of joint motion, and late fracture. But, the overall goal of lengthening usually has been achieved without major functional compromise in most patients. Limb lengthening probably should not be considered for discrepancies under 5 cm and is best done between the ages of 8 and 16 years. Bone grafting is frequently necessary with internal fixation. The process is more easily accomplished when the shortening is due to polio or trauma and is much more difficult when on a congenital basis. In any event, the technique is demanding.

Lengthening by epiphyseal distraction can yield up to 10 cm but has been so sparsely reported as to be considered experimental at this time.

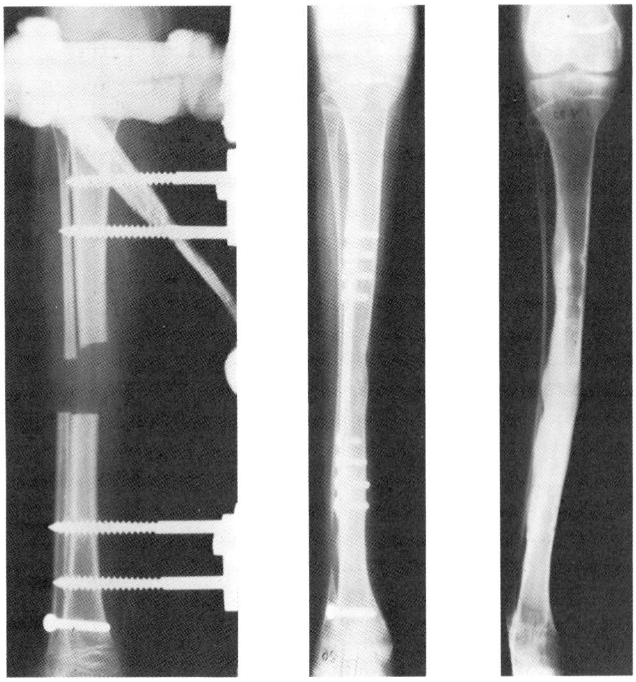

Figure 9-A Figure 9-B Figure 9-C

Figure 9: (A) Wagner lengthening device maintaining distraction of the tibia during tibial lengthening for shortening due to poliomyelitis. (B) Appearance 1 year after bone graft and plating for 5 cm gain in length. (C) Appearance 3 years postoperatively with plate removed.

ANNOTATED BIBLIOGRAPHY

Congenital and Developmental

Congenital Deficiency

Kruger, L.M.: Recent advances in surgery of lower limb deficiencies. Clin. Orthop. 148:97-105, 1980.

For major long bone deficiencies, amputation and prosthetic fitting are indicated to restore length and to avoid repetitive surgical procedures. This treatment is based on a better understanding of the natural history of major limb deficiencies.

Marquardt, E.: The Knud Jansen lecture. The operative treatment of congenital limb malformation. Part II, Case study. Prosthet. Orthot. Internat. 5:2-6, 1981.

A stump-capping procedure can be used in patients with bony overgrowth resulting from transdiaphyseal amputation. A cartilage-covered bone graft is attached to the end of the stump which is split into two pillars. This converts the diaphyseal amputation into one resembling a disarticulation that does not overgrow.

Congenital Angular Deformity

Morrissy, R.T.: A Symposium: Congenital Pseudarthrosis. Clin. Orthop. 166:1-61, 1982.

Eight papers outline the natural history, treatment results, recent clinical advances to include the fibula with internal fixation, the use of free vascularized bone graft, and pulsing electromagnetic fields to obtain union and more normal growth.

Patellar Instability

Chrisman, O.D.; Snook, G.A.; and Wilson, T.C.: A long-term prospective study of the Hauser and Roux-Goldthwait procedures for recurrent patellar dislocation. Clin. Orthop. 144:27-30, 1979.

In eighty-seven knees in seventy-five patients repaired consecutively and in random manner over an 8-year period, the authors compared the two procedures. Satisfactory long-term results were obtained in 72 percent with the Hauser technique and 93 percent with the Roux-Goldthwait technique.

McManus, F.; Rang, M.; and Heslin, D.J.: Acute dislocation of the patella in children: The natural history. Clin. Orthop. 139:88-91, 1979.

Reviewing fifty-five patients, only one child in six had recurrent dislocation of the patella after an acute dislocation. Two of six had minor symptoms, and three of six were asymptomatic. The majority of patients showed the radiological signs of patellofemoral dysplasia.

Medlar, R.C., and Lyne, E.D.: Sinding-Larsen-Johansson disease: Its etiology and natural history. J. Bone Joint Surg. 60A:1113-1116, 1978.

Eight patients with ten knees affected were identified to have Sinding-Larsen-Johansson disease by clinical and radiographic criteria. It appears to be a traction tendonitis of the proximal attachment of the patellar tendon to the inferior pole of the patella and is characterized by a self-limited, benign course.

Saunders, K.C.; Louis, D.L.; Weingarden, S.I.; and Waylonis, G.W.: Effect of tourniquet time on postoperative quadriceps function. Clin. Orthop. 143:194-199, 1979.

Forty-eight patients who underwent knee arthrotomy had postoperative electromyographic testing. Thirty of these patients (62.5 percent) developed abnormal postoperative EMG changes. Fewer EMG changes and more rapid clinical recovery were associated with decreased tourniquet time.

Developmental Angular Deformity

Langenskiöld, A.: Tibia vara: Osteochondrosis of deformans tibiae: Blount's disease. Clin. Orthop. 158:77-82, 1981.

Recommendations for treatment are based on age. Between 2 and 4 years of age with greater than 20 degrees of varus, osteotomy of the tibia and fibula is recommended. Beyond the age of 8 years, partial epiphyseal arrest occurs; epiphysiodesis and elevation of the medial condyle may be necessary.

Levine, A.M., and Drennan, J.C.: Physiological bowing and tibia vara: The metaphyseal-diaphyseal angle in the measurement of bowleg deformities. J. Bone Joint Surg. 64A:1158-1163, 1982.

The metaphyseal-diaphyseal angle is the measurement of the deviation from perpendicular of the proximal tibial metaphysis. When more than 11 degrees, twenty-nine of thirty affected extremities progressed to the typical radiographic changes of pathologic tibia vara. Only three of fifty-eight extremities with less than 11 degrees developed pathologic changes.

Vankka, E., and Salenius, P.: Spontaneous correction of severe tibiofemoral deformity in growing children. Acta Orthop. Scand. 53:567-570, 1982.

Twenty children with an exceptionally large angular deformity were followed from early childhood. Varus deformity as great as 33 degrees and valgus deformity of 20 degrees were noted to straighten spontaneously as late as 13 years of age. They encourage delaying osteotomy until at least 10 to 13 years of age.

Zuege, R.C.; Kempken, T.G.; and Blount, W.P.: Epiphyseal stapling for angular deformity at the knee. J. Bone Joint Surg. 61A:320-329, 1979.

Eighty-seven percent of fifty-six patients (eighty-two knees) treated by asymmetric epiphyseal stapling (sixty-four genu valgus and eighteen genu varus) over a 19-year period were satisfactory or improved at maturity. It is recommended that exaggerated physiological deformities not be stapled until skeletal age of 11 years for girls or 12 for boys and secondary deformities not before skeletal age 8 years.

Osteochondritis Dissecans

Guhl, J.F.: Arthroscopic treatment of osteochondritis dissecans. Clin. Orthop. 167:65-74, 1982.

Of fifty patients with osteochondritis dissecans of the knee, forty-four were treated by arthroscopic means either by drilling, pinning, reduction, or removal of fragments and bone grafting. Ninety percent healed in an average of 5 months.

Lindholm, T.S., and Osterman, K.: Long-term results after transfixation of an osteochondritis dissecans fragment to the femoral condyle using autologous bone transplants in adolescent and adult patients. Arch. Orthop. Trauma Surg. 97:225-230, 1980.

In sixteen adolescent patients with osteochondritis dissecans of the femoral condyle, the fragment was fixed in situ using autologous tibial graft. Union occurred in 90 percent, 60 percent were totally symptomfree, and the others improved. No immobilization or removal of bone fragments was needed.

Mubarak, S.J., and Carroll, N.C.: Juvenile osteochondritis dissecans of the knee: Etiology. Clin. Orthop. 157:200-211, 1981.

Seventy-three patients with osteochondritis dissecans of the knee were studied. One-half had multiple lesions, and thirty were of short stature. Trauma played a minor role. Constitutional factors such as heredity and abnormality of collagen or epiphysis frequently were associated and believed to be important in the etiology.

Inflammation and Infection

McCollough, N.C., III; Enis, J.E.; Lovitt, J.; Lian, E.C.; Niemann, K.N.; and Loughlin, E.C., Jr.: Synovectomy or total replacement of the knee in hemophilia. J. Bone Joint Surg. 61A:69-75, 1979.

The major lesion responsible for musculoskeletal disability in hemophilic patients is arthropathy of the knee. Synovectomy in young patients with recurrent hemarthrosis was successful in eight patients operated on at an average age of 16.4 years.

McNicol, K.; Taunton, J.E.; and Clement, D.B.: Iliotibial tract friction syndrome in athletes. Canadian J. Appl. Sport Sci. 6:76-80, 1981.

Fifty-two runners presented a typical clinical syndrome with tenderness over the lateral femoral epicondyle and sharp pain produced along the iliotibial tract during a varus extension stress test of provocation. Foot orthotics were used successfully in forty-two of fifty patients to improve the associated hyperpronation of the foot.

Stulberg, S.D.; Shulman, K.; Stuart, S.; and Culp, P.: Breaststroker's knee: Pathology, etiology and treatment. Am. J. Sports Med. 8:164-171, 1980.

Twenty-three breaststroke swimmers aged 6 to 30 years with painful knees were examined and studied with underwater movies. Medial knee pain was related to the technique used in performing the whip kick associated with the breaststroke. A strong treatment suggestion was to correct the technique of the swimmer's whip kick.

Trauma

Fractures

Czitrom, A.A.; Salter, R.B.; and Willis, R.B.: Fractures involving the distal epiphyseal plate of the femur. Internat. Orthop. 4:269-277, 1981.

Forty-two fractures are reported with the average age at injury of 11.2 years. The prognosis was related to the injury mechanism, displacement, and accuracy of reduction. Type I and II injuries had a shortening averaging 1.0 cm. Open injuries, severe displacement, and incomplete reduction gave poor or fair results.

Molander, M.L.; Wallin, G.; and Wikstad, I.: Fracture of the intercondylar eminence of the tibia: A review of 35 patients. J. Bone Joint Surg. 63B:89-91, 1981.

All the less severe and fourteen of seventeen severely displaced fractures were treated by cast immobilization. In follow-up radiographs, the authors found no significant loss of motion or discomfort, no instability, and no degenerative change. They recommend closed reduction.

Ogden, J.A.; Tross, R.B.; and Murphy, M.J.: Fractures of the tibial tuberosity in adolescents. J. Bone Joint Surg. 62A:205-215, 1980.

Fifteen physeal fractures of the tibial tuberosity were classified based upon displacement of the fracture fragments or extension into the joint. Results were good following accurate reduction (usually open) with no genu recurvatum in this group of patients near skeletal maturity.

Shelton, W.R., and Canale, S.T.: Fractures of the tibia through the proximal tibial epiphyseal cartilage. J. Bone Joint Surg. 61A:167-173, 1979.

In thirty-nine fractures treated over a 25-year period, two patients had disruption of the popliteal artery. Of the twenty-eight long-term follow-ups, twenty-four were satisfactory with unsatisfactory results due to chronic neurovascular insufficiency, growth disturbance, or traumatic arthritis.

Skak, S.V.: Valgus deformity following proximal tibial metaphyseal fracture in children. Acta Orthop. Scand. 53:141-147, 1982.

Seven children with primary valgus angulation showed medial cortical diastasis due to soft tissue in the fracture gap. The angulation progressed during the first year despite healing of the fracture but slowly regressed during the subsequent 2 years with corrective longitudinal growth.

Soft Tissue

Meniscus

Zaman, M., and Leonard, M.A.: Meniscectomy in children: Results in 59 knees. Injury 12:425-428, 1981.

Fifty-nine knees were examined at a mean follow-up of 7.5 years. The result was good in 68 percent of boys and 29 percent of girls, but only 27 percent had normal radiographs and 19 percent showed early osteoarthrosis. Meniscectomy is not a benign procedure in children, and preoperative arthroscopy is strongly recommended.

Knee Ligamentous Injuries

Clanton, T.O.; DeLee, J.C.; Sanders, B.; and Neidre, A.: Knee ligament injuries in children. J. Bone Joint Surg. 61A:1195-1201, 1979.

Of nine children, five had avulsion of the intercondylar eminence, four of whom had associated collateral ligament injuries. Despite surgical repair, all nine patients demonstrated some degree of postoperative ligament instability, which was worse in those having a meniscectomy.

Grana, W.A., and Moretz, J.A.: Ligamentous laxity in secondary school athletes. J. Am. Med. Assn. 240:1975-1976, 1978.

A prospective study tested ligamentous laxity in 198 male and 84 female athletes. These were compared to 167 male and 223 female high school students not involved in interscholastic sports. No correlation could be found between ligamentous laxity and the occurrence or type of injury.

Tumors

Campanacci, M., and Laus, M.: Osteofibrous dysplasia of the tibia and fibula. J. Bone Joint Surg. 63A:367-375, 1981.

Thirty-five patients presented with enlargement of the tibia associated with slight or moderate anterior or anterolateral bowing. Eccentric intercortical osteolysis seen on the radiograph is characteristic of the diagnosis. Marginal subperiosteal excision is suggested after 15 years of age as recurrence is common in younger patients.

Dunham, W.K.; Marcus, N.W.; Enneking, W.F.; and Haun, C.: Developmental defects of the distal femoral metaphysis. J. Bone Joint Surg. 62A:801-806, 1980.

A developmental defect often occurs in the posteromedial aspect of the distal femur in the area of insertion of the adductor magnus. This defect may be confused with osteosarcoma radiographically or even histologically. These defects are almost always incidental findings. The radiograph should be studied and biopsy avoided.

Limb Length Discrepancy (Anisomelia)

Ahmadi, B.; Akbarnia, B.A.; Ghobadi, F.; Ganjavian, M.S.; and Nasseri, D.: Experience with 141 tibial lengthenings in poliomyelitis and comparison of three different methods. Clin. Orthop. 145:150-153, 1979.

The average discrepancy was 5.2 cm, and lengthening obtained 4.8 cm. Comparing Anderson, Shafa, and Wagner apparatus, the latter was preferred because it was more comfortable, more accurate to apply, and more easily adjusted by the patient even at home.

Monticelli, G., and Spinelli, R.: Distraction epiphysiolysis as a method of limb lengthening. III. Clinical applications. Clin. Orthop. 154:274-285, 1981.

Traction epiphysiolysis of the proximal tibial epiphysis was performed in sixteen patients between 13 and 15 years of age. Five to 10 cm of length was obtained with minor and infrequent complications. Patients near the end of growth were chosen because of premature epiphyseal closure seen in experimental animals with the same technique.

Shapiro, F.: Developmental patterns in lower extremity length discrepancies. J. Bone Joint Surg. 64A:639-651, 1982.

The data on 803 patients obtained by serial radiographic measurement was used to define six patterns of discrepancy development. The patterns can be correlated with the conditions producing discrepancy and the time of occurrence. In conjunction with the Green and Anderson growth charts the patterns permit accurate projections of final discrepancy.

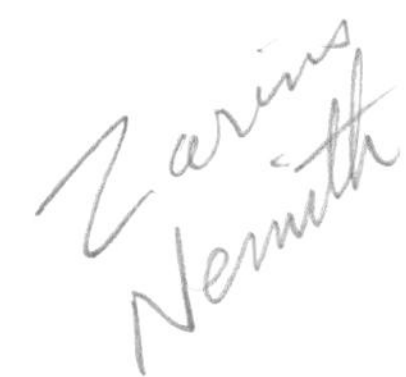

35 KNEE AND LEG: TRAUMA (SOFT TISSUE)

Subjects considered in this section include injuries to the cruciate and collateral ligaments and menisci, parapatellar injuries, muscle rupture, nonfracture-related compartment syndromes, and arthroscopy.

Knee

Introduction Diagnosis and treatment of knee injury have improved considerably over the past 5 years. Factors contributing to this improvement are better understanding of the mechanisms of injury, more precise physical diagnosis, and the use of arthroscopy. The most important new concepts relating to knee injuries are the recognition of: (1) the mechanism, incidence, and natural history of anterior cruciate ligament injury; (2) the importance of the menisci in load-bearing and joint stability; (3) the healing potential of menisci and the feasibility of meniscus repair; (4) the advantages of partial as opposed to total meniscectomy; (5) the benefits of early, protected knee motion following ligament injury, repair, and reconstruction; and (6) the length of time (1 year) required for repair collagen to attain sufficient tensile strength to prevent stretching.

Much of the current confusion about knee injury stems from variation in terminology. The word *laxity* is used here to describe increased physiologic motion of a joint in the absence of prior injury. This is often seen in loose-jointed individuals. The word *instability* describes a joint that has abnormal increase in motion as the result of an injury to a ligament or other stabilizing structure. If the patient has symptoms, such as giving way as the result of the instability, this is termed *functional instability*.

Instability can be quantified based on the degree of abnormal motion of the *tibia* in relation to the *femur* as follows: 1+—up to 5 mm; 2+—6-10 mm; 3+—11-15 mm; 4+—greater than 15 mm.

The term *pivot shift phenomenon* describes reduction or subluxation of the tibia on the femur under load at approximately 25 degrees flexion, regardless of the testing method used. There are a variety of tests that elicit the pivot shift phenomenon, including the jerk test, flexion-rotation drawer, ALRI (anterolateral rotatory instability) test, and Slocum's sidelying method. They differ in the way the leg is held, in whether the knee goes from a subluxated to a reduced position or vice versa, and whether the tibia is held in neutral or internal rotation.

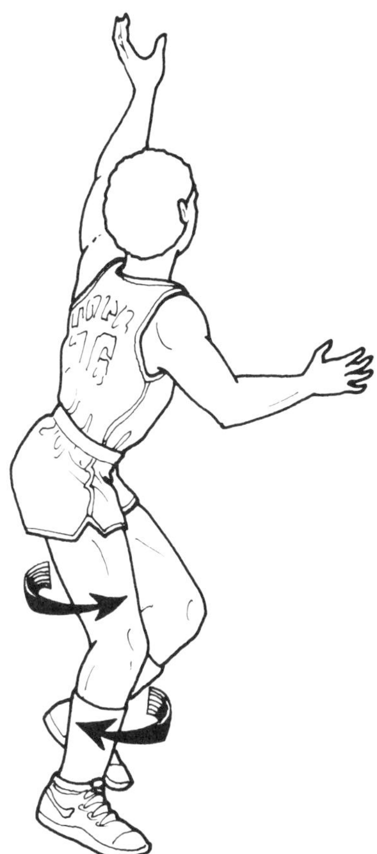

Figure 1: Most common mechanism of injury to anterior cruciate ligament: deceleration-valgus-external rotation, as in landing from a rebound in basketball on the right leg and twisting toward the left.

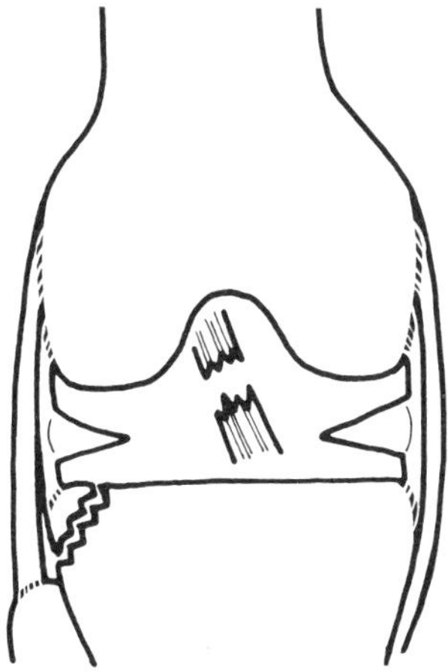

Figure 2: A small avulsion fracture of the lateral corner of the tibial condyle at the joint line seen on anteroposterior radiograph is highly suggestive of a torn anterior cruciate ligament and acute anterolateral rotatory instability. This is referred to as the lateral capsular sign. (Redrawn with permission from Lateral capsular sign: x-ray clue to a significant knee instability, by G.W. Woods, et al., Am. J. Sports Med. 7:27-33, 1979.)

They vary in sensitivity, but they do not test *different* phenomena. The ability to demonstrate one test and not another in a knee with a torn anterior cruciate ligament may be a function of the experience of the examiner, patient relaxation, or the degree of instability.

Anterior Cruciate Ligament Injury to the anterior cruciate ligament without associated gross disruption of other knee ligaments now is recognized as one of the most common major knee injuries related to athletics. The *mechanism* of injury is usually a noncontact deceleration-valgus-external rotation injury, such as in open field pivoting or in landing on the leg after jumping (Fig. 1). Less common mechanisms are deceleration-internal rotation and excessive hyperextension. The knee usually develops severe swelling within 2 hours after injury, indicating hemarthrosis. Many patients feel the whole knee momentarily "go out of place," and approximately one-third hear a "pop."

EXAMINATION: Physical examination following injury reveals a positive anterior drawer sign at 25 degrees knee flexion (Lachman test). This finding usually can be elicited in the swollen, painful knee without anesthesia. The anterior drawer sign at 90 degrees flexion is not a reliable test for a torn anterior cruciate ligament. The pivot shift phenomenon (a forward subluxation or reduction of the lateral tibial plateau in relation to the femur under load) usually is also positive although anesthesia may be required to elicit instability in a painful knee. The collateral ligaments are typically stable to stress testing, and the anterior drawer sign performed at 90 degrees knee flexion may be negative, especially if the menisci are intact.

Routine knee radiographs are usually negative. However, the presence of an avulsed fleck of bone adjacent to the lateral tibial articular surface on the anteroposterior view is highly suggestive of a torn anterior cruciate ligament and lateral capsular structures (Fig. 2).

Examination under anesthesia plus arthroscopy provides the most useful additional information for an accurate diagnosis of the underlying pathology in this type of knee injury. Approximately 75 percent of patients with acute traumatic hemarthrosis are found to have disruption of the anterior cruciate ligament. Two-thirds of these patients also have a torn meniscus, and one-fifth have a chondral fracture or surface defect.

NATURAL HISTORY AND BIOMECHANICS: Excessive anterior displacement of the tibia in relation to the femur can disrupt the anterior cruciate ligament. Loss of the anterior cruciate ligament allows the tibia to subluxate anteriorly. This results in an instability which is clinically manifested when changing direction during walking, running, or jumping especially with unexpected deceleration or twisting motion. The classic description is a "giving way" of the knee with pivoting motion. The athlete has a "trick knee" and a predictable instability.

Anterolateral rotatory instability (ALRI) is the term describing the knee that has a torn anterior cruciate ligament and exhibits a positive anterior drawer sign at 25 degrees flexion and a positive pivot shift. This term was chosen because there is excess anterior rotatory motion of the lateral tibial plateau in relation to the femur. There is some question whether the tibia does rotate significantly in the pivot shift. It is probable that the entire tibia subluxates forward in relation to the femur; however, greater excursion is apparent in the lateral compartment because of the small, round configuration of the lateral femoral condyle compared to the large, long, biconcave medial femoral condyle. However, excess rotation of the tibia in relation to the femur has been measured at 5 and 15 degrees flexion in knees with anterolateral instability.

The clinical test that reproduces the phenomenon of "giving way" is called the *pivot shift* phenomenon because of the patient's description that something is felt to "shift" in the knee when pivoting. There are a variety of ways to elicit the pivot shift phenomenon: the jerk test, ALRI test, flexion-rotation drawer test, and others. They all test the same phenomenon. A basic difference between the tests is whether or not the tibia is held internally rotated during the procedure. The test is more sensitive if the tibia is held in neutral or external rotation when the tibia is loaded and allowed to flex and extend. The pivot shift test and anterior drawer test carried out at 25 degrees flexion (Lachman) are not inherently dissimilar but, rather, are different manifestations of the same phenomenon, i.e., anterior subluxation of the tibia.

The knee with anterolateral instability tends to be injured frequently with activities requiring the pivoting motion. As the tibia subluxates forward under load, the menisci become trapped between the tibial and femoral condyles. The resultant shearing force can produce a vertical longitudinal tear in the posterior one-third of the medial and/or lateral meniscus (Fig. 3). The shearing force can also produce a chondral fracture, especially to the weight-bearing portion of the medial femoral condyle. After the meniscus tears, symptoms, such as popping, locking, swelling, and pain, can be present, in addition to that of giving way. Signs and symptoms of secondary joint pathology should be separated from those of the primary instability so treatment can be directed appropriately.

The anterior cruciate ligament is the primary ligamentous restraint preventing anterior subluxation of the tibia. The capsule, menisci, collateral ligaments, iliotibial tract, and bony contour are secondary restraints. A tear of the anterior cruciate ligament almost always results in some

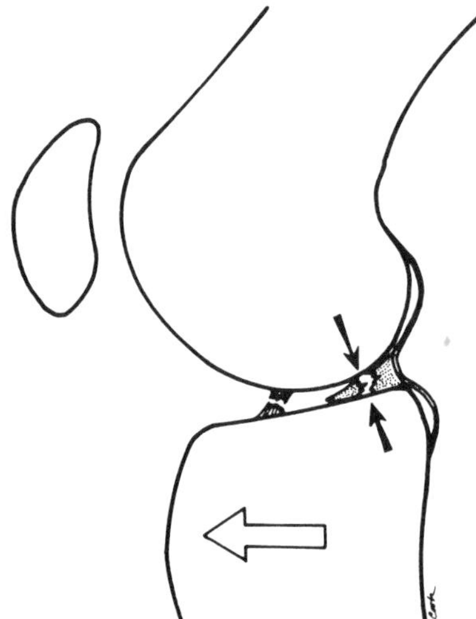

Figure 3: Forces involved in producing a vertical longitudinal tear of the posterior portion of the meniscus. The tibia subluxates forward tearing the anterior cruciate ligament. The meniscus is trapped between the femoral and tibial condyles and tears.

degree of ALRI. Experimental work on cadavers shows that division of the anterior cruciate ligament alone is sufficient to produce a positive pivot shift and anterior drawer test at 25 degrees flexion. Sequential division of additional capsular structures increases the instability. Therefore, if the knee has tight secondary restraints, the degree of instability will be mild, and the knee may function normally. If the secondary restraints are very lax, the knee will probably have marked anterolateral instability and resultant symptoms of giving way.

Laxity of secondary restraints can result from the initial knee injury, from reinjury, or can be physiologic as in loose-jointed individuals. This evidence correlates with the operative findings of no gross evidence of medial or lateral capsular injury in some knees that have complete disruption of the anterior cruciate ligament and have acute ALRI. On the other hand, a knee with a torn anterior cruciate ligament can be found to have a torn medial and/or lateral capsule but no disruption of the collateral ligaments. The explanation probably lies in the different degrees of importance of the anterior cruciate ligament to the stability of different knees and the relative contributions of secondary soft tissue restraints and bony configuration to the stability of an individual knee.

The knee with 1+ or 2+ ALRI frequently has no functional instability and a negative jerk test. The knee with a 3+ or 4+ pivot shift (i.e., moderate to severe ALRI) usually has a positive jerk test and functional instability.

Removing a torn meniscus can correct the symptoms resulting from the meniscal injury but usually does not improve the symptom of giving way, which is the result of the anterolateral instability. In fact, the symptoms of instability can be worsened by meniscectomy. Cadaver studies show that medial meniscectomy alone has no effect on anteroposterior motion. However, if the anterior cruciate ligament is cut and medial meniscectomy is then performed, anterior displacement significantly increases over that evident with anterior cruciate ligament cutting alone.

The disability resulting from a torn anterior cruciate ligament is related directly to the degree of ALRI, i.e., the severity of the pivot shift. Up to one-third of patients with a torn anterior cruciate ligament have a mild (1+) pivot shift phenomenon with minimal or no disability. Approximately one-third have moderate instability and are able to continue athletic activities but have frequent reinjuries and resultant meniscal injury. The final one-third have a marked pivot shift (3-4+) and are disabled in activities requiring pivoting.

TREATMENT OF ACUTE "ISOLATED" ANTERIOR CRUCIATE LIGAMENT TEAR: The young active patient who has an acute knee injury and resultant hemarthrosis usually should have examination under anesthesia and often arthroscopy. This is the best way to determine the nature of the intra-articular pathology and the degree of instability.

The role of primary repair of the "isolated" torn anterior cruciate ligament is controversial. The current consensus is that primary repair of the ligament alone is inadequate to stabilize a knee with significant anterolateral instability. Knees exhibiting torn anterior cruciate ligaments that do well after primary repair are probably those with mild instability which do equally well without surgery. If a young athletic patient sustains a torn anterior cruciate ligament and has marked ALRI, primary anterior cruciate ligament repair should be augmented with a transfer of tissue such as semitendinosus tendon, iliotibial tract, or a portion of the extensor mechanism as is done in intra-articular reconstructive procedures for chronic instability.

TREATMENT OF CHRONIC ANTEROLATERAL ROTATORY INSTABILITY: The treatment of this instability should be directed toward elimination of the pivot shift phenomenon. Symptoms of giving way directly correlate with the amount of pivot shift. Improvement following surgical reconstruction of the instability is related directly to reducing or eliminating the pivot shift phenomenon.

There are two broad categories of reconstructive procedures for ALRI: *intra-articular* transfers to replace the torn anterior cruciate ligament and *extra-articular* procedures to tighten lateral secondary restraints to prevent anterior subluxation of the lateral tibial plateau.

Intra-articular transfers commonly in use include transfer of a portion of the extensor mechanism (quadriceps tendon-patella-patellar tendon), semitendinosus tendon, or a portion of the iliotibial tract. A vascular pedicle attached to the transfer has been advocated, as well as covering the transferred tissue with a portion of the fat pad.

An intra-articular reconstructive procedure alone often is not adequate for severe anterolateral instability since secondary capsular structures are lax. Furthermore, tension studies show the transplant is weaker than a normal anterior cruciate ligament regardless of its source.

There are two different methods of routing intra-articular transfers for femoral attachment: *over-the-top* of the lateral femoral condyle or through a *drill hole* in the lateral femoral condyle. With the over-the-top method, the transfer courses across the knee joint, out of the joint through a posterior capsulotomy, and across the superior aspect of the rounded femoral condyle posteriorly. The over-the-top route has the advantages of easy, consistent placement near the anatomic attachment of the anterior cruciate ligament and a smooth surface. The arc of motion between the anterior cruciate ligament and femur is approximately 90 degrees compared to approximately 25 degrees between anterior cruciate ligament and tibia during full knee range of motion. Location of the tibial drill hole is less critical than placement of the femoral attachment.

Extra-articular reconstructive procedures create a restraining band extending from the lateral femoral epicondyle to Gerdy's tubercle in a line parallel to the intra-articular course of the anterior cruciate ligament. Extra-articular procedures avoid the problem of lack of vascularity to the intra-articular section of the transfer. Most extra-articular reconstructive procedures use variations of the iliotibial tract connecting the lateral epicondyle to Gerdy's tubercle. There is a trend toward *combining* intra-articular and extra-articular reconstructive procedures to improve results.

The validity of the concept of "dynamic" transfers to stabilize a knee with torn ligaments never has been proved scientifically and is open to question. The speed with which injury occurs is far greater than the ability of the reflex arc to protect the knee by active muscular contraction. Furthermore, the transfer of a muscle or

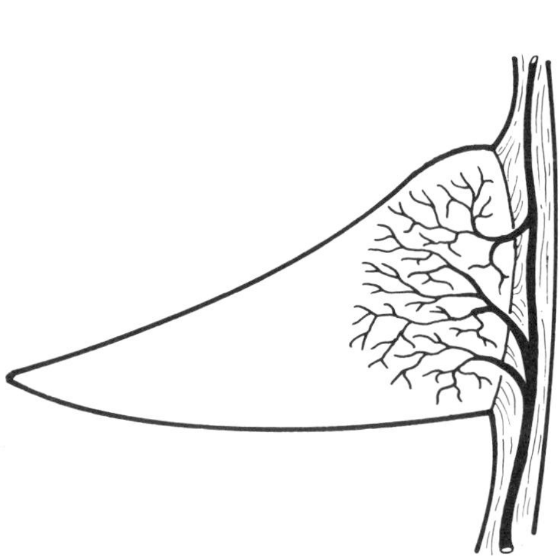

Figure 4: Vascular pattern in peripheral 10-30 percent of meniscus. This part of the meniscus has healing potential when repaired.

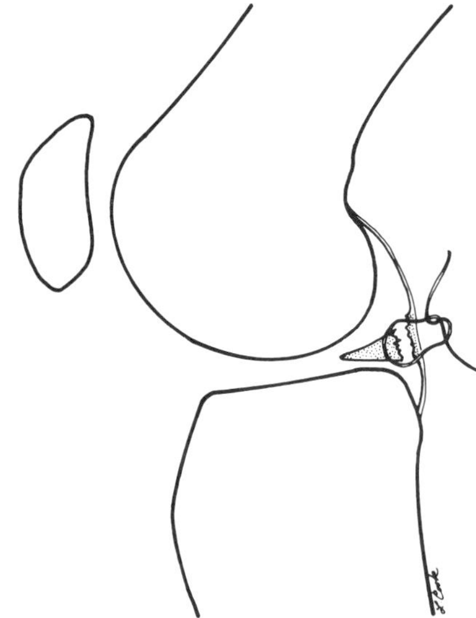

Figure 5: Method of meniscus repair. The suture penetrates the posterior capsule from the outside, passes through the peripheral edge of the meniscus, and exits through the posterior capsule. The knot is tied outside the capsule.

tendon usually weakens its strength by one grade. Critical analysis of the long-term results of pes anserinus transfer is not favorable. Thus, surgery for knee instability should be directed toward static stabilization.

In *postoperative treatment regimens* following knee ligament reconstruction, there is a trend toward early but limited knee motion. This can be accomplished safely following most types of surgery as early as 1 week by applying a functional brace that allows motion from 45 degrees to 90 degrees. If the collateral ligaments are intact, a simpler knee orthosis incorporating a posterior strap to limit extension or a dial-lock side hinge can be used. Strain is applied to the repair in most types of anterior cruciate ligament reconstruction procedures by extending the knee past 20 degrees flexion but not with valgus or varus stress. The goal of therapy is to regain full knee extension by not earlier than 6 months following surgery.

The emphasis placed on quadriceps strengthening exercises in the early postoperative period following anterior cruciate ligament reconstruction now is being questioned. The quadriceps muscles apply tension to the anterior cruciate ligament, especially as the knee extends, and could be disruptive to repair. Progressive resistive quadriceps exercises with the knee in flexion should not be instituted until approximately 6 months following surgery. By this time, the collagen of the repair has had more time to mature, and the knee has gained almost full range of motion. Delaying the use of resistive exercises also may decrease the incidence of postoperative chondromalacia of the patella.

Menisci The medial and lateral menisci play an important role in weight-bearing and joint stabilization and should be preserved whenever possible. A meniscus never should be sacrificed to achieve better capsular repair. Knee disability, instability, and progressive degenerative changes are directly related to loss of menisci.

ASSOCIATION WITH INSTABILITY: A vertical longitudinal tear of the posterior portion of a meniscus is caused by the meniscus being compressed between the femur and tibia. This can occur when the tibia subluxates forward under load, as in the pivot shift. With a displaced bucket handle tear of a meniscus, the torn inner section of meniscus remains displaced forward of the femoral condyle when the knee reduces. Most circumferential meniscal tears, including bucket handle tears, are associated with a torn anterior cruciate ligament. When removing a torn medial or lateral meniscus in the knee with anterolateral instability, it should be recognized that the instability will not be improved and, in fact, might be aggravated. However, symptoms of pain or locking caused by the torn meniscus may be relieved.

HEALING POTENTIAL OF MENISCI AND REPAIR: The peripheral 10-30 percent of the medial meniscus are vascularized and have the potential to heal if repaired (Fig. 4). The peripheral one-third of the lateral meniscus with the exception of a 2 cm distance at the posterolateral one-third (at the location of the popliteus tendon) has the same vascularity and healing potential.

Vertical longitudinal meniscal tears located in the peripheral one-fourth of the meniscus or at the meniscosynovial junction should be repaired by open suturing (Fig. 5). If the knee also has significant anterolateral instability (a common combination), the instability should

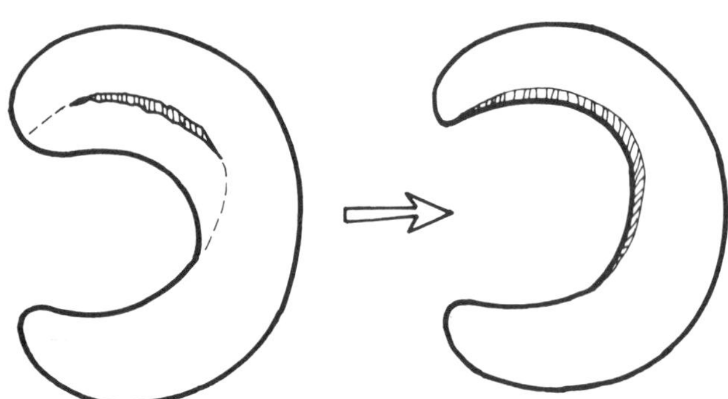

Figure 6: Vertical longitudinal meniscal tear treated by partial meniscectomy (dotted line) leaving a stable, symmetric meniscal rim.

be repaired to prevent subsequent reinjury of the meniscus.

PARTIAL MENISCECTOMY: Meniscal tears usually cause symptoms by becoming trapped between the femur and tibia during activity. The pain comes from traction on the remainder of the meniscus by the displaced fragment. Removal of the unstable portion of the meniscus usually relieves symptoms. For this reason, resection of the unstable portion of meniscus alone should be carried out, and the entire meniscus should not be sacrificed unless torn. A stable, symmetric "balanced" rim of meniscus should be left after partial meniscectomy (Fig. 6).

Degenerative Meniscal Tears As articular cartilage in the weight-bearing portion of the joint undergoes progressive wear and narrowing with age and use, the joint space narrows and pseudoligamentous laxity follows. The result is an increased shear on the menisci during knee motion.

Partial meniscectomy of degenerative meniscal tears gives good results if symptoms are due to mechanical causes, such as from an unstable meniscal piece. Results are not always predictable, however, and symptoms may, in fact, increase following meniscectomy. Regardless of whether the meniscectomy is done with arthroscopy or by open means, recovery time is much longer for knees with degenerative changes than those with nondegenerative tears. Disability lasting several months postoperatively is common.

Medial Collateral Ligament The medial collateral ligament usually tears as the result of a *contact* injury in which force is applied to the lateral or posterolateral aspect of the slightly flexed knee. If the knee has no effusion and is stable to anteroposterior stress on examination, the anterior cruciate ligament is probably not torn. The treatment for an "isolated" injury to the medial collateral ligament differs from that for the more extensive knee injury in which the anterior cruciate ligament is also injured.

Many "isolated" tears of the tibial collateral ligament can be treated nonoperatively. The results obtained using early motion are as good as those following operative repair. The knee should not be immobilized in a plaster cast but rather should be splinted for a few days or weeks until acute pain subsides at which time it can be replaced with a knee orthosis having side-hinges to prevent extremes of motion and valgus stress.

If the anterior cruciate ligament is injured in addition to tearing of medial capsular and collateral ligaments, the knee will usually have an effusion, positive anterior drawer sign at 25 degrees flexion, and a positive pivot shift, as well as instability on valgus stress. These injuries usually necessitate surgical repair.

Arthroscopy is usually not indicated for this type of injury for three reasons: excess extravasation of irrigation fluid into the extra-articular tissues occurs through the torn capsule; there is increased risk of infection during subsequent operative repair; and the intra-articular pathology will be identified when the knee is opened to repair the torn ligaments. It may be useful, however, to perform limited arthroscopy of the lateral compartment because there is a high incidence of torn lateral meniscus with this type of knee injury, and it is difficult to examine adequately the posterior portion of the lateral meniscus through a medial arthrotomy. Strict asepsis prior to medial arthrotomy must be maintained.

A single contrast knee *arthrogram* in the operating room just prior to making the incision helps to show the location of capsular tears. After sterile preparation and draping, 12 ml of Renografin mixed with 20 ml of saline is injected into the knee. An Esmarch bandage is wrapped around the knee at the joint line only, and the knee flexed to express intra-articular fluid through any synovial or capsular tears. A single large anteroposterior radiograph confirms the location of medial tears and often discloses unsuspected lateral tears.

A torn anterior cruciate ligament repaired at the same time as a medial collateral ligament should be augmented (reinforced) with a transferred semitendinosus tendon or iliotibial tract. A torn meniscus should be repaired whenever possible. Partial, rather than total, meniscectomy should be performed, leaving as much meniscus as possible to maintain a symmetric, balanced, stable meniscus rim.

A limited motion, functional brace (45 to 90 degrees flexion) applied at 1 week following surgery allows for joint motion in isometric range without stressing the repair. This avoids problems associated with prolonged or rigid immobilization. This postoperative regimen also minimizes the postoperative complication of joint stiffness and eliminates the necessity of joint manipulation to regain motion.

Posterior Cruciate Ligament A tear of the posterior cruciate ligament alone can occur from a dashboard injury or a fall on a flexed knee. The pathognomonic sign is a positive posterior drawer sign at 90 degrees of flexion or posterior "sag" of the tibia.

The role of primary repair of this tear without other associated ligamentous injury is controversial because of the technical difficulty in repairing the torn ligament and the poor results of primary repair. Therefore, the tendency is to treat this injury nonoperatively unless there is a flake of bone visible on a lateral radiograph, indicating an avulsion injury.

The functional impairment of a knee with a torn posterior cruciate ligament is *disability* whereas that of a knee with a torn anterior cruciate ligament is *instability*. The amount of disability a knee with a torn posterior cruciate ligament will have is difficult to predict since some knees function very well. Knees with posterior tibial subluxation appear to develop a higher incidence of patellofemoral symptoms because of the posterior displacement of the tibia, resulting in increased patellofemoral contact force. Meniscal tears are not as common with posterior cruciate ligament injury as with a torn anterior cruciate ligament.

A totally satisfactory reconstructive procedure to correct chronic posterior knee instability has not been described. Reconstructive procedures currently in use include medial head of gastrocnemius origin transfer with or without a femoral bone block. In this procedure, the transfer is moved forward between the femoral condyles into the intercondylar area to a new location near the femoral attachment of posterior cruciate ligament. There are problems with this transfer: difficulty in obtaining adequate length; the relative weakness of this transfer in relation to the normal strength of the posterior cruciate ligament; and the high failure rate. If the procedure is successful in holding the tibia forward (which is uncommon), it probably does so by scarring rather than by "dynamic" action.

Another reconstructive procedure used is transfer of both the semitendinosus and gracilis tendons. The tendons are divided at the musculotendinous junction and passed upward through a drill hole in the tibia to exit at the posterior tibia just below joint line in the midline. The transfers are then brought anteriorly through the intercondylar notch and through a drill hole in the medial femoral condyle where they are fixed to bone near the medial epicondyle. Transfer of a free graft taken from the extensor mechanism has also recently been advocated.

The knee with a torn posterior cruciate ligament that also has a torn anterior cruciate ligament and other major capsular and collateral ligaments injuries requires primary surgical repair. During surgery the tibiofemoral joint should be transfixed with a large smooth Steinmann pin through nonweight-bearing surfaces to hold the knee reduced. Otherwise, it may not be possible to hold the tibia in the proper relation to the femur postoperatively. The cast used following posterior cruciate ligament repair should be applied with the knee in 20 degrees flexion to help prevent posterior tibial subluxation.

As with augmentation of primary repairs of the anterior cruciate ligament, repair of the posterior cruciate ligament should be reinforced with a pedicle graft such as semitendinosus and/or gracilis tendon transfer.

Patella

Patellar Tendinitis (Jumper's Knee) This is an extremely common condition in athletes and is easily confused with chondromalacia of the patella. The lesion most commonly is located on the posterior surface of the patellar tendon origin from the inferior pole of the patella (Fig. 7).

Treatment of patellar tendinitis is usually nonoperative, including rest and avoidance of excess jumping or running with a toe-toe gait, application of ice, and use of oral anti-inflammatory medication. Injection of steroids into the area of maximum tenderness should be avoided because of its weakening effect on collagen and risk of subsequent patellar tendon rupture. Surgical excision of the involved portion of the patellar tendon and repair of the defect usually have favorable results in patients who do not respond to nonoperative treatment.

Chondromalacia of the Patella The etiology of this disease process is unknown. It may be due to trauma and/or mechanical overload due to malalignment of the extensor mechanism. It tends to be a self-limited process with a high incidence in young females and is usually not progressive.

Chondromalacia of the patella still is best treated nonoperatively in most patients. This program includes avoidance of activities that cause increased patellofemoral compression, isometric quadriceps exercises in extension, and oral anti-inflammatory medication. The early enthusiasm for the benefits of lateral retinacular release for chondromalacia is not substantiated in long-term studies.

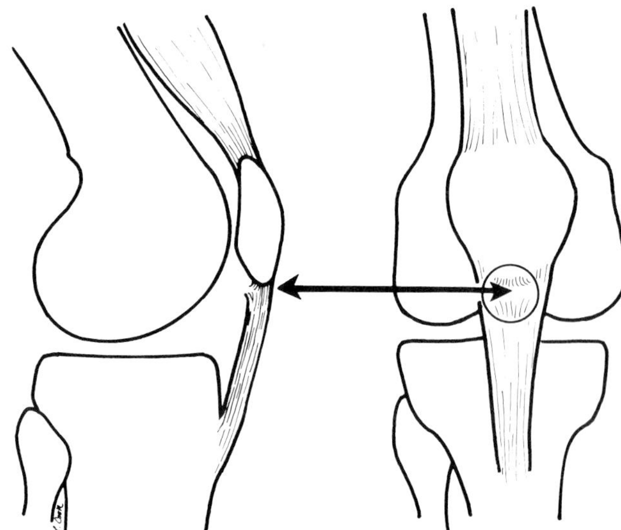

Figure 7: Location of pathology in patellar tendinitis at posterior aspect of patellar tendon origin from inferior pole of patella.

Lateral release occasionally is indicated for severe malalignment in which there is lateral patellar tilt with a tight lateral patelloepicondylar ligament (Fig. 8).

Anterior transposition of the tibial tubercle (Maquet procedure) has been shown experimentally to decrease patellofemoral compression force. The procedure is useful in eliminating patellofemoral pain in some patients with chondromalacia, but the role of this procedure in the treatment of patellofemoral disorders still awaits the results of long-term studies. The occasional complications of skin slough or sensitivity in the tibial tubercle region and tibial compartment syndrome detract from the more widespread use of this procedure.

Patellar debridement ("shaving") using arthroscopic means has recently been advocated for the treatment of chondromalacia of the patella. Short-term improvement has been reported following removal of fibrillated articular cartilage, although long-term results are unknown.

Subluxation and Dislocation In patients with recurrent patellar subluxation or dislocation requiring surgery, lateral retinacular release is usually the procedure of choice. The release can be performed percutaneously or under arthroscopic visualization. Lateral release alone is sufficient in approximately one-half of patients with patellar instability. The remaining patients who continue to have symptomatic patellar instability following lateral release

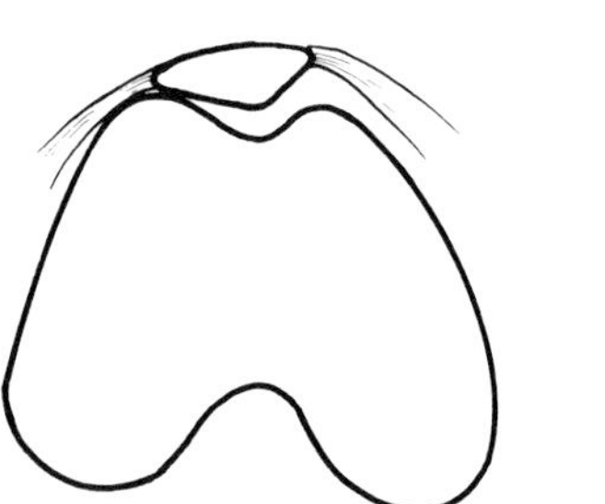

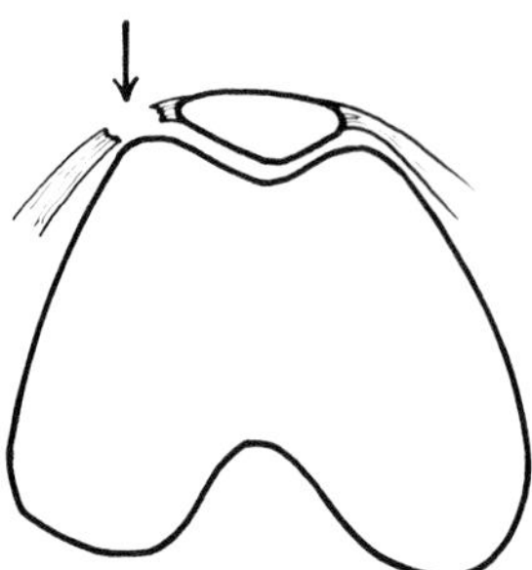

Figure 8: Lateral retinacular release for recurrent patellar instability. It is usually not successful for chondromalacia unless major malalignment exists.

can be treated with a formal proximal and/or distal extensor mechanism realignment as a second procedure. The use of the Hauser procedure that includes *distal* transfer of the patellar tendon insertion has a high incidence of complications and poor results.

Arthroscopy Diagnostic arthroscopy has become an important tool in the evaluation of internal knee derangements, allowing clear visualization of almost the entire interior of the knee. Most knee pathology with the exception of instability and severe joint degeneration or destruction now can be treated using arthroscopic surgical methods.

The single puncture method, with the arthroscope introduced through an anterolateral portal located near the inferior pole of the patella, has evolved into the standard approach for diagnostic arthroscopy. A 5 mm diameter arthroscope having 30 degree obliquity of the viewing angle is the instrument most commonly used. Ringer's lactate is more physiologic than saline for joint irrigation during arthroscopy. The use of a probe introduced from an anteromedial portal improves diagnostic accuracy by allowing palpation of intra-articular structures while viewing through the arthroscope. The method of triangulation has become standard as the best operative arthroscopic technique and has now replaced the operating arthroscope (Fig. 9).

In the treatment of meniscal lesions, partial arthroscopic meniscectomy is shown to have distinct advantages over standard knee arthrotomy and total meniscectomy. The short-term advantages of decreased morbidity and complications using arthroscopic means as well as the long-term advantages of partial over total meniscectomy appear to be withstanding critical analysis.

Arthroscopic treatment of patellar disorders remains controversial. The role of patellar debridement is questioned: although short-term improvements may be obtained with arthroscopic debridement of fragmented patellar articular cartilage, long-term advantages have not been demonstrated. Likewise, arthroscopic debridement of degenerative knee conditions is advocated; however, as yet there is no evidence of its long-term benefits.

Arthroscopy is not without complications. Infection or damage of articular surfaces from instrumentation may occur.

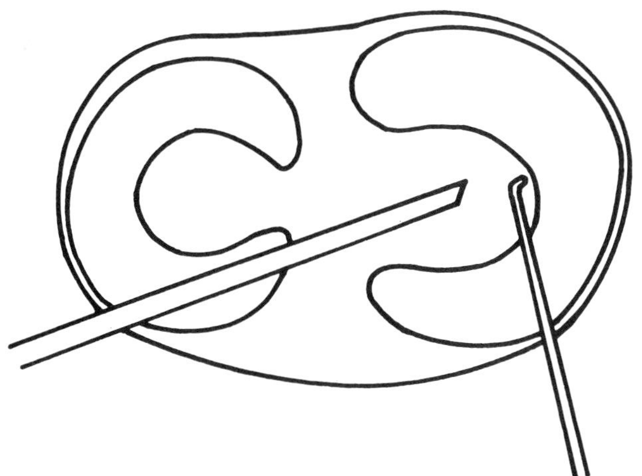

Figure 9: View of top of tibia and menisci showing technique of triangulation used for arthroscopic surgery.

Leg

The deleterious effects of *immobilization*, which include muscle atrophy and loss of strength in ligaments and tendons, are becoming better understood. Immobilization of uninvolved joints should be avoided whenever possible. The use of a limited motion functional brace or knee orthosis may avoid problems secondary to immobilization of a joint.

Electrical muscle stimulation is being considered as an adjunctive treatment of high performance athletes in whom prevention of disuse atrophy is important. Ongoing experimentation centers on the use of high voltage and high frequency electrical currents not only to retard atrophy but also to build muscle strength.

The significance of *eccentric* muscle contraction in normal function, in the causation of muscle strains, and in postinjury rehabilitation is now regarded as more important than previously believed. This muscle contraction involves elongation of the muscle while it is activated and generating tension.

Chronic exertional *compartment syndromes* are responsible for many chronic "shin splints." Symptoms are manifested as pain over the anterior or lateral leg after exercise. Tissue pressure measurements confirm excessive elevation of pressure within the compartment during exercise and prolonged delay of return to normal pressure in these patients. Treatment consists of fasciotomy with good results in properly selected patients. Chronic compartment syndromes of the leg should be differentiated from stress fractures and other causes of chronic leg pain in runners.

Rupture of the *plantaris* muscle or tendon had been believed to be the underlying pathology in calf muscle strains, but it is now suspected that this syndrome represents a rupture of the insertion of the medial head of the gastrocnemius into the common gastrocnemius-soleus tendon. Attention is directed toward the higher incidence of muscle strains in general, and hamstring strains in particular, in muscles with a higher percentage of type II or fast-twitch muscle fiber types.

ANNOTATED BIBLIOGRAPHY

Knee

Anterior Cruciate Ligament

Chick, R.R., and Jackson, D.W.: Tears of the anterior cruciate ligament in young athletes. J. Bone Joint Surg. 60A:970-973, 1978.

Thirty patients are followed 2.6 years after meniscectomy and surgically proven anterior cruciate deficiency. A negative pivot shift is present in all patients examined without anesthesia preoperatively. Eighty-three percent return to full activities with only six patients progressing to moderate instability with a positive pivot shift.

Clancy, W.G., Jr.; Narechania, R.G.; Rosenberg, T.D.; Gmeiner, J.G.; Wisnefske, D.D.; and Lange, T.A.: Anterior and posterior cruciate ligament reconstruction in rhesus monkeys. J. Bone Joint Surg. 63A:1270-1284, 1981.

Of twenty-nine rhesus monkeys with nineteen anterior cruciate and ten posterior cruciate ligament reconstructions using medial one-third patellar tendon, all are revascularized by 8 weeks. At 1 year the anterior cruciate ligament graft retains 80 percent and the posterior cruciate ligament 71 percent of the pretransfer tension strength. At 1 year the anterior cruciate ligament graft is equivalent to 52 percent of a normal anterior cruciate ligament while the posterior cruciate ligament graft is equivalent to 50 percent of a normal posterior cruciate ligament tension strength.

DeHaven, K.E.: Diagnosis of acute knee injuries with hemarthrosis. Am. J. Sports Med. 8:9-14, 1980.

Of 113 knees evaluated, none had demonstrable clinical laxity, but 90 percent were found to have a lesion of surgical significance. The incidence of anterior cruciate ligament tear was 72 percent with 70 percent of these knees also having a meniscal tear. Only 15 percent of knees had a meniscal tear without a torn anterior cruciate ligament.

Fetto, J.F., and Marshall, J.L.: Injury to the anterior cruciate ligament producing the pivot-shift sign. J. Bone Joint Surg. 61A:710-714, 1979.

The pathomechanics necessary to produce the pivot shift sign in 25 cadavers are studied. Thirty-three of the thirty-seven knees with a cut anterior cruciate ligament demonstrate a positive pivot shift. Cutting the iliotibial band, lateral collateral ligament, and popliteus tendon results in a positive pivot shift in only one of the nine knees, but if the anterior cruciate ligament is also cut, the pivot shift is enhanced.

Freeman, B.L., III; Beaty, J.H.; and Hayes, D.B.: The pes anserinus transfer. J. Bone Joint Surg. 64A:202-207, 1982.

This procedure is performed in forty-eight patients (fifty knees) with an average follow-up of 9 years. There is a high incidence of anteromedial and anterolateral instability with only 38 percent of patients having no limitation of function.

McDaniel, W.J., Jr., and Dameron, T.B., Jr.: Untreated ruptures of the anterior cruciate ligament. J. Bone Joint Surg. 62A:696-705, 1980.

In an average 10-year follow-up of fifty patients with surgically verified ruptures of the anterior cruciate ligament, there is a high incidence of instability with only eight of fifty-two patients with both menisci intact. Seventy-two percent of patients return to strenuous sports, and 47 percent believe they have no restrictions.

Noyes, F.R.; Bassett, R.W.; Grood, E.S.; and Butler, D.L.: Arthroscopy in acute traumatic hemarthrosis of the knee. Incidence of anterior cruciate tears and other injuries. J. Bone Joint Surg. 62A:687-695, 1980.

All eighty-five knees have negligible instability on initial examination. Further evaluation reveals a 72 percent incidence of anterior cruciate ligament disruption, a 62 percent incidence of a meniscal tear, and a 20 percent incidence of a chondral fracture or surface defect associated with a torn anterior cruciate ligament.

Woods, G.W.; Stanley, R.F.; and Tullos, H.S.: Lateral capsular sign: X-ray clue to a significant knee instability. Am. J. Sports Med. 7:27-33, 1979.

Four patients demonstrate fleck of bone near the tibial articular surface of lateral tibial plateau on anteroposterior radiograph. At surgery, all four patients have disruption of middle one-third of the lateral capsule and torn anterior cruciate ligament. These patients also have a tear in middle one-third of medial capsule.

Biomechanics

Butler, D.L.; Noyes, F.R.; and Grood, E.S.: Ligamentous restraints to arterior-posterior drawer in the human knee. J. Bone Joint Surg. 62A:259-270, 1980.

Fourteen cadaver knees in an Instron testing system are described. The anterior cruciate ligament supplies an average 86 percent of the total resisting force to anterior drawer. The posterior cruciate ligament supplies a mean 95 percent of restraining force to posterior drawer.

Fukubayaski, T.; Torzilli, P.A.; Sherman, M.F.; and Warren, R.F.: An in vitro biomechanical evaluation of anterior-posterior motion of the knee: Tibial displacement, rotation, and torque. J. Bone Joint Surg. 64A:258-264, 1982.

Nine cadaver knees in a designed apparatus are evaluated. In the intact knee anterior force produces internal tibial rotation which disappears with cutting anterior cruciate ligament. Posterior force produces external rotation which disappears with cutting of the posterior cruciate ligament.

Levy, I.M.; Torzilli, P.A.; and Warren, R.F.: The effect of medial meniscectomy on anterior-posterior motion of the knee. J. Bone Joint Surg. 64A:883-888, 1982.

Nine cadaver knees studied on an in vitro knee testing device revealed medial meniscectomy has no effect on anteroposterior motion. Anterior cruciate ligament cutting significantly increases anterior displacement which is further significantly increased with medial meniscectomy.

Zarins, B.; Rowe, C.R.; Harris, B.A.; and Watkins, M.P.: Rotational motion of the knee. Am. J. Sports Med. 3:152-156, 1983.

Passive range of rotational motion in the knee was measured to be approximately 70 degrees total rotation in positions of 30 to 90 degrees flexion. At 5 degrees flexion, total range of rotation was 33 degrees. Knees with torn anterior cruciate ligaments had 58 degrees rotational motion at 5 degrees flexion (significant increase) but normal rotation at angles greater than 30 degrees flexion.

Rehabilitation

Haggmark, T., and Eriksson, E.: Cylinder or mobile cast brace after knee ligament surgery. Am. J. Sports Med. 7:48-56, 1979.

Sixteen patients are treated postoperatively with 1 week in dorsal splint and 4 weeks in either cast brace or cylinder cast. Eight cast brace patients have no significant change in cross-sectional areas of type I or type II muscle fibers or in succinate dehydrogenase (SDH) activity in vastus lateralis. Eight cylinder cast patients have significant atrophy of type I muscle fibers and a significant reduction of SDH.

Paulos, L.; Noyes, F.R.; Grood, E.S.; and Butler, D.L.: Knee rehabilitation after anterior cruciate ligament reconstruction and repair. Am. J. Sports Med. 8:140-149, 1981.

This is a comparison and description of a rehabilitation program with a survey of forty knee experts. The survey reveals 38 percent recommend early motion at a mean starting time of 3.1 weeks postsurgery. The majority wants maximum range of motion by 6 months. The mean time to return to full activities is 9.4 months with a wide range.

Meniscus

Arnoczky, S.P., and Warren, R.F.: Microvasculature of the human meniscus. Am. J. Sports Med. 10:90-95, 1982.

An investigation of the microvascular anatomy of menisci from twenty cadaver knees demonstrates a perimeniscal capillary plexus supplies the peripheral 10 to 30 percent of the meniscus. No penetrating vessels are present in the posterolateral aspects of the lateral meniscus adjacent to the popliteus tendon.

Cassidy, R.E., and Shaffer, A.J.: Repair of peripheral meniscus tears. Am. J. Sports Med. 9:209-214, 1981.

Twenty-nine repairs of peripheral one-third meniscal tears are reported with no confirmed retears. Postoperative arthrograms in four patients show complete healing. Two repairs directly visualized are healed.

Hargreaves, D.J., and Seedhom, B.B.: On the bucket handle tear: Partial or total meniscectomy? A quantitative study. *In* Proceedings of the British Orthopaedic Research Society. J. Bone Joint Surg. 61B:381, 1979.

Load transmission of the meniscus in six cadaver knees using a four-spring model of the knee is studied. Load transmission is reduced from 85 percent to 35 percent for medial meniscus and from 75 to 50 percent for lateral meniscus after partial meniscectomy. The average stress in the area of direct contact doubles after partial meniscectomy but quadruples after total meniscectomy.

Jackson, R.W., and Rouse, D.W.: The results of partial arthroscopic meniscectomy in patients over 40 years of age. J. Bone Joint Surg. 64B:481-485, 1982.

The procedure is performed on 73 knees with 95 percent of patients having good or excellent results if no degenerative joint changes present. If degenerative changes are present, the results are 80 percent good or excellent but some patients having prolonged recovery periods. Patient age has no effect on result.

Noble, J., and Erat, K.: In defence of the meniscus: A prospective study of 200 meniscectomy patients. J. Bone Joint Surg. 62B:7-11, 1980.

Meniscal symptoms in 50 of 250 patients (20 percent) subside and surgery is deferred. At arthrotomy in the remaining 200 patients, no tear could be found in fifty-four (27 percent) patients.

Medial Collateral Ligament

Derscheid, G.L., and Garrick, J.G.: Medial collateral ligament injuries in football. Nonoperative management of grade I and grade II sprains. Am. J. Sports Med. 9:365-368, 1981.

Fifty-one grade I and II sprains are treated with active rehabilitation programs involving partial or no immobilization. The average time to return to unprotected participation is 10.6 days and 19.5 days in grade I and II injuries respectively with no appreciable increased likelihood of reinjury.

Hastings, D.E.: The non-operative management of collateral ligament injuries of the knee joint. Clin. Orthop. 147:22-28, 1980.

Twenty-six medial and four lateral isolated collateral ligament injuries are considered. The first seventeen patients are treated with cast for 2 weeks, then functional brace for 4 weeks. Only one patient does not return to full activities. No subsequent operations are required, and there is no apparent difference between the two groups in regard to stability.

Posterior Cruciate Ligament

Hughston, J.C.; Bowden, J.A.; Andrews, J.R.; and Norwood, L.A.: Acute tears of the posterior cruciate ligament: Results of operative treatment. J. Bone Joint Surg. 62A:438-450, 1980.

Of thirty-two acute posterior cruciate repairs, twenty are evaluated 5 to 16 years after operation. The results are good in thirteen, fair in four, and poor in three.

Patella

Ferguson, A.B., Jr.: Elevation of the insertion of the patellar ligament for patellofemoral pain. J. Bone Joint Surg. 64A:766-771, 1982.

One hundred eighty-four patients undergo modified Maquet procedure with a transverse incision and 1.25 cm elevation of the patellar ligament insertion. Eighty-five percent satisfactory results are reported with only one superficial wound infection. Fifty percent require over 4 months before symptoms decrease enough to return to full activities.

Ferguson, A.B., Jr.; Brown, T.D.; Fu, F.H.; and Rutkowski, R.: Relief of patellofemoral contact stress by anterior displacement of the tibial tubercle. J. Bone Joint Surg. 61A:159-166, 1979.

Tibial tubercle elevation of 1.3 cm in eight amputated lower limbs results in a 57 percent reduction in contact stress. Elevation to 2.5 and 3.8 cm produce additional decreases of 30 percent and 6 percent respectively.

Osborne, A.H., and Fulford, P.C.: Lateral release for chondromalacia patella. J. Bone Joint Surg. 64B:202-205, 1982.

In seventy-five patients, 87 percent achieve good results in grade I and II chondromalacia at 1 year. Results deteriorate to 37 percent by 3 years. Only 20 percent of patients with grade III and IV chondromalacia have good results at 1 year.

Patellar Tendinitis

Bassett, F.H.; Soucacos, P.N.; and Carr, W.A.: Jumper's knee: Patellar tendinitis and patellar tendon rupture. *In* AAOS Symposium on the Athlete's Knee, p. 96-106. St. Louis, C.V. Mosby, 1980.

Fifty-two patients after failure of nonoperative treatment undergo excision of the scar of granulation tissue in the patellar tendon under local anesthesia. Forty-two patients have complete relief of symptoms while eight patients require a second operation and only one patient has no relief.

Roels, J.; Martens, M.; Mulier, J.C.; and Burssens, A.: Patellar tendinitis (jumper's knee). Am. J. Sports Med. 6:362-368, 1978.

Thirty-six patients are separated into phase 1, 2, or 3 depending upon degree of symptoms. Treated nonoperatively, six of seven patients in phase 1 or 2 have good results, while only nine of sixteen in phase 3 have good results. In surgical group (resection of necrotic segment), all phase 3, ten of ten have very good or good results.

Leg

Butler, D.L.; Grood, E.S.; and Noyes, F.R.: Biomechanics of ligaments and tendons. Factors influencing tissue properties. Exercise and Sports Science Review 6:162-165, 1978.

Rhesus monkeys, immobilized for 8 weeks in either whole body or cylinder casts, are tested after 0, 5, or 12 months reconditioning. Stiffness decreases by 31 percent and returns to 93 percent of control value by 5 months. Maximum load at failure and energy absorbed to failure decreases by 39 percent and 32 percent respectively, returns to about 80 percent at 5 months, and shows no statistical differences from control values at 12 months.

Eriksson, E., and Haggmark, T.: Comparison of isometric muscle training and electrical stimulation supplementing isometric muscle training in the recovery after major ligament surgery. Am. J. Sports Med. 7:169-171, 1979.

Of eight patients having anterior cruciate ligament reconstruction, four are treated with plaster cast and isometric muscle exercises alone, and four also have percutaneous electrical stimulation. Clinically, the electrically stimulated group has better muscle function and less atrophy. Muscle biopsies done preoperatively, 1, and 5 weeks postsurgery show significantly higher levels of succinate dehydrogenase activity in the stimulated group.

Mubarak, S., and Hargens, A.: Exertional compartment syndrome. *In* AAOS Symposium, The Foot and Leg in Running Sports, pp. 141-159. St. Louis, C.V. Mosby, 1982.

The anterior exertional compartment syndrome is secondary to elevated intramuscular pressure for several possible causes. Acute exertional compartment syndromes are uncommon with fewer than 100 patients documented. In chronic exertional compartment syndrome, there is pain over the anterior or lateral compartment after exercise (75 percent bilaterally) with occasional hypesthesia on the dorsum of the foot. Resting compartment pressure is usually greater than 15 mm Hg, increases to about 75 mm Hg during exercise, and remains greater than 30 mm Hg for a minimum of 5 minutes. Following fasciotomy through a 5 cm skin incision, compartment pressures become essentially normal.

Severance, H.W., Jr., and Bassett, F.H., III: Rupture of the plantaris. Does it exist? J. Bone Joint Surg. 64A:1387-1388, 1982.

The literature dating back to the 1700s on the original description of the plantaris tendon rupture is reviewed. No autopsy or surgical evidence supports this diagnosis. The condition "plantaris rupture" probably does not exist but, in reality, is a rupture of all or part of the gastrocnemius muscle or tendon.

36 KNEE AND LEG: TRAUMA (BONE)

Topics covered in this section are fractures of the supra- and intercondylar regions of the femur, patella, tibial plateau, tibial shaft, and nonunion of fractures of the tibial diaphysis, as well as compartment syndrome associated with tibial fractures.

Knee

Supracondylar and Intercondylar Fractures of the Femur Supracondylar fractures are those involving the distal 9 cm of the femur, measured proximally from the articular surface of the femoral condyle. Intra-articular condylar fractures often are associated with a supracondylar fracture. There are several classifications for these injuries, and all are based upon the degree of comminution and the extent of the articular fracture (Fig. 1). These fractures may be difficult to manage due to marked comminution and/or displacement and articular surface involvement. Muscular forces acting about the fracture can impede the achievement and preservation of reduction. Restriction of knee motion is often a sequela of these injuries.

TREATMENT: Minimally displaced stable fractures can be managed with closed reduction and immobilization in a long-leg plaster or a functional brace. Closed reduction and skeletal traction with a proximal tibial pin, occasionally combined with a traction pin through the distal femoral fragment, has been employed with varying degrees of success. There is renewed interest in open reduction and rigid internal fixation of these injuries. Several studies show improved results with these methods. If accurate reduction and rigid fixation can be attained, followed by early knee motion, success is achieved in most patients. The most common cause of failure is incomplete reduction and stabilization of the fracture. Infection remains a potential complication.

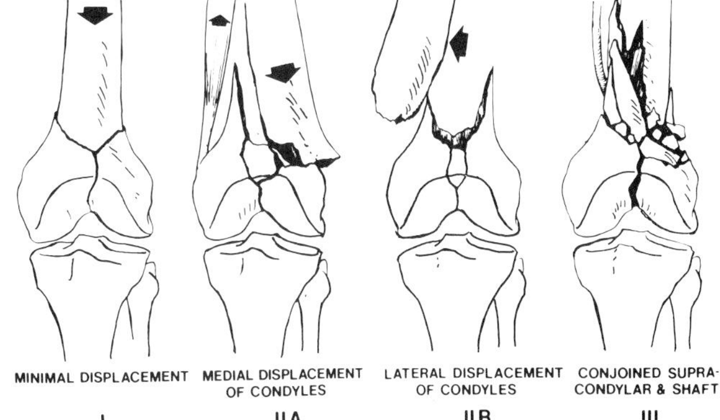

Figure 1: Anatomic classification of supracondylar fractures of the adult femur as proposed by Neer. Group I fractures occur in osteoporotic bone, are impacted or minimally displaced, spare the extensor mechanism, are never open, and unite rapidly. Group II-A fractures result from an anterolateral force on the flexed knee, lacerate the extensor tendon, and when open are associated with an anterolateral wound. Group II-B fractures are produced by violent trauma on the lateral side of the extended thigh, spare the quadriceps tendon, and when open are associated with a medial wound. Group III fractures result from extreme violence on the flexed knee. (Reprinted with permission from Supracondylar fracture of the adult femur, by Neer, et al., J. Bone Joint Surg. 49A:591-613, 1967, and from Surgical treatment of displaced comminuted fractures of the distal end of the femur, by R.D. Mize, et al., J. Bone Joint Surg. 64A:872, 1982.)

Patellar Fractures The functions of the patella are to increase the mechanical advantage of the quadriceps tendon, to aid in the nourishment of the articular surface of the femur, and to protect the femoral condyles from injury. Fractures of the patella constitute about 1 percent of all skeletal injuries, occur more frequently in males (2:1), and can occur in all age groups but more commonly between the ages of 40 and 50 years.

TREATMENT: Fractures of the patella with less than 2 mm of displacement and an intact quadriceps mechanism can be managed with early weight-bearing in a cylinder plaster for 3 to 6 weeks. Transverse fractures with more than 2 mm of displacement and disruption of the lateral expansion of the quadriceps mechanism are best treated with open reduction and tension band wires with two Kirschner wires introduced vertically across the fracture and a wire loop passed behind the tips of the wires and over the anterior surface of the patella (Fig. 2). Accurate repair of the patellar retinaculum also should be undertaken. Early postoperative motion can be allowed with this method of fixation.

Comminuted displaced fractures of the patella are best treated surgically. Partial patellectomy with repair of the patellar tendon or quadriceps insertion generally is successful provided that at least one-half of the gliding surface of the patella is intact. Complete patellectomy may be required when there is extensive comminution and displacement of the fracture fragments. There should be careful attention to operative repair when performing a total patellectomy to prevent loss of strength of the quadriceps mechanism and extension lag.

Fractures of the Tibial Plateau Vehicular accidents and falls cause most tibial plateau fractures. The normal knee is in slight valgus, and usually the lateral plateau of the tibia is split or crushed by the lateral femoral condyle. Fractures of the medial condyle are less common because falls usually impose a valgus stress on the knee joint. The bone usually gives way before excessive stress is placed on

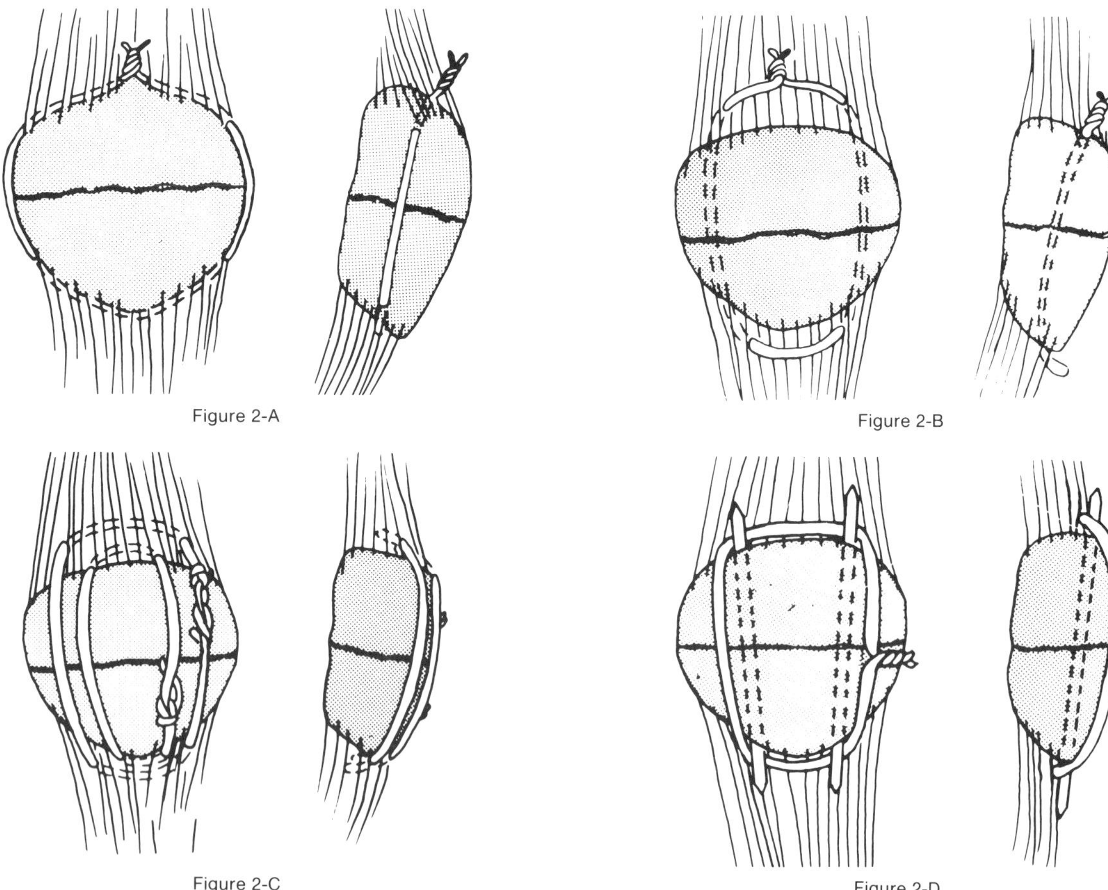

Figure 2: Four wiring techniques used to repair transverse patellar fractures of twenty-five fresh cadaver knees mounted in machines capable of measuring quadriceps force, flexion angle, and fracture separation simultaneously. (A) Circumferential; (B) Magnuson; (C) Standard tension band; (D) Modified tension band, the only technique in which there was no measurable separation of the fragments throughout a complete range of motion of the knees. (Reprinted with permission from Efficacy of various forms of fixation of transverse fractures of the patella, by M.J. Weber, et al., J. Bone Joint Surg. 62A:217, 1980.)

the ligaments, but concomitant injuries to the medial knee ligaments are estimated to occur in 10 to 30 percent of patients. Arterial and nerve complications are rare but may be overlooked without careful evaluation. To visualize the extent of comminution and displacement, anteroposterior and lateral radiographs are necessary. Tomograms particularly help in assessing the extent of depression of the articular fragments. CT scans soon may replace tomography since assessment of the location of the fractures and the degree of depression is more accurate. Stress films under anesthesia are useful, and if the medial joint space opens more than 1 cm, significant ligamentous injury is present. If operative repair of tibial plateau fractures is undertaken, careful planning of the surgical approach and handling of the soft tissue are essential. Knee stiffness frequently develops following surgery, and prolonged rehabilitation is often necessary. Late traumatic arthritic changes may develop.

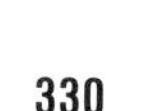

CLASSIFICATION AND TREATMENT: Type I is the pure cleavage fracture (Fig. 3A). The lateral femoral condyle is driven into the articular surface of the tibia creating a typical wedge-shaped fragment that is split off and displaced outward and downward. If the displacement can be reduced, these fractures may be treated with either cast immobilization or open reduction and internal fixation with equally good results.

Type II is cleavage combined with depression (Fig. 3B). A lateral wedge is split as in Type I, but also varying portions of the remaining lateral tibial plateau and articular surface are comminuted and depressed downward into the metaphysis. It is believed by some that if there is less than 1 cm depression, especially if the posterior aspect of the tibial plateau is involved, these fractures can be treated with closed reduction with the knee manipulated in varus and immobilized in plaster for 4 to 5 weeks with the knee in extension. But, if the depression is more than 1 cm, especially if in the anterior tibial plateau in a young patient, the procedure of choice is open reduction and internal fixation with a buttress plate and cancellous screws with supplemental bone grafts placed under the elevated tibial plateau fracture.

Type III is the pure central depression (Fig. 3C). The articular surface of the lateral tibial plateau is depressed and driven into the lateral tibial condyle. There is no lateral wedge and the lateral cortex is intact. This fracture, seen in older osteoporotic patients, is commonly due to simple falls with pure axial loading of the plateau. If the depression is less than 1 cm and the knee is stable on examination under anesthesia, these injuries can be treated with cast immobilization. If depression is greater than 1 cm, especially in young patients, or if significant valgus instability exists on examination, surgical treatment is recommended. Elevation and packing of bone graft beneath the elevated fragments should be done. Fixation

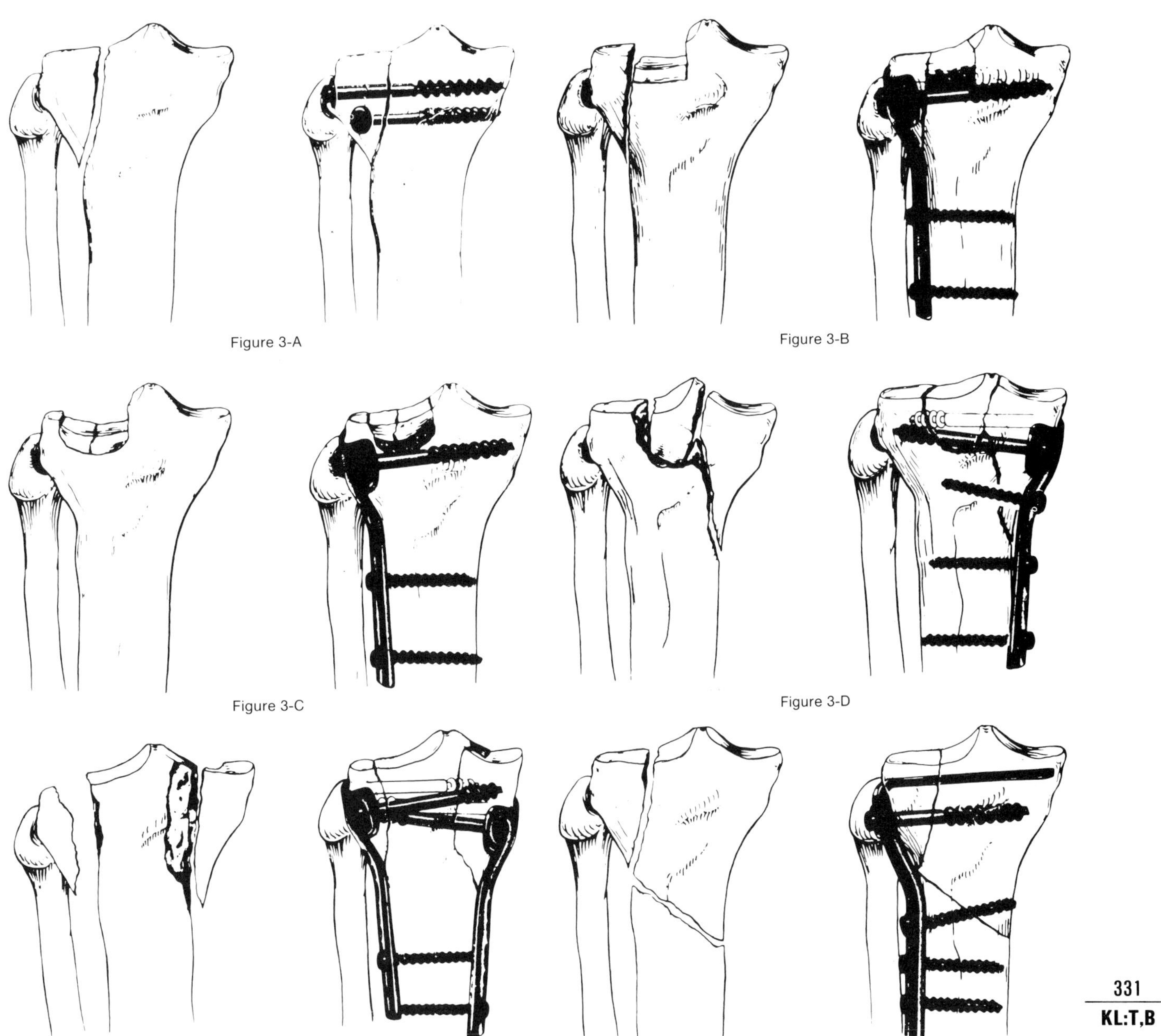

Figure 3: Classification of tibial plateau fractures. (A) Type I: Pure cleavage fracture. (B) Type II: Cleavage combined with depression. Reduction requires elevation of fragments with bone grafting of the resultant hole in the metaphysis. The lateral wedge is lagged on the lateral cortex and protected with a buttress plate. (C) Type III: Pure central depression. There is no lateral wedge. The depression may also be anterior or involve the whole plateau. After elevation of the depression and bone grafting, the lateral cortex is best protected with a buttress plate. (D) Type IV: Fracture of the medial plateau. The medial condyle is either split off as a wedge or it may be crumbled, depressed, and comminuted. There is often associated fracture of the tibial spines. (E) Type V: Pure bicondylar or inverted Y-fracture. Note the continuity of the metaphysis and diaphysis. Both sides must be protected with buttress plates. (F) Type VI: Tibial plateau fracture with dissociation of the tibial metaphysis and diaphysis. The essence of this fracture is the fracture line which dissociates the metaphysis from the diaphysis. The fracture pattern is variable, and all types can occur. If both condyles are involved, the proximal tibia should be buttressed on both sides. (Reprinted with permission from The tibial plateau fracture, by J. Schatzker, et al., Clin. Orthop. 138:94-104, 1979.)

with lag screws and/or buttress plate is also advocated.

Type IV is a fracture of the medial plateau (Fig. 3D). There are two distinct types. There is the pure cleavage fracture of the medial tibial plateau which occurs in younger people with severe trauma. If these are undisplaced, they may be treated with a long-leg plaster for 4 to 6 weeks. If they are displaced more than 2 mm, they should be reduced and internally fixed with cancellous screws. There also is a depression fracture of the medial tibial plateau. These fractures usually occur in older people as a result of minor trauma and carry a guarded prognosis. They often have associated injury to the anterior cruciate ligament complex. They are best managed with open reduction, elevation of the depressed plateau, and bone grafting and internal fixation with a buttress plate. If there is anterior cruciate instability or if anterior cruciate ligament reconstruction has been carried out, a functional brace with a stop should be used postoperatively to allow early restricted knee motion and protection to the ligamentous repair.

Type V is a pure bicondylar or inverted Y-fracture (Fig. 3E). This is a rare fracture pattern. Although closed reduction and traction through a distal tibial pin have been suggested for treatment, results have been less than satisfactory in many series. This is due to the inability to control varus and valgus angulation and the fact that these are high-velocity injuries with significant soft-tissue injury and subsequent fracture instability. Utilization of medial and lateral buttress plates after accurate open reduction and supplemental bone grafting yield superior results as compared with closed methods.

Type VI is a tibial plateau fracture with dissociation of the tibial metaphysis and diaphysis (Fig. 3F). The essence of this fracture is the transverse or oblique fracture of the proximal tibia. This makes it unsuitable for any type of traction. Despite marked displacement and instability, surgical elevation of the fracture, the addition of supporting bone graft, and fixation with long buttress plates can achieve good results.

Tibia

Tibial Shaft Fractures The tibia is the most frequently fractured long bone. Although union is generally rapid in children, there is a significant incidence of complications including delayed union, malunion, nonunion, and infection in adults. The single most important factor causing delayed healing is the extent of initial fracture displacement. A fractured tibia with major initial displacement greater than the diameter of its shaft has an incidence of delayed union (i.e., greater than 20 weeks) of 50 percent. For a fracture to undergo this degree of displacement, much energy must be expended with associated major soft-tissue and bone damage. Open wounds and comminution have a similar, but less pronounced, effect on bone healing. Tibial fractures with minimal displacement, usually resulting from indirect violence and low-energy trauma, heal more rapidly. The fracture sites most associated with delay in healing are the middle third and the junction between the middle and proximal thirds. This is because direct trauma most often is applied to the bone at these levels. The widely held belief that fractures in the distal third heal more slowly has not been substantiated. However, healing in malalignment is more common in this location. There is no conclusive evidence to prove that an intact fibula delays healing. In fact, the reverse may be true.

Classification: Open fractures are classified into three categories according to the extent of associated soft-tissue damage. Grade I fractures have skin perforation from the inside (usually caused by indirect violence). Grade II includes those with skin contusion or perforation from outside (usually caused by direct violence). Grade III are those with laceration of the skin and soft tissues with or without damage to blood vessels and/or nerves (caused by direct, high-energy violence).

Treatment: Most stable, closed, low-energy fractures are treated successfully with closed reduction and plaster immobilization with or without early weight-bearing in a long-leg plaster cast, a below-knee functional cast, or a functional brace. Recent studies show that loss of bone mineral from the upper ends of the tibia and fibula does not differ for patients with tibial shaft fractures allowed weight-bearing in a functional below-knee brace and those treated with a long-leg plaster cast without weight-bearing. Also, by using load cells placed under the heel, there is no difference between the forces transmitted by the same subject wearing a below-knee functional cast, a conventional below-knee cast, or an above-knee cast. Consequently, casts must be chosen for other reasons (e.g., maintenance of knee motion).

There are few well-controlled, randomized studies comparing open plate fixation with closed reduction and plaster immobilization for treatment of closed, stable tibial shaft fractures. One study indicates that open reduction and internal fixation resulted in faster healing, less ankle joint restriction, and earlier return to normal activities. This is true even when additional temporary disability accompanying removal of the implant is taken into consideration. Conversely, the factors of operating time and duration of hospitalization favor the nonsurgical method. The most important difference between the two methods of treatment is the infection rate, virtually nil in the nonsurgical group and between 0 and 15 percent in the group treated by open reduction and plate fixation. Another study indicates that with closed functional bracing the nonunion rate was less than 1 percent with 92 percent of the fractures healing with less than 1 cm shortening and 96 percent with angular deformity less than 10 degrees (Fig. 4).

The management of open (grade II and grade III) tibial fractures can be difficult. The extent of soft-tissue damage in these patients is as or more important than the injury to the underlying osseous tissue. External fixation is increasingly used with these injuries (Fig. 5). Anatomical reduction and stabilization can be accomplished with such devices. This allows access to the site of the soft-tissue damage for necessary dressing, local debridement, and coverage procedures. Significant advances have been made recently in the treatment of major soft-tissue defects following severe trauma. Muscle and musculocutaneous flaps are being used to cover these large defects. Initial reports are encouraging.

With the use of external fixators under both bending and torsional loads, rigidity is greatly increased when compression can be applied to the fracture site. The bone-pin interface is the least rigid link in the entire structure, particularly in the anteroposterior bending mode. Rigidity of the external fixator can be improved

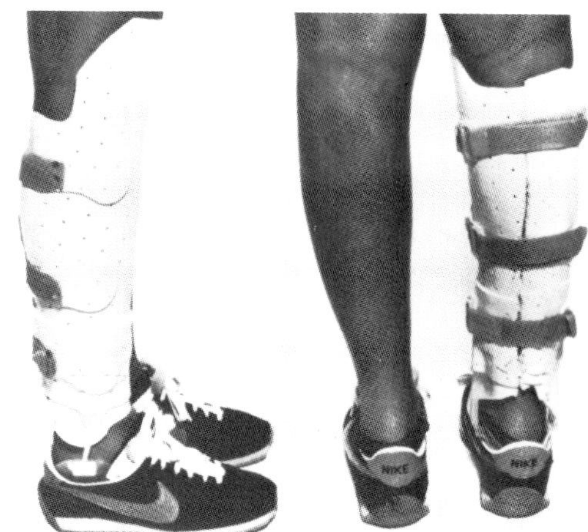

Figure 4: Prefabricated functional brace for tibia fractures. (Reprinted with permission from Closed Functional Treatment of Fractures, by A. Sarmiento, et al., pp. 95, New York, Springer-Verlag, 1981.)

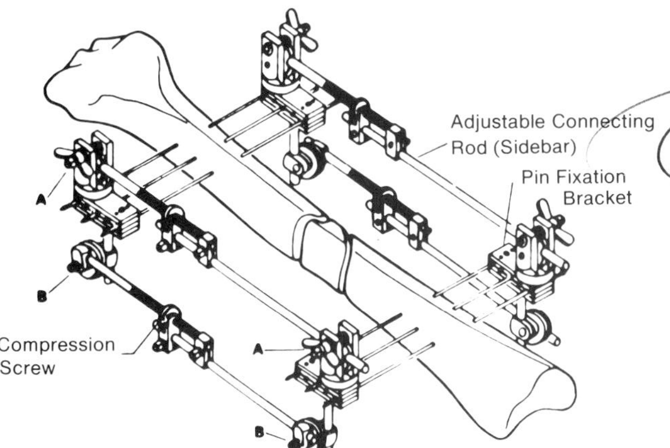

Figure 5: The standard Hoffman-Vidal quadrilateral apparatus for tibial application. (A) The universal ball-joint. (B) The articulation coupling. (Reprinted with permission from The mechanical performance of the standard Hoffmann-Vidal external fixation apparatus, by B.T. Briggs, et al., J. Bone Joint Surg. 64A:567, 1982.)

substantially by increasing the number of pins, using fullthreaded pins with large diameters, decreasing the side connecting rod distances, and increasing the pin separation distance in each pin group.

There are some disadvantages of bilateral external fixation frames when applied to the tibia, namely the possibility of injury to the neurovascular structures and transfixion of the ankle dorsiflexors and possibly the peroneii while inserting the pins. To prevent the transfixion of musculotendinous units and to reduce the risk of neurovascular injury, the use of two-plane unilateral frames has been advocated (Fig. 6). These half-frames can be modified by the addition of pins and rods to provide improved two-plane rigidity and accommodate particular mechanical and clinical needs.

In most reports of open fractures treated by plate fixation, there has been a higher incidence of deep sepsis and delayed healing than in those managed by closed reduction and external fixation. The use of intramedullary fixation of unstable tibial fractures has been advocated. However, to obtain good stability with this method requires reaming of the medullary canal to insert a nail large enough to obtain torsional and bending stability. This affects the healing potential of the endosteum. Intramedullary fixation with small flexible wires does not provide rigid fixation and often requires a supplemental cast to maintain reduction.

Nonunion of Tibial Diaphyseal Fractures Nonunion is that condition existing in a fractured bone in which the effective reparative processes have ceased, and bone continuity has not been restored. The extent of the initial fracture displacement, comminution, soft-tissue damage or interposition, and infection increase the incidence of nonunion.

TREATMENT: Many methods of treatment of nonunions of the tibia have been advocated. When the fibula remains intact or fractures but heals prior to the tibia, it may prevent effective compression at the tibial fracture site. In this situation, partial fibulectomy and controlled weight-bearing in a well-molded plaster cast are reported to result in union in nearly 77 percent of patients. Hypertrophic, reactive nonunions often unite once stabilized by intramedullary nailing or compression plating without excision of the interposed pseudarthrosis tissue, bone grafting, or postoperative cast immobilization.

Treatment of established nonunions of the tibia with electricity, using invasive, semi-invasive, and noninvasive (electromagnetic pulsing field) methods reportedly yields approximately the same overall success rate of 80 to 85 percent. All three methods require application of the principles of good fracture treatment. The mechanism by which electricity induces osteogenesis is largely unknown. But, it is known that when a cathode is used, there is oxygen consumption and the production of hydroxyl radicals (OH). Thus, the local oxygen tension is lowered, and the local tissue pH is raised in the vicinity of the cathode. Low oxygen tension is believed to promote bone formation. The rather high pH (7.70 ± 0.05) of the growth

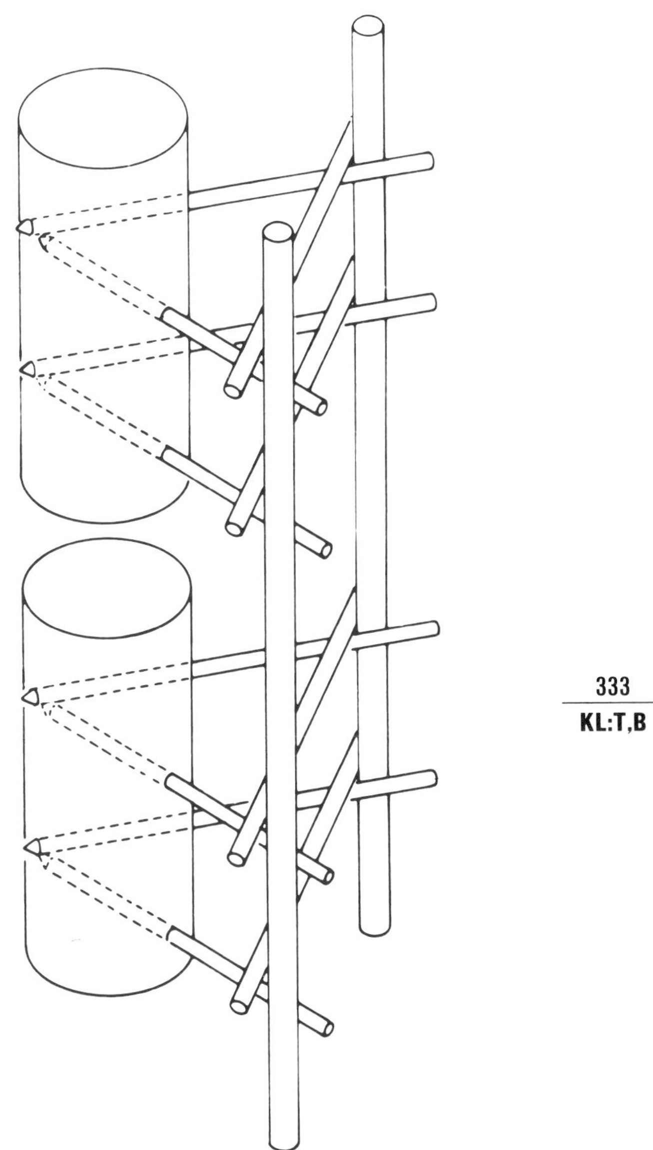

Figure 6: Diagram of a two-plane unilateral frame. Altered pin and rod arrangements permit the construction of many different unilateral frames. (Reprinted with permission from Unilateral external fixation for severe lower extremity lesions: Experience with the ASIF (AO) tubular frame, by F. Behrens. Edited by D. Seligson and M. Pope. *In* Concepts in External Fixation, pp. 279-291, New York, Grune and Stratton, 1982.)

plate at the calcifying front suggests that an alkaline environment is favorable to calcification.

Electricity also may act directly on bone and cartilage cells. Such an effect may activate the cyclic AMP system of the cell which, in turn, may activate various enzyme systems within the cell to trigger its specific physiologic response.

Electricity is not successful when there is an established fluid-filled pseudarthrosis at the fracture site or there is a nonunion in which the fracture gap is greater than one-half the diameter of the bone. The presence of metal at the fracture site does not interfere with semi-invasive or invasive systems. It may interfere with the noninvasive system if the metal is highly magnetic. The presence of active draining infection contraindicates usage of invasive and semi-invasive but not the noninvasive system.

In tibial nonunions with extensive soft-tissue damage anteriorly, segmental bone loss, and active infection in the anterior compartment, cancellous bone grafting from the posterior lateral approach is an effective method of obtaining fracture stability by creating a tibiofibular synostosis. In most patients once a stable tibiofibular synostosis is created above and below the fracture site, the tibial fracture unites, and drainage, if present, diminishes or ceases.

Compartment Syndromes Associated with Tibial Fractures One inevitable consequence of tibial fractures (open as well as closed) is increase in tissue pressure in the closed fascial compartments of the leg. If intracompartmental tissue pressure exceeds capillary pressure, there will be no tissue perfusion which causes ischemia and muscle anoxia and ultimately may result in necrosis of all elements in the involved compartment. The diagnosis of compartment syndrome usually can be made clinically with these findings: (1) local pain disproportional to the injury; (2) palpably swollen muscle compartments; (3) pain on passive stretching of the involved muscles; (4) diminished simple touch perception; (5) decreased strength of the involved compartmental muscles; and (6) hypesthesias or anesthesia in the sensory distribution of nerves in the involved compartment. Distal pulses usually are palpable unless there is associated vascular injury.

Several investigators recommend the measurement of intracompartmental pressures either by infusion or Wick catheter technique to determine when a compartmental syndrome is imminent so a decompression fasciotomy can be performed. However, there is no consensus on the exact tissue pressure above which a compartmental syndrome occurs. Some advocate fasciotomy if the intracompartmental pressure is above 30 mm Hg, but others do not until it reaches 50 mm Hg. Compartmental pressure measurements are particularly useful when assessing an unreliable, uncooperative, or unresponsive patient or one with a fracture associated with contusion and nerve deficit in which there are difficulties in eliciting or interpreting clinical findings. The treatment of compartment syndromes is complete fasciotomy of all the involved compartments. This should be performed with dispatch because the warm ischemia time is 6 hours, after which there is irreversible muscle necrosis. In the leg the preferred method is release of all four compartments through a single posterolateral parafibular incision or combined medial and lateral incisions. Because of problems with possible injury to the peroneal and/or posterior tibial artery and loss of fracture stability, fibulectomy has lost favor as a method of decompression. The presence of an intact fibula may be necessary for later posterolateral bone grafting, and the fibula should not be sacrificed.

ANNOTATED BIBLIOGRAPHY

Knee

Supracondylar and Intercondylar Fractures of the Femur

Giles, J.B.; DeLee, J.C.; Heckman, J.D.; and Keever, J.E.: Supracondylar-intercondylar fractures of the femur treated with a supracondylar plate and lag screw. J. Bone Joint Surg. 64A:864-870, 1982.

Of twenty-six patients with supracondylar intercondylar fractures of the femur treated with a supracondylar plate and lag screw to achieve two-plane fixation, all fractures were united in an average of 4 months with an average range of knee motion of 120 degrees. There were no infections.

Mize, R.D.; Bucholz, R.W.; and Grogan, D.P.: Surgical treatment of displaced, comminuted fractures of the distal end of the femur: An extensile approach. J. Bone Joint Surg. 64A:871-879, 1982.

Excellent or good results were achieved in twenty-four of thirty limbs with severely displaced comminuted supracondylar and intercondylar fractures of the femur stabilized with ASIF techniques. An extensile surgical approach with elevation of the tibial tuberosity was successfully utilized to facilitate the exposure of multiplanar intra-articular fractures in eight patients.

Schatzker, J., and Lambert, D.C.: Supracondylar fractures of the femur. Clin. Orthop. 138:77-83, 1979.

Eighteen patients with internal fixation of supracondylar femur fractures that failed to obtain a satisfactory result were analyzed. The most common causes of failure using this method were incomplete reduction of the fracture, failure to achieve interfragmental compression, and failure to use autogenous cancellous bone graft to fill defects associated with comminuted fractures.

Patellar Fractures

Böstman, O.; Kiviluoto, O.; and Nirhamo, J.: Comminuted displaced fractures of the patella. Injury 13:196-202, 1981.

In this retrospective analysis of sixty-four comminuted displaced fractures of the patella, the results of anterior tension band wire fixation were acceptable even in severe comminuted fractures. Partial excision showed satisfactory results provided that at least three-fifths of the patella could be preserved.

Haajanen, J., and Karaharju, E.: Fractures of the patella: One hundred consecutive cases. Ann. Chir. et Gynaec. Fenniae 70:32-35, 1981.

Based on the results of treatment of 100 consecutive patella fractures, partial excision of the patella was the best procedure for comminuted fractures in which at least one-half of the patella's gliding surface was intact. Tension band wiring fixation was effective in dealing with transverse fractures but not with comminuted fractures.

Weber, M.J.; Janecki, C.J.; McLeod, P.; Nelson, C.L.; and Thompson, J.A.: Efficacy of various forms of fixation of transverse fractures of the patella. J. Bone Joint Surg. 62A:215-220, 1980.

The patellae of twenty-five fresh cadaver knees were fractured transversely after the knees were mounted in machines capable of measuring quadriceps force, flexion angle, and fracture separation simultaneously. The fractures were fixed using techniques of circumferential wiring, tension band wiring, Magnuson wiring, and modification of tension band wiring. Fracture separation was less in those patellae fixed with modified tension band wiring (which consisted of a wire loop passed behind two Kirschner wires which had been introduced vertically across the fracture).

Fractures of the Tibial Plateau

Burri, C.; Bartzke, G.; Coldewey, J.; and Muggler, E.: Fractures of the tibial plateau. Clin. Orthop. 138:84-93, 1979.

In a collective review of the German study group of 342 patients with displaced tibial plateau fractures treated surgically, 278 were available for evaluation at an average of 32 months postoperatively. Good results were obtained when accurate reduction and internal fixation with a buttress plate was accomplished, and supplemental bone grafting employed.

Schatzker, J.; McBroom, R.; and Bruce, D.: The tibial plateau fracture: The Toronto experience, 1968-1975. Clin. Orthop. 138:94-104, 1979.

Ninety-four patients with fractures of the tibial plateau were evaluated at an average follow-up of 28 months. Stable fractures with minimal displacement did not require surgery. Displaced fractures required anatomic reduction, autogenous cancellous bone grafting, fixation of the fracture with cancellous screws, and buttressing of the cortex to prevent collapse.

Waddell, J.P.; Johnston, D.W.; and Neidre, A.: Fractures of the tibial plateau: A review of ninety-five patients and comparison of treatment methods. J. Trauma 21(5):376-381, 1981.

In ninety-five patients with tibial plateau fractures, adequacy of reduction was as important as early motion in obtaining a satisfactory result regardless of the type of fracture treated. Tibial plateau fractures with depressions or widening of less than 1 cm did well when treated nonoperatively. If open reduction was undertaken, both internal fixation and bone grafting were required to obtain optimal results.

Tibia

Tibial Shaft Fractures

Allum, R.L., and Mowbray, M.A.S.: A retrospective review of the healing of fractures of the shaft of the tibia with special reference to the mechanism of injury. Injury 11:304-308, 1980.

A retrospective study of 500 fractures of the tibia confirmed Nicoll's finding (1964) that major initial displacement is the most potent single cause of poor bone healing. Compounding and comminution have a similar but less pronounced effect on bone healing.

Austin, R.T.: The Sarmiento tibial plaster: A prospective study of 145 fractures. Injury 13:10-22, 1981.

Of 145 tibial fractures seen between 1973 and 1979, 132 were treated with Sarmiento below-knee functional casts (PTB). In 116 fractures, the cast was applied within 4 weeks of injury. All but one fracture united. The maximum angular deformity was 14 degrees, and 96 percent of the fractures healed with deformity less than 10 degrees. The maximal shortening was 2.8 cm, and 99 percent had less than 2 cm whereas 92 percent had less than 1 cm of shortening.

Batten, R.L.; Donaldson, L.J.; and Aldridge, M.J.: Experience with the AO method in the treatment of 142 cases of fresh fracture of the tibial shaft treated in the UK. Injury 10:108-114, 1978.

A prospective study was carried out in 142 fresh fractures of the tibial shaft treated by internal fixation according to AO principles. Ninety-five fractures were closed and forty-three open. In patients with closed fractures the minor infection rate (erythema and increased local temperature) was 4.1 percent, and major infection (pus present) was 4.1 percent. In open fractures, the overall infection rate was 14 percent with 7 percent being major.

Briggs, B.T., and Chao, E.Y.S.: The mechanical performance of the standard Hoffman-Vidal external fixation apparatus. J. Bone Joint Surg. 64A:566-573, 1982.

A standard Hoffman-Vidal quadrilateral fixation system for tibial fractures was analyzed using different geometric and material variations of the basic configuration. The results show that the bone-pin interface is the least stiff link in the entire structure, particularly in the anteroposterior bending mode. Under both bending and torsional loads, the stiffness values are greatly increased when compression occurs at the fracture site. Rigidity of the device can be substantially improved by increasing the number of pins, using fullthreaded pins with a large diameter, decreasing side connecting rod distance, and increasing pin separation distances in each group.

Hasenhuttl, K.: The treatment of unstable fractures of the tibia and fibula with flexible medullary wires: A review of 235 fractures. J. Bone Joint Surg. 63A:921-931, 1981.

A retrospective study of 235 closed and open unstable fractures of the tibia treated with flexible intramedullary wires was carried out. Primary healing of soft tissues and bone occurred in 99 percent of the closed fractures and 65.7 percent of the open fractures.

Lawyer, R.B., Jr., and Lubbers, L.M.: Use of the Hoffman apparatus in the treatment of unstable tibial fractures. J. Bone Joint Surg. 62A:1264-1273, 1980.

The Hoffman apparatus was employed in the treatment of thirty-four complex tibial fractures considered to have a poor prognosis with conventional forms of treatment. All fractures united within an average of 5.8 months. This time seems directly related to the accuracy of reduction.

Van Der Linden, W., and Larsson, K.: Plate fixation versus conservative treatment of tibial shaft fractures. J. Bone Joint Surg. 61A:873-878, 1979.

One hundred consecutive patients with displaced fractures of the tibial shaft were randomly assigned to two groups. One was treated with AO plate fixation and the other with nonoperative methods. Comparison of the two groups showed that a longer duration of hospital stay was needed in the AO plate group, and there were also more complications in that group. However, the median healing time was shorter and the anatomic end results were better than in the patients treated nonoperatively. Closed longitudinal fractures were found to be suitable for AO plate fixation, but open fractures were not. In the group that was treated nonsurgically, most fractures that healed in malalignment were located in the distal third of the tibial shaft.

Nonunion of Tibial Diaphyseal Fractures

Bassett, C.A.L.; Mitchell, S.N.; and Gaston, S.R.: Treatment of ununited tibial diaphyseal fractures with pulsing electromagnetic fields. J. Bone Joint Surg. 63A:511-523, 1981.

The overall success rate in treating 127 ununited tibial diaphyseal fractures with pulsating electromagnetic fields was 87 percent. The exact mechanism by which they affect fracture healing is unknown.

Brighton, C.T.: Current concepts review. The treatment of nonunions with electricity. J. Bone Joint Surg. 63A:847-851, 1981.

The treatment of nonunions with electricity using invasive, semi-invasive and noninvasive electromagnetic pulsing fields reportedly gives the same overall success rate of 80 to 85 percent. All require the principles of good fracture treatment with adequate fracture reduction and immobilization. The presence of actively draining osteomyelitis is not a contraindication for the use of the noninvasive system but is a contraindication for the semi-invasive and invasive systems.

Brighton, C.T.; Black, J.; Friedenberg, Z.B.; Esterhai, J.L.; Day, L.J.; and Connolly, J.F.: A multicenter study of the treatment of nonunion with constant direct current. J. Bone Joint Surg. 63A:2-13, 1981.

One hundred nine of 136 (80 percent) established nonunions of the tibia were successfully treated with semi-invasive constant direct electrical current. The unsuccessful cases were believed to be due to inadequate electricity, the presence of synovial pseudarthrosis, infection, or dislodgement of the electrodes.

DeLee, J.C.; Heckman, J.D.; and Lewis, A.G.: Partial fibulectomy for ununited fractures of the tibia. J. Bone Joint Surg. 63A:1390-1395, 1981.

Partial fibulectomy proved to be a relatively effective and simple method of achieving union in thirty-seven of forty-eight patients with established tibial nonunions. Failure of union after fibulectomy was associated with either failure of the patient to bear weight postoperatively, the presence of a pseudarthrosis at the fracture site, or previous prolonged treatment of the initial fracture with external fixation.

Reckling, F.W., and Waters, C.H., III: Treatment of nonunions of fractures of the tibial diaphysis by posterolateral cortical cancellous bone grafting. J. Bone Joint Surg. 62A:936-941, 1980.

Union was obtained in forty-three of forty-four tibial nonunions utilizing cancellous bone grafts inserted from the posterolateral approach. Three fractures required a second bone grafting. The majority of the fractures had been complicated by severe soft-tissue damage, segmental bone loss or infection and multiple previous attempts had been made to obtain union prior to the posterolateral bone grafting procedure.

Compartment Syndromes Associated With Tibial Fractures

DeLee, J.C., and Stiehl, J.B.: Open tibia fracture with compartment syndrome. Clin. Orthop. 160:175-184, 1981.

Of 104 open tibia fractures, six developed compartment syndromes involving all four compartments of the lower leg. All had four compartment fasciotomies performed within 8 to 17 hours of the onset of symptoms. All had some residual foot drop as well as sensory deficits.

Halpern, A.A., and Nagel, D.A.: Anterior compartment pressures in patients with tibial fractures. J. Trauma 20:786-790, 1980.

Twenty patients with tibial fractures had measurements of tissue pressure in the anterior compartment acutely and for the first 72 hours following injury. Measurements were made using a mercury manometer indicator. In normotensive patients in this series, fasciotomy was not necessary for tissue pressure less than 50 mm Hg in the absence of any sensory or motor compromise.

Matsen, F.A., III; Winquist, R.A.; and Krugmire, R.B., Jr.: Diagnosis and management of compartmental syndromes. J. Bone Joint Surg. 62A:286-291, 1980.

Of thirty-one compartments at risk for compartmental syndrome, the patients varied in their tolerance for increased tissue pressure. Thus, there was a range of intracompartmental pressure in which some demonstrated neurovascular deficits.

Mubarak, S.J.; Owen, C.A.; Hargens, A.R.; Garetto, L.P.; and Akeson, W.H.: Acute compartment syndrome: Diagnosis and treatment with aid of the Wick catheter. J. Bone Joint Surg. 60A:1091-1095, 1978.

Most compartment syndromes can be diagnosed clinically. However, there are three groups of patients in whom the measurement of intracompartmental pressures is particularly valuable as a criteria for determining when a decompression fasciotomy should be performed. They are uncooperative, unreliable, or unresponsive patients and patients with fractures or contusions and nerve deficit.

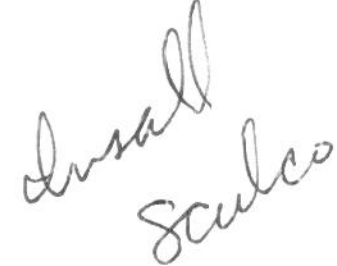

37 KNEE AND LEG: RECONSTRUCTION

Subjects covered in this section include osteotomy and total knee replacement.

Introduction The knee is commonly involved in degenerative and inflammatory joint diseases. Damage to joint surfaces in the osteoarthritic knee tends to be focal (medial, lateral tibiofemoral, or patellofemoral compartment), particularly in its early stages. Associated patellofemoral involvement is common in patients with medial tibiofemoral damage. Varus and valgus deformities may result from severe compartmental degeneration and produce secondary soft-tissue alterations about the knee joint. Problems of instability on the convex side of the deformity and fixed contractures on the concave side are then present.

Patients with rheumatoid arthritis manifest more universal panarticular damage with symmetrical joint space narrowing secondary to articular cartilage loss in all compartments of the knee joint. Persistent synovial hyperplasia with associated pain and alteration of knee joint function (particularly limitation of flexion and inability to achieve full extension) may be present prior to significant cartilage damage. In later stages when persistent damage occurs to the joint surface, malalignment and associated soft-tissue problems may arise in the rheumatoid as in the osteoarthritic knee.

Patellofemoral Joint Although degenerative disease of the patellofemoral joint generally occurs with tibiofemoral involvement, it may be the predominant source of pain to the patient. If nonsurgical treatment (e.g., anti-inflammatory medication, exercise program, activity alteration, bracing) has proved unsuccessful, surgery is a consideration for the patient with significant disability.

The procedures available for the treatment of patellofemoral arthritis include debridement, excisional arthroplasty, or replacement arthroplasty. Attempts to reduce the load on the patellofemoral joint by the elevation of the tibial tubercle have also been advocated by Maquet.

Debridement procedures for patellofemoral arthritis may provide relief in patients with localized and early patellar surface changes. Removal of osteophytic spurs and damaged cartilage with drilling of subchondral bone may result in production of fibrocartilage and some improvement in knee function. However, results are unpredictable, and patellofemoral joint degeneration tends to recur.

Patellectomy has also produced mixed results. The continuity of the extensor mechanism must be preserved during patellectomy, requiring its careful removal from the patellar surface. Failure to do so often leads to an incompetent and lengthened quadriceps mechanism with a persistent extension lag. Patellectomy can result in reduced power of knee extension, and patients may complain of difficulty on arising from a seated position as well as ascending and descending stairs. Tibial tuberculoplasty has been recommended in patellectomy patients to lengthen the extension moment arm and increase quadriceps force. Problems may also arise in the remaining quadriceps tendon that must articulate with the distal femur, and degenerative changes are commonly seen in the tendon after patellectomy. In females the cosmetic appearance of the knee after removal of the patella may be objectionable. Patients who progress to more symptomatic tibiofemoral arthritis and require total knee replacement may have a less satisfactory result if a previous patellectomy has been performed. Despite these considerations, patients with isolated or predominant patellofemoral arthritis may benefit from this procedure. Ninety percent good to excellent results with patellectomy for patellofemoral arthritis have been reported when a tube is fashioned from the remaining quadriceps mechanism.

There are two varieties of isolated patellofemoral replacement: a hemiarthroplasty, usually metal, which is implanted in the posterior surface of the patella; and various designs which replace both the patellar surfaces with polyethylene and incorporate a metal flange cemented into the anterior femur. The hemiarthroplasty design has the inherent problems of a metal implant articulating on a damaged joint surface. Progressive hyaline cartilage deterioration on the femur has resulted in these patients. Total replacement of the patellofemoral joint is difficult without the implant affecting the tibiofemoral joint. If a later total knee replacement is required, revision of these implants produces a considerable defect in the anterior femur that must be filled with cement or bone graft. Clinical experience with total patellofemoral replacement is limited.

Anterior displacement of the tibial tubercle lessens patellofemoral compression load. This reduction in force approaches 50 percent if anterior displacement is 12 to 15 mm (Fig. 1). Results have been mixed with these procedures, and complications including wound problems, nonunion, and proximal tibial fracture have been reported.

Knee Joint (Except Replacement Arthroplasty)

Synovectomy This procedure is recommended for intractable proliferative synovitis of longer than 6 months duration in patients with good preservation of articular cartilage. Synovectomy is recommended earlier if knee

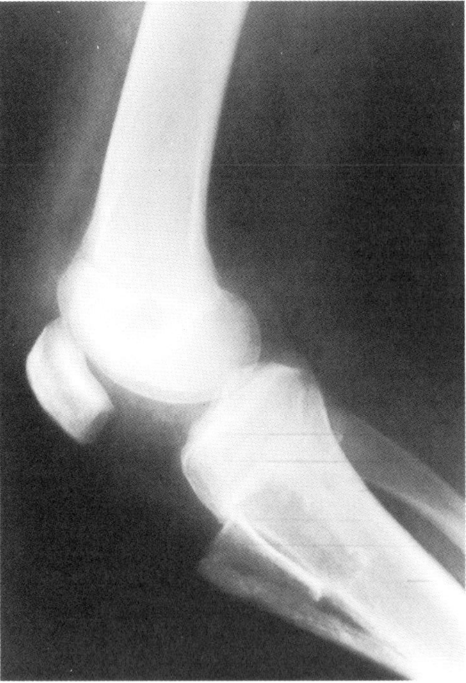

Figure 1-A

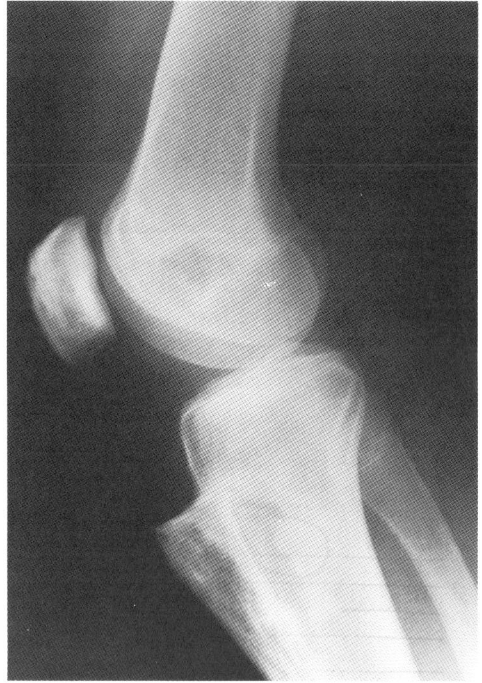

Figure 1-B

Figure 1: (A) Immediate postoperative radiograph of a Maquet-type anterior displacement of tibial tubercle. (B) One-year follow-up showing filling in of defect created in anterior tibia.

function, particularly loss of motion and flexion contracture, is developing rapidly. The release of lysozymes from inflammatory cells in a chronic synovitis may lead to accelerated articular cartilage destruction.

The beneficial results of synovectomy for rheumatoid arthritis tend to be temporary, however. Histologically and chemically, typical rheumatoid synovium tends to recur in 3 to 6 months. In the majority of patients, clinical synovitis has reappeared within 2 years.

Knee synovectomy may be performed through a single medial parapatellar incision, but generally the lateral and posterior compartments are better visualized if two incisions are used. The bulk of this tissue should be removed sharply en bloc, and a rongeur can be used to extirpate more adherent synovium.

Postoperative return of knee motion may be slow if surgical dissection is extensive. Early motion assisted by a

Figure 2: (A, B) Technique of high tibial osteotomy. (Reprinted with permission from Tibial osteotomy for gonarthrosis of the knee, by G.C.H. Bauer, et al., J. Bone Joint Surg. 51A:1549, 1969.)

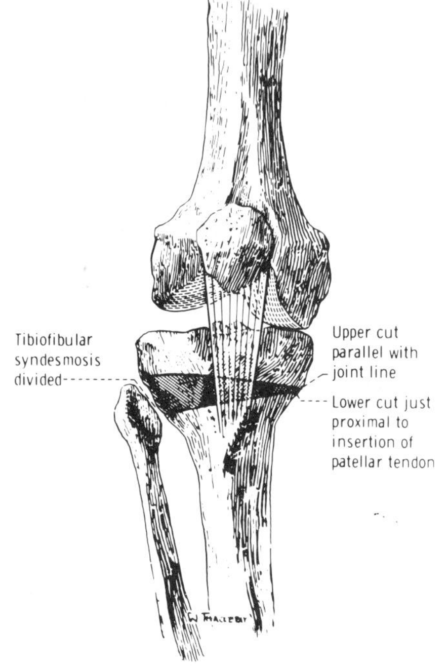

Figure 2-A

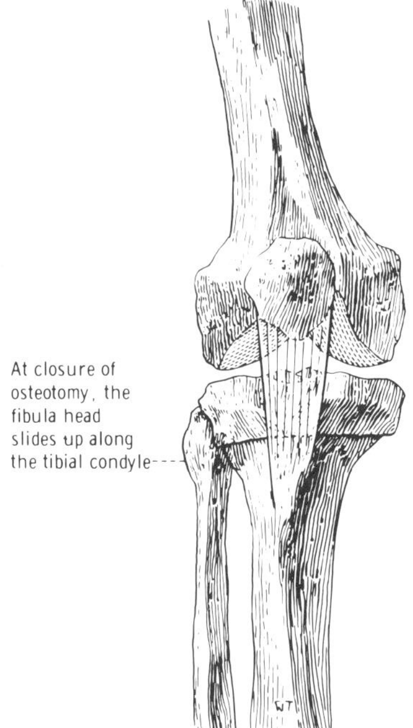

Figure 2-B

Figure 3-A

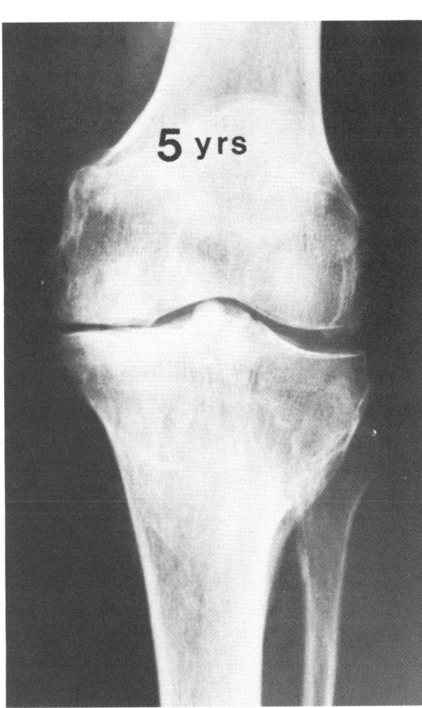

Figure 3-C

Figure 3: (A) Preoperative standing radiograph demonstrating medial compartment osteoarthritis. (B) Three months after high tibial osteotomy. (C) Five-year follow-up radiograph. Patient with some recurrent medial compartment narrowing but clinically doing well.

physical therapist is recommended. A passive motion device applied in the recovery room also may improve resultant range of motion. Wound healing may be delayed if the patient has been on steroids or immunosuppressive medication.

Debridement Procedures Open debridement procedures in which osteophytes, loose bodies, and joint debris

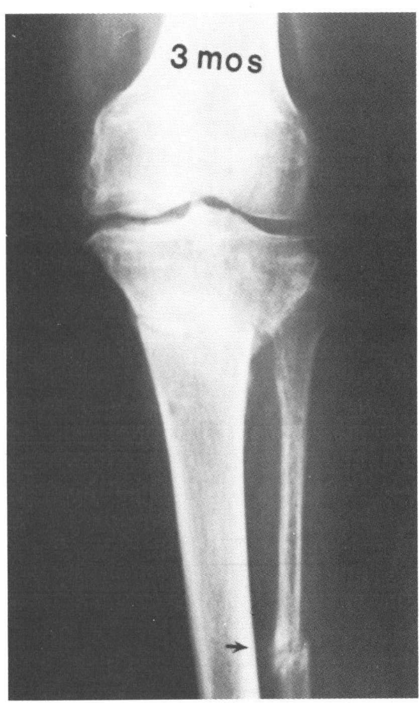

Figure 3-B

are removed and subchondral bone is drilled have met with limited success. Good results generally have been transient, particularly in the older patient. Formal open debridement procedures frequently result in knee stiffness and a prolonged convalescence. Although morbidity is less, arthroscopic debridement procedures also have been employed with limited success, and patients with crystal synovitis benefit from the copious irrigation. In the older patient with advanced degenerative knee disease, total knee replacement is a more predictable procedure.

Osteotomy In patients with predominantly unicompartmental arthritic involvement (medial or lateral), either distal femoral or proximal tibial osteotomy can provide excellent long-term benefits. The resultant mechanical axis of weight-bearing should be restored, however, for the procedure to be successful. This requires careful preoperative planning to realign the tibiofemoral axis to a 5 to 8 degree valgus angle. The benefit of osteotomy is probably twofold: unloading of the degenerative compartment and an alteration of intraosseous vascular pressure in the proximal tibia.

In patients with medial compartment degeneration and a varus deformity, high tibial osteotomy is recommended. This can be performed through a transverse lateral incision, and a lateral-based bone wedge can be removed above the insertion of the patellar tendon. The proximal tibiofibular syndesmosis must be released sharply to close this osteotomy (Figs. 2 and 3). Alternative methods are to remove the head of the fibula or a segment of fibula. Postoperative immobilization with a cylinder cast is required, and early weight-bearing is allowed. A compression-type plate may be used to fix the osteotomy if early range of motion is required. Percutaneous pins with external fixation have been associated with a high incidence of peroneal palsy, nonunion, and pin tract infection and should be avoided.

Arthrotomy at the time of the osteotomy may lead to

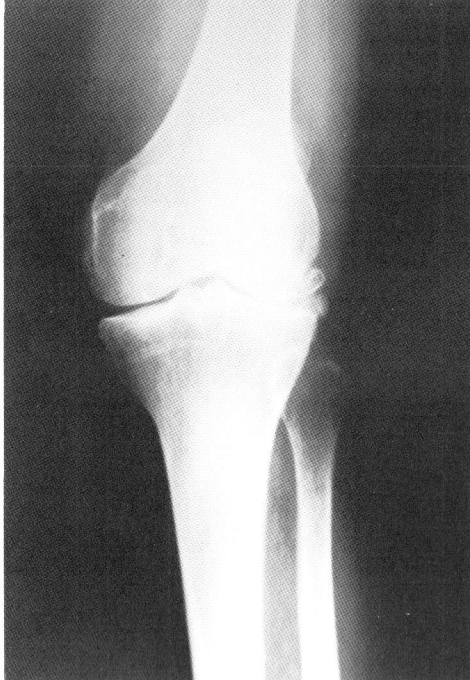

Figure 4-A

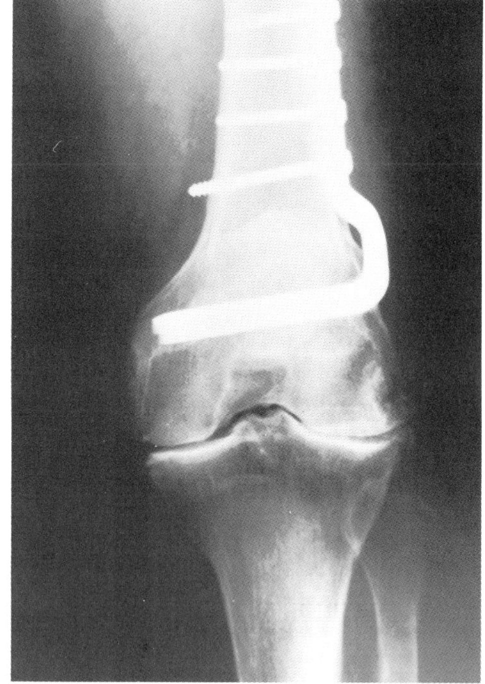

Figure 4-B

Figure 4: (A) Preoperative standing radiograph demonstrating lateral compartment osteoarthritis. (B) One-year follow-up radiograph after femoral osteotomy.

limitation of knee motion and generally is unnecessary. Experience is being gained with the combination of arthroscopic evaluation, drilling, and abrasion of the lateral compartment, followed immediately by proximal tibial osteotomy. Nonunion is uncommon if the osteotomy is performed through the predominantly cancellous metaphysis of the tibia and proximal to the patellar tendon insertion.

In the patient with a valgus deformity and lateral compartment osteoarthritis, osteotomy should be performed in the supracondylar area of the femur. This may be fixed with a blade plate (Fig. 4). Plaster is not required postoperatively, and range of motion is begun within 5 to 7 days after surgery. Protected weight-bearing is advised for 4 to 8 weeks. Since the intercondylar femoral osteotomy of Debeyre has had only fair results, it is performed infrequently. Patellofemoral problems are common.

Proximal tibial osteotomy for a valgus deformity may lead to obliquity of the knee joint and later medial femoral

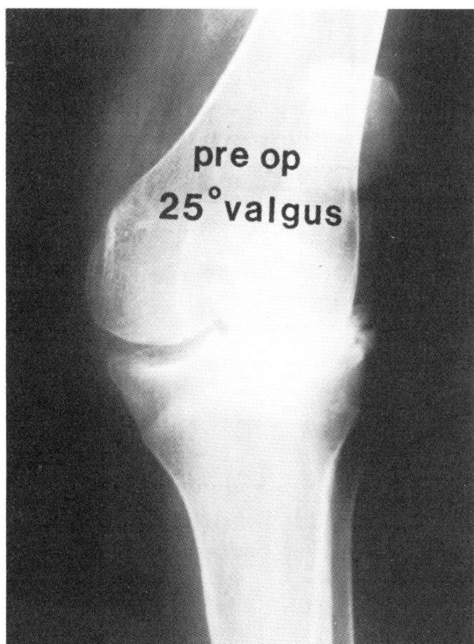

Figure 5-A

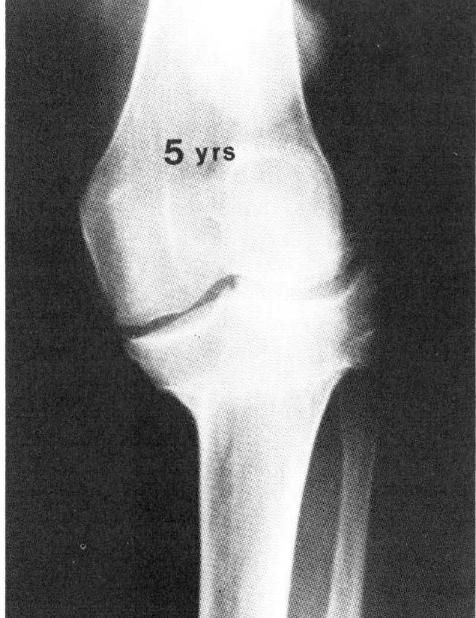

Figure 5-B

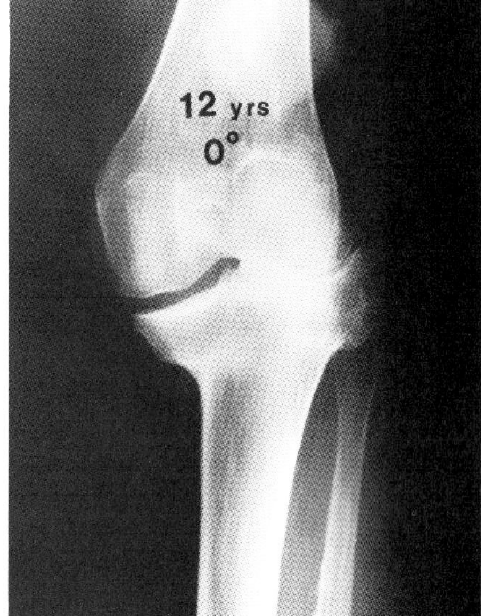

Figure 5-C

Figure 5: (A) Preoperative standing radiograph demonstrating lateral compartment osteoarthritis and 25 degree valgus deformity. (B) Five-year follow-up demonstrating obliquity of joint line and early subluxation. (C) Twelve-year follow-up showing marked recurrent lateral compartment destruction and progressive obliquity and subluxation.

subluxation (Fig. 5). There is also a tendency toward undercorrection when the medial tibial wedge is removed.

Results of osteotomy have been good if deformity is corrected and weight-bearing shifted to provide more symmetrical load distribution across both tibiofemoral compartments. Sixty to 70 percent of patients followed 5 to 10 years report continued benefit from this procedure in several large series.

Arthrodesis Currently this procedure is rarely performed as a primary procedure because patients are reluctant to accept it. It may be used in young laborers with diffuse knee joint damage that is disabling and intractable to other medical and surgical treatment. Young patients with persistent knee instability despite adequate bracing and multiple surgical procedures may also be candidates for arthrodesis.

Knee arthrodesis removes one of the primary energy-conserving mechanisms of gait, i.e., knee flexion during stance phase. Thus, about 20 percent more energy is required to walk with a fused knee joint. Other activities of daily living also differ (e.g., ascending and descending stairs). Other treatment alternatives should be sought when knee disease is bilateral as the prospect of bilateral knee fusions is unattractive.

It is best performed using an external fixation apparatus with multiple pins through the distal femur and proximal tibia, with the knee placed in 10 to 15 degree flexion and 5 to 10 degrees valgus.

Most commonly, arthrodesis is a salvage procedure for an infected total knee replacement. Union may be difficult in these patients, and augmentation of osteogenesis with electrical stimulation may promote arthrodesis.

Total Knee Replacement

Background The development of knee arthroplasty has followed two parallel paths.

RESURFACING DESIGNS: Campbell reported the successful use of a metallic interposition femoral mold in 1940. MacIntosh used a different type of hemiarthroplasty inserting tibial plateau prostheses into the medial and lateral femorotibial compartments to restore stability and relieve pain. Gunston, carrying MacIntosh's ideas a step further, substituted metallic runners embedded in the femoral condyles, articulating against polyethylene troughs attached to the tibial plateau. These latter components were the first to be fixed by acrylic cement. Freeman and Swanson had a great influence upon the evolution of prosthetic design, employing a two-part femorotibial replacement based on the principle of a "roller in a trough." The early cemented resurfacing designs suffered from a number of problems, most notably patellofemoral pain and tibial component loosening. Thus, a second generation of resurfacing models were developed, such as the total condylar device (which required excision of the cruciate ligaments), the Townley, and duopatellar prostheses (which retained the cruciate ligaments). These three designs all provided for patellofemoral resurfacing and formed the basis of current prosthetic designs. Subsequent modifications include right and left components with different radii of curvature of medical and lateral femoral condyles, cruciate substitution, anatomic patellar resurfacing, porous coating, and various stems or posts to enhance fixation.

Unicompartmental replacement of the femorotibial joint also has some advocates, using the modified Gunston or polycentric design or more anatomic components such as the Marmor or unicondylar designs.

CONSTRAINED PROSTHESES: The second line of development in knee arthroplasty was begun by Walldius who developed a hinged prosthesis in 1951 that was initially made of acrylic and later of metal. Shiers described a similar device with even simpler mechanical characteristics. Later designs, such as the Guepar, used acrylic cement fixation. Hinged prostheses have a considerable appeal for some situations because they are in part self-aligning and substitute for inadequate ligaments. However, simple metallic hinges suffer from high infection rates and frequent loosening. To reduce these problems, more sophisticated constrained designs with metal-on-polyethylene bearing surfaces have been developed. The most widely used are the spherocentric, Attenborough, Sheehan, and rotating kinematic hinge prostheses.

Classification and Selection of Prostheses All total knee prostheses can be divided into two categories, each with subdivisions (Table I).

Table I
Classification of Knee Prostheses

I. Surface Replacements
  A. Unicondylar
  B. Bicondylar
    1. Cruciate Retaining
    2. Cruciate Excising
    3. Cruciate Substituting
II. Constrained Prosthesis
  A. Loose—some degree of rotation and varus/valgus rock is permitted
  B. Rigid fixed axis hinges

It generally is agreed that a bicondylar design is more applicable for the majority of knees requiring replacement. There is debate about the need to preserve cruciate ligaments. It is argued that preservation of the posterior cruciate ligament prevents posterior subluxation and also may dissipate forces that otherwise would be absorbed at the bone-cement interface. But, cruciate excision (according to some) makes the operation easier and more precise, particularly with reference to soft-tissue balancing. In addition, cruciate excision allows correction of greater deformities by collateral ligament release.

The role of unicompartmental replacement is also controversial because the reported clinical results are conflicting. Most knees with unicompartmental disease are suitable for treatment by osteotomy (except, perhaps, in elderly people with bilateral knee involvement).

Constrained designs are needed in a small number of knees, particularly in revision cases. One to 10 percent of patients may need a prosthetic device of this type.

Description of Bicondylar Prosthesis Although originally the name of a specific prosthesis, *total condylar* recently has been expanded to describe a generic class of prostheses.

The femoral component has a grooved anterior (patellar) flange, separating posteriorly into condylar runners. In most designs these runners have a decreasing radius of curvature in the posterior portion (sagittal plane) and a convex curvature in the coronal plane.

The tibial component is made of high-density polyethylene which is in one piece containing two separate tibial plateaus that are biconcave and separated by an intercondylar eminence to prevent translocation. A posterior cutout for the posterior cruciate ligament may be provided, and most current designs have a stiff metallic backing of the polyethylene. The deep surface of the tibial component has either a central peg or multiple post fixation.

The polyethylene patellar component may be either dome-shaped so that rotary alignment is not required or anatomic with medial and lateral facets. The latter type requires careful rotary alignment to prevent binding in the femoral groove. Both types of patellar components may have one or multiple fixation lugs.

When the bicondylar prosthesis is designed for posterior cruciate retention, the tibial component must be flattened posteriorly in the sagittal plane to allow "roll back" of the femoral condyles when the knee is flexed.

The controversy over cruciate retention probably has received excessive emphasis as both cruciate-excising and cruciate-retaining designs give very similar clinical results when properly inserted. However, one group of investigators has found that stair-climbing gait is better with cruciate-retaining designs.

Cruciate substitution (as in the posterior stabilized condylar knee) recently has been introduced. The function of the posterior cruciate ligament is assumed by a polyethylene cam component which causes a controlled femoral roll back with flexion.

Indications and Contraindications Symptoms and disability must be severe to warrant knee joint replacement. A frank discussion with the patient concerning the possible consequences of prosthetic failure is essential, and alternative techniques such as tibial or femoral osteotomy should be selected when feasible.

INDICATIONS: Rheumatoid panarthritis regardless of age is one indication for knee joint replacement.

With gonarthrosis the age of the patient, occupation, level of activity, weight, and sex are factors. Arthroplasty generally should be avoided in patients under 60 years of age, and in manual laborers, athletes, and the grossly overweight. Males tend to abuse the arthroplasty more than females.

In posttraumatic osteoarthritis knee replacement in the younger patient rarely may be indicated following intra-articular fractures or other traumatic injuries to the joint.

No adverse effects with regard to tibial fixation have been reported when knee replacement was performed following failure of high tibial osteotomy.

CONTRAINDICATIONS: Generally these include genu recurvatum associated with muscular weakness, gross quadriceps insufficiency, neuropathic joint, active sepsis, and a sound, painless arthrodesis.

Surgical Technique Component placement, overall alignment of axis, and soft-tissue balance are critically important in determining the success of knee arthroplasty.

PRINCIPLES: Regardless of the prosthesis selected, there are some common surgical principles that apply to the use of surface replacements whether or not the cruciate ligaments are excised. Most prostheses, however, have femoral components of varying sizes and tibial components of varying thicknesses so that component size can be roughly adjusted to the dimensions of the knee being replaced. A gross mismatch in size between the components and the bones makes the arthroplasty difficult and

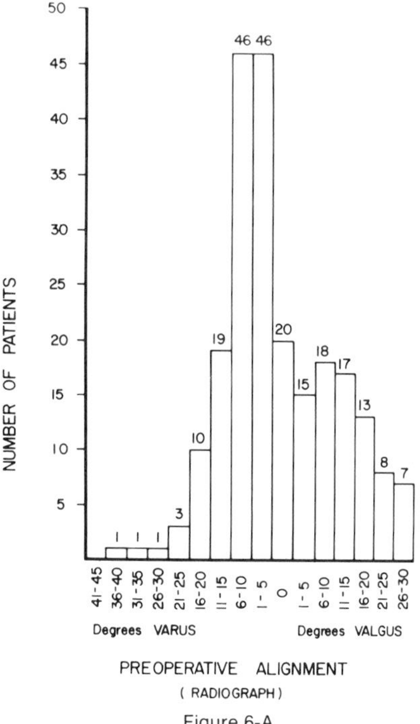

Figure 6-A

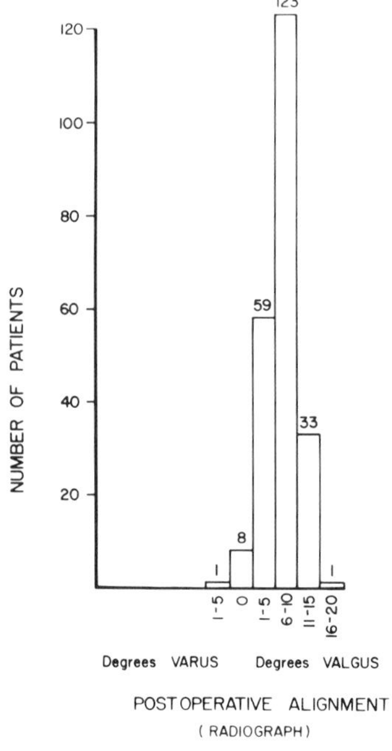

Figure 6-B

Figure 6: (A) Preoperative alignment of the tibia with respect to the femur as determined from a weight-bearing radiograph. (B) Postoperative alignment as determined from a weight-bearing anteroposterior radiograph. (Reprinted with permission from The correction of knee alignment in 225 consecutive total condylar knee replacements, by R.W. Hood, et al., Clin. Orthop. 160:96, 99, 1981.)

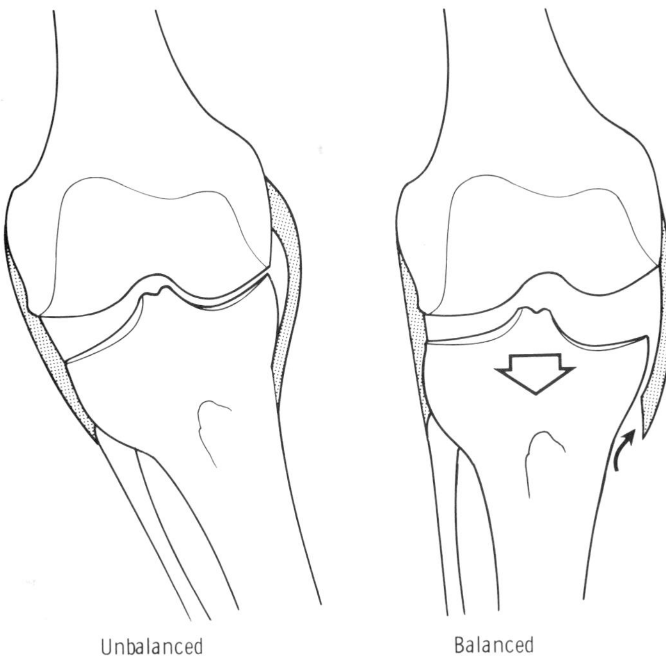

Figure 7: Ligament asymmetry in a knee with varus deformity is corrected by medial release so that the knee is balanced. (Reprinted with permission from The total condylar knee prosthesis: A report of 220 cases, by J. Insall, et al., J. Bone Joint Surg. 61A:174, 1979.)

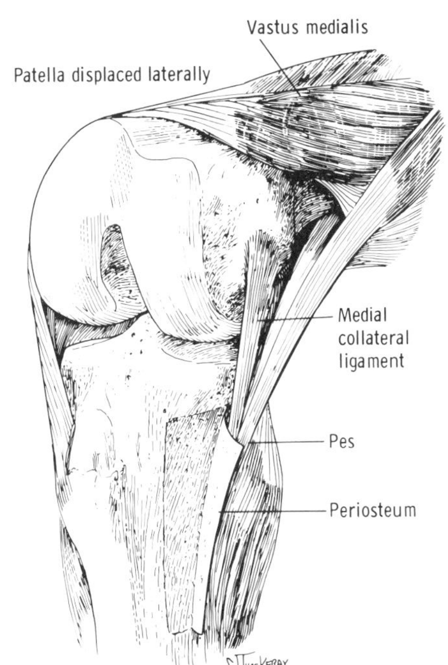

Figure 8: Medial release for fixed varus deformity. The medial capsule, periosteum, insertion of the pes anserinus, and superficial medial collateral ligament are developed as a flap from the upper medial surface of the tibia. The distal insertion of the superficial medial collateral ligament need not be elevated unless the deformity is severe. Medial osteophytes, when present, are removed. By progressive external rotation the proximal end of the tibia can be buttonholed forward, allowing when necessary the division of the posterior capsule and the semimembranous insertion. (Reprinted with permission from The total condylar knee prosthesis: A report of 220 cases, by J. Insall, et al., J. Bone Joint Surg. 61A:174, 1979.)

unsatisfactory so that an adequate inventory of component parts is essential.

The simplest knee to replace is one in which only the

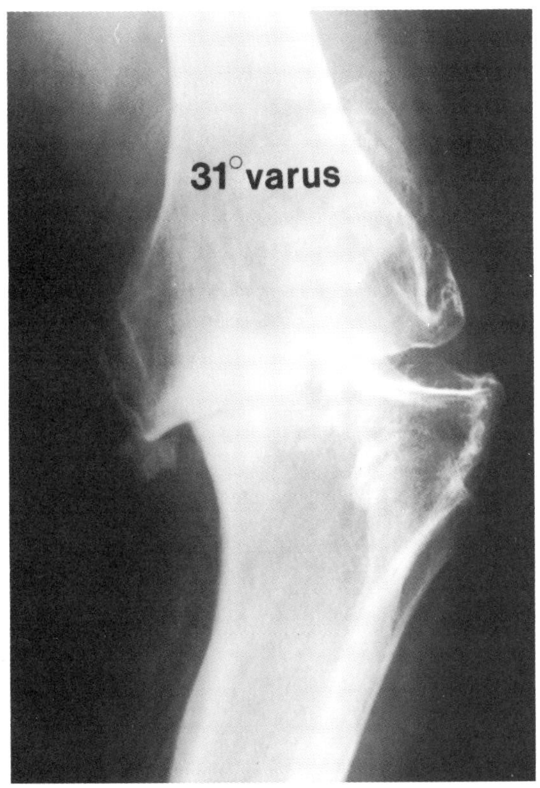

Figure 9-A

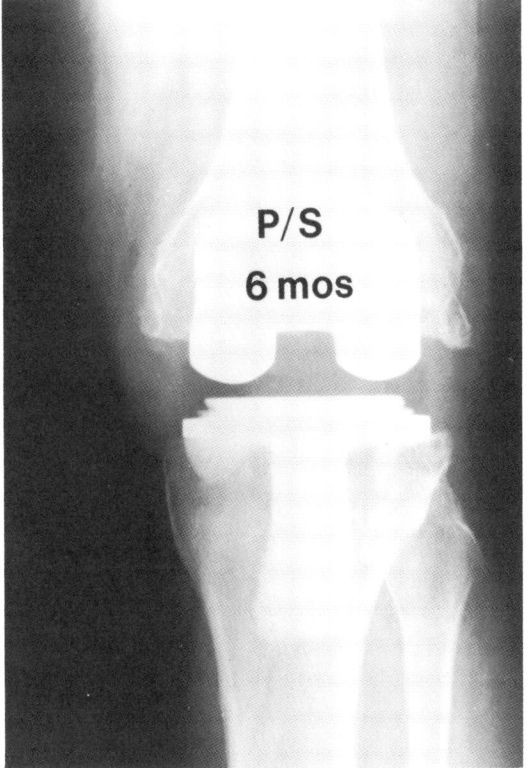

Figure 9-B

Figure 9: (A) Preoperative radiograph of a female with degenerative arthritis with severe varus deformity. (B) Postoperative radiograph after correction by medial release. A medial cement build-up was used to compensate for the bony defect.

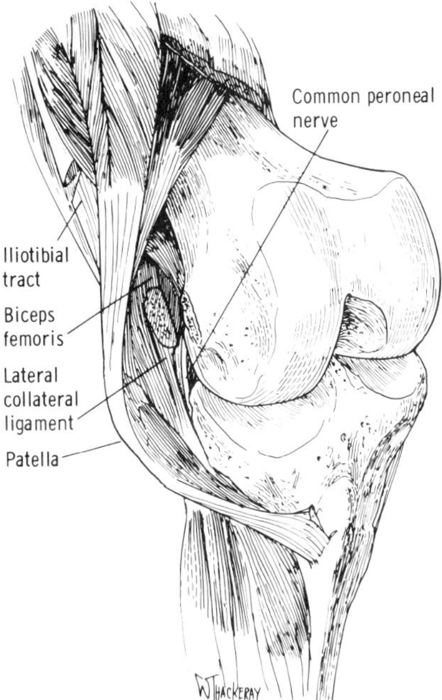

Figure 10: Lateral release for fixed valgus deformity. A lateral parapatellar skin incision allows access to the lateral side of the knee. The iliotibial band is divided transversely about 10 cm above the joint line. A lateral patellar release is accomplished by longitudinal division behind the iliotibial band. The joint is opened through a medial parapetallar capsular incision, and the patella is dislocated laterally. The lateral capsule, lateral ligament, and popliteus tendon are cut from the lateral femoral condyle, and division of the posterior capsule from the femur sometimes is necessary. If full correction still is not possible, a search should be made for remaining fibrous bands. (Reprinted with permission from The total condylar knee prosthesis: A report of 220 cases, by J. Insall, et al., J. Bone Joint Surg. 61A:175, 1979.)

articular cartilage is damaged so that normal alignment is retained, the ligaments are unaltered, and there are no bone defects. Bone ends should be reshaped so that they may be capped by the components. Sufficient bone should be removed so that the components fit in such a manner that the new prosthetic geometry will be compatible with existing ligament lengths throughout the range of motion.

Steps: The *flexion gap* is created by femoral condyle excision. Templates are used to select the prosthesis which roughly approximates the original size of the femur, particularly in its anteroposterior dimensions. The flexion gap is created by removing the posterior femoral condyles and the tibial plateau so that the resulting space can be filled by the combined bulk of the femoral and tibial components. When the cruciate ligaments are excised, the flexion gap is of critical importance because too loose a fit will result in a posterior subluxation.

Because it is desirable for the anterior femoral flange to fit flush with the anterior femoral shaft, the point of reference for beginning the bone cut is the anterior femoral cortex. After its creation, the flexion gap is sized with a spacer.

The *extension gap* is created with the knee extended and distracted using laminar spreaders or a tensor instrument. The gap is completed by resection of bone from the distal femoral condyles so that the spacer chosen for the flexion gap fits snugly in extension.

Bone trimming is the final stage of bone end preparation and consists of shaping the bone to receive the components.

Component positioning and limb axis are the next step. For most prostheses the recommended positioning for the

Figure 11-A

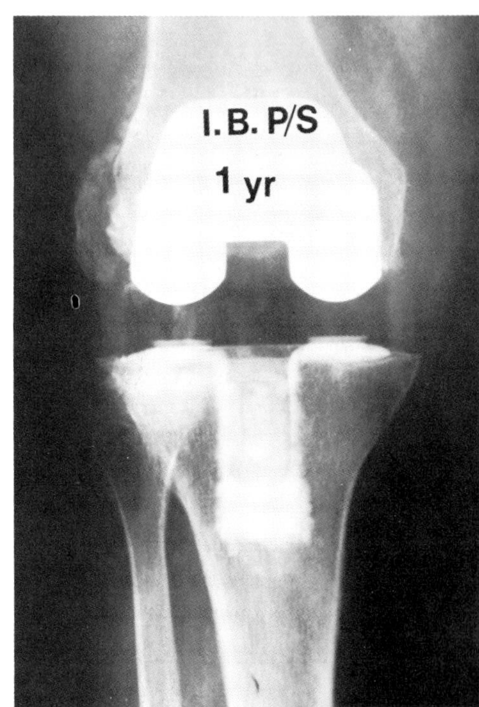

Figure 11-B

Figure 11: (A) Radiograph of a 77-year-old female with a 25-year history of right knee pain and severe genu valgus measuring 30 degrees; the preoperative Hospital for Special Surgery Knee Score was 34. (B) One year postoperation showing correction to 2 degrees of valgus employing the posterior stabilized condylar prosthesis; knee score at this visit was 89. The bone lateral to the lateral femoral condylar is due to subperiosteal soft tissue release required to balance this 30 degree valgus knee. (Reprinted with permission from The correction of knee alignment in 225 consecutive total condylar knee replacements, by R.W. Hood, et al., Clin. Orthop. 160:98, 1981.)

tibial components is 90 degrees to the long axis of the tibia. For the femoral component a positioning in 7 degrees of anatomic valgus is recommended. Thus, the overall axis of the limb is also 7 degrees (Fig. 6). Most instrument systems align to the mechanical axis (center of hip, center of knee, and the center of ankle) using an alignment rod. The center of the ankle and the center of the knee are readily identified, but unless the hip joint is identified radiographically, its position must be estimated so that an ill-defined proximal landmark is the most frequent source of alignment error.

In some knees, ligament releases may be necessary. In most pathological knees, some ligament asymmetry will exist. Unless a constrained prosthesis is to be used, ligament asymmetry should be corrected by a ligament release (Fig. 7).

In varus deformity, the medial soft-tissue structures become contracted. A medial release (Fig. 8) consists of subperiosteal stripping from the medial tibia and excision of all medial osteophytes. When this is insufficient to correct ligament asymmetry, the distal insertion of the superficial medial ligament is elevated from the tibia by a subperiosteal dissection. A laminar spreader is inserted into the medial compartment and the bones gradually separated. The distal connections progressively "give way" until the correct alignment is reached (Fig. 9).

For valgus deformity, lateral release is required (Fig. 10). For anatomical reasons, this is done on the femur. The first stage of this release is division of the lateral capsule, lateral ligament, and popliteus tendon, followed, if necessary, by the lateral posterior capsule. A laminar spreader is inserted in the lateral compartment, and the overall ligament balance assessed. If the deformity has not yet been corrected, a transverse incision is made through the iliotibial tract and lateral intramuscular septum. This incision is done from "inside out" about 10 cm proximal to the knee joint (Fig. 11).

Minor degrees of flexion contracture can be overcome by removing relatively more bone from the distal femur. However, significant flexion deformities require a posterior release. To gain access to the posterior capsule, it is necessary to produce the flexion gap and excise the cruciate ligaments. The posterior capsule is then visible and can be divided transversely with a knife.

In long-standing stiffness of the knee, adaptive shortening may have occurred in the quadriceps muscle resulting in extension contractures. This may cause difficulties in exposure, resulting in an inadvertent avulsion of the tibial tubercle. An inverted V-Y quadriceps turndown can be used, dividing the quadriceps tendon and turning the patella distally and laterally. This approach is often valuable for revision surgery.

The surgeon must be familiar with these soft-tissue techniques to successfully employ a surface replacement.

Patella resurfacing is now provided by most prosthetic designs, although occasionally when the patellar articular surface is well preserved, it may not be necessary to use the patellar prosthesis. Patellar tracking at the conclusion of surgery must be correct. The patella should remain in place throughout the range of knee motion without being passively held in place. If it does not, a lateral retinacular release is indicated. Patellar tracking is also affected by incorrect rotary placement of the tibial component which should always face the tibial tubercle.

Fixation of prosthetic components depends partially upon their design. There is clinical and theoretical evidence to suggest that the short central stem on the tibial component improves load distribution on the tibial bone, enhances fixation, and prevents sinkage. Stems on the femoral component are probably unnecessary. Adequate exposure is essential, and the tibia should be fully displaced anterior to the femoral condyle. Bone surfaces should be thoroughly cleaned, preferably with pulsatile water lavage or a brush to remove blood, marrow, and fat. The bone should be dried before applying cement to the exposed cancellous surface. With standard cementing techniques, penetration of 2 to 3 mm into the cancellous bone can be obtained. All exposed and excess cement should be removed.

Greater penetration into the bone can be achieved using low viscosity cement and pressurization "guns." There is a danger of excessive penetration that makes cement removal difficult in the event of infection, malposition, or subluxation. A technique of cementless press fit fixation using finned polyethylene studs has been devised.

Coating the prosthetic surfaces with cobalt chrome beads providing a pore size of between 100 and 200 μ allows biological fixation by porous bone ingrowth. As with any cementless technique, this method requires bone cuts of great accuracy and precision. Bone ingrowth has been demonstrated experimentally. However, the mean follow-up time is still very short, and clinical data is lacking. A porous surface of cobalt chrome also has raised concern because of possible metallic ion release and toxicity.

Aftercare Intravenous antibiotics (usually oxacillin or a cephalosporin) are administered immediately preoperatively and for 48 hours postoperatively. Thromboembolism is not considered a major threat after knee arthroplasty although fatal pulmonary emboli have been reported. Most surgeons rely on early ambulation and muscle activity, perhaps with the use of aspirin. Routine postoperative venography is practiced in some centers, and intermittent compression stockings also may prove valuable. Total knee patients are allowed to walk on the third or fourth postoperative day with weight-bearing as tolerated using a walker or crutches. Quadriceps exercises are not stressed early because of the risk of capsular disruption. Range of motion is begun about the fourth day when wound healing permits. Mechanized passive flexion recently has been advocated, and early reports indicate success in reducing pain and improving motion. Use of a stationary bicycle as an aid in gaining flexion also is recommended. For resistant knees, manipulation under anesthesia is done 2 to 3 weeks after surgery. One study demonstrated, however, that manipulation does not affect the range of flexion at 1 year.

Complications Urinary retention and urinary tract infections are the most frequent general complications. Venography has shown frequent calf vein thrombophlebitis, and fatal cases of pulmonary embolism have been reported. Fat embolism also has occurred.

Local complications include wound problems, neurovascular problems, stress fractures, component loosening, instability, and infection.

Wound problems, including delayed healing and drainage, are seldom serious but require delaying flexion therapy until the wound is healed. Wound drainage should not be treated with antibiotics to avoid masking a deep infection. Skin necrosis is very likely in previously operated knees.

Vascular complications are rare, and the absence of peripheral pulses is not necessarily a contraindication to surgery.

Nerve palsy (usually involving the peroneal nerve) may follow correction of severe valgus and flexion deformities. If it occurs, early removal of the dressing and flexion of the knee may hasten recovery.

Stress fractures may occur in the patella, femur, and tibia. Patellar fractures can be treated expectantly and, unless the patellar prosthesis is loosened, usually heal well after a few weeks' immobilization.

Stress fractures of the lower femur are most likely if the femur was violated at operation by notching of the anterior femoral cortex. Although internal fixation is sometimes required, these fractures usually can be managed by applying skeletal traction.

Avulsion of the tibial tubercle can occur during intraoperative maneuvers, and reconstruction is difficult and often unsatisfactory. A quadriceps turndown will avoid this complication. Stress fractures of the tibia beneath the component may occur, particularly with such designs as the polycentric device.

Component breakage is rare and usually restricted to hinges and linked designs. For example, breakage in the Guepar prosthesis may occur in the femoral stem about 3 cm proximal to the joint.

Component wear of clinical significance has not yet been demonstrated with current resurfacing designs. Retrieval analysis of removed total joint implants consistently has revealed polyethylene particles in the synovium. Inspection of removed components often shows embedded cement particles with scratching, pitting, and burnishing of the articular surfaces.

Component loosening may now be restricted to constrained devices. Most current surface replacements demonstrate acceptably low short-term loosening rates. Recent modifications, such as metal backing of the polyethylene and improved cement techniques, should further reduce this rate. Malalignment of the arthroplasty or soft-tissue imbalance predisposes loosening.

Instability after knee arthroplasty can be categorized as extension instability, flexion instability, rotary instability, translocation, and genu recurvatum.

Instability after a surface replacement is usually a technical problem that should be recognized and corrected in the operating room. If proper stability cannot be obtained, it is better to convert to a constrained design rather than to expect the ligaments to tighten. Adherence to sound surgical principles and complete ligament releases to correct deformities usually ensures a stable arthroplasty. When there is significant bone loss, the defect should be built up with screws, wire mesh, a bone graft, or a custom component rather than cutting back bone excessively. Longer fixation stems may also be required.

Infection should be considered when symptoms persist in the absence of a clear mechanical explanation. Infection is more common in rheumatoid arthritis and when metal-on-metal constrained hinged prostheses are selected.

Early infection occurring in the first 3 months after surgery can sometimes be successfully treated by debridement, leaving the prosthetic components in situ if they are not loose. Intravenous antibiotic therapy is begun. Antibiotic blood levels are monitored against cultures of the infecting organism with the objective of maintaining mean inhibitory concentrations at a minimum eightfold dilution. If the wound is not benign and cultures negative after 2 weeks, the prosthetic components and all cement should be removed.

Late infection is more common than early, and the diagnosis is usually straightforward unless antibiotics have been given previously. Aspiration usually provides the diagnosis. Treatment for proven or suspected late deep infection is incision, drainage, debridement of the involved tissue, and removal of the prosthetic components along with the acrylic cement. Appropriate antibiotic therapy is given intravenously for 6 weeks. After the infection has been cured or controlled, there are three courses available.

One is prolonged immobilization in a supportive orthosis, allowing a fibrous ankylosis to develop. Often a satisfactory and painless knee results. Another is formal arthrodesis using an external fixator or a long, slightly curved, intramedullary Küntscher rod. Finally, there is reimplantation of another prosthesis. For success the antibiotic therapy must have been adequate at bactericidal levels as demonstrated by monitoring the blood levels against the organism. The wound must have been completely benign for 6 weeks. Usually only infections due to gram-positive organisms can be managed in this manner. At reoperation, frozen tissue sections are obtained to assess tissue information as well as Gram stains and cultures of the tissues. The macroscopic appearance of the wound should be completely benign. Usually the new prosthesis can be a surface design, but bony defects may demand custom components. Antibiotic-impregnated cement has been recommended (see also Section 13: Polymethyl Methacrylate).

Revision Although component loosening was the major cause of failure with early prosthetic designs, with later models of resurfacing prostheses the causes of failure are divided equally among malposition, loosening, infection, and subluxation.

Subperiosteal exposure of the tibia and sometimes of the distal femur also can be done if exposure is still inadequate or there is difficulty in removing articulated components. Special devices to remove the component and cement are useful. A large sliding hammer with various gripping devices is invaluable, particularly for the extraction of hinge-type prostheses. A high-speed, low-matic drill is useful for cement removal.

All patients must be carefully reviewed preoperatively, considering the type of prosthesis required for the revision and any special components that must be ordered. Bone loss is the major problem in revision surgery, and although small bone defects of the tibial plateau may be managed with screws, titanium mesh, or a bone graft, larger defects require custom-designed metal trays. Femoral components are modified with posterior, anterior, or distal augmentation.

Although most revision surgery can be done with a surface replacement, it is necessary to have a constrained design to allow for ligament substitution when required.

Results of revision surgery are nearly as good as those of the primary operation. However, there are fewer excellent and more good results, and pain relief is not quite so complete. Extensor mechanism problems, such as patellar subluxation, quadriceps weakness, and extension lag, are relatively more common. Radiographic radiolucent lines are much more frequent in revision cases and may reflect the difficulty of cleaning the bone ends after removing the previous component.

Results Several investigators have stated that a 2-year follow-up is of little value in predicting long-term results of a nonconstrained surface replacement. In one series, 86 percent good results were reported at 2 years. This subsequently deteriorated so that after 7 years good results were noted in only 64 percent. Causes of failure were loosening of tibial components, settling, unexplained pain, lax ligaments, dislocation, and patellar problems.

There is reason to believe that current resurfacing designs will not deteriorate in the same manner. In a study of the first 100 consecutive arthroplasties using the total condylar prosthesis, 91 percent were rated excellent or good after an average follow-up of 6.6 years (with a range of 5 to 9 years). This differs little from an earlier report on the same prosthesis.

In one study of 100 knees after unicondylar replacement followed for 2 to 6 years, pain relief was satisfactory in 92 of the 100 knees. However, in another series of twenty-two unicondylar knee replacements with a 5- to 7-year follow-up, only 36 percent remained in the excellent and good category, and 28 percent had been revised. A report on fifty-nine knees after unicompartmental replacement with a minimum follow-up of 4 years showed 75 percent of these patients with good to excellent results. However, another study found that the Marmor modular prosthesis gave results that were inferior to bicompartmental replacement.

A report on cemented Guepar prostheses showed that 15 percent of the patients had aseptic loosening at 5 years, and there was a deep infection rate of 6.6 percent. A review of eighty-two consecutive spherocentric arthroplasties with an average follow-up of 4 years showed a 10 percent incidence of aseptic loosening and a 4 percent infection rate. Eight patients with confirmed or suspected loosening in thirty-six spherocentric arthroplasties followed for an average of 3 years have been reported. A long-stem modification of the prosthesis was recommended.

ANNOTATED BIBLIOGRAPHY

Patellofemoral Joint

Compere, C.; Hill, J.; Lewinnek, G.; and Thompson, R.: A new method of patellectomy for patellofemoral arthritis. J. Bone Joint Surg. 61A:714-719, 1979.

This describes a new method of handling quadriceps mechanism after patellectomy and reports 90 percent good to excellent results in twenty-six patients.

Maquet, P.: Mechanics and osteoarthritis of the patellofemoral joint. Clin. Orthop. 144:70-73, 1979.

A description of patellofemoral forces and rationale for forward and medial displacement of tibial tubercle is provided. The technique of the procedure is described.

Knee Joint (Except Replacement Arthroplasty)

Osteotomy

Coventry, M.B.: Upper tibial osteotomy for gonarthrosis. Orthop. Clin. North America 10:191-210, 1979.

Long-term results of tibial osteotomy are reviewed. Results were best when 7 degrees of valgus alignment (anatomical) was obtained.

Ha'eri, G.B., and Wiley, A.M.: High tibial osteotomy combined with joint debridement: A long-term study of results. Clin. Orthop. 151:153-159, 1979.

A technique of open joint debridement and tibial osteotomy in which internal fixation plate is used yielded 83 percent satisfactory results with average follow-up of 6 years.

Kettelkamp, D.B.; Wenger, D.R.; Chao, E.Y.S.; and Thompson, C.: Results of proximal tibial osteotomy. J. Bone Joint Surg. 58A:952-960, 1976.

Best results after osteotomy were found in patients with tibiofemoral angles greater than 5 degrees genu valgum. Medial tibial plateau force was calculated from radiographs and best results were obtained if force reduced to 50 percent body weight or less.

MacIntosh, D.L., and Welsh, R.P.: Joint debridement: A complement to high tibial osteotomy in the treatment of degenerative arthritis of the knee. J. Bone Joint Surg. 59A:1094-1097, 1977.

This describes use of pin fixation for tibial osteotomy to allow early motion when arthrotomy also is performed.

Vainionpää, S.; Läike, E.; Kirves, P.; and Tiusanen, P.: Tibial osteotomy for osteoarthritis of the knee: A five to ten-year follow-up study. J. Bone Joint Surg. 63A:938-946, 1981.

In a long-term follow-up (average 6.9 years) of tibial osteotomy, 83.5 percent of results were satisfactory. Fifteen percent of patients underwent revision to total knee arthroplasty at an average 7.6 years from osteotomy.

Total Knee Replacement

Bicondylar Prosthesis

Andriacchi, T.P., Galante, J.O.; and Fermier, R.W.: The influence of total knee-replacement design on walking and stair-climbing. J. Bone Joint Surg. 64A:1328-1335, 1982.

Gait characteristics in twenty-six patients with asymptomatic total knee replacements are described. The less constrained prosthesis with cruciate retention had more normal gait during stair climbing.

Bartel, D.L.; Burstein, A.H.; Santavicca, E.A.; and Insall, J.N.: Performance of the tibial component in total knee replacement: Conventional and revision designs. J. Bone Joint Surg. 64A:1026-1033, 1982.

The advantage of metal trays for tibial component is demonstrated especially if supporting tibial bone is insufficient. A custom design prosthesis also is presented.

Insall, J.N.; Lachiewicz, P.F.; and Burstein, A.H.: The posterior stabilized condylar prosthesis: A modification of the total condylar design. Two to four years clinical experience. J. Bone Joint Surg. 64A:1317-1323, 1982.

Posterior cruciate ligament function was provided by tibial polyethylene spine and transverse femoral cam. Ninety-one patients (118 arthroplasties) followed 2 to 4 years had improved results when compared with a similar series of patients with a Total Condylar prosthesis.

Surgical Technique

Blaha, J.D.; Insler, H.P.; Freeman, M.A.R.; Revell, P.A.; and Todd, R.C.: The fixation of a proximal tibial polyethylene prosthesis without cement. J. Bone Joint Surg. 64B:326-335, 1982.

Fixation of polyethylene to bone utilizing peg system for tibial component is described. In fifty-two patients fixed without cement, no prosthesis was loose at follow-up.

Aftercare

Fox, J.L., and Poss, R.: The role of manipulation following total knee replacement. J. Bone Joint Surg. 63A:357-362, 1981.

Patients 1 year after total knee replacement had similar range of motion regardless if postoperative manipulation was performed.

Complications

Brodersen, M.P.; Fitzgerald, R.H., Jr.; Peterson, L.F.A.; Coventry, M.B.; and Bryan, R.S.: Arthrodesis of the knee following failed total knee arthroplasty. J. Bone Joint Surg. 61A:181-185, 1979.

An 81 percent arthrodesis rate after condylar-type replacement and 56 percent after hinge-type prosthesis are described. The technique of arthrodesis did not influence fusion rate.

Revision

Barger, W.L.; Cracchiolo, A., III; and Amstutz, H.C.: Results with the constrained total knee prosthesis in treating severely disabled patients and patients with failed total knee replacements. J. Bone Joint Surg. 62A:504-512, 1980.

This reviews fifty-six constrained total knee replacements in severely disabled patients. Good pain relief was found in only 64 percent, and more than one-half had patellofemoral pain. There was a 16 percent reoperation rate.

Results

Convery, F.R.; Minteer-Convery, M.; and Malcom, L.L.: The spherocentric knee: A reevaluation and modification. J. Bone Joint Surg. 62A:320-327, 1980.

Complications with the spherocentric knee and a 30 percent failure rate are reviewed. Modification in design is described.

Gibbs, A.N.; Green, G.A.; and Taylor, J.G.: A comparison of the Freeman-Swanson (ICLH) and Walldius prosthesis in total knee replacement. J. Bone Joint Surg. 61B:358-361, 1979.

Long-term follow-up of 75 Mark I Freeman-Swanson (ICLH) total knee replacements showed 80 percent success.

Scott, R.D., and Santore, R.F.: Unicondylar unicompartmental replacement for osteoarthritis of the knee. J. Bone Joint Surg. 63A:536-544, 1981.

There was 92 percent good to excellent pain relief in patients undergoing unicompartmental replacement. Pes anserinus bursitis was the most common complication occurring in 12 percent of knees.

38 ANKLE AND FOOT: PEDIATRIC

These afflictions have been organized into congenital and developmental, infectious, traumatic, and neuromuscular categories.

Congenital and Developmental

Congenital Ball-and-Socket Ankle This condition is associated with a short extremity and is asymptomatic. It appears to be a congenital abnormality of the ankle, and it is often associated with tarsal coalition.

Hypermobile Flatfoot (Pes Planus) Longitudinal arch formation continues during the first 5 years of life. Normally, there is progressive narrowing of the heel as compared to forefoot width and of the talocalcaneal angle as viewed on standing or simulated standing anteroposterior radiographs. This does not occur in the hypermobile flatfoot.

The deformity is best quantified on standing or simulated standing anteroposterior and lateral radiographs of the foot. They demonstrate an increased talocalcaneal angle and plantar convexity of the first metatarsal-talar angle. Because construction of these angles is somewhat inexact, development of new measurement methods continues.

There is no documentation from population studies that failure of formation of the longitudinal arch leads to long-term disability as long as the foot remains flexible. Also, there is no convincing data that treatment, such as shoe modifications or custom-fabricated orthoses, alters the normal growth and development of the longitudinal arch. For these reasons, treatment remains empirical. In general, physicians most aware of the natural history are the least likely to prescribe shoe modifications as a form of treatment. However, there are some patients with severe deformity whose function and, perhaps, structure appear to be improved with support of the longitudinal arch. Indications may include functional disability in the child, leg pain in the juvenile, and rapid wearing out of shoes. If a foot orthosis (such as a UCBL type) is prescribed, it should be checked to be certain that heel position is being controlled.

Long-term results of surgical management are generally not available except following extra-articular subtalar arthrodesis. These have not been satisfactory, apparently because of alteration in gait mechanics.

Accessory Navicular (Os Tibiale Externum) This sesamoid bone is located in the posterior tibial tendon at its insertion on the navicular and is present in approximately 12 percent of the population. It is not a cause of hypermobile flatfoot, but, because both are common, they may present together. In a few patients, the accessory navicular may be prominent enough to cause pressure symptoms. Simple excision appears to be effective. However, if hypermobile flatfoot is associated, the Kidner procedure is preferred.

Vertical Talus These patients usually have a neurologic deficit, such as cerebral palsy, or associated abnormalities, such as arthrogryposis. However, vertical talus may occur as an isolated deformity. If so, there frequently is a familial incidence.

The deformity is characterized by a fixed lateral and superior displacement of the talocalcaneonavicular complex. The peroneals, ankle extensors, and Achilles tendon as well as the superior talonavicular and the posterior tibiotalar capsules are shortened. The plantar calcaneonavicular ("spring") ligament is elongated.

The deformity is fixed and cannot be reduced completely by manipulation. This can be confirmed by a stress lateral radiograph of the foot and ankle, in which plantar flexion of the forefoot and the os calcis fail to reduce the lateral talocalcaneal angle or align the first metatarsal with the talus.

Postnatal manipulation and serial casting, placing the transverse talar joint in plantar flexion, the subtalar joint in inversion, and the ankle in calcaneus, are recommended to control and improve the deformity. However, permanent correction is very seldom achieved. Surgical treatment is best performed from about 6 to 12 months of age and is less successful after approximately 3½ years of age. As the deformity involves anterior, lateral, posterior, and medial structures, correction is best performed in one stage. This includes anterior, lateral, and posterior release with medial reefing and fixation of the reduced talonavicular joint with a Kirschner wire. Excision of the navicular is not advocated. Neurologic imbalance should be corrected by appropriate transfer or release, such as transfer of the anterior tibial tendon to the neck of the talus or the peroneus longus or brevis to the posterior tibialis tendon.

Idiopathic Equinovarus Congenital equinovarus is the result of polygenetic inheritance modified by environmental factors. The incidence among whites is 1.2 per thousand live births and increases to 2.1 percent for first degree relatives (siblings and parents). The threshold number of genes is lower for boys, as the younger brother of an affected male has a 2.3 percent chance of being affected whereas the risk to a younger brother of an affected female sibling is 6.3 percent.

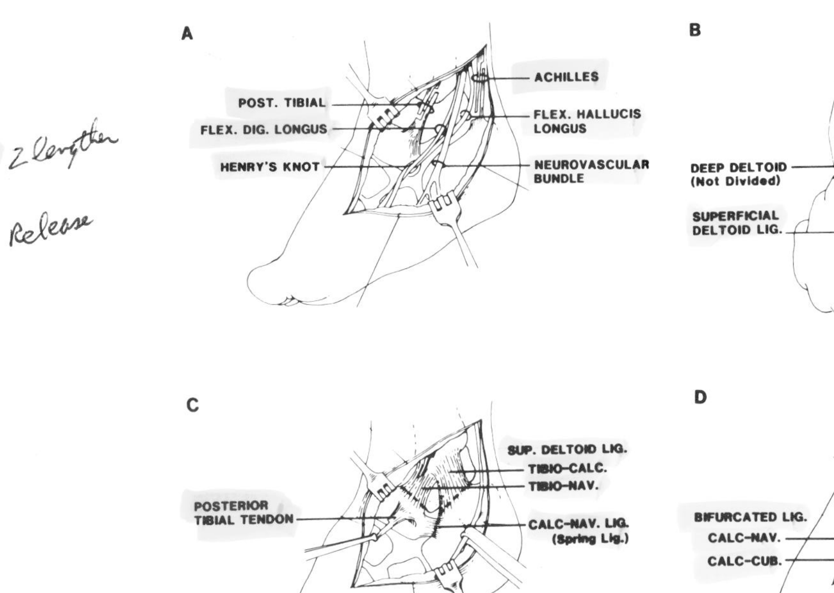

Figure 1: Techniques for the one-stage posterior medial release. (A) Exposure. (B) Posterior release. (C) Superficial medial release. (D) Deep medial release. (Adapted with permission from Surgical correction of the resistant club foot, by V. Turco, J. Bone Joint Surg. 53A:481-482, 1971.)

The pathological changes involve the posterior and medial ligaments, muscles, tendons and tendon sheaths, and the tarsal bones. Histological study of the short, thick ligaments reveals myofibroblast and mast cells, similar to the findings in Dupuytren's contracture. Muscle abnormalities include decreased fiber number and increased type I fibers, at least in the soleus. This implies an early maturation of the soleus. There is increased fibrous connective tissue in the sheaths of the short, thick Achilles tendon and posterior tibial tendons. As a result of these soft-tissue changes, the os calcis apparently rotates through the subtalar joint and moves toward the fibula posteriorly, while simultaneously tilting into varus. Altered tarsal bone shape, size, and relationship appear to be secondary to the soft-tissue changes. Careful documentation of the pathological changes has aided treatment but has not clarified the pathogenesis of the disorder.

The deformity consists of ankle equinus, hindfoot varus, and midfoot and forefoot adduction, but almost never internal tibial torsion. These findings are best confirmed and quantitated by standing or simulated standing lateral and anteroposterior radiographs. Ankle equinus is demonstrated by the calcaneotibial angle. Subtalar varus, which includes inversion and adduction, is best inferred from the lateral talocalcaneal angle. The anteroposterior talocalcaneal angle is helpful but is less accurate. Adduction occurs at the talonavicular joint and is demonstrable by medial displacement of the navicular. Prior to ossification of the navicular at ages 1 to 5 years, this is best quantitated by the talar-first metatarsal angle, which normally should be approximately zero degrees.

Treatment: Corrective manipulation and serial cast application (usually above-knee) beginning in the immediate postnatal period remain the treatment of choice. This is effective in approximately one-half of the patients and reflects the variable severity of the deformity. If correction is not complete, as documented by clinical and radiographic evaluation, surgical correction is necessary.

Occasionally, a posterior soft-tissue release coupled with continued serial cast correction may be indicated in the infant. However, one-stage posterior medial release is the most effective surgical procedure and results in a higher percentage of satisfactory results. This is because the deformity involves posterior, medial, and plantar structures.

The one-stage posterior medial release is a demanding surgical exercise (Fig. 1) and includes the following: (1) Achilles tendon Z-lengthening with secure reconstruction; (2) posterior release of the ankle and subtalar joint, including the calcaneofibular and the posterior talofibular ligaments; (3) Z-lengthening (or release) of the posterior tibial tendon; (4) medial release of the subtalar joint, the superficial deltoid which includes the calcaneotibial and tibionavicular ligaments, the calcaneonavicular (spring) ligament, the talonavicular ligament dorsally, the bifurcated ligament (calcaneonavicular and calcaneocuboid), the anterior talocalcaneal capsule, and release of only enough of the talocalcaneal interosseous ligament to allow rotation of the os calcis on the talus; and (5) occasionally, plantar release, including the abductor hallucis, plantar fascia, short toe flexors, and abductor digiti minimi. An extended transverse incision designed to facilitate the extensive exposure necessary for this procedure (and others) recently has been described.

The most opportune age for performing a one-stage posterior medial release is controversial. Surgical correction in the neonatal period has been reported recently. However, patient selection may be difficult as many of these feet will correct with conventional serial cast treatment, and well-developed neonatal and orthopaedic surgical techniques are necessary. Thus, this approach cannot be recommended without reservation.

Best results have usually been in those patients operated

Figure 2-A

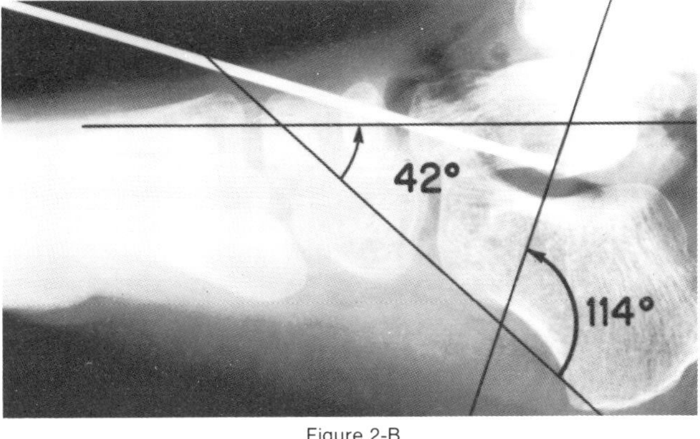

Figure 2-B

Figure 2: Radiographs before and after one-stage posterior medial release for residual idiopathic equinovarus of the right foot of a 6-year, 5-month-old girl. (A) Preoperative standing lateral view of abnormal lateral talocalcaneal angle (N = 35-50 degrees) and marginally normal lateral calcaneotibial angle (N = 95-125 degrees). (B) Postoperative view of deformity correction.

on between 1 and 2 years of age. More complications and poor results are encountered in younger infants, possibly because of the difficulty of maintaining correction in the preambulation patient. For these reasons, delay of the one-stage posterior medial release until the patient is approximately 8 months old seems wise at this time. Serial cast application to contain the deformity while awaiting surgery is desirable although difficult because of the small high heel. Increasing age up to 6 years does not seem to compromise the yield of satisfactory results, and the procedure may be performed, if necessary, up to ages 8 or 10 years. In the older child, calcaneocuboid fusion, partial cuboid body excision, or excision of the distal part of the calcaneus (to shorten the lateral column of the foot) is also occasionally necessary.

The result of one-stage posterior medial release correlates best with correction of the lateral talocalcaneal and the lateral calcaneotibial angles to normal (Fig. 2). The correction should be confirmed by postoperative radiographs. Unsatisfactory results commonly are associated with persistent medial subluxation of the navicular or with overcorrection of the navicular laterally resulting in a planovalgus deformity. Positioning the navicular on the talar head with a smooth Kirschner wire is, therefore, recommended.

Postoperative maintenance of the foot in the corrected position with serial plaster of paris casts for 4 months or longer is important to prevent recurrent deformity. Hyperpronation of the forefoot should be avoided. Nighttime maintenance of correction and passive stretching for an additional several months is desirable. A splint worn while sleeping is appropriate until the child is running and jumping. Following this program, residual metatarsus adductus and cavovarus deformity should not be significant problems.

In the older child with mild or moderate residual deformity and evidence of muscle imbalance, satisfactory salvage may at times be accomplished by transfer of the anterior tibial tendon to the third cuneiform unless the posterior tibial tendon has been divided. Transfer of the posterior tibial tendon through the interosseous membrane may be indicated occasionally, such as when the subtalar joint can barely be brought to neutral and the posterior tibial muscle-tendon unit is clearly a major deforming force. Persistent intoeing is usually the result of incompletely corrected subtalar varus and less commonly due to forefoot adduction. Persistent intoeing is very seldom the result of internal tibial torsion but may be the result of femoral anteversion. Treatment is determined by clinical severity and is directed at correction of the deformity as documented by clinical and radiographic evaluation.

COMPLICATIONS: Salvage of the foot overcorrected into planovalgus is very difficult. If the subtalar joint can be reduced adequately, extra-articular subtalar arthrodesis may be helpful. Poor push-off, resulting from overlengthening of the Achilles tendon, may be improved by shortening the tendon. For the occasional young adolescent with unacceptable residual deformity, triple arthrodesis remains the treatment of choice. This may be very difficult, especially if there is residual rocker-bottom deformity and/or residual equinus.

Cavovarus This developmental deformity may be idiopathic but usually is associated with residual congenital equinovarus or some neuromuscular disease, such as Charcot-Marie-Tooth or spinal dysrhaphia. A diagnostic work-up is necessary.

The deformity consists of tight plantar fascia, forefoot pronation with depression of the first ray (Fig. 3), and heel varus. Some observers consider the forefoot to be in supination. However, correction of the hindfoot varus by placing a block under the lateral side of the foot demonstrates the forefoot supination to be apparent rather than real.

The deformity is usually progressive and nonoperative treatment is not effective. Operative treatment should be tailored to the deformity. If the subtalar varus is flexible, a plantar or plantar medial release followed by serial cast applications promoting hindfoot eversion and forefoot inversion is satisfactory. If the hindfoot or forefoot deformity is fixed, appropriate corrective osteotomy is indicated in addition to the plantar release. If the os calcis varus alone is fixed, lateral closing osteotomy of the Dwyer type may be employed. If plantar flexion of the first ray persists, either first metatarsal or first cuneiform, dorsal closing or volar opening osteotomy may be performed. Osteotomy of the lateral four metatarsals may be necessary if forefoot adduction is a significant portion of the deformity. Finally, it may be necessary to add long toe extensor transfers to provide dynamic support of the metatarsal necks, especially the first.

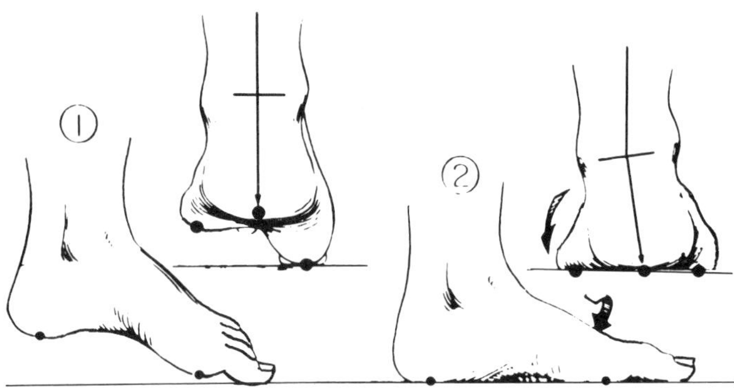

Figure 3: With a fixed, plantar-flexed first metatarsal, for the foot to be plantigrade on weight-bearing, the hind part of the foot must assume a varus position to compensate for the pronated fore part. (Reprinted with permission from Pes cavovarus: Review of a surgical approach using selective soft-tissue procedures, by L. Paulos, et al., J. Bone Joint Surg. 62A:943, 1980.)

Rigid deformity in patients approaching skeletal maturity may be treated by a tarsometatarsal resection arthrodesis or triple arthrodesis.

Tarsal Coalition Tarsal coalition appears to result from a failure of segmentation of primitive mesenchyme and exhibits an autosomal dominant inheritance pattern. Symptoms, if present, almost always appear in the second decade and consist of pain, limited subtalar motion, and, occasionally, spasm of the peroneals with attempted subtalar inversion. Patients commonly present with rigid, painful flat feet.

Calcaneonavicular (CN) and talocalcaneal (TC) middle facet coalitions are the most common. CN coalition is demonstrated by an oblique foot radiograph and TC middle facet coalition by the Harris view, a 45 degree posterior plantar view showing the posterior and medial TC facets. Lateral tomography may be necessary to confirm the diagnosis. Also a positive polyphosphate bone scan in the region of the subtalar joint can be expected in patients with a symptomatic coalition.

Most patients with tarsal coalition do not become symptomatic and do not require treatment. However, these patients appear to be at greater risk of ankle sprain than the normal population. Symptomatic patients are sometimes permanently relieved by temporary cast immobilization. Manipulation is not helpful. For patients with a cartilaginous CN coalition who remain symptomatic, excision of the coalition and interposition of the origin of the extensor digitorum brevis into the defect have been established as a successful procedure. Results are correlated with the degree of restoration of subtalar motion. Excision of the TC middle facet coalition with fat graft interposition is being tried but cannot be considered an established procedure at this time. Satisfactory results have been reported following calcaneal osteotomy, although the procedure does not appear to be widely practiced. Symptoms may warrant triple arthrodesis.

Metatarsus Adductus This deformity is usually present at birth but may not become apparent for a year. As with all substantial or structural foot deformities, careful examination of the hip is necessary because of the reported increased incidence of hip dysplasia.

The forefoot is adducted and slightly supinated, and the hindfoot is in neutral or mild valgus. The deformity may be secondary to abnormal muscle action with over-pull of the abductor hallucis or anomalous insertion of the posterior tibial tendon distally most frequently suspect. The deformity may or may not be passively correctable. Anteroposterior radiographic evaluation reveals the adduction to occur mainly at the tarsometatarsal joints.

Although most appear to resolve spontaneously, no factors predictive of the outcome have been identified. About 4 percent of the feet appear to remain stiff and fixed by the age of 4 years. Because of the variable natural history and relatively benign nature of the problem, it is difficult to determine which feet require treatment. As treatment outcome is most reliably predicted by the patient age at which it is begun, it seems wise to treat babies whose feet cannot be passively corrected at about 6 to 8 months of age. The feet usually respond to four or five serial corrective cast applications, placing the heel in neutral or some varus and forefoot in maximum abduction and slight pronation. If there is a marked dynamic component, the possibility of muscle over-pull should be considered. Recurrence or residual deformity usually responds to tenotomy of the abductor hallucis tendon at the first metatarsal neck followed by corrective cast application for 6 or more weeks.

Hallux Valgus This developmental deformity has a familial predisposition. Wearing closed-toe shoes has been implicated in its development. This apparently encourages lateral luxation of the superior, medial, and plantar dynamic stabilizers of the first metatarsophalangeal joint. Metatarsus primus varus may or may not be present.

Examination reveals valgus of the first metatarsophalangeal joint, pronation of the large toe, and varying degrees of varus alignment of the first metatarsal. There also may be varying degrees of loss of transverse arch with widening of the forefoot. Deformity quantitation is best performed on a standing anteroposterior radiograph taken with the beam 15 degrees to perpendicular (Fig. 4A).

Nonoperative treatment is unsuccessful. Operative treatment in the adolescent has been followed by a higher recurrence rate than in adults. Therefore, if possible, it seems best to postpone operative treatment until the child becomes older. Pain and difficulty with shoe fitting are indications for surgery. Appearance is a relative indication.

To be successful, operative treatment must restore normal muscle balance at the first metatarsophalangeal joint, and this is most reliably accomplished by including in the operation an osteotomy of the first metatarsal to reduce the first and second intermetatarsal, as well as the first metatarsophalangeal joint alignment to well within normal limits (Fig. 4B). It is important to avoid dorsal displacement of the first metatarsal head. Excision of the lateral sesamoid and transfer of the adductor hallucis tendon to the metatarsal neck may result in hallux varus.

Miscellaneous *Osteochondrosis of the tarsal navicular* (Köhler's disease) is a mild self-limiting disease that can be expected to heal without treatment. However, a below-knee walking cast for approximately 8 weeks appears to speed the resolution of symptoms.

Multiple hereditary exostoses may result in either epiphyseal disturbances or mechanical problems. Surgery is

Figure 4-A

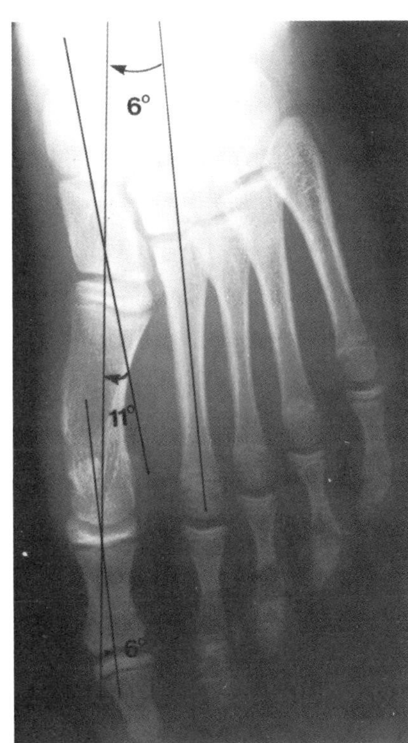

Figure 4-B

Figure 4: (A) Standing preoperative anteroposterior foot radiograph of a 10-year, 4-month-old male with left hallux valgus. (B) Standing anteroposterior foot radiograph 2 years, 9 months following surgical reconstruction (Mitchell type). Angles used to describe the deformities are:

Angle	Patient Pre-op	Patient Post-op	Normal
A. Hallux valgus	43 degrees	6 degrees	(n = 9–17)
B. 1-2 Intermetatarsal angle	15	6	(n = 9–5)
C. Metatarsus primus varus angle	19	11	(n = 18)

only necessary for those causing mechanical problems. Valgus tilt of the ankle is well tolerated.

Camptodactyly of the toes (curly toes) is usually mild and does not progress to severe deformity. With severe deformity, tenotomy of the long flexor tendon is usually satisfactory.

Infection

Foot infections may result from heel puncture in the neonate, hematogenous-seeding, or from puncture wounds. All these causes are unusual and have in common a delay in diagnosis, local signs of infection with absence of early systemic systems, and usually an elevation in sedimentation rate. In other ways there are significant differences between these patient groups.

The most common age of involvement for the hematogenous and the puncture wound groups is about 11 years. The posteroinferior portion of the os calcis most commonly is involved in the heel puncture and hematogenous patients, whereas the rays are most commonly involved in puncture wounds. Trauma is not usually a factor in hematogenous patients. Puncture wounds are fairly common in children, and problems are usually prevented by the usual treatment of wound toilet, tetanus prophylaxis, and an antibiotic against gram-positive organisms. However, 3 to 15 percent develop an infection which is almost always caused by *Pseudomonas aeruginosa.* The source of the infecting organism is not known, but it does not appear to be a result of inoculation of normal skin flora. In heel puncture and hematogenous patients, *Staphylococcus aureus* is the most common infecting organism.

Treatment for heel puncture and hematogenous infections involves appropriate parenteral antibiotics with incision and drainage if response is not prompt or if there is evidence of soft-tissue or bony abscess. Treatment of puncture wounds infected with Pseudomonas requires thorough surgical debridement and curettage of all infected tissue, including involved cartilage and bone, followed by usually 10 to 14 days of sensitivity-based parenteral anti-Pseudomonas antibiotic therapy. Staphylococci also may be present requiring addition of a penicillinase-resistant anti-staphylococcal antibiotic.

Trauma

Fractures and Dislocations In children under 10 years of age, rotational trauma of the lower leg usually results in tibia and fibula fractures, whereas in older children ankle fractures are more frequent. By far the most common ankle fractures are either supination-adduction or supination-eversion (external rotation) injuries. The former results in transverse fracture of the lateral malleolus and/or tear of the lateral anterior talofibular and calcaneofibular ligaments, plus/minus fracture of the medial malleolus. As a group, the latter (supination-eversion injuries) are more troublesome and have received the most attention recently.

There are four stages of a *supination-eversion* injury. In stage 1 there is fracture of the anterior lateral corner of the distal tibial epiphysis (Tillaux fragment) at the site of insertion of the anterior tibiofibular ligament. Stage 2

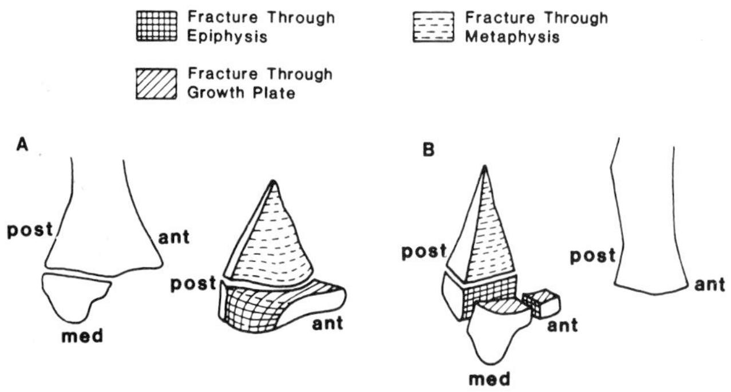

Figure 5: Diagram shows three-dimensional configuration of two different triplane fractures viewed anterior medially. (A) Two-fragment fracture. Note the curved shape of the epiphyseal fracture. (B) Four-fragment fracture. (Reprinted with permission from Computed tomography of intra-articular supination: Eversion fractures of the ankle in adolescents, by J. Kärrholm, et al., J. Pediat. Orthop. I:186, 1981.)

includes periosteal detachment of the distal tibia superior to the anterior tibiofibular ligament and may include physeal fracture of the distal fibula. In stage 3, the so-called triplane fracture, there may be two to four fragments (Fig. 5). In stage 4, the distal fibular metaphysis is fractured.

Treatment consists of a nonweight-bearing, long-leg cast with the foot in internal rotation. Most do not require reduction or can be adequately reduced manually. In approximately 10 percent, displacement of more than 2 mm persists, and open reduction is indicated.

Fractures of the talar neck can be overlooked in children and become apparent only after the onset of osteonecrosis. Revascularization occurs, but the patient should be kept nonweight-bearing during healing.

In *tarsometatarsal joint injuries*, the focus is on the base of the second metatarsal which is fractured and displaced. Closed reduction with percutaneous pin fixation to secure the reduction, which is usually unstable, is almost always adequate.

Bicycle spoke fractures may result in a displaced varus and anteriorly angulated buckle fracture of the distal tibia and fibula. In motorcycle spoke injuries, there is more likely to be avulsion of the heel.

Because of its proximity to the nail matrix, a Salter-Harris type I *epiphyseal fracture of the distal phalanx of the large toe* frequently may be open. If so, there is blood at the edge of the cuticle. Prophylactic antibiotics are probably indicated.

Amputations Partial traumatic foot amputations in children occur most commonly following lawn mower injuries. Length and epiphyses should be preserved as much as possible. If the amputation is through the Chopart joint, equinus may develop requiring revision to a Syme's amputation (see Section 8, General: Amputations and Prosthetics). The possibility of reimplantation should be kept in mind for those unusual situations when the amputation is "clean."

Soft Tissue Tendon and sensory nerve injuries about the ankle and foot should be repaired primarily, except for the long extensors and flexors of the toes, which do not require repair. However, following flexor digitorum longus laceration, the toe should be splinted in a functional position during healing to avoid late hyperextension deformity.

Neuromuscular Disease

Cerebral Palsy Ankle equinus is the major ankle and foot problem for cerebral palsy patients. Because of the difficulties of assessment, surgery is generally not recommended until the patient has been followed for some time.

Selection of surgical management and postoperative care remain controversial. The main surgical choices are Achilles tendon lengthening (TAL) or gastrocnemius lengthening. The Silfverskiöld test, positive when ankle dorsiflexion increases to normal or more with knee flexion, has been used to select patients for selective gastrocnemius lengthening. Its accuracy has been questioned, and recent reports suggest that TAL is more reliable with fewer recurrences. Recurrence seems to depend more upon the pathophysiology of the muscle than on the type of lengthening performed. The muscles may be short, spastic, or both; the differentiation is difficult to make. However, in most patients there is shortening to some extent, and in this group recurrence is quite likely. In addition to recurrence, complications include overlengthening which results in a calcaneus deformity. Thus, the ankle should be placed in only 5 to 10 degrees of dorsiflexion postoperatively and a long-leg cast applied with the knee in extension. Finally, lengthening of the Achilles tendon should not be performed on patients who have no active push-off as this will encourage a crouched gait.

Whether or not to prescribe postoperative night bracing and physical therapy until puberty is controversial but would certainly seem to be desirable in recurrent cases.

In addition to equinus, there may be either subtalar varus or valgus. The varus may be due to spasm of the triceps surae or of the posterior tibial tendon or both. If due to posterior tibial spasticity, the deformity will be present without weight-bearing. Tenotomy has not produced consistently satisfactory results. Transfer through the interosseous membrane is most likely to be satisfactory if the posterior tibial muscle is active in swing phase. Z-lengthening has been more satisfactory, although overcorrection or recurrence occasionally has occurred. For these reasons, split posterior tibial transfer, performed at the time of TAL, is being evaluated as a means of balancing the foot.

Extra-articular arthrodesis has been satisfactory in managing subtalar valgus, and late triple arthrodesis has been avoided. However, significant residual deformity exists, the longitudinal arch does not develop, and the results have not been as satisfactory as had been desired. Malposition is a common cause of failure, and internal fixation with a talocalcaneal positioning screw is being utilized more frequently. The proper position is 5 degrees of subtalar valgus.

Hallux valgus is a developmental deformity in the valgus foot. Management is difficult but includes correction and stabilization of the subtalar joint followed by realignment of the first ray. (See preceding discussion of hallux valgus.)

Hallux flexis, a sagittal plane deformity, may occur alone or in conjunction with hallux valgus. If the metatarsophalangeal cartilage is intact, muscle balance should be restored, but, if not, first metatarsophalangeal arthrodesis is recommended.

Triple arthrodesis is indicated for the older child with fixed deformity. Success is correlated with correction of the deformity, and skeletal fixation with either Steinmann pins or staples is preferable to cast immobilization alone.

Poliomyelitis Long-term results continue to become available for the various treatments provided for deformities secondary to poliomyelitis.

Calcaneocavus is a progressive disabling deformity resulting from weakness of the triceps surae muscles. Orthotic management is not successful. Between the ages of 5 and 12 years, a two- or three-stage operation is necessary. It consists of: (1) stabilization of the hindfoot by extra-articular subtalar arthrodesis; (2) correction of calcaneus deformity by displacement osteotomy and plantar release; and (3) muscle transfers as necessary to balance the foot. In children over 12 years of age, the steps are corrective triple arthrodesis and appropriate tendon transfer.

Ankle arthrodesis is a time-honored procedure with many technical pitfalls, the most common being pseudarthrosis and poor joint position. Intraoperative radiographs are recommended to identify technical faults. The transfibular arthrodesis has been associated with a high failure rate. Another common cause of failure is subtalar pain. This may be the result of excessive equinus, disruption of the subtalar joint at the time of ankle arthrodesis, or preoperative disease of the subtalar joint. In the growing child, the distraction compression bone graft arthrodesis with iliac-crest bone graft interposition (Chuinard) has been especially successful. Preservation of distal epiphyseal growth has been confirmed.

The extra-articular subtalar arthrodesis (Grice) was designed for subtalar valgus deformity occurring after poliomyelitis and has been most successful when used for this indication. Failure is most commonly related to overcorrection into varus, loss of position due to displacement or resorption of the graft postoperatively, or development of ankle valgus.

Myelomeningocele It has been shown experimentally that normal levels of repetitive mechanical stress are more likely to cause plantar ulceration in the denervated foot than the normal foot. Thus, in these patients it is especially important to maintain plantigrade feet and good skin hygiene and to provide custom-made insoles of a foam material with memory such as Plastazote.

The most common deformities are paralytic equinovarus in the young child and subtalar and ankle valgus and ankle calcaneus in the older child.

Lasting correction of paralytic equinovarus with nonoperative methods cannot be expected, but control of the magnitude of the deformity can be achieved. One-stage posterior medial release has been successful with failures primarily related to technical problems. (See preceding discussion of idiopathic equinovarus.) Because of the paralysis, long-term position control is necessary.

Progressive subtalar valgus may be associated with growth and ambulation. If caused by spastic peroneals, tenotomy is indicated. It is often accompanied by ankle valgus with associated pressure ulceration over the medial malleolus. Correction of subtalar valgus alone is not successful if there is associated ankle valgus. Both deformities can be evaluated radiographically. Ankle valgus is related to fibular shortening which is, at least partially, due to paralysis of the soleus. In addition, there is usually increased ankle dorsiflexion. If the fibula shortening is less than 10 mm, Achilles tendon tenodesis to the fibula is indicated. If ankle valgus is greater than this, supramalleolar tibia and fibula valgus correction osteotomy is indicated (Fig. 6).

If the patient has calcaneus deformity and a grade 4 or 5 tibialis anterior tendon, transfer through the interosseous membrane combined with Achilles tenodesis may improve gait. This result may be further improved by ankle-foot orthotic support.

Except for low-level sacral paraplegics, these patients perform best with ankle-foot orthoses. This provides alignment control, sensory feedback from skin below the knee, and partial load transfer to the leg.

Muscular Dystrophy Progressive paralytic equinovarus is an important reason for premature gait deterioration in patients with Duchenne muscular dystrophy. Properly timed, posterior tibial tendon transfer through the interosseous membrane to the lateral cuneiform can add an average of 3 years functional ambulation and is, therefore,

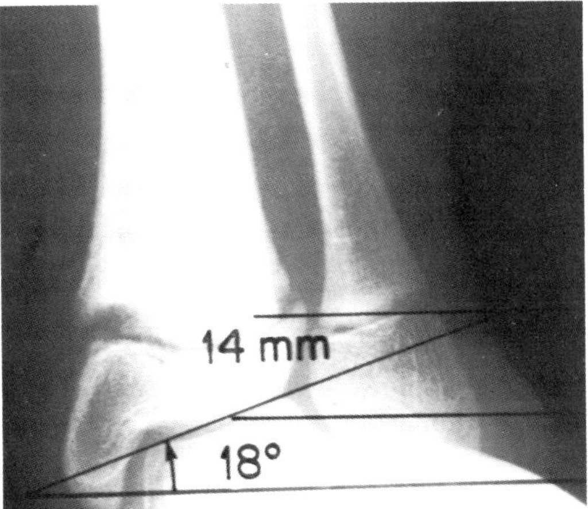

Figure 6-A

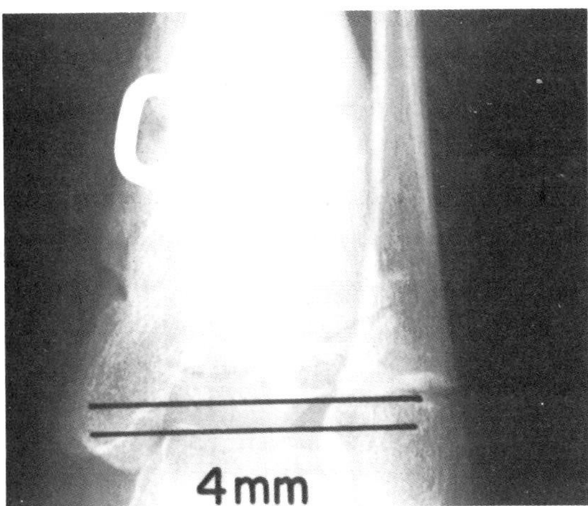

Figure 6-B

Figure 6: (A) Standing preoperative anteroposterior angle radiograph of a 9-year, 10-month-old girl with lumbar, four-level paraplegia. Fibular shortening and ankle valgus are demonstrated. (B) Comparable standing postoperative supramalleolar tibial and fibular osteotomy radiograph of the same patient demonstrating deformity correction.

a useful procedure. Sometimes Achilles tendon lengthening is necessary as well.

Degenerative Neuropathy Charcot-Marie-Tooth disease is the most common disease in this category and usually is associated with a progressive claw toe and cavus deformity. Triple arthrodesis at maturity often is necessary to correct the deformity. During the growing years, plantar fasciotomy, long toe extensor transfer to the metatarsal necks with PIP fusion, and posterior tibial tendon transfer through the interosseous membrane to the lateral cuneiform (if the muscle is active in swing phase) may help to retard the development of the deformity.

ANNOTATED BIBLIOGRAPHY

General

Coleman, S.S.: Complex foot deformities in children. Philadelphia, Lea & Febiger, 1983.

An illustrated text discussing the etiology and pathogenesis, symptomatology, natural history, and primary and salvage treatment options for idiopathic equinovarus, congenital vertical talus, cavovarus, calcaneocavus, severe flatfoot, and paralytic and teratogenic deformities.

Congenital and Developmental

Congenital Ball-and-Socket Ankle

Pappas, A.M., and Miller, J.T.: Congenital ball-and-socket ankle joints and related lower-extremity malformations. J. Bone Joint Surg. 64A:672-679, 1982.

Of fifty-one patients, fifty were followed because of congenital shortening of the lower extremity, and thirty had some degree of osseous coalition. None were symptomatic.

Accessory Navicular (Os Tibiale Externum)

Sullivan, J.A., and Miller, W.A.: The relationship of the accessory navicular to the development of the flat foot. Clin. Orthop. 144:233-237, 1979.

Accessory navicular does not appear to correlate with an increased incidence of flatfoot. Simple excision of the ossicle is adequate when nonoperative management fails.

Vertical Talus

Adelaar, R.S.; Williams, R.M.; and Gould, J.S.: Congenital convex pes valgus: Results of an early comprehensive release and a review of congenital vertical talus at Richmond Crippled Children's Hospital and the University of Alabama in Birmingham. Foot Ankle 1:62-73, 1980.

Results of nonoperative treatment were poor in twelve of twelve feet. Comprehensive release resulted in ten satisfactory and five poor results. Poor results were associated with operation after 3½ years of age, arthrogryposis, cerebral palsy, and plantar diastasis of the calcaneocuboid joint.

Idiopathic Equinovarus

Cowell, H.R., and Wein, B.K.: Current concepts review. Genetic aspects of club foot. J. Bone Joint Surg. 62A:1381-1384, 1980.

Idiopathic talipes equinovarus is the result of a multifactorial inheritance system modified by environmental factors. Male risk is greater because of a lower gene threshold number.

Crawford, A.H.; Marxen, J.L.; and Osterfeld, D.L.: The Cincinnati incision: A comprehensive approach for surgical procedures of the foot and ankle in childhood. J. Bone Joint Surg. 64A:1355-1358, 1982.

A satisfactory experience using a transverse incision at the level of the tibiotalar joint in ninety-nine patients (154 feet) with a variety of problems is described.

Gray, D.H., and Katz, J.M.: A histochemical study of muscle in club foot. J. Bone Joint Surg. 63B:417-423, 1981.

The muscle structure was normal except for a reduction in muscle fiber numbers in the calf and an increase in type I fiber in the soleus (61 percent compared to 44.3 percent normal).

Ippolito, E., and Ponseti, I.V.: Congenital club foot in the human fetus. A histological study. J. Bone Joint Surg. 62A:8-22, 1980.

Pathologic anatomy was demonstrated in five clubfeet and compared to three normals. Soft-tissue alterations were posterior and medial and included ligament shortening and thickening, muscle atrophy, and increased fibrous connective tissue. The tarsal bones were altered in shape, size, and relationships.

Karube, S.; Shoji, H.; D'Ambrosia, R.; Roberts, J.; Bruns, J.; Zimmy, M.; and Willig, S.: Biochemical and ultrastructural observation of soft tissue changes in clubfeet. Trans. Orthop. Res. Soc. 6:235, 1981.

Connective tissue at the tibiotalonavicular junction demonstrated increase in type 3 collagen and the presence of mast and myofibroblast-like cells.

McKay, D.W.: New concept of and approach to clubfoot treatment: Section I—Principles and morbid anatomy. J. Pediat. Orthop. 2:347-356, 1982.

Based on operative material, the concept is presented that the major deformity is the inward rotation and varus angulation of the whole foot on the talus, with the os calcis pivoting on the interosseous ligaments.

Ryöppy, S., and Sairanen, H.: Neonatal operative treatment of club foot. A preliminary report. J. Bone Joint Surg. 65B:320-325, 1983.

Minimum 2-year follow-up of sixty-four patients (eighty-nine feet) operated upon between 1974 and 1979 using an operative technique under development since 1959. Ninety percent (eighty feet) were satisfactory after the primary treatment, although nine feet required one or more additional operations. Of the 10 percent (nine feet) with unsatisfactory results, all but one foot became satisfactory after secondary treatment.

Turco, V.J.: Resistant congenital club foot—One-stage posteromedial release with internal fixation: A follow-up report of a 15-year experience. J. Bone Joint Surg. 61A:805-814, 1979.

The results were excellent or good in 83 percent and failed in 5 percent of 149 feet. Loss of correction was associated with operative age of less than 1 year, no pin fixation, and effective cast immobilization of less than 4 months. Overcorrection was associated with complete release of the talocalcaneal interosseous ligament and lateral displacement of the navicular.

Cavovarus

Jahss, M.H.: Tarsometatarsal truncated-wedge arthrodesis for pes cavus and equinovarus deformity of the fore part of the foot. J. Bone Joint Surg. 62A:713-722, 1980.

The operation was performed on thirty-four feet in twenty-five skeletally mature patients, mostly between ages 16 and 19 years. Its advantages are avoidance of the subtalar joint and selective correction of deformity combinations.

Paulos, L.; Coleman, S.S.; and Samuelson, K.M.: Pes cavovarus: Review of a surgical approach using selective soft-tissue procedures. J. Bone Joint Surg. 62A:942-953, 1980.

The deformity is defined as a plantar-flexed first ray resulting in forefoot pronation. Treatment is based on the flexibility of the deformity. Twenty patients, average age 7 years (6 months to 15 years), obtained 85 percent acceptable results in twenty-seven feet followed 2 years or more.

Sherman, F., and Westin, G.: Plantar release in the correction of deformities of the foot in childhood. J. Bone Joint Surg. 63A:1382-1389, 1981.

Residual cavovarus from clubfoot or poliomyelitis was treated by plantar release followed by serial casts. The technique improved forefoot adduction and cavus but improved equinus only in paralytics. Subtalar alignment remained unchanged. The operation was contraindicated in the presence of calcaneus deformity.

Watanabe, R.; Hillman, D.; and Brummett, S.: Metatarsal

osteotomy for cavus foot. AAOS Videotape 44, 1981.

Pes cavus is considered to be a problem of forefoot plantar flexion. Satisfactory results were obtained in 81 percent of thirty-eight feet treated by plantar fasciotomy, first metatarsal and sometimes two to five metatarsal osteotomies and toe extensor tenotomies with PIP resection and fibrous ankylosis.

Tarsal Coalition

Chambers, R.B.; Cook, T.M.; and Cowell, H.R.: Surgical reconstruction for calcaneonavicular coalition. Evaluation of function and gait. J. Bone Joint Surg. 64A:829-836, 1982.

Nineteen patients with thirty-one involved feet were analyzed 3 to 14 years postoperatively. All had pain preoperatively, and none did postoperatively. Function correlated with subtalar motion and was normal when motion was good.

Metatarsus Adductus

Bleck, E.E.: Metatarsus adductus: Classification and relationship to outcomes of treatment. J. Pediat. Orthop. 3:2-9, 1983.

Retrospective study of 160 children with 265 involved feet (259 treated) followed for more than 12 months. Plaster cast treatment was most effective if begun before age 8 months. Severity and flexibility did not seem to effect the treatment outcome.

Rushforth, G.F.: The natural history of hooked forefoot. J. Bone Joint Surg. 60B:530-532, 1978.

Of 130 feet in eighty-three children followed an average of 7 years, 86 percent satisfactorily resolved without treatment and 4 percent remained deformed and stiff. Resistant cases could not be detected before age 4 years. The deformity is not always apparent at birth, although the most severe ones are.

Hallux Valgus

Gottschalk, F.A.B.; Beighton, P.H.; and Solomon, L.: The prevalence of hallux valgus in three South African populations. South African Med. J. 60:655-656, 1981.

The hallux angle is less for young white than for black girls. However, by age 10 years, the angle is significantly greater for the white girls, a difference that increased throughout the second decade of life. It is postulated that the wearing of closed-toe shoes may be partially responsible.

Helal, B.: Surgery for adolescent hallux valgus. Clin. Orthop. 157:50-63, 1981.

An analysis of the results of several British orthopaedic surgeons reveals the best results following the Wilson (shaft) osteotomy, 94 percent; Golden (base) osteotomy, 91 percent; and Mitchell (neck) osteotomy, 80 percent. The fewest satisfactory results followed soft-tissue procedures such as McBride (46 percent) and Joplin (60 percent).

Houghton, G.R., and Dickson, R.A.: Hallux valgus in the younger patient: The structural abnormality. J. Bone Joint Surg. 61B:176-177, 1979.

The frontal plane bony alignment was determined from the standing anteroposterior radiographs of fifteen normal young adults. The hallux angle was 16.7 degrees, the first-second intermetatarsal angle 9.5 degrees, and the metatarsus primus varus 18.1 degrees.

Miscellaneous

Browning, W.H., and McKinnon, B.: Camptodactyly of the toes: A simple surgical treatment. Foot Ankle 1:291, 1981.

This abstract describes the indications and results of long toe flexor tenotomy in eight patients (fifteen feet, forty toes).

Jahss, M.H., and Olives, R.: The foot and ankle in multiple hereditary exostoses. Foot Ankle 1:128-142, 1980.

Epiphyseal disturbance resulted in ankle valgus, shortened metatarsals, and angular deformities of the metatarsal. Mechanical problems related to the exostoses resulting in localized tenderness, synostosis of the medial subtalar facet, and asymptomatic lower tibial fibular synostosis. Surgery was only necessary for exostosis producing local tenderness.

Williams, G.A., and Cowell, H.R.: Köhler's disease of the tarsal navicular. Clin. Orthop. 158:53-58, 1981.

Sixteen males (average presentation age of 6 years, 2 months) and four females (average age 4 years, 6 months) were reviewed. Treatment with a short-leg walking cast for 8 weeks decreased symptom duration from 15 to 3.2 months.

Infection

Canale, S.T., and Manugian, A.H.: Neonatal osteomyelitis of the os calcis: A complication of repeated heel punctures. Clin. Orthop. 156:178-182, 1981.

Three neonates developed osteomyelitis of the right heel, possibly secondary to heel punctures. All had a swollen lower extremity, and extension to proximal areas may occur. Treatment is with appropriate antibiotics and surgical drainage if response is not prompt.

Jacobs, R.F.; Adelman, L.; Sack, C.M.; and Wilson, C.B.: Management of Pseudomonas osteochondritis complicating puncture wounds of the foot. Pediatrics 69:432-435, 1982.

Thirteen patients with an average age of 11.2 years (6-16) and an average duration of symptoms of 6 days (2-21) were studied. All responded to thorough surgical debridement and curettage of necrotic and infected tissue, including cartilage and bone and 10.8 days (5-14) of anti-Pseudomonas antibiotic therapy. Anti-Pseudomonas antibiotic therapy without debridement or with soft-tissue debridement alone was not successful.

Morrey, B.F.; Bianco, A.J.; and Rhodes, K.H.: Hematogenous osteomyelitis at uncommon sites in children. Mayo Clin. Proc. 53:707-713, 1978.

Of twenty patients, the os calcis was involved in four. Patient age was 11 to 13 years, delay in treatment was 2 to 24 weeks, and *Staphylococcus aureus* was isolated in all four. Treatment consisted of parenteral antibiotics and incision and drainage of soft-tissue or bony abscess.

Trauma

Kärrholm, J.; Hansson, L.I.; and Laurin, S.: Supination-eversion injuries of the ankle in children: A retrospective study of radiographic classification and treatment. J. Pediat. Orthop. 2:147-159, 1982.

Of 457 ankle fractures in children up to 18 years of age, 176 (39 percent) were supination-eversion injuries. These included the juvenile Tillaux fracture and "triplane" fractures. Open reduction was performed in 10 percent.

Letts, R.M., and Gibeault, D.: Fractures of the neck of the talus in children. Foot Ankle 1:74-77, 1980.

Of twelve patients ranging in age from 1 year, 7 months to 13 years, 11 months, none had significant displacement. Three developed osteonecrosis of the body and in two of these the fracture was not recognized until osteonecrosis became radiographically apparent.

Pinckney, L.E.; Currarino, G.; and Kennedy, L.A.: The stubbed great toe: A cause of occult compound fracture and infection. Radiology 138:375-377, 1981.

Four children with Salter-Harris type I fracture of the distal phalanx of the great toe developed infection caused by Staphylococcus in three and Staph plus Enterobacter in the other. Prophylactic antibiotic treatment for this injury is recommended.

Roffman, M.; Moshel, M.; and Mendes, D.G.: Bicycle spoke fracture. Clin. Orthop. 144:230-232, 1979.

Of twenty-nine children, five had a nondisplaced varus anteriorly angulated fracture of the distal tibia and fibula. Healing was uneventful.

Wicks, M.H.; Harbison, J.S.; and Paterson, D.C.: Tendon injuries about the foot and ankle in children. Australian New Zealand J. Surg. 50:158-161, 1980.

In sixty-four patients, the Achilles tendon was involved in one-third and sensory nerves were frequently severed. Early repair yielded good results and late repair was less satisfactory. The long extensors and flexors of the toes did not require repair.

Wiley, J.J.: Tarso-metatarsal joint injuries in children. J. Pediat. Orthop. 1:255-260, 1981.

The mechanism of injury was landing in the "tip toe" position in ten, heel to toe compression in three, and backward fall with pinned forefoot in four. Fracture of the second metatarsal base was the distinguishing feature.

Neuromuscular Disease

Cerebral Palsy

Goldner, J.L.: Hallux valgus and hallux flexus associated with cerebral palsy: Analysis and treatment. Clin. Orthop. 157:98-104, 1980.

This combined developmental deformity was usually seen in equinovalgus feet with: (1) weak extensor hallucis longus; or (2) over-pull of the tibialis anterior; and/or (3) spasticity or contracture of the flexor hallucis longus or brevis. It was not from a weak peroneus longus.

Gräbe, R.P., and Thompson, P.: Lengthening of the Achilles tendon in cerebral paresis: Basic principles and follow-up study. South African Med. J. 56:993-996, 1979.

Fifty children had eighty lengthenings at an average age of 7.5 years with an average follow-up of 4.5 years. Results were good in 87 percent, and nine children had postoperative improvement of scissor gait without adductor surgery. Night AFO's were utilized until puberty.

Green, N.; Griffin, P.; and Shiavi, R.: Split posterior tibial tendon transfer in cerebral palsy. J. Bone Joint Surg. 65A:748-754, 1983.

Sixteen children between ages 4.5 and 10 years with equinovarus and a posterior tibial muscle active in both swing and stance phase were treated. Fifteen had concurrent sliding heel cord lengthening and two had calcaneal osteotomies. After 3 or more years, all had a heel toe or flat foot gait without recurrence of deformity.

Holstein, A.: Hallux valgus—An acquired deformity of the foot in cerebral palsy. Foot Ankle 1:33-38, 1980.

Thirty ambulatory patients were studied. Feet in equinovalgus all developed hallux valgus. Hallux valgus did not develop in equinovarus feet but did follow varus overcorrection associated with posterior tibial lengthening.

Keats, P.: Extra-articular subtalar fusion in cerebral palsy: Long-term clinical x-ray follow-up. Foot Ankle 2:357-358, 1982. (Abstract)

Nineteen patients had thirty-five feet operated at an average age of 4.8 years. Feet were not painful, and triple arthrodesis had been avoided. Twelve feet had significant residual deformity, and a longitudinal arch did not develop.

Lee, C.L., and Bleck, E.E.: Surgical correction of equinus deformity in cerebral palsy. Devel. Med. Child Neurol. 22:287-292, 1980.

Extremities with a positive Silfverskiöld test (fifty-one) had gastrocnemius lengthening and those with a negative test (seventy-one) had Achilles tendon lengthening. The recurrence rate was 29 percent for the first group and 9 percent for the second group. Neither group had postoperative bracing or heel cord stretching.

Truscelli, D.; Lespargot, A.; and Tardieu, G.: Variation in the long-term results of elongation of the tendoachillis in children with cerebral palsy. J. Bone Joint Surg. 61B:466-469, 1979.

Short muscles without spasticity (forty-three) were temporarily improved, but equinus deformity recurred. Results for short spastic muscles (forty-one) were variable and depended upon the balance between dorsiflexion and plantar flexion spasm. Spastic muscles (forty-one) results were unpredictable.

Poliomyelitis

Bradley, G.M., and Coleman, S.S.: Treatment of the calcaneocavus foot deformity. J. Bone Joint Surg. 63A:1159-1166, 1981.

The deformity develops from a neural disorder causing weakness of the triceps surae muscles. Staged surgical management is necessary, the details depending upon patient age, deformity severity, the underlying neurological disorder, and the pattern of muscle imbalance.

Lance, E.M.; Pavel, A.; Fries, I.; Larsen, I.; and Patterson, R.L., Jr.: Arthrodesis of the ankle joint. A follow-up study. Clin. Orthop. 142:146-158, 1979.

Of 183 patients, 75 were under 16 years of age and most had had poliomyelitis. Unsatisfactory results (25 percent) were usually the result of nonunion which was associated with neurologic disorder and technical shortcoming.

Southwell, R.B., and Sherman, F.C.: Triple arthrodesis: A long-term study with force plate analysis. Foot Ankle 2:15-24, 1981.

Results were satisfactory in 89 percent (good or ideal in 58 percent) and failed in 11 percent. Residual varus, calcaneovalgus and forefoot supination all resulted in painful feet. Use of skeletal fixation to avoid pseudarthrosis and position loss is supported.

Myelomeningocele

Banta, J.V.; Sutherland, D.H.; and Wyatt, M.: Anterior tibial transfer to the os calcis with Achilles tenodesis for calcaneal deformity in myelomeningocele. J. Pediat. Orthop. 1:125-130, 1981.

Both extremities in seven L5 or SI level paraplegics were treated. Gait analysis revealed improved function in all patients. Improvement was enhanced by the use of an ankle-foot orthosis.

Dias, L.S.: Ankle valgus in children with myelomeningocele. Devel. Med. Child Neurol. 20:627-633, 1978.

Normally the distal fibular growth plate is slightly proximal to the dome of the talus before age 5 years after which it moves to approximately 3 mm below. Shortening is related to age and soleus weakness and in eighty-six ankles ranged from 5 to 18 mm.

Manley, M.T., and Darby, T.: Repetitive mechanical stress and denervation in plantar ulcer pathogenesis in rats. Arch. Phys. Med. Rehab. 61:171-177, 1980.

Normal levels of repetitive mechanical stress caused plantar ulceration more readily in the denervated than the normal foot. Foot pad temperature during stimulation increased more in the normal than the denervated foot, suggesting better removal of the by-products of traumatized tissue.

Menelaus, M.B.: The orthopaedic management of spina bifida cystica. Ed. 2, pp. 92-118. New York, Churchill Livingstone, 1980.

To facilitate this comprehensive discussion, foot deformities were arranged into three groupings: Group A with varus, equinovarus, equinus, cavovarus, and internal tibial torsion deformities; Group B with calcaneus, calcaneovalgus, calcaneovarus, adductovalgus, and external tibial torsion deformities; and Group C, the miscellaneous group.

Muscular Dystrophy

Miller, G.M.; Hsu, J.D.; Hoffer, M.M.; and Rentfro, R.: Posterior tibial tendon transfer: A review of the literature and analysis of 44 procedures. J. Pediat. Orthop. 2:363-370, 1982.

Results were most satisfactory in patients with Duchenne muscular dystrophy and least satisfactory in idiopathic equinovarus. In cerebral spastic patients, satisfactory results correlated with the presence of swing phase activity of the posterior tibialis muscle.

39 ANKLE AND FOOT: TRAUMA

Subjects in this section include Achilles tendon injuries, ankle sprains, and fractures and dislocations of the foot.

Ankle Joint

Achilles Tendinitis and Partial Tendon Rupture Achilles tendinitis presents with a vague but well-localized pain in the Achilles tendon. Poor training habits may produce this condition in a runner. Tendinitis may result if the runner trains in shoes with heels lower than street shoes or competes in shoes with heels lower than the training shoes. Regardless of etiology, an increased stress on the Achilles tendon initiates the problem. On physical examination, tenderness along the course of the tendon and limited dorsiflexion are noted. Treatment should be directed toward reducing inflammation, reducing the excess pull on the Achilles tendon, and increasing flexibility of the gastrocsoleus complex. Specific management includes oral anti-inflammatory medication, 3-cm heel lift, and heel cord stretching three times a day by either backing away from a wall or walking downstairs backward.

Partial rupture of the Achilles tendon often occurs suddenly as the result of a load increase on the tendon in young, skeletally mature individuals. The patient complains of a sharp stabbing pain in the lower calf (distinctly different from the ache of tendinitis). The gait is antalgic, and an intensely painful area of irregular thickening of the Achilles tendon can be detected. If the diagnosis is in doubt after an examination, ultrasonography can be helpful by demonstrating decreased echoes in the area of partial rupture.

Bursography demonstrating encroachment of the retroachilles bursa into the Achilles tendon may help with diagnosis. Nonoperative treatment should be attempted first with icing, strapping, and a heel lift. Steroid injection should be avoided because of the possibility of masking symptoms which might allow complete rupture to occur. If this program does not relieve symptoms, surgical repair is indicated.

A standard posteromedial skin incision exposes the defect at the site of injury. The peritenon is incised longitudinally, thus freeing the tendon dorsally and ventrally. All granulation tissue and devitalized tendon should be excised. The gap is sutured side-to-side with synthetic absorbable sutures. The repair can be augmented by transferring the plantaris into the defect and suturing it to the distal end of the rupture. Postoperatively, the patient should wear a short-leg walking cast with the foot in moderate plantar flexion for 3 weeks. This is followed by a short-leg walking cast with the foot in neutral position for another 3 weeks. A heel lift should be used for the first 3 months after casting is discontinued.

Achilles Tendon Rupture Complete rupture of the Achilles tendon most commonly occurs during the third to fifth decades of life. The patients often report hearing a loud pop and feeling a sudden, sharp pain near the heel. Often they try to continue walking and delay seeking medical attention. The diagnosis may be missed in as many as 20 to 25 percent of the patients unless a high level of suspicion is maintained. Although patients limp, palpation of a tendon defect may be obscured by the presence of blood within the tendon sheath. Careful observation reveals that the patient with complete rupture will plantar flex the ankle by leading with plantar flexion of the great toe. By maintaining the great toe in neutral, the examiner can block plantar flexion of the ankle.

The "squeeze test" remains the definitive test for complete rupture of the Achilles tendon. During examination, the patient should lie prone or kneel on a chair. The examiner squeezes the patient's calf in the middle third, just below the place of widest girth. The examiner's hand should be distal to the apex of the curve of the soleus since a normal ankle does not plantar flex when compressed proximal to the apex of the soleus curve. Failure of plantar flexion of the ankle when the calf is squeezed signifies a complete rupture.

Treatment of complete ruptures should be individualized. A recent prospective study used a protocol that divided a group of patients with complete ruptures between nonoperative and operative treatments. Plantar flexion power was reduced in both groups. Despite apparently less power in the group treated by cast immobilization, Cybex testing failed to reveal a statistically significant difference in plantar flexion power between the two groups. The incidence of tendon rerupture was 8 percent in the cast immobilization group, compared to 4 percent in the operated group. Because of the lesser morbidity and lower cost, the study concluded that nonsurgical treatment was preferable.

However, when treating a competitive athlete by cast immobilization, reapproximation of the ruptured ends of the tendon should be documented under fluoroscopic control to achieve the best results. Five ml of contrast medium are injected into the tear gap. After exercising the ankle, the patient rests the foot on a chair with the ankle at 90 degrees. The calf is wrapped with an elastic wrap from the knee down to force the retracted upper end of the tendon distally. If the tendon ends are opposed, as verified by fluoroscopic examination, nonoperative treatment should be successful. If not opposed, the patient will lose strength and push-off power and be at a higher risk of rerupture. In the competitive athlete, surgical repair is justified in most instances.

Ankle Sprains Ankle sprains are frequent injuries and can be divided into anterior capsular, medial eversion, and lateral sprains.

Anterior Capsular Sprain When a player performs a hook-slide in baseball or suffers an impact on a plantar flexed ankle in football, the anterior capsule may tear. Examination reveals pain on resisted dorsiflexion and passive plantar flexion. A long course of rehabilitation is required to restore full function.

Medial Eversion Sprain External rotation and abduction at the ankle produce a medial eversion sprain. Continuation of the force can tear the syndesmosis. Stress radiographs should be taken if there is tenderness along the anterior tibiofibular ligament and tenderness medially to determine if a diastasis of the syndesmosis has occurred. If the deltoid ligament has ruptured completely, it can be trapped between the talus and tibia, widening the ankle mortise. Surgical repair is necessary.

Lateral Sprain A lateral ankle sprain is the most common type. Because the talus normally adducts during walking and the lateral ligaments are weaker, a patient is more inclined to invert than evert. These sprains often occur when walking or running on an irregular surface. A tight heel cord predisposes to a lateral sprain by forcing the foot into inversion and turning the foot under. Most lateral sprains involve the anterior talofibular ligament. A careful history of the mechanism of injury can help diagnose more severe ligament disruptions. Total inversion of the ankle, in which the plane of the sole of the foot is parallel with the sagittal plane of the tibia and the lateral border of the foot is flush with the ground, accompanied by an audible or palpable pop, probably signifies disruption of both anterior talofibular and calcaneofibular ligaments. The posterior talofibular ligament rarely is injured.

Measuring talar tilt radiographically in plantar flexion and dorsiflexion can help determine the integrity of the anterior talofibular ligament and calcaneofibular ligament, respectively. A wide range of "normal" tilt measurements exists. However, tilting of the talus greater than 5 degrees may represent a significant injury to healthy young adult patients without a previous injury. In less active patients, who may have suffered previous injury but remain functionally normal, wider variability of talar tilt should be expected with a range up to 18 degrees at neutral and 13 degrees in plantar flexion. In these patients, an anterior drawer test of the ankle can be a more reliable indicator of injury to the lateral ligaments, particularly the anterior talofibular. Anterior shift greater than 3 mm probably represents a significant injury (Fig. 1).

A well-organized, practical approach to ankle sprains is available and provides safe guidelines for return to activity (Fig. 2).

Treatment of severe sprains should be individualized. Patients with lateral ankle sprains who show talar tilts of 5 degrees or more, have an anterior drawer greater than 3 mm, and are physically and athletically active are candidates for repair of their lateral ligaments.

Ankle Fractures Most ankle fractures occur when a force applied to the foot is transmitted through the talus displacing it beyond the normal elasticity of the ligaments of the ankle. If the force is in an axial direction, fractures of the tibial plafond (the so-called pilon fracture) with variable amounts of compression occur. If the force involves less axial load but more rotational movement of the talus on the tibia, malleolar fractures occur. The work by Lauge-Hansen remains the most definitive classification correlating mechanism of injury with anatomic structures involved (Fig. 3).

Diagnosis of fractures of the medial and lateral malleolus usually can be established on the basis of a careful physical examination. However, fractures of the posterior lip of the tibia are best confirmed by radiograph because

Figure 1-A

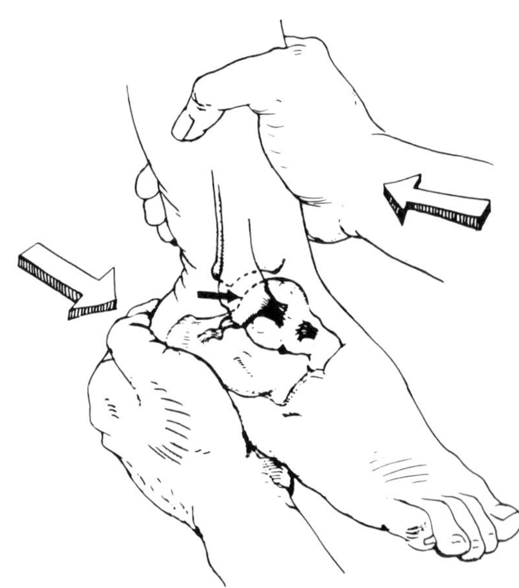

Figure 1-B

Figure 1: (A) Anterior draw sign test to evaluate the status of the anterior talofibular and calcaneofibular ligaments. (B) Positive anterior draw sign. (Reprinted with permission from Physical Examination of the Spine and Extremities, by S. Hoppenfeld, Chapter 8, pg. 222, Norwalk, Appleton-Century-Crofts, 1976.)

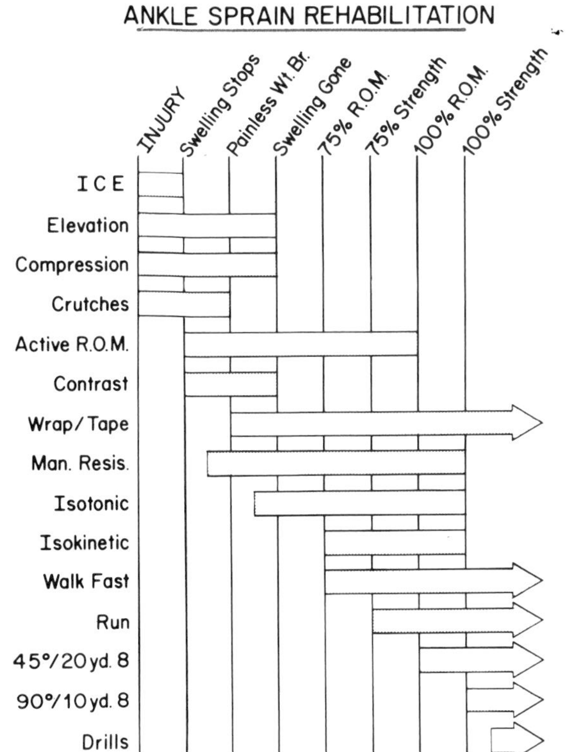

Figure 2: Treatment items. Ice: A minimum of 20 minutes of cold application (crushed ice) once every 4 waking hours. **Elevation:** Elevation at or above waist level of the injured part at all times when not actively using it, e.g., range of motion exercises, ambulation, etc. **Compression:** Elasticized stockinette over felt donut or horseshoe. **Crutches:** Nonweight-bearing or partial painless weight-bearing with a heel-toe gait. **Active ROM:** Having patient "write the alphabet" in letters as large as possible with forefoot. **Contrast:** Contrast baths (100 to 102 Fahrenheit and slush) at least three times daily. Range of motion exercise during the warm bath. **Wrap/Tape:** Louisiana wrap or ankle taping with all ambulation. **Man. Resis.:** Manual resistance in all planes of ankle and subtalar motion. **Isotonic:** Surgical tubing resistance in all planes of ankle and subtalar motion. **Isokinetic:** Cybex II reciprocal training in plantar-dorsiflexion and inversion-eversion. **Walk fast:** A nonlimping heel-toe gait. **Run:** Progression from jogging to running to sprinting. **45 degrees/20 yd. 8:** 45 degree cutting-turning both directions; figure 8 patterns with the total height of the 8 being 20 yards; going from jog to sprint speed. **90 degrees/10 yd. 8:** 90 degree cutting-turning both directions; figure 8 height of 10 yards; jog to sprint speed. **Drills:** Specific for sport in question.

Rehabilitation steps. Injury: Period from time of trauma to next stage ("swelling stops"). **Swelling stops:** Swelling no longer worsening. **Painless Wt. Br.:** Normal weight-bearing (slow), heel-toe gait with no limp. **Swelling gone:** No appreciable swelling. **75 percent ROM:** 75 percent painless motion (all planes) compared to uninjured ankle subtalar joint. **75 percent strength:** As estimated by manual resistance testing or documented by Cybex II test. **100 percent ROM:** Full motion equal to uninjured side. **100 percent Strength:** Equal to opposite side by manual resistance testing or Cybex II test. (Reprinted with permission from When can I? A practical approach to rehabilitation illustrated by treatment of an ankle injury, by J. Garrick, et al., Am. J. Sports Med. 9:68, 1981.)

of the overlying soft-tissue cover. Fractures of the medial malleolus with tenderness of the midshaft or proximal fibula may indicate a possible Dupuytren's or Masson-neiuve injury involving a diastasis of the distal tibiofibular syndesmosis. Examination of the mortise relationship, including comparison or stress radiographs is indicated. Similarly, a fracture of the lateral malleolus with tenderness medially over the deltoid ligament may indicate an unstable injury if the deltoid is torn completely. If no lateral shift of the talus is present, stress radiographs are indicated to determine the integrity of the deltoid ligament. Lateral shift of the talus greater than 2 mm probably indicates a torn deltoid.

The most satisfactory long-term results following treatment of displaced bimalleolar fractures are obtained by anatomical restoration. Displacement of fracture fragments of more than 2 mm, mortise widening of more than

	Description
Supination-eversion	
Stage	
1	Disruption of anterior tibiofibular ligament.
2	Oblique or short spiral fracture of lateral malleolus.
3	Fractured posterior lip of tibia.
4	Fractured medial malleolus or tear of deltoid ligament.
Supination-adduction	
Stage	
1	Transverse fracture of lateral malleolus or tear of fibular collateral ligaments.
2	Vertical fracture of medial malleolus at joint level.
Pronation-eversion	
Stage	
1	Fracture of medial malleolus or tear of deltoid ligament.
2	Disruption of anterior tibiofibular ligament and interosseous membrane.
3	Short oblique fracture of fibula 8 or more cm proximal to lateral malleolus.
4	Disruption of posterior tibiofibular ligament and fracture of posterior lip of tibia.
Pronation-abduction	
Stage	
1	Fracture of medial malleolus or tear of deltoid ligament.
2	Disruption of anterior and posterior tibiofibular ligaments.
3	Oblique fracture of lateral malleolus with comminution of the lateral cortex. This fracture is horizontal on the lateral view.
Pronation-dorsiflexion	
Stage	
1	Fracture of medial malleolus.
2	Fracture of tibial plafond.
3	Fracture of posterior lip of tibia.
4	High transverse or oblique fracture of fibula.

Figure 3-A

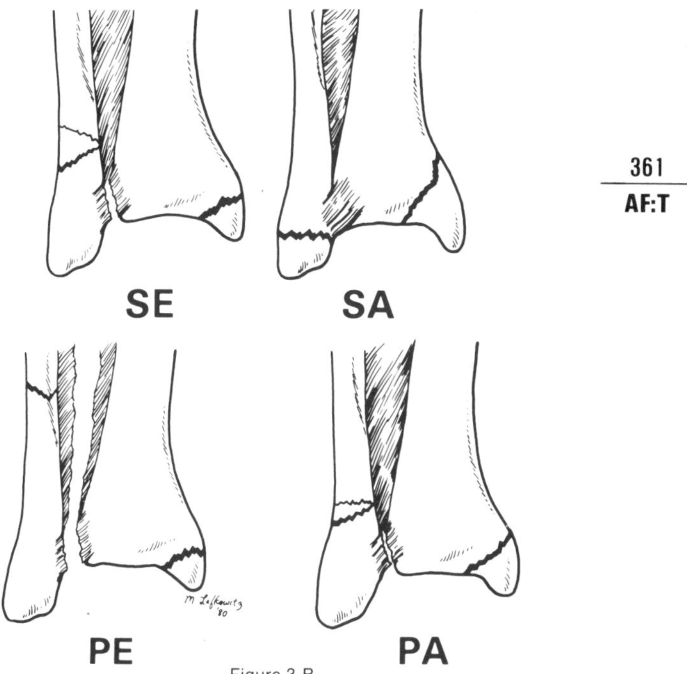

Figure 3-B

Figure 3: (A) Classification of ankle injuries according to Lauge-Hansen. (The terms supination and pronation refer to the position of the forefoot. Adduction and abduction describe the direction of the force. Eversion and inversion designate the direction of rotation of the ankle on the tibia.) (B) Illustration of ankle injuries according to Lauge-Hansen. SE = supination-eversion; SA = supination-adduction; PA = pronation-abduction; PE = pronation-eversion. (Reprinted with permission from I. Yablon, et al., Ankle Injuries, pp. 32, 33, New York, Churchill Livingstone, 1983.)

1 mm, displaced posterior lip fragments of more than 25 percent, and any talar tilt are, generally, not associated with good results. Exact reductions can be achieved and maintained more predictably by open reduction and internal fixation than by closed methods (Fig. 4).

Despite rigid internal fixation, supplementary plaster immobilization often is required in the postoperative management of patients with fibular fractures above the syndesmosis. The use of a below-knee orthosis (Fig. 5) that permits plantar flexion and dorsiflexion but restricts rotation in such patients may eliminate the need for postoperative plaster casts. A clinical trial has been carried out in over eighty patients with unstable ankle fractures treated by open reduction, exact anatomic restoration, and rigid internal fixation followed postoperatively by immediate weight-bearing in a below-knee orthosis. Sound healing without displacement of the mortise and fixation failure and return of joint motion beyond 10 degrees of dorsiflexion have been reported.

Major trauma to the foot and ankle resulting in massive soft-tissue loss and complex fractures can be managed more effectively by external fixation. Unless uncontrollable deep sepsis becomes established, it is reasonable to expect to salvage a severely damaged limb and to achieve acceptable function after healing. Indications for use of external fixation include stabilization of grade III open fractures or dislocations of the ankle, maintenance of length when bone has been lost, prevention of contracture, and control of joint position in highly comminuted articular injuries. Using an external fixator provides unobstructed access for skin care, but it should not be used unless there has been extensive soft-tissue loss.

Intra-articular fractures of the tibial plafond, the pilon fracture, present a formidable treatment challenge. Best results have been achieved by following the principles established by a study group: (1) reconstruction of the correct length of the fibula; (2) reconstruction of the articular surface of the tibia; (3) introduction of a cancellous autograft to fill metaphyseal defects of the tibia; and (4) stabilization of the medial aspect of the tibia by a plate. Inadequate reconstruction of the articular surfaces or unstable internal fixation predispose the patient to progressive degenerative arthritis.

Hindfoot

The talus and calcaneus compose the major structures of the hindfoot. The talocalcaneal joint allows eversion and inversion of the heel. Simultaneously, anteroposterior rocking of the calcaneus on the talus also can occur. The action of the subtalar joint simulates a torque converter changing pronation and supination of the foot into external and internal rotation of the leg. The interosseous ligament provides primary stability to the subtalar joint, while medially the deltoid ligament and laterally the fibular collateral ligament provide secondary stability. The Achilles tendon inserts halfway down on the posterior aspect of the calcaneus. The upper posterior portion of the calcaneus is separated from the Achilles tendon by a bursa, and another bursa separates the Achilles tendon from the overlying skin. After insertion on the os calcis, the Achilles tendon thins and broadens. It sweeps under the posteroinferior aspect of the heel and projects forward as the plantar fascia inserts distally on the metatarsal heads and proximal phalanges of the toes.

Subtalar Dislocation Subtalar dislocation occurs when the calcaneus is displaced medially or laterally beneath the talus. An often unrecognized associated subluxation of the talonavicular joint occurs at the time of dislocation. Medial subtalar dislocation occurs most frequently and

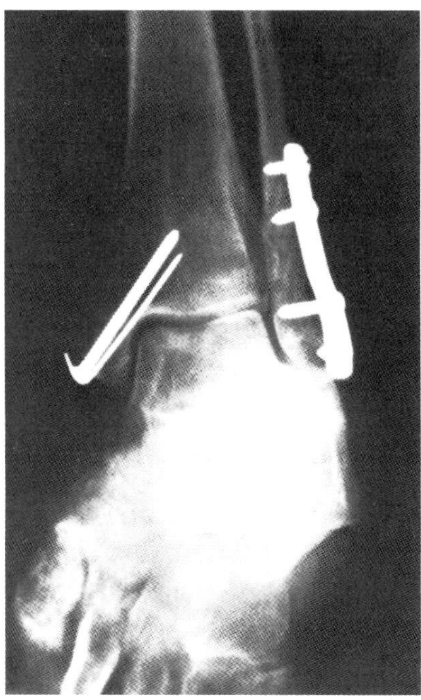

Figure 4: Anatomic reduction of medial and lateral malleolus. Note bending of the plate to fit configuration of the fibula. (Reprinted with permission from Displaced ankle fractures treated surgically and postoperative management, by D. Segal, *In* AAOS Instructional Course Lectures XXVIII:81, St. Louis, C.V. Mosby, 1979.)

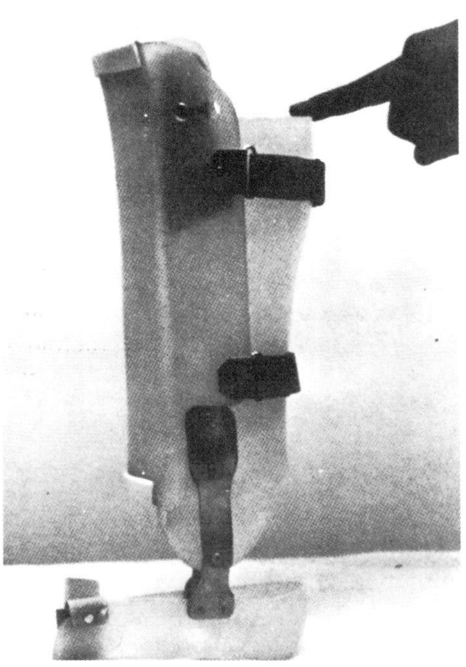

Figure 5: Below-knee brace with its three components. (Reprinted with permission from Displaced ankle fractures treated surgically and postoperative management, by D. Segal, *In* AAOS Instructional Course Lectures XXVIII:85, St. Louis, C.V. Mosby, 1979.)

usually results in minimal long-term disability if there is no fracture. Lateral subtalar dislocations are frequently open and may require operative intervention to obtain a reduction. These injuries need to be immobilized for only 3 weeks, followed by vigorous ankle and subtalar exercise to regain good motion. Poor results usually are seen in patients who do not regain full subtalar joint motion or have an associated unrecognized fracture involving the subtalar joint. If such fractures are recognized early, more satisfactory results are obtained by instituting early joint motion.

Os Calcis

Plantar Fasciitis Syndrome Pain at the plantar surface of the heel is common in adults. Usually the patient localizes the pain to the plantar medial tuberosity of the calcaneus near the origin of the plantar fascia. Multiple episodes of microtrauma create this painful disabling condition.

The precise etiology of pain is unknown. Plantar fasciitis, periostitis of the medial tuberosity leading to heel spurring, and entrapment of the calcaneal branch of the posterior tibial nerve in the tarsal tunnel have been implicated. The patient first notices pain upon awakening and beginning weight-bearing. The first few steps of the day and a morning shower alleviate the pain.

An examiner can elicit tenderness when palpating the plantar medial tuberosity. Marked limitation of dorsiflexion of the ankle, signifying tightness of the gastrocsoleus complex, frequently accompanies this syndrome. Usually the ankle can be dorsiflexed to only 10 degrees.

Treatment includes vigorous heel cord stretching by backing away from the wall or walking downstairs backward at least three times a day. Also, because of the link between the gastrocsoleus complex and the plantar fascia, elevation of the heel by 1.25 to 2.0 cm will relieve tension on the plantar fascia. If the patient has severe pain, oral anti-inflammatory agents can be administered. If, after 3 weeks, little or no relief has occurred, orthotics should be considered to cushion the heel and support the arch. Plastic heel cup inserts are usually tried first, but Plastazote, cork leather, and soft rubber can be molded into a device that cups and cushions the heel and supports the arch. Flexible, soft devices are particularly appropriate in the treatment of long distance runners. With refractory patients, rigid acrylic inserts lined with Plastazote may have to be used to eliminate stretch on the plantar fascia. A patient must wear the orthosis until no tenderness of the medial calcaneal tuberosity remains. Steroid injections usually should be administered only once. Steroids can cause atrophy of the heel fat pad, leading to further loss of cushioning.

Occasionally for a runner it may be necessary to recommend alternate physical activity until the pain subsides. Bicycling and swimming provide good opportunities for maintaining aerobic conditioning and psychological well-being until heel pain is gone. Surgery remains a last resort and should be considered only if a specific cause for heel pain can be identified that will respond to operation. Operation may include release of plantar fascia from the medial tuberosity of the calcaneus, excision of a heel spur, and/or release of a compressed medial calcaneal nerve. If a specific cause cannot be identified, all three procedures may have to be considered. Full return to preoperative activity levels cannot be assured.

Retrocalcaneal Bursitis Pressure caused by a heel counter-rubbing against the posterolateral prominence of the calcaneus creates a bursitis that causes posterior heel pain. The point of inflammation centers on the retrocalcaneal bursa which separates the upper posterior portion of the calcaneus from the Achilles tendon.

Initial treatment consists of removal of pressure from the posterior aspect of the calcaneus. This can be done by lowering the counter of the shoe, by wearing a heel cup that relieves pressure in the area, or by temporarily wearing a clog. Aspiration of the bursa can be helpful, especially if pain is severe and persists despite treatment. Cortisone injection should be avoided. If pain persists despite these measures, surgical excision of the superior prominence of the calcaneus that causes pressure against the Achilles tendon can relieve the symptoms.

Calcaneal Stress Fracture A stress fracture also can produce plantar calcaneal heel pain. However, the pain appears suddenly and remains constant, unlike the fluctuating pain of plantar fasciitis. Medial and lateral compression of the tuberosity of the calcaneus produce severe pain. Initial radiographs are normal. Subsequent radiographs at 4 to 6 weeks reveal a radiodense condensation running posterosuperior to anteroinferior. Treatment requires rest, elevation, and range of motion exercises for 2 to 3 weeks. Runners are encouraged to stop running and begin swimming to maintain conditioning. When tenderness subsides and subtalar motion returns, the patient may resume normal recreational activities.

Calcaneal Fracture Fractures of the anterior process, the posterior inferior tuberosity, the beak of the tuberosity and the body not involving the subastragalar joint are best treated by early compression dressings in conjunction with elevation of the foot for several days, followed by a short-leg cast with early weight-bearing. This usually results in union of the fracture, although the anterior process fractures of the calcaneus do progress to nonunion in some patients. It has been found that early recognition and prolonged plaster immobilization lead to a high percentage of satisfactory results. Late excision of the fragment is recommended and may lead to a fairly high salvage rate.

Treatment of fractures of the body of the os calcis with subastragalar joint involvement remains controversial. Most os calcis fractures are of this variety and often have gross deformities. The standard closed treatment by early motion or plaster immobilization results in satisfactory union but with residual deformities and often long periods of subtalar pain. The use of percutaneous pins for traction or reduction of tuberosity angle has not been particularly satisfactory either for reduction or for subtalar pain prevention. Operative methods of open reduction from the lateral side with the use of iliac-bone grafts, subtalar arthrodesis, and triple arthrodesis have yielded about 75 percent satisfactory results.

Recently a classification and a surgical method of treatment, based on an experience with over 90 patients, have been suggested. This method is reported to eliminate both the early pain of the patient and severe deformities of the posterior calcaneal facet by lifting the fragments and securing them with two- and three-prong staples. Bone grafts have not been necessary. Operative intervention is recommended within the first 24 hours after the injury. The fracture is approached through a medial incision, but occasionally this needs to be combined with a lateral incision. The technique seems promising for complex fractures with depression of the posterior facet and reversal of Boehler's angle. The results have not yet been verified by other investigators, thus more experience with this technique is necessary to establish its role in the management of complex fractures of the calcaneus.

The occasional proximal avulsion fracture with displacement by the Achilles tendon requires internal screw fixation to regain satisfactory plantar flexion.

Talus

Os Trigonum Syndrome The os trigonum, an accessory ossicle united to the posterior aspect of the talus by a synostosis, can be separated from the talus by plantar flexion and inversion. This mechanism also can cause a sprain of the lateral ligaments of the ankle. Therefore, this syndrome typically presents as persistent pain behind the ankle on plantar flexion after a lateral ankle sprain has healed. Radiographs reveal the trigonum separated from the talus by a vertical line. Nonoperative treatment is usually not helpful, and excision of the os trigonum usually will eliminate pain.

Dome Fracture Over one-half the papers dealing with talus fractures published during the past 3 years concern osteochondral dome fractures. These fractures are generally classified as: stage I, a small area of compression; stage II, a partially detached fragment; stage III, a completely detached fragment remaining in the crater; and stage IV, a displaced osteochondral fragment. Plaster immobilization remains the treatment of choice for stages I and II. In stages III and IV an alternative to operative excision is under investigation. This technique involves the use of a concentrated fibrinogen adhesive to glue the osteochondral fragments into place. Subchondral cysts seen beneath an osteochondral lesion in the dome of the talus suggest osteochondritis dissecans rather than trauma as the cause for the lesion. The mechanism of injury continues to be related to inversion and eversion injuries.

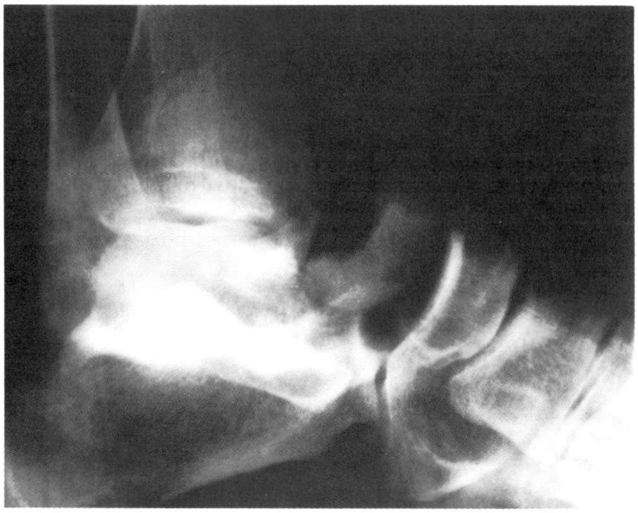

Figure 6: Type IV fracture-dislocation with subluxation of the head of the talus from the talonavicular joint. (Reprinted with permission from Fractures of the neck of the talus, by S.T. Canale, et al., J. Bone Joint Surg. 60A:144, 1978.)

When the osteochondral fragment presents on the medial margin of the dome of the talus, it appears to be located more on the posterior third of the dome. When the osteochondral fragment presents on the lateral margin of the dome, it seems to be located most commonly in the middle third of the dome.

Lateral Process Fracture Lateral body fractures involve the posterior talocalcaneal facet and can present late with bony overgrowth limiting valgus in the hindfoot, degenerative changes in the posterior facet of the subtalar joint, nonunion, and weight-bearing pain. This fracture, if recognized early, is best treated by immobilization. Since the mechanisms of dorsiflexion and inversion are frequently associated with this fracture, two views of this area frequently are necessary to make the correct diagnosis.

Neck Fracture Dorsiflexion of the ankle is associated with talar neck fractures. A generally accepted classification of these injuries is: type I, vertical fracture with no displacement of the fracture and a normal ankle and subtalar joint; type II, vertical fracture with displacement of the talar neck and subluxation or dislocation of the posterior facet of the subtalar joint; and type III, displaced neck fracture with both ankle and subtalar joint dislocation. Recently an infrequently encountered fracture-dislocation with subluxation of the talar head from the talonavicular joint has been described and is now classified as a type IV (Fig. 6).

There have been no recent reports on osteonecrosis. It has been suggested that rigid fixation with cancellous bone screws may make the recognition of osteonecrosis more difficult. A posterior approach to the talus has been recommended with screws being inserted from posterior to anterior. Results in additional patients having a Blair (tibiotalar) arthrodesis for osteonecrosis of the talus are available. The most favorable results in this series were in those patients who attained nearly 20 degrees of tibial pedal motion and had successful arthrodesis between the tibia and the neck of the talus.

Posterior Process Fracture This fracture involves the posterior eminence of the body of the talus and is best seen on the lateral radiograph. This fracture must be differentiated from an os trigonum resulting from a separate secondary ossification center of this eminence. This fracture may result in disability secondary to a painful arthrosis when it involves the posterior talocalcaneal joint.

Body Fracture It has been suggested that compression and sagittal shearing fractures of the body of the talus, which are displaced, require anatomic reduction to obtain favorable results. Crush injuries of the body of the talus have a poor prognosis, usually resulting in functional disability. Nonweight-bearing is recommended until solid healing has occurred.

Midfoot

The navicular, cuboid, and cuneiforms compose the bony structures of the midfoot. Chopart's joint, bordered anteriorly by the navicular and cuboid and posteriorly by the calcaneus and talus, locks and unlocks in response to inversion and eversion of the calcaneus. Since this relative motion exists, the joint can be subjected to injury. The cuneiforms, navicular, and cuboid are bound by very strong ligaments. The tibialis posterior, the principle muscle acting on the midfoot, inserts primarily on the medial aspect of the navicular and also onto the cuneiform and the bases of the second, third, and fourth metatarsals.

Posterior Tibial Tendinitis Chronic pain over the medial aspect of the foot just inferior and distal to the medial malleolus can follow a twisting injury to the foot. Posterior tibial tendinitis, partial avulsion of the insertion of the tendon from the navicular, partial tendon rupture of the substance of the tendon, and accessory navicular can be responsible for these symptoms. In addition to localized tenderness along the course of the posterior tendons, these patients have difficulty raising up on the ball of the foot with the heel locked in inversion. The hindfoot appears to be in valgus while the forefoot may be slightly abducted.

Nonoperative treatment consisting of rest, 0.3 cm medial heel wedge, posterior calf stretching, and strengthening of the posterior tibialis muscle should be tried first and usually provides relief. Few patients require revision of the origin of the tendon, excision of degenerated midsubstance of the tendon, or excision of accessory navicular.

Navicular Fracture The insidious onset of vague pain on the dorsum or the medial aspect of the arch in a patient suggests a stress fracture of the navicular. Local tenderness is usually present, and activity increases the pain. This sagittal plane fracture occurs in the middle third of the navicular where the blood supply is limited (Fig. 7). A negative radiograph should be followed by a radionuclide scan. If the scan is positive, tomograms usually reveal the fracture site. The treatment recommended in these patients is nonweight-bearing in a plaster cast for 6 to 8 weeks, followed by weight-bearing in plaster cast for 4 weeks, after which limited activity can be begun. Fracture healing can usually be expected.

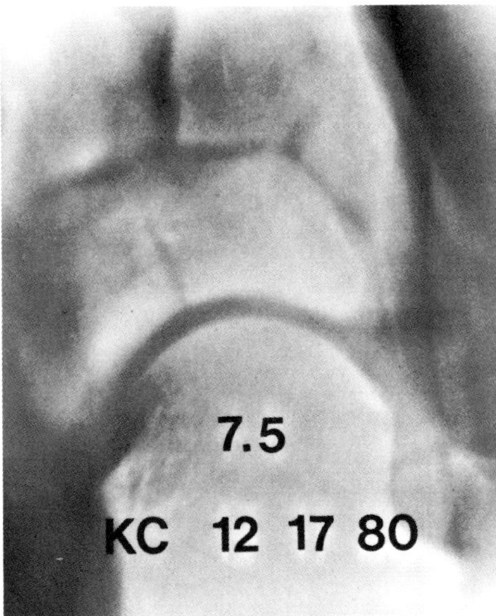

Figure 7: A 27-year-old professional basketball player with bilateral partial proximal stress fracture of the navicular. An anteroposterior tomogram of the right foot made 1 month after the onset of symptoms shows a partial stress fracture involving the proximal articular border of the tarsal navicular, but the distal articular border showed no evidence of fracture. Deeper sections also showed that the fracture was limited to the dorsal aspect of the bone. (Reprinted with permission from Stress fractures of the tarsal navicular: A retrospective review of 21 cases, by J.S. Torg, et al., J. Bone Joint Surg. 64A: 701, 1982.)

Tarsometatarsal Fracture-Dislocation This uncommon and often unrecognized injury is recognizable because of widening of the first metatarsal interspace, a fracture-dislocation at the base of the second metatarsal, and/or associated crush fractures of the cuboid. In patients in whom this injury is suspected, comparable weight-bearing films may allow the more subtle injuries to be recognized. The recent literature emphasizes the difficulty in reduction by closed methods as the anterior tibial tendon may become interposed, often necessitating an open reduction. It has been suggested that a successful closed manipulative reduction can be prevented by a fracture fragment in the second metatarsal intermediate cuneiform joint. A stable reduction by open reduction and internal fixation may avoid later fusion. Superior results are reported in teenage patients. Gangrene following injury to the dorsalis pedis artery in the first intermetatarsal space has been reported only rarely.

Spontaneous Dislocation in Diabetic Neuropathy The foot remains the area most frequently involved with neuropathic joints in diabetes. Spontaneous fractures in tarsals and metatarsals occur frequently in patients with diabetic neuropathy. These fractures often progress to nonunion and early, prolonged immobilization remains the best treatment. It has been reported that in a series of six patients with diabetic neuropathy severe ligamentous weakening allowed spontaneous dislocation to occur (Fig. 8). The joints involved were ankle, talonavicular, first cuneiform, and tarsometatarsal. Early fusion followed by prolonged immobilization was recommended. Even if fusion was not obtained, the foot seemed to remain stable in a satisfactory position.

Forefoot

Metatarsophalangeal Injuries

Forefoot Problems in Runners Running can aggravate a myriad of forefoot disorders. Hammer toe, mallet toe, hallux valgus, interdigital neuromas, and corns are among the more common conditions. These should be treated according to standard methods. Metatarsalgia, metatarsal stress fractures, and sesamoiditis involve the most common forefoot overuse syndromes for runners. Metatarsalgia, which is pain across the metatarsophalangeal articulation with plantar callouses, is best treated by distributing weight-bearing forces more evenly. Total contact molded inserts with a metatarsal bar that lies proximal to the metatarsal head accomplishes the purpose. The runner seems to tolerate flexible inserts like cork leather or Plastazote best. Metatarsal stress fractures occur particularly after an increase in length and intensity of training. Treatment consists solely of limitation of activity with resumption as pain allows.

Sesamoiditis, or stress fractures of the sesamoids, are common injuries. If pads and cushioning fail to relieve symptoms, excision may be necessary.

Metatarsal Fractures Normal function of the forefoot requires weight-bearing distributed between the two sesamoids of the first metatarsal and the lateral four metatarsal heads. Basic treatment for single shaft and neck fractures continues to be alignment with adjacent metatarsals in a well-molded plaster dressing with early weight-bearing.

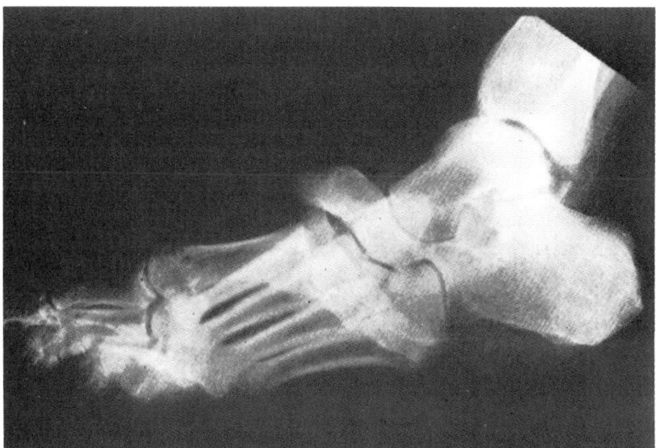

Figure 8: Initial radiograph demonstrating dislocations of the medial cuneiform and the tarsometatarsal joint. (Reprinted with permission from Spontaneous dislocation in diabetic neuropathy, by J. Newman, et al., J. Bone Joint Surg. 61B:485, 1979.)

Open reduction and anatomic reduction of metatarsals associated with severe trauma to the forefoot have been recommended by some. The possibility of a compartment syndrome in the deep posterior compartment of the leg or in the foot should be constantly considered.

Stress is a frequent cause of a transverse diaphyseal fracture of the base of the fifth metatarsal (Fig. 9). A high incidence of delayed union in young patients is associated with functional disability. Intramedullary screw fixation is useful in treating nonunion and has been recommended as the initial treatment. This fracture should be differentiated from avulsion fracture of the base of the fifth metatarsal resulting from an inversion injury.

Metatarsophalangeal Fractures Various combinations of metatarsophalangeal fracture-dislocations have been recorded in the recent literature. Most emphasis has been placed on the dorsal, closed, irreducible dislocations. Dislocations of the first metatarsophalangeal joint often can be successfully reduced by closed methods. Later follow-up, however, has indicated that a high number of patients develop degenerative arthritis in this joint. Fracture of the fibular sesamoid at the first metatarsophalangeal joint has been reported to be associated with dislocations of this joint. Stress has been suggested as a causative factor in fractures involving the fibular sesamoid.

Lawn Mower Injuries

Power lawn mowers can produce severe disabling injuries because the standard 26-inch rotary blade turning at 3,000 rpm supplies three times the energy of a .357 magnum pistol.

Most of these injuries can be prevented. Although design improvements have lessened the risk, it is the user who is best able to minimize the chance for injury. Precautionary steps include: using as low a blade velocity as necessary to cut grass; maintaining a sharp blade so that the mower can run at low speeds; removing potential missles from the lawn; prohibiting bystanders; filling the gas tank with the engine off; using extreme caution when riding a mower on a slope; not allowing children to operate a mower; not allowing passengers to ride on a mower; wearing sturdy shoes with a tread sole (no tennis shoes); and not mowing wet grass.

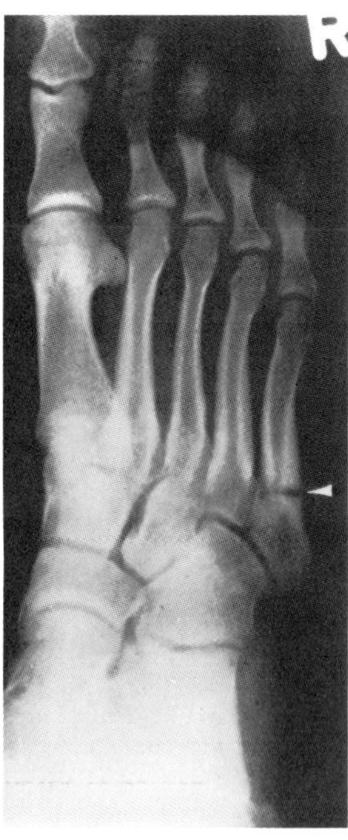

Figure 9: Radiograph of the foot of a college recreational athlete with a Jones fracture bilaterally. The radiograph was made 2 months after refracture of the right foot. This lesion actually occurred 1 year before this radiograph as the patient was hurling a discus. The fracture initially caused only mild discomfort. Despite restriction of active sports activities, the patient continued to complain of mild aching in the foot. Months after the original injury, the patient had sudden, severe pain while running, and a refracture was diagnosed. This so-called refracture was treated with a short cast, nonweight-bearing, for 4 weeks, following which he was ambulatory, weight-bearing without external immobilization. Internal fixation is not being considered. (Reprinted with permission from The Jones fracture revisited, by J.H. Kavanaugh, et al., J. Bone Joint Surg. 60A:777, 1978.)

Treatment of these contaminated wounds requires immediate copious irrigation, thorough debridement and packing the wounds open. Intravenous antibiotic prophylaxis should be given for 72 hours. For minimally contaminated wounds, a broad spectrum cephalosporin should be sufficient. However, for heavily contaminated, extensively crushed wounds an aminoglycoside also should be used to provide gram-negative coverage. In heavily contaminated patients, intravenous penicillin should be given as protection against Clostridium. These wounds often require multiple debridements and reconstructive procedures to achieve adequate skin coverage.

ANNOTATED BIBLIOGRAPHY

Ankle Joint

Achilles Tendinitis and Partial Rupture

Denstad, T., and Roaas, A.: Surgical treatment of partial Achilles tendon rupture. Am. J. Sports Med. 7:15-17, 1979.

Fifty-eight patients with Achilles tendon pain at the beginning of strenuous exercise, who were unsuccessfully treated, underwent surgical excision of degenerative tissue and reapproximation of the tendon. Few required modified Lindholm repair for defects. Forty-four patients who engaged in competitive sports preoperatively resumed their previous activities.

Vazelle, F.; Rochcongar, P.; Masse, M.; and Ramée, A.: Achilles tendon lesion: An unexpected application of mammography. J. Radiol. 62:299-307, 1981.

Distinctions between simple, chronic, and nodular tendinitis, total or partial ruptures, and localized bursitis are presented. In 75 percent of patients, clinical diagnosis was confirmed or errors of assessment elucidated.

Achilles Tendon Rupture

Nistor, L.: Surgical and non-surgical treatment of Achilles tendon rupture. A prospective randomized study. J. Bone Joint Surg. 63A:394-399, 1981.

Forty-five patients were treated surgically and sixty by cast immobilization. Both treatment groups demonstrated loss of plantar flexion power, but no statistically significant difference existed. The nonoperated group had a slightly higher rerupture rate of 8 percent as compared to 4 percent.

Ankle Sprain

Brand, R.; Collins, M.; and Templeton, T.: Surgical repair of ruptured lateral ankle ligament. Am. J. Sports Med. 9:40-44, 1981.

Fifty-two patients with lateral ankle ligament injuries repaired by interrupted nonabsorbable suture followed by short-leg cast for 6 weeks were reevaluated 3 to 56 months following surgery. Indications for surgery were talar tilt greater than 25 degrees, functional instability with recent injury, avulsion fracture with talar tilt 15 degrees, and osteochondral fracture of the talus. At follow-up 98 percent were functionally stable.

Cox, J., and Hewes, T.: "Normal" talar tilt angle. Clin. Orthop. 140:37-41, 1979.

Two hundred two midshipmen with 404 ankles were studied. Three hundred sixty-five out of 404 ankles (90.4 percent) tested showed no talar tilt. Thirty-two ankles (7.9 percent) showed tilting between 1 and 5 degrees. Only seven ankles (1.7 percent) tilted greater than 5 degrees. Tilting of the talus greater than 5 degrees probably represents a significant injury.

Garrick, J.: "When can I ...?" A practical approach to rehabilitation illustrated by treatment of an ankle injury. Am. J. Sports Med. 9:67-68, 1981.

Progression through a rehabilitation program based on an athlete's progress as a reflection of the physiology of healing and severity of the injury. It avoids the time trap (e.g., "You said I would be running in two weeks").

Niedermann, B.; Andersen, A.; Andersen, S.; Funder, V.; Jorgensen, J.P.; Lindholmer, E.; and Vuust, M.: Rupture of the lateral ligaments of the ankle: Operation or plaster cast? Prospective study. Acta Orthop. Scand. 52:579-587, 1981.

Two hundred and nine patients were treated randomly with either plaster cast for 5 weeks or surgical repair followed by nonweight-bearing plaster for 5 weeks. Good results were obtained in 76 percent of the nonoperative group and 81 percent of the operative group. This is not a statistically significant difference.

Seligson, D.; Gassman, J.; and Pope, M.: Ankle instability: Evaluation of the lateral ligaments. Am. J. Sports Med. 8:39-42, 1980.

In functionally normal ankles, the range of inversion tilt was 0 degrees to 18 degrees while the maximum anterior displacement was 3 mm. The anterior drawer appears to evaluate the lateral ligaments more critically.

Ankle Fractures

Kenzora, J.E.; Edwards, C.; Browner, B.; Gamble, J.; and DeSilva, J.: Acute management of major trauma involving the foot and ankle with Hoffman external fixation. Foot Ankle 1:348-361, 1981.

Massive trauma involving the foot and ankle was treated by external fixation in thirty-three patients. After treatment, twenty-six patients had a functional painfree foot. Five patients had injuries so extensive that amputation was necessary.

Lund-Kristensen, J.; Greiff, J.; and Riegels-Nielsen, P.: Malleolar fractures treated with rigid internal fixation and immediate mobilization. Injury 13:191-195, 1981.

Twenty-eight consecutive patients with displaced bimalleolar fractures were treated by anatomically exact open reduction, rigid internal fixation, and immediate postoperative exercises. Weight-bearing was delayed 9 weeks. All fractures healed within 6 to 10 weeks with no late displacement. Twenty-one of twenty-three had normal ankle motion at an average of 39 months after injury.

Segal, D.: Displaced ankle fractures treated surgically and postoperative management. *In* AAOS Instructional Course Lectures. XXVIII:79-88. St. Louis, C.V. Mosby, 1979.

Only 10 percent of weight-bearing forces transmit to the distal fibula during plantar flexion and dorsiflexion; this is higher with rotation. A below-knee orthosis with a free ankle allows immediate postoperative motion with weight-bearing following open reduction and internal fixation of displaced ankle fractures.

Yablon, I.: Reduction of displaced bimalleolar ankle fractures. *In* AAOS Instructional Course Lectures. XXVIII:72-79. St. Louis, C.V. Mosby, 1979.

This cadaver study demonstrated more instability of the ankle when sectioning the lateral collateral ligaments and osteotomy of the fibula distal to the syndesmosis. It is important to reduce the fibula exactly as well as the medial malleolus.

Hindfoot

Subtalar Dislocation

DeLee, J.C., and Curtis, R.: Subtalar dislocation of the foot. J. Bone Joint Surg. 64A:433-437, 1982.

Of seventeen subtalar dislocations reported, four were lateral. Associated intra-articular fractures were present in six patients, but polytomography was required to make the diagnosis in two patients. Thirteen of the seventeen dislocations were reduced closed and four required open reduction, including three of four lateral dislocations. Lateral dislocation and the presence of associated injuries were associated with a higher incidence of poor results.

Monson, S.T., and Ryan, J.R.: Subtalar dislocation. J. Bone Joint Surg. 63A:1156-1158, 1981.

Eleven medial subtalar dislocations showed loss of subtalar motion but no major fracture of the talus. A method to clinically measure subtalar motion is presented.

Os Calcis

Calcaneal Fractures

McReynolds, I.S.: The case for operative treatment of fractures of the os calcis. *In* Controversies in Orthopaedic Surgery, edited by R.E. Leach and F.T. Hoaglund pp. 232-254. Philadelphia, W.B. Saunders, 1982.

Based on experience with more than 90 fractures of the os calcis treated operatively through a medial approach, the author describes his technique for operative repair of comminuted os calcis fractures. A triangular staple secures the impacted superior medial fragment. Bone grafts are infrequently used.

Talus

Dome Fracture

Alexander, A.H., and Lichtman, D.M.: Surgical treatment of transchondral talar-dome fractures (osteochondritis dissecans): Long-term follow-up. J. Bone Joint Surg. 62A:646-652, 1980.

A long-term follow-up of forty-nine surgically treated lesions concludes that early excision and curettage of fragments gives a high percentage of good results and postponing the operation does not seem to adversely affect the results.

Neck Fractures

Canale, S.T., and Kelly, F.B., Jr.: Fractures of the neck of the talus. J. Bone Joint Surg. 60A:143-156, 1978.

A detailed review of seventy-one fractures of the neck of the talus. The incidence of osteonecrosis appears related to the classification of the fractures. In a high percentage of patients, surgical treatment was utilized.

Dennis, M.D., and Tullos, H.S.: Blair tibiotalar arthrodesis for injuries to the talus. J. Bone Joint Surg. 62A:103-107, 1980.

Delayed Blair fusions for group II and group III fractures are reviewed. Five patients had good results, and each had 16 to 20 degrees of tibiopedal motion. The technique is modified and pseudarthrosis is discussed.

Lemaire, R.G., and Bustin, W.: Screw fixation of fractures of the neck of the talus using a posterior approach. J. Trauma 20:669-673, 1980.

After closed reduction under fluoroscopic control, a lag screw was inserted through the posterior tubercle stabilizing the fracture in five patients. A posterior lag screw was used after open reduction in two patients.

Midfoot

Navicular Fracture

Torg, J.S.; Pavlov, H.; Cooley, L.H.; Bryant, M.H.; Arnoczky, S.P.; Bergfeld, J.; and Hunter, L.Y.: Stress fractures of the tarsal navicular: A retrospective review. J. Bone Joint Surg. 64A:700-712, 1982.

Stress fracture of the tarsal navicular was diagnosed late in twenty-two young male distance runners. Localized pain and a positive bone scan are indications for tomograms if plain films fail to show the fracture.

Tarsometatarsal

Spontaneous Dislocation in Diabetic Neuropathy

Newman, J.: Spontaneous dislocation in diabetic neuropathy: A report of six cases. J. Bone Joint Surg. 61B:484-488, 1979.

Six diabetic patients with ankle or intertarsal dislocations were studied. Ligament involvement allowed dislocations at the ankle and intertarsal area. Arthrodesis was offered as a method of obtaining a stable foot in satisfactory position.

Forefoot

Metatarsophalangeal

Metatarsal Fracture

Kavanaugh, J.H.; Brower, T.; and Mann, R.V.: The Jones fracture revisited. J. Bone Joint Surg. 60A:776-782, 1978.

A series of twenty-three displaced fractures of the proximal base of the fifth metatarsal were studied. Delayed union was frequent. Stress as the cause of the fracture in these young athletic patients was suggested.

Lawn Mower Injuries

Thurston, A.J.: Foot injuries caused by power lawn mowers. New Zealand Med. J. 91:131-133, 1980.

Foot injuries resulting from power lawn mowers in seventeen patients are studied. In this group, all were wearing inadequately protective footwear at the time of injury. The types of and problems with the injuries are discussed.

40 ANKLE AND FOOT: RECONSTRUCTION

Subjects covered in this section include ankle arthrodesis and arthroplasty, hallux valgus, tarsal tunnel syndrome, rheumatoid arthritis, affliction of the forefoot, and management of the diabetic foot.

Functional Anatomy and Biomechanics

The anatomy of the foot and ankle provides a specialized and complex arrangement of joints and soft tissues that plays an extremely important role in the function of the lower extremity. Whereas static gross anatomy has been well documented, more recently the dynamic function of the foot has been delineated. Newer surgical approaches to disorders of the ankle and foot are being based on these biomechanical principles, and, as a result, more predictable and improved surgical results are being achieved.

During the normal gait cycle, significant degrees of axial rotation occur in the lower extremity. The degree of rotation is increased progressively from the pelvis to the ankle. With the foot fixed on the walking surface during the stance phase of gait, the foot and ankle articulations must accommodate for the degree of transverse or axial rotation in the lower extremity. The anatomic design of the ankle allows for a small degree of correction, but the subtalar complex absorbs most of the rotation. These rotational and compensatory principles must be understood to plan surgical treatment of either the ankle or subtalar complex.

Most painful disorders of the ankle and foot are manifested during the stance phase of gait. The very complex structural and functional anatomy of the heel pad provides a means of absorbing both the direct and torsional stresses occurring at heel strike. Internal rotation of the lower limb follows ground contact until the foot is flat in the midstance phase. During this initial rotation phase, the subtalar joint is in an everted and "unlocked position" which provides for maximal flexibility to help absorb the longitudinal forces of body weight and simultaneously accommodates to the walking surface. Shortly after the foot flat position, there is external rotation of the foot on tibia until toe-off. During the external rotation phase, the subtalar complex undergoes inversion, and the midtarsal complex is locked into a more rigid position, thus allowing the entire weight of the body to be transferred to the forefoot.

During 40 percent of stance phase, the forefoot carries the entire body load. Like the heel pad, the soft tissues of the plantar aspect of the forefoot form a very specialized structure capable of absorbing the repetitive, direct, and shear stresses applied during ambulation. The bony architecture provides the stable scaffolding needed to accept body weight. Deformity or surgical procedures involving the hard- and soft-tissue structures of the forefoot may alter the function to a degree that the weight-bearing stresses are abnormally localized to certain areas, thus resulting in painful conditions about the forefoot.

Acquired Disorders

Ankle Joint Degeneration Although injuries to the ankle are common, they rarely become chronic, disabling conditions. Since the large forces borne across the ankle are well tolerated mechanically, primary degenerative disease of the ankle is extremely rare. Rheumatoid arthritis, degenerative joint disease secondary to ankle trauma, synovial osteochondromatosis, and talar injury secondary to osteonecrosis or osteochondritis dissecans are the disease processes that most commonly lead to chronic pain and disability of the ankle. Once ankle joint pathology becomes disabling, there are a number of palliative mechanical measures that can be considered. The simplest of these is a rocker bottom shoe with a SACH type of heel (Fig. 1). The cushioned heel provides excellent absorption of the forces at heel strike and also accommodates inversion-eversion stresses encountered on uneven ground. The rocker sole reduces dorsiflexion stresses across the ankle joint during the late stance phase. Patients failing to obtain relief with shoes may be placed into more rigid devices such as ankle lacers, double-upright steel braces, or the newer custom-molded polypropylene ankle-foot orthosis (Fig. 2). These devices limit ankle motion, thereby relieving the stresses occurring in a degenerative ankle in extremes of motion.

TREATMENT: From a surgical standpoint, several factors

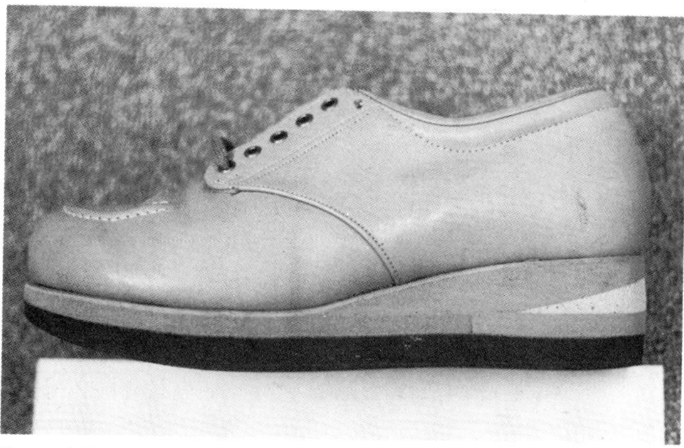

Figure 1: Rocker bottom shoe with a SACH type of heel.

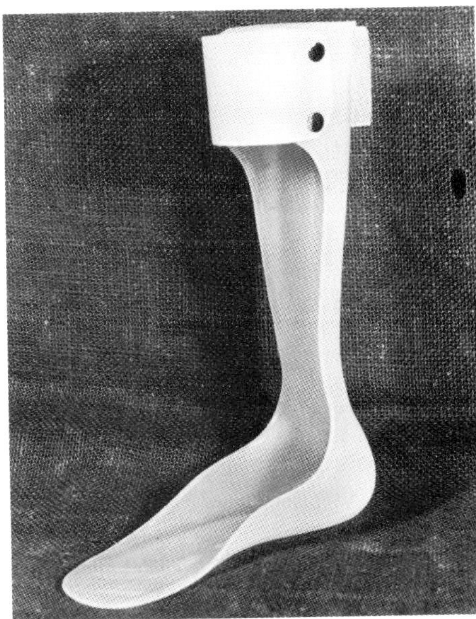

Figure 2: Custom-molded polypropylene ankle-foot orthosis.

must be considered. In the less involved ankle with an osteochondritic lesion, excision of the fragment or pinning and bone grafting the lesion may be the treatment of choice. In the active or athletic individual with disease limited primarily to the anterior aspect of the ankle joint, simple excision of the osteophytes from the talus and tibia may provide relief and allow the patient to resume full function. In those patients with more disabling conditions, the operative choice is between ankle fusion and total ankle arthroplasty.

Arthrodesis of the tibiotalar joint has been a commonly performed procedure. In the past, the Charnley type of resection arthrodesis probably has been the most popular procedure. Results, however, have been reported with complication rates as high as 60 percent. Complications may include pseudarthrosis, malunion, delayed union, pin track infection, and loss of motion in the subtalar joints. Several modifications have been described that improve on the technique of the Charnley-type fusion. Using a medial and lateral approach allows for better visualization of the joint surfaces to ensure that the resected surfaces of the tibia and talus have maximal contact. These surfaces should be as flat as possible to prevent "rockering" of the fusion site. Also, the talus should be displaced posteriorly to reduce forces across the midtarsal joint that may lead to subsequent degenerative changes. The two-incision approach also allows for easier access to resect the malleoli if needed. Radiographic confirmation of pin and fusion positions in the operating room should lessen the incidence of malalignment and subsequent malunion.

A less complicated approach is an in situ fusion rather than a resection type of arthrodesis. The advantages are several: (1) less trauma to the tissues with less postoperative morbidity; (2) maintenance of more normal contours about the ankle and hindfoot; (3) minimization of stiffness of the subtalar complex; (4) inherent stability with less likelihood of loss of position and subsequent malunion; (5) probable lower incidence of nonunions. This type of procedure is only applicable to an ankle without gross deformity.

Deformity secondary to soft-tissue contractures must be corrected by adequate soft-tissue releases so that the talus may be replaced in the ankle mortise in an appropriate position prior to fusion. The position of the fusion should be a neutral or slight degree of dorsiflexion. Numerous studies show this to be the best position for functional gait and minimization of stresses on the midtarsal and forefoot region as well as the ipsilateral knee. An equinus position at the ankle occasionally may be desirable in a patient with a limb length discrepancy or in a paralytic condition to provide for better knee stability.

In an in situ fusion, the talus is stabilized in the ankle mortise by either large threaded Steinmann pins or large cancellous screws. Prior to placing the fixation device, the foot should be placed in a neutral or minimal degree of dorsiflexion as measured by the plane of the plantar aspect of the foot and the anterior surface of the tibia. With the foot held in the proper position, the fixation device is placed across the tibiotalar joint, thereby securing the talus in the ankle mortise. Either a dowel-type fusion using iliac-crest graft or a sliding anterior tibial graft into the talus may be performed. The major surfaces of the joint do not need to be resected.

In patients with severe deformity and/or soft-tissue abnormality, the rate of failure may be significantly increased. Supplemental bone grafting improves results of fusion rates. A solid ankle fusion usually will result in a satisfactory outcome in 80 to 85 percent of patients. Once fusion has been obtained in an optimal position the good results do not appear to deteriorate with time.

Disadvantages of ankle arthrodesis include the necessity for 4 to 6 months of postoperative cast immobilization, the persistence of a limp and need for an assistive device in approximately 30 percent of patients, pseudarthrosis rates of nearly 20 percent, and subsequent degenerative changes in the subtalar and midtarsal joints.

Total ankle arthroplasty has been proposed as an alternative to arthrodesis in the management of painful conditions of the tibiotalar joint. The procedure still must be considered in the developmental stage. It is not indicated in the young and active patient due to a high likelihood of loosening and failure with the concomitant increased stresses. Best results with arthroplasty have been obtained in the rheumatoid and older individual with posttraumatic arthritis. Earlier mobilization and less stress on other joints are the suggested major advantages of arthroplasty over fusion for the elderly. Relative contraindications to arthroplasty are: (1) patients with osteoarthritis with significant ligamentous laxity, varus or valgus deformity of 20 degrees, or history of prior infection; (2) rheumatoid arthritis patients on long-term steroid therapy or with significant bone erosion; (3) patients with failed fusion; and (4) patients with osteonecrosis of the talus. In general, ankle fusion remains the procedure of choice for most painful conditions of the ankle, particularly if the subtalar and midtarsal joints are normal and the patient is involved in high levels of activity. Future developments with total ankle arthroplasty should be aimed at improving the design to allow for greater motion, reducing the constraining forces on the prosthesis, and improving the component bone fixation. As these improvements are developed, the indications for arthroplasty may be broadened.

Chronic Ankle Instability Although lateral ligamentous

* need to have good motion in rest of foot / LE to consider a fusion

injuries to the ankle are common, surprisingly few patients have symptomatic chronic laxity (see also Section 39, Ankle and Foot: Trauma). Diagnosis of the condition is not usually difficult. In addition to a history of chronic giving way of the ankle, physical examination usually reveals increased inversion and/or increased anterior drawer sign. Inversion stress radiographs may be used. The degree of talar tilt considered normal is debatable. Recent studies indicate that anything in excess of 5 degrees is abnormal. But, greater than 5 degrees of inversion instability by radiograph does not necessarily indicate that the patient has chronic symptoms of instability. Dynamic, muscular control of the ankle may compensate for loss of ligament constraints.

Treatment initially should consist of the following nonoperative means: lateral heel and sole wedges to the shoes, physical therapy to improve muscle tone and strength, and external bandages or orthotic devices. If unsuccessful, surgery may be considered. There are several surgical procedures available, and reports suggest similar outcomes in all. Most procedures that attempt to reconstruct both the anterior talofibular and calcaneofibular ligaments limit subtalar motion. Subtalar instability may exist in addition to ankle instability; if so, a procedure should be chosen which limits the talocalcaneal motion. Reconstruction of the lateral ligaments using the medial one-third of the Achilles tendon has been described. The method can be used in the treatment of combined talar and subtalar instability. However, the extensive dissection required may limit the usefulness of this procedure.

Hallux Valgus Numerous articles address the etiology and surgical correction of the hallux valgus deformity.

Although the deformity may occur successively in multiple generations, as yet no true genetic link has been discovered. Improperly fitting shoes appear to play an important role in the progress of the deformity. It is likely that patients with hallux valgus have some underlying functional anatomic deviation predisposing the great toe to abnormal forces with the resulting development of a progressive deformity.

The degree of splaying between the first and second metatarsals (primus varus deformity) closely parallels the degree of valgus deviation of the great toe. Once the deformity occurs, its progression can be explained from a biomechanical standpoint due to the medially directed component of force on the first metatarsal head from the base of the proximal phalanx. The increased medially directed force from the great toe causes attenuation of the medial capsule, thus allowing more valgus deformity of the great toe. With deformity progression, the abductor hallucis, which normally occupies a plantar medial position, is displaced laterally into a more plantar position. The base of the proximal phalanx remains firmly anchored to the adductor hallucis and lateral sesamoid. Pronation or axial rotation of the great toe occurs as the metatarsal head drifts more medially while the sesamoid sling is subluxated laterally. Some contend that there may be an initial pronation deformity of the first metatarsal predisposing to the development of the hallux valgus deformity.

Treatment: The goals of surgery for the hallux valgus deformity should be relief of pain, restoration of foot function to as nearly normal as possible, and adequate correction of the cosmetic deformity.

Recent articles have pointed out potential biomechanical problems with some of the numerous procedures described in the past. With progression of the hallux valgus deformity, the function of the first ray becomes increasingly impaired. Weight-bearing is shifted laterally and frequently results in an intractable plantar keratotic lesion beneath the second or third metatarsal. Because the first metatarsal is shorter than the second metatarsal in most individuals, the only means of fully involving the first ray in weight-bearing is for it to act independently of the second and third rays during the latter portion of the stance phase of gait.

This is accomplished by the windlass mechanism. With progressive dorsiflexion of the great toe, the plantar aponeurosis is partially wrapped around the metatarsal head (like a windlass). As a result the first metatarsal is driven into a more plantar direction, thus elevating and stabilizing the medial side of the foot. For this mechanism to be present there must be an intact insertion of the plantar aponeurosis into the base of the proximal phalanx of the great toe. With resection of the base of the proximal phalanx of the great toe, there may be a significant lateral shift of weight-bearing stresses to the second and third metatarsal regions. Shortening of the first metatarsal that may occur after some osteotomies may result in improper tension and function of the windlass mechanism and therefore further transfer of pressure to the lateral metatarsals. All functional aspects of anatomy about the great toe should be considered when planning a surgical procedure.

Distal metatarsal osteotomy has been a generally successful procedure. The Mitchell (Fig. 3A) and the Chevron (Fig. 3B) are the two most common types. The Mitchell osteotomy has more room for error from a technical standpoint. Dorsal displacement of the osteotomy or significant shortening through the osteotomy may lead to transfer metatarsalgia. The osteotomy should be done near the cancellous portion of the metatarsal head to minimize the incidence of nonunion. The Chevron osteotomy is a distal one that uses principles similar to the Mitchell. The design of the Chevron osteotomy tends to lessen the chances of displacement, instability, dorsal angulation, and nonunion that are potentially more likely with the Mitchell. Although the Chevron has some theoretical advantages, there are still some significant potential problems. Because of the very distal nature of this procedure, osteonecrosis and resorption of the first metatarsal head have been reported. If close attention to technical detail is not observed, malalignment of the metatarsal head also may occur. Excessive shortening with transfer metatarsalgia and hallux varus are also reported. Most procedures described result in approximately 85 percent

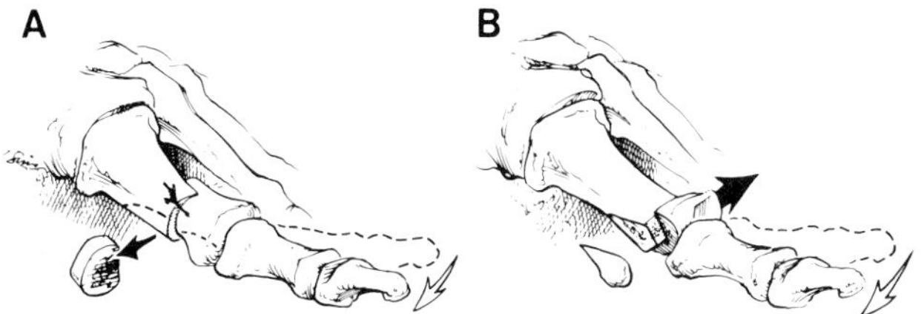

Figure 3: Distal metatarsal osteotomies. (A) Mitchell. (B) Chevron.

good to excellent outcomes. Close attention to the technical aspects of the surgical procedure in the postoperative period will improve results.

All components of the hallux valgus and bunion deformity may be corrected by the modified McBride procedure. The advantages of this procedure are that it eliminates the possibility of a nonunion or malunion of an osteotomy, allows for easier salvage if the surgery fails, and minimizes chances of developing a transfer metatarsalgia. Disadvantages include an increased incidence of hallux varus and a higher incidence of recurrent valgus deformity in the more severely deformed foot. If the intermetatarsal angle between the first and second metatarsals exceeds 15 degrees, an osteotomy at the base of the metatarsals in combination with the McBride procedure should be considered.

The Keller procedure has been very popular and generally has been considered the procedure of choice in the more elderly age group with hallux valgus deformities. The major problem with this procedure is the potential for development of transfer metatarsalgia secondary to the destabilizing effect of the first ray occurring after the base of the proximal phalanx is excised. In the nondysvascular foot in the elderly, recent studies have shown that successful results can be obtained with the distal metatarsal osteotomies and the modified McBride, provided the first metatarsophalangeal joint is free of disease.

Hallux Rigidus Hallux rigidus is a slowly progressing degenerative disease of the great toe metatarsophalangeal joint. Numerous etiologies have been proposed. Recently repeated episodes of minor trauma have been implicated. Progressive ridging on the dorsal, medial, and lateral aspects of the first metatarsal head and proximal phalanx are common radiographic findings. With enlargement of the ridges, the soft tissues passing dorsal to the joint may be compressed by shoe wear and thus initiate and aggravate the symptoms. There is a progressive loss of dorsiflexion of the great toe. Nonsurgical treatment attempts to lessen the dorsiflexion stresses on the great toe by the use of rigid-soled rocker bottom shoes. Adequate room in the toe box of the shoe is necessary to avoid direct pressure against the bony ridge.

Basic surgical goals are to remove both the impingement occurring between the dorsal aspect of the proximal phalanx and the first metatarsal head and the bony ridge that may irritate the overlying soft tissue. Resection arthroplasty, metatarsophalangeal joint arthrodesis, silicone interposition arthroplasty, phalangeal and metatarsal osteotomy, and cheilectomy have been used in the treatment of hallux rigidus. The simplest procedure appears to be a cheilectomy, in which the dorsal one-third of the metatarsal head is removed, thus eliminating the bony mass that impinges on the proximal phalanx (Fig. 4). Enough bone is excised to allow for 45 degrees of dorsiflexion. There is minimal postoperative morbidity. The procedure affords satisfactory results without producing an unstable metatarsophalangeal joint or necessitating the implantation of a foreign body. Failure from an initial cheilectomy can be salvaged easily with any of the other techniques.

A silicone implant in the base of the great toe proximal phalanx is an equally successful procedure. In the hallux rigidus deformity, a transfer metatarsalgia to the second

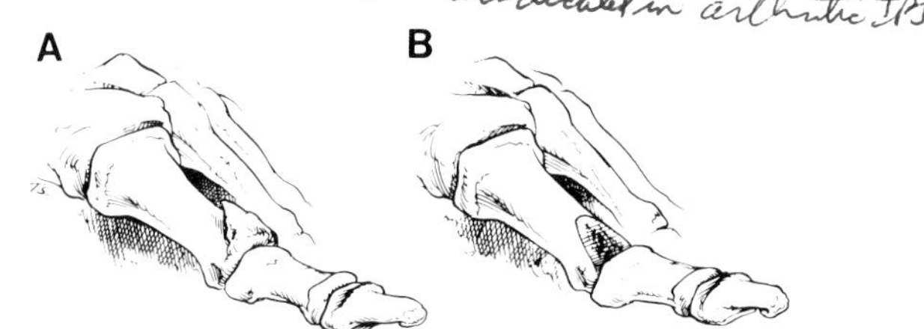

Figure 4: Cheilectomy for hallux rigidus. (A) Preoperative. (B) Postoperative.

metatarsal, which can result from the use of this implant for a routine hallux valgus deformity, usually does not occur.

Metatarsalgia As the term denotes, metatarsalgia is pain in the metatarsal region of the forefoot. Many disorders may produce such pain. Any disturbance which can affect the foot from a circulatory, metabolic, neurogenic, static, traumatic, or infectious process can be manifested by pain in the plantar or dorsal metatarsal region. The most common causes of metatarsalgia are disturbances of the sesamoids, plantar keratotic lesions, Morton's neuroma, pes cavus, pronated feet, and hallux valgus. Diagnosis of the etiology responsible for discomfort is essential for appropriate treatment selection.

If no etiology can be found other than a thinned plantar fat pad with prominent metatarsals, one should pursue a nonsurgical treatment. Initially this may be a very simple metatarsal pad placed proximal to the metatarsal region to lessen pressure. If this fails, a more formal inlay may be used to provide cushion to the metatarsal region while simultaneously attempting to redistribute pressure away from the metatarsal head. Pedorthists are especially helpful in providing shoe modifications and fabricating specialized shoe inlays that are valuable in the nonoperative treatment of these disorders. Patients with metatarsalgia secondary to generalized callousing and pressure beneath all the metatarsal heads are not good candidates for surgical correction and generally should be treated nonsurgically.

Ingrown Toenail (Onychocryptosis) The large toe of young adults is most commonly involved. Believed most commonly related to the use of closed-toe shoes or faulty toenail care, the distal nail edge traumatizes the distal nail groove, resulting in nail groove and fold swelling, inflammation, infection, and hypertrophy. If untreated, these changes progressively involve the full length of the lateral nail fold, including the groove and the wall.

Treatment is designed to decrease the trauma between the distal nail edge and the nail groove. In the early stages this can often be accomplished by elevating the distal nail edge out of the groove by inserting a small piece of cotton between the groove and the nail, and by measures to decrease local inflammation, infection, and soft-tissue hypertrophy (i.e., soaks, topical and systemic antibiotics, and silver nitrate cauterization of granulation tissue).

Surgery to relieve chronic nail groove trauma is frequently necessary. There are two general approaches: (1) to reduce the width of the nail, and (2) to redirect the nail groove peripheral to the nail edge. The first is easier and more commonly performed. The lateral nail edge is excised and the lateral germinal matrix proximal to the nail bed is carefully and completely excised. A small longitudinal excision in the eponychium is often but not always necessary to allow visualization of the germinal matrix. In addition, the epithelium on the bottom and lateral nail groove and in the proximal nail fold is excised to remove all possible germinal cells.

The second approach, redirection of the nail groove peripheral to the nail (DuVries), involves full-length excision of the hypertrophied lateral nail fold (including the wall and groove), elevation of the full length of the lateral nail edge, and suture of the lateral skin edge under the nail. This procedure is not recommended if there is marked plantar curving of the nail edge.

Surgical treatment of ingrown toenail is, however, associated with a high incidence of recurrence. Avulsion of the nail edge or the total nail is not recommended. Excision of the entire germinal matrix, and therefore elimination of the nail, is not recommended as a primary procedure but may be necessary when the nail has been severely deformed. Excision of the central nail bed is not recommended. Terminal Syme amputation is seldom necessary.

Neurologic Disorders

Interdigital Neuroma Morton's toe or Morton's neuroma is a well-known pathologic condition. The term *neuroma* is a misnomer since many studies have shown it is a perineural type of fibrosis. The deep fibers of the plantar aponeuroses form two marginal and eight intermediate sagittal septa, which penetrate beneath the flexor tendons, the nerves, and vessels to the sides of the fibrous flexor sheaths and the plantar ligaments. The sagittal septa have sharp proximal edges which the digital nerves must pass behind before they can proceed anteriorly from the central compartment. This anatomic arrangement forces the nerve of the third interspace to follow an oblique course on the surface of the flexor digitorum brevis. The nerve bends anteriorly on the edge of this flexed septum, predisposing to entrapment. This anatomic arrangement explains the fact that interdigital neuromas commonly are found in the third interspace.

Initial symptoms are usually vague and intermittent in nature. The diagnosis is established by pain and discomfort when compressing the involved interspace. When the diagnosis is unclear, 3 cc of 1 percent plain Xylocaine can be injected into the interspace and the patient allowed to ambulate for 10 to 15 minutes wearing a shoe. If a neuroma is present, the block should relieve the discomfort totally. When symptoms are of short duration, steroid injections may provide some relief. Shoe corrections are usually unsuccessful in patients with long-standing symptoms. Surgical resection remains the treatment of choice.

Most surgeons prefer the dorsal approach for patients without prior surgery. An adequate incision must be made, and the transverse metatarsal ligament should be released to allow clear visualization of the proximal nerve trunk. Recent studies on releasing the transverse metatarsal ligament rather than resecting the nerve have shown similar success. In an extremely thickened and enlarged nerve trunk, excision of the nerve would be preferable to surgical decompression.

Patients with failed neuroma surgery or recurrence of pain should have the interspace explored from a plantar approach. The incision should be longitudinal between the metatarsal heads. Dissection in the proximal portion of the incision allows the proximal nerve trunk to be identified. Distal dissection usually demonstrates a postsurgical neuroma stump which is scarred down to the transverse metatarsal ligament. The plantar approach in these patients provides much better visualization of the pathology than the dorsal approach. Only the skin is closed and no deep sutures are placed. The patient should be kept nonweight-bearing for the first 3 weeks and then gradually allowed to weight-bear on a well-padded, rigid-soled shoe for the following 3 weeks. This will minimize scar formation about the plantar incision.

Tarsal Tunnel Syndrome This is a symptom complex arising from compression of the posterior tibial nerve or its branches as they pass beneath the flexor retinaculum at the ankle. Posttraumatic fibrosis, engorgement of the venous plexus, tenosynovitis of the flexor digitorum longus, accessory hypertrophic abductor hallucis muscles, valgus deformity of the foot, rheumatoid arthritis, and neurilemoma of the nerve have been described as etiologic agents in this syndrome. In many patients no etiology can be identified. Unlike carpal tunnel syndrome, reports of bilateral tarsal tunnel syndrome are rare. First recorded in children less than 16 years of age in 1964, the syndrome is much more common in girls.

Symptoms consist of burning pain and paresthesias in the plantar region of the foot. The pain may worsen at night and be relieved by ambulation. Physical exam may reveal decreased sensation in the distribution of the posterior tibial nerve. All patients demonstrate tenderness to palpation in the tarsal canal region. A positive Tinel's sign should also be present.

Further diagnostic confirmation of the syndrome usually is obtained by electrodiagnostic measures. Determination of the distal motor latencies in the medial and lateral plantar nerves has been the basis for diagnosis. More recently, the amplitude and duration of the motor-evoked potentials have been shown to be a more sensitive indication of neuropathy. The lateral plantar branch of the posterior tibial nerve probably is affected earlier than the medial. Electrodiagnostic evaluation is useful in distinguishing a tarsal tunnel syndrome from a compression of the first sacral nerve root at the spinal level.

Injection of the tarsal canal with steroids may be beneficial in some patients. If this fails, surgical decompression usually is required. This involves release of the flexor retinaculum as far posteriorly as possible to prevent posterior tibial subluxation.

Anterior Tarsal Tunnel Syndrome Compression of the deep peroneal nerve as it crosses the anterior aspect of the ankle joint has been reported. Numbness and paresthesias may be noted in the first web space region. Aching and tightness about the ankle and dorsum of the foot may be the chief complaints.

Both motor and sensory signs may be present with tenderness over the anterior region of the ankle. Electrodiagnostic studies rule out a more proximal neural involvement.

Treatment consists of avoiding footwear and activity that compress or unduly stretch the deep peroneal nerve. Infiltration of the anterior tarsal tunnel with steroids may be used to relieve the symptoms. In some patients surgical exploration will be required. If the deep peroneal nerve is

Figure 5: Extra-depth shoe with composite inlay of Plastazote and sponge rubber.

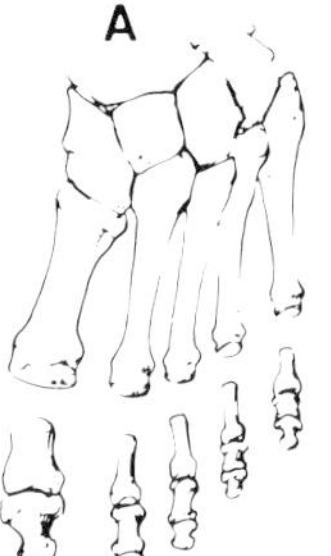

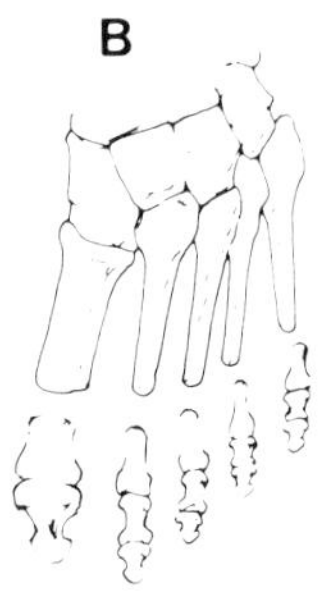

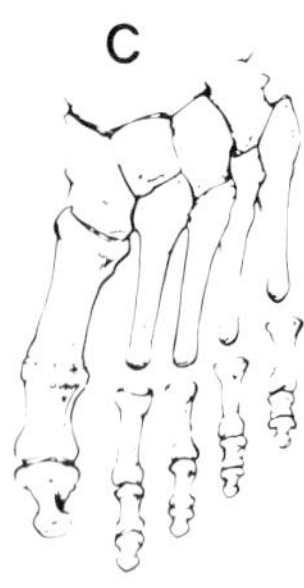

Figure 6: Various types of forefoot resections. (A) Section of bases of proximal phalangeal. Lack of resection of the major bony prominences (metatarsal heads) makes this procedure less effective. (B) Section of metatarsal heads and bases of proximal phalanges. Procedure adequately decompresses the bony deformity but may result in significant forefoot instability and recurrence of the toe deformities. (C) Fusion and head resections. Stabilizing the first ray minimizes recurrence of the deformity, and maintaining the bases of the proximal phalanges provides for a more stable forefoot.

explored, care should be taken to visualize the nerve from several centimeters above the inferior extensor retinaculum, as well as underneath it, to eliminate pathologic adhesions that may alter the mobility of the nerve.

Arthritis

Rheumatoid Forefoot Rheumatoid arthritis frequently affects the forefoot region. Early in the disease there may be only a synovitis about the metatarsophalangeal joints with resultant pain and swelling in the forefoot. But, with time, many patients may develop severe hallux valgus and dorsal dislocation of the metatarsophalangeal joints of the lesser toes.

Initial treatment in the minimally deformed foot is primarily medical. Control of the synovitis is the initial concern and may involve oral medications and/or local injections of steroid into the metatarsophalangeal joints. Properly sized shoes with cushioned inlays may also provide relief. As the deformity progresses, mechanical abnormalities develop that can lead to severely altered weight-bearing patterns.

In the severely deformed foot, conservative footwear is indicated. Although footwear does not correct the deformity, it can relieve the associated pain from the altered mechanical function of the foot. The extra-depth oxford, combined with a liner of a polyethylene foam, is effective in the treatment of the painful rheumatoid forefoot (Fig. 5). While Plastazote was the initial material used in several studies, there are other similar polyethylene foams available. A composite inlay of foam material backed by sponge rubber may be superior to the foam by itself. The sponge rubber will provide for a longer life for the inlays while simultaneously providing more cushion and less stress to the forefoot region.

In patients with deformities so severe that fitting any shoe is difficult, surgical alternatives may be considered. Many operations have been used to treat the deformed rheumatoid forefoot. Almost all excise some portion of the bony structure in the metatarsophalangeal joint (Fig. 6). The great toe may be treated similarly to the lesser toes, or the great toe metatarsophalangeal joint may be fused. Initial results with all types of forefoot resections are satisfactory. However, several long-term follow-up series have documented a high rate of recurrence of deformities and metatarsalgia. With too much bony resection, patients may complain of forefoot instability and imbalance.

Implant arthroplasty of the great toe has been useful (Fig. 7). In the severely deformed forefoot, recurrence of the deformity may be a problem. It is suggested that if a metatarsus primus varus deformity of greater than 15 degrees is present, corrective osteotomy of the metatarsal should be considered. More recently a double-stemmed implant has been recommended as a replacement arthroplasty. Smaller double-stemmed implants have been developed for the lesser toe metatarsophalangeal joints. Long-term follow-up studies with the double-stemmed implants in all of the forefoot metatarsophalangeal joints are not available.

Maintaining motion in the great toe metatarsophalangeal joint with the use of silicone arthroplasty may provide some theoretical advantages over fusion. From a practical standpoint, however, most patients with a severely deformed forefoot do not require any motion at the metatarsophalangeal joint to be functional and wear conservative footwear. Reports of patients with fusions of the great toe metatarsophalangeal joint have been generally satisfactory. Potential complications of fusion are malunion, nonunion, and prolonged immobilization in the postoperative period. Successful fusion rates in rheumatoid arthritic patients are high. The position of fusion should be approximately 15 to 20 degrees of dorsiflexion relative to the first metatarsal (Fig. 8). In the correct position, the toe should rest on the walking surface when the foot is in the flat position. A slight degree of valgus also is preferred to allow for better shoe fit. Numerous studies point out the improved weight-bearing pattern in the forefoot after fusion as compared to excisional arthroplasty as in a Keller procedure.

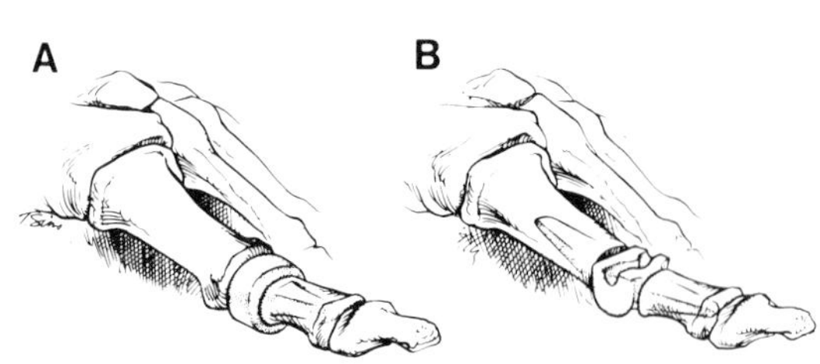

Figure 7: Implant arthroplasty of the great toe. (A) Single-stem silicone implant. (B) Double-stem, hinge-type, silicone implant.

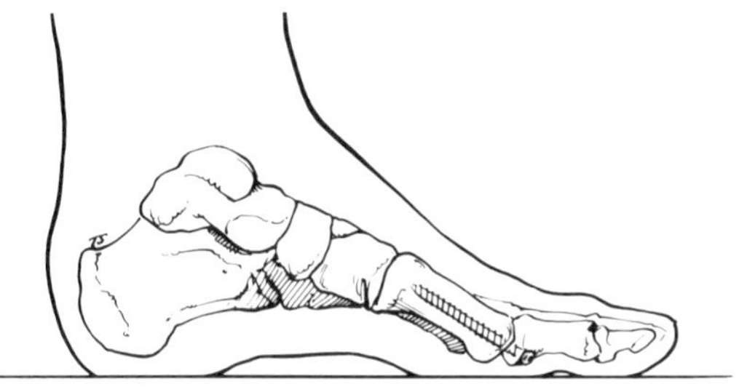

Figure 8: Desired position of fusion of the great toe MTP joint. (Note the great toe is resting flat on the walking surface.)

Metabolic

Diabetic Foot Care of the foot in the diabetic should begin with the initial diagnosis of diabetes. Although most diabetics do not develop significant insensitivity, all should be aware of this potential condition. Once the diagnosis of diabetic neuropathy is made, the patient must be educated in self-care of feet.

Office treatment of the insensitive foot is important. Adequate fitting shoes with protective insoles should be prescribed. Periodic debridement of calluses, corns, and nails should be carried out. With proper care, the development of open lesions can be prevented in most patients.

Ulcerations in the diabetic foot usually occur beneath the great toe, beneath the metatarsal heads, and on the dorsum of the proximal interphalangeal joints. The more superficial ulcers may be treated with debridement of the hypertrophic marginal skin and with use of a healing sandal or shoe with a composite type of inlay of polyethylene foam and sponge rubber. A total contact cast has been recommended for treatment of ulcers that have failed to heal by other means.

When deformity is present which results in significant localized pressures beneath certain areas, surgical correction of the deformity may be indicated to allow for healing. Surgical excision of the proximal one-half of the proximal phalanx of the great toe, followed by a split-thickness skin graft to the ulcer bed, has been used successfully to treat the resistant ulcer on the plantar aspect of the great toe. Studies have shown that diabetics with adequate blood flow heal most surgical wounds without difficulty. Doppler studies may be carried out to evaluate the status of blood flow in an extremity. Investigations suggest that toe pressure of 40 mm/Hg is needed for healing. Others have shown that satisfactory healing can be predicted if blood flow in the lower extremity is pulsatile and if the pressure index is greater than .45 and the systolic pulse pressure near 70 mm/Hg. The systolic pressure index is a ratio of lower extremity systolic pressure divided by the upper or brachial artery systolic pressure.

Charcot joints are another problem that may affect the diabetic patient with neuropathy. The diabetic with an insensitive foot may sustain an injury or combination of injuries that may not produce pain commensurate with the severity of the injury. Frequently these injuries will be unrecognized and may lead to an advanced degree of deformity and destruction. Successful treatment of this condition requires early diagnosis followed by prolonged immobilization and protection until the injury has had adequate time for healing. Immobilization may be required for two to three times longer than that required in treating a patient with normal sensation. The use of a custom-molded ankle-foot orthosis may be indicated for such a patient.

Infection is another common problem in the insensitive foot. Spread of infection often occurs before medical treatment is sought, due to the presence of minimal pain. Radical debridement is the best approach. This may involve both dorsal and plantar incisions. All infected tissue should be decompressed in an attempt to salvage the foot. Because of the frequent incidence of a mixed flora involving gram-negative rods and anaerobic bacteria, broad spectrum antibiotics are indicated. Cultures from surgical specimens are preferable to those from simple swabs from open wounds.

Amputation is a frequent result in severe infections and extensive ulcerations. Patients with large vessel disease may be candidates for vascular surgery to improve the blood flow and allow for a more conservative level of amputation. With adequate blood flow and control of the infection, partial amputations of the foot, including partial and total calcaneal excisions, can be successful. With improved diagnostic capabilities of determining the status of blood flow, single toe amputations or ray resections may be successfully performed. Amputations should be as far distal as possible because of the improved functional aspects of the more distal levels.

ANNOTATED BIBLIOGRAPHY

Functional Anatomy and Biomechanics

Bojsen-Mooller, F.: Anatomy of the forefoot, normal and pathologic. Clin. Orthop. 142:10-18, 1979.

The gross anatomy of the forefoot and its relationship to certain biomechanical principles are discussed in both normal and pathologic conditions.

Mann, R.A.: Surgical implications of biomechanics of the foot and ankle. Clin. Orthop. 146:111-118, 1980.

Basic biomechanics of the foot and ankle are reviewed and the functional aspects of the principles are related to specific surgical procedures involving the foot and ankle.

Acquired Disorders

Ankle Joint Degeneration

Morrey, B.F., and Wiedeman, G.P.: Complications and long-term results of ankle arthrodeses following trauma. J. Bone Joint Surg. 62A:777-784, 1980.

A review of sixty patients with ankle fusions shows relatively high complication rates but with eventual 83 percent patient satisfaction. Neutral varus-valgus and dorsiflexion plantar flexion is the optimum position of fusion.

Newton, St. E., III: Total ankle arthroplasty. J. Bone Joint Surg. 64A:104-111, 1982.

A review of fifty patients who had total ankle arthroplasty is presented. Best results were obtained in patients with degenerative arthritis whose ankles were stable and not deformed. Contraindications include osteonecrosis of the talus, pseudarthrosis of the site of a previous attempted fusion, and talar tilt of 20 degrees or more.

Stauffer, R.N.: Total joint arthroplasty: The ankle. Mayo Clin. Proc. 54:570-575, 1979.

The development of total ankle arthroplasty is reviewed. One hundred and two ankle arthroplasties were performed with reasonable results in patients with rheumatoid arthritis and older patients with posttraumatic degenerative arthritis. Younger patients had disappointing results.

Chronic Ankle Instability

Leach, R.E.; Namiki, O.; Paul, G.R.; and Stockel, J.: Secondary reconstruction of the lateral ligaments of the ankle. Clin. Orthop. 160:201-211, 1981.

Twenty-one athletically active patients (twenty-two ankles) with ankle pain and insecurity were treated. A well-described procedure designed to replace both the anterior talofibular and the calcaneofibular ligaments with all or a portion of the distal peroneus brevis tendon was utilized. All patients were able to return to their desired athletic activity.

Solheim, L.F.; Denstad, T.F.; and Roaas, A.: Chronic lateral instability of the ankle. Acta Orthop. Scand. 51:193-196, 1980.

Reconstruction of the lateral ankle ligaments using the medial one-third of the Achilles tendon as a vascularized graft is discussed. The results are good, and techniques are described.

Hallux Valgus

Johnson, K.A.; Cofield, R.H.; and Morrey, B.F.: Chevron osteotomy for hallux valgus. Clin. Orthop. 142:44-47, 1979.

All eighteen patients (twenty-six osteotomies) were improved at an average of 10 months postoperatively. The procedure offers the advantages of osteotomy stability, technical ease, and absence of secondary deformity such as transfer metatarsalgia.

Mann, R.A., and Coughlin, M.J.: Hallux valgus: Etiology, anatomy, treatment and surgical considerations. Clin. Orthop. 157:31-41, 1981.

A modified McBride procedure resulted in consistently satisfactory surgical results. Recommendations include fibular sesamoidectomy if the sesamoid is subluxated more than one-half of its width into the first intermetatarsal space, addition of a basilar metatarsal osteotomy if the hallux angle exceeds 40 degrees and the first intertarsal angle exceeds 15 degrees, and weekly dressing changes to ensure correct hallux position.

Stokes, I.A.; Hutton, W.C.; Stott, J.R.; and Lowe, L.W.: Forces under the hallux valgus foot before and after surgery. Clin. Orthop. 142:64-72, 1979.

Abnormalities in the hallux valgus foot and changes after surgery are investigated by measuring the distribution of load on the foot in walking. Pre- and postoperative studies show a decreased load on the medial aspect of the foot as compared to normal feet.

Hallux Rigidus

Mann, R.A.; Coughlin, M.J.; and DuVries, H.L.: Hallux rigidus: A review of the literature and a method of treatment. Clin. Orthop. 142:57-63, 1979.

The etiology of the hallux rigidus is discussed as well as the treatment by cheilectomy. The procedure involves resection of the proliferative bone at the metatarsophalangeal joint to allow for at least 45 degrees of passive dorsiflexion.

Ingrown Toenail (Onychocryptosis)

Dixon, G.L., Jr.: Treatment of ingrown toenail. Foot and Ankle 3:254-260, 1983.

Based on the stage of disease, the age of the patient, and the variety of treatment regimes available, the author provides a practical compendium of general and specific techniques to the treatment of any specific ingrown toenail.

Palmer, B.V., and Jones, A.: Ingrowing toenails: The results of treatment. British J. Surg. 66:575-576, 1979.

Two hundred and eight patients were studied for the rate of recurrence. Following avulsion of a strip of the nail, the recurrence rate was 83 percent, total avulsion of the nail was 70 percent, wedge resection was 29 percent, and total proximal nail bed ablation was 28 percent.

Neurologic Disorders

Interdigital Neuroma

Lassmann, G.: Morton's toe: Clinical, light and electron microscopic investigations in 133 cases. Clin. Orthop. 142:73-84, 1979.

Histologic studies on the tissues from surgical specimens point out that the syndrome appears to be an entrapment neuropathy. The most efficient treatment is resection of the interdigital nerve.

Tarsal Tunnel Syndrome

Albrektsson, B.; Rydholm, A.; and Rydholm, U.: The tarsal tunnel syndrome in children. J. Bone Joint Surg. 64B:215-217, 1982.

Ten patients, 9 to 15 years of age, were studied. Compared to affected adults, there was marked increase in female distribution, recurrent sharp pains, and inability to bear weight on the foot in some.

Kaplan, P.E., and Kernahan, W.T.: Tarsal tunnel syndrome. J. Bone Joint Surg. 63A:96-99, 1981.

Electrodiagnostic studies are used to show that reduced amplitude and increased duration of motor potentials are more sensitive indications of the presence of tarsal tunnel syndrome than the distal motor latency.

Anterior Tarsal Tunnel Syndrome

Borges, L.F.; Hallett, M.; Selkoe, D.J.; and Welch, K.: The anterior tarsal tunnel syndrome. J. Neurosurg. 54:89-92, 1981.

Report of two patients with anterior tarsal syndrome is presented along with a discussion of the various aspects of this underrecognized syndrome.

Arthritis

Rheumatoid Forefoot

Cracchiolo, A.: Management of the arthritic forefoot. Foot Ankle 3:17-23, 1982.

Evaluation and nonoperative care of the rheumatoid forefoot are discussed. Operative care, from excising all or part of the MTP joints to silicone implant arthroplasty of all MTP joints, is presented.

Lipscomb, P.R.: Arthrodesis of the first metatarsophalangeal joint for severe bunions and hallux rigidus. Clin. Orthop. 142:48-54, 1979.

Compression arthrodesis of the great toe metatarsophalangeal joint by the McKeever technique is presented. Advantages of this procedure over resection arthroplasty are discussed.

Swanson, A.B.; Lumsden, R.M.; and Swanson, G.D.: Silicone implant arthroplasty of the great toe. Clin. Orthop. 142:30-43, 1979.

A single-stem implant should probably not be used if the hallux angle exceeds 40 degrees. Corrective osteotomy of the base of the first metatarsal is recommended if the metatarsus primus varus angle is greater than 15 degrees. Twenty-four of the ninety-five rheumatoid feet required revision. A double-stemmed flexible hinge implant was developed and used in 105 great toes with the primary indication being rheumatoid arthritis.

Vahvanen, V.; Piirainen, H.; and Kettunen, P.: Resection arthroplasty of the metatarsophalangeal joints in rheumatoid arthritis. Scand. J. Rheumat. 9:257-265, 1980.

Follow-up results on 100 patients showed more than 50 percent had recurrences of the callosities and deformities of the toes. All patients with fusion of the great toe were satisfied.

Metabolic

Diabetic Foot

Jacobs, R.L., and Karmody, A.M.: Office care of the insensitive foot. Foot Ankle 2:230-237, 1982.

The most common cause of foot insensitivity is diabetes. Optimal treatment includes in-depth patient education, attentive foot care, and peripheral circulatory status monitoring. Walking tolerance and quantitative Doppler ultrasound measurements are emphasized.

Kwong, P.K.: Applications of Doppler ultrasound to foot and ankle care. Foot Ankle 2:220-223, 1982.

The use of systematic pressure measurements by means of Doppler ultrasound is beneficial in evaluating the diabetic or dysvascular foot for healing potential when planning surgery.

Wagner, F.W., Jr.: Transcutaneous Doppler ultrasound in the prediction of healing and the selection of surgical level for dysvascular lesions of the toes and forefoot. Clin. Orthop. 142:110-114, 1979.

Dysvascular lesions of the toes and forefoot are divided into five grades matched with appropriate treatment programs. Healing can be predicted with 90 percent accuracy when adequate blood flow is demonstrated by Doppler studies.

AUTHOR INDEX

Aaro, S., 226
Abdulla, D., 97
Abelson, H.T., 48
Abu Yousef, M.M., 131
Adams, J.P., 179, 188
Adelaar, R.S., 356
Adelman, L., 357
Afeiche, N., 216
Aglietti, P., 308
Ahlberg, A., 141
Ahlgren, S., 258
Ahmadi, B., 318
Ahmed, K.B., 224
Aidinis, S.J., 88
Akbarnia, B., 64, 318
Akeson, W.H., 7, 188, 336
Albin, D., 107
Albin, R., 188
Albrand, O.W., 244
Albrektsson, B., 376
Albright, J.A., 14, 207, 216
Albright, J.P., 131
Albright, T., 8
Aldridge, M.J., 335
Alexander, A.H., 367
Alho, A., 40
Ali, M.S., 141
Allen, B.L., Jr., 207, 225, 270
Allieu, Y., 141
Allum, R.L., 335
Almström, C., 70
Alon, G., 150
Altman, R.D., 38
Amadio, P.C., 187
Amato, J.J., 87
Ames, M.D., 269
Amiel, D., 7
Amos, W., 88
Amstutz, H.C., 97, 102, 130, 132, 309, 348
An, K.N., 161
Andersen, A., 367
Andersen, S., 367
Anderson, C.P., 236
Anderson, H.C., 26
Andersson, G., 257
Andrews, J.R., 327
Andriacchi, T.P., 77, 97, 347
Ansell, B.M., 114
Anthony, H., Jr., 257
Aracil, J., 151
Arafiles, R.P., 154, 161
Arden, G.P., 114, 132
Ariño, V.L., 151
Armstrong, G.W.D., 235
Arnoczky, S.P., 326, 368
Arnold, J.A., 132
Aromaa, A., 258
Arons, M.S., 179
Aronson, D., 187
Ashby, M.E., 124
Ashley, R.K., 141
Ashton, J.E., 39
Askew, L., 150, 161
Askew, M.J., 97
Athanasoulis, C.A., 88, 285, 309
Atkinson, J.R., 102
Austin, L.A., 27
Austin, R.T., 335
Avioli, L.V., 28
Axelgaard, J., 224
Badalamente, M.A., 184, 188
Bahnson, H.T., 70
Bailey, C., 5, 7
Bailey, H.L., 87
Bailey, S., 78
Baixauli, F., 151
Balfour, G.W., 124
Ball, J., 257
Bancel, P., 97
Bang, G., 64
Banta, J.V., 358
Barak, A.J., 88
Bardos, D.I., 96
Barger, W.L., 348
Barnes, G., 114
Barquet, A., 269
Barrett, A.J., 38
Barrington, T.W., 309
Bartel, D.L., 347
Bartlett, P., 57
Barton, N.J., 172
Bartzke, G., 335
Bashey, R.I., 39
Bassett, C.A.L., 236, 335
Bassett, F.H., 327
Bassett, R.W., 326
Batten, R.L., 335
Battista, A.F., 71
Baud, C.A., 26
Bauer, G.C.H., 338
Bauman, T.D., 188
Bazilevskaia, Z.V., 235
Beach, R.B., 187
Beals, R.K., 14
Beatty, M.E., 179
Beaty, J.H., 326
Beaupré, A., 269
Beck, R.J., 77
Beckenbaugh, R.D., 188, 295
Becker, D.A., 132
Becker, J.A., 284
Becker, R.O., 58
Beckstead, J.H., 48
Bedbrook, G.M., 207
Beeckman, C., 224
Behrend, A.J., 70
Behrens, F., 333
Beighton, P., 13, 14, 357
Bell, J.L., 187
Bell, R.S., 39
Benady, S.G., 77
Bendick, P.J., 216
Benjamin, A., 132
Benn, R., 257
Benner, B., 236
Bennett, E.L., 38
Bennett, J.B., 150
Bentivoglio, J., 243
Bentley, G., 39, 268
Bergfeld, J., 368
Bergfeld, M.A., 28
Bergmann, R., 107
Bernick, S., 257
Bert, J.M., 160, 162
Bertoni, F., 48
Bethea, 303
Bethem, D., 14, 225
Betts, H.B., 71
Bhuller, G.S., 152
Bianco, A.J., 114, 225, 357
Binder, W., 296
Binner, H., 243
Biovin, G., 26
Birnholz, J., 8
Bishop, J.O., 268
Bittinger, S., 179
Bittner, S., 64
Bivins, B.A., 70
Bjorklund, S., 224
Black, J., 26, 96, 335
Black, K., 102
Black, M., 64
Blackburne, J.S., 226
Blaha, J.D., 347
Blakemore, M.E., 152
Blanco, L.N., 38
Bleck, E., 77, 268, 357, 358
Blencke, B.A., 107
Bloom, M.H., 213, 216
Blount, W.P., 243, 317
Blowers, R., 58
Blum, C.E., 71, 152
Boardman, K.P., 87
Bobyn, J.D., 97
Bogduk, N., 215
Bogoch, E.R., 39
Bohart, P.G., 179
Böhler, J., 207
Bohlman, H.H., 207, 216, 236
Bojsen-Mooller, F., 375
Bolsen, B., 48
Bonnel, F., 141
Bonucci, E., 26
Borden, L.S., 308
Borges, L.F., 376
Bornstein, P., 13
Boskey, A.L., 26
Böstman, O., 334
Bouyala, J.M., 114
Bovill, E.G., Jr., 48, 124, 295
Bowden, J.A., 327
Bowers, W.H., 179, 188
Bowker, J.H., 71
Bowman, W.E., 295
Boxall, D., 226
Boychuck, L., 236
Boyd, R.D., 38
Boyer, D.W., 268
Braakman, R., 197
Bradford, D., 14, 224, 225, 226, 236, 244
Bradley, G.M., 358
Bradley, G.W., 107
Brady, P.G., 114
Brady, T., 257
Brain, L., 215
Brakenbury, P.H., 152
Brand, P.W., 187
Brand, R., 96, 308, 367
Brandt, K.D., 38
Braum, R., 123
Braun, R.M., 113, 179
Braune, M., 152
Brause, B.D., 309
Brickley-Parsons, D., 188
Briele, H.A., 48
Briggs, B.T., 132, 333, 335
Bright, D.S., 180
Bright, R.W., 64
Brighton, C.T., 12, 13, 14, 26, 39, 40, 335

Brodersen, M.P., 348
Brodeur, A.E., 140, 151
Brömer, H., 107
Bromley, J.W., 257
Bronson, M.L., 114
Brooks, A.L., 207
Brooks, D.H., 70
Brooks, H.L., 224
Brotman, S., 70
Broudy, A.S., 141
Brower, T.D., 87, 368
Brown, A., 88, 284
Brown, G.C., 308, 309
Brown, H.G., 172
Brown, J.C., 224
Brown, N., 40
Brown, P.W., 71
Brown, R.H., 236
Brown, S.A., 98
Brown, T.D., 285, 327
Browne, E.Z., Jr., 187
Browne, R.S., 285
Browner, B., 70, 367
Browning, W.H., 357
Bruce, D., 335
Brumfield, R.H., Jr., 161
Brummett, S., 356
Brunet, M.E., 127
Brunner, C., 296
Bruns, J., 356
Brunton, F.J., 215
Bryan, R.S., 161, 179, 348
Bryan, W.J., 216, 286, 309
Bryant, L., 114
Bryant, M.H., 368
Buchholz, H.W., 107, 308
Bucholz, R.W., 261, 286, 334
Budzilovich, G.N., 71
Bufan, D., 47
Buhl, O., 151
Bullen, B., 8
Bunnell, W.P., 224
Buonanno, F., 257
Burchardt, H., 26
Burdick, D.C., 295
Burgess, E.M., 70
Burke, F., 172
Burkhalter, W.E., 187
Burri, C., 335
Bursens, H., 97
Burssens, A., 327
Burstein, A.H., 347
Burwell, R.G., 268
Buskirk, E.R., 7
Bustin, W., 368
Butler, D.L., 326, 327
Buyse, M., 197
Buzzard, B., 141, 161
Byers, D.H., 13
Byrnes, D.P., 207
Cacavio, A., 48
Cailliet, R., 257
Caine, K., 70
Callahan, R.A., 207, 216
Calver, R., 268
Cameron, H.U., 97
Campanacci, M., 48, 318
Campbell, D., 113
Campbell, R., 225
Canale, S.T., 197, 270, 317, 357, 364, 367
Cannell, L.B., 38
Capanna, R., 48
Caparros, B., 48
Carlson, J.M., 224
Carol, M., 207
Carollo, J., 225
Carr, W.A., 224, 327
Carroll, N., 269, 317
Carroll, R.E., 187
Carson, W.G., 113
Carter, D.R., 308
Carter, V.S., 124
Cary, J.M., 71
Casey, M.J., 296
Caspari, R.B., 131
Cassidy, R.E., 326
Castle, M.E., 269
Catterall, A., 262, 268
Cederberg, P.A., 70
Cerny, K., 78
Chaganti, R.S.K., 27
Chai, Y.B., 48
Chambers, R.B., 357
Chandler, H.P., 39
Chao, E.Y.S., 150, 161, 309, 335, 347
Chapman, G.K., 197
Chapman, M.W., 295, 296
Chappuis, J.P., 113
Charlesworth, D., 70
Charnley, J., 102
Chaudhuri, P.K., 48
Chekofsky, K.M., 309
Chen, P.Q., 97
Cheng, P.T., 38
Chesney, R.W., 27
Chick, R.R., 325
Childers, S.J., 70
Chou, S.N., 236, 244
Chow, S.P., 179
Chrestian, P., 114
Chrisman, O.D., 316
Chryssanthou, C., 87
Chung, S.M.K., 109, 110, 112, 113, 198
Cicek, R.Z., 102
Cimino, W.R., 102
Clancy, W.G., Jr., 325
Clanton, T.O., 296, 318
Clarke, I.C., 97, 102, 132
Clawson, D.K., 267
Clayton, M.L., 188
Clement, D.B., 317
Clements, N., 39
Cleveland, R.J., 87
Clippinger, F.W., 71
Cloward, R.B., 207
Cochran, T.P., 243
Cofield, R.H., 124, 131, 132, 376
Cohen, A.W., 114
Cohen, M.M., 141
Coker, T.P., 132
Colapinto, V., 285
Coldewey, J., 335
Coleman, S.S., 268, 356, 358
Collert, S., 308
Collins, H.R., 124
Collins, M., 367
Colwill, J.C., 216
Comeaux, L.J., Jr., 87
Compere, C., 347
Conlogue, G.J., 114
Conn, K.M., 27
Connolly, J.F., 88, 335
Conrad, J., 7
Convery, F.R., 348
Cook, T.M., 357
Cooke, T.D.V., 38
Cooley, L.H., 368
Cooney, W.P., III, 57, 180
Cooper, L., 77, 78
Cooper, R.R., 172
Copeland, S.A., 132, 161
Corbett, M., 124
Corea, J.R., 148, 152
Corkill, G., 244
Corkill, J.A., 107
Coskey, R.J., 170, 172
Costanza, M., 256
Costanzo, G., 224
Coster, I., 97
Coughlin, M.J., 376
Coventry, M.B., 309, 347, 348
Cowell, H.R., 356, 357
Cowley, R.A., 70
Cox, J., 8, 367
Cracchiolo, A., 58, 348, 376
Crandall, R.C., 88
Crane, D.B., 88
Cravioto, H.M., 71
Crawford, A.H., 356
Crider, R.J., 268
Crilly, R.G., 244
Cristofaro, R.L., 77
Cronemeyer, R.L., 142
Crout, D.H.G., 107
Crowninshield, R.D., 96, 297, 308
Cruess, R.L., 132, 269, 295
Crugnola, A., 102
Csongradi, J., 77, 295
Cuckler, J., 258
Culp, P., 317
Cummine, J.L., 244
Cumming, W.A., 114
Cummings, B.J., 142
Cupic, Z., 102
Currarino, G., 357
Curtis, L.E., 88
Curtis, R., 367
Curtis, R.M., 179
Cyron, B., 257
Czitrom, A.A., 317
D'Ambrosia, R., 356
Dabrowski, W., 114
Dahmer, C., 88
Dal Monte, A., 48
Dallas, T.G., 268
Daly, M.J., 70
Dameron, T.B., Jr., 151, 326
Dan, B.B., 57
Daniel, D., 77
Daniel, R.K., 88, 161
Daniels, A.U., 235
Danielsson, L.G., 141
Danoff, J.V., 150
Darby, T., 358
Dardik, H., 70
Dardik, I., 70
Daruwalla, J.S., 152
Das Gupta, T.K., 48
Das, M., 114
Das, S.K., 172
Daube, J.R., 162
Daudet, M., 113
Daussange, J., 197
Davidovits, P., 216
Davidson, R.I., 215
Davis, P., 257
Davis, R.E., 187
Davis, R.F., 188
Dawe, C., 141
Dawson, E.G., 142, 197, 236
Day, L.J., 124, 295, 335
De Korompay, V., 258
De Mauroy, J.C., 224
DeHaven, K.E., 326
Del Sel, H.J., 88
DeLaTorre, J.C., 235
DeLee, J.C., 87, 151, 296, 318, 334, 335, 336, 367
Dell, P.C., 141
DeLuca, F., 258
Denis, F., 227, 235
Dennis, M.D., 367
Denstad, T., 366, 376
DeOrio, J.K., 225
Derby, R., 258
Derscheid, G.L., 327
DeSilva, J., 367
DeSmet, A.A., 114, 142
Desnick, R.H., 141
DeSousa, A., 225
Deutsch, S.D., 77
Deutscher, K.K., 107
Devogelaer, J.P., 27
Dewerpe, P., 258
Dias, L.S., 358
Dickinson, D., 284
Dickson, J., 236
Dickson, R.A., 357
Dickstein, H., 152
Dieppe, P.A., 38
Dignan, P.St.J., 14
Dimeglio, A., 141
Dimnet, J., 225
Dines, D., 131
Dingeldein, E., 107
DiNubile, N.A., 39
DiStefano, V., 114
Dixon, G.L., Jr., 376
Dobyns, J.H., 57, 161, 179, 180, 188
Donaldson, L.J., 335
Donovan, R.M., 114
Donovan, W.H., 207
Doppelt, S.H., 48
Dorgan, J., 268
Dorr, L.D., 87, 309

Dowden, R.V., 132
Dowling, J.M., 102
Dowling, S.V., 188
Doyle, J.R., 141
Draenert, K., 310
Draganich, L.F., 97
Drake, D., 124
Dran, G., 224
Drayer, B.P., 236
Drennan, D.B., 150
Drennan, J.C., 77, 225, 317
Drezner, M.K., 27
Drinker, H., 295
Droegenmueller, W., 64
Drummond, D.S., 269
Dubois, P.J., 236
Dubousset, J., 225
Ducheyne, P., 97
Ducker, T.B., 207
Dumbleton, J.H., 102
Duncan, J.W., 269
Dunham, W.K., 318
Dunn, E.J., 215, 216
Dunn, H.K., 235
DuPont, B., 27
Dustman, J.A., 187
Dutton, R.O., 142
DuVries, H.L., 376
Eady, J.L., 26
Eaton, B., 26
Eaton, R.G., 187
Ebskov, B., 70
Ecker, M., 114
Eckhardt, W.A., 180
Edmonson, A.S., 224
Edwards, C., 367
Edwards, W.T., 236, 257
Ege, W., 107
Eidman, D.K., 114
Eilber, F.R., 48
Eismont, F.J., 207, 216, 236
Ejeskär, A., 179
El-Khoury, G.Y., 131, 197
Eldevik, P., 258
Eliopoulos, G.M., 57
Ellenberg, S.S., 87
Ellis, H.A., 27
Ellis, J., 187
Elmstedt, E., 87
Elson, R.A., 105, 107, 308
Emery, F.E., 270
Eng, G.D., 114
Engel, J., 180
Engelbrecht, E., 107, 308
Engh, C.A., 97
Engkvist, O., 40, 180
English, P., 87
Enis, J.E., 87, 317
Enneking, W.F., 26, 47, 48, 318
Enzinger, F.M., 48
Epner, R.A., 188
Epstein, H.C., 295
Erat, K., 326
Erickson, D.L., 236
Ericson, R., 180
Eriksson, E., 326, 327
Erkkila, J.C., 236
Ernst, C.B., 70
Erwin, W.E., 224
Esterhai, J.L., Jr., 26, 335
Evans, G.A., 77, 225
Evans, J.P., 161, 180
Evans, L.E., 70
Evarts, C.M., 309
Eversmann, W.W., Jr., 151, 161, 187
Evrard, J., 58
Ewald, F.C., 155, 161
Ezaki, M., 286
Fahey, J.T., 269
Fahmy, N.R., 87
Fair, W.R., 88
Fairbank, J., 257, 258
Fallstrom, K., 243
Farfan, H., 257, 258
Farine, I., 58, 180
Farrar, E.L., III, 150
Fazzalari, N., 295
Fearns, M., 141, 161
Feest, T.G., 27
Feffer, H.L., 87
Feingold, M., 141
Feltner, J.B., 309
Fen, G., 47
Ferguson, A.B., Jr., 327
Ferguson, R.L., 207, 225
Ferlic, D.C., 188
Fermier, R.W., 77, 347
Fernando, L., 179
Ferrer, J., 151
Fetto, J.F., 326
Fidler, M.O., 172
Fielding, J.W., 190, 193, 197, 198, 295
Filipovic, M., 113
Finsterbush, A., 13, 142
Fischer, R.P., 284
Fitzgerald, B., 150
Fitzgerald, R.H., Jr., 57, 58, 348
Flamant, R., 58
Flanigan, D.P., 70
Flatt, A., 172
Flesch, J.R., 236
Flint, L.M., Jr., 88, 284
Flye, M.W., 70
Folkers, K., 187
Fonseka, N., 114
Ford, W.F., 77
Fornasier, V.L., 142
Foster, B.K., 268
Foster, C.R., 124
Fowles, J.V., 151
Fox, E.L., 2, 3, 7
Fox, J.L., 347
Frankel, H.L., 236
Franklin, B.A., 7
Franklin, J.D., 172
Fraser, M., 269
Frazier, J.K., 78
Fredericks, G.R., 40
Freeman, B.L., III, 326
Freeman, M.A.E., 97
Freeman, M.A.R., 104, 107, 347
Frei, E., III, 48
Freitag, J.J., 27
Friedenberg, Z.B., 26, 335
Fries, I., 358
Frisch, R.E., 8
Froimson, A.I., 157, 162
Frymoyer, J., 256
Fu, F.H., 327
Fuji, T., 216
Fujisawa, Y., 39
Fukubayaski, T., 326
Fulford, G.E., 141
Fulford, P.C., 327
Fuller, D.J., 152
Fuller, S., 295
Fullerton, R., 27
Funder, V., 367
Galante, J.O., 77, 96, 97, 107, 347
Galleno, H., 64
Gallico, G.G., III, 58
Gallop, P.M., 27
Gamble, J., 367
Ganel, A., 58, 180
Gangemi, M., 197
Ganjavian, M.S., 318
Garetto, L.P., 336
Garfin, S., 152, 268
Garland, D.E., 77, 78, 152, 162
Garrett, R., 295
Garrick, J., 327, 361, 367
Garside, H., 285
Gartsman, G.M., 150
Garver, D.F., 151
Gassman, J., 367
Gaston, S.R., 335
Gaul, J.S., Jr., 179
Geehr, R.B., 197
Geist, R.W., 296
Gelberman, R.H., 114, 150, 152, 179, 187, 188
Gelfan, S., 236
Ger, E., 171
Ger, R., 58
Ghista, D.N., 236
Ghobadi, F., 318
Gibbs, A.N., 348
Gibeault, D., 357
Gilbert, A., 168, 172
Giles, J.B., 334
Gillström, P., 308
Gimlette, T., 268
Gitelis, S., 48
Glatstein, E., 48
Glaubiger, D., 48
Glenn, W., 258
Glimcher, M.J., 26, 87, 141, 188
Glogovac, S.V., 179
Glover, J.L., 216
Gmeiner, J.G., 325
Goald, H., 257
Goggin, J., 256
Gold, R.H., 48
Goldberg, I., 150
Goldberg, M.J., 197
Goldberg, N.H., 172
Goldie, I.F., 284
Goldman, A., 258
Goldman, M., 257
Goldner, J.L., 358
Goldner, R.D., 64
Goldsand, E.M., 267
Gomez, J.G., 257
Gomez, M.A., 7
Gomis, R., 141
Goncalves, R.P., 39
Gonon, G.P., 224
Good, R.A., 27
Goode, G.L., 27
Goodman, M.J., 188
Goodman, S.H., 101
Goodwin, C.A., 38
Goorin, A.M., 48
Goossen, C., 27
Gottlieb, N.L., 39
Gottschalk, F.A.B., 357
Gotz-Welbergen, A.V., 8
Gould, J.S., 356
Gräbe, R.P., 358
Grace, T.G., 151, 156, 161
Graf-Radford, A., 309
Graham, C.B., 141
Graham, D.R., 57
Gramse, R.R., 162
Grana, W.A., 318
Granberry, W.M., 169, 172
Graviss, E.R., 140, 151
Gray, D.H., 356
Gray, J.E., 224
Gray, R.G., 39
Green, B.A., 207
Green, G.A., 348
Green, J.F., 161
Green, N.E., 268, 358
Green, W.T., 141
Green, W.T., Jr., 39
Greene, G., 14
Greene, W.B., 71
Greenfield, A.J., 88
Greer, R.B., III, 39
Gregg, J.R., 114
Greiff, J., 367
Griffen, W.O., Jr., 70
Griffin, D.W., 197
Griffin, P.P., 268, 358
Griss, P., 309
Gristina, A.G., 129, 132
Griswold, D.M., 207
Grogan, D.P., 334
Grood, E.S., 326, 327
Grosfeld, J.L., 141
Gross, A., 107
Gross, A.E., 37, 40
Gross, R.H., 257
Grossman, J.A.I., 179
Gruber, R., 152
Gruen, T., 97
Gruenwald, C., 187
Gschwend, N., 161
Guess, V., 224
Guhl, J.F., 317
Gui, P.L., 216
Guilford, W.B., 188
Gupta, S.K., 70
Gustilo, R.B., 87
Guyer, R., 258

Gwathmey, F.W., 87, 172
Ha'eri, G.B., 131, 347
Haajanen, J., 334
Haas, L.M., 88
Haase, G., 64
Habener, J.F., 27
Habig, T., 77
Haderspeck, K., 257
Haggmark, T., 326, 327
Hakkinen, S., 284
Hall, J.E., 197, 225
Hall, J.G., 14, 141
Hall, P., 225
Hall, P.V., 216
Hall, V., 224
Haller, J.A., Jr., 286
Hallett, M., 376
Halley, D.K., 102
Halpern, A.A., 149, 152, 336
Hamilton, P.J., 141, 161
Hampton, S.J., 97
Hancock, D.O., 236
Hanissian, A.S., 114
Hansen, S.T., Jr., 285, 296
Hansen, T., 258
Hansen-Leth, C., 71
Hanson, C.T., 150
Hansson, L.I., 357
Harbison, J.S., 357
Hardy, A.E., 152
Hargens, A., 187, 327, 336
Hargreaves, D.J., 326
Harley, J.D., 285
Harmon, S.L., 97
Harrelson, J.M., 71
Harrington, K.D., 216, 244, 295
Harrington, P., 236
Harris, B.A., 326
Harris, E.D., 38
Harris, L.J., 295
Harris, M.B., 27
Harris, W.D., 132
Harris, W.H., 88, 97, 285, 308, 309
Harris, W.R., 123
Harrison, M.H.M., 268
Harrison, P., 187
Hart, D.L., 207
Harty, M., 114
Hartz, C.R., 162
Harwood, A.R., 142
Hasenhuttl, K., 335
Haskell, S.S., 132
Hastings, D.E., 327
Haughton, V., 258
Haun, C., 318
Hauschka, P.V., 27
Hawkins, R.J., 131, 197, 198
Hayes, D.B., 326
Hayes, W., 7, 236, 257
Heath, H., III, 27
Heath, J.C., 97
Heckman, J.D., 334, 335
Hedley, A.K., 97, 309
Hedström, S., 107
Heger, H., 71
Heimke, G., 309
Heinz, E.R., 236
Heiple, K.G., 64
Helal, B., 357
Helbig, F.E., 295
Helfer, R., 64
Helikson, M.A., 286
Hellberg, S., 151
Hempton, R.F., 188
Hench, L.L., 97
Hennig, W., 107
Henriksson, J., 7
Henry, R.E., 70
Hensinger, R.N., 197
Herbert, V., 7
Herberts, P., 70
Hergenroeder, P.T., 152
Herman, R., 224
Hermann, H., 8
Hermansen, L., 7
Hernborg, J.S., 39
Herr, B., 224
Herring, J., 225
Herrington, J., 27
Heslin, D.J., 316
Hewes, T., 367
Hill, C., 58
Hill, J.A., 124, 347
Hillman, D., 356
Hilton, R., 257
Hirabayashi, K., 212
Hirsch, J.F., 197
Hirschowitz, D., 132
Hislop, H., 78
Ho, E., 179
Hodgson, S.F., 27
Hoffer, M.M., 77, 78, 123, 140, 358
Hoffman, A.D., 224
Holliday, P., 71
Hollister, D.W., 13
Holmes, J.C., 197
Holmström, T., 40
Holstein, A., 358
Holstein, P., 70
Hood, R.W., 342, 344
Hooper, G., 141
Hoppenfeld, S., 360
Horan, F., 13
Horne, G., 150
Horne, J.G., 70
Horoszowski, H., 58
Horsman, A., 27, 244
Hotokebuchi, T., 87
Houghton, G.R., 357
House, J.H., 172
Howard, R.C., 132
Howell, D.S., 38
Howson, D.C., 224
Hoyt, W.A., 269
Hrubec, Z., 71
Hruska, K.A., 27
Hsu, J., 77, 123, 358
Huaux, J.P., 27
Hubbard, C.N., 197
Hubbard, D.D., 267
Hughston, J.C., 327
Hui, F.C., 180
Hulth, A., 38
Hultman, E., 7
Hungerford, D.S., 81, 82, 87, 97
Hunninghake, D.B., 7
Hunter, G.A., 71, 309
Hunter, L.Y., 71, 162, 368
Hurst, L.C., 187, 188
Husby, O.S., 64
Huskisson, E.C., 38
Husseini, N., 142
Hussey, R.W., 76
Huston, C.C., 70
Hutton, W.C., 257, 376
Huvos, A.G., 48
Hyslop, G., 236
Ibrahim, I.M., 70
Ilardi, C.F., 39
Ilstrup, D.M., 295
Immenkamp, M., 216
Inglis, A.E., 131, 155, 161, 216, 309
Inoue, K., 257
Insall, J., 343, 344, 347
Insler, H.P., 347
Ippolito, E., 224, 269, 356
Irstram, L., 243
Ito, H., 236
Iwano, K., 161
Jablon, M., 132
Jackson, D.W., 325
Jackson, J.L., 77
Jackson, M.A., 269
Jackson, R.P., 243
Jackson, R.W., 326
Jacobs, R.F., 357
Jacobs, R.L., 376
Jacobs, R.R., 236
Jacquemeir, M., 114
Jaeger, S.H., 172
Jahss, M.H., 356, 357
James, M.L., 107
James, P.M., 141
Janecki, C.J., 334
Jardon, O.M., 88
Jaroma, H., 284
Jarrah, M., 70
Jaslow, B., 150
Javech, N., 224
Jenkin, R.D., 142
Jenkins, E.B., 207
Jensen, J.S., 295
Jimenez, S.A., 39, 40
Jobe, F.W., 124
Johansson, J.E., 309
Johansson, S.H., 40
Johnson, K.A., 376
Johnson, L.L., 131
Johnson, R.K., 162
Johnson, R.M., 207, 215, 216
Johnson, R.P., 180
Johnston, D.W., 335
Johnston, R.C., 96, 308
Johnston, R.M., 285, 295
Jolley, M.N., 308, 309
Jones, A., 376
Jones, F., 258
Jones, P., 141, 161
Jorgensen, J.P., 367
Josefsson, G., 309
Joseph, R.B., 179
Josephsen, P., 70
Joyce, J.W., 70
Judet, R., 275, 285
Judice, D.J., 123
Julkunen, H., 258
Jungbluth, K.H., 285
Kacy, S.S., 70
Kagan, A., II, 97
Kaijser, L., 7
Kaiser, T.E., 47
Kalamchi, A., 71, 198, 267
Kalsbeck, J., 225
Kamhin, M., 58
Kaplan, F., 39
Kaplan, P.E., 376
Kaplan, S.S., 145, 146, 152
Kapoor, N., 27
Karagancheva, S., 179
Karaharju, E., 285, 334
Karle, A., 71
Karmody, A.M., 376
Kärrholm, J., 354, 357
Karube, S., 356
Kassab, M.T., 151
Katsuki, I., 87
Katz, J., 88
Katz, J.M., 356
Kaufer, H., 151, 295
Kaufman, B., 215
Kavanaugh, J.H., 366, 368
Kay, L., 141, 161
Kaye, J., 258
Keagy, R.D., 71
Keating, T.M., 71, 162
Keats, P., 358
Keever, J.E., 334
Keggi, K, 216
Kehl, D.K., 224, 268
Keifer, T., 70
Kellam, J., 284
Kelly, E.G., 78
Kelly, F.B., Jr., 367
Kelly, W.N., 38
Kelsey, J., 257
Kempe, C.H., 64
Kempken, T.G., 317
Kenmore, P.I., 87
Kenna, R.V., 97
Kennedy, J.C., 131
Kennedy, L.A., 357
Kenner, G.H., 97
Kenzora, J.E., 87, 367
Kerlan, R.K., 124
Kernahan, W.T., 376
Kerr, D.N.S., 27
Ketcham, A.S., 71
Kettelkamp, D.B., 347
Kettunen, P., 376
Khang-Cheng, H., 258
Kier, E.L., 197
Kikuchi, S., 215
Kilcoyne, R.K., 180
King, H., 224
Kirchmer, N.A., 142
Kirkaldy-Willis, W., 257, 258
Kirkpatrick, D., 27
Kirkpatrick, J., 64

Kirves, P., 347
Kiss, A., 151
Kistler, J., 257
Kiviluoto, O., 334
Klahr, S., 27
Klassen, R.A., 64
Klawitter, J.J., 107
Kleerekoper, M.B., 27
Kleinert, H.E., 161, 172, 188
Kleinman, H.K., 27
Kleinman, R.G., 268
Kleinman, W.B., 188
Klimach, O., 70
Kliman, M., 142
Kline, D.G., 114, 123
Klinger, J., 236
Klisic, P., 113
Knekt, P., 258
Knutsson, F., 246
Koch, B., 114
Koffman, M., 77
Kohler, R., 113
Komaroff, A., 257
Koogle, T.A., 236
Koskinen, E.V.S., 40
Koskinen, M., 77
Kosloff, C., 48
Kostuik, J.P., 243
Kott, J., 114
Kozinn, S.C., 97
Kramer, G., 97
Kreutner, A., 97
Krick, H.J., 71
Kristaphonis, J., 27
Kruger, L.M., 316
Krugmire, R.B., Jr., 336
Kudo, H., 161
Kuei, S.C., 7
Kunee, J., 179
Kuo, D.P., 48
Kuo, K.N., 77
Kutz, J.E., 161
Kwok, D.C., 295
Kwong, P.K., 376
Labosky, D., 114
Lachiewicz, P.F., 347
Läike, E., 347
Lambert, D.C., 334
Lamberta, F.J., 188
Lance, E.M., 358
Lane, J.M., 26, 27, 48, 295
Lange, T.A., 325
Langenskiöld, A., 64, 317
Langer, F., 40, 142
Langer, L.O., 14, 225
Langlais, F., 39
Lansinger, O., 284
LaRocca, H., 215
Laros, G.S., 296
Larsen, I., 358
Larsen, L.J., 141, 268
Larson, S., 258
Larsson, K., 335
Lassmann, G., 376
Latta, L., 224
Laurin, S., 357
Laus, M., 318
Lavalette, R., 152
Lawyer, R.B., Jr., 335
Leach, J., 78
Leach, R.E., 124, 375
Leape, L.L., 197
Ledbetter, C.A., 71
Lee, A.J., 103, 104, 107
Lee, C.K., 215
Lee, C.L., 358
Lee, Y.F., 187
Leffert, R.D., 123, 162
Lehmann, T.R., 207
Leibel, S.A., 48
Leider, L.L., 236
Lemaire, R.G., 368
Lendeen, F.H., 88
Lennox, D.W., 64
Lenz, H.W., 8
Lenzi, W.D., 142
Leon, A.S., 7
Leonard, M.A., 318
Lereim, P., 107
Lespargot, A., 358
Letournel, E., 275, 285
Lettin, A.W.F., 132
Letts, R.M., 357
Levine, A.M., 313, 317
Levinson, E.M., 258
Levy, I.M., 326
Levy, M., 150, 187
Levy, R.N., 48
Lewinnek, G., 347
Lewis, A.G., 335
Lewis, J., 97
Li, S.M., 48
Li, W.K.P., 26
Lian, E.C., 87, 317
Lian, J.B., 27
Liang, M., 257
Libman, R.H., 88
Lichter, A., 48
Lichtman, D.M., 161, 367
Lidgren, L., 107
Lidström, J., 224
Lidwell, O.M., 58
Lindberg, L., 309
Lindholm, T.S., 161, 317
Lindholmer, E., 367
Lindseth, R., 225, 269
Lindstrom, J.R., 268
Ling, R.S., 107
Linscheid, R.L., 161, 162, 177, 179, 180, 188
Lippert, F.G., III, 150
Lipscomb, P.R., 376
Lipscomb, R., 285
Lipton, D.E., 172
Liskova-Kiar, M., 96
Lister, G.D., 188
Liu, C.C., 48
Liyanage, I.S., 114
Lloyd-Roberts, G.C., 269
Lluch, E.E., 151
Lodenkämper, H., 107, 308
Lombardo, S.J., 124
Lonstein, J.E., 14, 224, 225, 244
Lopez, C., 27
Lord, G., 97
Lorig, R.A., 236
Lotke, P., 114
Loughlin, E.C., Jr., 87, 317
Louis, D.L., 317
Louis, D.S., 71, 162, 179
Lovell, W.W., 113, 224
Lovitt, J., 87, 317
Low, W.G., 161
Lowbury, E.J., 58
Lowe, D., 58
Lowe, L.W., 376
Lubahn, J.D., 309
Lubbers, L.M., 335
Lucas, J.T., 207
Lucie, R.S., 295
Lugli, T., 132
Luisiri, A., 140, 151
Lukash, F.N., 58
Lumsden, R.M., 376
Lund-Kristensen, J., 367
Lundborg, G., 180, 187
Lunde, O., 88
Luque, E.R., 225
Lüscher, J.N., 296
Luthy, D.A., 141
Lutter, L., 14, 225
Lyles, K.W., 27
Lyne, E.D., 316
MacCarty, C.S., 197, 225
MacDonald, R.I., 161
MacEwen, G.D., 14, 114, 198, 224, 267
MacIntosh, D.L., 347
Mack, G.R., 161
Mack, L.A., 285
Mackay, I., 150
MacKenzie, I.G., 268
Macleod, A.M., 172, 188
MacNab, I., 208, 215
Magerl, F., 296
Mai, L.L., 309
Makin, M., 243
Malawer, M.M., 48
Malcom, L.L., 348
Maldague, B., 27
Malerich, M.M., 187
Malghem, J., 27
Malone, J.M., 70
Mangum, G.L., 172
Mankin, H.J., 40, 45, 48
Manley, M.T., 358
Mann, R.A., 375, 376
Mann, R.J., 187
Mann, R.V., 368
Manske, P.R., 141
Mansour, M.J., 77
Manugian, A.H., 357
Maquet, P., 39, 347
Marberry, T.A., 124, 131
Marcove, R.C., 48
Marcus, N.W., 318
Margolies, M.N., 88
Margolis, R.N., 216
Markand, O.M., 216
Markolf, K.L., 236
Marks, K.E., 308
Marks, M.I., 57
Maroudas, A., 38
Marquardt, E., 70, 316
Marshall, D.H., 27, 244
Marshall, J.L., 326
Martens, M., 97, 327
Martin, G.R., 27
Martin, K.J., 27
Martin, R.B., 38
Martins, A.N., 215
Martos, F., 151
Marxen, J.L., 356
Mason, J.A., 87
Masse, M., 366
Massiah, K.A., 285
Mast, J.W., 151
Masuhara, K., 39
Matalon, T.S., 88
Matev, I.B., 167, 168, 172, 179, 187, 188
Matsen, F.A., III, 70, 336
Matthews, J.G., 151
Matthews, L.S., 151
Maulucci, R., 224
Maxwell, G.M., 71
May, J.W., Jr., 58, 88
Mayfield, J.K., 180, 225, 236
Maylahn, D.J., 150
Mazas, F., 58
McArthur, J.W., 8
McBroom, R., 309, 335
McCall, I., 258
McCann, V.J., 187
McCarroll, H.R., Jr., 141
McCarthy, J.C., 39, 97
McCaskill, B.L., 309
McClelland, C.Q., 64
McClinton, M.A., 179
McCollough, N.C., III, 87, 224, 317, 87
McComas, A.J., 187
McCracken, G.H., Jr., 57, 269
McCraw, J.B., 132
McCullough, C.J., 152
McDaniel, W.J., Jr., 326
McElfresh, E., 162
McElhaney, J.H., 71
McFarlane, R., III, 267
McGarvey, M.L., 27
McGlynn, F.J., 131
McKay, D.W., 141, 356
McKee, N.H., 40
McKenzie, R., 257
McKibbin, B., 17, 26
McKinney, R.V., Jr., 107
McKinnon, B., 268, 357
McKusick, V.A., 14
McLaughlin, R.E., 107
McLeod, P., 334
McManus, F., 316
McMaster, M.J., 225
McMurty, R., 284
McNicol, K., 317
McPhee, I.B., 226
McReynolds, I.S., 367
Meachim, G., 97
Mears, D.C., 96, 285

Medlar, R.C., 316
Medsger, T.A., Jr., 27
Meek, E.S., 39
Mehta, B., 48
Meir, I., 150
Melby, A., 269
Melkonian, G.J., 77
Mellencamp, D.D., 243
Melton, L.J., III, 295
Melzack, O.J., 236
Memoli, V.A., 97
Menczel, J., 243
Mendes, D.G., 357
Menelaus, M.B., 269, 358
Menon, J., 152, 188
Merlini, L., 216
Merritt, K., 98
Messer, H.H., 26
Metzmaker, J.N., 215
Meyers, M.H., 40
Michaelis, L.S., 236
Mickelson, M.R., 268, 269
Mikanagi, K., 257
Mikelberg, R., 78
Milinkovic, Z., 113
Millender, L.H., 187, 188
Miller, E.A., 14
Miller, F., 236
Miller, G.K., 150
Miller, G.M., 358
Miller, J.H., 150
Miller, J.T., 356
Miller, S.E., 88
Miller, W.A., 356
Milroy, J.C., 308
Minster, R.R., 39
Minteer-Convery, M., 187, 348
Mirra, J.M., 48
Mital, M.A., 139, 141, 142
Mitani, M., 123
Mitchell, J.E.I., 26
Mitchell, S.N., 335
Miura, T., 171
Mize, R.D., 329, 334
Mnaymneh, W., 71
Moe, J.H., 14, 224, 225, 226, 243, 244
Moellering, R.C., Jr., 57
Mohler, J.G., 87
Moiel, R., 236
Molander, M.L., 317
Molster, A., 295
Monson, S.T., 367
Montgomery, S., 224, 225
Montgomery, W.J., 131
Monticelli, G., 14, 318
Montique, F., Jr., 26
Mooney, V., 124, 296
Moore, E.E., 285
Moore, W.S., 70
Moreau, M., 269
Moreau, P., 215
Moretz, J.A., 318
Morisaki, N., 257
Morrey, B.F., 114, 161, 309, 357, 375, 376
Morrey, B.V., 150
Morrison, W.A., 172, 188
Morrissy, R.T., 197, 316
Morse, T., 64
Moses, J.M., 172
Moshel, M., 357
Moskovitz, P.A., 87
Moskowitz, A., 243
Moskowitz, R.W., 38
Moulton, A., 295
Mowbray, M.A.S., 335
Mubarak, S., 77, 114, 152, 260, 268, 317, 327, 336
Muggler, E., 335
Muir, H., 38
Mulier, J.C., 97, 327
Mullan, G.B., 285
Murphy, M.J., 317
Murphy, W.A., 28
Murr, P.C., 285
Murray, W.R., 295
Musher, D.M., 58
Mut, T., 151
Myers, R.A.M., 87
Nabai, H., 172
Nachemson, A., 224, 243, 257, 258
Nagant de Deuxchaisnes, C., 27
Nagel, D.A., 152, 236, 336
Nalebuff, E.D., 188
Namiki, O., 375
Narakas, A., 123
Narbaitz, R., 225
Narechania, R.G., 325
Nasca, R., 269
Nash, C.L., Jr., 236
Nashold, B.S., Jr., 236
Nasseri, D., 318
Neer, C.S., II, 120, 121, 122, 124, 131, 132
Neff, J.R., 142
Neff, R.S., 87
Nehil, J.L., 179
Neidre, A., 318, 335
Nelson, C.L., 131, 334
Nelson, D.D., 285
Nelson, J.D., 57, 269
Nelson, M., 14
Nelson, R.P., 224
Neviaser, J.S., 124
Neviaser, R.J., 87, 116, 124
Neviaser, T.J., 124
Newberger, E., 64
Newhouse, J., 257
Newman, J., 366, 368
Newton, St. E., III, 375
Nicholson, J.T., 198
Nickel, V.L., 78
Niedermann, B., 367
Niemann, K.N., 87, 317
Nilsson, B.E., 39
Nirenberg, A., 48
Nirhamo, J., 334
Nirschl, R.P., 159, 162
Nissenbaum, M., 109, 110, 112, 113, 188
Nistor, L., 367
Noble, J., 326
Nordesjö, L.O., 114, 132
Nordgren, B., 114, 132
Nordin, B.E., 27, 244
Nordt, J.C., 197
Nordwall, A., 224
Norlin, R., 77
Northmore-Ball, M.D., 71
Northrup, B.E., 216
Norwood, L.A., 327
Novelline, R.A., 88
Noyes, F.R., 326, 327
Noyes, J.D., 268
Nusbaum, H.J., 102
Nutt, J.N., III, 172
Nuzzo, R.M., 77
O'Brien, B.M., 172, 188
O'Brien, E.T., 269
O'Brien, J., 226, 257, 258
O'Brien, R.P., 207
O'Connor, J.C.B., 14
Odenrick, P., 77
O'Fallon, W.M., 27
Ogata, K., 267
Ogden, J.A., 114, 197, 286, 317
Ohno, O., 38
Ohtsuka, K., 225
Ojina, S., 216
Okade, F., 216
Oley, T.J., 268
Olives, R., 357
Olshen, R., 77, 78
Omar, M.M., 258
Önnerfält, R., 107
Ono, K., 216
Ooi, Y., 257
Oppenheim, W.L., 64
O'Reilly, R.J., 27
Örtengren, R., 224, 257
Ortiz, V., 64
Osborne, A.H., 327
Osborne, D.R.S., 236
Osebold, W.R., 221, 225
Oster, Z., 180
Osterfeld, D.L., 356
Österman, K., 161, 317
Otis, J.C., 150
Otsuka, A.S., 27
Otto, S.R., 114
Owen, C.A., 336
Owen, J.R., 207
Owen, P., 141, 161
Paccola, C.A., 39
Palmer, A.K., 179, 180, 188
Palmer, B.V., 376
Pang, D., 236
Panjabi, M.M., 215
Pankovich, A.M., 296
Pankratz, D.G., 162
Pappas, A.M., 142, 356
Pardo, V., 38
Parfitt, A.M., 27
Park, J.B., 97
Park, J.P., 128, 132
Park, W., 258
Parkinson, I.S., 27
Pasquet, A., 225
Patel, D.G., 87
Patel, M.E., 172
Patel, M.K., 48
Paterson, D.C., 268, 357
Patterson, R.L., Jr., 358
Patton, D., 70
Paul, G.R., 375
Paul, I., 38, 102
Paulos, L., 326, 352, 356
Pavel, A., 358
Pavlov, H., 368
Pearlman, H.S., 172
Pedersen, D.R., 96
Pedley, R.B., 97
Pedras, C.V., 225
Peiro, A., 151
Pelleray, B., 258
Pellicci, P.M., 161, 300, 309
Pennal, G.F., 285
Pennel, B.M., 107
Perkash, I., 236
Perry, J., 77, 78
Perry, J.F., 284
Person, D.A., 39
Peterson, H.A., 59, 64, 197, 224, 225
Peterson, L.F.A., 348
Peterson, L.J., 88, 107
Petruson, B., 224
Pettersson, H., 141
Pettrone, F.A., 162
Petty, W., 58
Pfister-Goedeke, L., 152
Philips, C.A., 188
Phillips, T.L., 48
Pho, R.W.H., 156
Picci, P., 48
Piero, D.L., 216
Piirainen, H., 376
Pilliar, R.M., 97
Pinckney, L.E., 357
Pinto, W.C., 244
Pipkin, G., 287
Piziali, R.L., 236
Pogrund, H., 13
Pohost, G., 257
Polayes, I.M., 179
Polk, H.C., 88, 284
Pollack, M.S., 27
Pollak, R., 87
Pollock, F.H., 124
Ponseti, I.V., 224, 243, 268, 269, 356
Pope, M., 152, 256, 367
Poppen, N.K., 132
Porter, I., 258
Porter, R.W., 285
Poser, J.W., 27
Posner, A.S., 26
Posner, I., 236, 257
Poss, R., 161, 309, 347
Post, M., 129, 132
Post, M.J.D., 207
Price, P.A., 27
Prietto, C.A., 151
Pritchard, D.J., 47, 48, 70
Pritzker, K.P.H., 38, 40
Protzman, R.R., 124
Purcell, G.A., 236
Pyeritz, R.E., 14
Pykett, I., 257

Quencer, R.M., 207
Quinlan, W.R., 114
Quinnell, R., 248, 257
Quirt, I., 142
Radin, E.L., 38, 102, 150
Rae, T., 98
Rahbari, H., 172
Ramaherison, P., 114
Raman, N., 27
Rambach, B.E., 70
Ramee, A., 366
Ramenofsky, M.L., 197
Ramirez, A.M., 151
Ranawat, C.S., 216, 309
Rand, J.A., 180
Raney, F.L., Jr., 216
Rang, M., 316
Raugstad, T.S., 295
Raunio, P., 132
Rauschning, W., 114, 128, 132
Reckling, F.W., 152, 335
Reed, R.B., 8
Reed, S.D., 14
Regan, B.F., 114
Reger, S.I., 107, 236
Reichard, S.A., 286
Reid, S., 78
Reineck, F.T., 39
Reingold, A.L., 57
Renier, D., 197
Renlund, R.C., 38
Rennie, C., 102
Renshaw, T.S., 268
Rentfro, R., 358
Reuss, K., 107
Revell, P.A., 107, 347
Reynolds, D.A., 270
Rhinelander, H.F., 87
Rhoades, K.H., 114
Rhodes, K.H., 357
Richardson, E.G., 70
Richardson, J.D., 88, 284
Riegels-Nielsen, P., 367
Ries, M., 102
Rigault, P., 197
Riggs, B.L., 27, 295
Riley, W.B., Jr., 187
Rills, B.M., 71
Rimoin, D.L., 14
Riseborough, E.J., 150
Riska, E.B., 284
Ritsick, J.A., 187
Ritts, R.E., Jr., 47
Rivard, C., 225
Roaas, A., 366, 376
Roberts, A., 141
Roberts, J., 356
Roberts, J.B., 160, 162
Robin, G.C., 243
Robinson, R.A., 214, 216
Roca, R.P., 58
Rochcongar, P., 366
Rockwood, C.A., Jr., 87, 151, 296
Rodrigo, J.J., 39
Rodriguez, L., 151
Roeckel, I.E., 87
Roels, J., 327
Roffman, M., 357
Rogers, L.F., 151
Romanus, B., 284
Rombouts-Lindemans, C., 27
Ronnigen, H., 97
Roos, D.B., 215, 216
Root, L., 269
Rorabeck, C.H., 70, 123
Rose, J.S., 27
Rose, R.M., 38, 99, 100, 102
Rosen, G., 41, 48
Rosen, J., 256
Rosen, J.F., 27
Rosenberg, T.D., 325
Rosenthal, R.K., 77
Roski, R.A., 215
Rostoker, W., 97, 107
Rothenberger, D.A., 284
Rothman, R., 258
Rothman, S.L.G., 197
Rothschild, B.M., 114
Röttger, J., 107, 308
Roure, J.L., 39
Rouse, D.W., 326
Rowe, C.R., 118, 119, 124, 326
Rubash, H.E., 285
Rubenfire, M., 7
Rubin, B.D., 295
Rubin, B.E., 87
Ruddy, S., 38
Rüedi, T.P., 296
Rushforth, G.F., 357
Russell, R.C., 179
Russman, B.S., 77, 225
Rutkowski, R., 327
Ryan, J.R., 367
Rybka, V., 132
Rydholm, A., 376
Rydholm, U., 376
Ryer, R.A., 71
Ryöppy, S., 114, 356
Sabsay, B., 27
Sack, C.M., 357
Sage, F.P., 161
Sahlstedt, B., 114, 132
Sahlstrand, T., 224
Sairanen, H., 356
Sajadi, K., 161
Sakellarides, H.T., 142
Sakimura, I., 87
Salamon, P.B., 179
Salenius, P., 40, 317
Salman, N.N., 97
Salmons, S., 7
Salter, R.B., 39, 317
Saltin, B., 7
Salvati, E.A., 302, 308, 309
Salzman, E.W., 309
Samilson, R.L., 113
Samson, R.H., 70
Samuelson, K.M., 356
Sanders, B., 318
Sandlund, B., 77
Santavicca, E.A., 347
Santore, R.F., 348
Sarant, J.B., 197
Sarmiento, A., 332
Satoh, Y., 257
Sauer, H.D., 285
Saunders, K.C., 317
Sauser, D., 258
Savage, J.P., 268
Savini, R., 216
Scales, J.T., 132
Scanlon, P.W., 309
Schaad, U.B., 269
Schajowicz, F., 48
Schatzinger, L.A., 236
Schatzker, J., 331, 334, 335
Scheinberg, R.D., 161
Scheller, A.D., Jr., 309
Schenkar, D.L., 87
Schepsis, A., 124
Scher, L.A., 70
Schiffman, E., 207
Schmidt, D., 114
Schneider, C., 269
Schneider, H., 102
Schoch, E.P., III, 270
Schöttle, H., 285
Schrantz, J., 269
Schuler, J.J., 70
Schultz, A., 257
Schultz, M., 224
Schultz, P., 78
Schuster, J.H., 285
Schwab, G.H., 150
Schwartz, S.S., 101
Schweigel, J.F., 207
Sclafani, S.J., 284
Scott, R.D., 161, 348
Scott, W.N., 39
Sculco, T.P., 150, 216, 295
Seaber, A.V., 71
Seedhom, B.B., 326
Seeman, E., 27
Segal, D., 362, 367
Seligson, D., 367
Selinger, D.S., 57
Selkoe, D.J., 376
Semon, R., 258
Septimus, E.J., 58
Serfass, R., 7
Sevastikoglou, J.A., 226
Severance, H.W., Jr., 327
Sew Hoy, A.L., 132
Sfakianakis, G., 64
Shaffer, A.J., 326
Shah, K.J., 114
Shahriaree, H., 161
Shanmugasundaram, T.K., 114
Shannon, R., 258
Shaperman, J., 70, 114
Shapiro, F., 142, 318
Sharp, J.T., 39
Sharwood, P.F., 268
Sheikholeslamzadeh, S., 161
Shelton, W.R., 161, 317
Shemeta, D.W., 286
Shen, C., 102
Sheppard, J.E., 141
Sheridan, G.W., 270
Sherk, H.H., 198, 269
Sherman, F.C., 268, 356, 358
Sherman, M.F., 326
Shiavi, R., 358
Shields, C.L., Jr., 124
Shiomi, S., 39
Shirahama, T., 40
Shives, T.C., 188
Shizukuishi, S., 187
Shoji, H., 356
Shorter, N., 286
Shrewsbury, M.M., 162
Shu, W.P., 48
Shulman, K., 317
Siegal, A., 107, 308
Siegel, I.M., 77
Siff, S.J., 114
Silberstein, M.J., 140, 147, 148, 151
Sillence, D.O., 14
Silva, J., 224
Silver, C.M., 161
Silver, H.K., 64
Silver, J.W., 172
Silverman, F.N., 64
Simmons, C.W., 70
Simmons, E.H., 216, 243, 244
Simon, S.R., 77, 102, 142, 269
Simonis, R.B., 215
Simpson, M., 27, 244
Skak, S.V., 317
Sklower, S.L., 141
Slabaugh, P., 77
Slätis, P., 285
Slatopolsky, E., 27
Sledge, C.B., 38, 161, 309
Slovis, T., 64
Smith, C.A., 39
Smith, G.R., 224
Smith, L., 197
Smith, N.J., 7
Smith, R.J., 141, 187, 188
Smith, W., 141
Smith, W.L., 197
Smokvina, M., 114
Smyth, H.S., 216
Snook, G.A., 316
Sokoloff, L., 39
Solheim, L.F., 376
Solomon, L., 38, 357
Solonen, K.A., 114
Sonnabend, D.H., 197
Sonne-Holm, S., 295
Sonstegard, D.A., 151
Soreide, O., 295
Sorell, M., 27
Soucacos, P.N., 327
Southwell, R.B, 358
Southwick, W.O., 207, 215, 216
Spadaro, J.A., 58
Span, Y., 243
Spanger, J.W., 14
Spangfort, E., 226
Spanier, S.S., 48
Spear, C.V., 87
Spector, M., 97
Spencer, C., 258
Spengler, D., 258
Spero, C.R., 269
Spetzler, R.F., 215

Spierings, E.L., 197
Spinelli, R., 14, 318
Spinner, M., 162
Stagnara, P., 224
Staheli, L.T., 267, 270
Stainsby, D., 141, 161
Stamp, W.G., 107, 236
Stanley, R.F., 326
Stanley, S.J., 58
Stanton, F.J., 132
Stauffer, E.S., 78, 197, 208
Stauffer, R.N., 308, 375
Steed, D., 285
Steel, H.H., 14
Steele, B.F., 64
Steichen, J.B., 187, 188
Stein, R.E., 87
Steinberg, R., 243
Stelzer, L., Jr., 187, 225
Stephen, I.B., 151
Stephenson, C.T., 268
Stern, L., 188
Stern, P.J., 158, 188
Stetler-Stevenson, W., 27
Stiehl, J.B., 336
Stock, J.R., 85, 88, 285
Stockdale, H., 257
Stockel, J., 124, 375
Stokes, I.A., 376
Stokes, N.A., 207
Stoltenberg, J.J., 87
Stoltz, M., 151
Stone, B., 224
Stone, J.P., 285
Stott, J.R., 376
Stratigos, J.S., 71
Strickland, J.W., 179, 187, 188
Stromberg, W.B., 187
Stuart, S., 317
Stulberg, S.D., 317
Stuyck, J., 224
Sudmann, E., 58, 64
Sugioka, Y., 87
Sullivan, J.A., 356
Sullivan, T.R., 48
Sumida, C.T., 70, 114
Sung, H.W., 48
Sussman, B., 70
Sussman, M.D., 64
Sussman, S., 64
Sutherland, A.D., 268
Sutherland, C.J., 299, 308
Sutherland, D., 77, 78, 268, 358
Svahn, T., 87
Swank, S., 244
Swanson, A.B., 140, 171, 187, 376
Swanson, G.D., 141, 187, 376
Swanson, K., 141
Swanson, S.A.V., 97
Swischuck, L.E., 197
Tague, B., 88
Takagi, Y., 27
Takemura, K., 187
Taleisnik, J., 176, 180
Tamai, S., 180
Tank, G.W., 57
Tanzer, T.L., 70
Tarabishy, I.E., 296
Tardieu, G., 358
Tarlov, I.M., 236
Tator, C.H., 208
Taunton, J.E., 317
Taves, D.R., 27
Taylor, J.G., 161, 348
Taylor, T.K.F., 197
Taylor, W.F., 41
Tchang, S., 258
Teague, M.A., 187
Teipner, W.A., 151
Teitelbaum, S.L., 28
Telaranta, T., 114
Temes, K., 123
Temple, W.J., 71
Templeton, T., 367
Tenenbaum, J., 38, 39
Tepper, J., 48
Termine, J.D., 27
Terrin, B.N., 27
Tetzlaff, T.R., 57
Thakkar, D.H., 285
Thomas, B.J., 309
Thomas, V.J., 40
Thomas, W.H., 161
Thompson, C., 347
Thompson, D.E., 187
Thompson, D.M., 150
Thompson, E., 39
Thompson, J.A., 334
Thompson, P., 358
Thompson, R., 162, 347
Thurston, A.J., 368
Tibone, J.E., 151
Tile, M., 284, 285, 286
Tirman, R.M., 126, 131
Tirman, W.S., 131
Tiusanen, P., 347
Todd, R.C., 347
Toledo, L.C., 114, 171
Tolia, K., 27
Tomford, W.W., 40, 48
Tondevold, E., 295
Torell, G., 224
Torg, J.S., 64, 365, 368
Torholm, C., 107
Torzilli, P.A., 326
Trafton, P.G., 124, 295
Tranbaugh, R.F., 48
Travis, C., 39
Trichkova, P., 179
Troisier, O., 258
Tross, R.B., 317
Truscelli, D., 358
Tsai, T., 172
Tsekov, P., 179
Tsuyama, N., 258
Tubiana, R., 71
Tuck, S.L., 131
Tucker, A.K., 38
Tullos, H.S., 114, 143, 144, 150, 268, 286, 309, 326, 367
Turco, V., 350, 356
Turner, D., 216
Turner, R.H., 309
Turner, T.M., 97
Uhthoff, H., 96, 225
Ulrich, R., 187
Ungar, G.H., 236
Unger, G., 258
Unis, G.L., 296
Upadhyay, S.S., 295
Upton, A.R.M., 183, 187
Urban, C., 48
Urban, R.M., 97
Urbaniak, J., 87, 179, 180
Uzelac, O., 113
Vahvanen, V., 172, 376
Vainio, K., 132
Vainionpää, S., 347
Vakili, F., 308
Van Beek, A.L., 179
Van Dam, B.E., 268
Van Der Linden, W., 180, 335
Vance, R., 268
Vandell, R.F., 179
Vangala, S.S., 107
Vankka, E., 161, 317
Varma, V.M., 87
Vasey, H., 58
Vasu, R., 308
Vavoulis, G., 236
Vazeery, A.K., 88
Vazelle, F., 366
Veidlinger, O.F., 216
Veis, A., 27
Veith, F.J., 70
Velikas, E.P., 226
Venn, M., 38
Venugopal, V., 268
Verbiest, H., 216
Vernon, J.D.S., 236
Vernon-Roberts, B., 295
Vickers, D.W., 64
Videman, T., 7
Vigorita, V.J., 27
Vincze, J., 151
Vine, D., 27
Vitale, S., 236
Volz, R.G., 161
Von Bonsdorff, H., 284
Von Laer, L.R., 152
Von Recum, A.F., 97
Vuust, M., 367
Wackenhut, J., 48
Waddell, J.P., 285, 335
Wadsworth, T.G., 150
Wagner, F.W., Jr., 88, 376
Wahlig, H., 106, 107
Waldvogel, F.A., 58
Walker, P.S., 97, 101, 132
Wallach, S., 27
Wallin, G., 317
Walsh, J.J., 236
Walters, R., 263, 269
Waltman, A.C., 88, 309
Walton, D., 284
Wang, G.J., 107, 236
Wanninger, M.H., 224
Wanters, M., 225
Wara, W.M., 48
Ward, M.K., 27
Warren, M.P., 8
Warren, R.F., 131, 326
Washington, J.A., II, 57
Watanabe, B.M., 268
Watanabe, R., 356
Watanabe, S., 161
Waterhouse, G.M., 27
Watermeier, J.J., 187
Waters, C.H., III, 335
Waters, R.L., 77, 78, 152, 162
Watkins, M.P., 326
Watson, H.K., 172, 188
Watson, K.C., 132
Watson, M., 131
Waylonis, G.W., 317
Weatherly, G.C., 97
Webb, L.X., 132
Weber, A.H., 225
Weber, M.J., 330, 334
Weber, R.J., 216
Weber, T.R., 141
Webster, M.W., 70
Wedge, J., 258
Weeks, P.M., 179
Weems, W.L., 285
Weidner, A., 216
Weiland, A.J., 27, 161, 188
Wein, B.K., 356
Weinberg, E.H., 97
Weiner, D.S., 269
Weingarden, S.I., 317
Weinstein, A.M., 107
Weinstein, S.L., 243, 268
Weisl, H., 308
Weisman, M.H., 187
Weiss, A.B., 215
Weiss, S.W., 48
Welch, K., 376
Welsh, R.P., 347
Wenger, D.R., 225, 268, 347
Werner, C., 162
Werner, F.W., 188
Westerlund, M., 172
Westin, G., 356
Westin, G.W., 268
White, A.A., III, 209, 215, 236, 257
White, A.H., 258
White, F.C., 7
White, R.E., Jr., 97, 268, 286
Whitesides, T.E., Jr., 113, 216, 236
Whitson, S.W., 27
Whyte, M.P., 28
Whyte, W., 58
Wichterman, K.A., 57
Wicks, M.H., 295, 357
Wickstrom, J., 141
Wiedeman, G.P., 375
Wiedemann, H.R., 14
Wientroub, S., 269
Wiesel, S., 258
Wigh, R., 257
Wigren, A., 114, 132
Wiklander, B., 309
Wikstad, I., 317
Wilberger, J.E., 236
Wilde, A.H., 308
Wilde, D., 256
Wiley, A.M., 347

Wiley, J.J., 357
Wilgis, E.F.S., 179
Wilkes, E., 39
Wilkins, K.E., 151
Wilkinson, J.A., 113, 215
Wilkinson, M., 215
Williams, D.F., 97
Williams, G.A., 357
Williams, L.R., 70
Williams, P.F., 14
Williams, R.M., 356
Williamson, S.R., 87
Willig, S., 356
Willis, R.B., 317
Willner, J.P., 141
Wilmore, J.H., 8
Wilson, C.B., 357
Wilson, H.J., Jr., 295
Wilson, J.G., 268
Wilson, P.D., Jr., 308, 309
Wilson, T.C., 316
Wiltse, L., 245, 249, 253, 256, 258
Wingard, D.W., 88
Winquist, R.A., 285, 296, 336
Winter, R.B., 14, 220, 222, 224, 225, 226, 236, 243, 244
Wise, K.S.H., 215
Wisnefske, D.D., 325
Witschi, J., 8
Wixson, R.L., 39, 97
Wolf, J.W., 179
Wolma, F.J., 70
Woo, R.Y.G., 309
Woo, S.L., 7, 77
Wood, M., 285
Wood, R.W., 78
Wood, V.E., 171
Woodman, J.L., 97
Woods, G.W., 150, 319, 326
Worley, R.J., 27
Worth, R.M., 216
Wray, R.E., Jr., 179
Wroblewski, B.M., 88
Wu, Y., 71
Wyatt, M., 78, 358
Wynne, G., 258
Wynne-Davies, R., 14, 141, 268
Wyss, A., 296
Wyss, C.R., 70
Xavier, C.A., 39
Yablon, I., 40, 361, 367
Yamamoto, H., 224
Yasuoka, S., 197, 225
Yngve, D.A., 269
Yocum, L.A., 124
Yong-Hing, K., 14, 198, 258
Yoshikawa, T.T., 58
Yoshimura, M., 141
Yousefzadeh, D.K., 197
Zaffer, Z., 14
Zahrawi, F., 162
Zaltzman, S., 58
Zaman, M., 318
Zancolli, E.A., 172
Zancolli, E.J., 172
Zannis, V.J., 285
Zarins, B., 124, 326
Zavala, D.C., 243
Zeide, M., 258
Zickel, R.E., 296
Zimmy, M., 356
Zizic, T.M., 87
Zolan, S., 295
Zook, E.G., 179
Zuege, R.C., 317

SUBJECT INDEX

Page numbers in italics indicate illustrations.

Accessory navicular, 349
Acetabular fractures. *See also* Pelvis injuries
  anatomy, 271
  initial management, 282
  pathophysiology, 271-272
  pediatric, 284
  surgical approaches, 281-284, *281*
  surgical reconstruction, 282-284
  treatment principles, 280-282, *283*
Achilles tendon
  rupture, 359-360
  stroke, and, 76-77
  tendinitis, 359
Achondroplasia, 11-12, *12*
Acromioclavicular joint
  separations, adult, 127, 128, *128*
  separations, pediatric, 112
Adenosine triphosphate (ATP), 1-3
Adriamycin, 41-43, *41*
Adult respiratory distress syndrome, 83
Aerobic conditioning, 5
Aerobic glycolysis, 1
Airflow systems, 53, 301-302, *302*
Alcoholism
  foetal alcohol syndrome, 13
  osteonecrosis, 81-82, *81, 82*
Alkaline phosphatase
  matrix vesicles, 17
  mineralization, 16
  Paget's disease, 25
Alloying, 89-90
Aluminum
  osteomalacia and renal dialysis, 24
Aminoglycosides, 51-53, 55, 301
Amputations and prosthetics
  complications, 65, 69, 158
  diabetes, 375
  Ewing's sarcoma, 43
  general considerations, 65
  lower extremities, 68-69, 354
  myoelectric, 66-67, 134
  myoplastic closure, 65, 67-69
  osteosarcoma, 42
  upper extremities, 67-68, 134
  vascular disease, 65-66
Anaerobic energy systems, 1
Anaerobic infection, 49-50, *50*
Anal reflex, 229-230
Anatomy
  ankle and foot, 369
  elbow, 143, *143*
  fibula, vascularized transfer of, 156, *156*
  latissimus dorsi musculocutaneous flap, 158-159, *158*
  pelvis and acetabulum, 271
  thoracic outlet syndrome, 213-214
  wrist
    triangular fibrocartilage complex (TFCC), 184-185, *185*
Anesthesia, 84-85
Aneurysmal bone cyst, 223, *223*
Angiography
  fluorescein, 66
  pulmonary, 79
  therapeutic embolism, and, 84-85, 272, 274, *85*
Ankle. *See also* Foot
  anatomy, 369
  arthritis, 369-370, *369, 370*
  arthroplasty, 370
  biomechanics, 369
  cerebral palsy, 354-355
  congenital ball and socket, 349
  fractures, 353-354, 360-362, *354, 361, 362*
    classification, 360-361, *361*
    supination-eversion, pediatric, 353-354, *354*
  multiple hereditary exostoses, 352-353
  muscular dystrophy, 355-356
  myelomeningocele, 355, *355*
  sprains
    acute, 360-361, *360, 361*
    chronic, 370-371
  stroke, 76-77
Ankylosing spondylitis, 213, 241
Anterior cord syndrome, 76
Anterolateral rotatory instability (ALRI), 319-322
Anteversion, increased femoral, 259
Antibiotics, 50-55, 266, *52*
  adverse effects, 51-53
  aminoglycosides, 51-53, 55, 301
  cephalosporins, 50-55, 176, 266
  human bite, 176
  polymethyl methacrylate impregnation, 105-106, *105, 106*
  prophylactic in hip fractures, 288
  prophylactic in THR, 301
Anticoagulants, 79-80, 288, 302
Anti-inflammatory, nonsteroidal, agents, 34
Approach. *See* Surgical approach
Arachnoiditis, 250
Artery
  popliteal
    injury to, 314
  superior gluteal injury, pelvis/posterior column fracture, 272
Arthritis. *Refer also* to specific anatomical reconstruction sections on Contents page
  ankylosing spondylitis, 213, 241
  inflammatory associated with infectious agents, 33
  juvenile rheumatoid
    hip, 305
    knee, 314
    shoulder, 113, *113*
    wrist and hand, 169-170, *169*
  Lyme disease, 33
  osteoarthritis
    general, 31-33, 36, *34, 35*
  pyogenic
    hip, pediatric, 266
    knee, pediatric, 313
  rheumatoid
    forefoot, 374-375, *374, 375*
    general, 33-36
    spine, cervical, 213
  traumatic, 36-37, *36, 37*
  treatment, general comments
    nonoperative, 33-34, *34*
    operative, 34-36, *34, 35*
  tuberculosis
    elbow, 154
    knee pediatric, 313, 314
Arthrochalasis multiplex congenita, 10
Arthrodesis
  ankle, 355, 370
  elbow, 154, *154*
  foot, 354-355
    metatarsophalangeal, 374, *374, 375*
    subtalar, extra-articular, cerebral palsy, 354-355
    tarsal, 365, 366
    triple, 354-355
  general, 34-35, *34*
  knee, 341
  shoulder, 67, 130-131, *131*
  spine, cervical
    atlantooccipital, 192
    Cloward procedure, 213
    occiput to C2, 192
    Smith-Robinson technique, 213, *213*
    strut grafts, 213, *214*
  spine, lumbosacral
    anterior interbody, 255
    herniated intervertebral disc, and, 249-250, *250*
  spine, thoracolumbar
    segmental spinal instrumentation (Luque), 221
  thumb carpometacarpal joint, 181-182, *182*
  wrist
    scapho-trapezio-trapezoid, 186, *186*
Arthrography. *See* Diagnostic radiology
Arthrogryposis multiplex congenita, 13, 138
Arthroplasty
  ankle, 370
  elbow
    excisional, 153-154

total, 154-155, *155*
foot
metatarsophalangeal, first, 372, 374, *374*
general
biological, 34, 36-38, *34, 36, 37*
excision, 34, 35, *34*
infected total joint, 57
prosthetic, 34-36, *34*
hand
metacarpophalangeal joint, 181
proximal interphalangeal joint, 181, *181*
thumb carpometacarpal joint, 181-182, *182*
hip
total replacement, 299-306, *300, 301, 302, 303, 304, 305, 306*
knee
total replacement, 341-347, *343, 344*
patellofemoral, 337, 345
shoulder
acromioplasty, anteroinferior, 116-117, 127
total, 128-130, *129, 130*
wrist
centralization for radial clubhand, 135-136, *135, 136*
prosthetic, 185, *185*
Arthroscopy
elbow, 153
knee, 313, 315, 320-321, 323-325, *313, 314, 315, 325*
anterior cruciate ligament, 320
menisci, 315, 325, *315, 325*
osteochondritis dissecans, and, 313-314, *313, 314*
patellar shaving, 324
shoulder, 119, 125
spine
intervertebral discectomy, 249
Aspirin
anticoagulant action, 79, 80, 288, 302
anti-inflammatory action, 34
Athletics. *See* Training programs
Atlantooccipital fusion; occipitalization or assimilation of the atlas, 192, *192*
Back pain
acute low, 254
epidemiology, 245
leg length discrepancy, and, 245
Bacteria. *See* Microbiology
Bacteroides fragilis, 49, 50
Bankart
lesion, 118, *118*
procedure, 119-120, *119*
Basilar impression, 191-192, *191*
Battered child syndrome, 61, 63, 64, *63*
Beta-lactam agents, 52, 54
Biceps tendinitis, 126. *See* Shoulder, rotator cuff and biceps tendon
Bilhaut-Cloquet procedure, 164, 165, *165*
Biofeedback, prosthetics, and, 67
Biomechanics
ankle and foot, 362, 364, 369
anterior cruciate ligament, 320-321
hip, 297-298
intervertebral disc, 246-247
nonnewtonian, characteristic of synovial fluid, 31
shoulder
total replacement arthroplasty, 128
Biopsy, bone
Ewing's sarcoma, 43
osteosarcoma, 41
transiliac, 22-24, *22, 23*
Bleomycin, 41, 42, *41*
Blood
anticoagulants, 79-80, 288, 302
platelet deficiencies, 84
Blount's disease, 312-313, *313*
Bone and bone metabolism
calcium and phosphate hemeostasis, 18-19
calcium-binding proteins, 19-20
gamma-carboxyglutamic acid-containing proteins, 19-20
phosphoproteins, 19
osteonectin, 19
cells
osteoblasts, 15
osteoclasts, 15-16
osteocytes, 15
endochondral formation and mineralization, 16
endocrine effect, 20-21
calcitonin, 20-21
estrogens and corticosteroids, 21
parathyroid hormone, 20
thyroid hormones, 21-22
ingrowth, 93-95
lengthening, 167, 183, *167, 168*
neoplasms. *See* Neoplasms
osteodensity, increased
osteopetrosis, 25-26
Paget's disease, 25
osteogenesis
electrically induced, 333-334
grafting, 18
repair and fracture biology, 16-18, *17*
osteopenia
osteomalacia, 23-24, *23*
osteoporosis, 22-23, *22*
vitamin D, 18-19
metabolic pathways, 19
target organs, 19
Bone cement. *See* Polymethyl methacrylate
Bone graft. *See* Grafting, bone
Bone matrix gelatin (BMG), 18
Bone morphogenetic protein (BMP), 18
Braces. *See* Orthotics
Brachial plexus
injuries, 67, 115
paralysis
elbow, effect on, 159-160
obstetrical, 112-113, *113*
thoracic outlet syndrome, 213-214
Bristow procedure, 119
Brown-Séquard syndrome, 76
Bulbocavernosus reflex, 229-230
Burns test, 247-248, *248*
Bursitis
retrocalcaneal, 363
subacromial, 126
Bursography
retroachilles, 359
subacromial, 125
Calcaneocavus, 335
Calcaneus. *See* Os calcis
Calcitonin
effect on bone mineral metabolism, 20-21
Paget's disease, treatment, 25
Calcium. *See also* Bone, metabolism
daily requirements, 18
treatment of postmenopausal osteoporosis, 22-23
Calcium and phosphate, homeostasis, 18-19
Callus. *See* Fracture, biology of repair
Camptodactyly, 353
Cancer. *See* Neoplasms
Capsulorrhaphy
hip, 260
shoulder, 119, 121-122, *119, 121, 122*
Carbohydrate metabolism, 1-2
Cardiac arrest
polymethyl methacrylate, 104-105
Cardiac output, 5
Carpal tunnel syndrome, 183, *183*
Carpometacarpal joints
arthroplasty, first, 181-182, *182*
fracture-dislocations, 174-175
Cartilage metabolism, 29-32, *29, 30*
Cauda equina syndrome, 248
Caudal regression syndrome, 13
Cavovarus, 351-352, *352*
Central cord syndrome, 76
Central hand deficiency, congenital, 166-167, *166*
Cephalosporins, 50-55, 176, 266
Ceramic prostheses, 308
Cerebral palsy
ankle and foot, 75, 354
elbow, 139, *139*
general and gait, 73, 75
hand, 170-171
hip, 75, 265-266
knee, 75
spine, 220
Chance fracture, 228-229, *229*
Charcot-Marie-Tooth disease, 356
Chemonucleolysis, 249
Chemotherapy
Ewing's sarcoma, 43, 139
osteosarcoma, 41-42
Child abuse, 61, 63, 64, *63*
Cholecalciferol (vitamin D_3), 19
Chondrocytes, 16, 29, *29*
Chondroitin-4-sulfate and -6-sulfate, 29, 30, 31, *29, 30*
Chondrolysis
idiopathic, 264
slipped capital epiphysis, and, 264
Chondrosarcoma, 43-44, *44*
Chymopapain, 249
Cisplatin, 42
Citrovorum factor, 41-42, *41*
Clavicle, 110-111
congenital pseudarthrosis, 110-111, *110, 111*
fractures, 111
Clay shoveler's fracture, 206, *206*
Clinodactyly, 166, *166*
Clubfoot. *See* Equinovarus
CMW, 105
Cobalt-chrome alloy. *See* Metals
Cobalt-nickel-chromium-molybdenum alloy. *See* Metals
Collagen
Ehlers-Danlos, 9
intervertebral disc, 246
metabolism, 29-30, *29, 30*
osteogenesis imperfecta, 11
Collagenase, 32, 249
Compartment syndromes
forearm, 149-150, *149, 150*
leg
associated with fractures, 334
chronic exertional, 325
Conditioning, physical
exercise, 1-5
training, 6-7
Condylocephalic nails, 290-292, *291, 292*
Congenital. *See also* anatomic locations
angular deformity, tibia, 311

ball and socket, ankle, 349
central hand deficiency, 166-167, *166*
cervical block vertebra, 210-211, *211*
contractural arachnodactyly, 9-10
deficiency
femur, 311
fibula, 311, *311*
radial, 134-136, *135, 136*
thumb, 167-168, *167, 168*
tibia, 311, *311*
ulnar, 136
dislocation of the hip, 259-261, *260, 261*
pseudarthrosis. *See* Pseudarthrosis, congenital
spine deformity, 218-219, *220*
Connective tissue disorders, 9-11
Constriction rings, congenital, of hand, 165-166
Continuous passive motion. *See* Passive motion
Contractures
deltoid, 111
elbow, acquired flexor spasticity, 158-159
forearm rotation, 160, *160*
quadriceps, 312
Corrosion, 89-90
Corticosteroids
effect on bone mineral metabolism, 21
rheumatoid arthritis, and, 34
Craniosynostosis, 134
Creep, polyethylene, 99
Crystal deposits, cartilage, 32
Cubital tunnel syndrome, 156-157
Curly toes, 353
Cyclic adenosine monophosphate (cAMP), 15
Cyclophosphamide, 41-43, *41*
Dactinomycin, 41-43, *41*
Dantrolene sodium, 85
Dead arm syndrome, 118
Decubitus ulcer, 86-87
Dextran, 79, 288
Diabetes mellitus
embryopathy, 13
foot, 365-366, 375, *366*
Diagnostic radiology
arthrography
hip, 260
shoulder, 116, 125, *117, 126*
wrist, 177, *178*
computed tomography. *See* specific problem
conventional radiography
bending, spine, 246, 250, *250*
myelography
arachnoiditis, 250
cervical, 201, 210
congenital spine deformity, 219
metrizamide, 201, 250, 253
neurofibromatosis, 221-222
thoracolumbar, intraoperative, 233
nuclear magnetic resonance (NMR), 248
radiation exposure, 217
radionuclide scans
battered child syndrome, and, 63, *63*
infection, spine, 241
osteosarcoma, 41
pulmonary, 79
thrombophlebitis, 79
venography, intraosseous, 81, *82*
Dilantin
osteomalacia, 24
Diphosphonates
heterotopic bone, prevention of, 303
Paget's disease, treatment of, 25
Disc. *See* Intervertebral disc
Discography, spine
cervical, 210
lumbar, 238, 247-248, *248*
Discoid lateral meniscus, 315
Dislocations. *See also* anatomic locations
Ehlers-Danlos, 9
elbow, 144, 154, *144*
foot
diabetic neuropathy, 365-366, *366*
hip
congenital, 259-261, *260, 261*
total replacement, following, 302-303
traumatic, 266, 287-288
metacarpophalangeal joint, 175
patella, 312, 324-325
shoulder
chronic unreduced, 123
recurrent anterior, 117-120, *118, 119*
spine, cervical
with spinal cord injury, 204
without spinal cord injury, 203, 204, 206, *203*
spine, thoracolumbar, 234
subtalar, 362-363
Doppler ultrasound
amputation level selection, 66
Double crush syndrome, 157, 183, *183*
Down's syndrome
atlantoaxial subluxation, 189, *189*
Ductility, 89
Dupuytren's contracture, 184, *184*
Eccentric muscle contraction, 3-4, 325
EHDP. *See* Diphosphonates
Ehlers-Danlos syndrome, 9-10
Elbow
acquired flexor spasticity, 158-159
anatomy, 143, *143*
arthrodesis, 154, *154*
arthrogryposis multiplex congenita, 138
arthroplasty, 153-155, *155*
arthroscopy, 153
cerebral palsy, 138-139, *138, 139*
dislocations, 144, *144*
hemophilia, 137-138
heterotopic ossification, 150, 160, *160*
normal development, 133-134, *133*
osteochondritis dissecans, 140, 153
poliomyelitis, 138
surgical approach, 153
synovectomy, 153
tendon transfers, 159-160
tennis, 158, 160, *159*
Electricity
fracture healing, 18, 333-334
muscle stimulation, 218, 325
piezoelectric effect, 15, 17
silver ions, generation of, 55
Electrodiagnostic studies
thoracic outlet syndrome, 213
Embolism
fat embolism syndrome, 82-83
therapeutic, 84-85, 272, 274, *85*
thromboembolism, 79-80, 288, 302
Environment
congenital skeletal abnormalities with environmental cause, 13
Epidemiology
back pain, 245
hip fractures, 288
Epiphyseal plate. *See* Growth plate
Epiphysiodesis, 312, 316
Equinovarus and equinus
arthrogryposis, 13
cerebral palsy, 354
idiopathic, 349-351, *350, 351*
muscular dystrophy, 355
myelomeningocele, 355
stroke, 76-77
Erb's palsy, 112-113
Ergocalciferol (vitamin D_2), 19
Escherichia coli, 53, 57
Estrogens, 21-23
Ewing's sarcoma. *See* Neoplasms
Excision
growth plate bars, 60-62, *60, 62*
Exercise, 1-2, *2*
External fixation
femur, chronic osteomyelitis, *56*
limb lengthening, 167, 183, 316, *167, 316*
radius, 176
tibia, 332-333, *333*
Eye
Ehlers-Danlos, 10
homocystinuria, 10
Marfan's syndrome, 9
Facet
fractures, 254
tropism, 245
Fanconi's syndrome, 134
"Far out" syndrome, 253, *253*
Fasciitis, plantar, 363
Fat embolism syndrome, 82-83
Fat metabolism, 2
Femur
anteversion, increased, 259
congenital deficiency, 311
Legg-Calvé-Perthes disease, 261-263, *262, 263*
slipped capital femoral epiphysis, 264, *263*
Femur fractures
diaphyseal
adult, 292-295, *293*
below-head prostheses, 293-294, *294*
following total hip replacement, 303, *303*
intramedullary nailing, 294-295, *294*
ipsilateral knee ligament damage, 293
ipsilateral neck fractures, 293
pediatric, 267
plating, 294
traction and functional bracing, 293-294
distal
chondral, 314
growth plate, 314
supra- and intercondylar, 329, *329*
general
battered child syndrome, and, 63, *63*
head injuries, and, 293
neoplasms, metastatic, 289, *289*
Paget's disease, and, 293, *293*
proximal
general considerations, 288-289
intertrochanteric, 290-291, *290, 291*
intracapsular, 289-290
pathological, 289, *289*
pediatric, 266-267
subtrochanteric, 291-292, *292*
Fibrous cortical defect, 315
Fibrous dysplasia
tibia and fibula, 315
Fibula
congenital deficiency, 311, *311*
vascularized transplant, 156, *156*
Fingers. *See also* anatomic location
congenital absence, 166-167
tip injuries
adult, 173, *173*

pediatric, 168
Fluorides, 22-23
Foetal alcohol syndrome, 13
Foot. *See also* Ankle; Toes
accessory navicular, 349
anatomy, 369
biomechanics, 369
cavovarus, 351, *352*
cerebral palsy, 354-355
Charcot-Marie-Tooth disease, 356
diabetic, 375
equinovarus
arthrogryposis, 13
cerebral palsy, 354
idiopathic, 349-351, *350, 351*
muscular dystrophy, 355
myelomeningocele, 355
stroke, 76-77
forefoot problems in runners, 365-366, *366*
fractures and dislocations. *See* anatomic locations
hallux rigidus, 372, *372*
hallux valgus
adult, 371-372, *371*
pediatric, 352-353, *353*
hypermobile flat (pes planus), 349
infection, pediatric, 353
ingrown toenail, 372-373
lawn mower injuries, 354, 366
metatarsalgia, 372
metatarsus adductus, 352
Morton's neuroma, 373
myelomeningocele, 355
nerve injuries, pediatric, 354
osteochondrosis of navicular (Köhler's disease), 352
plantar fasciitis syndrome, 363
poliomyelitis, 355
rheumatoid arthritis, 373, 375, *375*
tarsal coalition, 352
tendon injuries, pediatric, 354
vertical talus, 349
Forearm
compartment syndromes, 149-150, *149, 150*
nodular (pseudosarcomatous) fasciitis, 160-161
rotation contracture, 160, *160*
Forefoot
rheumatoid, 374, *374*
trauma, 365-366, *366*
Fractures. *See also* anatomic locations
amputations, and, 69
biology of repair, 16-18, *17*
electricity, 18, 333-334
growth plate
paraplegic children, and, 314
partial arrest, following, 59-62, *59, 60, 62*
pathological, 46-47
radiation therapy, following, 43
stress, 314
sesamoids, 365
tarsal navicular, 365, *365*
Fracture-dislocations. *See* anatomic locations
Functional bracing. *See* Orthotics
Gait
cerebral palsy, 73, 75
normal, 73, 369, *74*
stroke, 76
Galeazzi fractures, 149
Gamekeeper's thumb. *See* Metacarpophalangeal joint
Gastrointestinal system
hemorrhage, 86
injuries associated with pelvic trauma, 272
osteomalacia, and, 24
Genitourinary system
injury from pelvic trauma, 274
urinary tract infection, 86
Gentamicin. *See* Aminoglycosides
Genu
recurvatum, 312-314
valgus, 312, 340-341, *312, 340*
varus, 11, 312, 339, *312, 313, 338, 339*
Giant cell tumors, 44-45, *44, 45*
Gla-proteins, 19-20
Gluten sensitive enteropathy, 22-24, *22, 23*
Glycosaminoglycans, 29-31, *29, 30*
Grafting
arterial, 65
bone
biology, 18
free toe phalanx to thumb or finger, 167-168, *168*
microvascularized toe to thumb or finger, 167-168, *168*
vascularized, 156, *156*
bone marrow transplantation
osteopetrosis, 26
combination (compound), 86
composite
femur, chronic osteomyelitis and, 55, *56*
free bone microvascular "wrap-around," 183-184, *184*
fat
spine, lumbosacral, 249
muscle and myocutaneous flaps, 86, 332
latissimus dorsi, 131, 159, *158*
pectoralis, 131
osteochondral, 36-38, 45, *35, 36, 37, 45*
Growth plate
bar excision, 60-62, *60, 62*
epiphysiodesis, 60, 312, 316
fractures. *See* anatomic locations
partial arrest, 59-62, *59, 60, 62*
structure and function, 12-13, 16, *12, 13*
G-suit. *See* MAST
Haemophilus influenzae, 50, 266
Hallux
rigidus, 372, *372*
valgus
adult, 371, 372, *371*
cerebral palsy, 354
pediatric, 352
Hand. *See also* anatomic locations
arthritis, juvenile rheumatoid, 169-170, *169*
central deficiency, congenital, 166-167, *167*
cerebral palsy, 170-171
clinodactyly, 166, *166*
constriction rings, congenital, 165-166
dislocations. *See* anatomic locations
Dupuytren's contracture, 184, *184*
fingers
congenital absence, 166-167
tip injuries, 168, 173, *173*
fractures and fracture-dislocations. *See* anatomic locations
infections, 175-176
macrodactyly, 171
nail bed injuries, 173, *174*
neoplasms
lipofibromatous hamartoma of the median nerve, 171, *171*
recurrent digital fibrous tumor, 171, *170*
nerve injuries, 174
opponensplasty, 182-183, *182*
pollicization, 168, 183
replantation, 169, 178
ring avulsion injuries, 178-179
syndactyly, 163, *163, 164*
tendon injuries, flexor, 173-174
tendon transfers, 182-183, *182*
thumb, congenital absence of, 167-168, *167, 168*
thumb, duplication, 163-165, *164, 165*
thumb, pollicization, 168, 183
thumb, reconstruction
composite free bone; microvascular "wrap-around," 183-184, *184*
free toe phalanx transfer, 167
metacarpal lengthening, 167, *167, 168*
microvascularized toe transfer, 167-168, *168*
Hangman's fracture, 202, 204
Hastings frame, 249, *249*
Head injury, 75
Health maintenance, 6-7
Heel avulsion, motorcycle spoke, 354
Hemangioma, 315
Hemophilia
elbow, 137-138
general, 83-84
knee, 314
Heparin, 79-80, 288, 302
Herniated intervertebral disc
cervical, 211
lumbosacral, 247-250, *247, 248, 249, 250*
thoracic, 243
Heterotopic ossification
elbow, 150, 160, *160*
hip, following total joint replacement, 303
Hindfoot, trauma, 362-364, *364*
Hip
biomechanics
prosthetic reconstruction, and, 297-298
cerebral palsy, and, 265-266
dislocations, congenital, 259-261, *260, 261*
dislocations, traumatic
anterior, 287
pediatric, 266
posterior, 287
posterior, with femoral head fractures, 287-288
fractures, 288-292, *289, 291, 292*
infection
arthroplasty, and, 300-302, *301, 302*
fractures, and, 288
pediatric, 266
irritable, syndrome, 261
Legg-Calvé-Perthes disease, 261-263, *262, 263*
neoplasms
chondrosarcoma, 44, *44*
metastatic, 46, *46*
osteotomy, 298
prosthetic replacement
cementless arthroplasty (porous materials), 307-308, *307*
surface, 307
total, 299-307, *299, 300, 301, 302, 303, 304, 305, 306, 307*
slipped capital femoral epiphysis, 264, *363*
stroke, 76
HLA-DR4 antigens, 33
Holt-Oram syndrome, 134
Homocystinuria, 9-10
Hoover test, 247
Hormonal therapy
neoplasms, 46
osteoporosis, 22, *23*
Hot isostatic pressing (HIP), 90
Human bite, 176
Humerus

normal development, distal, 133, 134, 147, *133, 147*
unicameral bone cyst, 45, *45*
Humerus fractures
diaphyseal, 123
distal
growth plate separation, 145-146, *145, 146*
lateral condyle, 146, *146*
lateral epicondylar, 147
medial condyle, 146-147
medial epicondylar, 145-146
supracondylar, adult, 143-144
supracondylar, pediatric, 145
proximal
adult, 123
growth plate, 111-112
Hydroxyapatite, 16
cartilage crystal deposits, 32
Hyperthermia, malignant, 85
Hypotensive anesthesia, 84
Idiopathic
chondrolysis, 264
equinovarus, 349-351, *350, 351*
scoliosis, 217-219, *218, 219*
vertebral sclerosis, 250-251, *251*
Iliotibial friction syndrome, 313
Immobilization, deleterious effects, 325
Immunology
neoplasms, and, 42
rheumatoid arthritis, 33-34
Impingement syndrome. *See* Shoulder, rotator cuff and biceps tendon
Incision. *See* Surgical approach
Infantile cortical hyperostosis, 139
Infection
foot, 353
hand, 175-176
hip
pediatric, 266
prosthetic replacement, and, 57, 300-301, *301*
intervertebral disc, 223
knee
pediatric, 313
prosthetic replacement, 346
prevention of
antibiotics, 54
hip fractures, 288
hip, total replacement arthroplasty, 301-302
open fractures and joint injuries, 54-55
ultraviolet irradiation, 302
unidirectional airflow systems, 53
shoulder, 111
spine, cervical, 212-213
spine, thoracolumbar, 241
tuberculosis
elbow, 154, *154*
knee, 313-314
spine, 223
urinary tract, 86
Ingrown toenail, 372-373
Instability. *See also* Subluxation
ankle, 360, 370-371, *360*
knee, 319-322, *319, 320*
total replacement arthroplasty, and, 346
patella, 312, 324-325, *324*
shoulder, 117-123, *118, 119, 120, 121, 122*
spine, cervical
atlantoaxial, 189-190, *189, 190*
definition, 209
pseudosubluxation of C2 on C3, 191, *191*
spine, lumbosacral, 246-247, *246*
spine, thoracolumbar
posttraumatic, 231, 234-235
wrist
posttraumatic carpal, 176-178, *176, 177, 178*
Interphalangeal joints (fingers)
arthroplasty, proximal, 181, *181*
fracture-dislocations, 175, *175*
Intervertebral disc
cervical
acute disc protrusion, 211
painful segments, 211-212
congenital
end plate defects, 245
inadequate, 251-252, *252*
degeneration, 245-247
infection, 223
lumbar
herniation, 222, 247-250, *247, 248, 249, 250*
thoracic
herniation, 243
Irritable hip syndrome, 261
Isokinetic exercises, 3-4
Isometric exercises, 3-4
Isotonic exercises, 3-4
Jerk test. *See* Pivot shift phenomenon
Joints. *See also* anatomic locations
lubrication, 31
normal, 29-31, *29, 30*
Jones fracture, 366, *366*
Jumper's knee, 324
Juvenile rheumatoid arthritis
hip, 305
knee, 314
shoulder, 113
wrist and hand, 169-170
Keller procedure, 372
Kenny-Howard sling, 127
Keratan sulfate, 29-31, *29, 30*
Kienböck's disease, 186-187, *186*
Klippel-Feil syndrome, 193-195, *194*
Klumpke's paralysis, 112-113
Knee
angular deformity, congenital and developmental, 312-313, *312, 313*
anterior cruciate ligament injury, 320-322, *319, 320*
arthrodesis, 341
arthroplasty, total replacement, 341-347, *342, 343, 344, 345, 346*
debridement, 339
fractures, 314
iliotibial friction syndrome, 313
ligamentous injuries, pediatric, 315
medial collateral ligament injury, 323
menisci, 314-315, 322-323, *315, 322*
osteochondral allografts, 37, *37*
osteochondritis dissecans, 313, *313, 314*
osteochondroma, 315
osteotomy, 338-341, *338, 339, 340*
patella and patellofemoral joint. *See* Patella and patellofemoral joint
patient evaluation, 319-321
posterior cruciate ligament injury, 323-324
stroke, 76
synovectomy, 337-339
Knutsson test, *246*
Köhler's disease, 352
Krukenberg's amputation, 67, 134
Kyphosis (hyperkyphosis)
achondroplasia, 11-12, *12*
ankylosing spondylitis, 213, 241
osteoporosis, 240-241
posttraumatic, 231, 234
Scheuermann's disease, 218-219, 240, *219*
Lachman test, 320
LaCroix, perichondrial ring of, 16
Lactic acid, 1-3, 6, *2*
Laminar airflow, 53, 301-302, *302*
Laminectomy
cervical, 212
lumbar, 248-249, *249*
spine deformity following, pediatric, 222
spine fractures, thoracolumbar, problems with, 231
Latissimus dorsi musculocutaneous flap, 159, *158*
Lauge-Hansen classification of ankle fractures, 360-361, *361*
Lawn mower injuries, 354, 366
Leg
compartment syndromes
chronic exertional, 325
tibial fractures, and, 334
immobilization, deleterious effects, 325
"plantaris rupture," 325
Legg-Calvé-Perthes disease, 261-263, *262, 263*
Leukemia, 315
Ligaments. *See also* anatomic locations
sprains, definition of, 201-202
Limb length discrepancy
lower extremity, back pain, and, 245
management, 60, 315-316, *316*
metacarpal lengthening, 167, *167, 168*
radial clubhand, and, 135
Limb salvage, 42-43
Link proteins, 29-30, *29, 30*
Lipofibromatous hamartoma of the median nerve, 171, *171*
Looser's zones, 23
Lubrication, 31
Lunatomalacia, 186-187, *186*
Luque technique, 221, *222*
Lyme disease, 33
Lymphocytes, T and B, 33
Macrodactyly, hand lipofibromatous hamartoma, and, 171
McBride procedure, 372
Madelung's deformity, 137
Malabsorption, 24
Malignant hyperthermia, 85
Malunion. *See* Pseudarthrosis
Maquet procedure, 324, 337-338, *338*
Marfan syndrome, 9-11
MAST (Military Antishock Trousers), 272, 274
Matrix vesicles, 15-17, *17*
Median nerve. *See* Nerve
Menisci
knee, 314-315, 322-323, *315, 322*
Menopause
osteoporosis, and, 22-23, *22*
Metacarpophalangeal joint
arthroplasty, 181
dislocation, 175
ligamentous injury of first, 175, *175*
Metals
biocompatibility, 95-96
chrome-cobalt, 90
cobalt-nickel-chromium-molybdenum, 91
failure, 91-93, *92, 93*
porous, 93-95, 307-308, *94*
stainless steels, 89-90
titanium, 90-91
Metastases. *See* Neoplasms

Metatarsalgia, 365, 372
Metatarsals
  fractures, 365-366, *366*
    battered child syndrome, *63*
Metatarsophalangeal joints, fractures and/or dislocations, 366
Metatarsus adductus, 352
Methotrexate, 41-43, *41*
Methyl methacrylate. *See* Polymethyl methacrylate
Methylprednisolone, 45-46, *45*
Microbiology, 49-51, 55
Microdiscectomy, lumbar, 249
Midfoot, 364-365, *365*
Mineral metabolism, 18-22
Minimal bactericidal concentration (MBC), 50
Minimum inhibitory concentration (MIC), 53
Mithramycin
  Paget's disease, treatment, 25
Mitral valve prolapse syndrome, 9-10
Monteggia fractures, 149
Morton's neuroma, 372-373
Mucopolysaccharidoses, 11
Multiple hereditary exostoses, 139-140, *140*
Muscle
  anconeus, 143
  contraction, 3-4, 325, *3*
  deltoid, fibrotic bands, 110-111, *112*
  disease, general, 75
  electrical stimulation, 325
  fiber types, 4, 325
  "plantaris rupture," 325
  quadriceps
    myofibrosis, 312
    sarcoma, 47, *47*
  strength training, 4-5
  structure and function, 3, *3*
Muscle and myocutaneous flaps
  general, 86, 332
  latissimus dorsi, 131, 159, *158*
  pectoralis, 131
Muscular dystrophy, 75, 355-356
Myelography. *See* Diagnostic radiology
Myeloma, 212, 241
Myelomeningocele
  ankle and foot, 355, *355*
  general, 75
  hip, 264-265
  spine, 220-221, *221*
Myelopathy, cervical, 212
Myocutaneous flaps. *See* Muscle and myocutaneous flaps
Myoelectric prostheses, 66-67, 134
Myofibrosis, quadriceps, 312
Nail bed injuries, 173, 354, *174*
Nail, ingrown, 372-373
Navicular bone, carpal. *See* Scaphoid
Navicular bone, tarsal
  accessory, 349
  fracture, stress, 365, *365*
  osteochondrosis (Köhler's disease), 352
Neoplasms
  aneurysmal bone cyst, 223, *223*
  chemotherapy, 42, 43, *41*
  chondrosarcoma, 43-44, *44*
  eosinophilic granuloma, 197
  Ewing's sarcoma, 42-43, 139, 197, *43*
  fibrous cortical defect, 315
  fibrous dysplasia, 315
  giant cell tumor, 44-45, *44, 45*
  hemangioma, 315
  infantile cortical hyperostoses, 139
  irradiation sarcomas, 43
  leukemia, 315
  lipofibromatous hamartoma of the median nerve, 171, *171*
  metastases
    bone, 42, 46-47, 289, *46, 289*
    pulmonary, 42
    spine, cervical, 212
    spine, thoracolumbar, 241-243
  multiple hereditary exostoses, 139-140, 352-353, *140*
  myeloma, 212, 241
  neurofibromatosis, 197, 315
  nodular (pseudosarcomatous) fasciitis, 160-161
  Ollier's disease, 315
  osteoblastoma, 223
  osteochondroma, 315
  osteoid-osteomas, 139, 223
  osteosarcoma, 41-42, *41, 42*
  radiation therapy, 43, 45-47, 139, 289, *46, 47*
  recurrent digital fibrous tumor, 171, *170*
  soft-tissue
    nodular (pseudosarcomatous fasciitis, 160-161
    pigmented villonodular synovitis, 161
    sarcoma, 47
  spinal cord, 223
  spine, thoracolumbar, 241-243, *242*
  unicameral bone cyst, 45-46, *45*
Nerve. *See also* Nerve compression syndromes; Neuromas
  injury repair, 174
  median
    lipofibromatous hamartoma of, 171
  musculocutaneous
    neurectomy, 159
    phenol block, 158-159
  peroneal
    total knee replacement, and, 346
  posterior tibial block, 76-77
  radial
    humeral shaft fractures, and, 123
  sciatic palsy
    acetabular fracture, and, 272
    total hip replacement, and, 302
Nerve compression syndromes
  carpal tunnel, 183
  cubital tunnel, 156-157, *157*
  double crush, 157, 183, *183*
  peroneal, deep, 373
  posterior interosseous nerve entrapment, 158
  posterior tibial nerve, 373
  pronator teres, 157-158
  thoracic outlet syndrome, 213-215
Neurofibromatosis, 221-222, 315
Neuromas, amputation
  below-elbow, 158
  Morton's, 373
Nodular (pseudosarcomatous) fasciitis, 160-161
Nonnewtonian, characteristics of synovial fluid, 31
Nonsteroidal anti-inflammatory agents, 34
Nonunion. *See* Pseudarthrosis
Nuclear magnetic resonance (NMR). *See* Diagnostic radiology
Nucleus pulposus. *See* Intervertebral disc
Nutrition, 2-3
Obstetrical paralysis, 112-113
Odontoid
  congenital anomalies, 192-193, 210, *193*
  fractures, adult, 202
Ollier's disease, 315
1,25-hydroxycholecalciferol, 19
Onychocryptosis, 372-373
Opponensplasty, 182-183, *182*
Orthotics
  ankle and foot, 349, 362, 369-370, *362, 369, 370*
  foot, 374, *374*
  functional fracture bracing
    ankle, 362, *362*
    femur, 293-294
    humerus, 123
    tibia, 332, *332*
  spine
    achondroplasia, 11-12, *12*
    adolescent idiopathic scoliosis, 217-218, *218*
    fractures and fracture-dislocations, 234
    Marfan's syndrome, 10
    Scheuermann's disease, 218-219, 240, *219*
Os calcis
  fracture, 363-364
  plantar fasciitis, 363
  retrocalcaneal bursitis, 363
Os odontoideum, 192-193, 210, *193*
Ossification, heterotopic, 150, 160, 303, *160*
Ossification of posterior longitudinal ligament (OPLL), 212, *212*
Osteoarthritis, 31-34, *34, 35, 36. See also* anatomic locations
Osteoblasts, 15
Osteocalcin, 20
Osteochondritis dissecans
  elbow, 140, 153
  knee, 313, *313, 314*
Osteochondroma, 315
Osteoclasts, 15-16
Osteoclast activating factor (OAF), 16
Osteoconduction, 18
Osteocytes, 15
Osteodensity, increased, 25-26
Osteogenesis. *See* Bone
Osteogenesis imperfecta, 9, 11
Osteoid-osteomas, 139
Osteoinduction, 18
Osteomalacia, 23-24, *23*
Osteomyelitis. *See also* Antibiotics; Microbiology; Infection
  acute hematogenous, 55, *56*
  chronic, 55
  pelvis, pediatric, 266
  spine, cervical, 212-213
Osteonecrosis
  etiology, 80-81, *81, 82*
  femoral head
    congenital dislocation, and, 260-261, *261*
    hip fractures, and, pediatric, 267
    rotational osteotomy for, 298
    slipped capital epiphysis, and, 264
  treatment, 81-82
Osteopenia, 22-24, *22, 23*
Osteoporosis, 22-23, 240-241, *22*
Osteosarcoma. *See* Neoplasms
Osteotomy
  femur
    distal, 340
    proximal, 260, 263, 298
  general, 34-35, *34*
  growth plate arrest, and, 60, 62, *62*
  metatarsal, hallux, 352-353, 371, *353, 371*

os calcis, 351
pelvis, 260, 263, 298
radioulnar synostosis, 137
radius, Madelung's deformity, 137
shoulder, 131
spine, thoracolumbar, 238-240
tibia, 338-341, 355, *338, 339, 340*
Os trigonum syndrome, 364
Oxygen utilization (VO_2), 5-6
Paget's disease, 25, 293, *293*
Painful arc syndrome. *See* Shoulder, rotator cuff and biceps tendon
Palacos R, 105-106, *105, 106*
Papineau procedure, 55
Paraplegia. *See* Spinal cord injuries
Parathyroid hormone, 20
Parkinson's disease, hip fractures in, 288-289
Partial meniscectomy, 323
Passivation process, 90
Passive motion
flexor tendon injuries, and, 174
knee synovectomy, and, 338-339
total knee replacement, and, 345
Patella and patellofemoral joint
arthritis, 337
chondromalacia, 312-324
debridement, 337
fractures, 329-330, *330*
instability, 312, 324-325, *324*
patellectomy, 337
prosthetic replacement, 337
shaving, 324
Sinding-Larsen-Johansson's disease, 312
subluxation and dislocation, 324-325
tendinitis (jumper's knee), 324, *324*
Pelvis
injuries, 271-280, 284, *272, 273, 274, 276, 277, 278, 279*. *See also* Acetabular fractures
acute resuscitation, 272-275
anatomy, 271
associated injuries, and, 272
classification and treatment, 279-280
nonunion and malunion, 280
pathophysiology, 271
radiographic assessment, 273, 275, *273*
stabilization techniques, 275-279
surgical approaches, 276-279
neoplasms, 44, 46, *44, 46*
osteomyelitis, pediatric, 266
Peroneal nerve. *See* Nerve
Pes planus, 349
Phalanges and interphalangeal joints (fingers)
arthroplasty, proximal, 181, *181*
fracture-dislocations, 175, *175*
growth plate fracture, 168
Phenol injection, 158-159
Phlebography, 79
Phosphate, metabolism, 19
Phospholipids, 16
Physis. *See* Growth plate
Piezoelectric effect, 15, 17
Pigmented villonodular synovitis, 161
Pipkin's classification, 287-288, *287*
Pivot shift phenomenon (jerk test, flexion-rotation drawer, ALRI, Slocum's sidelying method), 319-321
Plaster burns, 150
Poliomyelitis
ankle and foot, 355
elbow, 138
spine, *239*
Pollicization, 183
Polydactyly, thumb, 163-165, *165*
Polyethylene, 99-101, *99, 100*
Polymethyl methacrylate (PMMA)
adjunctive applications, 106-107, 213, 243
cervical spine, 213
femur, 47, 289
pelvis, *44, 46*
thoracolumbar spine, 243
antibiotic impregnated, 105-106, *105, 106*
bone-cement interface, 104, *104*
carbon reinforced, 304, *304*
effects on cardiac physiology, 104-105
giant cell tumor, 45
mechanical properties, 103-104, *103, 104*
neutrophil chemotaxis, inhibition of, 57
polyethylene wear, debris and, 101, *101*
techniques, surgical, 304, *304*
Porous materials and implants, 93-95, 307-308, *94, 307*
Posterior cord syndrome, 76
Posterior interosseous nerve entrapment, 158
Posterior tibial tendinitis, 365
Posttraumatic carpal instability, 176-178, *176, 177, 178*
Po_2 measurements, segmental transcutaneous, 66
Pregnancy
scoliosis, effect on, 237-238
Pressure ulcers, skin, 86
Pronator teres syndrome, 157-158
Prophylactic antibiotics, 54, 288, 302
Prostaglandins, 32
Prostheses. *See also* Metals; Polyethylene
ankle, 370
ceramic, 308
custom, 42
elbow
radial head, 144, *144*
total replacement, 154-155, *155*
foot, 372, 374, *374*
hand, 181-182, *182*
hip
cementless (porous materials), 95, 307-308, *307*
hemiarthroplasty, 290
surface replacement, 307
total replacement, 297-298, *297*
knee
total replacement, 95, 341, 342
porous, 95, 307-308, *94, 307*
shoulder, 128-130, *129, 130*
wrist, 185, *185*
Prosthetics. *See* Amputations and prosthetics
Proteoglycans
bone, 16
cartilage, 29-31, *29, 30*
intervertebral disc, 246
Protrusio acetabuli
Marfan's syndrome, 10-11
Proximal focal femoral deficiency (PFFD), 65, 311
Pseudarthrosis
congenital
clavicle, 110-111, *110, 111*
radius and/or ulna, 137
tibia, 311
greater trochanter, 303
pelvic, 280
radiotherapy, following, 43
spine, thoracolumbar, 240
tibia, 333-334
Pseudomonas aeruginosa, 52, 53, 55
Pseudomembranous entercolitis, 51
Pulmonary embolism. *See* Embolism
Pulmonary metastases
osteosarcoma, 42
sarcoma, soft-tissue, 47
Quadriplegia. *See* Spinal cord injuries
Radial aplasia (radial clubhand), 134-136, *135, 136*
Radial nerve. *See* Nerve
Radiation
exposure, 217
spine deformity following therapy, 222
sterilization, polyethylene, 101
Radiology. *See* Diagnostic radiology
Radiotherapy
Ewing's sarcoma, 43, 139
giant cell tumors, 45
metastatic neoplasms, 46-47, 289, *46*
sarcoma, soft-tissue, 47, *47*
Radioulnar synostosis, 13, 136-137
Radius
aplasia (radial clubhand), 134-136, *135, 136*
Madelung's deformity, 137
Radius fractures
distal, 176
Galeazzi, 149
head, adult, 144, *144*
head and neck, pediatric, 148, *147, 148*
Radius and/or ulna
pseudarthrosis, congenital, 137
radioulnar synostosis, 136-137
Radius and ulna fractures
diaphyseal
adult, 148
pediatric, 149
reconstruction, 155, *156*
Ranvier, ossification groove of, 16
Recurrent digital fibrous tumor, 171, *171*
Rehabilitation
amputation, 65-69
ankle sprains, 360-361, *361*
flexor tendon injury, hand, 174
general, 6-7
knee, 312, 322, 325, 345
shoulder, rotator cuff, 117, 127
spinal cord injury, 75-76
stroke, 76-77
Renal failure, 24
Replantation
wrist and hand, 169, 178
Respiratory distress syndrome, adult, 83
Respiratory system. *See also* Embolism
injuries associated with pelvic trauma, 272
Rheumatoid arthritis. *See also* Arthritis and anatomic locations
general, 33-36
hip fractures, and, 288
Rickets, 24
Ring avulsion injuries, 178-179
Rotator cuff. *See* Shoulder
Roundback. *See* Kyphosis
Running
Achilles tendinitis, 359
forefoot problems, 365-366, *366*
plantar fasciitis, 363
Sacrohorizontal angle (Ferguson's angle), 245
Sarcoma. *See* Neoplasms
Scaphocapitate fractures, 177
Scaphoid fracture
adult, 176
pediatric, 168-169
Scheuermann's disease, 218-219, 240, *219*
Sciatic nerve. *See* Nerve

Scoliosis
adolescent idiopathic, 217-218, *218, 219*
adult, 237-240, *237, 240*
congenital, 218-219
Ehlers-Danlos, 9
Marfan's syndrome, 9
neurofibromatosis, 221-222
neuromuscular, 219-221, *239*
osteogenesis imperfecta, 11
posttraumatic, pediatric, 235
Seat belt injury, 228-229, *229*
Segmental spinal instrumentation, 221, *222*
Sesamoid fracture, 365
Sesamoiditis, 365
7-dehydrocholesterol, 19
Shin splints, 325
Shock
hemorrhagic, 84, 272, 274
spinal, 229
Shoulder
adhesive capsulitis, 126
arthritis, juvenile rheumatoid, 113, *113*
arthrodesis, 67, 130-131, *131*
arthroplasty, total, 128-130, *129, 130*
biceps tendon. *See* Shoulder, rotator cuff and biceps tendon
debridement, 130
embryology and growth, 109
fibrotic bands of deltoid, 111
infection, 111
instability
chronic unreduced dislocations, 123
involuntary multidirectional, 120-122, *120, 121, 122*
recurrent anterior dislocation and subluxation, 117-120, *118, 119*
voluntary subluxation, 117, 119
osteotomy, double, 131
patient evaluation, 125-126, *126*
rotator cuff and biceps tendon, disorders of (impingement syndrome, supraspinatus syndrome, painful arc syndrome, subacromial syndromes), 115-116, 126-127, *127*
rotator cuff tears, 116-117, 125-126, *116, 117, 126*
examination, 116, 125-126, *126*
treatment, 117
Sprengel's deformity, 109-110, *109, 110*
synovectomy, 130
Sickle cell anemia, 84
Simplex P, 105, *105*
Sinding-Larsen-Johansson's disease, 312
Skeletal dysplasias, 11-12
Skin
Ehlers-Danlos, 9-10
perfussion pressure, 66
pressure ulcers, 86
Slipped capital femoral epiphysis, 264, *263*
Soft-tissue neoplasms. *See* Neoplasms
Spina bifida cystica. *See* Myelomeningocele
Spinal. *See also* Spine
cauda equina, 230
compression, experimental, 232
conus medullaris, 230
cord injury, 75-76, 199, 201, 204, 229-232, 234-235, *200*
muscular atrophy, 219-220, *222*
shock, 229
stenosis, 11, 234, 251-254, *253*
Spine, cervical
achondroplasia, 11-12
arthrodesis
atlantooccipital, 192
Cloward procedure, 213
occiput to C2, 192
Smith-Robinson technique, 213, *213*
strut grafts, 213, *214*
biomechanics, 209
congenital abnormalities
atlantooccipital fusion, 192, *192*
basilar impression, 191-192, *191*
block vertebra, 210-211, *211*
Klippel-Feil syndrome, 193, 195, *194*
odontoid, 192-193, 210, *193*
dislocation, traumatic
with spinal cord injury, 204
without spinal cord injury, 203, 204, 206, *203*
examination, 199-201, 210, *200*
fractures
C1, 201-202, *201*
C2 (hangman's fracture), 202, 204
C3-7 (burst fracture), 205-206, *205*
odontoid, 202
pediatric, 196-197
spinous processes, 206, *206*
infection, 212-213
instability and subluxation
atlantoaxial, 189-190, *189, 190*
C1-2, 202
C3-4, 206, *204*
definition, 209, *209*
occipital C1 separation, 202
painful intervertebral segments, and, 211-212
pseudosubluxation of C2 on C3, 191, *191*
intervertebral disc, 211-212
myelopathy, 212
neoplasms, 197, 212
os odontoideum, 192-193, 210, *193*
sprains, 201-202
strains, 201
torticollis, 195-196, *195, 196*
vertebral disc calcification, 196
Spine, lumbosacral
arachnoiditis, 250
arthrodesis, 249-250
end plate injuries, 254
facet
arthrosis, 251
fractures, 254
tropism, 245
intervertebral disc
congenitally indequate, 251-252, *252*
degeneration, 245-247
herniation, 247-250, *247, 248, 249*
idiopathic vertebral sclerosis, 250-251, *251*
spinal stenosis, 251, 253-254, *253*
spondylolisthesis, 223, 254-256, *223, 256*
transitional vertebra, 245
Spine, thoracic
intervertebral disc herniation, 243
Spine, thoracolumbar
cerebral palsy, 220
congenital deformity, 218-219, *220*
deformity
following irradiation, 222
following laminectomy, 222
dwarfism, 11-12, 222, *12*
fractures and fracture-dislocations
chronic stage, 234-235
classification, 227-230, *227, 228, 229, 230, 231*
patient evaluation, 230-232
pediatric, 235
treatment, 232-234, *233*
infection, 223, 241
kyphosis (hyperkyphosis)
achondroplasia, 11-12, *12*
ankylosing spondylitis, 241
osteoporosis, 240-241
posttraumatic, 231, 234
Scheuermann's disease, 218-219, 240, *219*
neoplasms, 223
metastatic, 47, 241-242, *242*
neurofibromatosis, 221-222
neurological injury, 229-235
neuromuscular, 220-221, *221, 239*
radiation
deformity following therapy, 222
exposure, 217
scoliosis
adolescent idiopathic, 217-218, *218, 219*
adult, 237-240, *237, 240*
spinal muscle atrophy, 219-220, *222*
Split anterior tibialis transfer (SPLATT), 77
Spondylolisthesis, 223, 254-256, *223, 256*
Sports. *See* Training programs
Sprains
ankle, 360-361, *360, 361*
spine, cervical, 201-202
Sprengel's deformity, 109-110, 193, *109, 110*
Staging, soft-tissue sarcoma, 47
Stainless steels. *See* Metals
Staphylococcus aureus, 49, 50, 52, 53, 54, 57
Steroids
arthritis, and, 34
osteonecrosis, 80-81
spinal cord injury, and, 232
Strains
spine, cervical, 201
Stroke, 76-77
acquired elbow flexor spasticity, in, 158-159
Subacromial bursitis, 126
Subacromial syndromes, 126-127, *127. See also* Shoulder, rotator cuff and biceps tendon, disorders of
Subluxation. *See also* anatomic locations
acromioclavicular joint, 127-128, *128*
elbow, 154
knee, 319-322
patella, 312, 324-325
shoulder, 117-123, *118, 119, 120, 121, 122*
spine, cervical, 202, 204, 206, *204*
wrist, 178
Subtalar joint
arthrodesis, 354-355
dislocation, 362-363, *364*
Supraspinatus syndrome. *See* Shoulder, rotator cuff and biceps tendon
Surgical approach
acetabulum, 281-284, *281*
elbow, 153
pelvis, 276-279, *278*
Syndactyly, 163, *163, 164*
Synostosis
radioulnar, 136-137
tarsal coalition, 352
Synovectomy
elbow, 137-138, 153
general, 34
knee, 337, 338, 339
shoulder, 130
Synovium, 31
Syringomyelia, posttraumatic, 234
Talonavicular subluxation, 364, *364*
Talus

fractures
adult, 364, *364*
pediatric, 354
os trigonum syndrome, 364
vertical, 349
Tarsal coalition, 352
Tarsal tunnel syndrome, 373-374
Tarsometatarsal
fracture-dislocation, 354, 365
Tendinitis
Achilles, 359
biceps, long head, lesions of, 115-116, 126-127
patellar (jumper's knee), 324, *324*
posterior tibial, 365
Tendon injuries
foot and toes, pediatric, 354
hand, flexor, 173-174
Tendon transfers
extensor pollicis brevis opponensplasty, 182-183
extensor pollicis longus opponensplasty, 182, *182*
flexor carpi ulnaris, 170
flexor digitorum longus, 77
flexor hallucis longus, 77
latissimus dorsi, 159, *158*
pectoralis major, 138, 159-160
posterior tibial, 354
split anterior tibialis, 77
Steindler flexorplasty, 138
triceps brachii, 138
Tennis elbow, 158, 160, *159*
Thoracic outlet syndrome, 213-215
Thrombocytopenia absent radius syndrome (TAR), 134
Thromboembolism. *See* Embolism
Thumb. *See* Hand
Thyroid hormones, 21-22
Tibia
angular deformity, 312-313, *312, 313*
congenital deficiency, 311, *311*
fibrous dysplasia, 315
posteromedial angular deformity, 311
pseudarthrosis, 311
tubercle elevation, 337, *338*
Tibia fractures
battered child syndrome, and, 63, *63*
bicycle spoke, 354
diaphyseal
adult, 332-333
compartment syndromes associated with, 334
nonunion, 333-334
pediatric, 314
distal
growth plate, partial arrest, 59, 62, *59, 62*
proximal
osteochondral, 314
plateau, 329-332, *331*
Tillaux fragment, 353
Titanium. *See* Metals
Toes. *See also* Foot
camptodactyly, 353
growth plate fracture, 354
ingrown toenail, 372-373
tendon injuries, pediatric, 354
Torticollis, 195-196, *195, 196*
Tourniquet time, 312
Toxic shock syndrome, 50
Training programs, 6-7
Transitional vertebra, 245
Transplant. *See* Grafting
Trapezium fracture, ridge, 176-177
Tuberculosis
elbow, 154
knee, pediatric, 313, 314
spine, thoracolumbar, 223, 241
Tumors. *See* Neoplasms
Turco-type procedure, 350, *350*
25-hydroxycholecalciferol, 19
Ulna
aplasia, 136
radioulnar synostosis, 136-137
Ulna fractures
diaphyseal, adult, 148-149, *148*
Monteggia, 149
olecranon
adult, 144
pediatric, 147-148, *147*
Ulna and/or radius
pseudarthrosis, congenital, 137
Ulna and radius. *See* Radius and ulna
Ulnar nerve. *See* Nerve compression syndromes, cubital tunnel
Ultraclean air systems, 301-302, *302*
Ultrahigh molecular weight polyethylene (UHMWPE), 99
Ultraviolet irradiation, 302
Unicameral bone cyst. *See* Neoplasms
Unidirectional airflow systems, 53
Upper extremity plaster burns, 150
Urinary tract infections, 86
VATER association, 134
Vertebral cervical disc calcification, 196
Vertical talus, 349
Vincristine, 41, 43, *41*
Vitamin D
deficiency, 24
metabolism, 18-19
treatment of postmenopausal osteoporosis, 22-23
Warfarin, 79, 288, 302
Water
cartilage, and, 31, *29*
nutrition, 2
Wear
polyethylene, and, 99-101
Weaver-Dunn technique, 128, *128*
"West Point view," 118
Wrist
arthrodesis, limited; scapho-trapezio-trapezoid, 186, *186*
arthroplasty, 185, *185*
centralization for radial clubhand, 135-136, *135, 136*
prosthetic, 185, *185*
instability, posttraumatic, 176-178, *176, 177, 178*
Kienböck's, 186-187, *186*
replantation, 169, 178
subluxation
distal radioulnar joint, 178
extensor carpi ulnaris tendon, 178
triangular fibrocartilage complex (TFCC), 184-185, *185*
Xenon 133 skin clearance, 66
Z-plasty
constriction rings, congenital, of hand, 166
syndactyly, hand, 163
thumb duplication, 165